616
853
ENG
2013

D1758906

✳

INFORME
MEDICO·MORAL
DE LA PENOSISSIMA,
Y RIGOROSA ENFERMEDAD
DE LA EPILEPSIA,
QUE A PEDIMENTO

DE LA M. R. M. ALEXANDRA BEATRIZ
de los Dolores, dignifsima Priora del Convento
de Religiofas del Gloriofo, y Maximo Doctor
Señor San Geronymo,

HACE

EL BACHILLER PEDRO DE HORTA,
Medico revalidado por el Real Tribunal del Protho-Medi-
cato de efta Nueva-Efpaña, y proprietario del Hofpital
Real del Señor San Pedro, y del Convento de Señoras
Religiofas Capuchinas de efta Ciudad de la Puebla
de los Angeles, en la Nueva-Efpaña.

CON LICENCIA.

En MADRID : En la Oficina de Domingo Fernandez
de Arrojo, Calle del Carmen. Año de 1763.

Title page of the book **A Medical-Moral Account of the Most Painful and Rigorous Illness of Epilepsy,** written in 1754 by Pedro de Horta, owner of the Royal Hospital of St. Peter and physician to the Capuchin convent in the village of Los Angeles, New Spain. This is the earliest known text devoted entirely to epilepsy written in the Western Hemisphere. (Courtesy of the Francis A. Countway Library of Medicine, Boston, Massachusetts.)

SERIES EDITOR

Sid Gilman, MD, FRCP
William J. Herdman Distinguished University Professor of Neurology
University of Michigan

Contemporary Neurology Series

62 ISCHEMIC CEREBROVASCULAR
DISEASE
Harold P. Adams, Jr., MD,
Vladimir Hachinski, MD, and
John W. Norris, MD

65 MIGRAINE: MANIFESTATIONS,
PATHOGENESIS, AND
MANAGEMENT
Second Edition
Robert A. Davidoff, MD

67 THE CLINICAL SCIENCE OF
NEUROLOGIC REHABILITATION
Second Edition
Bruce H. Dobkin, MD

68 NEUROLOGY OF COGNITIVE AND
BEHAVIORAL DISORDERS
Orrin Devinsky, MD, and
Mark D'Esposito, MD

69 PALLIATIVE CARE IN NEUROLOGY
Raymond Voltz, MD, James L. Bernat, MD,
Gian Domenico Borasio, MD, DipPallMed,
Ian Maddocks, MD, David Oliver, FRCGP,
and Russell K. Portenoy, MD

70 THE NEUROLOGY OF EYE
MOVEMENTS
Fourth Edition
R. John Leigh, MD, FRCP, and
David S. Zee, MD

71 PLUM AND POSNER'S DIAGNOSIS
OF STUPOR AND COMA,
Fourth Edition
Jerome B. Posner, MD,
Clifford B. Saper, MD, PhD,
Nicholas D. Schiff, MD, and
Fred Plum, MD

72 PRINCIPLES OF DRUG THERAPY
IN NEUROLOGY
Second Edition
Michael V. Johnston, MD, and
Robert A. Gross, MD, PhD, Editors

73 NEUROLOGIC COMPLICATIONS
OF CANCER
Second Edition
Lisa M. DeAngelis, MD, and
Jerome B. Posner, MD

74 NEUROLOGIC COMPLICATIONS
OF CRITICAL ILLNESS
Third Edition
Eelco F.M. Wijdicks, MD, PhD, FACP

75 CLINICAL NEUROPHYSIOLOGY
Third Edition
Jasper R. Daube, MD, and
Devon I. Rubin, MD, Editors

76 PERIPHERAL NEUROPATHIES
IN CLINICAL PRACTICE
Steven Herskovitz, MD,
Stephen N. Scelsa, MD, and
Herbert H. Schaumburg, MD

77 CLINICAL NEUROPHYSIOLIOGY
OF THE VESTIBULAR
SYSTEM
Fourth Edition
Robert W. Baloh, MD, FAAN, and
Kevin A. Kerber, MD

78 THE NEURONAL CEROID
LIPOFUSCINOSES (BATTEN
DISEASE)
Second Edition
Sara E. Mole, PhD,
Ruth D. Williams, MD, and
Hans H Goebel, MD, Editors

79 PARANEOPLASTIC
SYNDROMES
Robert B. Darnell, MD, PhD, and
Jerome B. Posner, MD

80 JASPER'S BASIC MECHANISMS
OF THE EPILEPSIES
Jeffrey L. Noebels, MD, PhD,
Massimo Avoli, MD, PhD,
Michael A. Rogawski, MD, PhD,
Richard W. Olsen, PhD, and
Antonio V. Delgado-Escueta, MD

81 MYASTHENIA GRAVIS AND
MYASTEHNIC DISORDERS
Second Edition
Andrew G. Engel, MD, Editor

82 MOLECULAR PHYSIOLOGY AND
METABOLISM OF THE
NERVOUS SYSTEM
Gary A. Rosenberg, MD

SEIZURES AND EPILEPSY

Second Edition

Jerome Engel, Jr., MD, PhD
*Jonathan Sinay Distinguished Professor of Neurology, Neurobiology,
  and Psychiatry and Biobehavioral Sciences*
University of California, Los Angeles
Los Angeles, CA

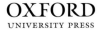

OXFORD
UNIVERSITY PRESS

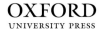

Oxford University Press is a department of the University of Oxford. It furthers the University's
objective of excellence in research, scholarship, and education by publishing worldwide.

Oxford   New York
Auckland   Cape Town   Dar es Salaam   Hong Kong   Karachi
Kuala Lumpur   Madrid   Melbourne   Mexico City   Nairobi
New Delhi   Shanghai   Taipei   Toronto

With offices in
Argentina   Austria   Brazil   Chile   Czech Republic   France   Greece
Guatemala   Hungary   Italy   Japan   Poland   Portugal   Singapore
South Korea   Switzerland   Thailand   Turkey   Ukraine   Vietnam

Oxford is a registered trademark of Oxford University Press in the UK and certain other
countries.

Published in the United States of America by
Oxford University Press
198 Madison Avenue, New York, NY 10016

© Oxford University Press 2013

All rights reserved. No part of this publication may be reproduced, stored in a retrieval
system, or transmitted, in any form or by any means, electronic, mechanical,
photocopying, recording, or otherwise, without the prior permission of Oxford University Press.

You must not circulate this work in any other form
and you must impose this same condition on any acquirer.

Library of Congress Cataloging-in-Publication Data
    Engel, Jerome. Seizures and epilepsy / Jerome Engel Jr. — 2nd ed.
        p. ; cm. — (Contemporary neurology series ; 83)
    Includes bibliographical references and index.
    ISBN 978–0–19–532854–7 (hardcover : alk. paper)
    I. Title.   II. Series: Contemporary neurology series; 83. 0069–9446
    [DNLM: 1. Epilepsy. W1 CO769N no.83 2013 / WL 385]
    616.85'3 — dc23   2012014268

The science of medicine is a rapidly changing field. As new research and clinical experience broaden our knowledge,
changes in treatment and drug therapy occur. The author and publisher of this work have checked with sources believed
to be reliable in their efforts to provide information that is accurate and complete, and in accordance with the standards
accepted at the time of publication. However, in light of the possibility of human error or changes in the practice
of medicine, neither the author, nor the publisher, nor any other party who has been involved in the preparation or
publication of this work warrants that the information contained herein is in every respect accurate or complete. Readers
are encouraged to confirm the information contained herein with other reliable sources, and are strongly advised to check
the product information sheet provided by the pharmaceutical company for each drug they plan to administer.

9 8 7 6 5 4 3 2 1
Printed in China
on acid-free paper

For Catherine

Preface to the Second Edition

It has been almost a quarter of a century since the first edition of *Seizures and Epilepsy* was published. Writing a second edition after such a long delay has offered a unique opportunity to appreciate how profoundly the field has changed during this time. In 1989, there were very few molecular neurobiological or genetic studies being carried out on epilepsy, modern neuroimaging was in its infancy, and we were essentially using only four first-line medications: phenytoin, carbamazepine, valproate, and ethosuximide, although phenobarbital was still considered a first-line drug by some workers. At that time, it was possible to envision a relatively small but still comprehensive textbook that organized and synthesized current knowledge, highlighting certain provocative areas ripe for future research. It became apparent, as preparations for the second edition began, that the state of knowledge today is so overwhelming compared with what was known in 1989 that a major challenge would be not only how to capture everything of importance but also how to decide what should be excluded. This challenge could only be met with the help of numerous experts who kindly offered valuable advice and reference material, as noted in the acknowledgments.

The organization of the four parts and 17 chapters in the second edition follows that of the first; however, the second edition is not an update but rather a complete revision with several new sections. There is extensive cross-referencing for those readers who wish to use this volume as a reference source. As with the first edition, I have attempted to be provocative and to speculate on areas where future research is necessary. It is interesting, however, to note what has become of the three points of view that were identified in the preface to the first edition as particularly controversial: (1) enhanced inhibition underlies certain types of epilepsy, (2) epilepsy itself can induce enduring cerebral dysfunction, and (3) surgical treatment for epilepsy is underutilized. All are now fully accepted concepts.

There has been much recent work on classification and terminology. In this volume, the classification structure and terminology adhere to the latest recommendations of the International League against Epilepsy. Although it was admittedly a challenge to write an entire book without using the term *complex partial seizure* once, except for historical purposes, the new, more accurate terminology eventually became familiar and easy to use. Consequently, although much discussion persists, I believe that not only will the new terminology be adopted universally but also that it will support more rational dialogue and research directions.

It has been an extremely enlightening and rewarding experience to appreciate the enormous extent of new knowledge and methodological advances of the past two-and-a-half decades. These seminal accomplishments are poised to have a greater positive impact on the lives of people with epilepsy than have past advances, presenting an exciting challenge for future translational research to fully realize the ultimate goal, that no person's life will be compromised by epilepsy. However, there is much yet to do. Tremendous insights into the disturbances that underlie epileptic phenomena at the molecular and genetic levels have yet to explain mechanisms of epileptogenesis and seizure generation at the systems level. This important deficit will likely be addressed soon by innovative multidisciplinary developments in the burgeoning new field of connectomics. Whereas identification of specific dysfunctions of ion channels, neurotransmitter receptors, and other important membrane and intracellular processes has provided novel targets for the design of new antiseizure medications, most of the new effective drugs appear to owe their success predominantly to other, largely unidentified mechanisms. The 17 new antiseizure drugs added to the market since 1989 offer important advantages with respect to side effects and dosing parameters; however, there is no evidence that the percentage of patients who are medically intractable has decreased as a result. Elucidation of the fundamental neuronal mechanisms underlying pharmacoresistance, as opposed to those responsible for epileptogenicity per se, will be essential for identifying novel treatments for the drug-refractory population. The demonstration that several psychiatric comorbidities, autism, and sudden unexplained death have an integral relationship with epilepsy has been a major contribution, and elucidation of shared underlying substrates will suggest interventions to avoid consequent disability and mortality. Prevention and cure remain elusive objectives. The explosion of technologies for structural and functional neuroimaging has led to a revolution in neurodiagnostics, specifically the visualization of lesions, such as hippocampal sclerosis and focal cortical dysplasia, that are amenable to surgical treatment. Furthermore, the safety and efficacy of surgical therapy have improved greatly, as a result of transformative advances not only in diagnosis but also in microsurgical techniques. However, the percentage of potential surgical candidates referred to epilepsy surgery centers has not changed appreciably since 1990, and the delay from onset of epilepsy to surgical referral, if anything, has increased. This appears to be a cultural problem that must be resolved by more effective education rather than additional research. Finally, there is an overriding need to address the burden of epilepsy in the developing world, where 80% of people with epilepsy live and 90% of these have little or no access to modern diagnosis and treatment. Concerted efforts on the part of the Global Campaign Against Epilepsy and the World Federation of Neurology are achieving inspiring results in these parts of the world. Solving problems of affordable, sustainable health care delivery in countries with limited resources could also provide insights that will help create more cost-effective approaches in the industrialized world, where resources are also rapidly becoming limited.

Another major advance since 1989 is the Internet. A value of older textbooks was to provide comprehensive, often difficult-to-obtain references to the literature. Today, with easy Internet access to information with search engines such as Google, and sites such as PubMed, and Wikipedia, extensive databases are no longer necessary. Consequently, this second edition is not referenced as thoroughly as the first; citations are limited for the most part to books, review articles, seminal papers, web sites, and very recent work (from within the past year or two). However, many original references from the first edition have been retained, both for historical purposes and because they are not always easy to find on the Internet.

It is appropriate to repeat here a sentence from the last paragraph of the preface to the first edition: "The most important message to be derived from this volume is not contained in the facts that represent our current state of knowledge, but rather in the appreciation of our level of understanding as a constantly evolving process." With the lightning pace of knowledge evolution in our field, much of this text will become out of date during the time it takes for publication. It should, therefore, be viewed as a snapshot in time, perhaps to be updated periodically in the future.

Jerome Engel, Jr.
Los Angeles
May, 2012

Preface to the First Edition

By an interesting coincidence, the earliest known New World book devoted entirely to epilepsy, *A Medical-Moral Account of the Most Painful and Rigorous Illness of Epilepsy*, by Pedro de Horta, was written in 1754 in a village in New Spain called Los Angeles (see frontispiece). De Horta was physician to the capuchin convent of Los Angeles, and his book, which was eventually published in Madrid in 1763, was a treatise on epilepsy as possession by demons. Should de Horta return today, he would be as amazed by the following account of epilepsy as he would be by the modern appearance of Los Angeles from which it came. Although the specter of evil surrounding a diagnosis of epilepsy may not yet be completely dispelled, this disorder has been given a firm neurobiological basis, and most people with epilepsy now clearly benefit from modern medical and surgical intervention.

The present monograph on current concepts of epileptic seizures, epileptic disorders, and the problems of persons with epilepsy was undertaken primarily as a comprehensive text for practicing physicians and physicians in training. The objective, however, was not to compile an encyclopedia, but rather to synthesize current knowledge of both basic and clinical science into a cohesive overview of the field. In this regard, opportunities were taken to develop novel or proactive concepts that would also be of interest to epileptologists and perhaps influence their research. There are four parts. Part I introduces the terminology and classification schemes used in the study of epilepsy, and places this disorder in historical and epidemiological perspective. Part II discusses basic mechanisms of epileptic phenomena and causes of human epilepsy. Part III describes the phenomenology of epileptic seizures, epileptic syndromes, and other epilepsy-related disturbances. Part V presents the management of problems caused by epilepsy and considers diagnosis, treatment, and psychosocial intervention. The chapters are organized to be read in succession, and concepts are presented in logical order. However, for those who may prefer to read only parts, or use the volume as a reference source, frequent cross-indexing identifies chapters in which additional relevant details can be found.

Although a single-authored text of this sort offers certain advantages of consistent style and integrated content, there is a need to compensate for the author's necessarily limited personal experience and conceptual biases. For this reason, a number of colleagues (noted in the acknowledgements) graciously agreed to review parts or all of the manuscript. With their help, definitive statements have been made where appropriate; but since biomedical science is a rapidly advancing dynamic field, emphasis is often placed on the existence of conflicting views and potential directions for future change. A few personal biases have been unavoidably interjected, and indeed are often essential to whatever synthesis has been achieved. In all fairness to the reader who is using this volume as an introduction to epileptology, four specific areas where content may deviate from prevailing thought are here listed:

1. Some of the terms in this book are new (such as *reactive seizures*) or currently out of favor (such as *temporal lobe epilepsy*), but they convey important information when used as specifically defined in Chapter 1.
2. References to the neuronal substrates of epilepsy not only consider disinhibition and increased excitation as important mechanisms of epileptogenicity, but also stress the growing evidence that *enhanced inhibition* underlies certain epileptiform phenomena, such as hypersynchronization.
3. Serious attention is given to experimental evidence for epilepsy-induced enduring cerebral dysfunction, such as *secondary epileptogenesis*, suggesting that certain human ictal and interictal symptoms might be progressive. Although mechanistic relationships between these animal phenomena and aspects of clinical epilepsy remain hypothetical, such potential

opportunities to identify reversible or preventable causes of disability should not be overlooked.

4. The role of *surgical treatment for epilepsy* is emphasized. Primary care physicians have no identified tens of thousands of epileptic patients who might be candidates for surgical treatment, and patients who are referred to epilepsy surgery centers often would have been better served this had referral been made 10 or 20 years earlier.

The most important message to be derived from this volume is not contained in the facts that represent our current state of knowledge, but rather in the appreciation of our level of understanding as a constantly evolving process. With de Horta's treatise in mind, this monograph may be viewed with a sense of geographic continuity, as a testament to continuing progress in the field of epileptology.

Jerome Engel, Jr., MD, PhD

Acknowledgments

I am grateful to the many patients, students, teachers, and colleagues who have taught me much that is contained in this book. The faculty, postdoctoral fellows, students, and other staff at the UCLA Seizure Disorder Center who sat with me weekly to read and critique these chapters for the better part of a year are too numerous to mention by name, but their often valuable input is appreciated. In particular, however, I would like to thank the following colleagues who offered advice, at times even helped me rewrite sections, and provided voluminous references and other materials, including figures and tables: Joan Austin, Alon Avidan, Ann Berg, Sam Berkovic, Ingmar Blümcke, Susan Bookheimer, Christine Bower Baca, Anatol Bragin, Pedro Churchman, Lyn Clarito, Hanneke de Boer, Sunita Dergalust, Sandi Dewar, Sandy Finucane, Robert Fisher, Aristea Galanopoulou, David Gloss, Mark Hallett, Dale Hesdorffer, Christine Hung, Margaret Jacobs, Andy Kanner, Curt LaFrance, Wolfgang Löscher, Rohit Marawar, Eli Mizrahi, Istvan Mody, Nico Moshé, Amanda Newaira, Viet Nguyen, Doug Nordli, Marc Nuwer, Tomis Panayiotopoulos, Emilio Perucca, Fabienne Picard, Noriko Salamon, Raman Sankar, Phil Schwartzkroin, Simon Shorvon, Mike Sperling, Rick Staba, Jim Stables, John Stern, Paul Thompson, David Treiman, Roberto Tuchman, Paul Vespa, Harry Vinters, Claude Wasterlain, Steve White, and Karen Wilcox. Their numerous corrections and suggestions have significantly increased my comfort level with the quality and accuracy of this text. I am also greatly indebted to Sabrina Hubbard for her administrative assistance, Alex Hoang for help with figures, and particularly to Dale Booth not only for typing the manuscript but for the editorial partnership that made this work possible.

Original research discussed here was supported in part by grants NS02808, NS15654, GM24839, NS33310, NS37897, NS42372, NS65877, and NS71048 from the National Institutes of Health, contract DE-AM03–76-SF00012 from the Department of Energy, and grants from Citizens United for Research in Epilepsy, the Epilepsy Foundation of America, the Epilepsy Therapy Project, the Milken Family Foundation, the Oppenheimer Foundation, and the Resnick Foundation.

Contents

Abbreviations   **xxi**

PART 1   INTRODUCTION

1.   TERMINOLOGY AND CLASSIFICATIONS   3

TERMINOLOGY   3
Epileptic Seizures • Epilepsy Disorders • Epileptic and Epilepsy • Ictal, Postictal, and Interictal • Epileptogenesis and Epileptogenicity • Epileptic Spike Focus, Epileptogenic Lesion, and Epileptogenic Zone or Region • Control, Cure, and Drug Resistance • Antiepileptogenesis, Prevention, and Disease Modification • Nonepileptic Seizures

CLASSIFICATIONS   14
Older Classifications of Epileptic Seizures • Older Classifications of the Epilepsies • Recent Efforts to Revise the International Classifications • Practical Considerations

SUMMARY AND CONCLUSIONS   31

2.   PERSPECTIVES   33

EPILEPSY THEN—HISTORICAL PERSPECTIVE   34
Medical History • Epilepsy and Religion • Epilepsy and Genius

EPILEPSY NOW—EPIDEMIOLOGICAL PERSPECTIVE   45
Definitions of Incidence and Prevalence • Methodological Considerations • Estimates of Incidence and Prevalence • Global Burden of Disease

SUMMARY AND CONCLUSIONS   49

PART 2   PATHOPHYSIOLOGY

3.   MECHANISMS OF NEURONAL EXCITATION AND SYNCHRONIZATION   55

THE NEURON   56
The Excitable Membrane and Its Microenvironment • Intracellular Processes • Structure-Function Relationships of Neuronal Elements • Interneuronal Connections

GLIAL INFLUENCES   73

NEURONAL NETWORKS   73
Intrinsic Organization of Ammon's Horn • Intrinsic Organization of the Neocortex • Subcortical
and Interhemispheric Connections

PHYLOGENY AND ONTOGENY   82
Species Differences • Cortical Development • Maturational Effects on Excitability

SYSTEMIC INFLUENCES   84

NEURONAL BASIS OF EEG ACTIVITY   86

METHODOLOGICAL DEVELOPMENTS   87

SUMMARY AND CONCLUSIONS   89

4.   BASIC MECHANISMS OF SEIZURES AND EPILEPSY   99

EXPERIMENTAL MODELS OF SEIZURES AND EPILEPSY   100
Acute Models • Chronic Models

STUDIES OF HUMAN EPILEPSY   122
Electrophysiological Investigations • Investigations Using Brain Imaging
Techniques • Microanatomical Investigations • Biochemical and Molecular Investigations

MOLECULAR GENETIC INVESTIGATIONS   135
Gene Discovery • Acquired Genetic Disturbances

POSSIBLE MECHANISMS OF HUMAN EPILEPTIC PHENOMENA   138
Epileptogenesis • Interictal State • Ictogenesis • Ictus • Ictal Termination • Postictal
Period • Possible Consequences of Epileptic Seizures

SUMMARY AND CONCLUSIONS   143

5.   CAUSES OF HUMAN EPILEPSY   157

NONSPECIFIC PREDISPOSING FACTORS   159
Genetic Factors • Environmental Factors • Dynamic Aspects of Threshold

SPECIFIC EPILEPTOGENIC DISTURBANCES   163
Genetic Causes of Epilepsy Disorders • Acquired Causes of Epilepsy Disorders

PRECIPITATING FACTORS   182
Nonspecific Precipitating Factors • Specific Precipitating Factors

SUMMARY AND CONCLUSIONS   185

PART 3   PHENOMENOLOGY

6. EPILEPTIC SEIZURES   193

NEUROBIOLOGICAL CONSIDERATIONS FOR THE DIAGNOSIS OF EPILEPTIC
SEIZURE TYPES   194
Anatomical Substrates • Pathophysiological Mechanisms • Pharmacological Considerations

TYPES OF EPILEPTIC SEIZURES   199

FOCAL SEIZURES   204
Neocortical Seizures • Limbic Seizures • Focal Seizures Evolving into Secondarily
Generalized Seizures

GENERALIZED SEIZURES   216
Tonic-Clonic Seizures • Typical Absence Seizures • Atypical Absence Seizures • Myoclonic
Absences • Eyelid Myoclonia • Myoclonic Seizures • Myoclonic Atonic Seizures • Myoclonic
Tonic Seizures • Clonic Seizures • Tonic Seizures • Atonic Seizures

UNCLASSIFIED SEIZURES   228
Epileptic Spasms • Reflex Seizures • Neonatal Seizures

MYOCLONUS   233

SUMMARY AND CONCLUSIONS   237

7. EPILEPSY SYNDROMES   243

NEONATAL PERIOD   244
Benign Familial Neonatal Epilepsy • Early Myoclonic Epilepsy • Ohtahara Syndrome

INFANCY   245
Epilepsy of Infancy with Migrating Focal Seizures • West Syndrome • Myoclonic Epilepsy
in Infancy • Benign Infantile Epilepsy and Benign Familial Infantile Epilepsy • Dravet
Syndrome • Myoclonic Encephalopathy in Nonprogressive Disorders

CHILDHOOD   250
Febrile Seizures Plus • Panayiotopoulos Syndrome • Epilepsy with Myoclonic-Atonic
Seizures • Benign Epilepsy with Centrotemporal Spikes • Autosomal Dominant Nocturnal
Frontal Lobe Epilepsy • Late Childhood Occipital Epilepsy (Gastaut Type) • Epilepsy with
Myoclonic Absences • Lennox-Gastaut Syndrome • Epileptic Encephalopathy with Continuous
Spike-and-Wave During Sleep • Landau-Kleffner Syndrome • Childhood Absence Epilepsy

ADOLESCENCE-ADULT   263
Juvenile Absence Epilepsy • Juvenile Myoclonic Epilepsy • Epilepsy with Generalized Tonic-Clonic
Seizures Alone • Progressive Myoclonus Epilepsies • Autosomal Dominant Epilepsy with Auditory
Features • Other Familial Temporal Lobe Epilepsies

SYNDROMES WITH LESS SPECIFIC AGE RELATIONSHIP   268
Familial Focal Epilepsy with Variable Foci • Reflex Epilepsies

DISTINCTIVE CONSTELLATIONS   269
Mesial Temporal Lobe Epilepsy with Hippocampal Sclerosis • Rasmussen Syndrome • Gelastic
Seizures with Hypothalamic Hamartoma • Hemiconvulsion-Hemiplegia-Epilepsy • Head Nodding
Syndrome

CONDITIONS WITH EPILEPTIC SEIZURES THAT ARE TRADITIONALLY NOT
DIAGNOSED AS FORMS OF EPILEPSY PER SE   278
Benign Neonatal Seizures • Febrile Seizures • Reactive Seizures • Neonatal Seizures Due to
Structural and Metabolic Disorders

MYOCLONIC SYNDROMES   283

SUMMARY AND CONCLUSIONS   285

8.   EPILEPTOGENESIS   296

THE DEVELOPMENT OF EPILEPSY   297
Phenomenology • Character of the Lesion • Location of the Lesion • Genetic Factors •
Practical Considerations

THE PROGRESSIVE NATURE OF EPILEPSY   307
Secondary Epileptogenesis • Clinical Evidence for Progression • Practical Considerations

EPILEPTIC SEIZURES AND BRAIN DEVELOPMENT   312
Epileptic Susceptibility of the Immature Brain • Evolution of Syndromes • Migration of the
Interictal EEG Spike • Practical Considerations

SUMMARY AND CONCLUSIONS   314

9.   PERIICTAL PHENOMENA   320

ICTAL INITIATION   320
Mechanisms • Clinical Considerations

SLEEP-WAKE CYCLES AND CHRONOBIOLOGY   326

METABOLIC AND TOXIC INFLUENCES   329

PSYCHOLOGICAL STRESS   330

POSTICTAL SYMPTOMS   331
Mechanisms • Clinical Considerations

MORTALITY   335
Comorbidity • Sudden Unexpected Death • Drowning

SUMMARY AND CONCLUSIONS   337

10. STATUS EPILEPTICUS 342

GENERALIZED CONVULSIVE STATUS EPILEPTICUS 344
Clinical Description • Incidence • Etiology • Treatment • Prognosis

ABSENCE STATUS EPILEPTICUS 358
Clinical Description • Incidence • Etiology • Differential Diagnosis • Treatment • Prognosis

EPILEPSIA PARTIALIS CONTINUA 360
Clinical Description • Incidence • Etiology • Differential Diagnosis • Treatment • Prognosis

FOCAL DYSCOGNITIVE (COMPLEX PARTIAL) STATUS EPILEPTICUS 360
Clinical Description • Incidence • Etiology • Differential Diagnosis • Treatment • Prognosis

SUBTLE STATUS EPILEPTICUS 366

FEBRILE STATUS EPILEPTICUS 367

NEONATAL STATUS EPILEPTICUS 367

EPILEPTIC BRAIN DAMAGE 368

SUMMARY AND CONCLUSIONS 369

11. CHRONIC BEHAVIORAL DISTURBANCES 374

EPIDEMIOLOGY OF PSYCHIATRIC COMORBIDITY IN EPILEPSY 375

PHENOMENOLOGY OF BEHAVIORAL DISTURBANCES IN EPILEPSY 376
Ictal and Periictal Behavior • Psychosocial Adaptation • Neurological, Intellectual, and Cognitive
Function • Personality • Mood and Affect • Anxiety • Attention Deficit Hyperactivity
Disorder • Psychosis • Classification of Neuropsychiatric Disorders in Epilepsy • Autism
Spectrum Disorders

MECHANISMS OF INTERICTAL BEHAVIORAL DISTURBANCES
IN EPILEPSY 387
Psychosocial Factors: The Predicament • Neuropathological Factors • Effects of
Treatment • Epilepsy-Induced Neurobiological Factors

SUMMARY AND CONCLUSIONS 395

PART 4   MANAGEMENT

12. DIAGNOSTIC EVALUATION 405

HISTORY 405
Seizure History • Antiseizure Drug History • Past Medical History • Family
History • Psychosocial History

PHYSICAL EXAMINATION   411
General Physical Examination • Neurological Examination • Epileptic Seizure Observation

LABORATORY EXAMINATION   415
Clinical Laboratory Tests • Electroencephalography • Magnetoencephalography • Transcranial Magnetic Stimulation • Structural Neuroimaging • Functional Neuroimaging

PSYCHOLOGICAL EVALUATION   439

BIOMARKERS   440

SUMMARY AND CONCLUSIONS   441

13. DIFFERENTIAL DIAGNOSIS   449

DIFFERENTIAL DIAGNOSIS OF NONEPILEPTIC PAROXYSMAL EVENTS   450
Systemic Disturbances • Neurological Disturbances • Psychogenic Disturbances

DIFFERENTIAL DIAGNOSIS OF REACTIVE (ACUTE SYMPTOMATIC, PROVOKED) EPILEPTIC SEIZURES   467
Alcohol Withdrawal Seizures • Recurrent Reactive Seizures

DIFFERENTIAL DIAGNOSIS OF CHRONIC EPILEPSY   468

USE OF THE EEG IN THE DIFFERENTIAL DIAGNOSIS OF EPILEPSY   468
Avoiding an Inappropriate Diagnosis of Epilepsy • EEG Contributions to a Positive Diagnosis of Epilepsy • EEG Contributions to Diagnosis of the Type of Epilepsy

USE OF FUNCTIONAL IMAGING IN THE DIFFERENTIAL DIAGNOSIS OF EPILEPSY   486

SUMMARY AND CONCLUSIONS   487

14. GENERAL PRINCIPLES OF TREATMENT   493

PHARMACOLOGICAL TREATMENT   494
Pharmacological Principles • Adverse Side Effects • Drug Monitoring • Choosing the Appropriate Drug • Discontinuation of Medication • Special Considerations

MEDICALLY REFRACTORY SEIZURES   529

ALTERNATIVE THERAPY   530

PSYCHOSOCIAL CONSIDERATIONS   530

USE OF EEG IN ASSESSING TREATMENT   530

MANAGEMENT AFTER A SINGLE SEIZURE   531

EMERGENCY TREATMENT   532

SUMMARY AND CONCLUSIONS   532

15. ANTISEIZURE DRUGS   541

STANDARD OLDER DRUGS   543
Phenobarbital (PB) • Phenytoin (PHT) • Primidone (PRM) • Ethosuximide
(ESM) • Benzodiazepines • Carbamazepine (CBZ) • Valproic Acid (VPA)

NEWER DRUGS   561
Eslicarbazepine Acetate (ESL) • Ezogabine (EZG) • Felbamate (FBM) • Gabapentin
(GBP) • Lacosamide (LCM) • Lamotrigine (LTG) • Levetiracetam (LEV) • Oxcarbazepine
(OXC) • Pregabalin (PGN) • Rufinamide (RUF) • Tiagabine (TGB) • Topiramate
(TPM) • Vigabatrin (VGB) • Zonisamide (ZON)

SPECIAL AND RARELY USED DRUGS   578
Acetazolamide • ACTH and Adrenocorticosteroids • Barbiturates • Benzodiazepines •
Bromides • Hydantoins • Oxazolidinediones • Paraldehyde • Phenacemide •
Piracetam • Progabide • Propofol • Stiripentol • Succinimides • Sulthiame

NEW-DRUG DEVELOPMENT   590
Identification of New Compounds • Preclinical Evaluation • Clinical Evaluation

DRUGS UNDER INVESTIGATION   594
Drugs in Phase III Trials • Drugs in Preclinical Development

SUMMARY AND CONCLUSIONS   596

16. NONPHARMACOLOGICAL THERAPY OF SEIZURES   603

SURGICAL THERAPY   604
Historical Perspectives • Surgical Therapy Continues to Be Underutilized • Misconceptions About
Surgical Candidates • Arguments for Early Surgical Intervention • Surgically Remediable Epilepsy
Syndromes • Therapeutic Surgical Procedures • Surgical Protocols • Outcome • Development of
New Centers

VAGUS NERVE STIMULATION   628

HORMONE THERAPY   629

IMMUNE THERAPY   629

COMPLEMENTARY AND ALTERNATIVE MEDICINE   630
Diet • Traditional and Folk Medicine • Behavioral Therapies • Physical
Interventions • Nonallopathic Medical Systems

SUMMARY AND CONCLUSIONS   636

17. SOCIAL MANAGEMENT   644

STIGMA   645

QUALITY OF LIFE   647

ACTIVITIES OF DAILY LIVING   647
Driving • Participation in Sports • Alcohol and Drugs • Specific Hazards

FAMILY   652
The Child with Epilepsy • The Parent with Epilepsy

SCHOOL   654

EMPLOYMENT   654

LEGAL RIGHTS   655

INSURANCE   655

FINANCIAL AID   657

RESOURCES   657

HEALTH CARE DISPARITIES   660

SUMMARY AND CONCLUSIONS   662

Index   665

Abbreviations

2DG 2-deoxyglucose
4AP 4-aminopyridine
AAN American Academy of Neurology
ACh acetylcholine
ACTH adrenocorticotropic hormone
AD Alzheimer's disease
ADD Antiepileptic Drug Development
  program
ADEAF autosomal dominant epilepsy with
  auditory features
ADHD attention deficit hyperactivity disorder
ADNFLE autosomal dominant nocturnal
  frontal lobe epilepsy
AES American Epilepsy Society
AHP afterhyperpolarization
AHRQ Agency for Healthcare Research and
  Quality
AIDS acquired immunodeficiency syndrome
AMPA α-amino-3-hydroxy-5-methyl-4-isoxazo
  le propionic acid
AMT ^{11}C-α-methyl-tryptophan
AMT α-methyl-tryptophan
AQP4 aquaporin-4
ARX aristaless-related homeobox gene
ASP Anticonvulsant Screening Project
ATP adenosine triphosphate

BDNF brain-derived neurotrophic factor
BECTS benign childhood epilepsy with
  centrotemporal spikes
BETS benign epileptiform transients of sleep
BFIE benign familial infantile epilepsy
BFNE benign familial neonatal epilepsy
BIE Benign infantile epilepsy
BNS Benign neonatal seizures
BOLD blood oxygenation level–dependent
BRAC basic rest activity cycle

CA carbonic anhydrase
CADASIL cerebral autosomal dominant
  arteriopathy with subcortical infarcts and
  leukoencephalopathy
CAE childhood absence epilepsy
CAM complementary and alternative
  medicine
CaM-KII calmodulin-dependent protein
  kinase II

cAMP cyclic adenosine 3,5-monophosphate
CAP cyclic alternating pattern
CBT cognitive behavioral therapy
CBZ carbamazepine
CDC Centers for Disease Control
cDNA complementary DNA
cGMP cyclic guanosine 3,5-monophosphate
CLB clobazam
CLN clonazepam
CNS central nervous system
CNV copy number variant
COX-2 cyclooxygenase-2
CP centroparietal
CRF corticotropin-releasing factor
CRH corticotropin-releasing hormone
CSA compressed spectral array
CSF cerebrospinal fluid
CSWS epileptic encephalopathy with
  continuous spike-and-wave during sleep
CT X-ray computed tomography
CTA CT arteriography
CTV CT venography
Cx36 connexin 36

DAG diacylglycerol
DALY disability-adjusted life year
DEXA dual-energy X-ray absorptiometry
DMN default mode network
DNA deoxyribonucleic acid
DNET dysembryoplastic neuroepithelial
  tumor
DOD Department of Defense
DPT diphtheria-pertussis-tetanus
DREADD designer receptors exclusively
  activated by designer drugs
DS Dravet syndrome
DTI diffusion tensor imaging
DWI diffusion-weighted imaging
DZP diazepam

EAAC-1 excitatory amino acid carrier-1
ECD (99m)Tc-ethylcysteinate dimer
ECG electrocardiography
ECoG electrocorticography
ECS electroconvulsive shock
ECT electroconvulsive shock therapy
EEG electroencephalography

EF Epilepsy Foundation
EFMR epilepsy and mental retardation limited to females
EIEE early infantile epileptic encephalopathy
EMA epilepsy with myoclonic absences
EMAS epilepsy with myoclonic-atonic seizures
EME early myoclonic encephalopathy
EMG electromyography
EPSP excitatory postsynaptic potential
ERG electroretinogram
eSAM etomidate speech and memory test
ESES epilepsy with electrical status epilepticus during slow sleep
ESI-55 Epilepsy Surgery Inventory-55
ESL eslicarbazepine acetate
ESM ethosuximide
EZG ezogabine

FBM felbamate
fcMRI functional connectivity magnetic resonance imaging
FDA US Food and Drug Administration
FDG ^{18}F-fluorodeoxyglucose
FDG-PET positron emission tomography with ^{18}F-fluorodeoxyglucose
FIRES febrile infection–related epilepsy syndrome
FLAIR fluid-attenuated inversion recovery
fMRI functional magnetic resonance imaging
FPP fast prepotential
FS febrile seizures
FS+ febrile seizures plus

GABA γ-aminobutyric acid
GABA-T GABA transaminase
GAD glutamic acid decarboxylase
GAD-7 Patient's Health Questionnaire–Generalized Anxiety Disorder-7
GAERS genetic absence epilepsy rat from Strasbourg
GAT-1 GABA transporter-1
GBP gabapentin
GCAE Global Campaign Against Epilepsy
GEFS+ genetic epilepsy with febrile seizures plus
GEPR genetically epilepsy-prone rat
GERD gastroesophageal reflux disease
GKS gamma knife surgery
GLUT1 glucose-transporter-1
GO gene ontology
GPFA generalized paroxysmal fast activity

GWAS genome-wide association studies
HCN hyperpolarization-activated cyclic nucleotide–gated cation channel
HFO high-frequency oscillation
HHE hemiconvulsion-hemiplegia-epilepsy
HIV human immunodeficiency virus
HM-PAO (99m)Tc-hexamethylpropyleneamine oxime
HRQOL health-related quality of life
HRSA Health Resources and Services Administration
HVA high-voltage-activated

IAP intracarotid amobarbital procedure
IBE International Bureau for Epilepsy
ICA independent component analysis
ICD International Classification of Diseases
ICSD-II International Classification of Sleep Disorders, second edition
ICV intracerebroventricular
IDIC 15 inversion duplication 15 syndrome
IEG immediate early gene
IFN-alpha interferon
IGE idiopathic generalized epilepsy
iGluR ionotropic glutamate receptor
IL interleukin
ILAE International League against Epilepsy
IMSD independent multifocal spike discharges
IP$_3$ inositol triphosphate
iPSC induced pluripotent stem cell
IPSP inhibitory postsynaptic potential
ISW initial slow wave
IVIg intravenous immunoglobulin

JAE juvenile absence epilepsy
JME juvenile myoclonic epilepsy

KA kainic acid
KAP knowledge attitudes and practice
L-5-HTP L-5-hydroxytryptophan

LCM lacosamide
LEV levetiracetam
LGI1 leucine-rich, glioma-inactivated 1 gene
LGS Lennox-Gastaut syndrome
LIFUP low-intensity focused ultrasound pulsation
LKS Landau-Kleffner syndrome
lod log of the odds ratio
LTD long-term depression
LTG lamotrigine
LTP long-term potentiation

LVA low-voltage-activated
LVF low-voltage fast (referring to an ictal
   onset pattern)
LZP lorazepam

MAM methylazoxymethanol acetate
MCD malformation of cortical development
MCT medium-chain triglyceride
MDR multidrug resistance
MEG magnetoencephalography
MEI myoclonic epilepsy in infancy
MELAS mitochondrial encephalomyopathy,
   lactic acidosis, and stroke-like episodes
MERRF myoclonic epilepsy with ragged red
   fibers
MES maximal electroshock seizure
mGluR metabotropic glutamate receptor
MHD 10-monohydroxy derivative
MMPI Minnesota Multiphasic Personality
   Inventory
MPSI migrating partial seizures in infancy
MRA magnetic resonance arteriography
MRI magnetic resonance imaging
mRNA messenger ribonucleic acd
MRS magnetic resonance spectroscopy
MRV magnetic resonance venography
MSI magnetic source image
MSLT Multiple Sleep Latency Test
MST multiple subpial transection
MTLE mesial temporal lobe epilepsy
MTLE with HS mesial temporal lobe epilepsy
   with hippocampal sclerosis
mTOR mammalian target of rapamycin

NAA *N*-acetyl-aspartate
NDA New Drug Application
NFκB nuclear factor-κB
NGF nerve growth factor
NIH National Institutes of Health
NINDS National Institute of Neurological
   Disorders and Stroke
NMDA *N*-methyl-ᴅ-aspartic acid
NP3 neurotrophin 3
NPY neuropeptide Y
NREM non-REM
NSE neuron-specific enolase

OCD obsessive-compulsive behavior
OS Ohtahara syndrome
OXC oxcarbazepine

PAS+ periodic acid–Schiff-positive
PB phenobarbital
PCDH19 protocadherin 19 gene

PCr phosphocreatine
PDS paroxysmal depolarization shift
PE phenytoin-equivalent
PEMA phenylethylmalonamide
PET positron emission tomography
PGN pregabalin
PGP P-glycoprotein
pHFO pathological high-frequency oscillation
PHT phenytoin
PLED pseudoperiodic lateralized
   epileptiform discharge
PLMS periodic leg movements of sleep
PME progressive myoclonus epilepsies
PML progressive multifocal
   leukoencephalopathy
PNES psychogenic nonepileptic seizures
POLG polymerase gamma gene
POSTS positive occipital sharp transients of
   sleep
PPF paired pulse facilitation
PRM primidone
PS Panayiotopoulos syndrome
PSA prostate-specific antigen
PTE posttraumatic epilepsy
PTP posttetanic potentiation
PTZ pentylenetetrazol
PWE person with epilepsy

QOLIE Quality of Life in Epilepsy

r14 Ring 14 syndrome
r20 Ring 20 syndrome
RBD REM sleep behavior disorder
REM rapid eye movement
RLS restless legs syndrome
RMTD rhythmic midtemporal discharge
RNA ribonucleic acid
RSDHI Retirement, Survivors, Disability, and
   Health Insurance
RTG retigabine
rTMS repetitive transcranial magnetic
   stimulation
RT-PCR reverse transcription polymerase
   chain reaction
RUF rufinamide

SANAD Standard and New Antiepileptic
   Drug study
SAR structure-activity relationship
SEEG stereotactic depth electrode
   electroencephalography
SEM simultaneous EEG and fMRI
SEP somatosensory evoked potential
SIDS sudden infant death syndrome

SISCOM subtraction ictal SPECT with
coregistration on MRI
SMAP 2-sulphamoylacetyl-phenol
SMEI severe myoclonic epilepsy of infancy
SMR sensory motor rhythm
SNP single-nucleotide polymorphism
SNRI serotonin norepinephrine reuptake
inhibitor
SPECT single-photon emission computed
tomography
SPM statistical parametric mapping
SREDA subclinical rhythmic EEG discharge
of adults
SSI Supplemental Security Income
SSRI selective serotonin reuptake inhibitor
SSS small sharp spikes
SSSE self-sustained status epilepticus
STXBP1 syntaxin binding protein 1 gene
SUD sudden unexpected (or unexplained)
death
SUDEP SUD in epilepsy
Sv2a synaptic vesicle protein 2a

TBI traumatic brain injury
TE echo time
TGB tiagabine
TIA transient ischemic attacks
TIRDA temporal intermittent rhythmic delta
activity

TMS transcranial magnetic
stimulation
TNF-α tumor necrosis factor-α
TNS trigeminal nerve stimulation
TPM topiramate
TPO temporal-parietal-occipital
TR repetition time
TSC tuberous sclerosis complex

UCLA University of California,
Los Angeles
UDS up-down state

Vd volume of distribution
VEM video-EEG monitoring
VEP visual evoked potential
VGB vigabatrin
VGKC voltage-gated K+ channel
VNS vagus nerve stimulation
VPA valproic acid
VZ ventricular zone

WFN World Federation of Neurology
WHO World Health Organization
WPSI Washington Psychosocial Seizure
Inventory
WS West syndrome

ZON zonisamide

PART 1

Introduction

Chapter 1

Terminology and Classifications

TERMINOLOGY
Epileptic Seizures
Epilepsy Disorders
Epileptic and Epilepsy
Ictal, Postictal, and Interictal
Epileptogenesis and Epileptogenicity
Epileptic Spike Focus, Epileptogenic Lesion, and Epileptogenic Zone or Region
Control, Cure, and Drug Resistance
Antiepileptogenesis, Prevention, and Disease Modification

Nonepileptic Seizures

CLASSIFICATIONS
Older Classifications of Epileptic Seizures
Older Classifications of the Epilepsies
Recent Efforts to Revise the International Classifications
Practical Considerations

SUMMARY AND CONCLUSIONS

The literature on epilepsy has been plagued by ambiguous and inconsistent language, which has contributed greatly to current controversy and confusion. It is necessary, therefore, to begin by establishing a basic understanding of the terminology and classifications to be used in this book.

TERMINOLOGY

This section considers important terms and concepts. Specific definitions are provided for only the most essential terms. Each definition is followed by a discussion of related terms and concepts that are often used imprecisely or incorrectly. These discussions are intended to identify, if not always resolve, sources of confusion and to minimize semantic inconsistencies in this volume. Some terms will be used here in ways that deviate slightly from their use elsewhere, and a few unique terms are used to facilitate the presentation of material in subsequent chapters. Other terms that cannot be defined simply serve to raise questions addressed in more detail later in the book.

3

Epileptic Seizures

DEFINITION

The International League Against Epilepsy (ILAE) has defined an epileptic seizure as "a transient occurrence of signs and/or symptoms due to abnormal excessive and synchronous neuronal activity in the brain" (Fisher et al., 2005).

DISCUSSION

This definition takes into account basic research in recent years that contradicts an older view that epileptic seizures result from increased excitation and decreased inhibition. Rather, synchronization appears to be a more important underlying neuronal mechanism, and in some situations inhibition may be increased (Chapter 4). Many types of epileptic seizures occur. The behavioral features of an epileptic seizure reflect the functions of the cerebral areas where the abnormal neuronal activity originates and spreads (Chapter 6). An epileptic seizure can consist of impaired higher mental function or altered consciousness (a *dyscognitive* state), involuntary movements or cessation of movement, sensory or psychic experiences, or autonomic disturbances; it often occurs as a combination of dysfunctions and a progression of signs and symptoms. Epileptic seizures have electrophysiological correlates that usually, but not always, can be recorded by a scalp electroencephalogram (EEG).

The word *epilepsy* derives from the Greek word επιλαμβανεν (*epilambanein*), meaning "being seized," and refers to the seizure of a person undergoing an epileptic attack. It is correct to say that a patient *had a seizure* but incorrect to say that a patient *seized* or to speak of a *seizing* patient. The word *seizure* is used loosely in medicine to refer to a sudden, often catastrophic event. Like the words *fit*, *attack*, *spell*, and *turn*, the term *seizure* can be applied nonspecifically when the exact nature of the event it describes remains in doubt, or it can be modified (e.g., *psychogenic nonepileptic seizure* or *cardiac seizure*) to indicate a specific nonepileptic phenomenon. Epileptic seizures are so commonly referred to simply as seizures, however, that care must be taken to ensure that the word *seizure* alone is not mistaken to mean

"epileptic seizure" when this specific definition is not intended or warranted.

Epileptic seizures occur with a variety of diseases and disorders that alter neuronal function to produce epileptogenic activity. Over 100 years ago, John Hughlings Jackson defined this alteration as an "excessive neuronal discharge" (Jackson, 1870). This concept is still accepted, although the neuronal mechanisms of some seizures involve increased synchrony rather than increased firing per se (Chapter 4). Simply, the nervous system has a limited repertoire of responses to injury and noxious stimuli: The activity of neurons either decreases or increases. Destructive insults depress or abolish neuronal activity and generally lead to hypofunctional (negative) symptoms such as paralysis, blindness, or coma. Neuronal destruction can also release hyperfunctional (positive) symptoms such as rigidity or hemiballismus. Irritative insults cause excessive or synchronous neuronal activity and positive symptoms. Pain is the most common positive symptom when the peripheral nervous system is irritated, whereas epileptic seizures are the most common positive symptoms when the brain is irritated.

In reality, most neurological disorders produce a combination of positive and negative symptoms, such as spasticity and weakness or paresthesias and numbness. Epileptic seizures can arise from specific neurological disturbances that are both irritative and destructive (e.g., a stroke or brain tumor), causing intermittent positive symptoms (seizures) superimposed on chronic negative symptoms (e.g., paresis). Moreover, epileptic seizures often disrupt function in such a way that neuronal activity is transiently depressed after the seizure is over (Chapter 9). Although some epileptic seizures actually consist of a cessation or decrease in certain behaviors, such as loss of muscle tone (*atonic seizure*) or impaired consciousness (*absence*), to be consistent with the definition of the epileptic seizure as an excessive or synchronous activation of neurons, these behaviors can be viewed as the result of excessive or synchronous inhibitory neuronal activity until data prove otherwise.

Many types of epileptic seizures occur, as discussed later in this chapter and in Chapter 6. *Generalized tonic-clonic seizures* (sometimes referred to as *convulsions*) and *absences*, for instance, are particular classes of epileptic seizures that appear to reflect different pathological mechanisms (Chapter 4). The pharmacological agents used to treat epileptic seizures are commonly called *antiepileptic drugs*, when in fact they are *antiseizure* drugs. The term *antiepileptic* is nondescriptive and inaccurate (to many, an epileptic is a person with epilepsy). It is replaced by the term *antiseizure* throughout this book. When a more general term is required, *antiepilepsy* is more appropriate. A*nticonvulsant drugs* and *antiabsence drugs* are specifically effective against convulsions and absences, respectively. The terms *convulsion* and *anticonvulsant* should not be used as synonyms for *epileptic seizure* and *antiseizure*. Because the term *convulsion* has been inconsistently applied to mean focal as well as generalized motor seizures, its use has been discouraged (Engel, 2001); however, it is useful to denote generalized tonic-clonic motor activity.

Traditionally, epileptic seizures are divided into *partial seizures*, originating in a part of one hemisphere, and *generalized seizures*, originating simultaneously in both hemispheres (Commission on Classification, 1981). This is a false dichotomy, because all seizures need to begin somewhere and even after they are fully developed, very few, if any, involve the entire brain. Nevertheless, this division has been useful for teaching purposes and has been preserved, as will be discussed later in this chapter; however, *partial seizures* are now referred to as *focal seizures* (Engel, 2001; Berg et al., 2010). The term *focal seizure* was initially discouraged, because it created the misconception that epileptic seizures are due to a discretely localized focal abnormality. The word *partial*, however, has also created confusion, because it connotes incomplete rather than localized. Because the epilepsy community has now generally accepted that epilepsy, even when the abnormality involves only a part of one hemisphere, is a distributed disturbance, the ILAE has considered it safe to officially return to the older terminology of *focal seizures*.

Most human epileptic seizures involve abnormalities of the cerebral cortex (Chapter 4). However, normal or abnormal subcortical influences facilitate or even provoke epileptic activity, and propagation of epileptic discharges through subcortical structures is usually important for the clinical manifestation of epileptic seizures. Although the old concept of a purely *centrencephalic* (meaning deep brain) source of epileptic seizures is not supported by current data, we now know that the thalamus is important for the generation of absences and that certain *gelastic seizures* originate in hypothalamic hamartomas (Chapter 5). Cortical involvement may not be necessary for an apparent seizure to be considered epileptic (Chapter 6).

Epileptic phenomena cannot always be clearly distinguished from a variety of nonepileptic signs and symptoms produced by abnormal neuronal activity in subcortical structures (Chapter 4). In particular, certain forms of myoclonus that appear to be cortically generated are often referred to as epileptic myoclonus, while other forms of myoclonus that reflect subcortical dysfunction may involve neuronal mechanisms similar to those of epilepsy or be more closely related to movement disorders or other nonepileptic neurological symptoms (Chapter 6). Because there are many abnormal nonepileptic intermittent behavioral symptoms, appropriate EEG changes are useful for making a definite diagnosis of an epileptic seizure (Chapter 12). Simultaneous observations of both behavioral and EEG abnormalities indicative of an epileptic seizure allow confirmation with a high degree of confidence (Chapter 6). Such *electroclinical* correlations usually are not obtained, however, because patients only rarely have epileptic seizures during routine EEG recordings, few require inpatient video EEG monitoring, and this technology is not available in most parts of the world. Furthermore, some forms of epileptic seizure are associated with electrical discharges that cannot be detected by scalp EEG electrodes.

Characteristic EEG abnormalities that occur during seizures and also between seizures are referred to as *epileptiform*, when they appear to reflect epileptic disturbances. Such EEG discharges do not, in themselves, constitute an epileptic seizure, which requires a behavioral change. Single or repeated epileptiform *spike-and-wave* EEG discharges, which characteristically occur in most patients with epilepsy when they are not having epileptic seizures, are referred to as *interictal spikes*, but with sophisticated testing, behavioral correlates can sometimes be identified. Consequently, these events might be considered fragments of seizures (Chapter 4). More prolonged EEG discharges that are indistinguishable from those seen during epileptic seizures can be recorded, most commonly using intracranial electrodes, without associated recognizable clinical manifestations. Such events are called *electrographic seizures* or *subclinical seizures*. Moreover, brief and prolonged epileptiform EEG events are occasionally seen in persons who have never had and never will have epileptic seizures (Chapter 13). Consequently, epileptiform EEG abnormalities alone should not be considered definitive evidence for a diagnosis of epilepsy, which depends most heavily on an appropriate history (Chapter 12).

It is not uncommon, particularly when reporting in vivo and in vitro research on acute animal models, for authors to use the term *epileptic seizure* incorrectly when referring to an electrical event only (Chapter 4). This has led to considerable confusion, because some experimental treatments can produce EEG changes that resemble those seen during epileptic seizures but are generated by nonepileptic pathophysiological mechanisms.

Afterdischarge refers to an epileptiform electrical neuronal discharge produced by and outlasting a specific perturbation. The provocative event is usually, but not necessarily, electrical stimulation of the brain. The term *afterdischarge* is often used incorrectly to describe any epileptiform EEG pattern. Spontaneous epileptiform EEG events are not the same as provoked afterdischarges.

In general, epileptic seizures can be characterized as *brief, intermittent, spontaneous*, and *paroxysmal*, but important exceptions must be noted. Epileptic seizures are usually self-limiting but not always brief. In some situations, such as *epilepsia partialis continua* and *spike-wave stupor*, epileptic seizure activity appears to be continuous for periods that can last days or, rarely, even years (Chapter 10). The term *intermittent* is not appropriate for isolated events that can be diagnosed as epileptic seizures even if they do not recur. *Provoked, acute symptomatic*, or *reactive epileptic seizures* that are not spontaneous can be induced in persons without epilepsy by transient noxious events, for instance, the use of convulsant drugs or alcohol withdrawal (Chapters 5 and 7). Epileptic seizures can be described as spontaneous to emphasize the presence of an inherent seizure generator. However, patients with certain forms of *reflex epilepsy* have epileptic seizures that are triggered only by specific stimulation and never occur spontaneously

(Chapter 9). *Paroxysmal* implies a sudden and severe event, but many epileptic seizures are subtle and can begin insidiously (Chapter 6).

Epilepsy Disorders

DEFINITION

Epilepsy disorders are referred to simply as *epilepsy* or, more correctly, *the epilepsies*. The ILAE has defined epilepsy as "a chronic condition of the brain characterized by an enduring propensity to generate epileptic seizures, and by the neurobiological, cognitive, psychological, and social consequences of this condition. The definition of epilepsy requires the occurrence of at least one epileptic seizure" (Fisher et al., 2005).

DISCUSSION

Surprisingly, there was no formal agreed-upon international definition of epilepsy prior to 2005, although the general concept was that epilepsy is a condition of recurrent epileptic seizures, and the operant definition used, for instance, for epidemiological studies, was two or more unprovoked seizures occurring more than 24 hours apart (Thurman et al., 2011). The 2005 ILAE definition initially engendered considerable controversy, particularly among epidemiologists, who were concerned that it might inflate incidence measures because epilepsy could now be diagnosed after one seizure. In fact, the intention of this definition is to communicate the essence of the disorder and to codify what physicians do in practice. Indeed, if patients presenting with a single epileptic seizure are evaluated and an enduring epileptogenic abnormality is identified, indicating a high risk of subsequent seizures, treatment is usually instituted and the patient then carries a diagnosis of epilepsy.

The issue here is the difference between a conceptual definition and an operational definition. The ILAE definition is as close as we can come at this time to a conceptual definition of epilepsy, one that is not intended to be operationalized. The epidemiological operational definition works for certain epidemiological studies, but numerous other operational definitions of epilepsy can be devised for other research or even clinical purposes that do not detract from the importance of a conceptual definition. It is important to note that epilepsy is not only the occurrence or risk of occurrence of epileptic seizures but also the adverse consequences associated with these events.

Many types of epilepsy disorders exist. Some are sufficiently well defined according to characteristic electrophysiological and behavioral features of ictal events, as well as other clinical signs and symptoms, age of onset, family history, and course, to constitute symptom complexes referred to as *epilepsy syndromes* (Chapter 7). Whereas all patients with chronic recurrent epileptic seizures have an *epilepsy disorder*, not all have disorders that can be considered an epilepsy syndrome. Epilepsy syndromes, which are defined most importantly by the epileptic phenomena, are different from pathologically defined syndromes or diseases that are usually but not invariably associated with epileptic seizures (e.g., tuberous sclerosis and Aicardi's syndrome). Although many, maybe most, patients with epilepsy disorders cannot be diagnosed as having a specific epilepsy syndrome, recognition of these syndromes when present often informs prognosis, etiology, and therapy.

Traditionally, when epileptic seizures occur as the sole manifestation of a genetic disturbance, the epileptic disorder or syndrome is said to be *primary*, *idiopathic*, or *essential*. When epileptic seizures occur as symptoms of specific structural or metabolic pathology, either acquired or inherited, the epileptic disorder or syndrome is said to be *secondary*, *symptomatic*, or *acquired*. The term *idiopathic epilepsy* derives from the Greek word for "self" and means "epilepsy itself," sui generis. In other areas of medicine, *idiopathic* connotes an unknown cause; consequently, the term *idiopathic epilepsy* is often used incorrectly to define a secondary epilepsy disorder in which available diagnostic tests have not demonstrated the specific lesion. These conditions in epilepsy were referred to as *cryptogenic*, but there was confusion in the literature as to whether *cryptogenic* refers only to presumed *symptomatic* conditions for which no specific etiology has been determined or also applies when it is uncertain whether conditions are idiopathic *or* symptomatic. Consequently, it is now recommended that the term *cryptogenic* no longer be used and that conditions be more specifically described as *presumed symptomatic, presumed*

idiopathic, or simply *unknown* (Engel, 2001, 2006; Berg et al., 2010).

The dichotomy between *idiopathic* and *symptomatic*, however, is artificial; many, maybe most, epilepsy conditions involve both genetic and acquired components (Chapters 5 and 7). It is no longer recommended, therefore, to attempt to force all epilepsy syndromes into idiopathic or symptomatic categories. However, it is difficult to avoid the use of these terms altogether when they occasionally communicate well-known conditions, such as the *idiopathic generalized epilepsies* (Engel, 2001, 2006; Berg et al., 2010). When an etiological designation is appropriate, recommended terminology is now *genetic* rather than *idiopathic*, and *structural/metabolic* rather than *symptomatic* (Berg et al., 2010), recognizing that these concepts are not dichotomous. Genetic in this sense is defined as conditions that are the direct result of a known or presumed genetic defect in which seizures are the core symptom of the disorder. Genetic diseases such as tuberosclerosis, where the primary consequence of the genetic defect is a structural or metabolic condition that causes epilepsy, albeit not consistently, would be considered structural/metabolic (Berg et al., 2010).

Although epileptic seizures are always abnormal events, not all reflect chronic neurological disturbances. Some types of epileptic seizures can be a natural reaction of the normal brain to physiological stress or transient systemic insult (Chapter 5). Single, isolated generalized tonic-clonic seizures (Chapter 6) with documented transient causes, such as sleep deprivation, alcohol or sedative drug withdrawal, use of convulsant drugs, fever, and acute head trauma, do not reflect chronic epileptic neurological dysfunction and therefore do not constitute an epilepsy disorder. A similar situation exists for recurrent epileptic seizures induced by reversible infectious, toxic, or metabolic processes. Such seizures will be referred to here as *reactive epileptic seizures*, but are also called *provoked seizures* and *acute symptomatic seizures*. Although *benign febrile seizures* constitute a recognized syndrome, they are characterized by the occurrence of reactive epileptic seizures (Chapter 7) and children with this disorder are not considered to have epilepsy. The duration of illness for the syndrome of benign neonatal seizures is so short that babies with the syndrome also are no longer considered to have epilepsy (Engel, 2006; Berg et al., 2010).

Clinical management and research into pathophysiological mechanisms require that chronic epilepsy disorders be distinguished from disorders characterized by reactive epileptic seizures. Diagnostic difficulties arise, however, for a number of reasons: (1) Immediate antiseizure drug treatment after a single, isolated epileptic seizure can make it impossible to determine whether or not a chronic disorder exists; (2) endogenous or exogenous precipitating factors can produce several reactive epileptic seizures within a short time; (3) repeated exposure to a particular insult can cause recurrent reactive epileptic seizures widely spaced in time; and (4) enduring but remediable disturbances (e.g., a brain tumor) can give rise to recurrent epileptic seizures that stop when the disturbance is removed. Features of the events and the circumstances under which they occurred often permit a diagnosis of reactive epileptic seizures (Chapter 12).

Distinguishing between a *provoked* and an *unprovoked* epileptic seizure can be important when one is considering the management of a single, isolated event (Chapter 14). The term *provoked seizure*, however, is not exactly synonymous with the term *reactive seizure*, as used here. Reactive seizures may appear to be unprovoked if the precipitating factors go unnoticed, whereas provoking stimuli may induce the first seizure of an epileptic disorder. The term *acute symptomatic epileptic seizure* is also used only when there is an identifiable cause. The term *reactive epileptic seiz*ure will be used in this text to include provoked and acute symptomatic events, as well as isolated events with no identifiable provocation or cause that do not warrant a diagnosis of epilepsy.

Epileptic and Epilepsy

DEFINITION

The word *epileptic*, in the general sense, is used to define a class of signs and symptoms, such as epileptic seizures. In the specific sense, the word *epilepsy* is used to refer only to those chronic conditions with enduring epileptogenic brain dysfunction that can be considered epilepsy disorders. Because there are many types

of epilepsy disorders, it is more correct to refer to them as *the epilepsies*.

DISCUSSION

Confusion arises when the adjective *epileptic* is used to define particular phenomena that are not indicative of an epilepsy disorder. For instance, reactive neurological symptoms that are correctly called epileptic seizures (in the general sense) can occur in people who do not have epilepsy (in the specific sense) (Chapters 5, 6, and 7). Not all people who have epileptic seizures associated with electroclinical epileptic abnormalities have epilepsy (e.g., febrile seizures; Chapter 7), and epileptiform EEG discharges can occur in patients who do not have epileptic seizures (Chapter 13). Individuals who suffer from epilepsy disorders have been referred to as "epileptics," but this unfairly identifies individuals with their affliction. The term *person with epilepsy* (PWE) acknowledges that one is defined by much more than one's illness and is preferred today to the historically pejorative term "epileptic."

Because there are many types of epilepsy disorders, referred to as *the epilepsies*, epilepsy itself has been referred to as a *disorder* and not a *disease*. For some people, the term *disease* is considered a pejorative, and for this reason it also has been avoided. Conversely, it is argued that failure to refer to epilepsy as a disease diminishes its importance and could contribute to the lack of recognition and resources devoted to this condition compared with other diseases that represent a comparable global health burden (Engel, 2010).

Ictal, Postictal, and Interictal

DEFINITION

The terms *ictus* and *ictal event* refer to the epileptic seizure itself, as identified clinically or electrophysiologically. The term *ictogenesis* can be used to refer to the generation of an epileptic seizure. Postictal phenomena are transient clinical or electrophysiological abnormalities in brain function that result from the ictus and appear after the ictal event has ended. The time during which postictal symptoms persist (usually seconds to a few days) is referred to as the *postictal period* (Chapter 9). The *interictal period* is the time between the resolution of postictal abnormalities and the beginning of the next ictal event. The term *interictal*, therefore, is applicable only for patients with recurrent epileptic seizures.

DISCUSSION

Ictus, like *seizure*, is a nonspecific word used in the medical context to indicate a sudden attack. *Ictus* means an epileptic seizure only when specifically indicated. Consequently, when doubt exists about the epileptic nature of a particular event, it can still be correctly referred to as an ictus.

Ictal, *postictal*, and *interictal* are used to describe these distinct phenomena even though the exact point of transition from one stage to the next is usually uncertain (Fisher and Engel, 2010). For some epileptic seizures, the end of the ictal event is well demarcated behaviorally and electrographically, but in many cases it is unclear when to attribute abnormal behaviors and EEG patterns to postictal rather than ictal neuronal mechanisms. Similarly, the transition between postictal and interictal periods cannot be rigorously defined, and so-called interictal abnormalities can occasionally reflect prolonged or delayed postictal changes. For example, it is commonly stated that postictal paralysis (*Todd's paralysis*), and therefore postictal phenomena in general, should not last longer than 48 hours (Chapter 9). However, there is no experimental evidence establishing such a rigid time limit on the transient disruption of neuronal function caused by epileptic seizures, and postictal psychosis typically occurs days after the ictal event, following a lucid interval (Chapter 9).

Postictal symptoms, in the currently accepted usage (and as used in this book), are manifestations of seizure-induced reversible alterations in neuronal function but not structure (Chapters 4 and 9). Some epileptic seizures can also cause structural brain damage and enduring neurological deficits (Chapter 10), which are technically distinct from postictal symptoms. Such deficits, however, are not necessarily irreversible; neuronal reorganization can result in long-term recovery of function, which accounts for the fact that some apparent postictal symptoms can last many months or even years but eventually disappear (Chapter 9).

It is impossible at times to identify the interictal state accurately. Epileptiform EEG abnormalities that occur between obvious epileptic seizures can represent (1) ictal events with clinical manifestations too brief or subtle to identify, as in some forms of absence seizures; (2) postictal phenomena reflecting a specific neuronal reaction to a seizure; or (3) truly interictal events generated by pathophysiological mechanisms different from those generating ictal and postictal EEG discharges (Chapter 4). Furthermore, apparent interictal behavioral disturbances can be seizures with EEG correlates that are not visible on scalp recordings (Chapter 11). Even the most advanced monitoring techniques cannot always distinguish among ictal, postictal, and interictal events. Although these terms have valid and useful clinical applications, more specific, evidence-based definitions are often necessary for research communications (Chapter 4).

An *aura* is typically regarded as a warning that precedes an epileptic seizure, although auras are actually the beginning of the ictal event (Chapter 6). When epileptic seizures begin with ictal phenomena perceived by the patient alone and then progress to include more obvious motor disturbances or impairment of cognitive function, the initial ictal symptoms constitute the aura. These same auras can also occur without progression to more obvious clinical seizures (*auras in isolation*). Some patients, however, experience less well-defined sensations or mood changes that can begin hours before the seizure onset and are not associated with ictal EEG discharges even when intracranial electrodes are used. These are not auras and are referred to as *prodromes*. Such prodromes are not likely to be ictal events but rather reflect the development of a systemic or neurological state that predisposes to the occurrence of epileptic seizures (Chapter 9).

Epileptogenesis and Epileptogenicity

DEFINITION

The term *epileptogenesis* has been defined as the development and extension of tissue capable of generating spontaneous behavioral or electrographic seizures (Pitkänen, 2010). It includes both the development of an epileptic condition and progression after the condition is established. The term *epileptogenicity* refers to the capacity to generate epileptic seizures.

DISCUSSION

The incorrect use of the term *epileptogenesis* to refer to the initiation of an epileptic seizure blurs the distinction between two separate phenomena with independent pathophysiological mechanisms (Chapters 4 and 8). The development of an epilepsy disorder implies abnormal neuronal reorganization occurring over a long period following a specific cerebral insult, whereas an epileptic seizure can be provoked in normal as well as abnormal brain.

The term *ictogenesis* is now preferred to describe the many mechanisms that might underlie the generation of individual epileptic seizures. The term *epileptogenicity*, however, connotes the presence and severity of epileptic seizure–generating capability. Thus a structural disturbance, such as a tumor or scar, that gives rise to chronic epileptic seizures is called an *epileptogenic lesion*, and the area of brain tissue from which epileptic seizures arise is referred to as the *epileptogenic zone* or *region*. The adjective *epileptogenic* is also applied in a more general sense to any cause of epileptic seizures. *Epileptogenic agents* are drugs or toxic substances that produce acute reactive as well as chronic epileptic seizures. It is technically incorrect to speak of epileptogenic agents or lesions as epileptic. Seizures are *epileptic*, meaning they have the characteristic features of epilepsy, whereas agents and lesions that cause epilepsy are *epileptogenic*. Technically, agents or lesions that only cause acute seizures are *ictogenic*.

Under certain conditions, epilepsy can be a progressive disorder, because recurrent epileptic seizures can themselves promote epileptogenesis. *Secondary epileptogenesis* is the term applied when focal epileptogenic abnormalities give rise to distant epileptogenic zones. This process is best exemplified experimentally by *kindling* and the *mirror focus* (Chapters 4 and 8). Controversy exists concerning the clinical importance of secondary epileptogenesis in humans, although there is no doubt that certain epilepsy syndromes, referred to as *epileptic encephalopathies*, are progressive (Chapter 8). Progression of these disorders involves nonepileptic as well as epileptic disturbances.

As noted previously, drugs or mechanisms that prevent epileptic seizures will be referred to as *antiseizure agents* and not *antiepileptic agents* in this book. More specific terms can be used to describe interventions that prevent specific types of seizures, such as *anticonvulsant* and *antiabsence*. Although no drugs or mechanisms currently exist that prevent the development or progression of epilepsy, such *antiepileptogenic* agents are an active area of research. All these interventions together can be referred to as *antiepilepsy treatments*.

Epileptic Spike Focus, Epileptogenic Lesion, and Epileptogenic Zone or Region

DEFINITION

An *epileptic spike focus* is defined electrophysiologically as the brain area that appears to be the major source of interictal epileptiform EEG discharges. EEG epileptiform discharges can be *focal*, indicating a single epileptic spike focus; *bilateral* and *independent*, indicating epileptic spike foci in two hemispheres; *multifocal*, indicating three or more epileptic spike foci; or *diffuse* (either widespread or generalized), in which case there is no apparent epileptic focus. An *epileptogenic lesion* is a structural abnormality responsible for the generation of epileptic seizures. The *epileptogenic zone* or *region* is defined as the area of brain necessary and sufficient for generation of spontaneous seizures. This area can be well circumscribed, multiple, or diffuse, although the term has practical value only with respect to focal epilepsies.

DISCUSSION

An epileptic spike focus is determined electroencephalographically and does not necessarily correspond to an area of brain capable of generating epileptic seizures (Chapters 4 and 16). It is usually localized by an analysis of the spatial distribution of interictal EEG spike-and-wave discharges. When this information is supplemented by localization derived from ictal EEG recordings, neuroimaging, and other diagnostic tests, an epileptogenic zone might be defined but is generally too extensive to be referred to as a "focus." More information about the spatial extent of interictal spiking can be derived from *intracranial electrode recordings, magnetoencephalography (MEG),* simultaneous EEG and *functional magnetic resonance imaging (fMRI),* and computerized analysis of EEG (Chapters 12 and 16). All of these techniques, however, record epileptiform electrical abnormalities that could reflect propagation from distant sites or epileptically abnormal brain regions incapable of initiating epileptic seizures and so, by themselves, do not delineate the epileptogenic zone.

The area of brain where an epileptogenic lesion is experimentally created by various techniques is often referred to as an *experimental epileptic focus* (Chapter 4). In most acute experimental models of epilepsy, electrophysiological studies indicate that the area of cerebral disturbance does become the major source of epileptiform electrical discharges. This use of the term *epileptic focus* is unfortunate, however, because it does not distinguish between the lesion and the electrically defined area of functional disruption, nor does it take into account the processes of epileptogenesis that take place over time in chronic experimental animal models as well as in patients.

The concept of a discrete epileptic focus derived from studies of local application of convulsants to the cortex of experimental animals is too simplistic to be relevant to most clinical epilepsy conditions. Therefore, use of the terms *epileptic focus* or *seizure focus* to refer to the epileptogenic zone in patients is misleading and should be avoided. Detailed electrophysiological investigations of patients who clinically appear to have a single well-localized epileptogenic lesion usually reveal the existence of multiple sources of interictal epileptiform EEG discharges and occasionally more than one site of ictal onset (Chapter 4). As more is becoming known about chronic focal epilepsy, it appears less and less likely ever to be associated with a single, discretely circumscribed area of functionally disturbed cerebral cortex (Chapter 4).

The epileptic spike focus is an electrophysiological concept and must be clearly distinguished from the epileptogenic lesion, a structural concept, and the epileptogenic zone or region, a theoretical concept the boundaries of which can only be approximated by comparing the results of multiple diagnostic testing approaches (Chapter 16). These three terms do not always define topographically congruent cortical areas. An epileptic spike focus is

often transient and shifting, and there can be multiple such foci. Not all epileptic spike foci generate seizures. A well-defined epileptogenic lesion can exist in the absence of an epileptic spike focus, because a localized structural abnormality can cause diffuse interictal EEG discharges or produce no interictal EEG transients at all (Chapters 12 and 13). The epileptogenic zone, where seizures actually begin, is rarely defined solely by interictal EEG spikes and can be within the epileptogenic lesion (as in *hippocampal sclerosis*), adjacent to it, or rarely at some distance from it (Chapters 4 and 16). A *primary epileptogenic zone* may give rise to *secondary epileptogenic zones* (Chapters 4 and 8).

Relationships among the epileptogenic lesion, the epileptic spike focus, and the epileptogenic zone are complex and poorly understood, but these areas can be clearly distinguished with proper diagnostic techniques. The epileptic spike focus is identified as the area where epileptiform EEG discharges are occurring (Chapters 12 and 13). The epileptogenic lesion usually can be visualized in situ by structural imaging techniques (Chapter 12) and positively identified by microscopic analysis of brain that is surgically resected or taken at autopsy (Chapter 5). The location and extent of the epileptogenic zone might be presumed from the correlation of electrophysiological and structural and functional neuroimaging studies, including intracranial EEG recordings, and by the disappearance of epileptic seizures after surgical resection; however, it is rarely proven definitively (Chapters 12 and 16). These three terms are not applicable in generalized epilepsy disorders.

Control, Cure, and Drug Resistance

DEFINITION

The term *control* is applied when the frequency or severity of epileptic seizures (or both) is reduced by treatment to some acceptable level for some period. Specific criteria have not been established for either the degree of seizure reduction or the period of time required to define *good control*, and criteria will vary depending on patient circumstances. *Complete control* means that the patient is seizure-free. Patients are technically *seizure-free* when they no longer have epileptic seizures, but definitions of seizure and the duration of the seizure-free period can vary, for pragmatic reasons (Chapters 16 and 17). A seizure-free patient who is not being treated for epilepsy might at some point be considered *cured*. For epidemiologic purposes, a patient is usually considered to have *active epilepsy* until seizure-free and off medications for five years (Chapter 2). Because no general definitions exist, the terms *seizure control* and *seizure-free* need to be defined for specific purposes each time they are used. *Drug resistance* is defined by the ILAE as failure of two appropriate drug trials because of inefficacy and not intolerance (Kwan et al., 2010), although some patients can become seizure-free after many trials (Luciano and Shorvon, 2007). Patients whose seizures can be controlled by antiseizure medications are referred to as *pharmacosensitive*, and those whose seizures continue despite adequate treatment as *pharmacoresistant*.

DISCUSSION

The term *seizure-free* is not always used to mean free of all epileptic seizures, although that is the logical assumption. Reports on outcome from many clinical studies, particularly surgical series, refer to patients as seizure-free if they no longer suffer from epileptic seizures that impair function or are apparent to an observer, even though they may continue to experience auras and may still require antiseizure medication (Chapter 16). This incorrect usage of the term *seizure-free* serves a practical purpose but encourages physicians to ignore auras that are disturbing to the patient. For instance, health-related quality of life (HRQOL) is reduced for patients who continue to have auras postoperatively compared with those who are completely seizure-free (Vickrey et al., 1995) (Chapter 16). Epileptiform EEG discharges without associated behavioral signs or symptoms are never considered seizures, and except for patients with typical absences, there is a poor correlation between seizure control and the occurrence of interictal EEG abnormalities (Chapter 14).

A longer duration of complete seizure control is undoubtedly associated with a lower risk of seizure recurrence, but this relationship is inadequately defined. Consequently, there are no guidelines for using the length of a seizure-free period to predict a lasting effect. For instance, all states in the United States and many other countries allow patients with epilepsy to obtain driver's licenses if they have been free of seizures that impair driving functions for some time, but the required seizure-free period varies from three months to three years (Chapter 17). Clinically, decisions regarding termination of medical therapy are usually made after a patient has been seizure-free for two years (Chapter 14). Two years is also generally accepted as the minimum time necessary for considering a patient seizure free when one is assessing the effectiveness of surgical therapy, although seizures can recur much later (Chapter 16). Because patient reports can be unreliable, there is a need for more objective means of determining whether a patient has been seizure-free (Chapter 12). Whenever the term *seizure-free* is used, the period of time should be stated and the manner of determination should be indicated.

Clearly, epileptic seizures are controlled when they no longer occur; however, epileptic seizures are often said to be under *good control* when less than a seizure-free state has been achieved. *Good control* usually means that epileptic seizures do not seriously interfere with activities of daily living. What constitutes serious interference often depends on the severity of the ictal events and the degree of functional impairment due to other causes. For instance, experiencing a brief generalized tonic-clonic seizure a few times a year might be considered by some to be good control for an institutionalized child with severe developmental delay who previously had many such epileptic seizures a day, but this would certainly be unacceptable for most individuals living independently and working in full-time jobs.

Because patients often experience a transient, nonspecific reduction or cessation of epileptic seizures when a new treatment is instituted, sufficient time must elapse before any improvement in the epilepsy condition can be attributed to a therapeutic intervention (Chapter 14). This period is obviously longer for patients who have infrequent seizures than for those with frequent seizures and should be at least three times the pretreatment interictal interval (Kwan et al., 2010). Knowledge of the causes of epileptic seizures is also important, because institution of antiseizure drug therapy following one or several reactive epileptic seizures would lead to the erroneous impression that they ceased as a result of this treatment.

Cure is a difficult word to use in association with epilepsy disorders, because patients can experience single or recurrent epileptic seizures many years after they have become seizure-free. This observation suggests that some patients with epilepsy disorders are never actually cured but rather enter remission while the underlying neurological disturbance continues to exist (Chapter 14). On the other hand, some of these patients can merely have an increased susceptibility to seizures, and an apparent recurrence actually reflects the consequences of a new epileptogenic insult. Certain genetic epilepsy disorders that occur in children and predictably disappear later in life, such as *benign epilepsy of childhood with centrotemporal spikes*, can appear to leave no traces of the underlying disturbance; however, more detailed analysis reveals that many such disorders are associated with some degree of behavioral comorbidity (Chapters 7 and 11). Most patients who have less benign epilepsy conditions but spontaneously stop having epileptic seizures or are successfully treated by surgical excision and then no longer require medication also will never experience another epileptic seizure. In this situation, however, it is impossible to predict the future and pronounce a cure a priori. Definitive diagnosis of cure awaits the development of a reliable biomarker of epileptogenicity (Chapter 12). If the definition of epilepsy given above, which includes its consequences, is accepted, a purist would not consider a patient cured unless all those consequences were also abolished.

The concept of *medically intractable epilepsy* no longer has practical meaning, because there are so many available antiseizure drugs that it would literally take a lifetime to perform adequate trials of each one alone and in all conceivable combinations. There are data, however, to suggest that seizure freedom becomes increasingly unlikely after failure of a few trials of antiseizure drugs due to inefficacy and not intolerance. Therefore, the ILAE has suggested a definition for *drug-resistant epilepsy* as "failure of adequate trials of two tolerated, appropriately chosen and used antiseizure drug schedules (whether as monotherapies or in combination) to achieve sustained seizure freedom" (Kwan et al., 2010). This criterion becomes important when one is deciding whether to abandon further antiseizure drug trials in a given patient and consider alternative therapies such as surgery. When patients continue to have seizures, their frequency can be expressed as seizure occurrence for a given period or, in some cases, as *seizure days*, meaning the number of days during which one or more seizures occurred for a given period.

Antiepileptogenesis, Prevention, and Disease Modification

DEFINITION

Antiepileptogenesis refers to any intervention that counteracts epileptogenesis, whether the development or progression of an epilepsy condition. *Prevention* occurs when a pathological process is reversed and completely eliminated. *Disease modification* refers to an intervention that reduces or prevents the progression of any neurological disturbances associated with an epilepsy disorder, both epileptic and nonepileptic (comorbidity). Antiepileptogenesis therefore is one aspect of disease modification.

DISCUSSION

Epilepsy conditions are generally not static. Whether they are genetic or acquired, there is a period of development before epileptic seizures appear, and in some instances there is a progression or a worsening of the epilepsy condition, even when treatment is instituted. Furthermore, epilepsy conditions can be associated with nonepileptic neurological and cognitive deficits, which may result from the underlying cause or from the epilepsy itself, as is presumed to be the case for the epileptic encephalopathies. The search for a reliable antiepileptogenic intervention remains a major goal of epilepsy research (Galanopoulou et al., 2012; Pitkänen 2010). Such a treatment could cause *seizure modification* by delaying the onset of epilepsy and by reducing the severity of consequent epileptic seizures, or it could completely prevent the development of the disorder. Prevention in this case could mean the failure of epileptic seizures to appear, but in a purer sense it could mean the absence of any trace of the underlying pathophysiological epileptogenic abnormality.

Once an epileptic condition appears, seizures can become more severe and more frequent. Antiepileptogenic interventions would be capable of preventing or reversing such a progression and could also result in cure, while antiseizure drugs may merely appear to halt progression by reducing or eliminating seizure recurrence. Therefore it could be difficult to distinguish between antiseizure and true antiepileptogenic effects unless the treatment is removed.

When epilepsy disorders are associated with neurological and cognitive deficits, it can be difficult to determine to what extent they are due to the underlying pathological process and to what extent to recurrent epileptic seizures. For the epilepsy disorders classified as epileptic encephalopathies, it is presumed that the recurrent seizures are the cause; however, because the underlying pathophysiology is unknown in these conditions, it is not possible to eliminate the etiological process as a cause of the nonepileptic disturbances. The term *disease modification* has been defined for epilepsy research as "a process that alters the development or progression of a disease, in this case epilepsy. Disease-modifying interventions may be antiepileptogenic. In addition, they could modify co-morbidity by reducing or preventing deleterious nonepileptic functional and/or structural changes in the brain, and can also modify the pathological changes underlying epileptogenesis or co-morbidities" (Pitkänen, 2010).

Nonepileptic Seizures

DEFINITION

Nonepileptic seizures are nonepileptic events resembling epileptic seizures that can have many causes. When there is an involuntary psychological cause, the event is referred to as a *psychogenic nonepileptic seizure* (*PNES*).

DISCUSSION

The term *pseudoseizure* has been used in reference to both PNES and all nonepileptic seizures regardless of the cause. This usage creates confusion. Therefore the term *pseudoseizure* is no longer recommended, and the term *nonepileptic seizure* should always be qualified as psychogenic or otherwise.

The phenomenology of PNES is not clearly understood, but many forms appear to exist (Chapter 13). The concept of PNES is purposely less precise than *hysteroepilepsy*, because not all PNES necessarily reflect hysterical conversion reactions. Voluntary events that represent *factitious disorders* or *malingering* (Chapter 13) are considered distinct from PNES.

CLASSIFICATIONS

When the underlying cause of epilepsy (Chapter 5) is either unknown or irreversible, treatment and prognosis usually depend on characteristics of the ictal events (Chapter 6). In some patients, treatment and prognosis may also be determined by diagnosis of a specific epilepsy syndrome based on seizure type and other clinical information (Chapter 7). Consequently, it has been useful to define specific epileptic seizure types and epilepsy syndromes for diagnosis of individual patients. In addition, efforts to devise a *classification of epileptic seizures* and a *classification of the epilepsies* involve organizing these seizure types and syndromes into logical categories for a variety of teaching, research, and clinical purposes. Diagnostic entities have evolved as more information has become available, but classifications based on natural classes with a firm biological basis remain elusive.

This section begins with a detailed discussion of the older classifications of epilepsy for historical purposes, to provide an understanding of how general concepts have developed and, perhaps more importantly, how attempts to simplify and catagorize can perpetuate misinformation and negatively influence both clinical practice and research. The current approaches of most immediate importance are discussed at the end of this section.

Older Classifications of Epileptic Seizures

Terminology for epileptic seizures has suffered from imprecision, characterized by the common early distinction between small events, *petit mal seizures*, and large events, *grand mal seizures*. Better understanding of anatomical substrates of some forms of epilepsy led to the differentiation of *focal*, or *local*, from *generalized* epileptic seizures. Certain types of focal seizures were recognized and given names, for instance, seizures characterized by a *jacksonian march* of motor symptoms, *uncinate fits* with olfactory symptoms, and *psychomotor seizures* with peculiar disturbances of mental and emotional function. Generalized seizures were divided into *convulsive* and *nonconvulsive* types, occasionally referred to as *major motor* and *minor motor*.

The term *petit mal seizure* has been variously used to refer to all minor motor seizures; all small seizures, whether focal or generalized; all seizures characterized by a brief lapse of consciousness, whether focal or generalized; only generalized seizures characterized by a brief lapse of consciousness, now called *absences*; and only a specific type of absence seizure associated with well-defined clinical and EEG features. Similarly, the term *grand mal* has been applied to all generalized seizures whether of focal or generalized onset, all motor seizures generalized from the start of the seizure, and only generalized motor seizures with both tonic and clonic components. Persistence of such imprecise terminology in clinical practice and even in the medical literature continues to create confusion. The attempts of the ILAE to categorize all identified epileptic seizures systematically according to descriptive phenomenology (Commission on Classification, 1981) have vastly improved the clarity of communication about epilepsy and signify a major advance; however, they remain a work in progress (Engel, 2001; 2006; Berg et al., 2010).

INTERNATIONAL CLASSIFICATION OF EPILEPTIC SEIZURES

The ILAE published the first International Classification of Epileptic Seizures in 1970 (Gastaut, 1970) and a revision in 1981 (Commission on Classification and Terminology, 1981). The latter classification (Table 1–1) is discussed briefly here and in more detail in Chapter 6. This classification scheme was based entirely on distinctive behavioral and electrophysiological features of the epileptic ictal events and purposely avoided implications of specific pathophysiological mechanisms or anatomical substrates, because these were largely unknown at the time. The objectives were to reduce descriptive ambiguity and to include all recognized ictal phenomena in logical categories. The terminology was considered transitional, meant to facilitate the communication of clinical information until research into fundamental mechanisms of epilepsy allowed a more pathophysiologically oriented classification.

According to this classification, seizures are termed *partial* when behavioral or EEG evidence indicates they begin in a part of the brain limited to one hemisphere and *generalized* when they appear to begin on both hemispheres at the same time. When partial seizures evolve into generalized tonic-clonic seizures, they are called *secondarily generalized seizures*.

Partial seizures are subdivided into *simple partial seizures*, without impairment of consciousness, and *complex partial seizures*, with impairment of consciousness. Simple partial seizures can progress to become complex. Simple partial seizures are further classified according to symptoms: *motor, sensory, autonomic,* and *psychic.* Simple partial seizures with sensory, autonomic, or psychic symptoms that precede progression to impaired consciousness or motor seizures of any type are commonly referred to as *auras.*

Generalized seizures are subdivided into lapses of consciousness, called *absences*; minor motor events (*myoclonic, atonic,* and some brief *tonic* seizures); and major motor events (*tonic-clonic* or *grand mal* seizures and purely *tonic* and purely *clonic* generalized seizures). Absences are further subdivided into those considered typical of *genetic absence epilepsies* (Chapters 6 and 7) and *atypical absences.*

Definition of terms for the 1981 International Classification of Epileptic Seizures (see Table 1–1) was more precise than for the previous classification, for two reasons. First, it used impairment of consciousness as the sole means of distinguishing between simple and complex partial seizures. Second, it addressed an important difficulty often encountered when attempting to assign dynamic ictal events to specifically defined categories, by taking into account the symptom progressions that characterize most epileptic seizures. The classification formally recognized categories of simple partial seizures that evolve into complex partial seizures as well as partial seizures that evolve into generalized seizures.

Table 1–1 1981 International Classification of Epileptic Seizures

I. Partial (focal, local) seizures
  A. Simple partial seizures
    1. With motor signs
    2. With somatosensory or special sensory symptoms
    3. With autonomic symptoms or signs
    4. With psychic symptoms
  B. Complex partial seizures
    1. Simple partial onset followed by impairment of consciousness
    2. With impairment of consciousness at onset
  C. Partial seizures evolving to secondarily generalized seizures
    1. Simple partial seizures evolving to generalized seizures
    2. Complex partial seizures evolving to generalized seizures
    3. Simple partial seizures evolving to complex partial seizures evolving to generalized seizures
II. Generalized seizures (convulsive or non-convulsive)
  A. Absence seizures
    1. Typical absences
    2. Atypical absences
  B. Myoclonic seizures
  C. Clonic seizures
  D. Tonic seizures
  E. Tonic-clonic seizures
  F. Atonic seizures (astatic seizures)
III. Unclassified epileptic seizures

From Commission on Classification, 1981, with permission; see also Chapter 6.

The 1981 International Classification of Epileptic Seizures directed considerable attention toward the diagnosis of impaired consciousness (Commission on Classification, 1981). This descriptive deviation from the 1970 International Classification of Epileptic Seizures (Gastaut, 1970) led to the major substantive criticism of the new taxonomy. Defining *complex partial seizure* phenomenologically meant that this term no longer could be used synonymously with *temporal lobe*, *psychomotor*, or *limbic seizure* (Chapter 6), a practice that had become common as a result of the 1970 classification. In the 1981 scheme, limbic ictal events with autonomic, psychic, olfactory, or gustatory symptoms *in clear consciousness* are called simple partial seizures, whereas ictal events with focal features and impaired consciousness that do not appear to be limbic are classified as complex partial seizures. The need for a more precise descriptive definition was given precedence over the need for a useful, but only implied, clinical concept (prominent participation of, but not always origin from, mesial temporal limbic structures) (Chapter 6).

OTHER SEIZURE CLASSIFICATIONS

A number of other classifications of epileptic seizures have been proposed, but each brings with it additional reasons for dissatisfaction (Chapter 6). An abbreviated classification of epileptic seizures and myoclonus can be based on practical therapeutic considerations, given that focal seizures respond to a particular group of antiseizure drugs, while absences and some other generalized seizures are responsive to a different group, and myoclonus to a third (Chapter 14). However, the most prevalent alternative classification system, which derives from the Cleveland Clinic, uses a descriptive system based entirely on observed clinical ictal signs and symptoms (Lüders et al., 1998). This system has been criticized for several reasons: (1) Semiological information does not necessarily have prognostic, etiologic, or therapeutic implications except where localization information is necessary when surgical treatment is contemplated; (2) semiological data are rarely well documented except in those few patients who are admitted for video-EEG monitoring; and (3) this is actually not a classification which permits seizures to be categorized into homogenic groupings useful for research into fundamental neuronal mechanisms and gene discovery. In certain situations, however, there is considerable merit in careful observation and reporting of epileptic seizure semiology. For this reason the ILAE has adapted this system and published a glossary of terminology that standardizes the description of ictal phenomena (Blume et al., 2001).

Older Classifications of the Epilepsies

Like epileptic seizures, all epilepsy disorders were originally divided into *petit mal* epilepsy and *grand mal* epilepsy. Further distinctions were also made between *focal* epilepsy and *generalized* epilepsy, and the specific disorder of *psychomotor* or *temporal lobe* epilepsy was later recognized. Etiologically, epilepsy disorders were commonly considered to be either *secondary* (*symptomatic, acquired*) or *primary* (*idiopathic, essential*).

There have been three officially accepted comprehensive international classifications of the epilepsies. The 1970 International Classification (Merlis, 1970) was superficial but provided some basic concepts that have proven useful. The World Health Organization (WHO) classification (World Health Organization, 1987; 1994)) was based largely on ictal symptoms and considered only a few syndromes. The 1989 International Classification (Commission on Classification and Terminology, 1989) is concerned primarily with syndromes.

THE 1970 INTERNATIONAL CLASSIFICATION

An International Classification of the Epilepsies (Table 1–2) based on the International Classification of Epileptic Seizures was approved by the ILAE in 1970 (Merlis, 1970) and provides insight into the evolution of current classification schemes. This classification asserted that almost all epilepsy disorders could be divided into *partial epilepsies*, characterized by partial epileptic seizures (with or without generalized seizures), and *generalized epilepsies*, characterized only by generalized epileptic seizures. The generalized epilepsies were

Table 1–2 **1970 International Classification of the Epilepsies**

I. Generalized epilepsies
   A. Primary generalized epilepsies
   B. Secondary generalized epilepsies
   C. Undetermined generalized epilepsies
II. Partial (focal, local) epilepsies
III. Unclassified epilepsies

From Merlis, 1970, with permission.

further divided into *primary* and *secondary* types. (All partial epilepsies were assumed to be secondary.) *Primary* indicated the presence of a nonprogressive, usually age-related, presumably genetically determined disturbance unassociated with structural or metabolic brain abnormalities. According to this classification, patients with primary generalized epilepsies have absences, bilaterally synchronous myoclonic seizures, tonic-clonic seizures, or some combination of these symptoms and no other neurological or psychological impairment. Their interictal EEGs are normal except for characteristic bilaterally synchronous epileptiform discharges. Their epileptic seizures begin in childhood or adolescence, usually respond to appropriate medication, and often disappear in adolescence or early adulthood. The term *secondary* indicated seizures due to diffuse or multifocal lesions of the brain or to metabolic disturbances that are so widespread or so severe that epileptic seizures are generalized from the start. According to this classification, patients with secondary generalized epilepsies have mixed seizures, including any type of generalized epileptic seizure, commonly with neurological and psychological signs and symptoms of diffuse cerebral lesions. Their typical interictal EEG patterns consist of irregular and often asynchronous epileptiform discharges superimposed on diffusely abnormal baseline rhythms, and their clinical seizures usually respond poorly to treatment and do not resolve with time.

This classification was useful because it defined categories of epilepsy disorders that were consistent with the terminology introduced by the 1970 International Classification of Epileptic Seizures and at the same time took into consideration additional clinical and EEG features that defined broad symptom complexes (but not syndromes). The concept of primary and secondary epilepsy was particularly important for clinical diagnoses, because in children these disorders can appear superficially similar early in their course, but the prognoses and indications for therapy are quite different.

Several shortcomings made this classification difficult to use and inaccurate. Considerable confusion was created by the similarity between the term *secondary generalized epilepsy*, which describes an epilepsy disorder, and *secondarily generalized epileptic seizure*, which refers to a partial seizure that has become generalized. To add to the confusion, the term *secondary generalization* is commonly used in reference to epileptiform EEG patterns that appear generalized but result from a single epileptogenic region, also called *secondary bilateral synchrony* (Chapter 13). This classification incorrectly limited the designations of *primary* and *secondary* to the description of generalized epilepsy disorders. Benign, age-related, genetic epilepsy disorders characterized by focal seizures also exist (Chapters 5 and 7) and are appropriately considered to be primary.

THE WHO CLASSIFICATIONS

Billing in the United States is based on the ninth version of the International Classification of Diseases (ICD-9) of the WHO (World Health Organization, 1987), which is periodically updated, most recently in 2008 (Table 1–3). Billing will change over to the ICD-10 (World Health Organization, 1994) (Table 1–4) in October 2013. These classifications allow disorders to be categorized by seizure type and etiology (if desired). A few syndromes are also included. These classifications do not take into account patients who do not have one of the syndromes listed but experience more than one type of seizure. The recognition of forms of *status epilepticus* as separate categories is a unique feature. Work is currently progressing on the ICD-11, with an effort to bring it more in line with the ILAE classifications.

THE 1985 AND 1989 INTERNATIONAL CLASSIFICATIONS

Many epilepsy syndromes are recognized, based on the combination of specific epileptic signs and symptoms; age of onset of seizures;

associated general physical, neurological, and mental abnormalities; the presence or absence of an inheritance pattern; and a characteristic course. Certain information about pathophysiology, anatomical substrates, and etiology sometimes can be inferred from this information. The International Classification of the Epilepsies and Epileptic Syndromes, accepted by the ILAE in 1985 and modified in 1989 (Commission on Classification and Terminology, 1989) (Table 1–5), represents the first major attempt to identify epilepsy syndromes and to organize them into cohesive groups. The characterization of epilepsy syndromes was determined after careful review of case histories and videotaped seizures by a panel of experts. Descriptions of syndromes were published in French in 1984 and English in 1985 (Roger et al., 1985). This book has come to be known as the *Blue Guide* (*Le Guide Bleu*), and updated editions have since appeared, the most recent in 2005 and 2012 (Roger et al., 2005; Bureau et al., 2012). Classification is based on three specific features: (1) whether seizures are partial or generalized, (2) whether the disorder is primary or secondary, and (3) the age of onset of habitual seizures (Chapter 7). By 1984, primary focal epilepsies were well recognized.

In an effort to avoid semantic difficulties, the term *localization-related* replaced *partial* because the latter seemed to imply that syndromes rather than seizures were partial or incomplete. The terms *idiopathic* and *symptomatic* replaced *primary* and *secondary* to avoid confusion with secondarily generalized seizures. Unfortunately, as noted earlier, the term *idiopathic* is commonly misused and introduced confusion with an earlier vocabulary.

Amendments accepted in 1989 included an expansion of the section on localization-related symptomatic epilepsies to include disorders defined by partial seizures of specific types, such as temporal lobe epilepsy and epilepsia partialis continua. The concept of cryptogenic epilepsy was introduced to define syndromes presumed to be symptomatic but with unknown etiology.

Two other major problems were perpetuated by the 1989 classification: The idiopathic/symptomatic and the localization/generalized dichotomies are simplistic and unsupportable. With respect to the former, there is reason to believe that the causes of most, perhaps

Table 1–3 Epilepsy Section of the Ninth International Classification of Diseases (ICD-9)

345 Epilepsy and recurrent seizures

> *EXCLUDES* progressive myoclonic epilepsy (333.2)

The following fifth-digit subclassification is for use with categories 345.0,.1, 4-.9:

> **0 without mention of intractable epilepsy**
> **1 with intractable epilepsy**

DEF: Brain disorder characterized by electrical-like disturbances; may include occasional impairment or loss of consciousness, abnormal motor phenomena and psychic or sensory disturbances.

345.0 Generalized nonconvulsive epilepsy

Absences:	Pykno-epilepsy
atonic	Seizures
typical	akinetic
Minor epilepsy	atonic
Petit mal	

345.1 Generalized convulsive epilepsy

Epileptic seizures:	Epileptic seizures:
clonic	tonic-clonic
myoclonic	Grand mal
tonic	Major epilepsy

> *EXCLUDES* convulsions
> > NOS (780.39)
> > infantile (780.39)
> > newborn (779.0)
> > infantile spasms (345.6)

DEF: Convulsive seizures with tension of limbs (tonic) or rhythmic contractions (clonic)

345.2 Petit mal status

Epileptic absence status

DEF: Minor myoclonic spasms and sudden momentary loss of consciousness in epilepsy

345.3 Grand mal status

Status epilepticus NOS

> *EXCLUDES* epilepsia partialis continua (345.7) status:
> > Psychomotor (345.7)
> > Temporal lobe (345.7)

DEF: Sudden loss of consciousness followed by generalized convulsions in epilepsy

345.4 Localization-related (focal) (partial) epilepsy and epileptic syndromes with complex partial seizures

Epilepsy:
  limbic system
  partial:
    secondarily generalized
    with impairment of consciousness
    with memory and ideational disturbances
  psychomotor
  psychosensory
  temporal lobe
Epileptic automatism

345.5 Localization-related (focal) (partial) epilepsy and epileptic syndromes with simple partial seizures

Epilepsy:
  Bravais-Jacksonian NOS
  Focal (motor) NOS
  Jacksonian NOS
  motor partial
  partial NOS:
    without impairment of consciousness

(continued)

Table 1–3 (Continued)

sensory-induced
somatomotor
somatosensory
visceral
visual

345.6 Infantile spasms

Hypsarrhythmia   Salaam attacks
Lightning spasms
EXCLUDES   *salaam tic (781.0)*

345.7 Epilepsia partialis continua

Kojevnikov's epilepsy

DEF: Continuous muscle contractions and relaxation; result of abnormal neural discharge

345.8 Other forms of epilepsy and recurrent seizures

Epilepsy   Epilepsy
cursive [running]   gelastic

345.9 Epilepsy, unspecified

Epileptic convulsions, fits, or seizures NOS
Recurrent seizures NOS
Seizure disorder NOS
EXCLUDES   *convulsion (convulsive) disorder (780.39)*
convulsive seizure or fit NOS (780.39)
recurrent convulsions (780.39)

NOS = not otherwise specified
From American Medical Association, 2011

Table 1–4 2012 International Classification of Diseases (10th Revision, Clinical Modification)* (2012 ICD–10–CM)

G40 Epilepsy and recurrent seizures

Note: the following terms are to be considered equivalent to intractable:
pharmacoresistant (pharmacologically resistant),
treatment resistant,
refractory (medically) and poorly controlled

Excludes: conversion disorder with seizures (F44.5)
convulsions NOS (R56.9)
hippocampal sclerosis (G93.81)
mesial temporal sclerosis (G93.81)
post traumatic seizures (R56.1)
seizure (convulsive) NOS (R56.9)
seizure of newborn (P90)
temporal sclerosis (G93.81)
Todd's paralysis (G83.8)

G40.0 Localization-related (focal) (partial) idiopathic epilepsy and epileptic syndromes with seizures of localized onset

Benign childhood epilepsy with centrotemporal EEG spikes
Childhood epilepsy with occipital EEG paroxysms
Excludes: adult onset localization-related epilepsy (G40.1-, G40.2-)

G40.00 Localization-related (focal) (partial) idiopathic epilepsy and epileptic syndromes with seizures of localized onset, not intractable

Localization-related (focal) (partial) idiopathic epilepsy and epileptic syndromes with seizures of localized onset without intractability

G40.001 Localization-related (focal) (partial) idiopathic epilepsy and epileptic syndromes with seizures of localized onset, not intractable, with status epilepticus

(continued)

Table 1–4 (Continued)

G40.009 Localization-related (focal) (partial) idiopathic epilepsy and epileptic syndromes with seizures of localized onset, not intractable, without status epilepticus
Localization-related (focal) (partial) idiopathic epilepsy and epileptic syndromes with seizures of localized onset NOS

G40.01 Localization-related (focal) (partial) idiopathic epilepsy and epileptic syndromes with seizures of localized onset, intractable

G40.011 Localization-related (focal) (partial) idiopathic epilepsy and epileptic syndromes with seizures of localized onset, intractable, with status epilepticus

G40.019 Localization-related (focal) (partial) idiopathic epilepsy and epileptic syndromes with seizures of localized onset, intractable, without status epilepticus

G40.1 Localization-related (focal) (partial) symptomatic epilepsy and epileptic syndromes with simple partial seizures
Attacks without alteration of consciousness
Epilepsia partialis continua [Kozhevnikof]
Simple partial seizures developing into secondarily generalized seizures

G40.10 Localization-related (focal) (partial) symptomatic epilepsy and epileptic syndromes with simple partial seizures, not intractable
Localization-related (focal) (partial) symptomatic epilepsy and epileptic syndromes with simple partial seizures without intractability

G40.101 Localization-related (focal) (partial) symptomatic epilepsy and epileptic syndromes with simple partial seizures, not intractable, with status epilepticus

G40.109 Localization-related (focal) (partial) symptomatic epilepsy and epileptic syndromes with simple partial seizures, not intractable, without status epilepticus
Localization-related (focal) (partial) symptomatic epilepsy and epileptic syndromes with simple partial seizures NOS

G40.11 Localization-related (focal) (partial) symptomatic epilepsy and epileptic syndromes with simple partial seizures, intractable

G40.111 Localization-related (focal) (partial) symptomatic epilepsy and epileptic syndromes with simple partial seizures, intractable, with status epilepticus

G40.119 Localization-related (focal) (partial) symptomatic epilepsy and epileptic syndromes with simple partial seizures, intractable, without status epilepticus

G40.2 Localization-related (focal) (partial) symptomatic epilepsy and epileptic syndromes with complex partial seizures
Attacks with alteration of consciousness, often with automatisms
Complex partial seizures developing into secondarily generalized seizures

G40.20 Localization-related (focal) (partial) symptomatic epilepsy and epileptic syndromes with complex partial seizures, not intractable
Localization-related (focal) (partial) symptomatic epilepsy and epileptic syndromes with complex partial seizures without intractability

G40.201 Localization-related (focal) (partial) symptomatic epilepsy and epileptic syndromes with complex partial seizures, not intractable, with status epilepticus

G40.209 Localization-related (focal) (partial) symptomatic epilepsy and epileptic syndromes with complex partial seizures, not intractable, without status epilepticus
Localization-related (focal) (partial) symptomatic epilepsy and epileptic syndromes with complex partial seizures NOS

G40.21 Localization-related (focal) (partial) symptomatic epilepsy and epileptic syndromes with complex partial seizures, intractable

G40.211 Localization-related (focal) (partial) symptomatic epilepsy and epileptic syndromes with complex partial seizures, intractable, with status epilepticus

G40.219 Localization-related (focal) (partial) symptomatic epilepsy and epileptic syndromes with complex partial seizures, intractable, without status epilepticus

G40.3 Generalized idiopathic epilepsy and epileptic syndromes
Code also MERRF syndrome, if applicable (E88.42)

G40.30 Generalized idiopathic epilepsy and epileptic syndromes, not intractable
Generalized idiopathic epilepsy and epileptic syndromes without intractability

(continued)

Table 1–4 (**Continued**)

G40.301 Generalized idiopathic epilepsy and epileptic syndromes, not intractable, with status epilepticus

G40.309 Generalized idiopathic epilepsy and epileptic syndromes, not intractable, without status epilepticus

Generalized idiopathic epilepsy and epileptic syndromes NOS

G40.31 Generalized idiopathic epilepsy and epileptic syndromes, intractable

G40.311 Generalized idiopathic epilepsy and epileptic syndromes, intractable, with status epilepticus

G40.319 Generalized idiopathic epilepsy and epileptic syndromes, intractable, without status epilepticus

G40.A Absence epileptic syndrome

Childhood absence epilepsy [pyknolepsy] Juvenile absence epilepsy

Absence epileptic syndrome, NOS

G40.A0 Absence epileptic syndrome, not intractable

G40.A01 Absence epileptic syndrome, not intractable, with status epilepticus

G40.A09 Absence epileptic syndrome, not intractable, without status epilepticus

G40.A1 Absence epileptic syndrome, intractable

G40.A11 Absence epileptic syndrome, intractable, with status epilepticus

G40.A19 Absence epileptic syndrome, intractable, without status epilepticus

G40.B Juvenile myoclonic epilepsy [impulsive petit mal]

G40.B0 Juvenile myoclonic epilepsy, not intractable

G40.B01 Juvenile myoclonic epilepsy, not intractable, with status epilepticus

G40.B09 Juvenile myoclonic epilepsy, not intractable, without status epilepticus

G40.B1 Juvenile myoclonic epilepsy, intractable

G40.B11 Juvenile myoclonic epilepsy, intractable, with status epilepticus

G40.B19 Juvenile myoclonic epilepsy, intractable, without status epilepticus

G40.4 Other generalized epilepsy and epileptic syndromes

Epilepsy with grand mal seizures on awakening

Epilepsy with myoclonic absences

Epilepsy with myoclonic-astatic seizures

Grand mal seizure NOS

Nonspecific atonic epileptic seizures

Nonspecific clonic epileptic seizures

Nonspecific myoclonic epileptic seizures

Nonspecific tonic epileptic seizures

Nonspecific tonic-clonic epileptic seizures

Symptomatic early myoclonic encephalopathy

G40.40 Other generalized epilepsy and epileptic syndromes, not intractable

Other generalized epilepsy and epileptic syndromes without intractability

Other generalized epilepsy and epileptic syndromes NOS

G40.401 Other generalized epilepsy and epileptic syndromes, not intractable, with status epilepticus

G40.409 Other generalized epilepsy and epileptic syndromes, not intractable, without status epilepticus

G40.41 Other generalized epilepsy and epileptic syndromes, intractable

G40.411 Other generalized epilepsy and epileptic syndromes, intractable, with status epilepticus

G40.419 Other generalized epilepsy and epileptic syndromes, intractable, without status epilepticus

G40.5 Epileptic seizures related to external causes

Epileptic seizures related to alcohol

Epileptic seizures related to drugs

Epileptic seizures related to hormonal changes

Epileptic seizures related to sleep deprivation

Epileptic seizures related to stress

(continued)

Table 1–4 (Continued)

Use additional code for adverse effect, if applicable, to identify drug (T36-T50 with fifth or sixth character 5)

Code also, if applicable, associated epilepsy and recurrent seizures (G40.-)

G40.50 Epileptic seizures related to external causes, not intractable

    G40.501 Epileptic seizures related to external causes, not intractable, with status epilepticus

    G40.509 Epileptic seizures related to external causes, not intractable, without status epilepticus

    Epileptic seizures related to external causes, NOS

G40.6 Grand mal seizures unspecified (with or without petit mal)°°

G40.7 Petit mal unspecified (without grand mal seizures)°°

G40.8 Other epilepsy and recurrent seizures

    Epilepsies and epileptic syndromes undetermined as to whether they are focal or generalized
    Landau-Kleffner syndrome

    G40.80 Other epilepsy

        G40.801 Other epilepsy, not intractable, with status epilepticus

        Other epilepsy without intractability with status epilepticus

        G40.802 Other epilepsy, not intractable, without status epilepticus

        Other epilepsy NOS

        Other epilepsy without intractability without status epilepticus

        G40.803 Other epilepsy, intractable, with status epilepticus

        G40.804 Other epilepsy, intractable, without status epilepticus

    G40.81 Lennox-Gastaut syndrome

        G40.811 Lennox-Gastaut syndrome, not intractable, with status epilepticus

        G40.812 Lennox-Gastaut syndrome, not intractable, without status epilepticus

        G40.813 Lennox-Gastaut syndrome, intractable, with status epilepticus

        G40.814 Lennox-Gastaut syndrome, intractable, without status epilepticus

    G40.82 Epileptic spasms, Infantile spasms Salaam attacks West syndrome

        G40.821 Epileptic spasms, not intractable, with status epilepticus

        G40.822 Epileptic spasms, not intractable, without status epilepticus

        G40.823 Epileptic spasms, intractable, with status epilepticus

        G40.824 Epileptic spasms, intractable, without status epilepticus

    G40.89 Other seizures

    Excludes: post traumatic seizures (R56.1)

        recurrent seizures NOS (G40.909)

        seizure NOS (R56.9)

G40.9 Epilepsy, unspecified

    G40.90 Epilepsy, unspecified, not intractable

    Epilepsy, unspecified, without intractability

        G40.901 Epilepsy, unspecified, not intractable, with status epilepticus

        G40.909 Epilepsy, unspecified, not intractable, without status epilepticus

    Epilepsy NOS

    Epileptic convulsions NOS

    Epileptic fits NOS

    Epileptic seizures NOS

    Recurrent seizures NOS

    Seizure disorder NOS

    G40.91 Epilepsy, unspecified, intractable

    Intractable seizure disorder NOS

        G40.911 Epilepsy, unspecified, intractable, with status epilepticus

        G40.919 Epilepsy, unspecified, intractable, without status epilepticus

NOS = not otherwise specified

Intended to be used in the United States for billing purposes after October 2014.

*Available online at http://www.cdc.gov/nchs/icd/icd10cm.htm

°°G40.6 and G40.7 are considered redundant and not included in the ICD-10-CM for billing purposes.

Table 1–5 1989 International Classification of the Epilepsies and Epileptic Syndromes

1. Localization-related (focal, local, partial)
   1.1 Idiopathic (with age-related onset)
        At present, the following syndromes are established, but more may be identified in the future:
        • Benign childhood epilepsy with centrotemporal spikes
        • Childhood epilepsy with occipital paroxysms
        • Primary reading epilepsy
   1.2 Symptomatic
        • Chronic progressive epilepsia partialis continua of childhood
   1.3 Cryptogenic (presumed to be symptomatic but with unknown etiology). The symptomatic and cryptogenic categories comprise syndromes of great individual variability that are based mainly on:
        • Seizure types (according to the International Classification of Epileptic Seizures)
        • Anatomical localization
          Temporal lobe epilepsies
          Frontal lobe epilepsies
          Parietal lobe seizures
          Occipital lobe epilepsies
          Bi- and multilobar epilepsies
        • Etiology (in symptomatic epilepsies)
        • Specific modes of precipitation
2. Generalized
   2.1 Idiopathic (with age-related onset, in order of age)
        • Benign neonatal familial convulsions
        • Benign neonatal convulsions
        • Benign myoclonic epilepsy in infancy
        • Childhood absence epilepsy (pyknolepsy)
        • Juvenile absence epilepsy
        • Juvenile myoclonic epilepsy (impulsive petit mal)
        • Epilepsy with grand mal (GTC) seizures on awaking
        • Other idiopathic generalized epilepsies not defined above
        • Epilepsies with seizures precipitated by specific modes of activation
   2.2 Cryptogenic or symptomatic (in order of age)
        • West syndrome (infantile spasms, Blitz-Nick-Salaam-Krampfe)
        • Lennox-Gastaut syndrome
        • Epilepsy with myoclonic-astatic seizures
        • Epilepsy with myoclonic absences
   2.3 Symptomatic
        2.3.1 Nonspecific etiology
               • Early myoclonic encephalopathy
               • Early infantile epileptic encephalopathy with suppression-burst
               • Other symptomatic generalized epilepsies not defined above
        2.3.2 Specific syndromes
3. Epilepsies and syndromes undetermined as to whether focal or generalized
   3.1 With both generalized and focal seizures
        • Neonatal seizures
        • Severe myoclonic epilepsy in infancy
        • Epilepsy with continuous spike-waves during sleep
        • Acquired epileptic aphasia (Landau-Kleffner syndrome)
        • Other undetermined epilepsies not defined above
   3.2 Without unequivocal generalized or focal features (e.g., many cases of sleep-grand mal)
4. Special syndromes
   4.1 Situation-related seizures (Gelegenheitsanfälle)
        • Febrile convulsions
        • Isolated seizures or isolated status epilepticus
        • Seizures due to acute metabolic or toxic factors such as alcohol, drugs, eclampsia, nonkinetic hyperglycemia, and so on

From Commission on Classification, 1989, with permission.

all, epilepsies are multifactorial, involving both genetically determined and acquired dysfunctions (Chapter 5) (Fig. 1–1). Most disorders can be viewed as lying on a continuum between the extremes; where they fall often determines prognosis and therapy. As a rule, the more the features of the disorder resemble primary epilepsy, the better the prognosis; the more they resemble secondary epilepsy, the worse the prognosis, although this is by no means absolute. Not all primary epilepsies are benign (e.g., *Dravet's syndrome*).

The boundaries between localization-related and generalized epilepsy disorders are also not well defined. This is most obvious for the secondary epilepsy conditions, where the location, extent, and severity of the lesion or lesions determine how generalized the behavioral and EEG features of an epileptic seizure appear to be at the start (Chapter 5). Consequently, a continuum also exists here, and conditions in between the extremes are characterized by epileptiform EEG discharges that are bilaterally independent, multifocal, and bilaterally synchronous with minor focal or lateralizing features (Fig. 1–2). It is not always easy to determine when epileptic seizures, as well as epilepsy disorders, should be classified as localization related or generalized. This distinction can be important when patients are candidates for surgical therapy (Chapter 16). Genetic factors also influence the degree of generalization for both idiopathic and symptomatic disorders, and overlap exists between idiopathic localization-related and idiopathic generalized epilepsies (Chapter 5).

Recent Efforts to Revise the International Classifications

In the late 1990s, for all of the reasons stated above, the ILAE began a concerted effort to revise the International Classifications of Epileptic Seizures and the Epilepsies. It was recognized that classifications are used for many purposes in addition to communication among physicians. Classification schemes are important for teaching; clear categorization of discrete clinical phenotypes is essential for basic research into fundamental mechanisms as well as gene discovery; other considerations need to be taken into account for clinical research purposes such as epidemiologic studies and clinical trials; and unique issues are important when evaluating surgical candidates. It was determined that any new classification would need to be seen as a flexible work in progress that could be modified as needed for different purposes and updated as new information became available. Finally, it was concluded that any new classification system should be considered a "testable working hypothesis, subject to verification, falsifications, and revisions" (Engel, 2001).

With respect to individual patients, however, organizing seizures and syndromes into comprehensive classification schemes is not

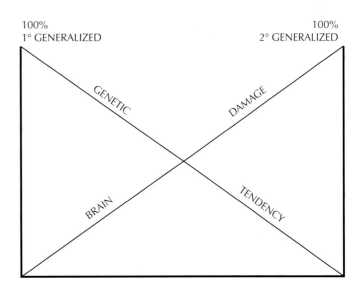

Figure 1–1. The multifactorial concept of generalized epilepsy. Although the primary generalized epileptic disorders are considered to be of genetic origin and secondary generalized epilepsy disorders are due to diffuse brain damage, patients often present with symptoms that reflect both features to some extent and cannot be definitively classified at one extreme or the other (after Gloor, 1977). (From Engel, 1984, with permission.)

100%
1° GENERALIZED

100%
2° GENERALIZED

GENETIC

DAMAGE

BRAIN

TENDENCY

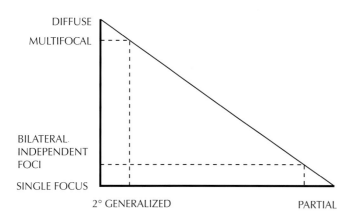

Figure 1–2. The spectrum of symptomatology along the continuum between secondary generalized and partial epilepsies depends on the extent and location of brain dysfunction. At the far right of this diagram, partial seizures may arise from discrete focal lesions, whereas bilaterally independent EEG spike foci are often seen with limbic involvements. As the extent of brain dysfunction increases, patients often demonstrate multifocal EEG and behavioral disturbances or generalized disturbances with focal features rather than the absolutely generalized symptomatology of secondary generalized seizures. (From Engel, 1984, with permission.)

necessarily a useful exercise compared with diagnosing discrete epilepsy syndromes and, when this is not possible, discrete seizure types. In a major departure from previous classifications of seizures, which were based on electroclinical features, it was determined that the state of knowledge regarding different types of ictal events is now sufficient to allow characterization of many epileptic seizures based on specific pathophysiological mechanisms and anatomical substrates. The intention is now to treat epileptic seizure types as diagnostic entities, so that when diagnosis of an epilepsy syndrome is not possible, the seizure diagnosis will have etiologic, therapeutic, and prognostic implications.

As a first step, a recommendation for a diagnostic scheme was published in 2001 (Table 1–6) (Engel, 2001). This is an approach to diagnosis in individual patients and is not a classification. Axis I is optional and consists of a description of ictal phenomenology according to a glossary of recommended terminology (Blume et al., 2001). Axis II is seizure types as diagnostic entities. Axis III is epilepsy syndromes, taking into account numerous advances in understanding these conditions since 1989, but without attempts to categorize epilepsies that did not fit into a recognized, well-defined syndrome. An updated list of syndromes was provided, which has subsequently been updated and organized by age (Berg et al., 2010). Axis IV is etiology and Axis V an optional classification of impairment, which is intended to be based on the WHO International Classification of Functioning and Disability (ICIDH-2, 1999).

The next attempt at revision (Engel, 2006) established "measurable criteria for recognizing epileptic seizure types and epilepsy syndromes as unique diagnostic entities or natural classes that can be reproducibly distinguished from all other diagnostic entities and natural classes." The intention is to move beyond signs and symptoms for identification of both epileptic seizures and epilepsy syndromes and to incorporate recent concepts of anatomical substrates, pathophysiological mechanisms, and genetics. Semiology alone is not a reliable basis for defining a discrete diagnostic entity, because seizures that look alike (e.g., absences and brief limbic seizures with impaired consciousness only) can represent entirely different diagnostic entities, whereas frontal lobe and occipital lobe seizures can be a single diagnostic entity when they reflect identical pathophysiological mechanisms even though their clinical appearances are entirely different.

Several other changes in terminology are now recommended as a result of these two reports. The term *focal* is now used for both seizures and syndromes to replace the terms *partial* and *localization-related*. The term *epileptic encephalopathy* has been introduced to describe conditions in which the epileptic processes themselves are believed to contribute to progressive disturbances in cerebral function. The terms *simple* and *complex partial seizures* are no longer recommended. It is acknowledged that ictal impairment of consciousness is important and should be described when appropriate for seizure patterns in individual patients, but this factor will not be used

Table 1–6 Proposed Diagnostic Scheme for People with Epileptic Seizures and with Epilepsy

Epileptic seizures and epilepsy syndromes are to be described and categorized according to a system that uses standardized terminology, and that is sufficiently flexible to take into account the following practical and dynamic aspects of epilepsy diagnosis:

1. Some patients cannot be given a recognized syndromic diagnosis.
2. Seizure types and syndromes change as new information is obtained.
3. Complete and detailed descriptions of ictal phenomenology are not always necessary.
4. Multiple classification schemes can, and should, be designed for specific purposes (e.g., communication and teaching; therapeutic trials; epidemiologic investigations; selection of surgical candidates; basic research; genetic characterizations).

This diagnostic scheme is divided into five parts, or Axes, organized to facilitate a logical clinical approach to the development of hypotheses necessary to determine the diagnostic studies and therapeutic strategies to be undertaken in individual patients:

Axis 1: Ictal phenomenology, from the Glossary of Descriptive Ictal Terminology, can be used to describe ictal events with any degree or detail needed.
Axis 2: Seizure type, from the List of Epileptic Seizures. Localization within the brain and precipitating stimuli for reflex seizures should be specified when appropriate.
Axis 3: Syndrome, from the List of Epilepsy Syndromes, with the understanding that a syndromic diagnosis may not always be possible.
Axis 4: Etiology, from a Classification of Diseases Frequently Associated with Epileptic Seizures or Epilepsy Syndromes when possible, genetic defects, or specific pathologic substrates for symptomatic focal epilepsies.
Axis 5: Impairment, this optimal, but often useful, additional diagnostic parameter can be derived from an impairment classification adapted from the WHO ICIDH-2.

From Engel, 2001, with permission.

to classify specific seizure types. According to the ILAE glossary, the correct terminology for focal seizures with impaired consciousness is *focal dyscognitive seizures* (Blume et al., 2001). For practical purposes, the distinction between focal and generalized seizures is maintained in the updated list of seizure types. In lieu of adequate evidence for categorizing epilepsy syndromes based on the two false dichotomies used in previous classifications, updated syndromes are now merely listed by age of onset, and it is acknowledged that many patients will have epilepsy disorders that cannot readily be diagnosed as a defined epilepsy syndrome (Berg et al., 2010).

The most recent ILAE recommendation for revision of terminology and concepts for organization of seizures and epilepsy was published in 2010 (Berg et al., 2010). Further effort has been made to clarify the focal/generalized dichotomy with respect to seizures. Generalized seizures are now defined as: originating at some point within, and rapidly engaging, bilaterally distributed networks. Such bilateral networks can include cortical and subcortical structures, but do not necessarily include the entire cortex. Although individual seizure onsets can appear localized, their location and lateralization are not consistent from one seizure to another. Generalized seizures can be asymmetric.

Focal epileptic seizures are defined as: originating within networks limited to one hemisphere, which may be discretely localized or more widely distributed. Focal seizures may originate in subcortical structures. For each seizure type, ictal onset is consistent from one seizure to another with preferential propagation patterns, which can involve the contralateral hemisphere. In some cases, however, there is more than one epileptogenic network, and more than one seizure type, but each individual seizure type has a consistent site of onset. Focal seizures do not fall into any recognized set of natural classes based on any current understanding of the mechanisms involved.

Electroclinical correlations may be necessary to identify ictal events as focal when there is rapid propagation or when they begin in silent areas of the brain and appear generalized behaviorally (Chapter 6). Although it has been considered useful to view limbic and neocortical focal seizures as distinct diagnostic entities (Engel, 2001; 2006), the current list of recognized seizure types (Table 1–7) includes only generalized seizures. The 2010 ILAE recommendation again acknowledges that impairment of consciousness is important for individual patients; however, this is not a useful criterion for classifying epileptic seizure types per se. An approach for categorization or classification for focal seizures has yet to be developed, but descriptors for use with individual patients are shown in Table 1–8.

With respect to epilepsies, the recommendation is that only recognized syndromes be considered. Previous attempts to fit all epilepsies into a comprehensive classification have been abandoned. The term *syndrome* is "restricted to a group of clinical entities that are reliably identified by a cluster of electroclinical characteristics." In practice, these are well-defined conditions that for the most part are genetic and in the past would have been identified as idiopathic. These conditions, however, are not necessarily benign. The

Table 1–7 **2010 Classification of Seizures***

Generalized seizures
    Tonic-clonic (in any combination)
    Absence
        Typical
        Atypical
        Absence with special features
            Myoclonic absence
            Eyelid myoclonia
    Myoclonic
        Myoclonic
        Myoclonic atonic
        Myoclonic tonic
    Clonic
    Tonic
    Atonic
Focal seizures
Unknown
    Epileptic spasms

*Seizures that cannot be clearly diagnosed into one of the categories above should be considered unclassified until further information allows their accurate diagnosis. This is not considered a classification category, however.
From Berg et al., 2010, with permission.

Table 1–8 **Descriptors of focal Seizures according to Degree of Impairment during Seizure***

Without impairment of consciousness or awareness
With observable motor or autonomic components. This roughly corresponds to the concept of "simple partial seizure." "Focal motor" and "autonomic" are terms that may adequately convey this concept depending on the seizure manifestations.
Involving subjective sensory or psychic phenomena only. This corresponds to the concept of an aura, a term endorsed in the 2001 Glossary.
With impairment of consciousness or awareness. This roughly corresponds to the concept of "complex partial seizure". "Dyscognitive" is a term that has been proposed for this concept (Blume et al., 2001).
Evolving to a bilateral, convulsive** seizure (involving tonic, clonic, or tonic and clonic components). This expression replaces the term "secondarily generalized seizure."

° For more descriptors that have been clearly defined and recommended for use, see Blume et al., 2001.
°° The term "convulsive" was considered a lay term in the Glossary; however, we note that it is used throughout medicine in various forms and translates well across many languages. Its use is therefore endorsed.
From Berg et al., 2010, with permission.

practice of referring to certain severe epilepsy syndromes as *catastrophic epilepsies* is discouraged. The dichotomies of focal/generalized and idiopathic/symptomatic are no longer considered valid or useful for the classification of epilepsy syndromes, which are listed by age in Table 1–9; however, several well-recognized epilepsy conditions that do not meet the current definition of electroclinical syndromes are also included as "constellations." The 2010 ILAE recommendation recognizes that certain conditions associated with epileptic seizures are not considered epilepsy syndromes because the epileptic seizures are either reactive or the duration of the disorder is short, and it acknowledges that epilepsies can be organized according to structural and metabolic causes. A more detailed etiological classification of the epilepsies has also been proposed (Shorvon, 2011) (Table 1–10), which could help resolve the difficulties in defining structural metabolic epilepsies that do not fit the concept of syndrome as described in this document.

Table 1–9 2010 Electroclinical Syndromes and Other Epilepsies

Electro-clinical syndromes arranged by age at onset°
    Neonatal period
        Benign familial neonatal epilepsy (BFNE)
        Early myoclonic encephalopathy (EME)
        Ohtahara syndrome
    Infancy
        Epilepsy of infancy with migrating partial seizures
        West syndrome
        Myoclonic epilepsy in infancy (MEI)
        Benign infantile epilepsy
        Benign familial infantile epilepsy
        Dravet syndrome
        Myoclonic encephalopathy in nonprogressive disorders
    Childhood
        Febrile seizures plus (FS+) (can start in infancy)
        Panayiotopoulos syndrome
        Epilepsy with myoclonic atonic (previously astatic) seizures
        Benign epilepsy with centrotemporal spikes (BECTS)
        Autosomal-dominant nocturnal frontal lobe epilepsy (ADNFLE)
        Late onset childhood occipital epilepsy (Gastaut type)
        Epilepsy with myoclonic absences
        Lennox-Gastaut syndrome
        Epileptic encephalopathy with continuous spike-and-wave during sleep (CSWS)°°
        Landau-Kleffner syndrome (LKS)
        Childhood absence epilepsy (CAE)
    Adolescence–adult
        Juvenile absence epilepsy (JAE)
        Juvenile myoclonic epilepsy (JME)
        Epilepsy with generalized tonic/clonic seizures alone
        Progressive myoclonus epilepsies (PME)
        Autosomal dominant epilepsy with auditory features (ADEAF)
        Other familial temporal lobe epilepsies
    Less specific age relationship
        Familial focal epilepsy with variable foci (childhood to adult)
        Reflex epilepsies
Distinctive constellations
    Mesial temporal lobe epilepsy with hippocampal sclerosis (MTLE with HS)
    Rasmussen syndrome
    Gelastic seizures with hypothalamic hamartoma
    Hemiconvulsion-hemiplegia-epilepsy
    Epilepsies that *do not* fit into any of these diagnostic categories can be distinguished first on the basis of the presence or absence of a known structural or metabolic condition (presumed cause) and then on the basis of the primary mode of seizure onset (generalized versus focal).
Epilepsies attributed to and organized by structural-metabolic causes
    Malformations of cortical development (hemimegalencephaly, heterotopias, etc.)
    Neurocutaneous syndromes (tuberous sclerosis complex, Sturge-Weber, etc.)
    Tumor
    Infection
    Trauma
    Angioma
    Peri-natal insults
    Stroke
    Etc.
Epilepsies of unknown cause
Conditions with epileptic seizures that are traditionally not diagnosed as a form of epilepsy per se.
    Benign neonatal seizures (BNS)
    Febrile seizures (FS)

° The arrangement of electro-clinical syndromes does not reflect etiology.
°° Sometimes referred to as epilepsy with status epilepticus in sleep (ESES).
From Berg et al., 2010, with permission.

Table 1–10 **Suggested Scheme for an Etiological Classification of Epilepsy**

Subcategory	Examples*
Epilepsies due to single-gene disorders	Benign familial neonatal convulsions; autosomal dominant nocturnal frontal lobe epilepsy; severe myoclonic epilepsy of childhood; benign adult familial myoclonic epilepsy
Epilepsies with complex inheritance	Idiopathic generalized epilepsy (and its subtypes); benign focal epilepsies of childhood; generalized epilepsy with febrile seizures plus
Epileptic encephalopathies	West syndrome; Lennox-Gastaut syndrome
Progressive myoclonic epilepsies	Unverricht-Lundborg disease; Dentato-rubro-pallido-luysian atrophy; Lafora body disease; mitochondrial cytopathy; sialidosis; neuronal ceroid lipofuscinosis; myoclonus renal failure syndrome
Neurocutaneous syndromes	Tuberous sclerosis; neurofibromatosis; Sturge-Weber syndrome
Other neurological single-gene disorders	Angelman syndrome; lysosomal disorders; neurocanthocytosis; organic acidurias and peroxisomal disorders; porphyria; pyridoxine-dependent epilepsy; Rett syndrome; urea cycle disorders; Wilson disease; disorders of cobalamin and folate metabolism
Disorders of chromosome function	Down syndrome; fragile X syndrome; 4p-syndrome; isodicentric chromosome 15; ring chromosome 20
Developmental anomalies of cerebral structure	Hemimegalencephaly; focal cortical dysplasia; agyria-pachygyria-band spectrum; agenesis of corpus callosum; polymicrogyria; schizencephaly; periventricular nodular heterotopia; microcephaly; arachnoid cyst
Hippocampal sclerosis	Hippocampal sclerosis
Perinatal and infantile causes	Neonatal seizures; postneonatal seizures; cerebral palsy; vaccination and immunization
Cerebral trauma	Open head injury; closed head injury; neurosurgery; epilepsy after epilepsy surgery; nonaccidental head injury in infants
Cerebral tumor	Glioma; ganglioglioma and hamartoma; dysembryoplastic neuroepithelial tumor; hypothalamic hamartoma; meningioma; secondary tumors
Cerebral infection	Viral meningitis and encephalitis; bacterial meningitis and abscess; malaria; neurocysticercosis; tuberculosis; HIV
Cerebrovascular disorders	Cerebral hemorrhage; cerebral infarction; degenerative vascular disease; arteriovenous malformation; cavernous hemangioma
Cerebral immunological disorders	Rasmussen encephalitis; systemic lupus erythematosus and collagen vascular disorders; inflammatory and immunological disorders
Degenerative and other neurological conditions	Alzheimer disease and other dementing disorders; multiple sclerosis and demyelinating disorders; hydrocephalus and porencephaly

*These examples are not comprehensive, and in every category there are other causes.
Adapted from Shorvon, 2011, with permission.

Practical Considerations

Efforts to create biologically based classifications continue, because understanding commonalities among epilepsy syndromes and among epileptic seizure types have value for the variety of potential uses stated above. Clinical care for individual patients, however, is not necessarily one of those uses. Such classifications cannot substitute for accurate diagnoses and indeed can have a detrimental effect. For instance, an attempt to diagnose all patients based on the double dichotomous system of the 1989 epilepsy classification creates a false sense of knowledge, discourages precision, and encourages diagnostic errors that lead to inappropriate treatment and poor outcomes. The primary clinical objective for each patient is to make a diagnosis of a specific epilepsy syndrome. When this is done, further classifying the patient as having an idiopathic generalized or symptomatic focal epilepsy serves no clinical purpose. Given the very real problem that a syndromic diagnosis is not possible in approximately half of children and the vast majority of adults with epilepsy, treatment and prognosis in such cases should be based on the underlying cause and the diagnosis of one or more specific epileptic seizure types. Productive future efforts, therefore, should come from using etiology, seizure semiology, and other factors to better define those epileptic seizure types that remain poorly characterized, particularly the diverse groups of focal seizures, as unique diagnostic entities that can inform etiology, treatment, and prognosis as least as well as the specific epilepsy syndromes do. In the meantime, diagnosis of the underlying cause in these cases is becoming increasingly possible with modern technology (Chapter 12). Consequently, current advice for the practitioner is: don't classify, diagnose. The ILAE has prepared a diagnostic manual for this purpose, which is available on the Internet at www.epilepsy.org.

Terminology in this text will adhere as closely as possible to that in the 2010 ILAE report (Berg et al., 2010).

SUMMARY AND CONCLUSIONS

Inconsistent terminology about epilepsy has contributed greatly to confusion and imprecision in the field. Important terms and concepts are presented here as they will be used in this book. *Epilepsy* is defined as a chronic condition of the brain characterized by an enduring propensity to generate epileptic seizures. The enduring epileptogenic abnormality distinguishes this condition from *reactive epileptic seizures*, which are a natural reaction of the normal brain to transient insults and do not indicate a chronic disorder. A drug that suppresses epileptic seizures is correctly called an *antiseizure agent*, and this term, rather than the less descriptive term *antiepileptic agent*, will be used in this book. An *epileptic spike focus* is defined electrophysiologically, an *epileptogenic lesion* is defined structurally, and the *epileptogenic zone* or *region* is a theoretical concept defined as the area necessary and sufficient for epileptic seizures to occur. EEG events will be referred to as *epileptiform* and can be interictal or ictal.

Epileptiform EEG transients can occur in individuals who do not have epileptic seizures. The old term *partial seizures* has been replaced by *focal seizures*. The concept of *idiopathic* versus *symptomatic* epilepsies is now understood to be a false dichotomy, but tradition dictates that these terms might still be used to define specific groupings such as the *idiopathic generalized epilepsies* and *symptomatic focal epilepsies*. With respect to etiology, however, *genetic epilepsies* are those for which the core manifestations are genetically determined, and *structural* or *metabolic epilepsies* are those caused by specific disturbances that may be acquired or genetic; not all epilepsies can be defined by these etiological terms. Similarly, although *focal* and *generalized seizures* are recognized, *epilepsy syndromes* cannot be easily defined by such a false dichotomy. The term *psychogenic nonepileptic seizure* will be used in place of the less precise term *pseudoseizure*.

Diagnosis of specific epileptic seizure types and, when possible, epilepsy syndromes in individual patients provides important information about etiology, treatment, and prognosis but is not the same as classification. Classification is categorization, preferably based on natural classes with a firm biological basis. Whereas such classifications are useful when discussing groups of patients for teaching, research, and clinical purposes, they are not necessary for diagnosis of individual patients.

Characterization of *epileptic seizure types* must be clearly distinguished from characterization of *epilepsy syndromes*. It is now possible to define certain seizure types as unique diagnostic entities that can inform treatment, etiology, and prognosis when an epilepsy syndrome diagnosis cannot be made. Although it is useful to distinguish limbic from neocortical seizures, the terms *simple partial* and *complex partial* seizures are no longer used. According to the new terminology, when it is necessary to refer to impaired consciousness during a focal seizure, this event is called a *focal dyscognitive seizure*.

Approaches to the classification of the *epilepsies* in the past took into consideration all epilepsies, but recent revisions concentrate on well-defined *epilepsy syndromes*, listed by age. As yet, there is no recommendation for categorization based on pathophysiological mechanisms or anatomical substrates. Most epilepsy disorders are multifactorial, and many, perhaps most, patients with epilepsy have disorders that cannot easily be diagnosed as specific syndromes. For these patients, management and prognosis are determined by diagnosis of their seizure type(s).

Precise classifications and terminology are important for teaching and communication, but they also inform concepts of mechanism and profoundly influence the direction of research. Epileptology benefits greatly from properly designed collaborative efforts to establish, validate, and regularly update the internationally agreed-upon terminology and systems of classification. For practical patient care, however, it is of primary importance to diagnose specific syndromes and seizure types that inform etiology, treatment, and prognosis. A diagnostic manual will be more valuable for this purpose than a classification system. The message for the clinical practitioner, therefore, is: don't classify, diagnose.

REFERENCES

American Medical Association (2011). ICD-9-CM, 2011, 12th Revision. Chicago, IL.

Berg, A.T., Berkovic, S.F., Brodie, M.J., Buchhalter, J., Cross, J.H., van Emde Boas, W., Engel, J. Jr., French, J., Glauser, T.A., Mathern, G.W., Moshé, S.L., Nordli, D. Jr., Plouin, P. and Scheffer, I.E (2010). Revised terminology and concepts for organization of seizures and epilepsies: Report of the ILAE Commission on Classification and Terminology, 2005–2009. Epilepsia 51:676–685.

Blume WT, Lüders HO, Mizrahi E, Tassinari C, van Emde Boas W, Engel J Jr (2001). Glossary of descriptive terminology for ictal semiology: Report of the ILAE Task Force on Classification and Terminology. Epilepsia 42:1212–1218,.

Bureau, MA, Genton, P, Dravet, C, Delgado-Escueta, A, Tassinari, CA, Thomas, P, Wolf, P (Eds) (2012). Epileptic Syndromes in Infancy, Childhood and Adolescence. London: John Libbey.

Commission on Classification and Terminology of the International League Against Epilepsy (1989). Proposal for revised classification of epilepsies and epileptic syndromes. Epilepsia 30:389–399.

Commission on Classification and Terminology of the International League Against Epilepsy (1981). Proposal for revised clinical and electroencephalographic classification of epileptic seizures. Epilepsia 22:489–501.

Engel, J. Jr (1984). A practical guide for routine EEG studies in epilepsy. J Clin Neurophysiol 1:109–142.

Engel J Jr (2001). A proposed diagnostic scheme for people with epileptic seizures and with epilepsy: Report of the ILAE Task Force on Classification and Terminology. Epilepsia 42:796–803.

Engel, J. Jr (2006). Report of the ILAE Classification Core Group. Epilepsia 47:1558–1568.

Engel, J. Jr (2010). Do we belittle epilepsy by calling it a disorder rather than a disease? Epilepsia 51:2363–2364.

Fisher, R.S. and Engel, J. Jr (2010). Definition of the post-ictal state: When does it start and end? Epilepsy and Behavior 19:100–104.

Fisher, R.S., van Emde Boas, W., Blume, W., Elger, C., Engel, J. Jr., Genton, P. and Lee, P (2005). Epileptic seizures and epilepsy. Definitions proposed by the International League against Epilepsy (ILAE) and the International Bureau for Epilepsy (IBE). Epilepsia 46: 470–472.

Galanopoulou, AS, Buckmaster, P, Staley, K, Moshé, SL, Perucca, E, Engel, J Jr., Löscher, W, Noebels, JL, Pitkänen, A, Stables, J, White, SH, O'Brien, TJ, and Simonato, M (2012). Identification of new epilepsy treatments: Issues in preclinical methodology. Epilepsia 53:571–582.

Gastaut, H (1970). Clinical and electroencephalographical classification of epileptic seizures. Epilepsia 11:102–113.

Gloor, P (1977). The EEG and differential diagnosis of epilepsy. In Current Concepts in Clinical Neurophysiology. Edited by H van Duijn, DNG Donker, and AC van Huffelen. The Hague: NV Drukkerij Trio, pp. 9–21.

ICIDH-2 Beta-2 Draft (1999). International Classification of Functioning and Disability. Geneva: World Health Organization.

Jackson, JH (1870). .A study of convulsions. Trans St Andrews Med Grad Assoc 3:1–45.

Kwan P, Arzimanoglou A, Berg AT, Brodie MJ, Hauser WA, Mathern G, Moshé SL, Perucca E, Wiebe S, French J (2010). Definition of drug resistant epilepsy: Consensus proposal by the ad hoc Task Force of the ILAE Commission on Therapeutic Strategies. Epilepsia 51:1069–1077.

Luciano AL, Shorvon SD (2007). Results of treatment changes in patients with apparently drug-resistant chronic epilepsy. Ann Neurol;62:375–381.

Lüders H, Acharya J, Baumgartner C, et al. (1998). Semiological seizure classification. Epilepsia 39:1006–1013.

Merlis, JK (1970). Proposal for an international classification of the epilepsies. Epilepsia 11:114–119.

Pitkänen A (2010). Therapeutic approaches to epileptogenesis—hope on the horizon. Epilepsia 51(Suppl. 3): 2–17.

Roger, J, Bureau, M, Dravet, C, Genton, P, Tassinari, CA, and Wolf, P (eds) (2005). Epileptic Syndromes in Infancy, Childhood and Adolescence. London: John Libbey.

Roger, J, Dravet, C, Bureau, M, Dreifuss, FE, and Wolf, P (eds) (1985). Epilepsy Syndromes in Infancy, Childhood and Adolescence. London: John Libbey.

Shorvon, SD (2011). The etiologic classification of epilepsy. Epilepsia 52:1052–1057.

Thurman, DJ, Beghi, E, Begley, CE, et al. (2011). Standards for epidemiologic studies and surveillance of epilepsy. Epilepsia 52 (Suppl 7) :1.

Vickrey, B., Hays, R., Engel, J. Jr., Spritzer, K., Rogers, W., Rausch, R., Graber, J. and Brook, R (1995). Outcome assessment for epilepsy surgery: The impact of measuring health-related quality of life. Ann Neurol 37:158–166.

World Health Organization (1987). Application of the International Classification of Diseases to Neurology ICD-NA (published for trial purposes). Geneva.

World Health Organization (1994) Application of the International Classification on Diseases to Neurology ICD-10. Geneva.

Chapter 2

Perspectives

EPILEPSY THEN—HISTORICAL PERSPECTIVE
Medical History
Epilepsy and Religion
Epilepsy and Genius

EPILEPSY NOW—EPIDEMIOLOGICAL PERSPECTIVE
Definitions of Incidence and Prevalence

Methodological Considerations
Estimates of Incidence and Prevalence
Global Burden of Disease

SUMMARY AND CONCLUSIONS

The place of epilepsy among the causes of human illness must be appreciated *historically* as well as *epidemiologically*. Although the impact of epilepsy disorders on world health today is considerable, epilepsy played a uniquely prominent role in medical matters of the past. The Greek word *epilambanein* initially referred to affliction by any disease (Temkin, 1945); the fact that it came to mean epilepsy implies this was "the disease" of antiquity. Lennox (1960) considered epilepsy "'distinguished'…with respect to its scientific interest and its place in the history of medicine" and noted that epilepsy accounts for 2.6% of "Hippocratic writings" (fifth century B.C.); 3.4% in Aretaeus (second century B.C.); 3% in John of Gaddesden (ca. 1314); but only 0.5% in the 1959 edition of Cecil's Medicine (Cecil and Loeb, 1959). Interestingly, epilepsy has more or less held its own in the past 50 years—the chapter on epilepsy in the 1988 edition of the *Cecil Textbook of Medicine*, prior to the first edition of *Seizures and Epilepsy*, constituted exactly 0.5% of the greatly expanded text (Engel, 1988) and slightly above 0.4% of the 2011 edition (Wiebe, 2011). However, the World Health Organization (WHO) determined that epilepsy accounts for 1% of the global burden of disease, equivalent to those of lung cancer in men and breast cancer in women (Murray and Lopez, 1994).

The reduced preoccupation of modern medical textbooks with epilepsy can be attributed in part to the demystification of epileptic

33

phenomena, but it also indicates that greater progress has been made in scientifically defining and managing many other medical conditions. The amount of space devoted to a disorder usually reflects more what is known about it than its importance as a cause of disability.

EPILEPSY THEN—HISTORICAL PERSPECTIVE

Lennox (Lennox, 1960) quotes an address delivered by Dr. Oliver Wendell Holmes in 1860: "If I wished to show a student the difficulties of getting a truth from medical experience, I would give him the history of epilepsy to read." Following Dr. Holmes's advice, much has since been written concerning the history of epilepsy (Daras et al., 2008), but the definitive text remains *The Falling Sickness*, by Owsei Temkin (1945).

Attitudes of past societies toward epilepsy and those who suffered from it, as well as past contributions to society of the study of epilepsy and of people with epilepsy, continue to be of interest to modern scholars. Often, however, the subjects of historical texts on epilepsy bear uncertain relevance to epilepsy disorders as they are known today. Prior to the mid-19th century, writings about epilepsy referred almost exclusively to generalized tonic-clonic seizures, or at least seizures associated with loss of consciousness and motor manifestations. Furthermore, in most cases, it is not possible to distinguish descriptions of epileptic seizures from other ictal events with similar characteristics, whether organic or psychogenic nonepileptic seizures. Hysteria, including mass hysteria, madness, and melancholia were frequently confused with epilepsy in older writings. Familiarity with epilepsy's past, therefore, does not necessarily elucidate the disorder of the present, but it does enable us to have an appreciation for the legacy it has left to those who are currently marked with the unfortunately pejorative label *epileptic*.

Medical History

ANCIENT AND MEDIEVAL PERIODS

The earliest references to epilepsy date back to late second millennium B.C. Mesopotamian

writings described *antasabbu*, literally "the falling disease," and *bel uri*, the name for a demon who was lord of the roof beams—presumably inspired by the patient's upward eye deviation. Kinnier Wilson cites remarkably accurate Mesopotamian descriptions of auras; versive, gelastic, and generalized tonic-clonic seizures; postictal paralysis; and epileptic psychosis (Kinnier Wilson, 1967a;b; Kinnier Wilson and Reynolds, 1990). Temkin (1945) notes that *bennu*, mentioned in the *Babylonian Law of Hammurabi*, might be epilepsy, but Kinnier Wilson argues that this term referred to heart attack. Indian Ayurvedic writings from roughly the same period also contained detailed clinical descriptions of epilepsy, called *ashepak* or *apasmara* (Mishra, 1987; Bharucha and Bharucha, 1989; Manyam, 1992). Ancient Chinese concepts of epilepsy have also been reported (Lai and Lai, 1991).

Temkin (1945) began his history with the first known attempt at a scientific explanation for epilepsy, a book entitled *On the Sacred Disease*, written by a physician of the school of *Hippocrates* in Greece about 400 B.C. At that time, epilepsy was known as "the sacred disease," because of a general belief that people who suffered from epileptic seizures were possessed by evil spirits or gods and should be treated by the invocation of religious, occult, and magical powers. *On the Sacred Disease* accused contemporary physicians of practicing sacrilege, using the gods as a cover for ignorance and fraud. The writer pointed out that epilepsy is hereditary and attributed it to dysfunction of the brain. Hippocrates and physicians of his school knew of the relationship between skull fractures and seizures beginning on the opposite side of the body. They believed, however, that convulsions were due to an excess of "cold phlegm," secreted by the pituitary body and accumulating in the ventricles.

After Hippocrates, those who advocated his teachings found "epilepsy" a more appropriate name for convulsive disorders than "the sacred disease." Five hundred years later, *Galen* made the next notable conceptual contribution by suggesting that some epileptic symptoms arose from influences on the brain from extracranial sources (Temkin, 1945). He called epilepsy originating in the brain *idiopathic* or *protopathic* and epilepsy originating outside the brain *sympathetic*. He defined two types of sympathetic epilepsy, one resulting from the body's attempt to remove irritating substances from the stomach and the other due to irritation rising up from the extremities. The latter was deduced from a patient's description of a sensation in his leg that gradually rose to his head before each convulsion. Galen assumed this to be a flow of pathological humors from the leg, because the patient could abort the convulsion by placing a ligature around the leg at the onset of the attack. He introduced the term *aura* for this phenomenon because it felt like a breeze to the patient.

In contrast to those who believed in possession by evil demons and chose religious, occult, and magical cures for epilepsy, physicians influenced by the views of Hippocrates and Galen practiced the scientific medicine of their time. This approach was considered *natural* rather than *supernatural*. Their more rational therapies included appropriate diet and hygiene, but their pharmacological and other manipulations were still based on superstition and not scientific method. Human blood was widely regarded as having curative powers, and people with epilepsy in Roman times were commonly seen sucking blood from fallen gladiators. Powdered skull, peony, mistletoe, garlic, and onion were also often prescribed. People with epilepsy were reasonably counseled to avoid baths but also were warned against wearing or sleeping on goatskins. A relationship between epileptic seizures and phases of the moon was not disproved until the 19th century (Leuret, 1843), although some patients still describe this phenomenon. *Trephining*, begun in primitive times, also continued into the 19th century, although it was used then primarily to remove specific skull deformities (Broca, 1867). More often practiced in earlier times was *cauterization*, usually of occiput or bregma. It was recommended that the cautery burn through the skull to the meninges. In some countries during the Middle Ages, cauterization was performed by laypersons. Mothers would cauterize their own infant children. Both trephining and cauterization seemed justified in the context of natural causes to remove excess phlegm and evil humors from the brain. Castration too was prescribed until the 19th century, not only to prevent genetic transmission of epilepsy but also because practitioners of natural medicine believed that some convulsions originated in the testes and that masturbation exacerbated epileptic seizures. The belief that onanism

caused seizures was the rationale for the use of *bromides* to treat women with *hysteroepilepsy* in the mid-19th century (Locock, 1857).

Probably because of the ineffectiveness of most natural therapies, and perhaps also the beneficial placebo effects of some supernatural interventions, the remarkable insights of Hippocrates and Galen were all but lost in Europe during the Middle Ages. Epilepsy became known as the *falling sickness*, and those who suffered from it were almost universally viewed as possessed by evil spirits, unclean, and contagious. Spitting at the sight of a person with epilepsy was commonly practiced to repel the infection. Although exorcism and other religious, magical, and occult treatments may have been less traumatic for people with epilepsy than many of the so-called scientific or natural therapies mentioned in the preceding paragraph, the stigma associated with a supernatural view of epilepsy made the poor sufferer's plight equally miserable.

A few European and Persian physicians did publish remarkably modern descriptions of epilepsy during the Middle Ages (Daras et al., 2008), and Temkin (1945) sums up this period by marveling at those few physicians who were able to keep alive the notion that epilepsy was a "natural disease caused by natural factors." By the 16th and 17th centuries, belief in the infectious nature of epilepsy was discarded, and physicians began to discuss openly the differential diagnosis of epilepsy and demonic possession. More humane treatment of people with epilepsy was advocated, notably by *Paracelsus* in 1530, on religious grounds, and by the anatomist and physician *Thomas Willis* in 1684, although even he still believed in demonic possession and witchcraft (Temkin, 1945). Insight into the social and political climate of the 17th century, when natural philosophers were evolving into scientists and modern brain research began with the work of Willis, can be found in Karl Zimmer's *Soul Made Flesh: The Discovery of the Brain—and How It Changed the World* (Zimmer, 2004). Syphilis, scurvy, smallpox, ergotism, and other diseases became recognized as responsible for epileptic seizures in some patients. The concept of irritation of the brain and its membranes by poisonous substances, rather than phlegm in the ventricles, was considered.

During the 18th century there was a gradual return to the natural explanations introduced by Hippocrates and Galen and a rejection of supernatural causes of epilepsy. Convulsions (generalized tonic-clonic seizures), however, were generally attributed to disturbances in the medulla oblongata. Nonconvulsive seizures became recognized as epileptic events, and patients no longer needed to fall to the ground to be considered epileptic. It was against this background of change that *de Horta*, writing in a village called Los Angeles in 1754 (de Horta, 1763) (see preface to the first edition of this book and frontispiece), offered his treatise on demonic possession among people with epilepsy. A more important 18th-century contribution was the *Traité de l'Épilepsie*, written by *Simon André Tissot* in 1770 (Tissot, 1770). Tissot recognized that chronic cerebral dysfunction acted as a *predisposing factor* for epilepsy and should be distinguished from the *provoking cause*. He defined *idiopathic* epilepsy, with a known brain injury, as different from *essential* epilepsy, with no definite etiology, presumably due to an epileptic disposition. Tissot's essential epilepsy corresponds to what in the 1970 and 1989 International Classifications (Merlis, 1970; Commission on Classification, 1989) was called *primary* or *idiopathic* epilepsy, whereas his idiopathic epilepsy corresponds to what was called *secondary* or *symptomatic* epilepsy. Finally, Tissot described two types of ictal events: generalized tonic-clonic seizures, which he called *grands accès*, and minor, probably absence, seizures, which he called *petits accès*.

In the beginning of the 19th century, the *Salpetrière* and *Bicêtre* Hospitals of Paris became centers for clinical research on epilepsy. Humanization of the treatment of the insane, which at the time included people with epilepsy (Berrios, 1984), resulted in hospital programs designed to benefit and not just isolate such patients. Many of the early 19th-century French physicians who contributed to our knowledge of epilepsy actually did so in pursuit of their research on psychiatric disorders. In 1815, *Esquirol* (Esquirol, 1838) defined *grand mal* and *petit mal* seizures. In 1824, *Calmeil* (Calmeil, 1824) described *absences* and *generalized convulsive status epilepticus*. In 1825, *Bouchet* and *Cazauvieilh* (Bouchet and Cazauvieilh, 1825) reported epidemiological studies on the causes of epilepsy that included the first description of *hippocampal sclerosis*. Unilateral motor seizures followed

by hemiplegia (*hemiplegic seizures*) were described in 1827 by *Bravais* (Bravais, 1827), although *postictal paralysis* would later bear the name of the Englishman *Todd*, who did not publish his descriptions until 30 years later (Todd, 1855). Meanwhile, in England, in 1822, *Pritchard* (Pritchard, 1822) preceded Bravais with his clear description of *focal seizures*, and in 1831, *Bright* (Bright, 1831) recognized that focal seizures were related to focal localized disease of the brain. In 1854, *Delasiauve* (Delasiauve, 1854) recognized that carrying out clinical studies required clear definitions and redefined *idiopathic* and *symptomatic* epilepsy in the same manner as those terms were used in the 1989 International Classification (Commission on Classification, 1989).

THE MODERN ERA

Building on progress made during the first half of the 19th century, a few men in London radically altered research and clinical practice with respect to epilepsy within 30 years. The first was a society physician named *Charles Locock*. On what appeared to be a whim, he tried bromides to treat hysterical seizures in women and in 1857 found them effective against epileptic seizures as well. Credit for popularization of the first effective pharmacotherapy for epilepsy, however, should go to *Samuel Wilks*, who completed more careful studies two years later (Temkin, 1945). The contributions of *John Hughlings Jackson* (Fig. 2–1) and *Victor Horsley*, on the other hand, were based on true scholarship and creativity (Engel, 2005; Taylor, 1987; Temkin, 1945; Tyler, 1984).

Jackson came to London in 1859, the same year the *National Hospital for the Paralysed and Epileptic at Queen Square* was founded there (because members of the British royal family had epilepsy). He was well aware of the publications of Pritchard, Bravais, Bright, and Todd, but at that time focal seizures were considered *epileptiform* and not epilepsy. Students of epilepsy investigated generalized tonic-clonic seizures and concentrated their attention on the medulla oblongata. Jackson parted from current thinking when he asserted that focal seizures were also epilepsy, that they originated in cerebral gray matter, and that generalized tonic-clonic seizures, therefore, were also mediated by the cerebral hemispheres. His first major contribution constituted a

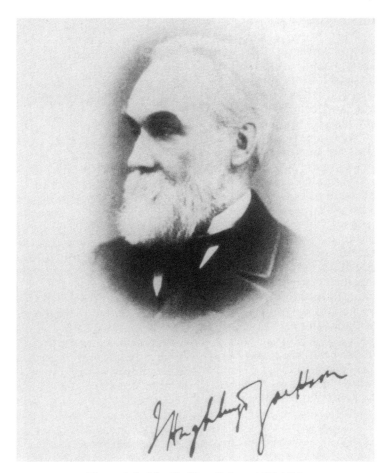

Figure 2–1. John Hughlings Jackson, 1835–1911.

strategy for attacking the problem: he made the study of epilepsy more manageable by focusing on epileptic seizures of localized origin. Jackson initially attributed ictal onset to the *corpus striatum* but speculated as early as 1866 that the epileptogenic tissue might be in the *convolutions*. By 1870, Jackson (Jackson, 1870) had formulated his hypothesis that epileptogenic gray matter was unstable as a result of *nutritional deprivation*. Although he was referring to impairment of local cerebral circulation, his speculation predicted the interictal hypometabolic zone seen on positron emission tomography (PET) (Chapters 4 and 12). Jackson viewed disturbances of the cortex as either *destructive*, causing negative symptoms, or *discharging*, causing positive symptoms such as epilepsy (Jackson, 1870). At about the same time, the German electrophysiologists *Fritsch* and *Hitzig* (Fritsch and Hitzig, 1870)

electrically stimulated the motor cortex of a dog and proved that discharging abnormalities could give rise to ictal manifestations. In 1873, *David Ferrier* (Ferrier, 1873) (Fig. 2–2) clearly demonstrated in monkeys that motor cortex, and not the medulla oblongata, initiated convulsive motor activity. By that year, Jackson (Jackson, 1873) had broadened his definition of epilepsy to include any "occasional, sudden, excessive, rapid and local discharges of gray matter." With this definition, he adopted the very modern concept that there is not one disease called epilepsy but many epilepsies with many manifestations, depending on the site of discharging gray matter.

By correlating careful observations of focal motor ictal onsets with postmortem pathological examinations of the brain, Jackson began to understand the localization of specific motor, as well as other, functions in the human

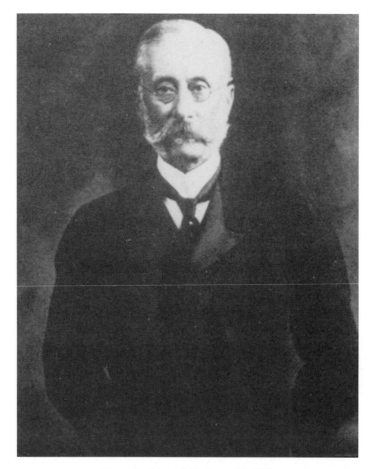

Figure 2–2. David Ferrier, 1843–1928.

cortex. This work included the first pathologically verified description of temporal lobe seizures (Jackson, 1898), as suffered by Jackson's famous patient and friend *Dr. Z* (Taylor and Marsh, 1980). Jackson had, therefore, developed revolutionary insights into the structural and functional substrates of epileptic activity and also acquired experience for localizing the sites of some epileptogenic lesions. This diagnostic capability would prove useful for a new approach to the treatment of focal epilepsy.

The neurosurgeon Victor Horsley (Fig. 2–3), emboldened by the clinical observations of the neurologist Jackson and confirmation of functional localization within the cerebral cortex by the electrophysiologist Ferrier and his own studies on monkeys, decided to attempt to cure epilepsy by surgically removing a region of epileptogenic cortical tissue. His first

procedure was performed on a patient who suffered from focal motor seizures secondary to a depressed skull fracture. Horsley resected a cortical scar in 1886, rendering the patient seizure-free. After two more patients, Horsley was able to publish his work that same year (Horsley, 1886). The initial surgical resection would probably not have taken place without the collaborative efforts of Jackson and Ferrier, both of whom were present in the operating theater to witness the historic event. These three men, a neurosurgeon, a neurologist, and an electrophysiologist, constituted a team that is still essential for surgical treatment of epilepsy today. Actually, another neurosurgeon, *William Macewen* (Macewen, 1879; 1881) preceded Horsley in treating focal epilepsy surgically based on Jackson's observations, but his work in Scotland received less attention than

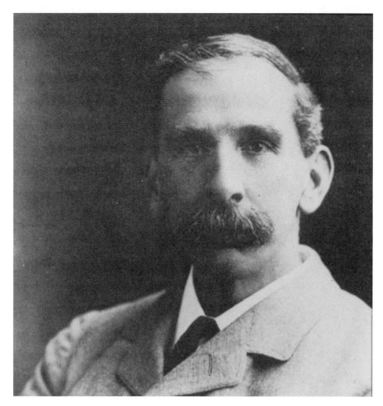

Figure 2–3. Victor Horsley, 1857–1916.

Horsley's. Even with Horsley's and Macewen's work, epilepsy surgery remained an extremely limited therapeutic modality until after electrophysiological localization became generally available in the mid-20th century (Engel, 2005) (Chapter 16).

One other major concept was put forth at the end of the 19th century. No clear distinction had been made between epilepsy and hysterical seizures until the seminal work of *Jean-Martin Charcot* (Charcot, 1886) (Fig. 2–4) and his Paris school on *hysteroepilepsy*. These workers differentiated seizures of psychogenic origin from epileptic seizures due to organic brain disturbances.

Jackson, Ferrier, Horsley, and Charcot had now defined a pathophysiology of epilepsy that was to become the foundation for modern scientific investigation. Except for bromides and the rare cortical resection, however, treatment of epilepsy remained medieval. *Gowers*, in his classic 1881 text *Epilepsy and Other Chronic Convulsive Diseases* (Gowers, 1881), lists among the potential treatments for epilepsy mistletoe,

turpentine, counterirritation (which was a later derivative of cauterization of the occiput), trephining, and castration (although Gowers preferred circumcision). To his credit, however, Gowers was the first to write that aggressive treatment might improve prognosis: "The tendency of the disease is to self-perpetuation; each attack facilitates the occurrence of another, by increasing the instability of the nerve elements" (Gowers, 1881). Thus he anticipated *kindling* and the progressive nature of some epilepsies (Chapters 4 and 8).

Further seminal advances occurred in the early 20th century. Pharmacotherapy came into its own with the introduction of phenobarbital in 1912 by *Hauptmann*, who sedated his patients at night so he could sleep and found it stopped their seizures (Hauptmann, 1912). After extensive testing of compounds with phenyl rings that resembled phenobarbital on experimental seizures in cats, *Merritt and Putnam* discovered phenytoin in 1937 (Merritt and Putnam, 1938) and demonstrated that antiseizure properties of drugs could be

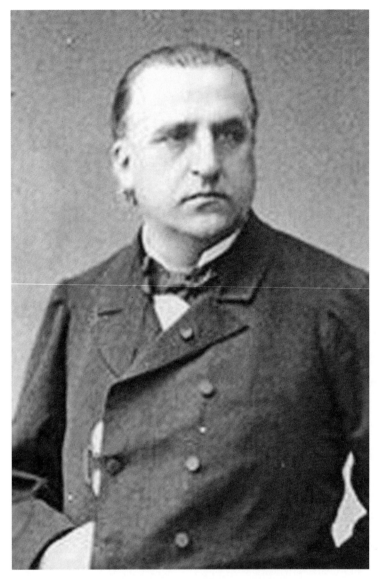

Figure 2–4. Jean-Martin Charcot, 1825–1893.

dissociated from their sedative and hypnotic properties. *Everett* and *Richards* (Everett and Richards, 1944; Richards and Everett, 1944) proved in 1944, with the antiabsence drug *trimethadione*, that antiseizure drugs could act selectively on specific epileptic symptoms. This was followed by enthusiastic efforts to identify effective antiseizure compounds (Shorvon, 2009) (Chapter 14).

Hans Berger's (Berger, 1929) (Fig. 2–5) invention of the *electroencephalogram* in 1929 had a revolutionary impact on the diagnosis of epilepsy that was not fully appreciated for another decade (Gibbs et al., 1938; Jasper and Kershman, 1941). This new methodology also permitted invasive neurophysiological research on the human brain, pioneered by *Penfield* and *Jasper* (Penfield and Jasper 1954). The tremendous progress that followed, since the middle of the 20th century, in defining the human epileptic condition, elucidating the basic mechanisms of epileptic phenomena, applying neuroimaging and genetics to diagnosis, and improving pharmacological, surgical,

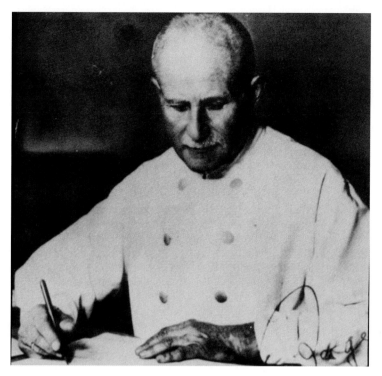

Figure 2–5. Hans Berger, 1873–1941.

and other treatments for people with epilepsy is the subject of the rest of this volume.

Epilepsy and Religion

Epilepsy, as "the sacred disease," has been profoundly intertwined with religious practices throughout the ages. This relationship between religion and epilepsy has been a complicated one. On the one hand, all Western religions at one time or another have perceived people with epilepsy as evil; on the other, many authors have considered the mystical experiences of some religious prophets and holy men to have been epileptic phenomena. Thus epilepsy may be viewed as both the bête noire and the inspiration of certain religious movements.

The religious persecution of people with epilepsy in the West as well as the use of religious practices as treatment has already been discussed in the preceding section. This view was prevalent in Judaism and Christianity. The most famous example is the thrice-repeated New Testament account of Jesus casting the evil spirit from an epileptic child. Matthew 17:14–18[1] recounts:

> And when they came to the crowd, a man came up to him and kneeling before him said, "Lord, have mercy on my son, for he is an epileptic and he suffers terribly; for often he falls into the fire, and often into the water. And I brought him to your disciples, and they could not heal him." And Jesus answered, "O faithless and perverse generation, how long am I to be with you? How long am I to bear with you? Bring him here to me." And Jesus rebuked him, and the demon came out of him, and the boy was cured instantly.

According to Mark 9:17–18, 20–22, 25–27:

> And one of the crowd answered him, "Teacher, I brought my son to you, for he has a dumb spirit; and wherever it seizes him, it dashes him down; and he foams and grinds his teeth and becomes rigid;

---

[1] Text for all biblical quotations is from the Oxford Revised Edition.

and I asked your disciples to cast it out, and they were not able....*" And they brought the boy to him; and when the spirit saw him, immediately it convulsed the boy, and he fell on the ground and rolled about, foaming at the mouth. And Jesus asked his father, "How long has he had this?" And he said, "From childhood...." And when Jesus saw that a crowd came running together, he rebuked the unclean spirit, saying to it, "You dumb and deaf spirit, I command you, come out of him, and never enter him again." And after crying out and convulsing him terribly, it came out, and the boy was like a corpse; so that most of them said, "He is dead." But Jesus took him by the hand and lifted him up, and he arose.

And Luke 9:38–39, 42 says:

And behold, a man from the crowd cried, "Teacher, I beg you to look upon my son, for he is my only child; and behold, a spirit seizes him, and he suddenly cries out; it convulses him till he foams, and shatters him...." While he was coming, the demon tore him and convulsed him. But Jesus rebuked the unclean spirit, and healed the boy, and gave him back to his father.

This child is depicted in at least two famous paintings, by Raphael (Fig. 2–6) and Rubens (Fig. 2–7).

Few Western sources reveal the extent to which practitioners of other religious groups identified epilepsy with evil powers. It would seem, however, that this belief was not universal. According to both Temkin (Temkin, 1945) and Lennox (Lennox, 1960), there is sufficient evidence to consider *Hercules*, the son of *Zeus*, to have epilepsy. It is unlikely that the ancient Greeks who conceived this myth would portray their hero of godly birth as a victim of epilepsy if they considered those afflicted with this disorder to be instruments of evil. At least one religion, *Siberian shamanism*, has been reported to recruit its religious leaders from among people with epilepsy (Temkin, 1945).

Conversely, a number of men and women who have attained religious prominence may have done so in spite of, or perhaps because of, their epileptic signs and symptoms. Although

Buddha has been considered to have epilepsy by some, there is no evidence that his mystical experiences were characteristic of epilepsy. Beran (Beran and Beran, 1987) cites many passages in both the Old and New Testaments that are questionable references to epileptic symptoms of prophets (Numbers 24:4; 1 Samuel 19:24; Ezekiel 1:28, 43:3; Daniel 8:17; Acts 9:4–18; Revelations 1:17). *St. Paul* has been most consistently considered to have epilepsy, because of the description of his suffering on the road to Damascus (Acts 9:4–18). Lennox (Lennox, 1960), however, questions even this, suggesting he may have had migraine, syncopy, and anorexia. Although *Mohammed* was reported to have had seizures since the age of 3 and to have admitted, "This is a common affliction of prophets, of whom you know I wish to be counted as one" (Lennox, 1960), Temkin (Temkin, 1945) wrote that Byzantine Christians might have called Mohammed epileptic to discredit him. *St. Ignatius*; *St. Teresa of Avila*; *Anne Lee*, founder of the Shaker sect; the Mormon prophet *Joseph Smith*; and the Hebrew prophets *Hosea, Isaiah, Jeremiah,* and *Ezekiel* all had mystical experiences that have been interpreted as epileptic (Beran and Beran, 1987; Lennox, 1960). It would seem impossible, however, to differentiate epilepsy from nonepileptic seizures, including perhaps divine phenomena, on the basis of any of these written descriptions.

St. Valentine is one of the better-known patron saints of epilepsy. Temkin (Temkin, 1945) suggests that this honor was accorded St. Valentine by the Germans because his name sounds like the German word *fallen*. There is more than one St. Valentine, and there is no evidence that any St. Valentine had epilepsy. Epilepsy was once known in France as *le mal de Saint-Jean* because *St. John* was considered a patron saint of this disorder—which St. John, however, is unknown, as is the reason for his connection with epilepsy (Temkin, 1945). *St. Vitus* and *St. Willibrord* are mentioned as patron saints of epilepsy, although their patronage rightfully belongs to the *dancing mania* known as *St. Vitus dance* (Temkin, 1945). Because the Three Wise Men *fell down* before Jesus, they also became patrons of epilepsy. In medieval times, merely speaking the names of *Gaspar, Melchior,* and *Balthazar* was believed to arouse patients from their ictal stupors (Temkin, 1945).

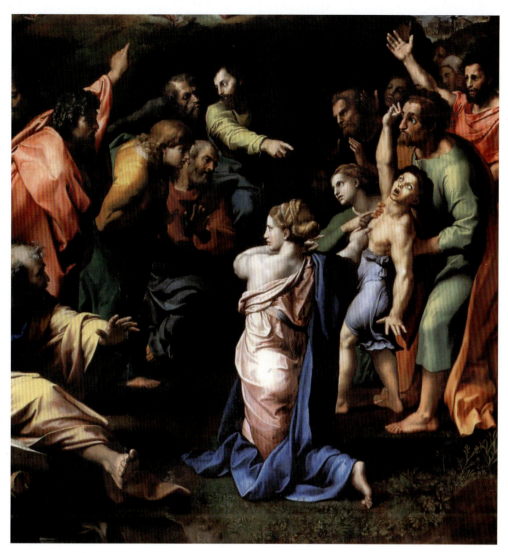

Figure 2–6. Detail of the epileptic boy from Raphael's *Transfiguration*. (Reproduced by permission from the Vatican Museum.)

Epilepsy and Genius

In addition to a belief that people with epilepsy gained prominence in religion because epileptic behaviors may have been mistaken for supernatural powers, epileptic seizures also have aspects of power and imagery that have suggested to some a relationship with unusual leadership abilities or creativity. There is no evidence, however, that either epileptic seizures or a predisposition to epilepsy is capable of engendering exceptional talents. Rather, the occasional concurrence of epilepsy and genius most likely reflects the probability that a common disorder will at times afflict people with uncommon potential. Lennox (Lennox, 1960) accepts the evidence that the following rulers and warriors had epilepsy: *Amenhotep, Drusus, Alexander the Great, Caligula, Julius Caesar, Peter the Great, William Pitt,* and *Napoleon Bonaparte*. Others whom he would consider as possibly having epilepsy include *Louis XIII of France, Charles V of Spain, Ferdinand V of Castile, Archduke Charles of Austria,* and the British rulers *Alfred the Great* and *William III*. Recently presented evidence suggests that

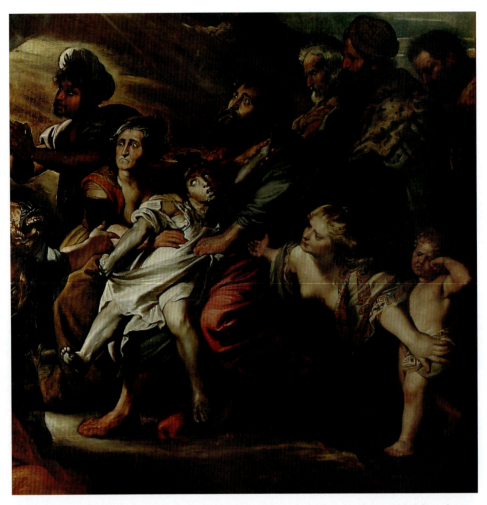

Figure 2–7. Detail of the epileptic boy from Rubens's *Transfiguration*. (Reproduced with permission from the Musée des Beaux-Arts, Nancy.)

Franklin Delano Roosevelt had epilepsy (Lomazow, 2011). Within the past few years, Chief Justice of the US Supreme Court John Roberts and Senator Edward Kennedy had epileptic seizures in public, but an official diagnosis of epilepsy was never mentioned in the media.

Among philosophers, artists, and scientists, Lennox accepts as epileptic *Francesco Petrarch, Charles Dickens, Molière, Blaise Pascal, Nicolo Paganini, Lord Byron, Feodor Mikhailovich Dostoyevsky, Gustave Flaubert, Algernon Charles Swinburne, Edward Lear, Vincent van Gogh, Alfred Nobel,* and *William Morris.* Also placed on this list by some are *Pythagoras, Empedocles, Socrates, Democritus, Brittanicus, Plotinus, Plutarch, Torquato Tasso,*

Isaac Newton, Jonathan Swift, Sir Walter Scott, Dante, Emanuel Swedenborg, George Frederick Handel, Peter Ilyich Tchaikovsky, Robert Schumann, Ludwig van Beethoven, Samuel Johnson, Leo Tolstoy, Guy de Maupassant, Emily Dickinson, and *Percy Bysshe Shelley.* More recent additions include *Truman Capote, Prince, Michael Wilding,* and *Neil Young.*

The most prominent contemporary public figure courageous enough to admit to having epilepsy is former US Representative and House whip *Tony Coelho* (Democrat from Merced, California). It was reported that Congressman Coelho may owe his first election to his spirited response when accused by an opponent of having epilepsy: "A lot of people have gone to Washington and had fits; at least

I'll have an excuse." The fact that a great many other men and women of considerable accomplishments have chosen to keep their epilepsy a secret attests to the continued stigma associated with this diagnosis.

Many famous people have had various types of attacks that were considered by some to be epileptic seizures, and one extensive evaluation of available data on 43 such individuals to document the evidence for or against a diagnosis of epilepsy concluded that 59% likely had other disorders (Hughes, 2005). Because epilepsy can be a symptom of a damaged brain, more persons with epileptic seizures have subnormal than supernormal capacity for achievement. Most, however, are ordinary men and women attempting to lead ordinary lives under the burden of their historically distinguished, but often oppressive, epileptic condition.

EPILEPSY NOW— EPIDEMIOLOGICAL PERSPECTIVE

It is estimated that every four minutes a person in the United States is diagnosed with epilepsy, and epilepsy is more common than autism, cerebral palsy, multiple sclerosis, and Parkinson's disease combined (Hirtz et al., 2007). In general, the risk of having at least one epileptic seizure in a normal lifetime is approximately 10%, and one-third of people experiencing a single seizure will eventually develop epilepsy (Hesdorffer et al., 2011). The average prevalence of active epilepsy is somewhere between 0.5% and 1%. The difference between this point prevalence figure and the lifetime incidence of about 3% predicted by the fact that one-third of those who experience a single seizure develop epilepsy is accounted for by remission and death. Based on these figures, 65 million people worldwide have epilepsy (Ngugi et al., 2010). Perhaps more than 40% of people with epilepsy in the United States have seizures that are not controlled by medication (Kobau et al., 2008). Although lower figures are cited in the literature, this measure depends on the definition of epilepsy and length of follow-up, which is usually short. The observation that it takes an average of nine years for focal epilepsies to become pharmacoresistant (Berg et al., 2003) suggests that the figure might be even higher.

No truly comprehensive epidemiological data on epilepsy are available, however, because existing studies have dealt with specific epileptic phenomena or conditions largely limited to selected populations. Furthermore, there are considerable methodological difficulties inherent in all investigations of this type (Hauser and Hesdorffer, 1990). A series of papers by Woodbury (Woodbury, 1977a-d), prepared in 1977 for the Commission for the Control of Epilepsy and Its Consequences, presents a thoughtful review of epidemiological methods and potential sources of error. Woodbury also used published data and logical assumptions in an attempt to extrapolate information on the epidemiology of epilepsy to the entire US population. Even if Woodbury's conclusions are accurate for the United States, however, they are not easily related to data from other countries and do not completely reveal the magnitude of the world health problem represented by epilepsy. The WHO has published an assessment of the global health burden represented by epilepsy and the resources available worldwide for its diagnosis and treatment (Murray and Lopez, 1994). Standards for epidemiological studies and surveillance of epilepsy have recently been published by the International League against Epilepsy (ILAE) (Thurman et al., 2011).

Definitions of Incidence and Prevalence

The *incidence* of epilepsy refers to the number of new cases of epilepsy occurring within a given period of time. Incidence is commonly reported as the *incidence rate*: the number of new cases divided by the population under observation and expressed as the incidence per 100,000 person-years. Because incidence rates for epilepsy vary considerably with age, *age-specific* incidence rates are more useful than overall figures. Age- and sex-adjusted incidence transforms the incidence rate derived from a given population to that of a standard population (e.g., the 2010 US population) so that incidence rates can be compared across geographic sites. *Sex-specific* incidence rates are of less interest for epilepsy in general because the difference between figures obtained for male and female populations are not usually significant, although incidence rates are almost always higher for males than for females (Hauser and Kurland, 1975). Significant sex differences do occur, however, for specific epilepsy disorders (Chapters 5 and 7). Incidence rates are useful for studies of epilepsy etiology and epilepsy prognosis. *Cumulative* incidence can be obtained by adding successive incidence rates for each year of age until a particular age of interest. This measures the risk for developing epilepsy. Consequently, the cumulative incidence for epilepsy at age 70 provides an estimate of the risk that an individual will develop epilepsy at any time between birth and age 70. The lifetime risk is also used to calculate the risk for developing epilepsy over a person's remaining lifetime. Unlike cumulative incidence, the lifetime risk considers the impact of the competing risk of death.

The *prevalence* for epilepsy usually refers to the number of cases of active epilepsy in a given population at a specific point in time. People with active epilepsy are defined as those either currently taking antiseizure drugs or who have had a seizure in either the past two years or the past five years (the ILAE uses five years). Prevalence is reported as a proportion for a specific population, expressed as a number per 1,000. The prevalence for epilepsy, therefore, indicates the magnitude of the disease burden presented by this disorder. Both age-specific and age-adjusted overall prevalence are useful. Prevalence is also occasionally reported for a period of time (e.g., one year) rather than for a specific point in time. Prevalence is a dynamic measure reflecting both the incidence and duration of a disorder, including, therefore, associated mortality: prevalence = incidence x duration.

Methodological Considerations

Measurements of incidence rates for epilepsy are subject to errors, particularly because of imprecise definitions of epilepsy and the inability to identify all persons with newly diagnosed epilepsy within a specified population over a specified time period. Incidence rates given for epilepsy are often underestimates: individuals do not admit they have epileptic seizures, do not recognize they have seizures, or do not seek medical attention, and physicians may miss the diagnosis of epilepsy. Incidence rates for epilepsy may occasionally be overestimated when

patients with reactive epileptic seizures or non-epileptic seizures are erroneously included. In balance, factors that lead to underestimation substantially outweigh those causing overestimation, and most figures reported in the literature are likely to be too low.

Measurements of prevalence for epilepsy are subject to the same errors as those for incidence rates but are even less reliable, because of variations in the definition of active epilepsy and the lack of accurate information concerning the duration of continued epileptic symptoms. Prevalence is commonly underestimated for the reasons stated in the previous paragraph and also because patients who have experienced only the first seizure of a chronic epileptic condition are excluded when epilepsy is defined as two unprovoked seizures, continued epileptic seizures may not be acknowledged or recognized by the patient or the physician, and patients are sometimes lost to follow-up. Consequently, prevalences for epilepsy reported in the literature may also be underestimates.

Estimates of Incidence and Prevalence

The most comprehensive epidemiological data on epilepsy were obtained from the population of Rochester, Minnesota, between 1935 and 1967 by Hauser and Kurland (Hauser and Kurland, 1975). Epilepsy was defined as more than one epileptic seizure, and patients with simple, febrile, and reactive seizures (Chapter 7) were excluded. Woodbury (Woodbury, 1977b) supplemented these data with those obtained from a population of children born between 1960 and 1967 in Oakland, California, by Van den Berg and Yerushalmy (Van den Berg and Yerushalmy, 1969. The latter study also excluded simple febrile seizures, but some of the children included had had only one epileptic seizure. The age-adjusted incidence rate for epilepsy in Oakland was estimated to be 46.7/100,000 per year, and the age-adjusted prevalence was estimated to be 6.25/1,000. From these data, Woodbury (Woodbury, 1977b) also calculated the average duration of epilepsy to be 13.4 years, but this figure varies considerably depending on the type of epilepsy disorder. An average duration has little meaning other than to indicate that the condition was considered to be resolved in some patients.

Implications derived from these classical studies are limited by the fact that they were carried out many years ago in geographically restricted populations with little racial or ethnic diversity. More diverse information has been obtained from studies of rural biracial (Haerer et al, 1986), inner-city racially and ethnically diverse (Benn et al, 2008), and Native American (Parko and Thurman, 2009) populations in the United States, but these were not nationwide. Large regional surveys carried out by the Centers for Disease Control and Prevention, and others (CDC 1994; Ferguson et al, 2005; Kobau and Condon, 2001; Kobau et al, 2004; 2007; 2008; Ottman et al, 2011) included large numbers of patients with prevalent epilepsy but asked relatively few questions. The need for a national surveillance system for epilepsy in the United States is recognized (Trevathan, 2011) and has been addressed by the Institute of Medicine (IOM, 2012). With respect to international studies, a recent meta-analysis suggests that the incidence rate of epilepsy in low- to middle-income countries may be twice that of high-income countries (Ngugi et al., 2011).

Although little has appeared to change over time with respect to data on the overall incidence and prevalence of epilepsy, there has been one important recent development in incidence rate plotted against age. The risk for epilepsy is greatest at the extremes of life: while in earlier studies incidence was highest in the first years of life, as the population has aged in the industrialized world, the incidence of epilepsy has now become greater in the elderly than in children (Banerjee and Hauser, 2008; Linehan and Kerr, 2010; Benn et al, 2008) (Fig. 2–8). Some studies have reported rates as high as 200 per 100,000 for people over 80 years of age compared with 70–80 per 100,000 for the first year of life (Jallon et al., 1997). However, in developing countries, prevalence remains high in the young (Fig. 2–9).

Woodbury (Woodbury, 1977b) used the data from the Rochester study (Hauser and Kurland, 1975) to plot prevalence of epilepsy against age and obtained a straight-line increase from 3.9/1,000 at 1 year of age to 9.1/1,000 at age 70. Although there are many problems with the interpretation of these data, an age-related increase in the prevalence of epilepsy indicates that more persons develop epilepsy with age than are cured or die. Additional information on the dynamic aspects of the prevalence of epilepsy is provided by the Rochester study (Hauser and Kurland, 1975), which demonstrated that remission rates were highest in persons whose epilepsy became evident between the ages of 1 and 9 years. This is generally believed to reflect resolution of symptoms in persons with the benign genetic epilepsies of childhood (Chapter 7), although this assumption is not necessarily consistent with the data. In the United States, 44% of adults with epilepsy reported having seizures within the past three months (Kobau et al., 2008).

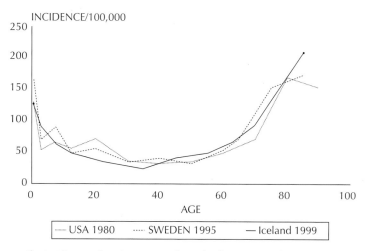

Figure 2–8. Age-specific incidence of epilepsy in industrialized countries. (From Banerjee and Hauser, 2008, with permission.)

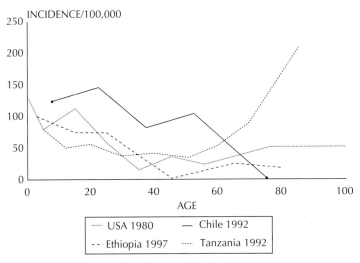

Figure 2–9. Age-specific incidence of epilepsy in developing countries. (From Banerjee and Hauser, 2008, with permission.)

The problem of underestimation in prevalence reflected in the cautious Rochester study (Hauser and Kurland, 1975) is revealed by comparing the expected prevalence rate at 8.5 years of age calculated from those data by Woodbury (Woodbury, 1977c) with that obtained by Rose and associates (Rose et al., 1973) in a study of third-grade children in Maryland. Both studies excluded simple but not complex febrile seizures. The prevalence for the former study, which was based on review of medical records, was estimated to be 4.46/1,000, whereas in the latter study, based on a questionnaire survey and selected examinations, it was 18.6/1,000. When the studies are more carefully matched for seizure type, however, the prevalence in the Rochester study is much closer to that calculated by Rose and associates. Whereas one-quarter of people with epilepsy escaped detection by the usual epidemiological methods practiced three decades ago (Woodbury, 1977c; Zielinski, 1974), approaches are more reliable today.

Accounting for the competing risk of death, Hesdorffer and colleagues (2011) used the Rochester data (Hauser and Kurland, 1975) to calculate the lifetime risk of epilepsy to be 1.6% to age 50, 3.0% to age 80, and 3.5% to age 87. Cumulative incidence was calculated to be 1.7% to age 50 and 3.4% to age 80 (Hesdorffer et al, 2011). Furthermore, allowance for the estimated percentage of people with epilepsy who were undetected by the Rochester study

(Woodbury, 1977c) could increase the lifetime risk of chronic epilepsy to close to 5%. The Rochester study (Hauser and Kurland, 1975) also indicates that for every two people with epilepsy, another has had one or more afebrile reactive epileptic seizures, and an additional 2% of all children have simple febrile seizures. This raises the percentage of the population that can expect to experience at least one epileptic seizure of any type during 80 years of life to almost 10%. Because these data were all gathered from a middle-class population who may be at relatively low risk for epilepsy, this is likely to be a conservative estimate of the problem (Banerjee and Hauser, 2008).

The circumstances for populations of urban areas and certain developing countries with reduced access to adequate health care and increased exposure to trauma and disease undoubtedly increase the risk of epilepsy, and worldwide figures could be two to four times higher than assumed from current data (Banerjee and Hauser, 2008; Diagana et al., 2010).

Global Burden of Disease

Perhaps more important than incidence and prevalence in understanding the impact of epilepsy as a worldwide health problem is the *global burden of disease*, as measured by *disability-adjusted life years (DALYs)*, the number of life years lost due to disability or premature death (Murray and Lopez, 1994). According to a WHO study, epilepsy accounts for 1% of the global burden of disease, which is equivalent to the respective burdens of the three other most important primary disorders of the brain: depression and other affective disorders, Alzheimer's disease and other dementias, and substance abuse (Murray and Lopez, 1994). Stroke is associated with a higher global burden of disease, but it is listed as a cardiovascular disorder by the WHO. The global burdens of disease for breast cancer in women and lung cancer in men in this study each was also similar to that of epilepsy, which can be explained by the fact that those disorders usually affect individuals late in life, while epilepsy often causes a lifetime of disability. Nonetheless, epilepsy receives much less public attention and resources than these other disorders, which could be due in part to the fact that it remains a stigmatized condition. This study was updated in 2004 (World Health Organization, 2008), but the figures for epilepsy in both studies are likely to be gross underestimates, because they identified individuals as having epilepsy only when the cause of the epilepsy was unknown. When the cause was known, individuals were listed according to the cause and not as epilepsy. The global burden of disease for epilepsy is highest in the developing world (see Fig. 17–1). Furthermore, twice as many people in the world will experience reactive seizures as have epilepsy, and little is known regarding the morbidity and mortality of those events. Early mortality, however, depends on the underlying cause, being highest with stroke, traumatic brain injury, and infection of the central nervous system (Hesdorffer et al., 2009).

SUMMARY AND CONCLUSIONS

Epilepsy can be put in perspective by an appreciation of its place in medical history and by epidemiological assessment of its importance today. Much has been written about the history of epilepsy in the West and Middle East, but little has reached the Western literature concerning the comparable history of this disorder elsewhere. In the Western literature, epilepsy occupied a considerably greater part of the deliberations of physicians and of the imagination of the general public in the past

than it does now. This can be attributed to its perceived religious significance; the mainstream of medical practice held the "sacred disease" to result from demonic possession or punishment for sins until the end of the 18th century.

The history of epilepsy has been described as distinguished and rightly concerns not only its perceived importance within the body of medicine but also the fascination of scholars with evidence that prominent prophets and other holy men, political leaders, philosophers, and many individuals who achieved greatness in the arts and sciences suffered from epilepsy. The epilepsy of their interest, however, was not the same as the epilepsy of today. Until the 19th century, the use of this word was confined almost exclusively to generalized tonic-clonic seizures characterized by loss of consciousness and falling, the "falling sickness" of medieval times. On the other hand, epileptic seizures were not well distinguished from other paroxysmal disturbances of organic or psychogenic origin, and some forms of madness and melancholia were also included within this category of disorders. Although a history of what was often erroneously considered epilepsy sheds little light on present-day epileptic seizures or epilepsy syndromes, ancient views of epilepsy as possession, evil omen, contagion, and insanity, as well as the horrible natural and supernatural therapies inflicted on the victims of epilepsy, are responsible for most of the stigma and damaging misconceptions that still contribute heavily to the disability suffered by persons with epilepsy.

The modern era of epilepsy began in the 19th century with major contributions to understanding the pathophysiology of epileptic seizures credited particularly to John Hughlings Jackson, David Ferrier, Victor Horsley, and Jean-Martin Charcot. Despite the tremendous progress made in this area during the last half of the 19th century, therapy for epilepsy remained essentially medieval until the introduction of phenobarbital in 1912.

Incidence rates and prevalence need to be age adjusted, because epileptic seizures and epilepsy disorders are most common at the extremes of age. As our population has aged, the incidence of epilepsy has become greater in the elderly than in children. Incidence rates and prevalence also depend on the definition of epilepsy. If one considers only individuals with chronic, recurrent epileptic seizures, the best available epidemiological data have suggested an age-adjusted incidence rate of 46.7/100,000 per year and an age-adjusted prevalence of 6.25/1,000 in the United States. However, based on information derived from urban and other largely underprivileged populations as well as documentation of the degree of underestimation due to failure to detect persons with epilepsy, the actual figures for incidence rates and prevalence may be two to four times higher. Even if one assumes the former, more conservative estimates, however, approximately 3–4% of persons living to the age of 80 will be given a diagnosis of a chronic epilepsy disorder at some time in their lives, and as many as 10% will experience at least one epileptic seizure. Incidence and prevalence of epilepsy is higher in the developing world than in industrialized countries, and it is estimated that 65 million people worldwide have active epilepsy.

Methodological difficulties have made it impossible at present to determine with certainty the current impact of epilepsy on world health. Epilepsy that cannot be attributed to a specific disease, most likely a small fraction of all epilepsy, is stated to account for 1% of the global burden of disease (almost certainly an underestimate), equivalent to those of lung cancer in men and breast cancer in women. Among primary disorders of the brain, it ranks with depression, dementia, and substance abuse.

Results of efforts to place epilepsy in perspective, both historically and epidemiologically, are of more than academic interest. An understanding of the roots of prejudice and misconceptions concerning epilepsy will help us realize and ultimately eradicate the suffering society inflicts on those with epilepsy. Epidemiological approaches also reveal the importance of environmental factors such as automobile accidents and poor hygiene in the development of epilepsy disorders and emphasize the role preventive medicine should play in reducing the impact of epilepsy on world health.

REFERENCES

Banerjee PN, Hauser WA (2008). Incidence and prevalence. In Engel J Jr, Pedley TA (Eds). Epilepsy: A Comprehensive Textbook, Second Edition. Philadelphia: Lippincott-Raven, pp. 45–56.

Benn, EK, Hauser, WA, Shih, T, Leary, L, Bagiella, E, Dayan, P, Green, R, Andrews, H, Thurman, DJ, and Hesdorffer, DC (2008). Estimating the incidence of first unprovoked seizure and newly diagnosed epilepsy in the low-income urban community of Northern Manhattan, New York City. Epilepsia 49:1431–1439.

Beran RG, Beran ME (1987). The way the gods used the sacred disease to make history fit. 17th Epilepsy International Congress, Jerusalem, September 1987. Book of abstracts, p. 10.

Berg, AT, Langfitt, J, Shinnar, S, Vickrey, BG, Sperling, MR, Walczak, T, Bazil, C, Pacia, SV, and Spencer SS (2003). How long does it take for partial epilepsy to become intractable? Neurology 60:186–190.

Berger, H (1929). Über das Elektrenkephalogram des Menschen. Arch Psychiatr Nervenkr 87:527–570.

Berrios, GE (1984). Epilepsy and insanity during the early 19th century: A conceptual history. Arch Neurol 41:978–981.

Bharucha EP, Bharucha NE (1989). Epilepsy in ancient Indian medicine. In Rose FC, Ed. Neuroscience Across the Centuries. London: Smith-Gordon & Nishimura, pp. 197–199.

Bouchet, C, and Cazauvieilh, JB (1825). De l'épilepsie considérée dans ses rapports avec l'aliénation mentale. Arch Gen Med 9:510–542.

Bravais, L-F (1827). Recherches sur les symptômes et le traitement de l'épilepsie hémiplégique, Paris (Thèse de Paris No. 118).

Bright, R (1831). Reports of Medical Cases, Vol II, Part II, London: Longman, Rees, Orme, Brown, Green, & Highley.

Broca, P (1867). Trépanation du crâne pratiquée avec succès dans un cas de fracture avec enfoncement. Bulletin de la Société Imperiale de Chirurgie de Paris pendant l'annee 1866, 2e serie 7:508–512.

Calmeil, LF (1824). De l'épilepsie étudiée sous le rapport de son siège et de son influence sur la production de l'aliénation mentale. Paris: Diderot.

CDC (1994). Current Trends Prevalences of Self-Reported Epilepsy—United States, 1986–1990. Atlanta: Centers for Disease Control and Prevention.

Cecil, R, and Loeb, RF (1959). A Textbook of Medicine. Philadelphia: Saunders.

Charcot, J-M (1886). Lecons sur les maladies du système nerveux, recueillies et publiées par Bourneville, t. I., Paris (Oeuvres complètes, I).

Commission on Classification and Terminology of the International League Against Epilepsy (1989). Proposal for revised classification of epilepsies and epileptic syndromes. Epilepsia 30:389–399.

Daras, MD, Bladin, PF, Eadie, MJ and Millett, D (2008). Epilepsy: Historical perspectives. In Engel, J Jr, and Pedley, TA (Eds.) Epilepsy: A Comprehensive Textbook, Second Edition. Philadelphia: Lippincott Williams & Wilkins, pp. 13–39.

de Horta, P (1763). Informe Medico Moral de la Penosissima y Rigorosa Enfermedad de la Epilepsia. Madrid: Domingo Fernandez de Arrojo.

Delasiauve (1854). Traité de l'épilepsie. Paris.

Diagana, M, Bhalla, D, Ngoungou, E, and Preux, P-M (2010). Epidemiology of epilepsies in resource-poor countries. In Atlas of Epilepsies, Volume 1. Edited by CP Panayiotopoulos. London: Springer, pp. 57–63.

Engel, J, Jr (1988). The epilepsies. In Cecil Textbook of Medicine, Ed 8. Edited by JB Wyngaarden and LH Smith, Jr, Philadelphia: WB Saunders, pp. 2217–2229. Esquirol, E: Des maladies mentales, 2 vols. Paris: Ballière.

Engel, J, Jr (2005). The emergence of neurosurgical approaches to the treatment of epilepsy. In Waxman, S. (Ed.). From Neuroscience to Neurology: Neuroscience, Molecular Medicine, and the Therapeutic Transformation of Neurology. Amsterdam: Elsevier, pp. 81–105.

Esquirol, E (1838). Des maladies mentales, 2 vols., Paris: Ballière.

Everett, GM, and Richards, RK (1944). Comparative anticonvulsant action of 3,5,5-trimethyloxazolidine-2,4-dione (tridone), dilantin and phenobarbitol. J Pharmacol Exp Ther 1:402–407.

Ferguson, PL, Selassie, AW, Wannamaker, BB, Dong, B, Kobau, R, and Thurman, DJ (2005). CDC. Prevalence of epilepsy and health-related quality of life and disability among adults with epilepsy—South Carolina, 2003 and 2004. MMWR 54:1080–1082.

Ferrier, D (1873). Experimental researches in cerebral physiology and pathology, The West Riding Lunatic Asylum Medical Reports 3:30–96.

Fritsch, G, and Hitzig, E (1870). Ueber die elektrische Erregbarkeit des Grosshirns, Berlin, n.d. [Reprinted from Reichert's und de BoisReymond's Archiv, Heft 3].

Gibbs FA, Gibbs EL, Lennox WG (1938). Cerebral dysrhythmias of epilepsy. Arch Neurol Psychiatr 39:298–314.

Gowers, WR (1881). Epilepsy and other chronic convulsive diseases, London.

Haerer, AF, Anderson, DW, and Schoenberg, BS (1986). Prevalence and clinical features of epilepsy in a biracial United States population. Epilepsia 27:66–75.

Hauptmann, A (1912). Luminal bei epilepsie. Munch Med Wochenschr 59:1907–1909.

Hauser, WA, and Hesdorffer, DC (1990). Epilepsy: Frequency, Causes and Consequences. New York: Demos Publications.

Hauser, WA, and Kurland LT (1975). The epidemiology of epilepsy in Rochester, Minnesota, 1935 through 1967. Epilepsia 16:1–66.

Hesdorffer, DC, Benn, EKT, Cascino, GD, and Hauser, WA (2009). Is a first acute symptomatic seizure epilepsy? mortality and risk for recurrent seizure. Epilepsia 50:1102–1108.

Hesdorffer, DC, Logroscino, G, Benn, EK, Katri, N, Cascino, G, and Hauser, WA (2011). Estimating risk for developing epilepsy: a population-based study in Rochester, Minnesota. Neurology 76:23–27.

Hirtz, D, Thurman, DJ, Gwinn-Hardy, K, et al. (2007). How common are the "common" neurologic disorders? Neurology 68:326–337.

Horsley, V (1886). Brain surgery. Br Med J 2:670–675.

Hughes, J (2005). Did all those famous people really have epilepsy? Epilepsy Behav. 6:115–139.

IOM (2012). Epilepsy Across the Spectrum: Promoting Health and Understanding. National Academy of Sciences. Washington, DC: The National Academies Press.

Jackson, JH (1898). Case of epilepsy with tasting movements and "dreaming state"—very small patch of softening in the left uncinate gyrus. Brain 21:580–590.

Jackson, JH (1873). On the anatomical, physiological, and pathological investigation of the epilepsies. West Riding Lunatic Asylum Medical Reports, Vol 3.

Jackson, JH (1870). A study of convulsions. Trans St Andrews Med Grad Assoc 3:1–45.

Jallon, P, Goumaz, M, Haenggeli, C, and Morabia, A (1997). Incidence of first epileptic seizures in the canton of Geneva, Switzerland. Epilepsia 38:547–552.

Jasper H, Kershman J (1941). Electroencephalographic classification of the epilepsies. Arch Neurol Psychiatr 45:903–943.

Kinnier Wilson, JV (1967a). Mental diseases of ancient Mesopotamia. In Diseases in Antiquity. Edited by D Brothwell and AT Sandison. Springfield, Ill: Charles C Thomas, pp. 723–733.

Kinnier Wilson, JV (1967b). Organic diseases of ancient Mesopotamia. In Diseases in Antiquity. Edited by D Brothwell and AT Sandison. Springfield, Ill: Charles C Thomas, p. 191–208.

Kinnier Wilson, JV, and Reynolds, EH (1990). Texts and documents: Translation and analysis of a cuneiform text forming part of a Babylonian treatise on epilepsy. Med Hist 34:185–198.

Kobau, R, and Condon, K (2001). Health-related quality of life among persons with epilepsy—Texas, 1998. MMWR 50:24–26.

Kobau, R, Dilorio, CA, Price, PH, et al. (2004). Prevalence of epilepsy and health status of adults with epilepsy in Georgia and Tennessee: Behavioral Risk Factor Surveillance System, 2002. Epilepsy Behav 5:358–366.

Kobau, R, Zahran, H, Grant, D, Thurman, DJ, Price, PH, and Zack, MM (2007). Prevalence of active epilepsy and health-related quality of life among adults with self-reported epilepsy in California: California Health Interview Survey, 2003. Epilepsia 48:1904–1913.

Kobau, R, Zahran, H, Thurman, DJ, Zack,MM, Henry, TR, and Schachter, SC, and Price, PH (2008). Epilepsy surveillance among adults—19 states. Behavioral Risk Factor Surveillance System MMWR 57 (SS-6):1–20.

Lai C-W, Lai Y-HC (1991). History of epilepsy in Chinese traditional medicine. Epilepsia 32:229–302.

Lennox, WG (1960). Epilepsy and Related Disorders, Vol 1–2. Boston: Little, Brown & Co.

Leuret, F (1843). Recherches sur l'épilepsie. Arch Gen Med (4e série) 2:32–50.

Linehan, C, and Kerr, M (2010). Epidemiology of epilepsies in developed countries. In Atlas of Epilepsies, Volume 1. Edited by CP Panayiotopoulos. London: Springer, pp. 51–56.

Locock, C (1857). Discussion of paper by EH Sieveking: Analysis of 52 cases of epilepsy observed by author. Lancet 1:527–528.

Lomazow, S (2011). The epilepsy of Franklin Delano Roosevelt. Neurology 76:668–669.

Macewen, W (1881). Intra-cranial lesions—illustrating some points in connexion with the localisation of cerebral affections and the advantages of aseptic trephining. Lancet ii, 544 and 581.

Macewen W (1879). Tumour of the dura matter removed during life in a person affected with epilepsy. Glas Med J 12:210.

Manyam BV (1992). Epilepsy in ancient India. Epilepsia 33:473–475.

Merlis, JK (1970). Proposal for an international classification of the epilepsies. Epilepsia 11:114–119.

Merritt, HH, and Putnam, TJ (1938). A new series of anti-convulsant drugs tested by experiments on animals. Arch Neurol Psychiatry 39:1003–1015.

Mishra, SK (1987). Concept of neurologic disorders in "Ayurveda" ancient Indian medical treatise (abstr). Neurology 37 (Suppl 1):240.

Murray CJL, Lopez AD (Eds) (1994). Global Comparative Assessment in the Health Sector; Disease Burden, Expenditures, and Intervention Packages. Geneva: World Health Organization.

Ngugi, AK, Bottomley, C, Kleinschmidt, I, Sander, JW, and Newton, CR (2010). Estimation of the burden of active and life-time epilepsy: a meta-analytic approach. Epilepsia 51:883–890.

Ngugi, AK, Kariuki, SM, Bottomley, C, et al. (2011). Incidence of epilepsy: a systematic review and meta-analysis. Neurology 77:1005–1012.

Ottman, R, Lipton, RB, Ettinger, AB, et al. (2011). Comorbidities of epilepsy: results from the Epilepsy Comorbidities and Health (EPIC) Survey. Epilepsia, 52:308–315.

Parko, K, and Thurman, DJ (2009). Prevalence of epilepsy and seizures in the Navajo Nation 1998–2002. Epilepsia 50:2180–2185.

Penfield, W, and Jasper, H (1954). Epilepsy and the Functional Anatomy of the Human Brain. Boston: Little, Brown & Co.

Pritchard, JC (1822). A treatise on diseases of the nervous system, Part the first, London.

Richards, RK, and Everett, GM (1944). Analgesic and anticonvulsive properties of 3,5,5-trimethyloxazolidine-2,4-dione (tridone) (abstr). Fed Proc 3:39.

Rose, SW, Penry, JK, Markush, RE, Radloff LA, and Putnam, PL (1973). Prevalence of epilepsy in children. Epilepsia 14:133–152.

Shorvon, S (2009). History of the drug treatment of epilepsy between 1955 and 1989 with special reference to the role of the International League Against Epilepsy (ILAE). In Shorvon, S, Perucca, E, and Engel, J Jr (Eds). The Treatment of Epilepsy, Third Edition. Chichester, UK: Wiley-Blackwell, pp. xxi–xxxviii

Taylor, DC (1987). One hundred years of epilepsy surgery: Sir Victor Horsley's contribution. In Surgical Treatment of the Epilepsies. Edited by Engel, J Jr. New York: Raven Press, pp. 7–11.

Taylor, DC, and Marsh, SM (1980). Hughlings Jackson's Dr. Z: The paradigm of temporal lobe epilepsy revealed. J Neurol Neurosurg Psychiatry 43:758–767.

Temkin, O (1945). The Falling Sickness. Baltimore: Johns Hopkins Press.

Thurman, DJ, Beghi, E, Begley, CE, et al. (2011). Standards for epidemiologic studies and surveillance of epilepsy. Epilepsia 52 (Suppl 7):1.

Tissot, SA (1770). Traité de l'épilepsie, faisant le tome troisième du traité des nerfs et de leurs maladies. Paris: PF Didot.

Todd, RB (1855). Clinical lectures on paralysis, certain diseases of the brain, and other affections of the nervous system. Philadelphia: Lindsay and Blakiston.

Trevathan, E (2011). "Flying blind" without epilepsy surveillance data. Neurology 76:10–11.

Tyler, KL (1984). Hughlings Jackson: The early development of his ideas on epilepsy. J Hist Med Allied Sci 39:55–64.

Van den Berg, BJ, and Yerushalmy, J (1969). Studies on convulsive disorders in young children. 1. Incidence of febrile and nonfebrile convulsions by age and other factors. Pediatr Res 3:298–304.

Wiebe, S (2011). The Epilepsies. In Goldman, L, and Shafer, AI, Eds. Cecil Textbook of Medicine, 24th edition. Philadelphia: Saunders, pp. 2283–2293.

Woodbury, LA (1977a). A brief consideration of the prognosis of epilepsy. In Plan for Nationwide Action on Epilepsy, Vol 4. Commission for the Control of Epilepsy and Its Consequences. Washington, DC: US DHEW, Public Health Service, NIH. DHEW Publ # (NIH)78–279, pp. 3–23.

Woodbury, LA (1977b). Incidence and prevalence of seizure disorders including the epilepsies in the United States of America: A review and analysis of the literature. In Plan for Nationwide Action on Epilepsy, Vol 4. Commission for the Control of Epilepsy and Its Consequences. Washington, DC: US DHEW, Public Health Service, NIH. DHEW Publ # (NIH)78–279, pp. 24–77.

Woodbury, LA (1977c). Prevalence of epilepsy: A continuing, dynamic process. In Plan for Nationwide Action on Epilepsy, Vol 4. Commission for the Control of Epilepsy and Its Consequences. Washington, DC: US DHEW, Public Health Service, NIH. DHEW Publ # (NIH)78–279, pp. 78–106.

Woodbury, LA (1977d). Shortening of the life span and mortality of patients with epilepsy. In Plan for Nationwide Action on Epilepsy, Vol 4. Commission for the Control of Epilepsy and Its Consequences. Washington, DC: US DHEW, Public Health Service, NIH. DHEW Publ # (NIH)78–279, pp. 107–114.

World Health Organization (2008). The Global Burden Of Disease, 2004 Update. Geneva: World Health Organization.

Zielinski, JJ (1974). Epileptics not in treatment. Epilepsia 15:203–210.

Zimmer, C (2004). Soul Made Flesh: The Discovery of the Brain—and How it Changed the World. New York: Free Press, pp. 367.

PART 2

Pathophysiology

Chapter 3

Mechanisms of Neuronal Excitation and Synchronization

THE NEURON
The Excitable Membrane and Its
  Microenvironment
Intracellular Processes
Structure-Function Relationships of
  Neuronal Elements
Interneuronal Connections

GLIAL INFLUENCES

NEURONAL NETWORKS
Intrinsic Organization of Ammon's Horn
Intrinsic Organization of the Neocortex

Subcortical and Interhemispheric
  Connections
PHYLOGENY AND ONTOGENY
Species Differences
Cortical Development
Maturational Effects on Excitability
SYSTEMIC INFLUENCES
NEURONAL BASIS OF EEG ACTIVITY
METHODOLOGICAL DEVELOPMENTS
SUMMARY AND CONCLUSIONS

Two factors predominantly determine the epileptogenic properties of neuronal tissue: excitability and synchronization. *Excitability* refers to an enhanced predisposition of a neuron or neuronal aggregate to discharge when stimulated or to discharge spontaneously. The enhanced response to stimulation may be a nonspecific susceptibility to all afferent input or a specific receptivity to input only along selected pathways. Hyperexcitability that results in increased random firing of individual neurons, however, does not result in increased behavioral activity (and may even reduce it). Neuronal firing must be organized appropriately within neuronal aggregates to constitute a functionally effective output. Patterned behavioral responses, both normal and abnormal, require a certain degree of *synchronization* of firing within the underlying neuronal substrate. Epileptic seizures result from excessive synchronization of neuronal firing. Therefore, epileptic behavior is modulated by mechanisms that alter both neuronal excitability and neuronal synchronization.

THE NEURON

Excitability of individual nerve cells in the brain is determined by many factors, including properties of the excitable membrane and its microenvironment, intracellular processes, structural features of neuronal elements, and effects of interneuronal connections. The most dramatic developments in neuroscience in the past two decades have come from a more detailed understanding of the molecular structure-function relationships of ion channels, neurotransmitter receptors, synthesis, and trafficking as well as other intracellular processes. Identification and isolation of genes that encode the protein structures underlying these mechanisms are important for studying normal brain function, and mutations in these genes are also responsible for epileptogenic dysfunction.

Molecular neurobiology, however, is an area of rapid and extensive research beyond the scope of this text; of necessity molecular mechanisms presented here must be incomplete. Nevertheless inclusion of certain concepts in the following discussion are necessary, because aberrations in several ion channels (referred to as *channelopathies*), neurotransmitter receptors, and important intracellular processes are responsible for many epilepsy disorders (Chapter 5) and will be the targets of future antiseizure drugs. Still, much more work is needed at the systems level to elucidate how these disparate molecular disturbances eventually give rise to the clinical manifestations of epilepsy.

The Excitable Membrane and Its Microenvironment

All excitable membranes, including the neuronal membrane, maintain an electrical charge, or *potential difference*, between the intracellular and extracellular spaces as a result of selective ion permeability. The membrane potential is determined by the ratios of internal to external concentrations of various ions, which in turn depend on (1) the flow of ionic currents across the membrane, particularly involving Na^+, K^+, Ca^{2+}, and Cl^-, and (2) the presence of large negatively charged molecules (*anions*) inside the cell that cannot pass

through the membrane. Permeable ions pass through specialized membrane pores, termed *channels* or *ionophores*. The ability of each ion to move across the membrane is referred to as the membrane's *conductance* for that ion. Conductance for a given ion species can be regulated by a variety of factors (Kandel et al., 2000; Nichollset al., 2001; Heinemann et al., 2008). *Voltage-gated channels* are activated by electrical signals, and *ligand-gated channels* by chemical signals.

Ion channels consist of pores surrounded by protein subunits that can be reconfigured in many ways to form a tremendous variety of structures with several different (*heteromeric*) or all the same (*homomeric*) subunits that confer vastly different properties. Great advances in molecular neurobiology over the past two decades have permitted researchers to clone and express ion channels in various nonneuronal systems, such as oocytes and HEK-29 cells, to study their physiological and pharmacological properties. Hypotheses regarding the function of these channels in the whole brain can be tested using *transgenic* mouse preparations and genetic engineering with *viral vectors*.

VOLTAGE-GATED CHANNELS

There are a number of voltage-gated K^+, Na^+, and Ca^+ channels, designated as K_v, Na_v, and Ca_v as well as by the genes that encode them (Kullmann and Schorge, 2008) (Table 3–1). The K_{v7} family of K^+ channels generates the *M-type current*, the first to be identified. This current is so called because it is completely suppressed by *muscarinic* effects of *acetylcholine (ACh)*. Multiple subunit types permit a wide variety of K^+ channels and currents, which are the most diverse of the voltage-gated channels. The first epilepsy channelopathy to be recognized was *benign familial neonatal seizures*, which are due to a missense mutation in the *KCNQ2* and *KCNQ3* K^+ channel–encoding genes. *4-Aminopiridine (4-AP)* blocks K^+ channels and is commonly used for inducing experimental epileptiform events in brain slices. The classes of Ca^{2+}- and Na^+-dependent K^+ channels that are selectively activated by influx of these ions are designated K_{Ca} and K_{Na}, and K^+ channels responsible for inverse rectifying currents are designated K_{ir}. Mutations of the *leucine-rich repeat protein (LGI1)* gene, which codes

Table 3–1 Some Important Ion Channel–Coding Genes

Gene	Channel	Relevance
KCNQ2	K⁺	Benign familial neonatal seizures
KCNQ3	K⁺	Benign familial neonatal seizures
LGI1	K⁺	Lateral temporal lobe epilepsy with auditory features, voltage-gated K⁺ channel complex
SCN1A	Na⁺	Dravet syndrome, GEFS⁺
SCN2A	Na⁺	GEFS⁺
SCN1B	Na⁺	GEFS⁺
NKCC2	Cl⁻	Increases intracellular Cl⁻
NCC1	Cl⁻	Decreases intracellular Cl⁻

GEFS⁺ = generalized epilepsy with febrile seizures plus.

for the *voltage-gated K⁺ channel (VGKC) complex* cause *lateral temporal lobe epilepsy with auditory features* (Chapter 7), but an autoimmune limbic encephalitis that targets this complex results in highly focal *faciobrachial* clonic seizures (Chapter 5).

There is considerable interest in voltage-gated Na⁺ channels. The channel $Na_{v1.1}$, encoded by the gene *SCN1A*, is highly concentrated in hippocampus and neocortex, and a mutation that appears to decrease interneuron firing is responsible for *Dravet syndrome*. Mutations of this gene and the genes *SCN2A* and *SCN1B* have been identified as causes of *genetic epilepsy with febrile seizures plus* (*GEFS+*), and a mutation of *SCN2A* has been implicated in *benign familial neonatal-infantile seizures*. Members of this family of genes are likely candidates for susceptibility genes that would increase the risk of developing a variety of genetic and acquired epilepsies (Chapters 5 and 7).

Voltage-gated Ca²⁺ channels are divided into *high-voltage-activated* (HVA) and *low-voltage-activated* (LVA) forms. There are a variety of HVA channels, which give rise to different types of Ca⁺ currents (*L, P/Q, N, R*), but the LVA channels which give rise to the *T-type currents* that can be de-inactivated by hyperpolarizing inhibitory input are of particular interest in epilepsy. They are responsible for rhythmic burst firing in the thalamus, and polymorphisms appear to be responsible for absence seizures (Chapter 4). There are other, *hyperpolarization-activated cyclic*

nucleotide–gated cation (HCN) channels which also promote epileptiform discharges and are upregulated in epileptogenic hippocampus (Chapter 4).

MEMBRANE PHYSIOLOGY

The *resting membrane potential* of nerve cells is negative inside, usually with a value of 60–80 mV. This potential is maintained by an active, energy-requiring process that extrudes Na⁺ from the intracellular space, coupled with an influx of K⁺ (*the Na⁺-K⁺ pump*), as well as other passive ionic currents and electrochemical equilibria. Transporter proteins responsible for this and other pump mechanisms have been identified. For most resting neurons, however, the only significant passive current is through K⁺ leak channels. The Na⁺ K⁺ pump depends on the action of an enzyme called *Na⁺ K⁺ ATPase*, which breaks down the high-energy *adenosine triphosphate (ATP)*. Consequently, under resting conditions, with adequate energy supplies, the concentration of intracellular Na⁺ is low and that of intracellular K⁺ is high compared with the extracellular concentrations of these ions.

When ion channels are opened, ions move passively across the membrane according to both *concentration* and *charge gradients*. An ion tends to move according to its electrochemical gradient, into the space where its concentration is lower and the charge is opposite to its own. If a specific ion channel is opened and free passage of that ion is allowed, a selective ionic current will occur. The ion will move down its concentration gradient as far as allowed by the charge separation across the membrane, resulting in a change in the membrane's potential that approaches the *equilibrium potential* for that ion. Under resting conditions in the normal adult brain, there are intracellular deficiencies in Na⁺, Cl⁻, and Ca²⁺, and opening any channels that permit their passage results in an influx. An influx of Na⁺ and Ca²⁺ brings positive charges into the cell and reduces the membrane potential (*depolarizes* the membrane), whereas an influx of Cl⁻ increases the membrane potential (*hyperpolarizes* the membrane). There is an excess of intracellular K⁺, however, and opening K⁺ channels leads to K⁺ efflux, which results in membrane hyperpolarization (Fig. 3–1).

Quantitative approaches allow calculation of equilibrium potentials for individual

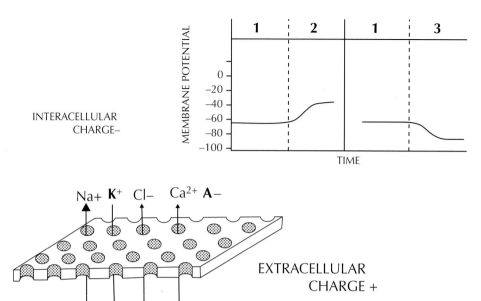

Figure 3–1. Membrane polarization in the adult brain. *Na+*, sodium ions; *K+*, potassium ions; *Cl–*, chloride ions; *Ca2+*, calcium ions; *A–*, negatively charged intracellular macromolecules (large anions). The size of the symbol indicates relative concentration. *Arrows* indicate the direction of ion flow if channels are open. *1:* The resting membrane potential is maintained at –65 mV by the Na+ K+ pump, which extrudes Na+, and by impermeability of the membrane to intracellular A–. *2:* Opening of Na+ or Ca2+ channels leads to influx of positive charges, causing depolarization of the membrane. *3:* Opening of K+ channels leads to efflux of positive charges, and opening of Cl– channels leads to influx of negative charges, both causing hyperpolarization of the membrane.

ions and of the membrane potential, which is the weighted average of the individual ionic potentials under various situations (Kandel et al., 2000; Nicholls et al., 2001; Heinemann et al., 2008). For purposes of this discussion, however, it is necessary to know only that the equilibrium potential for Na+ is approximately +55 mV (inside positive), for Cl– it is approximately –60 mV, for K+ it is approximately –75 mV, and for Ca2+ it can be as high as +200 mV (Krnjevic, 1980).

Chemical or electrical events that open some Na+ channels to allow Na+ influx cause a *graded* membrane depolarization, but this is countered by the Na+ K+ pump unless depolarization reaches a *threshold level*. At threshold, in selected regions of membrane, Na+ channels open that are responsible for generation of the *action potential*. This results in a rapid, *all-or-none regenerative* membrane depolarization approaching the equilibrium potential for Na+. The Na+ channels open rapidly for only a brief period and cannot reopen until the membrane repolarizes. Membrane depolarization also

opens K+ channels. This *voltage-dependent K+ current*, which is opposite in direction to the Na+ current, develops more slowly. As the membrane approaches the equilibrium potential for K+, there is a transient hyperpolarization before the resting potential is reestablished. This complete sequence of events is referred to as the *Na+ spike* or *action potential* (Fig. 3–2A).

In certain regions of the membrane, and under some conditions, depolarization can open voltage-dependent Ca2+ channels. This can produce a Ca2+ action potential that is of higher amplitude and longer duration than the Na+ action potential (Fig. 3–2B). Influx of Ca2+ can, in turn, open a second class of K+ channels to give rise to a *Ca2+-dependent K+ current*, which is longer lasting than the voltage-dependent K+ current. When membrane depolarization opens Ca2+ as well as Na+ channels, the result is a larger, longer-lasting depolarization followed by a more prolonged hyperpolarization (see Fig. 3–2B). The enhanced hyperpolarization can be followed by a transient rebound

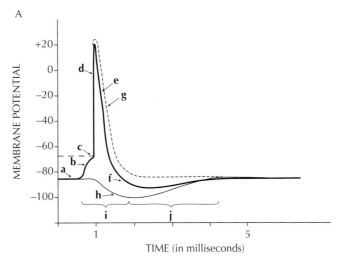

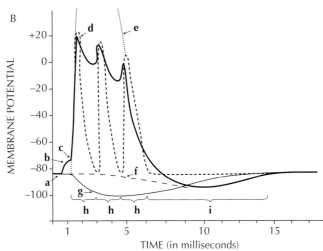

Figure 3–2. A. Na⁺ action potential. The *heavy solid line* shows Na⁺ action potential and afterhyperpolarization (AHP) recorded at soma. *a,* resting potential; *b,* graded Na⁺-mediated depolarization; *c,* threshold; *d,* "all or none" regenerative spike, rising phase; *e,* repolarization phase; *f,* AHP; *g,* Na⁺ current; *h,* voltage-dependent K⁺ current; *i,* absolute refractory period; *j,* relative refractory period. **B.** Ca²⁺ influx and the Ca²⁺ action potential. The *heavy solid line* shows voltage-dependent Ca²⁺ current–induced burst firing with prolonged two-phase AHP recorded at soma. *a,* resting potential; *b,* graded Na⁺-mediated depolarization; *c,* threshold; *d,* repetitive "all-or none" voltage-dependent Na⁺ spikes during prolonged depolarization due to *e; e,* voltage-dependent Ca²⁺ current; *f,* Ca²⁺-dependent K⁺ current; *g,* voltage-dependent K+ current; *h,* absolute refractory periods (for Na⁺); *i,* relative refractory period.

depolarization, causing the cell to be more excitable at a specific point in time. This mechanism underlies repetitive rhythmic firing of pacemaker neurons that can induce synchronized oscillatory activity.

Action potentials occur when the membrane depolarizes to some threshold level. Consequently, depolarizing influences increase and hyperpolarizing influences decrease the opportunity for a subsequent depolarization to trigger an action potential. Influences that open Na⁺ and Ca²⁺ channels to depolarize the membrane are called *excitatory*, while those that open K⁺ and Cl⁻ channels to hyperpolarize the membrane are called *inhibitory*. Excitatory neurotransmitters commonly act by transiently opening *ligand-gated* channels for Na⁺, Ca²⁺, or

both, while inhibitory neurotransmitters commonly act by opening channels for Cl⁻ or K⁺ (Fig. 3–3).

The Cl⁻ influx responsible for the hyperpolarizing inhibitory effect of Cl⁻ channel opening depends on the action of an outwardly directed Cl⁻ pump, mediated by a protein cotransporter encoded by the gene *KCC2*. Early in development, the protein encoded by the gene *NKCC1* transports Cl⁻ into cells, and the increased intracellular Cl⁻ concentration results in an excitatory depolarization in response to opening of the Cl⁻ channel (Macdonald and Mody, 2008; Heinemann et al., 2008). Consequently, in the neonatal brain and also in some pathological cells in epileptic brain, the inhibitory neurotransmitter γ-*aminobutyric acid (GABA)*,

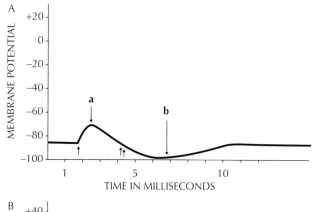

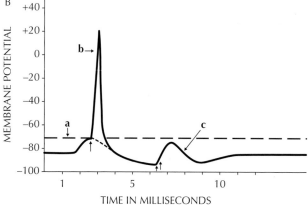

Figure 3–3. Postsynaptic potentials. **A.** *a*, excitatory postsynaptic potential (EPSP) due to Na⁺ influx (↑); *b*, inhibitory postsynaptic potential (IPSP) due to Cl⁻ influx or K⁺ efflux (↑↑). **B.** *a*, threshold; *b*, when EPSP reaches threshold and an all-or-none Na⁺ spike is generated (↑); *c*, when the same EPSP (↑↑) occurs during an IPSP, while the membrane is hyperpolarized, and so fails to reach threshold and generate an action potential.

which opens Cl⁻ channels, causes Cl⁻ efflux and a slight membrane depolarization that can be excitatory (Dzhala et al., 2005; Cohen et al., 2002; Ackermann and Moshé 2010).

Because Na⁺ channels are inactivated following a Na⁺ spike until repolarization occurs, there is an *absolute refractory period* when a second Na⁺ spike cannot be generated (see Fig. 3–2). Inactivation is usually caused by closing of a ball-like structure on the inside of the membrane, which blocks the channel to ion passage, determining rapidity of firing. The duration of inactivation determines the rate at which a neuron can fire repetitive action potentials. Interneurons, for instance, typically have fast recovery from inactivation permitting rapid burst firing. Mutations of the *SCN1A* and *SCN2A* genes, which code for the $Na_{v1.1}$ and $Na_{v1.2}$ channels, cause epilepsy conditions such as Dravet syndrome and GEFS+ (Chapters 5 and 7) by influencing β *subunits* to permit fast inactivation and rapid firing. Certain drugs like *phenytoin* and *carbamazepine* act to reduce excitability by slowing recovery from inactivation time, preventing rapid repetitive firing—commonly referred to as *use-dependent* block. During the *relative refractory period*, hyperpolarization due to endogenously generated K⁺ currents or to synaptically induced Cl⁻ or K⁺ currents (influences that normally open the Na⁺ channels) is effective, but a greater number of channels must be opened before the membrane reaches its threshold for producing a regenerative Na⁺ spike (see Fig. 3–2). Consequently, events that would ordinarily result in the production of an action potential may fail to reach threshold (Fig. 3–3). These hyperpolarizing currents, therefore, reduce the excitability of the neuronal membrane.

Extracellular ionic concentrations also contribute to neuronal excitability (Heinemann, 1987; Heinemann et al., 2008). Increased extracellular K⁺ concentration causes membrane depolarization and reduces inhibitory hyperpolarizing K⁺ currents. Extracellular K⁺ is increased during rapid neuronal firing, and K⁺ reuptake from the extracellular space (as well as maintenance of pH and water balance) is achieved to a large extent by glia. Neuronal excitability is enhanced by disturbances of glia that reduce their ability to perform these important functions (Van Gelder, 1983; Steinhauser et al., 2008).

Mg^{2+} ions block Ca^{2+} entry into cells at the resting membrane potential but are displaced by depolarization (MacDermott and Dale, 1987). Decreasing extracellular Mg^{2+} enhances membrane excitability, because less depolarization is necessary for Ca^{2+} currents to occur, while increasing extracellular Mg^{2+} has the opposite effect. A reduction in extracellular Ca^{2+} and Mg^{2+} also increases membrane excitability because these positive charges are removed from the extracellular surface of the membrane, regardless of the concentration gradient (Frankenhaeuser and Hodgkin, 1957; Heinemann et al., 2008).

Many pharmacological agents that alter neuronal excitability act by influencing these ionic mechanisms. For instance, *fluoroacetate*, *fluorocitrate*, and *methionine sulfoximine* are epileptogenic metabolic poisons that depolarize membranes by indirectly disrupting the function of the Na^+ K^+ pump. *Cardiac glycosides* such as *ouabain* directly inhibit this pump mechanism. *Perchlorate* and *thiocyanate* cause neuronal excitation by disrupting glial metabolism and interfering with the ability of glia to buffer ions in the extracellular space (Woodbury, 1980). For many common antiseizure drugs, on the other hand, one of the many possible mechanisms of action appears to involve modulation of voltage-gated conductance (Golden and Fariello, 1984; Macdonald and Rogawski, 2008; Walker et al., 2009) (Chapter 15).

Intracellular Processes

As with all cells, the operation of a neuron is controlled by genetic information contained in the nucleus. The *deoxyribonucleic acid (DNA)* code is expressed, via *ribonucleic acid (RNA)*, as protein synthesis. Anchoring filamentous and tubular proteins determine cell structure, while other proteins are responsible for energy metabolism and specialized functions such as neurotransmitter synthesis and release, receptor actions, and opening or closing of ion channels.

Important cellular functions include those that determine transport functions, such as transport of glucose into cells. Mutation of the gene *SLC2A1*, which encodes *glucose transporter-1 (GLUT1)*, results in *GLUT1 deficiency* characterized by severe metabolic encephalopathy associated with epileptic seizures (DeVivo et al., 1991) as well as other, more benign epilepsy conditions (Chapter 7). Another family of transporters that move molecules across the blood-brain barrier and function to expel toxins from the brain, such as *P-glycoprotein (PGP)* are of interest in epileptology, because they may also be activated by epileptic activity, reducing antiseizure drug levels in the epileptogenic region, resulting in *multidrug resistance (MDR)* (Sisodiya et al., 2008; Löscher and Schmidt, 2009) (Chapter 14). Other proteins maintain the intracellular milieu, including energy-generating molecules such as ATP, pH, and Ca^{2+} concentration, which determine dynamic alterations in neuronal excitability.

Neuronal excitability is preprogrammed in this manner, but both phasic and long-term changes can occur in response to environmental demands. The coupling mechanisms for inducing these functional and structural alterations are the subject of extensive research and appear to depend largely on ionic currents, particularly Ca^{2+} influx. Intracellular Ca^{2+} mediates changes in membrane and vesicular proteins to initiate neurotransmitter release and ion channel opening. Ca^{2+} activation of enzymes can also alter neuronal sensitivity without requiring protein synthesis by allowing neurons to rapidly insert or remove receptor sites in their membranes (*receptor trafficking*) and by influencing other processes such as phosphorylation/dephosphorylation (Lynch and Baudry, 1984, Wayman et al., 2008).

More persistent *plastic changes* in excitability require that neuronal experiences influence expression of genetic information. Activity-dependent gene expression is also mediated, in part, by Ca^{2+}. Influx of Ca^{2+} resulting from neuronal activation can selectively induce genes to synthesize protein for specific purposes. This was initially observed when administration of the convulsant drug *pentylenetetrazol* was shown to activate the *c-fos gene* to induce *c-fos protein* in cerebral neurons involved in an epileptic seizure (Morgan et al., 1987). Although the effects of this activation are unknown, such coupling phenomena provide a model mechanism by which neuronal excitation could influence cell growth and differentiation, provide a substrate for learning and memory, and perhaps mediate the development of chronic epilepsy (Chapter 4).

The past decade has witnessed tremendous advances in the study of activity-dependent alterations in gene expression as a result of the use of genome-wide microarrays that permit identification of altered expression profiles of tens of thousands of genes from a single sample (Lukasiuk et al., 2008). Such discovery-rather than hypothesis-driven investigative approaches to identifying candidate genes hold promise for elucidating molecular mechanisms underlying not only the development of epilepsy and the generation of epileptic seizures but also the adverse consequences of epilepsy on normal brain function (Lukasiuk et al., 2008; Parent et al., 2008) (Chapter 4).

Too much neuronal excitation can completely disrupt cell function (Chapter 10). Osmotic damage results from Cl⁻ influx, which also brings water into the cell; intracellular Ca^{2+} not only mediates gene expression but also activates *proteases* and *lipases*. Excessive Ca^{2+} influx causes *mitochondrial dysfunction* and cell death (Meldrum, 1983; Rothman and Olney, 1987) (Chapter 10).

Structure-Function Relationships of Neuronal Elements

The brain regions primarily involved in the pathophysiology of epilepsy are the neocortex and the hippocampus. The classical principal neuron in these regions is the *pyramidal cell*, characterized by an *apical* and several *basilar dendrites* appended to the cell body, or *soma*, and an *initial segment* or *axon hillock* close to the site of origin of the axon (Fig. 3–4). Many other neurons, however, such as *bipolar, fusiform*, and *stellate cells*, as well as a large variety of interneurons, have different morphological features. Membrane properties differ from one part of a neuron to another, allowing the various neuronal elements to subserve specialized physiological functions (see Fig. 3–4). Dendrites branch to a great degree and are often covered with processes called *spines*. Classical *excitatory synapses* are made primarily on these dendritic spines and along the dendritic shaft,

whereas classical *inhibitory synapses* are more concentrated on the soma and proximal dendrites, where they are most effective, although subtypes of *inhibitory interneurons* synapse on distal dendrites, and others on the midportion (Freund and Buzsáki, 1996). The shape and extent of dendritic arborizations and their spines confer variable capacities for spatial and temporal integration of afferent input, which determines their computational properties. Sophisticated neurophysiological techniques now permit investigations of the effect of excitation of a single spine, which reveal considerable differences in dendritic functions from one cell type to another and even between apical and basilar dendrites of the same cell (Krueppel et al., 2011).

Release of *excitatory neurotransmitters* from *presynaptic terminals* opens predominantly Na⁺ channels on *postsynaptic membranes*, giving rise to brief, graded depolarizing *excitatory postsynaptic potentials* (*EPSPs*). Release of *inhibitory neurotransmitters* opens Cl⁻ or K⁺ channels, giving rise to slightly longer-lasting hyperpolarizing *inhibitory postsynaptic potentials* (*IPSPs*) (see Fig. 3–3). The Cl⁻ channels opened by inhibitory neurotransmitters are also partially permeable to bicarbonate ions (HCO_3^-), causing an ionic current that is sensitive to carbonic anhydrase inhibitors. Synchronously occurring EPSPs and IPSPs, widely distributed over the surface of a neuron, summate to influence membrane potential at the axon hillock. The axon hillock membrane has a very high density of voltage-dependent Na⁺ channels, which give rise to a regenerative Na⁺ spike when the threshold is reached. *Saltatory conduction*—rapid progression from one unmyelinated node to the next along myelinated axons—and regenerative properties of unmyelinated axons allow the spike to be propagated without decay to the axon terminals. *Electrotonic conduction* along dendritic and some somatic membranes, however, results in spatial decay of graded postsynaptic potentials. Consequently, summation of EPSPs on distal dendrites is less likely than similar summation of EPSPs on proximal dendrites or soma to influence the membrane potential of the axon hillock and, therefore, less likely to affect spike generation at the axon hillock. IPSPs that cause hyperpolarization and shunting effects on somatic membrane are strategically placed

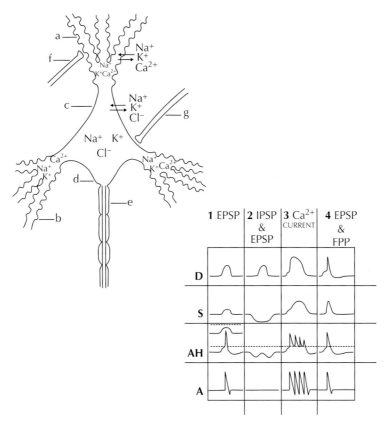

Figure 3–4. Structure-function relationships of the neuron. *a,* apical dendrite with spines; *b,* basilar dendrite with spines; *c,* soma; *d,* axon hillock; *e,* axon; *f,* excitatory input; *g,* inhibitory input. Also shown are distributions of Na$^+$, K$^+$, Cl$^-$, and Ca^{2+} channels over membrane. *1:* EPSP occurring at the dendrite (*D*) decays and may or may not generate an action potential at the axon hillock (*AH*) and propagate a spike down the axon (*A*). *2:* IPSP occurring at the soma (*S*) prevents the EPSP at the dendrite from generating an action potential at the axon hillock. *3:* EPSP-generated voltage-dependent Ca^{2+} current at the dendrite results in burst firing at the axon hillock. *4:* EPSP-generated fast prepotential (FPP) at the dendrite increases the probability of action potential generation at the axon hillock.

to powerfully prevent distant excitatory membrane events from generating spikes at the axon hillock.

In most instances, dendritic membranes remote from the axon hillock do not contain voltage-dependent Na$^+$ channels and do not have the ability to produce regenerative Na$^+$ action potentials. In some situations, however, *fast prepotentials* (FPPs) and other excitatory dendritic events such as backpropagating action potentials, dendritic Ca^{2+} spikes, and Na$^+$ channel hot spots have been recorded as rapid membrane depolarizations on dendrites at a distance from the axon hillock (Stuart et al., 2008). Backpropagating action potentials on dendrites are highly regulated by neurotransmitter and second-messenger systems (Johnston et al.,

1999). These events increase the ability of distant dendritic currents to influence spike generation at the axon hillock (See Fig. 3–4).

Ca^{2+} currents can be voltage-dependent or chemically induced and occur predominantly across proximal dendritic membranes. Regenerative Ca^{2+} currents are high-amplitude, prolonged membrane depolarizations with a high propensity for evoking rapid trains of Na$^+$ action potentials at the axon hillock. Ca^{2+} currents and Ca^{2+}-dependent K$^+$ currents are, therefore, associated with burst firing of Na$^+$ action potentials, followed by prolonged *afterhyperpolarization* (AHP) and cessation of neuronal firing (See Figs. 3–2 and 3–4). Although these Ca^{2+}-mediated membrane events are encountered in normal neurons, they also contribute to the *paroxysmal depo-larization shift* (*PDS*) and AHP that character-ize the epileptic *electroencephalogram* (*EEG*) spike-and-wave discharge (Matsumoto and Ajmone-Marsan, 1964) (see Fig. 3–19).

Alterations in neuronal morphology occur-ring spontaneously or in response to injury could enhance excitability. In addition to actual increases in the number of excitatory synapses and decreases in the number of inhibitory synapses, excitatory synaptic activity might be potentiated by (1) reduced dendritic branching, which would place excitatory synapses closer to the axon hillock, (2) changes in spine shape, including loss of spines, that would require excitatory synapses to terminate directly on the dendritic shaft, and (3) extension of the membrane distribution of voltage-dependent Na^+ and Ca^{2+} channels, which would allow long-lasting regenerative depolarization shifts to occur over wider areas of the cell.

Lesions of neuronal cell bodies or fiber tracts lead to degeneration of axon terminals, and new terminals may sprout from surviv-ing intact axons to make contact with vacated postsynaptic membrane (Cotman and Lynch, 1976; Raisman, 1969; Tsukahara, 1981). Such *axon sprouting* might also increase the excita-tory potential of a specific afferent influence on individual neurons as well as increase the sus-ceptibility of a neuronal aggregate to synchro-nous discharge (Messenheimer et al., 1979; Sutula et al., 1988; Tauck and Nadler, 1985) (Chapter 4).

Interneuronal Connections

Under normal circumstances, neurons are influ-enced by both synaptic and nonsynaptic neu-ronal interactions.

CHEMICAL SYNAPSES

The classical neuronal synapse consists of an *axon terminal*, or *presynaptic element*, that is separated by a *synaptic cleft* from the *postsyn-aptic membrane* on the postsynaptic neuron (Fig. 3–5). The postsynaptic membrane may be situated on a dendritic spine or may be part of the dendritic or somatic membrane. Membrane on either side of the synaptic cleft is specialized and can appear similar on both sides (*symmet-rical*) or not (*asymmetrical*) under the electron

microscope. Terminals that make symmetrical synapses, particularly when they contain flat-tened vesicles and end on somatic membrane (axosomatic), are usually inhibitory, whereas asymmetrical synapses with round presynaptic vesicles are likely to be excitatory (Gray, 1959; Jones and Cowan, 1983). This relationship is far from absolute, and more reliable informa-tion about synaptic function can be obtained by characterizing the postsynaptic receptor pharmacologically, histochemically, and molec-ularly. Ultimately, however, function must be determined electrophysiologically.

Classical chemical transmission between neurons involves a number of steps that can be selectively altered to influence neuronal excitability (see Fig. 3–5). The neurotransmit-ter itself must be synthesized, and this usu-ally requires axonal transport of substrates or the synthesized product to the axon ter-minal, the neurotransmitter is packaged into *vesicles* contained within the presynaptic ter-minal. Arrival of an action potential at the terminal opens voltage-dependent channels and allows Ca^{2+} influx. The exact mechanisms of Ca^{2+}-dependent neurotransmitter release are complex and not completely known, but the process involves additional molecules and protein phosphorylation (Erulkar, 1983; Heinemann et al., 2008). Ca^{2+} binds to intracel-lular proteins, including *calmodulin, calretinin,* and *parvalbumin*, that activate a *protein kinase*. Resultant changes in the protein structures cause neurotransmitter-containing vesicles to fuse with the presynaptic membrane and per-mit neurotransmitter to be released into the synaptic cleft (DeLorenzo, 1986). Complex proteins responsible for fusion of vesicles to the membrane and their recycling (*vesicle traf-ficking*) influence neurotransmitter release and are altered in models of epilepsy such as kindling (Matveeva et al., 2011). Genes have been identified that encode vesicle-trafficking proteins important in modulating neurotrans-mitter release. An example of the latter is *Sv2a*, which is upregulated in a model of epilepsy and is the target of the antiseizure drugs *levetirac-etam* and *brivaracetam* (Winden et al., 2011) (Chapter 15). *Calmodulin-dependent pro-tein kinase II* (*CaM-KII*) mediates long-term plastic changes of excitatory synapses (Wilcox et al., 2008).

The released neurotransmitter binds to a *receptor* on the postsynaptic membrane,

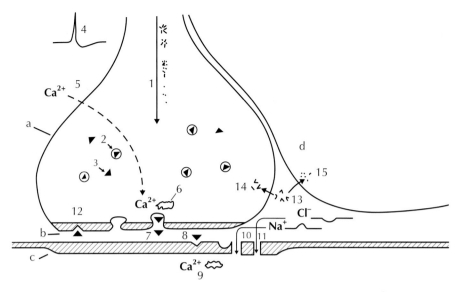

Figure 3–5. Schematic representation of the classical chemical synapse. *a,* presynaptic terminal at end of axon; *b,* synaptic cleft; *c,* postsynaptic membrane of the spine, dendritic shaft, or soma of a postsynaptic neuron; *d,* glia. Axon transport and transmitter synthesis (*1*) result in accumulation of transmitter in presynaptic terminal. Transmitter may be packaged in vesicles (*2*) or free (*3*). Arrival of action potential (*4*) at terminal results in opening of Ca^{2+} channels and Ca^{2+} influx (*5*). Ca^{2+} combines with calmodulin (*6*) to cause transmitter release into synaptic cleft (*7*). Transmitter binds with postsynaptic receptor (*8*) and may activate intracellular Ca^{2+} or other second messengers (*9*) or directly open Na^{2+} (*10*), Cl^- (*11*), or K^+ (not shown) channels to produce an EPSP or IPSP. Transmitter also binds to presynaptic autoreceptor (*12*) to regulate transmitter release. Transmitter is finally deactivated by breakdown in the synaptic cleft (*13*), uptake by the presynaptic terminal (*14*), and/or uptake by glia (*15*).

initiating a series of events within the postsynaptic neuron. Most synapses are *ionotropic*: the neurotransmitter-receptor complex directly regulates the opening or closing of ion channels on the postsynaptic membrane. Thus opening of Na^+ channels results in an EPSP, and opening of Cl^- or K^+ channels results in an IPSP. For *metabotropic* receptors, Ca^{2+} alone or with other molecules called *second messengers*, including *cyclic adenosine 3,5-monophosphate (cAMP)*, *inositol triphosphate (IP$_3$)*, and perhaps *cyclic guanosine 3,5-monophosphate (cGMP)* and *diacylglycerol (DAG)*, activates intracellular processes. These processes use protein kinases to open postsynaptic channels or initiate other intracellular functions. Therefore, both presynaptic and postsynaptic membrane events can be mediated by intracellular phosphorylation of specific proteins by protein kinases activated by Ca^{2+} and, in some cases, second messengers.

The neurotransmitter is finally deactivated by an enzyme that breaks it into inactive molecules, by reuptake into the axon terminal, or by uptake into glia. In all cases, transmitters or their metabolites are recycled to be released

again. *Autoreceptors* and *heteroreceptors* for neurotransmitters also exist on the presynaptic membrane, allowing neurotransmitters to provide feedback control over subsequent neurotransmitter release from the same or other terminals.

A few neurotransmitters are believed to act within classical synapses. The amino acids *glutamate* and *aspartate* can produce membrane depolarizations with a rapid time course and are the most important excitatory neurotransmitters in the central nervous system (Roberts et al., 1981; Wilcox et al., 2008). Excitatory amino acids are of particular interest because they can exert more profound excitatory influences under certain conditions by inducing Ca^{2+} currents (Cotman and Iversen, 1987; Heinemann et al., 2008; Wilcox et al., 2008).

Acetylcholine is the principal excitatory neurotransmitter in the peripheral nervous system and is the only neurotransmitter known to be enzymatically deactivated in the synaptic cleft. The deactivating enzyme is *acetylcholinesterase*. In contrast to the classical excitatory effect of ACh at the neuromuscular junction, its application in the hippocampus decreases excitability of principal cells by exciting inhibitory interneurons. This is followed by suppression of K⁺ conductance and prolonged depolarization of principal neurons (Benardo and Prince, 1982). The K⁺ channel responsible for the *M-type current* is encoded by *KCNQ* genes and is responsible for AHP following the action potential. Downregulation of these channels in transgenic mice results in epilepsy (Peters et al., 2005).

The primary inhibitory neurotransmitters in the central nervous system are the amino acids GABA and *glycine*. Glycine produces IPSPs by opening Cl⁻ channels, whereas GABA can open either Cl⁻ or K⁺ channels. Glycine synapses are mostly limited to the spinal cord and brain stem and produce fast IPSPs. GABA, on the other hand, produces slower hyperpolarizing membrane events. GABA is the predominant inhibitory neurotransmitter in the brain, but GABA synapses also occur in the spinal cord (Krnjevic, 1983; Macdonald and Mody, 2008). *Taurine* is another amino acid reported to have inhibitory properties (Van Gelder, 1978; Wu and Prentice, 2010).

The *biogenic amines* (*dopamine, norepinephrine,* and *serotonin*), as well as a large number of *peptides, proteins,* and *steroid hormones,* can act as neurotransmitters via classical synapses or exert neuromodulatory effects when released into the extracellular space. Neuromodulators can modify the action of neurotransmitters and other neuromodulators by directly altering the excitability of the postsynaptic membranes, blocking the receptor, or influencing neurotransmitter release. The effects of these agents are more prolonged than those of the classical neurotransmitters. The biogenic amines (Ferrendelli, 1986; Gale et al., 2008) and *adenosine* (Phillis and Wu, 1981; Gale et al., 2008) generally inhibit epileptiform activity, which explains why dopamine antagonists, such as *phenothiazines,* and adenosine antagonists, such as *aminophylline,* potentiate epileptic seizures. The *endogenous opioids* have an inhibitory action in most cerebral areas, including the neocortex (Nicoll et al., 1977), but excite the hippocampus, perhaps by attenuating inhibitory influences (Dingledine, 1981; Nicoll et al., 1980). Endogenous opioids have both proconvulsant and anticonvulsant properties (Caldecott-Hazard and Engel, 1987; Engel et al., 2008a). Paradoxically, the direct excitatory effect of opioids on the hippocampus can result in suppression of seizures, whereas proconvulsant effects of opioids involve interference with GABA-mediated inhibition (Caldecott-Hazard and Engel, 1987). A variety of other endogenous peptides have been found experimentally to excite neurons in an epileptiform manner as well as suppress epileptogenicity, but the exact mechanisms of these actions and their potential relevance to spontaneous epilepsy has not been established (Engel et al., 1984; Renaud, 1983; Scharfman and Schwarcz, 2008) (Table 3–2). *Adrenocorticotropic hormone (ACTH)* has effects on epileptic seizures that are specific for the developing brain, explaining its effectiveness against some childhood, but not adult, seizures (Holmes and Weber, 1986; Hrachovy and Frost, 2008). The inhibitory peptides *neuropeptide Y (NPY), somatostatin,* and *galanin,* as well as the excitatory peptide *cholecystokinin,* appear to play modulatory roles in the mediation of epileptic seizures (Chapter 4).

Presynaptic inhibition can result from certain types of *axoaxonic synapses* that depolarize the axon terminal. Because the amplitude of the axon potential is then reduced, less neurotransmitter is released (Fig. 3–6). Presynaptic terminal hyperpolarization can also have an inhibitory effect. *Dendrodendritic synapses, synaptic nests* or *glomeruli,* and *reciprocal synapses* in the central nervous system provide a wide variety of opportunities for neuronal interactions (Pappas and Purpura, 1972).

Neuronal excitability can be influenced by manipulation of any step in synaptic transmission, from neurotransmitter synthesis to postsynaptic potential generation. Certain convulsant drugs, such as *thiosemicarbazide, 3-mercaptopropionic acid,* and *allylglycine,* block the action of *glutamic acid decarboxylase (GAD),* an enzyme necessary for GABA synthesis. GAD exists in the brain in two isoforms, GAD65 and GAD67, encoded by the genes *GAD1* and *GAD2*. *Pyridoxine* deficiency results in convulsions because it is a cofactor in the synthesis of GABA. On the other hand, some GABA-mimetic drugs appear to exert an antiseizure action by interfering with *GABA transaminase (GABA-T),* an enzyme necessary for the metabolic breakdown of GABA (*valproic acid* has this effect); by irreversibly inactivating GABA-T (*vigabatrin*); and by antagonizing *GABA transporter-1 (GAT-1),* which is important for glial reuptake of GABA (*tiagabine* and *zonisamide*) (Chapter 15).

Table 3–2 **Neuropeptides**

POMC-derived neuropeptides
  Adrenocorticotropin (ACTH) (–)
  Melanocyte-stimulating hormone (MSH) (–)
  β-Lipotropin (β-LPH)
  Met-enkephalin (+)
  Leu-enkephalin (+)
  β-Endorphin (–)
  Dynorphin (–)
  Nociceptin (Orphanin FQ) (–)
Tachykinins
  Substance P (+)
  Neurokinin-A
  Neurokinin-B (+)
  Bradykinin (+/–)
Hypothalamic peptides
  Hormones
    Thyroid-stimulating hormone (TSH)
    Oxytocin (OT) (–)
    Luteinizing hormone (LH)
    Follicle-stimulating hormone (FSH)
    Vasopressin (AVP) or antidiuretic hormone (ADH) (+)
    Growth hormone
Releasing and inhibiting factors
  Corticotropin-releasing hormone (CRH or CRF) (+)
  Thyrotropin-releasing hormone (TRH) (–)
  Growth hormone–releasing hormone (GnRH)
  Luteinizing hormone–releasing hormone (LHRH or
    GHRH)
  Somatostatin growth hormone release–inhibiting
    hormone (–)
Gut peptides
  Motilin
  Cholecystokinin (CCK) (–)
  Vasoactive intestinal polypeptide (VIP)-glucagon family
    Secretin
    VIP (+)?
    Pituitary adenylate cyclase–activating peptide
      (PACAP) (+)
    Glucagon-like peptide 1 (GLP-1) (–)
  Neuropeptide tyrosine
    Neuropeptide tyrosine (NPY) (–)
    Pancreatic polypeptide (PP)
    Peptide tyrosine-tyrosine (PYY)
  Bombesin peptides
    Bombesin (gastrin-releasing peptide; GRP) (–)
    Gastrin
    Neuromedin B
    Galanin (–)
    Neurotensin
    Calcitonin gene–related peptide (CGRP)
Vascular peptides
  Natriuretic hormone family
    Atrionatriuretic hormone (ANH) or atriopeptin (+)
    Brain natriuretic hormone (BNP) (+)
    C-type natriuretic hormone (CNP) (+)
  Angiotensins I–IV (–)
Placental peptides
  Prolactin
  Chorionic gonadotropin
  Placental lactogen (choriomammotropin)

The major categories of neuropeptides are listed, with emphasis
on those that have been associated with seizures or epilepsy.
Peptides that have been shown to exert proconvulsant (+) or
anticonvulsant (–) activity are indicated; mixed effects are denoted
by +/–; a question mark indicates effects that are not clearly
proconvulsant or anticonvulsant.
Adapted from Scharfman and Schwarcz, 2008, with permission.

Repetitive stimulation of a presynaptic neuron can increase postsynaptic responsiveness. Enhancement after a single presynaptic pulse is referred to as *paired pulse facilitation* (*PPF*) and after a train of pulses as *posttetanic potentiation* (*PTP*). Under these conditions, the first pulse or train of pulses opens Ca^{2+} channels and increases Ca^{2+} concentration within the presynaptic terminal, enhancing the ability of a subsequent pulse to activate neurotransmitter release (Heinemann and Lambert, 1986). Repetitive stimulation can also lead to decreasing synaptic efficacy as a result of neurotransmitter depletion (*fatigue*).

Because Ca^{2+} influx plays a key role in mediating neurotransmitter release, coupling postsynaptic receptors to intracellular mechanisms, and also inducing burst firing at the axon hillock, drugs that block Ca^{2+} currents have been viewed as potential antiseizure agents (Meyer et al., 1986; Vanden Bussche et al., 1986; Witte et al., 1987), but these agents also have unacceptable side effects. Alterations in the concentration and function of calmodulin (DeLorenzo, 1986), other calcium-binding proteins (Miller et al., 1986), and specific protein kinases (Wasterlain et al., 1986) in the presynaptic terminal and the postsynaptic cell would also have profound effects on neuronal excitability, but such changes cannot yet be directly or specifically manipulated.

Neurotransmitters and neuromodulators all exert their effects by acting on receptors. Numerous receptors, with specific and nonspecific properties, have been identified through the use of agonist and antagonist drugs, some of which are convulsant or anticonvulsant agents. The classical example of multiple receptors for the same neurotransmitter is the division of acetylcholine receptors into *muscarinic* and *nicotinic* subtypes. $GABA_A$ receptors, which activate Cl^- currents, appear to be more important in mediating antiseizure events than $GABA_B$ receptors, which activate K^+ and other currents, and additional types of GABA receptors may also play a role in epilepsy (Enna, 1983; Macdonald and Mody, 2008; Zorn et al., 1986). Functional differences among the various recognized opiate receptor subtypes (Akil et al., 1984; Snead, 1986) may be important in understanding the mechanisms of some postictal behaviors (Caldecott-Hazard and Engel, 1987) (Chapter 9).

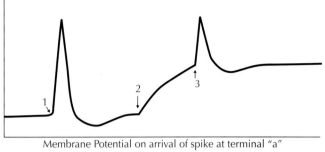

Membrane Potential on arrival of spike at terminal "a"

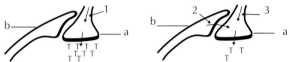

Figure 3–6. Presynaptic inhibition. *a*, presynaptic terminal on dendrite or soma; *b*, presynaptic terminal on *a* (axoaxonic synapse). Arrival of action potential at *a* (*1*) results in release of transmitter. The amount of transmitter released is determined by the height of the rising phase of the action potential. Activation of presynaptic inhibition by *b* results in depolarization of *a* (*2*). The rising phase of a subsequent action potential is reduced (*3*), and less transmitter is released.

Excitatory amino acid receptors are of particular interest. *Kainic acid (KA)*, α-*amino-3-hydroxy-5-methyl-4-isoxazole propionic acid (AMPA)*, and *N-methyl-D-aspartic acid (NMDA)* are the excitatory amino acid analogs used to define classes of receptors responsive to glutamate and aspartate (Meldrum and Chapman, 1986; Wilcox et al., 2008). *Ionotropic glutamate receptors (iGluRs)* open and close ion channels consisting of four subunits (Wilcox et al., 2008) (Fig. 3–7). There are three subfamilies of *NMDA receptors*, consisting of a large number of identified subunits with a variety of functions all related to Ca^{2+} permeability. There are four AMPA subunits, *GluA1–4*. Of particular interest is that AMPA receptors lacking a *GluA2* subunit are permeable to CA^{2+}. *KA receptors* have five subunits, *GluK5–7* and *KA1* and *KA2*. *KA autoreceptors* can increase or decrease glutamate release, and *GluK6* is responsible for death of pyramidal cells in area CA3 of the hippocampus following *kainate* administration, which is a commonly used model of chronic hippocampal epilepsy.

Metabotropic glutamate receptors (mGluRs) are coupled via second-messenger systems to biochemical pathways and ion channels made up of polypeptides rather than subunits (Wilcox et al., 2008). Channels are opened by activation of *G-proteins*. There are three groups and eight subtypes. Group I mGluRs consists of two types (1 and 5), Group II consists of three types (2, 3, and 8), and Group III consists of three types (4–7). Groups II and III are responsible for suppression of *forskolin-stimulated cAMP*

accumulation and decreased transmission at glutamate and GABA synapses. Postsynaptic metabotropic glutamate receptors are excitatory and presynaptic metabotropic receptors are inhibitory via axoaxonic synapses.

NMDA receptors are associated with cation channels that allow Ca^{2+} and Na^+ entry into the cell and mediate glutamate-induced Ca^{2+} currents (Heinemann et al., 2008; MacDermott and Dale, 1987). The NMDA receptor–cation channel complex has many regulatory sites, which allow modulation of Ca^{2+} current by a variety of mechanisms. Binding of both glutamate and glycine is necessary for an NMDA channel to remain open. *Competitive antagonists* bind to and block the glutamate site, *glycine antagonists* bind to and block the glycine site, *noncompetitive antagonists* bind to allosteric sites, and *uncompetitive antagonists* bind to an internal site. Most anesthetic and intoxicant NMDA antagonists are uncompetitive. Although NMDA antagonists are potential anticonvulsant drugs (Chapman, 1984; Meldrum and Chapman, 1986; Meldrum, 2008), interference with the diverse and essential functions of this receptor results in unacceptable side effects (Chapter 15).

Many features of the NMDA receptor place it in position to play a unique role in central nervous system function (Cotman and Iversen, 1987; MacDermott and Dale, 1987; Wilcox et al., 2008). The NMDA channel is blocked by Mg^{2+} ions, and therefore inactive, at the resting membrane potential. Because the displacement of Mg^{2+} is voltage-dependent, the effectiveness

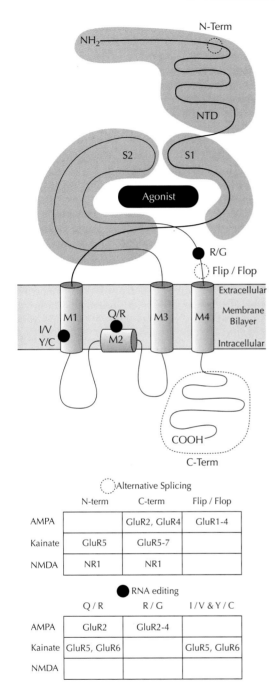

	Alternative Splicing		
	N-term	C-term	Flip / Flop
AMPA		GluR2, GluR4	GluR1-4
Kainate	GluR5	GluR5-7	
NMDA	NR1	NR1	

	RNA editing		
	Q / R	R / G	I / V & Y / C
AMPA	GluR2	GluR2-4	
Kainate	GluR5, GluR6		GluR5, GluR6
NMDA			

Figure 3–7. Schematic diagram of iGluR structure within the membrane. All these receptors have an extracellular N-terminus (*N-Term*), an intracellular C-terminus (*C-Term*), three transmembrane domains (M1, M3, M4), a membrane reentrant loop (M2) that forms a pore, and ligand-binding domains (S1 and S2). Subunits involved in the different components of the AMPA, kainate, and NMDA receptors are shown in the tables. (From Wilcox et al., 2008, with permission.)

of glutamate action on the NMDA receptor is directly related to the degree of depolarization of the postsynaptic membrane. In some instances, dual NMDA and KA or AMPA receptors allow glutamate to induce brief depolarizing Na^+ currents and thereby facilitate NMDA channel opening. Of more interest, however, is the possible situation where activation of the NMDA-cation channel complex can happen only when it is preceded by an independent (*conditioning*) depolarizing synaptic event on an adjacent area of postsynaptic membrane. The requirement for temporally related activation of two synaptic events would predispose to facilitated propagation along selected pathways and would make this receptor mechanism an ideal substrate for acquired behavioral change. Because the end result is Ca^{2+} influx, inputs with the proper temporal and spatial relationship not only would cause selective excitation of the postsynaptic membrane but also could initiate intracellular processes necessary for structural alterations (Collingridge and Bliss, 1987). For instance, Ca^{2+} activation of gene expression could cause protein synthesis (Morgan et al., 1987), resulting in redistribution of receptors and ion channels or the appearance of new synapses. Ca^{2+}-mediated cell death (Meldrum, 1986a; 1983; Rothman and Olney, 1987) could also contribute to behaviorally significant neuronal reorganization in an age-specific manner. Such mechanisms of *plastic change* underlie neuronal growth and differentiation during development, learning in the mature nervous system, and acquisition of certain neurological disorders, such as epilepsy (Bernard, 2008) (Chapters 4 and 8).

Multiple mechanisms contribute to synaptic plasticity that underlies behavioral change (Bernard, 2008). *Long-term potentiation* (*LTP*) and *long-term depression* (*LTD*) are experimental models of plastic change in the brain (Bliss and Lomo, 1973). In the classic example of LTP, tetanic stimulation is applied to the *perforant path*, a major excitatory afferent input to the hippocampus. Subsequent stimulation results in increased neurotransmitter release by the presynaptic terminal and enhanced responsiveness of the postsynaptic neuron (Bliss and Lomo, 1973; Collingridge and Bliss, 1987), although the primary change is believed by some to be presynaptic (Bernard, 2008). This effect can persist for weeks. The excitatory neurotransmitter at this synapse is glutamate. The postsynaptic changes with LTP can be accounted for, in part, by NMDA receptor mechanisms (Collingridge and Bliss, 1987), but AMPA receptors, other molecules, and perhaps structural changes also play a role (Bernard, 2008). The persistent changes in neuronal excitability in this model eventually disappear, however, and LTP alone cannot explain permanent acquired alterations in behavior. LTD is caused by low-frequency stimulation and also appears to reflect presynaptic changes in glutamate release (Bernard, 2008).

Glutamate and aspartate are also *excitotoxic neurotransmitters*, because their excessive release contributes to death of the postsynaptic neuron. Because this effect is Ca^{2+} dependent and can be blocked by NMDA antagonists (Rothman and Olney, 1987), it is believed to be mediated by the NMDA receptor–cation channel complex. Anoxic-ischemic, hypoglycemic, and epileptic brain damage all appear to depend on this mechanism and are age-specific. Therefore, drugs that interfere with activation of the NMDA receptor might eventually be *neuroprotective agents* used to protect against long-term neurological sequelae of cerebral insults such as stroke and status epilepticus (Chapter 10).

Considerable attention has been focused on the Cl^- channel, also referred to as the *Cl^- ionophore* (Fig. 3–8), because it is the site of action not only for the important inhibitory neurotransmitter GABA but also for a variety of convulsant, sedative, and depressant drugs (Olsen, 1981; Olsen et al., 1986; Macdonald and Mody, 2008). There are two main classes of GABA receptors, $GABA_A$ and $GABA_B$ (Macdonald and Mody, 2008). The $GABA_A$ receptor belongs to the *cys-loop* family of ionotropic ligand-gated ion channels related to the *nicotinic acetylcholine receptor*, the *glycine receptor*, and the *serotonin 5-HT_3 receptor* (Fig. 3–9). The Cl^- channel consists of eight subunit families: α, β, γ, δ, π, ε, θ, and ρ, of which α is the most important. Each has one to six subtypes, and altering the subunits to produce different receptor isoforms influences desensitization and the patterns of open and closed states. The $GABA_B$ receptor is metatropic, coupled to a K^+ or occasionally Ca^{2+} channel via a *guanosine triphosphate (GTP)*-binding protein. There are two subunits, $GABA_{B1}$ and $GABA_{B2}$. Postsynaptic $GABA_B$ receptors produce slow inhibition via K^+ currents, whereas presynaptic synapses reduce neurotransmitter release by decreasing Ca^{2+} influx. *Baclofen* is a specific agonist of $GABA_B$ receptors and *phaclofen* is a specific antagonist. GABA receptor mutations have been associated with *febrile seizures, childhood absence epilepsy, GEFS+, juvenile myoclonic epilepsy*, and *Dravet syndrome* (Chapters 5 and 7).

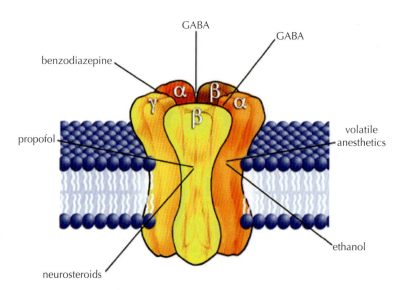

Figure 3–8. Stylized illustration of a GABA–Cl^- ion channel indicating sites where different pharmacological agents act. (From Lovinger, 2012, with permission.)

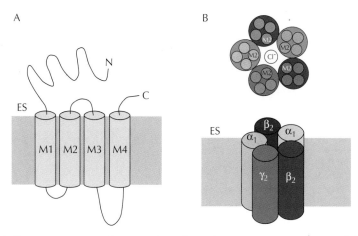

Figure 3–9. The GABA$_A$ receptor. **a.** Membrane topology of a single GABA$_A$ receptor subunit with four transmembrane segments (termed M1–4) and the extracellular NH$_2$ (N) and COOH (C) termini. M2 contributes to the ion-conducting pore. **b.** *Bottom:* Pentameric GABA$_A$ receptors composed of two α_1, two β_2, and one γ_2 subunits are the most abundant in the brain. *Top:* Cross section of the channel displays the Cl$^-$ pore formed by M2 helical elements. *ES*, extracellular space. (From Walker et al., 2009, with permission.)

The effect of GABA on the Cl$^-$ ionophore is antagonized in various ways by convulsant agents such as *picrotoxin*, *bicuculline*, and *penicillin*. *Strychnine*, however, exerts its convulsant action by blocking the inhibitory transmitter glycine. *Barbiturates* and *benzodiazepines* have anticonvulsant effects in part because they reinforce GABA action on the Cl$^-$ ionophore (Chapter 15). However, *progabide*, a GABA agonist that acts directly on the GABA receptor (Bartholini et al., 1985) was not successful as a clinical anticonvulsant (Chapter 15). Interestingly, some GABA agonists, such as the *convulsant* β-*carbolines* and *inverse agonists*, can cause epileptic seizures (Gloor and Fariello, 1988), and inhibition itself can cause some types of epileptic seizures (Engel et al., 2008a) (Chapter 4). Nevertheless, GABA agonists and glutamate antagonists remain the agents most actively investigated for potential clinical anticonvulsant action (Meldrum, 1986b; 1984; 2008) (Chapter 15).

Neuronal excitability is altered by disturbances in voltage- and Ca^{2+}-dependent K$^+$ currents, which are endogenous inhibitory mechanisms (Benardo and Pedley, 1985; Kullman and Schorge, 2008). ACh produces its prolonged excitatory effect on the hippocampus by decreasing K$^+$ conductance, which increases the opportunity for repetitive action potentials. In some neurons, neuromodulators such as norepinephrine, *histamine*, and *corticotropin-releasing factor* (*CRF*) can modify intracellular Ca^{2+} concentration and antagonize Ca^{2+}-dependent K$^+$ conductance, leading to increased excitation. Dopamine, on the other hand, appears to exert its prolonged inhibitory effect on the hippocampus in part by increasing K$^+$ conductance. Hyperpolarization mediated by GABA$_B$ receptors involves K$^+$ currents that are longer lasting than the fast Cl$^-$ hyperpolarizations mediated by GABA$_A$ receptors and helps synchronize neurons to produce rhythmic oscillations, including some hypersynchronized epileptiform abnormalities (Blumenfeld and Coulter, 2008; Engel et al., 2008a) (Chapter 4).

Receptor concentrations increase (*upregulation*) or decrease (*downregulation*) within hours or days because of processes influencing turnover, but much more rapid alterations can occur in some systems when active receptor sites are rendered more or less accessible by changes in protein configuration (Lynch and Baudry, 1984). Receptor availability fluctuates in response to various stimuli, most importantly neurotransmitter release. Consequently, decreased neurotransmitter release can result in an increase in receptors, whereas increased neurotransmitter release usually leads to a decrease in receptors. *Denervation supersensitivity* is a classical example of upregulation of receptors in the peripheral nervous system and can be seen in the *partially isolated cortical slab*, the postsynaptic neurons of which demonstrate increased responsiveness to ACh

(Echlin, 1959); however, there is not much additional evidence for this phenomenon in the central nervous system. Increased dopamine receptor sensitivity is responsible for some side effects of dopamine antagonists, whereas decreased benzodiazepine receptor sensitivity accounts for the development of tolerance to these agents.

Excitability can be increased by prolonging neurotransmitter contact with the receptor. For example, acetylcholinesterase inhibitors can be used to delay the breakdown of ACh within the synaptic cleft. For other neurotransmitters, however, the deactivation mechanism is reuptake, which is also important for replenishing stores. Consequently, drugs that act to block reuptake can result in neurotransmitter depletion, causing an acute increase and later a decrease in neurotransmitter action. This is demonstrated by the classical effect of *reserpine* on dopaminergic synapses. Because of the important role of glial uptake in deactivating some neurotransmitters, glial dysfunction can influence neurotransmitter efficacy.

Alterations in electrical transmission properties of the postsynaptic membrane affect synaptic control of neuronal excitability. This effect can occur as a result of changes in the ionic microenvironment as well as structural changes in the postsynaptic neuron. One intriguing observation has been swelling of the necks of dendritic spines after repetitive stimulation, which could facilitate spread of EPSPs from the postsynaptic membrane to the soma (Fifkova and Anderson, 1981; Van Harrveld and Fifkova, 1975).

ELECTROTONIC SYNAPSES

Electrotonic synapses, or *gap junctions*, serve an important role in neuronal synchronization in invertebrates (Bennett, 1977). *Electrotonic coupling* is not as rare in the mammalian brain as previously thought (Connors and Long, 2004; Richardson et al., 2008). Gap junctions act as bidirectional, low-pass filters that permit both excitatory and inhibitory influences to be rapidly communicated over long distances. Gap junction channels are formed of two hemichannels, each with six subunits (*connexins*). There are many isoforms of connexins, but only a few are expressed in the mammalian brain, and only *connexin 36 (Cx36)* appears to be important for neuron-to-neuron electrotonic transmission (Richardson et al., 2008).

In the adult neocortex, electrotonic coupling appears to be limited to interneurons, although gap junctions between pyramidal cells have been described in the pre- and postnatal brain (Richardson et al, 2008), and axoaxonal pyramidal cell gap junctions have been proposed as a mechanism for synchronizing *high-frequency oscillations (HFOs)* (Traub et al, 2001) (Chapter 4). Connexin coupling tends to occur between interneurons of the same type; for instance fast-spiking interneurons are connected to other fast-spiking interneurons, and slow-spiking interneurons to other slow-spiking interneurons. Opening and closing of gap junctions are regulated by cyclic nucleotide–coupled receptors and are influenced by pH (Lado and Moshé, 2008). Increased acidity during seizures could disrupt synchronization by blocking electrotonic conduction. Epileptiform discharges have been suppressed in some animal models of epilepsy with gap junction blockers such as *carbenoxolone* and *octanol* (Lado and Moshé 2008). Gap junctions have a potential role in neuronal synchronization underlying normal cerebral activity, as well as abnormal activity such as epileptiform discharges and HFOs (Chapter 4).

NONSYNAPTIC COMMUNICATION

Many chemically mediated alterations in neuronal activity result from release of neuromodulators into the extracellular space. The neuromodulatory effects of catecholamines, peptides, and certain protein and steroid hormones have already been discussed.

Activation within a population of neurons can take the form of a slow wave of excitation, similar to the *spreading depression* experimentally caused by increasing extracellular K^+ (Leao, 1972). In spreading depression, the wave of depolarization creates a transient front of excitation followed by depolarization block. Enhanced neuronal activity itself can alter the chemical microenvironment and lead to spreading depolarization (Heinemann, 1987). Rapidly firing neurons extrude large amounts of K^+, which may not be adequately taken up by surrounding glia. This can raise extracellular K^+ sufficiently to enhance excitability in neighboring neurons, which then fire rapidly, extrude K^+, and influence firing in their neighbors. Ca^{2+} influx in rapidly firing neurons can also decrease extracellular Ca^{2+} and increase excitability.

Electrical field potentials generated by neuronal discharges can directly influence ionic conductances in neighboring neurons (*ephaptic transmission*). This has been demonstrated in vitro (Jeffreys and Haas, 1982; Taylor and Dudek, 1982), and similar ephaptic influences on closely packed neurons in laminated structures such as cortex and hippocampus are theoretically possible in vivo (Dudek et al., 1986; Schwartzkroin, 1983a;b). During rapid neuronal firing, glia take up excess K$^+$ and swell; consequently, shrinkage of the extracellular space would increase this opportunity for direct electrical communication between adjacent neurons (Heinemann, 1987).

Under certain conditions neurons can be excited *antidromically* (Gutnick and Prince, 1972). With intense neuronal activity, afferent terminals can be depolarized to the point of action potential generation, which is then propagated backward along the axon to their cell bodies in thalamus or contralateral cortex. So far this effect has been demonstrated only for experimental epileptiform discharges in neocortex. Antidromic propagation cannot initiate an action potential at the axon hillock, but antidromic potentials can subsequently be propagated *orthodromically* along collaterals of the involved axon to other efferent synapses of the same neuron. Consequently, this *backfiring* could conceivably serve as an additional synchronizing mechanism.

GLIAL INFLUENCES

Astroglia play an important role in modulating neuronal excitability and synchronization (Steinhauser et al., 2008). Because the density of K$^+$ channels is much greater than that of Na$^+$ channels, glia are unable to generate action potentials, but they contain chemical receptors, and extensive glial networks are linked through gap junctions. Inwardly rectifying K$^+$ channels and the water channel *aquaporin-4 (AQP4)* are important for maintaining extracellular K$^+$ and water homeostasis. A main function of astrocytes is to remove neurotransmitters from the extracellular space. They take up glutamate released at axon terminals using glial-specific transporters (*EAAT1, EAAT2*) and deactivate

effects at the postsynaptic membrane. GABA is also taken up by active transport mechanisms and is metabolized to glutamate and *glutamine*. Astroglia release neuroactive agents (*gliotransmitters*), glutamate, ATP, and D-*serine* into the extracellular space, where they can act on neuronal membrane, as well as glutamate and glutamine to be taken up by neurons for the synthesis of GABA. These processes, mediated by intracellular Ca^{2+} waves across the extensive gap junction–coupled syncytium of glial filaments, help to mediate the synchronization essential for normal neuronal activity as well as the generation and spread of epileptic activity. *Microglia* play a principal role in immune and inflammatory reactions in the central nervous system (Vezzani et al., 2008) (Chapter 4). Considerable research is ongoing to elucidate the mechanisms of normal glial structure and function as well as disturbances that contribute to epileptogenicity.

NEURONAL NETWORKS

The intrinsic organization of *local circuits* of cerebral structures ultimately determines excitability and synchronization. In particular, the internal connections of the hippocampus and neocortex, together with the intrinsic properties of the elements that make up these circuits, uniquely predispose these structures to generate epileptiform activity. The manifestation of epileptic events is further mediated by broader networks involving subcortical and interhemispheric influences.

Epileptogenic networks in the mammalian brain can be divided into two broad systems. The limbic system, so called because it was envisioned as a rim bordering the ventricles and also referred to as *Papez's circuit* (Papez, 1937), was initially viewed as serving olfactory function but was later extended by Maclean (Maclean, 1952) as important for mediating emotional behavior. The limbic system consists of *Ammon's horn* and its subcortical connections to the *septal area, hypothalamus, anterior thalamus*, and *amygdala*; *parahippocampal structures (entorhinal, perirhinal,* and *piriform cortices)*; the *cingulate* and *orbital frontal cortex*, and the insula (Fig. 3–10). The neocortex can be broadly divided into posterior structures, which are largely responsible for

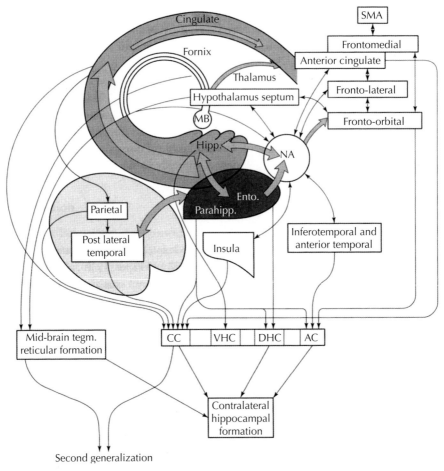

Figure 3–10. Diagrammatic representation of the human limbic system and its afferent and efferent connections. Note the major connections between the hippocampus, entorhinal cortex, and amygdala (*NA*), and the components of the Papez circuit, described in the text. *SMA*, supplementary motor area; *HIPP*, hippocampus; *ENTO*, entorhinal cortex; *MB*, mammillary body; *PARAHIPP*, parahippocampal gyrus; *CC*, corpus callosum; *VHC*, ventral hippocampal commissure; *DHC*, dorsal hippocampal commissure; *AC*, anterior commissure. (Adapted from Wieser, 1988, with permission).

receiving information, and anterior structures, largely responsible for executing functions.

Intrinsic Organization of Ammon's Horn

Sclerosis of Ammon's horn (*mesial temporal sclerosis, hippocampal sclerosis*) is the most common pathological substrate of epilepsy in patients (Mathern et al., 2008) and a specific cause of *mesial temporal lobe epilepsy (MTLE)* (Engel et al., 2008b) (Chapters 4, 5, and 7).

The organization of the neuronal interconnections within Ammon's horn, which consists of the *dentate gyrus (fascia dentata)* and the *hippocampus proper*, is shown schematically in Figure 3–11. The major input from entorhinal cortex is called the *perforant path* and ends primarily on *granule cells* of the dentate gyrus (Engel et al., 2002; McIntyre and Schwartzkroin, 2008). Granule cells then project via *mossy fibers* to pyramidal neurons and, to an even greater extent, interneurons in the *CA3 region*. The pyramidal neurons, in turn, have *Schaffer collaterals* that project to the *CA1 region* bilaterally. Glutamate or other excitatory amino acids are believed to serve as the neurotransmitter for these three synapses. Cholinergic excitatory inputs from the *nucleus of the diagonal band of Broca* and the septal

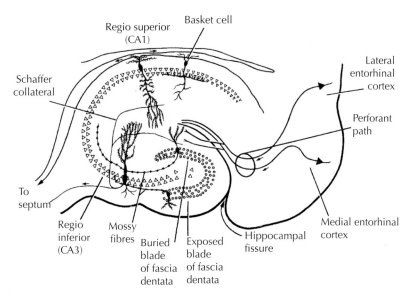

Figure 3–11. Schematic diagram of the intrahippocampal connections. Horizontal section through the right hippocampus. (From O'Keefe and Nadel, 1978, with permission.)

area enter the hippocampus via the *fornix* to end on pyramidal neurons as well as granule cells of the dentate gyrus. Mossy fibers of dentate granule cells also project to neurons in the *hilus*, located between the leaves of the dentate gyrus proximal to CA3. These axons end on inhibitory interneurons that also contain a variety of peptides, including somatostatin and NPY, as well as on principal *mossy cells*, which send their axons back to the inner molecular layer of the dentate gyrus, both ipsilaterally and contralaterally, where they make excitatory glutamatergic synapses with the proximal dendrites of granule cells, as well as with inhibitory interneurons. These feedback hilar influences, therefore, can provide powerful brakes on propagation of activity from the entorhinal cortex and dentate gyrus to hippocampus proper, a process referred to as the *dentate gate*.

Hippocampal pyramidal cells of CA1 send their axons to the *subiculum* and adjacent areas of the temporal cortex via the *alvear path* and into the *septum* and *mammillary bodies* via the fornix, and also to contralateral hippocampus via the *hippocampal commissure*. Interspersed between principal neurons are inhibitory interneurons, including *basket cells*, which receive excitatory input from afferent axons entering the hippocampus as well as from efferent axons exiting the hippocampus. Thus interneurons can inhibit principal neurons by

feedforward and *feedback (recurrent) inhibition* (Fig. 3–12A). The inhibitory effects of these interneurons are predominantly mediated by GABA and inhibitory peptides. Repeated activation of the interneuron can cause a decrement in the inhibitory response and, therefore, enhanced excitability of the principal neuron (Finch and Babb, 1977) (Fig. 3–12B).

The most common electrical manifestation of neuronal interactions in the central nervous system is the EPSP-IPSP complex, reflecting excitatory synaptic input, followed by inhibitory synaptic input, the latter due to feedforward or feedback inhibition. Feedback inhibition requires that the postsynaptic principal neuron generate an action potential, whereas feedforward inhibition is produced by the excitatory input's acting directly on inhibitory interneurons, even when the postsynaptic principal neuron fails to fire. Although the inhibitory interneurons are few compared with the principal neurons of the dentate gyrus and hippocampus, their axonal processes are widely distributed. Consequently, many neurons that are not involved in the initial excitatory event will be subsequently inhibited. Simultaneous inhibition of a large number of neurons plays a prominent role in synchronization, because all these neurons then become available at the same time to respond to a second excitatory input (Andersen and Sears, 1964; Spencer

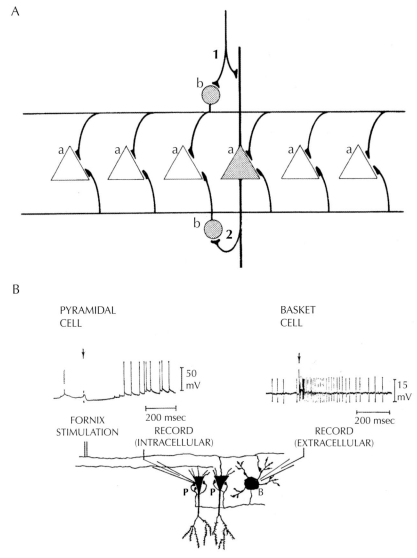

Figure 3–12. A. Feedforward and feedback inhibition. *a,* principal neurons; *b,* inhibitory interneurons. Excitatory afferent input (*1*) excites the principal neuron as well as the interneuron. The interneuron then inhibits the excited neuron and its neighbors (feedforward inhibition). Spike propagation down the axon of the principal neuron excites the inhibitory interneuron via axon collateral (*2*), which in turn inhibits the firing neuron and its neighbors (feedback inhibition). Feedforward and feedback inhibition may be mediated by the same interneuron. **B.** Schematic diagram of intrinsic circuit in the hippocampal pyramidal cell layer (*below*) and actual recordings obtained from such neuronal elements (*above*). Electrical stimulation of the fornix (*arrows*) produces excitation of the basket cell (*B*), which inhibits the pyramidal cell (*P*). (From Finch and Babb, 1977, with permission.)

and Kandel, 1961). If the second input occurs at the proper interval, just as the inhibited neurons all recover their resting potential and often undergo a transient rebound depolarization, they are all synchronously excited. Resultant postexcitation inhibition then increases the receptive neuronal pool even further (Fig. 3–13). Because of this inhibitory mechanism, excitatory input at the proper frequency is capable of recruiting greater and greater numbers of neurons into the synchronous discharge.

Excitability patterns differ from one region of the hippocampus to another (Schwartzkroin, 1984; 1986; McIntyre and Schwartzkroin, 2008). Spontaneous bursting occurs in CA3

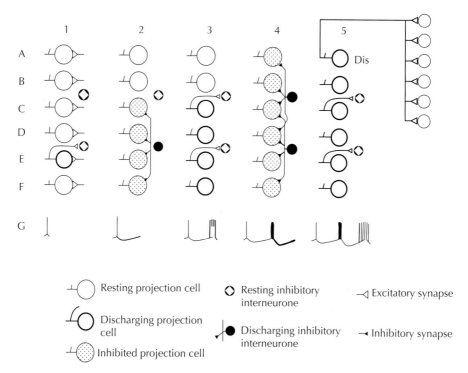

Figure 3–13. Diagrammatic representation of the neural events during the initiation of a thalamic spindle; note the key role of the inhibitory interneurons in "phasing" the discharges. Notice also how the distributor neuron (*Dis*) transmits spindle activity to other parts of the thalamus. (From Andersen and Sears, 1964, as modified by Kiloh et al., 1981, with permission.)

pyramidal cells and subiculum, as a result of dendritic *T-type* Ca^{2+} currents that sustain depolarization at the axon hillock. This results in repetitive action potentials until the burst is turned off by Ca^{2+}-dependent K^{+} currents and synaptic input from inhibitory interneurons. Under normal circumstances, bursting in CA3 pyramidal cells is asynchronous. One theory of the epileptogenic effect of convulsant agents such as penicillin on the hippocampus is that the CA3 bursting neurons become synchronized and act as pacemakers to drive CA1 pyramidal cells. CA1 neurons are not capable of generating bursts spontaneously but do generate bursts in response to afferent input from CA3 (Schwartzkroin, 1983a;b; 1986). Granule cells of the dentate gyrus do not generate burst discharges, even in the presence of penicillin.

Although penicillin is believed to act as a convulsant by blocking GABA-mediated inhibition, it is clear that synaptic inhibition is not blocked completely in this situation. Inhibition still plays a role in synchronization of epileptiform activity as well as other characteristic

aspects of the epileptic focus (Schwartzkroin, 1983b) (Chapter 4). Perhaps penicillin has a selective action on only some GABAergic synapses.

Hippocampal neurons in CA3 and CA1, dentate gyrus, and subiculum generate oscilatory patterns. The *theta rhythm* is a 4- to 6-Hz oscillation driven primarily by cholinergic input from the medial septal area (Petsche, 1962), although other synaptic interactions are involved and the true pacemakers are unknown (Buzsáki, 2006). It is most prominent during active motor behavior and rapid eye movement (REM) sleep. The hippocampal theta rhythm has been recorded in numerous animals, but its existence in humans remains controversial. Of more interest with respect to epilepsy are brief HFOs, because some are pathological and characteristic of epileptogenic tissue (Chapter 4). Normal HFOs in the frequency range of 100–200 Hz, however, are generated in CA3 and CA1 of hippocampus and are called *ripples*. Ripples are most prominent during slow-wave sleep and do not occur in dentate gyrus. Normal ripples reflect summated synchronous IPSPs that regulate discharges of principal cells and synchronize neuronal activity over long distances. This process mediates synaptic plasticity and is particularly important for episodic memory (Buzsáki, 2006). In contrast, *pathological HFOs (pHFOs)* have frequencies of up to 600 Hz; are generated in dentate gyrus as well as hippocampus proper, other limbic structures, and neocortex; and appear to reflect action potentials of synchronized bursting neurons (Engel et al., 2009; Staba and Bragin, 2011) (Chapter 4).

Intrinsic Organization of the Neocortex

The neuronal organization of the neocortex is in many ways similar to that of the hippocampus (Richardson et al., 2008). Input is predominantly from the thalamus and other cortical areas, with terminals from nonspecific thalamic nuclei ending on distal dendrites and from specific thalamic nuclei ending on more proximal dendrites and the soma of principal neurons. Thalamocortical inputs also terminate on other nonpyramidal neurons. GABAergic inhibitory interneurons provide feedforward and feedback inhibition on principal neocortical neurons and distribute their axons widely, as in the hippocampus (Houser et al., 1984). These inhibitory influences, therefore, serve to amplify responses to synchronizing afferent input and are at least partially responsible for the classical *recruiting* and *augmenting responses* (Dempsey and Morison, 1941a;b; Morison and Dempsey, 1942), discussed later in this chapter.

Spontaneously bursting principal neurons can be found in layers IV and V of the neocortex (Connors et al., 1983). These are the cell layers that appear to serve as a pacemaker for the development of synchronous burst discharges in a large population of neocortical neurons after application of a convulsant agent (Chatt and Ebersole, 1982). Consequently, similar mechanisms of neuronal interactions that lead to epileptiform excitability appear to be active in both neocortex and hippocampus. Neocortical networks are capable of generating HFOs in the ripple frequency range, and HFOs with a frequencies greater than 200 Hz

can be normal events in some cortical areas, such as the barrel sensory cortex of the rat and somatosensory cortex in humans (Staba and Bragin, 2011).

There are well-known structural variations from one area of human neocortex to another. The cortical regions delineated by the cytoarchitectural map of Brodmann (Brodmann, 1909) (Fig. 3–14) often correspond to functional specializations, the most important being *primary somatosensory* (areas 1, 2, and 3), *primary motor* (areas 4 and 6), *visual* (area 17), *auditory* (areas 41 and 42), *gustatory* (area 43), and *eye movement* (area 8). The *supplementary motor area* is rostral to areas 4 and 6 on the mesial surface of the brain. Epileptogenic properties can be influenced by these structural differences (Chapter 8), while manifestations of focal epileptic seizures are determined by the functional specialization of involved neocortex (Chapter 6). Cortical areas important in mediating limbic seizures include the entorhinal (areas 28 and 34), perirhinal (area 35), piriform (area 27), orbital frontal (areas 11 and 12), cingulate (areas 29–33) and insular (areas 13 and 14) cortices. Clinical diagnosis (and surgical treatment when indicated) requires familiarity with these cortical structure-function relationships as well as more specific anatomical representations of cortical motor and sensory function (Fig. 3–15) and localization of cortical language function in the dominant hemisphere (Fig. 3–16).

Subcortical and Interhemispheric Connections

A subcortical structure of particular interest for understanding basic mechanisms of epileptic excitability is the amygdala. As will be seen in the next chapter, stimulation of the amygdala is commonly used to induce experimentally *kindled* epileptic seizures (Chapter 4). This area also appears to be typically involved in human limbic seizures that originate from mesial temporal structures, as evidenced by prominent *oroalimentary* symptoms (Chapter 6). Mesial temporal sclerosis can involve cell loss and gliosis of the amygdala (Babb and Brown, 1987; Margerison and Corsellis, 1966; Mathern et al., 2008).

Some electrophysiological evidence from depth electrode recordings in patients suggests

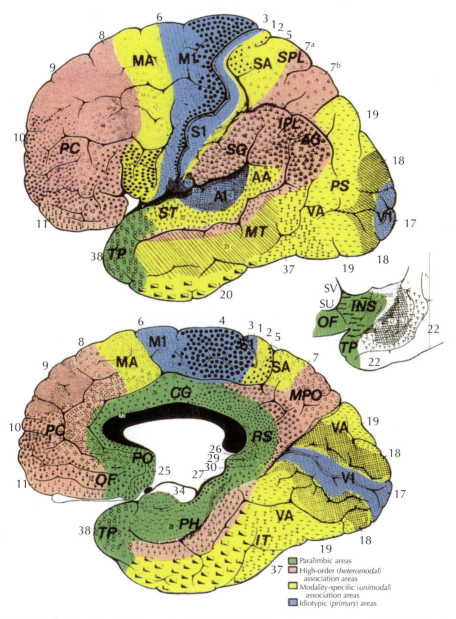

Figure 3–14. Distribution of functional zones in relationship to Brodmann's map of the human brain. The boundaries are not intended to be precise. Much of this information is based on experimental evidence obtained from laboratory animals and needs to be confirmed in the human brain. *A1,* primary auditory cortex; *AA,* auditory association cortex; *AG,* angular gyrus; *CG,* cingulate cortex; *INS,* insula; *IPL,* inferior parietal lobule; *IT,* inferior temporal gyrus; *M1,* primary motor area; *MA,* motor association cortex; *MPO,* medial parietooccipital area; *MT,* middle temporal gyrus; *OF,* orbitofrontal region; *PC,* prefrontal cortex; *PH,* parahippocampal region; *PO,* parolfactory area; *PS,* peristriate cortex; *RS,* retrosplenial area; *S1,* primary somatosensory area; *SA,* somatosensory association cortex; *SG,* supramarginal gyrus; *SPL,* superior parietal lobule; *ST,* superior temporal gyrus; *TP,* temporopolar cortex; *V1,* primary visual cortex; *VA,* visual association cortex. (From Mesulam, 1985, with permission.)

that limbic seizures might occasionally originate in the amygdala (Wieser, 1983); however, it has not been definitively proven that these electrographic ictal onsets represent primary discharges, as opposed to activity propagated from hippocampal or other (probably frontal) cortical areas not seen by recording electrodes. Selective amygdalotomy, which was once

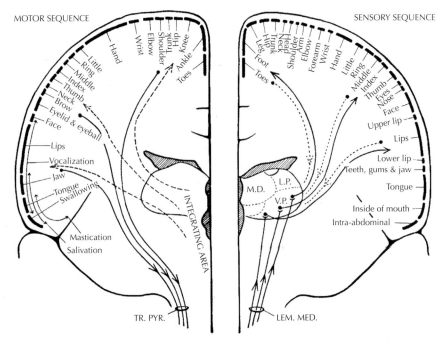

Figure 3–15. *Left:* Motor sequence in the rolandic cortex shown on a cross section of the hemisphere. The length of each black line in the cortex indicates the comparative extent of the representation of movement of each part. *Right:* Sensory sequence in the rolandic cortex shown on a cross section of the cerebral hemisphere. The lengths of each black line in the cortex indicate the approximate extent of the representation of sensation for each part. (From Penfield and Jasper, 1954, with permission.)

recommended as a treatment for some forms of human epilepsy (Narabayashi and Mizutani, 1970), has fallen out of favor (Chapter 16). Nevertheless, it is commonly agreed that anterior temporal lobe resections for the

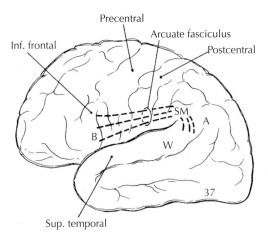

Figure 3–16. Diagrammatic view of the left hemisphere, indicating major cortical language areas. *A*, angular gyrus; *B*, Broca's area; *SM*, supramarginal gyrus; *W*, Wernicke's area; *37*, Brodmann area 37. (From Benson and Geschwind, 1985, with permission.)

treatment of epilepsy are more effective when the amygdala is removed (Vives et al., 2008). Consequently, an important role for the amygdala in the elaboration of certain human epileptic seizures, if not their initiation, must be acknowledged.

The amygdala complex (Ben Ari, 1981; McIntyre and Schwartzkroin, 2008) is a subcortical structure anatomically related to the *basal ganglia*, with cell types and connections similar to those of the *caudate nucleus*. It has major reciprocal connections with the *brain stem reticular formation*, hypothalamus, and septal area, as well as forebrain areas involved in olfaction (Lammers, 1972). Unlike in neocortex and hippocampus, the cytoarchitecture of the amygdala complex is poorly organized, with many cell types arranged into several nuclei. A *cortical medial* group appears to function predominantly in olfaction, whereas a *basolateral* group acts to modulate hypothalamic and brain stem functions.

Rhythmic stimulation of the amygdala at the proper frequency can induce recruiting responses in hippocampus via polysynaptic pathways (Gloor, 1955a;b) and can ultimately induce status epilepticus that continues when stimulation is terminated (Handforth and Ackermann, 1989; McIntyre et al., 1982). Repeated subthreshold amygdala stimulation results in *kindling*, the eventual development of limbic seizures, a commonly used animal model of limbic epilepsy (Goddard, 1967) (Chapter 4). However, ablation of the amygdala with kainic acid, which destroys cell bodies but not fibers of passage, does not abolish amygdala-kindled seizures, nor does it prevent the development of kindled seizures from stimulation in the region of the destroyed amygdala (Kaneko et al., 1981). Consequently, it is unclear to what extent these epileptogenic effects can be attributed to the amygdala itself rather than fibers that are near or pass through this structure.

Many brain stem and diencephalic structures have projections that alter hippocampal and neocortical excitability (Gale et al., 2008). These projection systems may be defined anatomically, chemically, or functionally. The old anatomical designation of *reticular formation* referred to the brain stem core that projects through thalamic structures to cortex. Today, brain stem and diencephalic projections are mapped according to the neurotransmitters involved (Moore and Bloom, 1979). Consequently, the *substantia nigra* and *ventral tegmental area* of the mesencephalon send *dopaminergic* projections to the forebrain (Bjorklund and Lindvall, 1984); the *locus coeruleus* and the *nucleus subcoeruleus* send *noradrenergic* projections (Moore and Card, 1984); the *raphe nuclei* send *serotonergic* projections (Parent et al., 1984); and the *lateral dorsal tegmental, pedunculopontine tegmental*, and *basal forebrain nuclei* send *cholinergic* projections (Butcher and Woolf, 1986). Some reciprocal projections from cortex to brain stem and diencephalon involve excitatory amino acids (Cotman et al., 1987), whereas the major GABAergic long-axon connections are subcortical (Fagg and Foster, 1983). Parts of these systems (e.g., the cholinergic nuclei of the dorsal pons) appear to be responsible for arousal, EEG desynchronization, and aspects of REM sleep, whereas others (e.g., noncholinergic projections of the basal forebrain nuclei) are involved in initiation of slow-wave sleep.

In general, brain stem and diencephalic influences that increase cortical neuronal synchronization, such as those that produce slow-wave sleep, increase the potential for epileptogenicity (Steriade 2003). Similarly, influences that desynchronize EEG activity and produce arousal or REM sleep reduce epileptiform excitability. These effects are not consistent, however, and also depend on the neurotransmitter systems involved. Consequently, the raphe nuclei may contribute to slow-wave sleep through a serotonergic mechanism (Jouvet, 1967), but serotonin inhibits epileptiform discharge, and raphe stimulation reduces epileptic excitability (Perryman et al., 1980). Noradrenergic and dopaminergic influences on forebrain, predominantly from locus coeruleus, substantia nigra, and the ventral tegmental area, also suppress epileptiform activity (Ehlers et al., 1980; Engel and Sharpless, 1977). The substantia nigra appears to play a role in the elaboration of some epileptic seizures (Engel et al., 1978; Gale, 1984; McNamara et al., 1984; Moshé et al., 1986), perhaps by limiting seizure recurrence and status epilepticus (Coppola and Moshé 2009). For the most part, its effects are mediated predominantly by modulation of GABAergic mechanisms in *pars reticulata* (Gale et al., 2008). Maturation and sex affect these functions (Velisek and Moshé, 2001). The thalamic reticular nucleus consists entirely of GABAergic inhibitory interneurons that play an important synchronizing role in the thalamus and mediate the generation of generalized 3-per-sec 3-Hz spike-and-wave discharges, as discussed in Chapter 4 (McCormick and Contras, 2001).

Synchronizing influences of subcortical structures on cortical neurons can be demonstrated by the classical augmenting and recruiting responses elicited by low-frequency electrical stimulation of specific diencephalic nuclei (Dempsey and Morison, 1941a;b; Morison and Dempsey, 1942). These synchronizing influences are important in generating some types of epileptiform discharges, because the same stimulation triggers generalized spike-and-wave discharges following systemic or cortical penicillin (Gloor et al., 1977). Subcortical structures that induce this epileptiform effect include the *nuclei centralis medialis, reticularis, ventralis anterior, lateralis posterior*, and *pulvinar* of the thalamus, as well as the *claustrum, putamen*, and *caudate*. It is clear that this experimental epileptiform phenomenon can be induced by normal afferent input acting on abnormal epileptogenic cortex (Chapter 4). Conversely, recurrent deep-brain stimulation of the anterior nucleus of the thalamus and other diencephalic structures reduces spontaneous seizure occurrence (Fisher et al., 2008) (Chapter 16).

The influence of the *cerebellum* on cortical excitability received some attention many years ago when chronic cerebellar stimulation was suggested as a treatment for epilepsy (Cooper et al., 1973). Electrical stimulation of the cerebellum can increase or decrease neocortical epileptic excitability in experimental animals (Dow et al., 1962). It has not been possible, however, to demonstrate a consistent beneficial effect of cerebellar stimulation on epileptogenesis, either experimentally or clinically, and cerebellar stimulation is no longer recommended as a treatment for epilepsy (Chapter 16). On the other hand, *vagus nerve stimulation* has become an important alternative for treatment of epilepsy, but the mechanisms by which stimulation of the vagus nerve reduces epileptic excitability are poorly understood. The vagus nerve is made up of fibers projecting both to and from the brain stem. Not only does stimulation of the nerve in the neck produce orthodromic afferent input to numerous brain stem structures, but cell bodies of the vagus nerve in the nodose ganglion have extensive collateral projections throughout the brain stem that can be activated by antidromic stimulation of efferent axons in the vagus nerve (Schachter and Boon, 2008) (Chapter 16).

The clinical use of section of the *corpus callosum* to control some forms of seizures indicates the importance of *interhemispheric influences* (Reeves, 1985; Roberts, 2008) (Chapter 16). In experimental animals, primary neocortical epileptic foci can give rise to secondary independent *mirror foci* in contralateral homotopic cortex, presumably as a result of the continuous bombardment across callosal pathways (Morrell, 1959/60) (Chapter 4). However, there is also evidence that callosal influences suppress epileptiform excitability: bilateral independent cortical epileptic foci appear to inhibit each other via callosal mechanisms and facilitate each other via subcortical connections (Mutani and Durelli, 1980); the predominant intracellular correlates of projected epileptiform discharges from a contralateral focus appear to be IPSPs (Crowell, 1970); and amygdaloid, but not hippocampal, kindling is facilitated in split-brain animals (McIntyre, 1975; McIntyre and Stuckey, 1985; Wada and Sato, 1975; Wada et al., 1981). Although corpus callosum section

can reduce the severity of some types of human epileptic seizures, worsening of epileptic seizures in a few patients has been reported (Spencer et al., 1984). Interhemispheric connections are not uniformly present for all cortical areas; for instance, they are absent for parts of primary motor and sensory cortex (Jones, 1985). There also does not appear to be a functional hippocampal commissure in the human brain (Wilson et al., 1987), at least for the anterior hippocampus.

Many descending projections from the neocortex and the hippocampus directly and indirectly influence the reticular core of the brain stem. Although epileptic excitability is considered to be a cortical phenomenon, investigations utilizing a wide variety of epileptic seizure models indicate that the *pontine reticular formation* plays an essential role in the manifestation of generalized tonic-clonic convulsions (Browning, 1985; Burnham, 1985). Any consideration of neuronal excitability pertinent to an understanding of motor seizures must take into account descending polysynaptic pathways from the cortex to the nonspecific core of the brain stem and spinal cord (Fromm et al., 1987; Gale et al., 2008) (Chapter 4).

PHYLOGENY AND ONTOGENY

Species Differences

Evidence from animal models, primarily kindling (Chapter 4), indicates that the development of epileptic phenomena takes longer with progression up the phylogenetic scale (Wada, 1978; Wilder et al., 1968; Galanopoulou and Moshé 2009), which suggests that the increased complexity of neuronal organization of cortical structures in higher animals militates against epileptogenicity. More specific information about the substrates of epileptic susceptibility is available from studies comparing epileptogenesis in the immature nervous system with that in the adult, because anatomical and physiological changes that occur with age are easier to define than species differences (Crino, 2008).

Cortical Development

An understanding of embryology has become important with the recent recognition that many forms of human epilepsy are due to *malformations of cortical development (MCD)* (Chapter 5). During the *embryonic period,* two to six weeks' gestation, the neural plate and neural tube form, and telencephalization occurs. Potentially epileptogenic disturbances associated with disruption at this stage include *anencephaly, encephalocele, Chiari malformation, holoprosencephaly,* and *Dandy-Walker malformation* (Vinters et al., 2008).

During the *fetal period,* 6–24 weeks, cell proliferation and migration occur (Sheen and Walsh, 2008) (Fig. 3–17). Neurogenesis and proliferation take place in the *ventricular zone* (VZ), and failure of proliferation causes microcephaly. Precursor neurons migrate into the cortical layers between 12 and 24 weeks, and disruption of this process causes *periventricular heterotopia, band heterotopia,* and *lissencephaly.* Population of the six-layered cortex begins from the deepest layers and ends in the superficial layers. Neuronal differentiation gives rise to the many neuronal subpopulations, and disruption of this process causes abnormal neuronal connectivity.

During the *perinatal period,* from 24 weeks' gestation to two years postnatal, organization and myelinization occur, and disruption of these processes gives rise to *polymicrogyria, schizencephaly, cortical dysplasias, microdysgenesis,* and *myelinization* disorders. Cerebral development is under the control of a large number of genes, and the genetic abnormalities that give rise to many recognized cortical malformations associated with epilepsy have been identified (Sheen and Walsh, 2008) (Chapter 5).

There is considerable variability in the timing of brain development in lower vertebrates (Schwartzkroin et al., 1995). These differences need to be considered when carrying out research on experimental models of epilepsy in the immature animal brain. Comparative developmental periods for human and rat brain maturation are shown in Table 3–3.

Maturational Effects on Excitability

Studies in laboratory animals, particularly the rat, and corroborated by clinical observations indicate that the immature brain is more susceptible to epileptic seizures and status epilepticus but less susceptible to the development of epilepsy and status-induced structural damage. Factors that appear to explain these maturational effects include the following: (1) excitatory processes develop before inhibitory processes; (2) there are differences in the ionic microenvironment between immature and mature brains; (3) delayed development of circuits modifies the expression of seizures; and (4) potentially epileptogenic stimuli such as fever, infection, and hypoxia are more common early in life (Velíseck and Moshé, 2001).

There are fewer neuroglial cells in the immature than in the mature cortex (Vernadakis and Woodbury, 1965), which should reduce K^+ buffering in the extracellular space (Hablitz and Heinemann, 1987). There is less dendritic arborization, and inhibitory synapses are poorly developed. There may also be more electrotonic coupling of cortical neurons in the immature brain (Connors et al., 1983). Inhibitory synapses appear early (Purpura, 1972), but EPSPs are better developed than IPSPs in immature hippocampus (Schwartzkroin, 1984) and neocortex (Kriegstein et al., 1987). As already discussed, GABA is depolarizing in the immature brain and hyperpolarizing in the mature brain (Mueller et al., 1984; Dzhala et al., 2005). There are also age-specific differences in neurotransmitter systems (Galanopoulou and Moshé, 2011).

Different mechanisms that control neuronal excitation and synchronization develop separately in the immature brain, which results in an increase and then a decrease in seizure susceptibility. Peak epileptogenicity occurs when all factors are maximally predisposed to both excitation and synchronization (Schwartzkroin, 1984; Crino, 2008). Extracellular potassium is high at birth and decreases as glial maturation occurs. Dendritic arborization and excitatory synaptic inputs increase with age, but functional synaptic inhibition develops late. Synchronization between distant structures is poor early and improves as myelinization develops (Mares et al., 1980). Thus early in development there is a lower threshold to epileptiform discharges, due to immature glial function and ineffective inhibition, but this activity is poorly organized, because of immature neuronal connections. As maturation progresses, the epileptiform activity becomes more organized, but the threshold for its induction increases (Schwartzkroin, 1984). Immature animals also appear to have a decreased refractory period for repetitive seizures, indicating an increased tendency toward status epilepticus (Moshé et al., 1983).

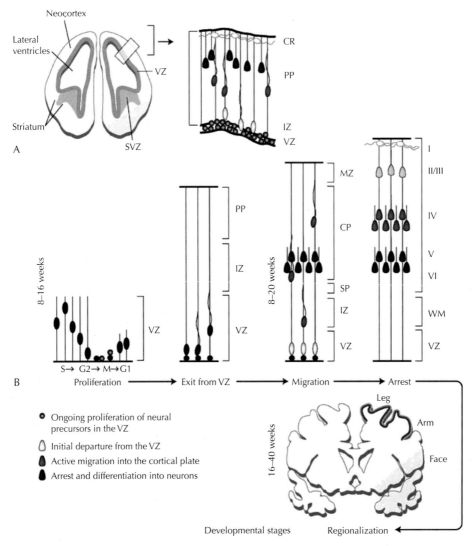

Figure 3–17. Diagram of the sequential developmental stages of the cerebral cortex. **A.** General anatomical overview of the developing cerebral cortex. Higher-magnification diagram (*right*) of inset (*left*) illustrates ongoing proliferation of neural precursors in the ventricular zone (VZ) (*circles*), initial departure from the VZ (*white ovals*), active migration into the cortical plate (*gray ovals*), and subsequent arrest and differentiation into neurons (*black ovals*). **B.** Temporal progression of human cerebral cortical development. During the first 8–16 weeks of development, neural progenitors undergo proliferation, with the period of neuronal migration extending from 8 to 20 weeks. By 16–40 weeks, regional specification with clear formation of sulci and gyri is apparent. Earlier-born neurons (*black*) become situated in deeper cortical layers (V and VI), and later-born neurons (*light gray*) are positioned more superficially in layers II and III. *CP*, cortical plate; *CR*, Cajal-Retzius cells; *IZ*, intermediate zone; *MZ*, marginal zone; *PP*, preplate; *SP*, subplate; *SVZ*, subventricular zone; *VZ*, ventricular zone; *WM*, white matter. (From Sheen and Walsh, 2003, with permission.)

Studies correlating the development of the various aspects of neuronal excitation and synchronization with the maturation of structural elements and neurotransmitter systems are providing clues to the neuronal mechanisms responsible for the generation of specific epileptiform events (Fig. 3–18).

SYSTEMIC INFLUENCES

A number of systemic physiological changes have nonspecific influences on excitability of cerebral neurons and can also precipitate certain forms of epileptic seizures. Any disturbance that results in a reduction of oxygen

Table 3–3 **Equivalency of Human and Rat Ages**

- Full-term infant = 7- to 8-day-old rat
- 2 months to 6 years = 2- to 3-week-old rats
- Adolescent = 5-week-old rat
- Aged = 2-year-old rat

Adapted from Velisek and Moshé, 2002, with permission.

and glucose delivery to the brain impairs the $Na^+ K^+$ pump and can cause membrane instability, leading to neuronal hyperexcitability. Acid-base imbalance also influences brain activity by causing complex alterations in the ionic microenvironment that are buffered by glial-specific *carbonic anhydrase* (White et al., 1986; Heinemann et al., 2008). Alkalosis enhances neuronal excitability, which may be

reversed by carbonic anhydrase inhibitors such as *acetazolamide* (Chapter 15). The prevailing view has been that hyperventilation precipitates epileptic seizures by causing hypocapnia, which results in both reduced energy substrates due to arterial constriction and also alkalosis. This concept has been challenged, however, and a direct effect of hypocapnia on the mesencephalic reticular formation has been suggested (Patel and Maulsby, 1987). Also, reducing CO_2 reduces adenosine, which has antiseizure properties (Dulla et al., 2005).

Stress and sleep deprivation precipitate epileptic activity, and some seizures demonstrate diurnal and other cyclical patterns of occurrence (Chapter 9). These effects are mediated in part by fluctuations in the blood levels of certain hormones. For example, neurosteroid metabolites of *progesterone* and *deoxycorticosterone*

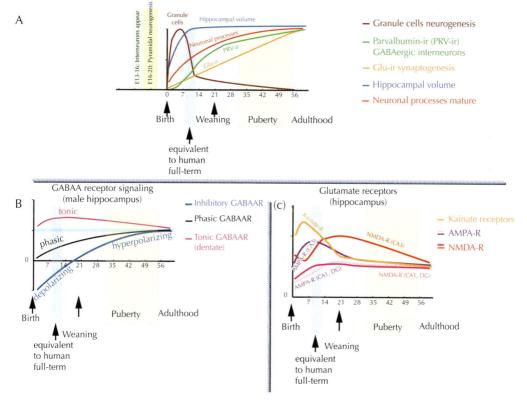

Figure 3–18. Schematic depiction of maturational changes in the male rodent hippocampus. **A.** Timeline of maturation of neurogenesis, excitatory (glutamatergic, *Glu-ir*) and GABAergic synaptogenesis, and hippocampal growth. **B, C.** Schematic depiction of maturational changes in the expression, function, and binding of GABA$_A$ receptors and glutamate receptors. Regional, sex, and cell type differences may occur that further augment the complexity of the observed effects of maturation on brain excitability and its susceptibility to seizures. (Based on data from Danglot et al., 2006; Dobbing et al., 1974; Galanopoulou, 2008; Galanopoulou and Moshé, 2011; Holter et al., 2010; Insel et al., 1990; Khazipor, 2004. (Reproduced with permission from Aristea Galanopoulou, MD, PhD, Albert Einstein College of Medicine, Bronx, NY. Modified from Danglot et al., 2006, with permission)

potentiate the action of GABA on the Cl⁻ ionophore to decrease neuronal excitability (Majewska et al., 1986), whereas *estrogen* classically enhances seizure susceptibility and may underlie the periodic exacerbation of epileptic seizures around the time of menses (*catamenial epilepsy*) (Hom and Butterbaugh, 1986; Veliskova and Velísek, 2007). The estrogen effect, however, is not entirely excitatory. There is evidence that β-*estradiol* potentiates NPY-mediated inhibition in the dentate gyrus (Veliskova and Velísek, 2007). These effects of neurosteroids appear to underlie the epileptogenic influences of stress and to play a role in the bidirectional relationship between epilepsy and certain interictal behavioral comorbidities, such as depression and anxiety disorders (Chapter 11).

Physiological disturbances and disease states that alter blood levels of Na^+, K^+, Ca^{2+}, Cl^-, and Mg^{2+}; increase levels of some toxic substances, such as ammonia; or induce cerebral edema all act to disrupt the ionic microenvironment of the brain and influence cerebral excitability (Chapter 5).

NEURONAL BASIS OF EEG ACTIVITY

The EEG is the most important clinical tool for measuring cerebral excitability and synchronization. An understanding of the neuronal basis of the electrical signals recorded by this technique is necessary for EEG interpretation (Buzsáki and Traub, 2008).

Each channel of an EEG measures potential differences between two electrodes oriented to record activity emanating from neural elements in the immediately underlying cerebral cortex (Cooper et al., 1965). The EEG records summated graded postsynaptic membrane potentials (EPSPs and IPSPs) resulting from axosomatic and axodendritic synaptic afferent input to cortical neurons (Creutzfeldt, 1974). The number of neuronal elements with similar dipoles synchronously generating these membrane events determines the amplitude of the potentials recorded at the surface. The duration of the summated EPSP-IPSP complex determines the frequency of the EEG rhythm. Desynchronization of neurons results in a *low-voltage fast* EEG pattern, whereas synchronization of neurons produces rhythmic, slower waves that become more prominent as the number of participating cortical elements increases (Fig. 3–19).

EPSP-IPSP complexes occurring on neurons located in thalamic structures regulate the rhythmic input to cortex, producing the cortical dendritic potentials underlying awake resting EEG rhythms. The typical 100-msec duration of the EPSP-IPSP complex in the pulvinar and other posteriorly projecting thalamic nuclei gives rise to the 10-Hz *alpha rhythm* in posterior cortical areas, while briefer repetitive EPSP-IPSP events in frontally projecting thalamic structures produce faster *beta rhythms* anteriorly (see Fig. 3–19).

The EEG pattern of deep sleep consists of 1- to 4-Hz *delta waves*, which correspond with slow oscillations occurring in deep (layer V) cortical layers (Buzsáki and Traub, 2008; Steriade et al., 1993). During the *up state*, there is depolarization and neuronal firing, reflected as negativity in the deep layers and positivity at the surface, while the *down state* reflects hyperpolarization and cessation of neuronal firing, recorded as positivity in the deep layers and negativity at the scalp. The neuronal substrates contributing to the *up-down state* are not completely known, but changes have been reported in epilepsy that could provide insights into epileptogenic mechanisms as well as provide a potential biomarker of epileptogenesis (Chapter 4).

EPSPs produced by axodendritic synapses in superficial cortical layers are negative extracellularly and are recorded by the scalp EEG as negative events. Because of the dipole effect of the neuron, EPSPs generated at axosomatic synapses are scalp-positive, whereas IPSPs generated from axosomatic synapses are scalp-negative. When a transient depolarization of apical dendrites is highly synchronized within a neuronal population, this event gives rise to a sharp negative *EEG spike*. The subsequent synchronized AHP produced by feedforward or feedback synaptic inhibition at the soma is seen on the EEG as an aftercoming negative slow wave (see Fig. 3–20). Large, presumably Ca^{2+}-mediated, dendritic PDSs, followed by prolonged somatic AHPs, are generated synchronously on neurons within experimental epileptic foci and are the neuronal substrate of the *EEG spike-and-wave* transient, the electrophysiological hallmark of epilepsy (Chapter 4). Sharp transients can also occur, however, in

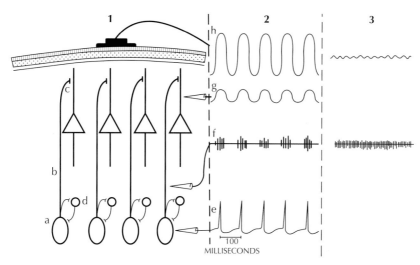

Figure 3–19. Generation of EEG rhythms. *1*: Thalamic neurons (*a*) discharge along fiber tracts (*b*) to dendrites of cortical neurons (*c*). Collateral axons also excite thalamic inhibitory interneurons (*d*). *2*: The intrinsic circuitry of the thalamus causes rhythmic neuronal discharges at a frequency determined by the EPSP-IPSP complex (*e*). When neuronal firing in the thalamus is synchronized, as indicated by multiple fiber recordings (*f*), synchronous EPSPs occur on cortical dendrites (*g*). These graded dendritic potentials summate to produce rhythmic EEG waves (*h*), the frequency of which is determined by the duration of the EPSP-IPSP complexes generated in the thalamus. In this example, a 100-msec interspike interval results in a 10-Hz EEG rhythm. *3*: When thalamic neurons are desynchronized, the resultant EEG pattern is not rhythmic (low-voltage fast activity).

the normal EEG (Chapter 13), and those transients reflect similar but nonpathological synchronous membrane events.

A spike-and-wave EEG discharge reveals the degree of synchrony of individual neuronal events within the underlying cortex but not the actual number of neurons involved. Consequently, hypersynchronous membrane events in a relatively small number of cortical neurons can give rise to high-amplitude EEG transients, whereas more active random activity in a much larger population of cortical neurons would give rise to desynchronized, low-voltage fast activity.

METHODOLOGICAL DEVELOPMENTS

The past two decades have witnessed tremendous advances in our understanding of neuronal excitability at the molecular and membrane level. In particular, the functional effects of specific genetic mutations can now be studied by using transgenic animal preparations, *in utero electroporation*, *viral vectors* to insert epileptogenic gene mutations

into adult animals (*viral transfection*) (Betley and Sternson, 2011), manipulation of genetic expression with pharmacological agents and light (Leung and Whittaker, 2005), and, most recently, the ability to reprogram somatic cells from patients with genetic diseases to a pluripotent state (*induced pluripotent stem cells, or iPSCs*), from which they differentiate into neuronal tissue with the same mutation for detailed in vitro investigations (Marchetto et al, 2011; Mattis and Svendsen, 2011). Results of such studies have contributed, and will continue to contribute, importantly to research in epilepsy and have provided targets for antiseizure drugs; however, synchronization, a basic substrate of epileptic seizures, is a function of neuronal networks. Elucidation of the fundamental neuronal mechanisms underlying normal brain behavior at the systems level and of potential disturbances in these mechanisms that could lead to hypersynchronization and epilepsy has been slow (Soltesz and Staley 2008). There is now a recent intensive effort to map the structural, functional, and effective connections of the entire brain, or *connectome* (Sporns, 2011; 2012). Future research in the new dynamic field of *connectomics* could help in the understanding of the emergence of

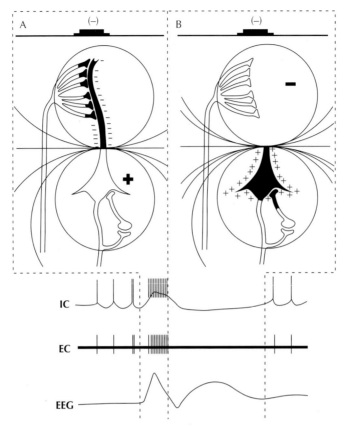

Figure 3–20. Neuronal basis of the EEG spike-and-wave discharge. **A.** Excitatory input opens channels on dendrite for Ca²⁺ entry, seen as a large PDS on intracellular recording (*IC*) and as burst unit firing on extracellular recording (*EC*). Summated outside-negative membrane events appear in the EEG as a negative spike. **B.** Prolonged AHPs caused not only by K⁺ currents but also by recurrent inhibition-induced Cl⁻ current at the soma are outside-positive membrane events (*IC*) but summate to appear as a slow negative wave in the EEG because of a dipole effect (the soma and apical dendrites maintain opposite polarity).

complex human behaviors, including abnormal behaviors such as epilepsy, as a result of the development of, and alterations in, the human connectome (www.humanconnectome.org).

Functional connectivity of the brain has traditionally been studied by direct electrical stimulation. Smaller and denser electrode arrays for intracranial use in awake and performing animals and patients facilitate this work, and a new flexible, high-density recording system for clinical use is now available (Viventi et al, 2011). Electrical stimulation, however, is imprecise, because it can both shut down and excite neurons at the point of stimulation, and these effects cannot easily be limited to the desired target (Borchers et al, 2012). Several new alternative methodological approaches suggest that major breakthroughs may be on

the horizon. *Optogenetics* is offering unique opportunities to delineate neurocircuits within complex networks. In the past, functional connectivity was determined by electrical stimulation, which activates all cell types as well as fibers of passage. Optogenetics is much more precise than direct stimulation, because it uses *microbial opsins*, which open ion channels in response to stimulation by colored light and can be delivered to populations of particular cell types using viral vectors and cell-specific promoters (Fenno et al., 2011). Three important *optogenetic tools* are *channelrhodopsins*, which open cation channels in response to blue light, causing depolarization; *hallorhodopsins*, which open chloride channels on exposure to yellow light, causing hyperpolarization; and *archirhodopsin,* which silences cells with yellow-green light, but does so by opening hydrogen channels without loading the cell with chloride. These tools are injected into selected areas of the brain, where the effect of excitation or inhibition of homogeneous neuronal populations can then be assessed by precise illumination with blue or yellow light. Such experiments have, for instance, confirmed the role of inhibition in synchronization by demonstrating the emergence of gamma oscillations with selective excitation of interneurons in vivo in normal animals (Sohal et al., 2009; Cardin et al., 2010) and could play a role in elucidating the fundamental mechanisms underlying pathological hypersynchronization in epilepsy. Another novel method for manipulating excitability of specific cell types, which is not yet widely used, employs designer receptors exclusively activated by designer drugs (DREADD) (Sasaki et al., 2011).

Computer modeling of neuronal networks, based on data derived from in vitro and in vivo electrophysiological experiments, is becoming an important tool for understanding how interconnections among thousands, perhaps hundreds of thousands, of neurons of different types function, both normally and abnormally (Jefferys, 2008; Soltesz and Staley, 2008). Functional connectivity among neurons is nonrandom, and computer modeling has identified *hub neurons*, which are neurons within a network that have increased input and output over long distances and therefore exert control over large populations of cells. (This concept derives from airline hubs, which provide a much more efficient approach to air travel than would connections from every airport to every other airport.) Hub neurons have so far been demonstrated only in hippocampus; they develop during maturation and can be altered by synaptic reorganization following injury (Bonifazi et al., 2009; Feldt et al., 2011). Whether the creation of pathological hub neuron circuits contributes to epileptogenesis remains to be determined.

Various modeling systems have been used to understand the dynamic interactions of neural interconnections, such as *graph theory* and *small-world networks* (Watts and Strogatz, 1998). Hub brain regions exist and constitute areas of concentrated traffic, referred to as *rich clubs* (Sporns, 2011; 2012). These approaches are now being applied to the analysis of *functional connectivity magnetic resonance imaging (fcMRI)* of whole brain in humans and animals,

in order to define normal and abnormal connectivity during the *resting state* (Meador, 2011). The *default mode network (DMN)*, areas of frontal and parietal cortex that are activated in the resting state, was originally conceptualized based on *positron emission tomography (PET)* (Raichle et al., 2001) but is now also apparent on resting fMRI. The DMN consists of the medial prefrontal cortex, posterior cingulate cortex, retrosplenial cortex including precuneus, inferior parietal lobules, lateral temporal cortices, and hippocampal formations. Studies of whole-brain connectivity can be carried out through *seeding*, where specific *regions of interest* are identified and their activity correlated with activity elsewhere in the brain (Morgan et al., 2011), or through *independent component analysis (ICA)*, where no presumptions are made and independent spatial maps are constructed and correlated with each other (Haneef et al., 2011). Application of fcMRI for clinical diagnosis is under investigation (Chapter 12). Finally, *diffusion tensor imaging (DTI)* MRI is being used to delineate white matter tracts, and this ability to perform *in vivo tractography* provides important structural information for correlation with the functional connectivity revealed by fcMRI in clinical studies where abnormal structure is anticipated (Chapter 12).

SUMMARY AND CONCLUSIONS

Over the past several decades, neuroscience has begun to reveal the incredible diversity of mechanisms available to neurons of the normal brain for transmitting and integrating information. The natural mechanisms that influence excitability and synchronization, in particular, have great relevance to epilepsy and are targets for most of the medical interventions currently used as treatments for this disorder.

At the membrane level, both excitatory depolarization caused by Na^+ and Ca^{2+} influx and inhibitory hyperpolarization caused by K^+ efflux and Cl^- influx are determined by movement of the respective ions through a variety of voltage-gated and ligand-gated ion channels with specific properties, as well as by the ionic microenvironment of the cell. Characteristics of a variety of channel types, passive and active mechanisms for altering the ionic microenvironment, and the complex nature of various classes of neurotransmitter receptors that regulate ionic current flow all contribute to the neuron's sophisticated capacity for integrating electrical and chemical information. It is likely that well-known mechanisms that influence membrane excitability, such as the $Na^+ K^+$ pump and the classical action potential, are less important to transient or long-term alterations leading to epileptiform excitability than are more subtle mechanisms that control or are controlled by Cl^- and Ca^{2+} currents.

The GABA receptor–Cl^- channel complex has been of considerable interest as the site of action for various convulsant drugs, such as picrotoxin and bicuculline, as well as for sedative and depressant drugs such as the barbiturates and benzodiazepines. It appears now that the properties of this receptor are sufficiently diverse to allow specifically designed pharmacological agents to potentiate inhibition of epileptiform phenomena without producing unwanted side effects.

Interest is also focused on the NMDA receptor–channel complex as the most logical substrate for plastic change within the nervous system. Not only are there many factors that determine the Ca^{2+} response to specific agonists and antagonists, but Ca^{2+} influx has a multiplicity of important consequences in addition to powerful membrane depolarization. Ca^{2+} couples membrane events to specific activities of neurons, such as neurotransmitter release by presynaptic terminals and gating of certain postsynaptic ion channels, as well as to more universal biological functions, such as genetic control of protein synthesis and cell death. These mechanisms allow experience to change neuronal structure and underlie acquired alterations in behavior. More research needs to be directed toward identifying NMDA antagonists that can selectively control epileptiform phenomena and prevent epileptic brain damage without inducing unacceptable disruption of normal brain function and structure.

A large number of neuromodulators, particularly peptides, hormones, adenosine, and the catecholamines, influence classical neurotransmitters and can also affect membrane excitability directly. Pharmacological manipulation of these chemicals and their receptors, as well as other nonsynaptic regulators of neuronal excitability, such as glial buffering, neurotransmitter inactivation, active transport, receptor trafficking, vesicle trafficking, and other subcellular processes, suggest possible avenues for preventing abnormal epileptiform events without disturbing normal neuronal function.

Tremendous advances in the past two decades in molecular neurobiology have resulted in the definition of molecular structures of ligand-gated and voltage-gated ion channels that determine their function in mediating neuronal excitability. In many cases, the genes encoding channel subunits are now known and specific gene mutations underlying certain channelopathies that give rise to epilepsy syndromes have been defined. Similar progress is being made at the receptor level. The genetic and molecular bases of other cellular processes, such as transporter molecules and vesicle trafficking, and the genes that code for these functions have helped to elucidate basic mechanisms of specific epileptogenic defects. These observations should reveal novel targets for antiseizure drugs. How these genetic and molecular disturbances alter neuronal interactions at the systems level to result in the manifestation of epileptic seizures and epilepsy, however, remains to be resolved.

The cytoarchitecture and functional integration of local neuronal circuits within the hippocampus and neocortex provide insights into the predisposition of those structures for the development of epileptiform activity. Susceptibility to epileptogenicity depends not only on excitatory interactions but also on the inhibitory connections responsible for synchronization. Both inhibition and excitation contribute to the abnormal but well-organized interactions of neuronal networks that underlie epileptiform events. Subcortical and endocrine systems regulate forebrain activity and undoubtedly help to initiate, maintain, or terminate epileptic events. They mediate the effects of nonspecific influences such as stress, sleep deprivation, and biorhythms on the pattern of occurrence of interictal and ictal phenomena.

There is considerable recent interest in elucidating the normal structure and function of the developing brain, which might explain disturbances resulting in epileptogenesis early in life. Researchers and clinicians need to appreciate how the immature brain differs from the adult brain. An understanding of normal embryology, and particularly processes of cortical development, is essential now that MRI has revealed that malformations of cortical development are common causes of epilepsy. Neuronal function early in life is age-dependent; the differential development of excitatory and inhibitory processes, changes in the ionic microenvironment, and incomplete development of circuits help explain why the immature brain is more susceptible than the mature brain to epileptic seizures and status epilepticus, but less susceptible to the development of chronic epilepsy and status-induced structural damage.

Until the specific pathophysiological substrates of individual chronic epilepsy conditions can be identified and individually corrected, the greatest hope for controlling epileptic seizures lies in manipulation of the mechanisms that regulate normal neuronal excitation and synchronization. Because this field is moving so quickly at the molecular level and because the use of new techniques such as optogenetics and fcMRI could revolutionize systems neurobiology, much of the material in this chapter will likely be out of date by the time it is published. With each new development in research on basic mechanisms of normal brain function, new concepts arise for more rational approaches to the management of human epilepsy.

REFERENCES

Ackermann, RF, and Moshé, SL (2010). Excitation/inhibition interactions and seizures: the brain's life-long balancing act. In Atlas of Epilepsies. Edited by CP Panayiotopoulos. London: Springer-Verlag, pp. 177–184.

Akil, H, Watson, SJ, Young, E, Lewis, ME, Khachaturian, H, and Walker, JM (1984). Endogenous opioids: Biology and function. Ann Rev Neurosci 7:223–255.

Andersen, P, and Sears, TA (1964). The role of inhibition in the phasing of spontaneous thalamo-cortical discharge. J Physiol 173:459–480.

Babb, TL, and Brown, WJ (1987). Pathological findings in epilepsy. In Surgical Treatment of the Epilepsies. Edited by J Engel, Jr, New York: Raven Press, pp. 511–540.

Bartholini, G, Bossi, L, Lloyd, KG, and Morselli, PL (Eds) (1985). Epilepsy and GABA Receptor Agonists: Basic and Therapeutic Research. New York: Raven Press.

Benardo, LS, and Pedley, TA (1985). Cellular mechanisms of focal epileptogenesis. In Recent Advances in Epilepsy, 2. Edited by TA Pedley and BS Meldrum. New York: Churchill Livingstone, pp. 1–17.

Benardo, LS, and Prince, DA (1982). Cholinergic pharmacology of mammalian hippocampal pyramidal cells. Neuroscience 7:1703–1712.

Ben Ari, Y (Ed) (1981). The Amygdaloid Complex. Amsterdam: Elsevier/North Holland.

Bennett, MVL (1977). Electrical transmission: a functional analysis and comparison with chemical transmission. In Handbook of Physiology, Section I: The Nervous System, Vol 1, Cellular Biology of Neurons, Part 1. Edited by ER Kandel. Bethesda, Md: American Physiological Society, pp. 357–416.

Benson, DF, and Geschwind, N (1985). Aphasia and related disorders: A clinical approach. In Principles of Behavioral Neurology. Edited by M Mesulam. Philadelphia: FA Davis, pp. 193–238.

Bernard, C (2008). Synaptic plasticity. In Epilepsy: A Comprehensive Textbook, Second Edition. Edited by J Engel Jr and TA Pedley. Philadelphia: Lippincott Williams & Wilkins, pp. 403–413.

Betley JN, Sternson SM (2011). Adeno-associated viral vectors for mapping, monitoring, and manipulating neural circuits. Hum Gene Ther. 22:669–677.

Bjorklund, A, and Lindvall, O (1984). Dopamine-containing systems in the CNS. In Handbook of Chemical Neuro-Anatomy, Vol 2, Part 1. Edited by A Bjorklund and T Hokfelt. Amsterdam: Elsevier/North Holland, pp. 55–122.

Bliss, TV, and Lomo, T (1973). Long-lasting potentiation of synaptic transmission in the dentate area of the anaesthetized rabbit following stimulation of the perforant path. J Physiol (Lond) 232:331–356.

Blumenfeld, H, and Coulter, DA (2008). Thalamocortical anatomy and physiology. In Epilepsy: A Comprehensive Textbook, Second Edition. Edited by J Engel Jr and TA Pedley. Philadelphia: Lippincott Williams & Wilkins, pp. 353–366.

Bonifazi, P, Goldin, M, Picardo, MA, Jorquera, I, Cattani, A, Bianconi, G, Represa, A, Ben-Ari, Y, and Cossart, R (2009). GABAergic hub neurons orchestrate synchrony in developing hippocampal networks. Science 326:1419–142.

Borchers, S, Himmelbach, M, Logothetis, N, Karnath, H-O (2012). Direct electrical stimulation of the human cortex—the gold standard for mapping brain functions? Nature Rev. 13:63–70.

Brodmann, K (1909). Vergleichende Lokalisationslehre der Grosshirnrinde in ihren Prinzipien dargestellt auf Grund des Zellenbaues. Leipzig, JA Barth.

Browning, RA (1985). Role of the brain-stem reticular formation in tonic-clonic seizures: Lesion and pharmacological studies. Federation of American Societies for Experimental Biology Proceedings 44:2425–2431.

Burnham, WM (1985). Core mechanisms in generalized convulsions. Fed Proc 44:2442–2445.

Butcher, LL, and Woolf, NJ (1986). Central cholinergic systems: Synopsis of anatomy and overview of physiology and pathology. In The Biological Substrates of Alzheimer's Disease. Edited by AB Scheibel and AF Wechsler. New York: Academic Press, pp. 73–86.

Buzsáki, G (2006). Rhythms of the Brain. Oxford: Oxford University Press, pp. 448.

Buzsáki, G, and Traub, RD (2008). Physiologic basis of the electroencephalogram and local field potentials. In Epilepsy: A Comprehensive Textbook, Second Edition. Edited by J Engel Jr and TA Pedley. Philadelphia: Lippincott Williams & Wilkins, pp. 797–807.

Caldecott-Hazard, S, and Engel, J, Jr (1987). Limbic postictal events: Anatomical substrates and opioid receptor involvement. Prog Neuropsychopharmacol Biol Psychiatry 11:389–418.

Cardin, JA, Carlen, M, Meletis, K, Knoblich, U, Zhang, F, Deisseroth, K, Tsai, L-H, and Moore, CI (2010). Targeted optogenetic stimulation and recording of neurons in vivo using cell-type-specific expression of Channelrhodopsin-2. Nature Protocols 5:247–254.

Chapman, AG (1984). Effect of anticonvulsant drugs on brain amino acid metabolism and GABA turnover. In Neurotransmitters, Seizures, and Epilepsy II. Edited by RG Fariello, PL Morselli, KG Lloyd, LF Quesney, and J Engel, Jr. New York: Raven Press, pp. 167–177.

Chatt, AB, and Ebersole, JS (1982). The laminar sensitivity of cat striate cortex to penicillin induced epileptogenesis. Brain Res 241:382–387.

Cohen, I, Navarro, V, Clemenceau, S, Baulac, M, and Miles, R (2002). On the origin of interictal activity in human temporal lobe epilepsy in vitro. Science 298:1418–1421.

Collingridge, GL, and Bliss, TVP (1987). NMDA receptors: Their role in long-term potentiation. Trends Neurosci 10:288–293.

Connors, BW, Benardo, LS, and Prince, DA (1983). Coupling between neurons of the developing rat neocortex. J Neurosci 3:773–782.

Connors BW, Long MA (2004). Electrical synapses in the mammalian brain. Annu Rev Neurosci. 27:393–418, .

Cooper, IS, Crighel, E, and Amin, I (1973). Clinical and physiological effects of stimulation of the paleocerebellum in humans. J Am Geriatr Soc 21:40–43.

Cooper, R, Winter, AL, Crow, HJ, and Walter, WG (1965). Comparison of subcortical, cortical and scalp activity using chronically indwelling electrodes in man. Electroencephalogr Clin Neurophysiol 18:217–228.

Coppola, A, and Moshé, SL (2009). Why is the developing brain more susceptible to status epilepticus (SE)? Epilepsia 50:25–26.

Cotman, CW, and Iversen, LL (1987). Excitatory amino acids in the brain: Focus on NMDA receptors. Trends Neurosci 10:263–275.

Cotman, CW, and Lynch, GS (1976). Reactive synaptogenesis in the adult nervous system: The effects of partial deafferentation on new synapses formation. In Neuronal Recognition. Edited by S Barondes. New York: Plenum Press, pp. 69–108.

Cotman, CW, Monaghan, DT, Ottersen, OP, and Storm-Mathiesen, J (1987). Anatomical organization of excitatory amino acid receptors and their pathways. Trends Neurosci 10:273–280.

Creutzfeldt, O (Ed) (1974). Electrical Activity From the Neuron to the EEG and EMG. The Neuronal Generation of the EEG. Handbook of Electroencephalography and Clinical Neurophysiology, Vol 2, part C. Series edited by A Rémond. Amsterdam: Elsevier.

Crino, PB (2008). Development of cortical excitability. In Epilepsy: A Comprehensive Textbook, Second Edition. Edited by J Engel Jr and TA Pedley. Philadelphia: Lippincott Williams & Wilkins, pp. 385–391.

Crowell, RM (1970). Distant effects of a focal epileptogenic process. Brain Res 18:137–154.

Danglot L, Triller A, and Marty S (2006). The development of hippocampal interneurons in rodents. Hippocampus 16:1032–1060.

DeLorenzo, RJ (1986). A molecular approach to the calcium signal in brain: Relationship to synaptic modulation and seizure discharge. Adv Neurol 44:435–464.

Dempsey, EW, and Morison, RS (1941a/2). The interaction of certain spontaneous and induced cortical potentials. Am J Physiol 135:301–308.

Dempsey, EW, and Morison, RS (1941b/2). The production of rhythmically recurrent cortical potentials after localized thalamic stimulation. Am J Physiol 135:293–300.

DeVivo, D, Trifiletti, RR, Jacobson, RI, Ronen, GM, Behmand, RA, Harik, SI (1991). Defective glucose transient across the blood-brain barrier as a cause of persistent hypoglycorrhchia, seizures, and developmental delay. N Engl J Med 325:703–709.

Dingledine, R (1981). Possible mechanisms of enkephalin action on hippocampal CA1 pyramidal neurons. J Neurosci 1:1022–1035.

Dobbing, J (1974). The later development of the brain and its vulnerability. In Scientific Foundations of Paediatrics. Edited by Davis, JA and Dobbing, J. New York: Raven Press.

Dow, RS, Fernandez-Guardiola, A, and Manni, E (1962). The influence of the cerebellum on experimental epilepsy. Electroencephalogr Clin Neurophysiol 14:383–398.

Dudek, FE, Snow, RW, and Taylor, CP (1986). Role of electrical interactions in synchronization of epileptiform bursts. Adv Neurol 44:593–617.

Dulla, CG, Dobelis, P, Pearson, T, Frenguelli, BG, Staley, KJ, and Masino, SA (2005). Adenosine and ATP link PCO2 to cortical excitability via pH. Neuron 48:1011–1023.

Dzhala, VI, Talos, DM, Sdrulla, DA, Brumback, AC, Mathews, GC, Benke, TA, Delpire, E, Jensen, FE, and Staley, KJ (2005). NKCC1 transporter facilitates seizures in the developing brain. Nat Med 11:1205–1213.

Echlin, FA (1959). The supersensitivity of chronically "isolated" cerebral cortex as a mechanism in focal epilepsy. Electroencephalogr Clin Neurophysiol 11:697–722.

Ehlers, CL, Clifton, DK, and Sawyer, CH (1980). Facilitation of amygdala kindling in the rat by transsecting ascending nonadrenergic pathways. Brain Res 189:274–278.

Engel, J, Jr, and Sharpless, NS (1977). Long-lasting depletion of dopamine in the rat amygdala induced by kindling stimulation. Brain Res 136:381–386.

Engel, J, Jr, Wolfson, L, and Brown, L (1978). Anatomical correlates of electrical and behavioral events related to amygdaloid kindling. Ann Neurol 3:538–544.

Engel, J, Jr, Caldecott-Hazard, S, Chugani, HT, and Ackermann, RF (1984). Neuropeptides, seizures and epilepsy. In Advances in Epileptology: XV Epilepsy International Symposium. Edited by RJ Porter, RH Mattson, AA Ward, and M Dam. New York: Raven Press, pp. 25–30.

Engel, J. Jr, Wilson, C., and Lopez-Rodriguez, F (2002). Limbic connectivity: anatomical substrates of behavioral disturbances in epilepsy. In Trimble, M., Schmitz, B (Eds), The Neuropsychiatry of Epilepsy. Cambridge: University Press, pp. 18–37.

Engel, J Jr, Dichter, MA, and Schwartzkroin, PA (2008a). Basic mechanisms of human epilepsy. In Epilepsy: A Comprehensive Textbook, Second Edition. Edited by J Engel Jr and TA Pedley. Philadelphia: Lippincott Williams & Wilkins, pp. 495–507.

Engel, J Jr, Williamson, PD, and Wieser, HG (2008b). Mesial temporal lobe epilepsy with hippocampal sclerosis. In Epilepsy: A Comprehensive Textbook, Second Edition. Edited by J Engel Jr and TA Pedley. Philadelphia: Lippincott Williams & Wilkins, pp. 2479–2486.

Engel, J Jr, Bragin, A, Staba, R, and Mody, I (2009). High-frequency oscillations: what's normal and what is not? Epilepsia 50:598–604.

Enna, SJ (Ed) (1983). The GABA receptors. Clifton, NJ: Humana Press.

Erulkar, SD (1983). The modulation of neurotransmitter release at synaptic junctions. Rev Physiol Biochem Pharmacol 98:63–175.

Fagg, GE, and Foster, AC (1983). Amino acid neurotransmitters and their pathways in the mammalian central nervous system. Neuroscience 9:701–719.

Feldt, S, Bonifazi, P, and Cossart, R (2011). Dissecting functional connectivity of neuronal microcircuits: experimental and theoretical insights. Trends Neurosci 34:225–236.

Fenno, L, Yizhar, O, and Deisseroth, K (2011). The development and application of optogenetics. Ann Rev Neurosci 34:389–412.

Ferrendelli, JA (1986). Roles of biogenic amines and cyclic nucleotides in seizure mechanisms. Adv Neurol 44:393–400.

Fifkova, E, and Anderson, CL (1981). Stimulation induced changes in dimensions of stalks of dendritic spines in the dentate molecular layer. Exp Neurol 74:621–627.

Finch, DM, and Babb, TL (1977). Response decrement in a hippocampal basket cell. Brain Res 130:354–359.

Fisher, RS, McKhann, GM II, Stern, JM, Quigg, MS, Régis, J, Schomer, DL, Schachter, SC, and Vezzani, A (2008). New therapeutic directions. In Epilepsy: A Comprehensive Textbook, Second Edition. Edited by J Engel Jr and TA Pedley. Philadelphia: Lippincott Williams & Wilkins, pp. 1415–1430.

Frankenhaeuser, B, and Hodgkin, AL (1957). The action of calcium on the electrical properties of squid axons. J Physiol 137:218–244.

Freund TF, Buzsáki G (1996). Interneurons of the hippocampus. Hippocampus. 6:347–470.

Fromm, GH, Faingold, CL, Browning, RA, and Burnham, WM (Eds) (1987). Epilepsy and the Reticular Formation: The Role of the Reticular Core in Convulsive Seizures. Neurology and Neurobiology, Vol 27. New York: Alan R Liss.

Galanopoulou, AS (2008). Dissociated gender-specific effects of recurrent seizures on GABA signaling in CA1 pyramidal neurons: role of GABA(A) receptors. J Neurosci 28:1557–1567.

Galanopoulou, AS, and Moshé, SL (2009). Pediatric/developmental aspects of epilepsy: treatment options/age specific responses to AEDs. In Encyclopedia of Basic Epilepsy Research, PA Schwartzkroin (Ed). Amsterdam: Elsevier, pp. 1025–1033.

Galanopoulou, AS, and Moshé, SL (2011). In search of epilepsy biomarkers in the immature brain: goals, challenges and strategies. In Biomarkers in Epilepsy. Edited by J Engel, Jr. Biomarkers in Medicine 5:615–628.

Gale, K (1984). The role of the substantia nigra in the anticonvulsant actions of GABAergic drugs. In Neurotransmitters, Seizures, and Epilepsy II. Edited by RG Fariello, K Lloyd, PL Morselli, LF Quesney, and J Engel, Jr. New York: Raven Press, pp. 57–79.

Gale, K., Proctor, M, Velíšková, J, and Nehlig, A (2008). Basal ganglia and brainstem anatomy and physiology. In Epilepsy: A Comprehensive Textbook, Second Edition. Edited by J Engel Jr and TA Pedley. Philadelphia: Lippincott Williams & Wilkins, pp. 367–384.

Gloor, P (1955a). Electrophysiological studies on the connections of the amygdaloid nucleus in the cat. I. The electrophysiological properties of the amygdaloid projection system. Electroencephalogr Clin Neurophysiol 7:243–264.

Gloor, P (1955b). Electrophysiological studies on the connections of the amygdaloid nucleus in the cat. II. The neuronal organization of the amygdaloid projection system. Electroencephalogr Clin Neurophysiol 7:223–242.

Gloor, P, and Fariello, RG (1988). Generalized epilepsy: Some of its cellular mechanisms differ from those of focal epilepsy. Trends Neurosci 11:63–68.

Gloor, P, Quesney, LF, and Zumstein, H (1977). Pathophysiology of generalized penicillin epilepsy in the cat: The role of cortical and subcortical structures. II. Topical applications of penicillin to the cerebral cortex and to subcortical structures. Electroencephalogr Clin Neurophysiol 43:79–94.

Goddard GV (1967). Development of epileptic seizures through brain stimulation at low intensity. Nature 214:1020–1023.

Golden GT, and Fariello, RG (1984). Epileptogenic action of some direct GABA agonists: Effects of manipulation of the GABA and glutamate systems. In Neurotransmitters, Seizures, and Epilepsy II. Edited by RG Fariello, PL Morselli, KG Lloyd, LF Quesney, and J Engel, Jr. New York: Raven Press, pp. 237–243.

Gray, EG (1959). Axo-somatic and axo-dendritic synapses of the cerebral cortex: an electron microscope study. J Anat 93:420–433.

Gutnick, MJ, and Prince, DA (1972). Thalamocortical relay neurons: Antidromic invasions of spikes from a cortical epileptogenic focus. Science 176:424–426.

Hablitz, JJ, and Heinemann, U (1987). Extracellular K^+ and Ca^{2+} changes during epileptiform discharges in the immature rat cortex. Dev Brain Res 36:299–303.

Handforth, A, and Ackermann, RF (1989). Electrically induced limbic status and kindled seizures. In Anatomy of Epileptogenesis. Edited by BS Meldrum, JA Ferendelli, and HG Wieser. London: John Libbey, 1989, pp. 71–87.

Haneef, Z, Lenartowicz, A, Yeh, HJ, Engel, J Jr, and Stern, J (in press). Functional connectivity MRI asymmetries in lateralized temporal lobe epilepsy. Epilepsy and Behavior (in press).

Heinemann, U (1987). Changes in the neuronal micro-environment and epileptiform activity. In Current Problems in Epilepsy, 3: The Epileptic Focus. Edited by HG Wieser, EJ Speckmann, and J Engel, Jr. London: John Libbey, pp. 27–44.

Heinemann, U, and Lambert, JC (1986). Changes in extracellular calcium and magnesium concentration and their consequences for the development of seizure activity. In Neurotransmitters, Seizures, and Epilepsy III. Edited by G Nistico, PL Morselli, KG Lloyd, RG Fariello, and J Engel, Jr. New York: Raven Press, pp. 65–74.

Heinemann U, Mody I, and Yaari Y (2008). Control of neuronal excitability. In Epilepsy: A Comprehensive

Textbook, Second Edition. Edited by J Engel Jr and TA Pedley. Philadelphia: Lippincott Williams & Wilkins, pp. 219–231.

Holmes, GL, and Weber, DA (1986). Effects of ACTH on seizure susceptibility in the developing brain. Ann Neurol 20:82–88.

Holter, NI, Zylla, MM, Zuber, N, Bruehl, C, and Draguhn, A (2010). Tonic GABAergic control of mouse dentate granule cells during postnatal development. The European J Neurosci 32:1300–1309.

Hom, AC, and Butterbaugh, GG (1986). Estrogen alters the acquisition of seizures kindled by repeated amygdala stimulation or pentylenetetrazol administration in ovariectomized female rats. Epilepsia 27:103–108.

Houser, CR, Vaughn, JE, Hendry, SHC, Jones, EG, and Peters, A (1984). GABA neurons in the cerebral cortex. In Cerebral Cortex, Vol 2, Functional Properties of Cortical Cells. Edited by EG Jones and A Peters. New York: Plenum Press, pp. 63–89.

Hrachovy, RA, Frost, JD Jr (2008). Adrenocorticotropic hormone and steroids. In Epilepsy: A Comprehensive Textbook, Second Edition. Edited by J Engel Jr and TA Pedley. Philadelphia: Lippincott Williams & Wilkins, pp. 1519–1529.

Insel, TR, Miller, LP, and Gelhard, RE (1990). The ontogeny of excitatory amino acid receptors in rat forebrain – I. N-methyl-D-aspartate and quisqualate receptors. Neuroscience 35:31–43.

Jefferys, JGR (2008). Epilepsy in vitro: Electrophysiology and computer modeling. In Engel J Jr, Pedley TA (Eds) Epilepsy: A Comprehensive Textbook, Second Edition. Philadelphia: Lippincott Williams & Wilkins, pp. 457–468.

Jefferys, JGR, and Haas, HL (1982). Synchronized bursting of CA1 hippocampal pyramidal cells in the absence of synaptic transmission. Nature 300:448–450.

Johnston, D, Hoffman, DA, Colbert, CM, and Magee, JC (1999). Regulation of back-propagating action potentials in hippocampal neurons. Curr Opin Neurobiol. 9:288–292.

Jones, EG (1985). Anatomy, development, and physiology of the corpus callosum. In Epilepsy and the Corpus Callosum. Edited by AG Reeves. New York: Plenum Press, pp. 3–20.

Jones, EG, and Cowan, WM (1983). The nervous tissue. In Histology: Cell and Tissue Biology, ed 5. Edited by L Weiss. New York: Elsevier Biomedical, pp. 282–370.

Jouvet, M (1967). Neurophysiology of the states of sleep. Physiol Rev 47:117–177.

Kandel, ER, Schwartz, JH, and Jessell, TM (Eds) (2000). Principles of Neural Science, ed 4. New York: McGraw-Hill.

Kaneko, Y, Wada, JA, and Kimura, H (1981). Is the amygdaloid neuron necessary for amygdaloid kindling? In Kindling 2. Edited by JA Wada. New York: Raven Press, pp. 249–264.

Khazipov, R, Khalilov, I, Tyzio, R, Morozova, E, Ben-Ari, Y, and Holmes, GL (2004). Developmental changes in GABAergic actions and seizure susceptibility in the rat hippocampus. European J Neurosci 19:590–600.

Kiloh LG, McComas, AJ, Osselton, JW, and Upton, ARM (1981). Clinical Electroencephalography, ed 4. London: Butterworths.

Kriegstein, AR, Suppes, T, and Prince, DA (1987). Cellular and synaptic physiology and epileptogenesis of developing rat neocortical neurons in vitro. Dev Brain Res 34:161–171.

Krnjevic, K (1980). Principles of synaptic transmission. Adv Neurol 27:127–154.

Krnjevic, K (1983). GABA mediated inhibitory mechanisms in relation to epileptic discharges. In Basic Mechanisms of Neuronal Excitability. Edited by HH Jasper and NM Van Gelder. New York: Alan R. Liss, pp. 249–280.

Krueppel, R, Remy, S, and Beck, H (2011). Dendritic integration in hippocampal dentate granule cells. Neuron 71:512–528.

Kullmann, DM and Schorge, S (2008). Voltage-gated ion channels: molecular biology and role of mutations in epilepsy. In Epilepsy: A Comprehensive Textbook, Second Edition. Edited by J Engel Jr and TA Pedley. Philadelphia: Lippincott Williams & Wilkins, pp. 253–265.

Lado, FA, and Moshé, SL (2008). How do seizures stop? Epilepsia 49:1651–1664.

Lammers, HJ (1972). The neural connections of the amygdaloid complex in mammals. In The Neurobiology of the Amygdala. Advances in Behavioral Biology, Vol 2. Edited by BE Eleftheriou. New York: Plenum Press, pp. 123–144.

Leao, AAP (1972). Spreading depression. In Experimental Models of Epilepsy—A Manual for the Laboratory Worker. Edited by DP Purpura, JK Penry, DB Tower, and RD Walter. New York: Raven Press, pp. 173–196.

Leung RK, and Whittaker, PA (2005). RNA interference: from gene silencing to gene-specific therapeutics. Pharmacol Ther. 107:222–239.

Löscher, W, and Schmidt, D (2009). Mechanisms of tolerance and drug resistance. In The Treatment of Epilepsy, Third Edition. Edited by S Shorvon, E Perucca, and J Engel, Jr. Oxford: Wiley-Blackwell, pp. 109–118.

Lovinger, DM (2012). Communication Networks in the Brain: Neurons, Receptors, Neurotransmitters, and Alcohol. National Institute on Alcohol Abuse and Alcoholism. http://pubs.niaaa.nih.gov/publications/arh313/196-214.htm.

Lukasiuk, K, Dingledine, R, Lowenstein, DH, and Pitkänen, A (2008). Gene expression underlying changes in network excitability. In Epilepsy: A Comprehensive Textbook, Second Edition. Edited by J Engel Jr and TA Pedley. Philadelphia: Lippincott Williams & Wilkins, pp. 307–322.

Lynch, G, and Baudry, M (1984). The biochemistry of memory: A new and specific hypothesis. Science 224:1057–1063.

MacDermott, AB, and Dale, N (1987). Receptors, ion channels and synaptic potentials underlying the integrative actions of excitatory amino acids. Trends Neurosci 10:280–284.

Macdonald, RL, and Mody, I (2008). $GABA_A$ and $GABA_B$ receptor-mediated inhibitory synaptic transmission. In Epilepsy: A Comprehensive Textbook, Second Edition. Edited by J Engel Jr and TA Pedley. Philadelphia: Lippincott Williams & Wilkins, pp. 245–252.

Macdonald, RL, and Rogawski MA (2008). Cellular effects of antiepileptic drugs. In Epilepsy: A Comprehensive Textbook, Second Edition. Edited by J Engel Jr and TA Pedley. Philadelphia: Lippincott Williams & Wilkins, pp. 1433–1445.

Maclean, PD (1952). Some psychiatric implications of physiological studies on frontotemporal portion of limbic system (visceral brain). EEG Clin Neurophysiol 4:407–418.

Majewska, MD, Harrison, NL, Schwartz, RD, Barker, JL, and Paul, SM (1986). Steroid hormone metabolites are barbituate-like modulators of the GABA receptor. Science 232:1004–1007.

Marchetto, MC, Brennand, KJ, Boyer, LF, and Gage, FH (2011). Induced pluripotent stem cells (iPSCs) and neurological disease modeling: progress and promises. Human Molecular Genetics 20:R109–R115.

Mares, P, Zouhar, A, and Brozek, G (1980). The electrocorticographic pattern of generalized seizures in rats during ontogenesis. Physiol Bohemoslov 29:193–200.

Margerison, JH, and Corsellis, JA (1966). Epilepsy and the temporal lobes: A clinical, electroencephalographic and neuropathological study of the brain in epilepsy, with particular reference to the temporal lobes. Brain 89:499–530.

Mathern, GW, Wilson, CL, and Beck, H (2008). Hippocampal sclerosis. In Epilepsy: A Comprehensive Textbook, Second Edition. Edited by J Engel Jr and TA Pedley. Philadelphia: Lippincott Williams & Wilkins, pp. 121–136.

Matsumoto, H, and Ajmone-Marsan, C (1964). Cortical cellular phenomena in experimental epilepsy: Interictal manifestations. Exp Neurol 9:286–304.

Mattis, VB, and Svendsen, CN (2011). Induced pluripotent stem cells: a new revolution for clinical neurology? Lancet Neurology 10:383–394.

Matveeva EA, Price DA, Whiteheart SW, Vanaman TC, Gerhardt GA, and Slevin JT (2012). Reduction of vesicle-associated membrane protein 2 expression leads to a kindling-resistant phenotype in a murine model of epilepsy. Neuroscience 202:77–86.

McCormick, DA, and Contreras, D (2001). On the cellular and network bases of epileptic seizures. Ann Rev Physiol 63:815–846.

McIntyre, DC (1975). Split brain rat: Transfer and interference of kindled amygdala convulsions. Can J Neurol Sci 2:429–437.

McIntyre, DC, and Schwartzkroin, PA (2008). Limbic anatomy and physiology. In Epilepsy: A Comprehensive Textbook, Second Edition. Edited by J Engel Jr and TA Pedley. Philadelphia: Lippincott Williams & Wilkins, pp. 337–352.

McIntyre, DC, and Stuckey, GN (1985). Dorsal hippocampal kindling and transfer in split-brain rats. Exp Neurol 87:86–95.

McIntyre, DC, Nathanson, D, and Edson, N (1982). A new model of partial status epilepticus based on kindling. Brain Res 250:53–63.

McNamara, JO, Rigsbee, LC, Galloway, MT, and Shin, C (1984). Evidence that activation of substantia nigra is necessary for limbic seizures. In Neurotransmitters, Seizures, and Epilepsy II. Edited by RG Fariello, K Lloyd, PL Morselli, LF Quesney, and J Engel, Jr. New York: Raven Press, pp. 44–55.

Meador, KJ (2011). Networks, cognition, and epilepsy. Neurology 77:930–931.

Meldrum, BS (1983). Metabolic factors during prolonged seizures and their relation to nerve cell death. Adv Neurol 34:261–275.

Meldrum, BS (1984). Amino acid neurotransmitters and new approaches to anticonvulsant drug action. Epilepsia 25(Suppl 2):S140–S149.

Meldrum, BS (1986a). Cell damage in epilepsy and the role of calcium in cytotoxicity. Adv Neurol 44:849–855.

Meldrum, BS (1986b). Pharmacological approaches to the treatment of epilepsy. In New Anticonvulsant Drugs. Edited by BS Meldrum and RJ Porter. London: John Libbey, pp. 17–30.

Meldrum BS (2008). Molecular targets for novel antiepileptic drugs. In Epilepsy: A Comprehensive Textbook, Second Edition. Edited by J Engel Jr and TA Pedley. Philadelphia: Lippincott Williams & Wilkins, pp. 1457–1468.

Meldrum, BS, and Chapman, AG (1986). Excitatory amino acid antagonists as anticonvulsant agents: Receptor subtype involvement in different seizure models. In Neurotransmitters, Seizures and Epilepsy III. Edited by G Nistico, PL Morselli, KG Lloyd, RG Fariello, and J Engel, Jr. New York: Raven Press, pp. 223–234.

Messenheimer, JA, Harris, EW, and Steward, O (1979). Sprouting fibers gain access to circuitry transsynaptically altered by kindling. Exp Neurol 64:469–481.

Mesulam, M (1985). Patterns in behavioral neuroanatomy: Association areas, the limbic system, and hemispheric specialization. In Principles of Behavioral Neurology. Edited by M Mesulam. Philadelphia: FA Davis, pp. 1–70.

Meyer, FB, Anderson, RE, Sundt, TM, Jr, and Sharbrough, FW (1986) Selective central nervous system calcium channel blockers—A new class of anticonvulsant agents. Mayo Clin Proc 61:239–247.

Miller, JJ, Baimbridge, KG, and Mody, I (1986). Calcium regulation in kindling-induced epilepsy. In Kindling 3. Edited by JA Wada. New York: Raven Press, pp. 301–318.

Moore, RY, and Bloom, FE (1979). Central catecholamine neuron system: Anatomy and physiology of the norepinephrine and epinephrine systems. Ann Rev Neurosci 2:113–168.

Moore, RY, and Card, JP (1984). Noradrenaline-containing neuron systems. In Handbook of Chemical Neuro-Anatomy, Vol 2, Part 1. Edited by A Bjorklund and T Hokfelt. Amsterdam: Elsevier/North Holland, pp. 123–156.

Morgan, JJ, Cohen, DR, Hempstead, JL, and Curran, T (1987). Mapping patterns of the *c-fos* expression in the central nervous system after a seizure. Science 237:192–197.

Morgan, VL, Rogers, BP, Sonmezturk, HH, Gore, JC, and Abou-Khalil, B (2011). Cross hippocampal influence in mesial temporal lobe epilepsy measured with high temporal resolution functional magnetic resonance imaging. Epilepsia 52:1741–1749.

Morison, RS, and Dempsey, EW (1942). A study of thalamocortical relations. Am J Physiol 135:281–292.

Morrell, F (1959/60). Secondary epileptogenic lesions. Epilepsia 1:538–560.

Moshé, SL, Albala, BJ, Ackermann, RF, and Engel, J, Jr (1983). Increased seizure susceptibility of the immature brain. Dev Brain Res 7:81–85.

Moshé, SL, Ackermann, RF, Albala, BJ, and Okada, R (1986). The role of substantia nigra in seizures of developing animals. In Kindling 3. Edited by JA Wada. New York: Raven Press, pp. 91–106.

Mueller, AL, Taube, JS, and Schwartzkroin, PA (1984). Development of hyperpolarizing inhibitory post-synaptic potentials and hyperpolarizing response to γ-aminobutyric acid in rabbit hippocampus studied in vitro. J Neurosci 3:860–867.

Mutani, R, and Durelli, L (1980). Mechanisms of interaction of asymmetrical bilateral epileptogenic foci in neocortex. Epilepsia 21:549–556.

Narabayashi, H, and Mizutani, T (1970). Epileptic seizures and the stereotaxic amygdalotomy. Confin Neurol 32:289–297.

Nicholls, JG, Martin, AR, Wallace, BG, and Fuchs, PA (2001). From Neuron to Brain: A Cellular and Molecular Approach to the Function of the Nervous System, Fourth Edition. Sunderland, Mass: Sinauer.

Nicoll, RA, Siggins, GR, Ling, N, Bloom, FE, and Guillemin, R (1977). Neuronal action of endorphins and enkephalins among brain regions: A comparative microiontophoretic study. Proc Natl Acad Sci 74:2584–2588.

Nicoll, RA, Alger, BE, and Jahr, CE (1980). Enkephalin blocks inhibitory pathways in the vertebrate CNS. Nature 287:22–25.

O'Keefe, JO, and Nadel, L (1978). The Hippocampus as a Cognitive Map. Oxford, England: Clarendon Press.

Olsen, RW (1981). GABA-benzodiazepine-barbiturate receptor interactions. J Neurochem 37:1–13.

Olsen, RW, Wamsley, JK, Lee, RJ, and Lomax, P (1986). Benzodiazepine/barbiturate/GABA receptor-chloride ionophore complex in a genetic model for generalized epilepsy. Adv Neurol 44:365–378.

Papez, JW (1937). A proposed mechanism of emotion. Arch Neurol Psychiat 38:725–743.

Pappas, GD, and Purpura, DP (1972). Structure and Function of Synapses. Raven Press: New York.

Parent, A, Poitras, D, and Dube, L (1984). Comparative anatomy of central monoaminergic systems. In Handbook of Chemical Neuro-Anatomy, Vol 2, Part 1. Edited by A Bjorkland and T Hokfelt. Amsterdam: Elsevier/North Holland, pp. 409–439.

Parent, JM, Coulter, DA, and Bertram EH (2008). The effect of seizures on the brain. In Epilepsy: A Comprehensive Textbook, Second Edition. Edited by J Engel Jr and TA Pedley. Philadelphia: Lippincott Williams & Wilkins, pp. 481–493.

Patel, VM, and Maulsby, RLs (1987). How hyperventilation alters the electroencephalogram: A review of controversial viewpoints emphasizing neurophysiological mechanisms. J Clin Neurophysiol 4:101–120.

Penfield, W, and Jasper, H (1954). Epilepsy and the Functional Anatomy of the Human Brain. Boston: Little, Brown & Co.

Perryman, KM, Babb, TL, Finch, DM, Brown, WJ, and Crandall, PH (1980). Effects of long-term raphe nucleus stimulation on chronic limbic seizures in monkeys. Epilepsia 21:479–487.

Peters HC, Hu H, Pongs O, Storm JF, and Isbrandt D (2005). Conditional transgenic suppression of M channels in mouse brain reveals functions in neuronal excitability, resonance and behavior. Nat Neurosci. 8:51–60.

Petsche, H, Stumpf, C, and Gogolak, G (1962). The significance of the rabbit's septum as a relay station between the midbrain and the hippocampus. I. The control of hippocampus arousal activity by the septum cells. Electroenceph Clin Neurophysiol 14:202–211.

Phillis, JW, and Wu, PH (1981). The role of adenosine and its metabolites in central synaptic transmission. Prog Neurobiol 16:187–239.

Purpura, DP (1972). Intracellular studies of synaptic organizations in the mammalian brain. In Structure and Function of Synapses. Edited by GD Pappas and DP Purpura. New York: Raven Press, pp. 257–302.

Raichle, ME, MacLeod, AM, et al. (2001). A default mode of brain function. Proc Natl Acad Sci USA 98:676–682.

Raisman, G (1969). Neuronal plasticity in the septal nuclei of the adult rat. Brain Res 14:25–48.

Reeves, AG (1985). Epilepsy and the Corpus Callosum. New York: Plenum Press.

Renaud, LP (1983). Role of neuropeptides in the regulation of neural excitability. In Basic Mechanisms of Neuronal Hyperexcitability, Neurology and Neurobiology, Vol 2. Edited by HH Jasper and NM van Gelder. New York: Alan R Liss, pp. 323–360.

Richardson, KA, Fanselow, EE, and Connors, BW (2008). Neocortical anatomy and physiology. In Epilepsy: A Comprehensive Textbook, Second Edition. Edited by J Engel Jr and TA Pedley. Philadelphia: Lippincott Williams & Wilkins, pp. 323–335.

Roberts, DW (2008). Corpus callosotomy. In J Engel Jr, TA Pedley (Eds), Epilepsy: A Comprehensive Textbook, Second Edition. Lippincott Williams & Wilkins, Philadelphia, pp. 1907–1913.

Roberts, PJ, Storm-Mathisen, J, and Johnson, GAR (Eds) (1981). Glutamate, Transmitter in the Central Nervous System. New York: John Wiley & Sons.

Rothman, SM, and Olney, JW (1987). Excitotoxicity and the NMDA receptor. Trends Neurosci 10:299–302.

Sasaki K, Suzuki M, Mieda M, Tsujino N, Roth B, and Sakurai T (2011). Pharmacogenetic modulation of orexin neurons alters sleep/wakefulness states in mice. PLoS One.6:e20360. Epub 2011.

Schachter, SC, and Boon, P (2008). Vagus nerve stimulation. In Epilepsy: A Comprehensive Textbook, Second Edition. Edited by J Engel Jr and TA Pedley. Philadelphia: Lippincott Williams & Wilkins, pp. 1395–1399.

Scharfman, HE, and Schwarcz, R (2008). Neuromodulation of seizures, epileptogenesis, and epilepsy. In Epilepsy: A Comprehensive Textbook, Second Edition. Edited by J Engel Jr and TA Pedley. Philadelphia: Lippincott Williams & Wilkins, 2008, pp. 289–305.

Schwartzkroin, PA (1983a). Local circuit considerations and intrinsic neuronal properties involved in hyperexcitability and cell synchronization. In Basic Mechanisms of Neuronal Hyperexcitability. Edited by HH Jasper and NM Van Gelder. New York: Alan R Liss, pp. 75–105.

Schwartzkroin, PA (1983b). Mechanisms of cell synchronization in epileptiform activity. Trends Neurosci 6:157–160.

Schwartzkroin, PA (1984). Epileptogenesis in the immature central nervous system. In Electrophysiology of Epilepsy. Edited by PA Schwartzkroin and H Wheal. New York: Academic Press, pp. 389–412.

Schwartzkroin, PA (1986). Hippocampal slices in experimental and human epilepsy. Adv Neurol 44:991–1010.

Schwartzkroin, PA, Moshé, SL, Noebels, JL, and Swann, JW, Eds (1995). Brain Development and Epilepsy. New York: Oxford University Press.

Sheen, VL, Walsh, CA (2003). Developmental genetic malformations of the cortex. Curr. Neurol. Neurosci. Reports 3:433–441.

Sheen, VL, and Walsh, CA (2008). Early events in the development of the cerebral cortex. In Epilepsy: A Comprehensive Textbook, Second Edition. Edited by J Engel Jr and TA Pedley. Philadelphia: Lippincott Williams & Wilkins, pp. 393–401.

Sisodiya, SM, Beck, H, Löscher W, and Vezzani, A (2008). Mechanisms of drug resistance. In Epilepsy: A Comprehensive Textbook, Second Edition. Edited by J Engel Jr and TA Pedley. Philadelphia: Lippincott Williams & Wilkins, pp. 1279–1289.

Snead, OC, III (1986). Seizures induced by morphine and enkephalin: μ or δ? In Neurotransmitters, Seizures, and Epilepsy III. Edited by G Nisticò, PL Morselli, KG Lloyd, RG Fariello, and J Engel, Jr. New York: Raven Press, 1986, pp. 331–339.

Sohal, VS, Zhang, F, Yizhar, O, and Deisseroth, K (2009). Parvalbumin neurons and gamma rhythms enhance cortical circuit performance. Nature 459:698–702.

Soltesz, I. and Staley, K (Eds) (2008). Computational Neuroscience in Epilepsy. San Diego: Elsevier, pp. 624.

Spencer, SS, Spencer, DD, Glaser, GH, Williamson, PD, and Mattson, RH (1984). More intense focal seizure types after callosal section: The role of inhibition. Ann Neurol 16:686–693.

Spencer, WA, and Kandel, ER (1961). Hippocampal neuron response to selective activation of recurrent collaterals of hippocampofugal axons. Exp Neurol 4:149–161.

Sporns, O (2011). Networks of the Brain. Boston: MIT Press.

Sporns, O (2012). Discovering the Human Connectome. Boston: MIT Press.

Staba, RJ, and Bragin, A (2011). High-frequency oscillations and other electrophysiological biomarkers of epilepsy: underlying mechanisms. Biomarkers Med 5:545–556.

Steinhauser, C, Haydon, PG, De Lanerolle, NC (2008). Astroglial mechanisms in epilepsy. In Epilepsy: A Comprehensive Textbook, Second Edition. Edited by J Engel Jr and TA Pedley. Philadelphia: Lippincott Williams & Wilkins, pp. 277–288.

Steriade, M (2003). Neuronal Substrates of Sleep and Epilepsy. Cambridge, Cambridge Press, pp. 522.

Steriade, M, McCormick, DA, and Sejnowski, TJ (1993). Thalamocortical oscillations in the sleeping and aroused brain. Science 262:679–685.

Stuart, G, Sprutson, N, and Hausser, M (Eds) (2008). Dendrites, Second Edition, Oxford: Oxford U. Press, pp. 560

Sutula, T, He, X-X, Cavazos, J, and Scott, G (1988). Synaptic reorganization in the hippocampus induced by abnormal functional activity. Science 239:1147–1150.

Tauck, DL, and Nadler, JV (1985). Evidence of functional mossy fiber sprouting in hippocampal formation of kainic acid-treated rats. J Neurosci 5:1016–1022.

Taylor CP, and Dudek, FE (1982). Synchronous neural after discharges in rat hippocampal slices without active chemical synapses. Science 218:810–812.

Traub, RD, Whittington, MA, Buhl, EH, et al. (2001). A possible role for gap junctions in generation of very fast EEG oscillations preceding the onset of, and perhaps initiating, seizures. Epilepsia 42:153–170.

Tsukahara, N (1981). Synaptic plasticity in the mammalian central nervous system. Ann Rev Neurosci 4:351–379.

Vanden Bussche, G, Wauquier, A, Ashton, D, and de Beukelaar, F (1986). Flunarizine. In Current Problems in Epilepsy, Vol 4, New Anticonvulsant Drugs. Edited by BS Meldrum and RJ Porter. London: John Libbey, pp. 125–145.

Van Gelder, NM (1978). Taurine, the compartmentalized metabolism of glutamic acid, and the epilepsies. Can J Physiol Pharmacol 56: 362–374.

Van Gelder, NM (1983). Metabolic interactions between neurons and astroglia: Glutamine synthetase, carbonic anhydrase, and water balance. In Basic Mechanisms of Neuronal Hyperexcitability. Edited by HH Jasper and NM Van Gelder. New York: Alan R Liss, pp. 5–27.

Van Harreveld, A, and Fifkova E (1975). Swelling of dendritic spines in the fascia dentata after stimulation of the perforant fibers as a mechanism of posttetanic potentiation. Exp Neurol 49:736–749.

Velísek, L, and Moshé, SL (2001). Pathophysiology of seizures and epilepsy in the immature brain: cells, synapses and circuits. In Pediatric Epilepsy, Diagnosis and Therapy, Second Edition. Edited by JM Pellock, WE Dodson, and BFD

Velísek, L, and Moshé, SL (2002). Effects of brief seizures during development. Prog Brain Res 135:355–364.

Bourgeois. New York: Demos Press, pp. 1–23.

Veliskova, J, and Velisek, L (2007). β-estradiol increases dentate gyrus inhibition in female rats via augmentation of hilar neuropeptide-Y. J. Neurosci. 27:6054–6063.

Vernadakis, A, and Woodbury, DM (1965). Cellular and extracellular spaces in developing rat brain: Radioactive uptake studies with chloride and inulin. Arch Neurol 12:284–293.

Vezzani, A, Peltola, J, and Janigro, D (2008). Inflammation. In Epilepsy: A Comprehensive Textbook, Second Edition. Edited by J Engel Jr and TA Pedley. Philadelphia: Lippincott Williams & Wilkins, pp. 267–276.

Vinters, HV, Salamon, N, Miyata, H, Khanlou, N, and Mathern, GW (2008). Neuropathology of developmental disorders associated with epilepsy. In Epilepsy: A Comprehensive Textbook, Second Edition. Edited by J Engel Jr and TA Pedley. Philadelphia: Lippincott Williams & Wilkins, pp. 137–160.

Viventi, J, Kim, D-H, Vigeland, L, Frechette, ES, Blanco, JA, Kim, Y-S, Arvin, AE, Tiruvadi, VR, Hwang, S-W, Vanleer, AC, Wulsin, DF, Davis, K, Gelber, CE, Palmer, L, Van der Spiegel, J, Wu, J, Xiao, J, Huang, Y, Contreras, D, Rogers, JA, and Litt, B (2011). Flexible, foldable, actively multiplexed, high-density electrode array for mapping brain activity in vivo. Nature Neuroscience 14:1599–1607.

Vives, K, Lee, G, Doyle W, Spencer DD (2008). Anterior temporal resection. In Epilepsy: A Comprehensive Textbook, Second Edition. Edited by J Engel Jr and TA Pedley. Philadelphia: Lippincott Williams & Wilkins, pp. 1859–1867.

Wada, JA (1978). The clinical relevance of kindling: Species, brain sites and seizure susceptibility. In Limbic Mechanisms. Edited by KE Livingston and O Hornykiewicz. New York: Plenum Press, pp. 369–388.

Wada, JA, and Sato, M (1975). The generalized convulsive seizure state induced by daily electrical stimulation of the amygdala in split brain cats. Epilepsia 16:417–430.

Wada, JA, Mizoguchi T, and Komai, S (1981). Cortical motor activation in amygdaloid kindling: Observations in nonepileptic rhesus monkeys with anterior two-thirds callosal bisection. In Kindling 2. Edited by JA Wada. New York: Raven Press, pp. 235–248.

Walker, MC, Surges, R, and Fisher, A (2009). Mechanisms of antiepileptic drug action. In The Treatment of Epilepsy, Third Edition. Edited by S Shorvon, E Perucca, and J Engel, Jr. Oxford: Wiley-Blackwell, pp. 91–108.

Wasterlain, CG, Bronstein, JM, Fairchild, MD, and Farber, DB (1986). Biochemical adaptations in kindled foci. In Neurotransmitters, Seizures, and Epilepsy III. Edited by G Nistico, PL Morselli, KG Lloyd, RG Fariello, and J Engel, Jr. New York: Raven Press, pp. 101–121.

Watts, DJ, and Strogatz, SH (1998). Collective dynamics of 'small world' networks. Nature 393:440–442.

Wayman GA, Lee YS, Tokumitsu H, Silva AJ, Soderling TR (2008). Calmodulin-kinases: modulators of neuronal development and plasticity. Neuron. 59:914–931.

White, HS, Woodbury, DM, Chen, CF, Kemp, JW, Chow, SY, and Yen-Chow, YC (1986). Role of glial cation and anion transport mechanisms in etiology and arrest of seizures. Adv Neurol 44:695–712.

Wieser, HG (1983). Electroclinical Features of Psychomotor Seizure. A Stereoelectroencephalographic Study of Ictal Symptoms and Chromatographical Seizure Patterns Including Clinical Effects of Intracerebral Stimulation. London: Butterworths.

Wieser, HG (1988). Human limbic seizures: EEG studies, origin, and patterns of spread. In Anatomy of Epileptogenesis. Edited by BS Meldrum, JA Ferrendelli, and HG Wieser. London, John Libbey, pp. 127–138.

Wilcox, KS, West, PJ, Dichter, MA (2008). Excitatory synaptic transmission. In Epilepsy: A Comprehensive Textbook, Second Edition. Edited by J Engel Jr and TA Pedley. Philadelphia: Lippincott Williams & Wilkins, pp. 233–244.

Wilder, BJ, King, RL, and Schmidt, RP (1968). Comparative study of secondary epileptogenesis. Epilepsia 9:275–289.

Wilson, CL, Isokawa-Akesson, M, Babb, TL, Engel, J, Jr, Cahan, LD, and Crandall, PH (1987). A comparative view of local and interhemispheric limbic pathways in humans: An evoked potential analysis. In Fundamental Mechanisms of Human Brain Function. Edited by J Engel, Jr, GA Ojemann, HO Lüders, and PD Williamson. New York: Raven Press, pp. 27–38.

Winden, KD, Karsten, S, Bragin, A, Kudo, L, Gehman, L, Ruidera, J, Engel, J, Jr. and Geschwind, D.H (2011). A systems level, functional genomics analysis of chronic epilepsy. PloS One 6: e2063.

Witte, OW, Walden, J, and Speckmann, EJ (1987). Antiepileptic effects of calcium antagonists in animal experiments. In Current Problems in Epilepsy, 3: The Epileptic Focus. Edited by HG Wieser, EJ Speckmann, and J Engel, Jr, London: John Libbey, pp. 193–207.

Woodbury, DM (1980). Covulsant Drugs: Mechanisms of action. Adv Neurol 27:249–303.

Wu, J-Y, and Prentice, H (2010). Role of taurine in the central nervous system. J Biomed Sci 17(Suppl 1)S1.

Zorn, SH, Willmore, LJ, Bailey, CM, and Enna, SJ (1986). A comparison of antinociceptive and anticonvulsant effects of GABAergic drugs: Evidence for a GABA receptor system unrelated to GABA$_A$ or GABA$_B$ sites. In Neurotransmitters, Seizures, and Epilepsy III. Edited by G Nisticò, PL Morselli, KG Lloyd, RG Fariello, and J Engel, Jr. New York: Raven Press, pp. 123–133.

Chapter 4

Basic Mechanisms of Seizures and Epilepsy

EXPERIMENTAL MODELS OF SEIZURES AND EPILEPSY
Acute Models
Chronic Models

STUDIES OF HUMAN EPILEPSY
Electrophysiological Investigations
Investigations Using Brain Imaging
Techniques
Microanatomical Investigations
Biochemical and Molecular Investigations

MOLECULAR GENETIC INVESTIGATIONS
Gene Discovery

Acquired Genetic Disturbances

POSSIBLE MECHANISMS OF HUMAN EPILEPTIC PHENOMENA
Epileptogenesis
Interictal State
Ictogenesis
Ictus
Ictal Termination
Postictal Period
Possible Consequences of Epileptic Seizures

SUMMARY AND CONCLUSIONS

As noted in the previous chapter, tremendous advances have been made in neuroscience in recent years, and this new knowledge as well as recently developed technologies is being applied to research on epilepsy (Schwartzkroin, 2009). The *National Institute of Neurological Disorders and Stroke (NINDS)* has established priorities, or *benchmarks*, for epilepsy research, which are being monitored and revised as the field progresses (Kelly et al., 2009, Jacobs et al.,

2001). Progress is posted annually at www. ninds.nih.gov/research/epilepsyweb.

There is no doubt that "the best model of a cat is another, or preferably the same, cat" (a statement attributed to Norbert Wiener). However, knowledge about the basic mechanisms of epilepsy (Schwartzkroin, 2009) derives mostly from studies of animal models. Biomedical research using animals requires an understanding of the relationships between these models of human disease and actual clinical situations (Engel and Schwartzkroin, 2006). Given that most human epilepsy disorders are much too complicated to be represented faithfully by any single animal model, it is necessary to dissect clinical epileptic phenomena into component parts that can be more reasonably approximated in the animal laboratory and then validated in patients. Thus it can be possible to identify physiological, anatomical, and molecular substrates of individual abnormal phenomena that when taken together make up those clinical conditions called epilepsy (Berkovic et al., 1996; Engel et al., 1992; Heinemann et al., 1996; Moshé et al; 2000; Schwartzkroin et al., 1998). Animal models of epilepsy are necessary not only for investigations into fundamental mechanisms but also for screening and testing potential antiepilepsy interventions (Galanopoulou et al., 2012) (Chapter 15).

EXPERIMENTAL MODELS OF SEIZURES AND EPILEPSY

Experimental models of epilepsy may be roughly categorized as acute or chronic (Avanzini et al., 2008; Engel, 1992; Pitkänen et al., 2006b). *Acute models* are essentially models of reactive epileptic seizures and usually involve systemic or topical administration of convulsant substances or sudden insults, such as electrical stimulation and metabolic or ionic derangements, that produce transient epileptiform activity. These models are appropriate for investigating mechanisms of epileptic seizure development, maintenance, and termination as well as postictal disturbances, but because the seizures are artificially provoked in a normal brain, these models do not provide opportunities to investigate enduring interictal epileptogenic abnormalities or mechanisms of spontaneous seizure generation (*ictogenesis*). *Chronic models* demonstrate enduring interictal epileptogenic abnormalities and therefore meet the definition of epilepsy (Fisher et al., 2005) (Chapter 1). These models usually involve the induction of permanent structural lesions of the brain or genetically epileptic animals. Chronic models can be used to study the development of epilepsy (*epileptogenesis*) and also allow investigation of those enduring

neuronal disturbances that exist interictally and account for intermittent spontaneous ictogenesis. Table 4–1 lists commonly used experimental models of epileptic phenomena according to their presumed clinical relevance.

Acute Models

Epileptic seizures or ictal discharges in vivo are usually produced acutely in the laboratory by *electrical stimulation* (Mares and Kubová, 2006) or *pharmacological agents* (Velísek, 2006; Cortez and Snead, 2006). These techniques, as well as manipulation of the ionic environment, are commonly used in in vitro preparations (Heinemann et al., 2006). In vivo interventions produce focal seizures when applied to localized areas of the brain and can produce generalized seizures when applied systemically or to bilateral or diffuse brain areas. Electrical stimulation is believed to act by depolarizing neurons until repeated action potentials are generated at the axon hillock as rapidly as the absolute refractory period allows (Gerin, 1960); internal circuitry of recurrent excitation and inhibition gives rise to continued synchronous firing, referred to as *afterdischarge*, which continues after the electrical stimulation is discontinued. This abnormal activity can then spread to become an epileptic seizure (Ajmone-Marsan, 1972; Swinyard, 1972). Convulsant drugs act by (1) enhancing excitation, (2) blocking inhibition, (3) disrupting cerebral metabolic processes, and (4) blocking active transport systems (Chapter 3). Table 4–2 shows the proposed mechanisms of action of commonly used convulsant drugs. Absence-inducing drugs have different mechanisms of action, often enhancing GABA-mediated inhibition (Cortez and Snead, 2006). Acute epileptic seizures can also be produced in the laboratory by local application of K^+, which induces neuronal depolarization and spreading epileptiform discharges as well as *spreading depression*; by *hypoxia* and *hyperbaric oxygen*; by *hypercarbia*; by *withdrawal from high carbon dioxide concentrations* (Withrow, 1972), and by *alcohol withdrawal* (N'Gouemo and Rogawski, 2006). Common mechanisms of inducing ictal-like discharges in vitro in slice preparations also include decreasing Mg^{2+}, which potentiates NMDA receptors, and

Table 4–1 **Commonly Used Experimental Models of Epileptic Phenomena**

I. Models of focal epileptic phenomena
  A. Neocortical
    1. Electrical stimulation
    2. Topical convulsant drugs (e.g., penicillin, bicuculline, picrotoxin, pentylenetetrazol)
    3. Partially isolated cortical slab
    4. Freeze lesion
    5. Metals (e.g., alumina, cobalt, tungstic acid, ferric chloride)
    6. Neocortical kindling
    7. Posttraumatic (could be limbic)
    8. Cortical dysplasia (*methylazoxymethanol acetate*, freeze, radiation)
  B. Limbic
    1. Electrical stimulation (acute)
    2. Long-term potentiation in hippocampus
    3. Metals
    4. Poststatus (kainic acid, pilocarpine, electrical stimulation)
    5. Amygdala and hippocampal kindling
  C. Neonatal
    1. Hypoxia
    2. Hyperthermia
II. Models of generalized epileptic phenomena
  A. Convulsive type
    1. Maximal electroshock seizure
    2. Maximal pentylenetetrazol seizure
    3. Maximal flurothyl-induced seizure
    4. Maximal audiogenic seizure
    5. Posttetanic potentiation in cat spinal cord
    6. Hyperthermia in immature animals
  B. Petit mal type
    1. Systemic pentylenetetrazol
    2. Feline-generated penicillin
    3. Intracerebroventricular opioids (e.g., enkephalins and endorphins)
    4. Systemic γ-hydroxybutyrate
    5. THIP model
    6. Subcortical stimulation, lesions, and convulsant drugs
    7. CO_2 withdrawal seizures
    8. Repetitive stimulation of cat spinal cord
  C. Genetic types (poorly classified)
    1. *Papio papio* baboon
    2. Audiogenic mice
    3. Genetically epilepsy-prone rat
    4. Seizure-prone gerbil
    5. Other mutant mouse models (e.g., totterer, reeler)
    6. Beagle
    7. Epileptic fowl
    8. Spontaneous spike-and-wave rat model

THIP = tetrahydroxyisoxozolopyridine.

application of *4-aminopyridine* (4AP), which blocks K^+ currents (Heinemann et al., 2006; Jefferys, 2008).

IN VIVO MODELS OF FOCAL SEIZURES

Much of the early research on acute seizures was carried out on the *penicillin-induced neocortical epileptic focus* (Matsumoto and Ajmone-Marsan, 1964a;b; Prince, 1968; Velísek, 2006). It remains useful to review the results of these classical studies. Investigations at the extracellular microelectrode level revealed at least two phenomena that can be considered characteristic of neuronal activity within this experimental epileptogenic cortex: abnormally hypersynchronous activity of large numbers of neighboring neurons, and paroxysmally bursting units with unusually rapid discharges.

Intracellular microelectrode recordings from neurons within these foci showed large *paroxysmal depolarization shifts (PDSs)* underlying the unit burst firing, followed by prolonged *afterhyperpolarizations (AHPs)* (Fig. 4–1). Paroxysmal depolarization shifts occur synchronously in over 90% of recorded neurons in the penicillin focus and summate to produce surface-recorded interictal EEG spikes, whereas the AHPs correspond to the EEG slow wave of the EEG spike-and-wave complex (Chapter 3). The mechanisms responsible for the development of synchronous, presumably Ca^{2+}-mediated PDSs in the acute epileptic focus are not completely known. Intrinsic bursting properties of neurons can interact with specific alterations in excitatory and inhibitory synaptic input to produce these membrane events (Prince and Connors, 1986), or they can result from abnormal synaptic influences alone (Johnston and Brown, 1981). Whether the PDS and AHP always reflect novel pathophysiological events unique to epilepsy or can be merely an exaggeration of normal interneuronal integration is still arguable. Some aspects of PDS development are intriguingly similar to changes recorded in neocortex during the *recruiting* and *augmenting* phenomena produced by nonspecific and specific thalamic stimulation of the normal brain (Andersen and Sears, 1964) (Chapter 3).

Although the prolonged AHP is due in part to Ca^{2+}-dependent K^+ currents (Schwartzkroin and Wyler, 1980), its magnitude and duration reflect enhanced synaptic inhibition (Engel

Table 4–2 Proposed Mechanisms of Action of Convulsant Drugs

Drugs	Proposed Actions
I. Enhance excitatory systems	
Pentylenetetrazol	Direct effect on membrane properties to increase spontaneous discharge by altering tonic conductance (also blocks effect of GABA; see below)
Anticholinesterases	Inhibit acetylcholinesterase and cause accumulation of acetylcholine
Flurothyl (hexafluorodiethyl ether)	Opens up Na^+ channels by an effect on membranes
Convulsant barbiturates (CHEB, DMBB)	Increase Ca^{2+} influx into nerve terminals and thereby increase release of excitatory transmitters
Homocysteic acid, kainic acid, N-methyl-aspartic acid, ibotenic acid	Stimulate excitant amino acid receptors (glutamate, aspartate); appear to increase Na^+ permeability by displacing Ca^{2+} from surface of the membrane or increase Ca^{2+} influx
Substance P	Unknown; probably same as glutamic acid
II. Block inhibitory systems	
A. Block effect of GABA at receptor	
Picrotoxin, penicillin, bicuculline, pentylenetetrazol	Block interaction of GABA with postsynaptic receptor; direct effect on chloride channel to prevent enhanced conductance of Cl^-; presynaptic and postsynaptic inhibition is blocked
B. Block GABA synthesis or release	
Tetanus toxin	Blocks release of inhibitory transmitter in spinal cord
Allylglycine	Inhibits GAD (probably acting via its metabolite, 2-keto-4-pentenoic acid); inhibits γ-glutamylcysteine and cystathionase
3-Mercaptopropionic acid	Inhibits GAD competitively; enhances GABA-aminotransferase
Oxygen at high pressure	Inhibits GAD and thereby decreases brain GABA
Thiosemicarbazide, semicarbazide, and other pyridoxal phosphate endings	Decrease synthesis of GABA by inhibiting GAD in presynaptic antagonists via an action on pyridoxal phosphate
C. Block effect of glycine at receptor	
Strychnine, brucine	Block postsynaptic inhibition at glycine receptor ionophore complex, probably by preventing glycine-induced increase in chloride conductance
III. Block energy metabolism	
Fluoroacetate, fluorocitrate, 2-deoxyglucose	Interfere with energy metabolism and thereby inhibit ion transport
Methionine sulfoximine	Inhibits glutamine synthetase, γ-glutamylcysteine synthetase, and protein synthesis; also promotes formation of abnormal methylated excitatory substances or enhances breakdown of S-adenosyl homocysteine to the excitatory substances homocysteine or homocysteic acid
IV. Ion transport inhibitors	
Cations (ouabain)	Inhibits Na^+-K^+-ATPase and thereby alters ion distribution across neurons
Anions (thiocyanate, perchlorate)	Inhibit glial cell anion transport system and HCO_3^- ATPase

CHEB = 5-(2-cyclohexylidene-ethyl)-5-ethyl barbituric acid; DMBB = 5-(1.3-dimethylbutyl)-5-ethyl barbituric acid; GAD = glutamic acid decarboxylase.

Adapted from Woodbury, 1980, with permission.

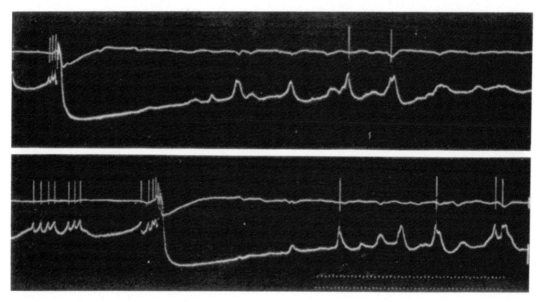

Figure 4–1. Two intracellular recording of PDSs, AHPs, and oscillations of membrane potential (lower trace of each panel) and surface EEG (upper trace of each panel). The PDSs are followed by long-lasting AHPs. As the latter decrease, transient depolarizations are possible, some of which are accompanied by spikes. The PDSs tend to occur preferentially at lower levels of membrane polarization. Calibrations: 10 mV (intracellular tracing) and 1 mV (surface tracing); 50 Hz. (From Matsumoto and Ajmone-Marsan, 1964a, with permission.)

and Wilson, 1986). Neurons in the region surrounding the penicillin epileptic focus produce large hyperpolarizing membrane events in the absence of preceding depolarization. This *inhibitory surround* (Prince and Wilder, 1967) is believed to act as a means of containing the epileptiform discharge, thereby maintaining the interictal state. Hyperpolarization of neurons in the inhibitory surround cannot be attributed to Ca^{2+}-dependent K^+ currents, because the Ca^{2+} depolarization does not occur there. Rather, this hyperpolarization reflects feedback synaptic input from inhibitory interneurons located within the experimental epileptic focus (Fig. 4–2). Furthermore, feedforward synaptic inhibition must occur in the deeper cortical layers of the penicillin focus, where hyperpolarization often precedes the PDS (Elger and Speckmann, 1983). Hyperpolarization involving the somatic membrane (Pollen, 1964), the region of predominant inhibitory synaptic input, accounts for the characteristically negative aftercoming slow wave seen on the EEG (Chapter 3).

Elements within penicillin foci have been observed to exhibit *fast prepotentials (FPPs)*, which represent action potentials occurring on dendrites (Loskata et al., 1974) (Chapter 3). The contribution of FPPs to the generation or maintenance of epileptiform activity is not known.

Transition of the penicillin focus from the interictal to the ictal state involves reversal of the AHP to prolonged depolarization with a consequent continuous burst of action potentials at the axon hillock (Matsumoto and Ajmone-Marsan, 1964b) (Fig. 4–3). Rapid neuronal firing leads to increased extracellular K^+, decreased extracellular Ca^{2+}, and shrinkage of extracellular space as glial swelling accompanies uptake of K^+ and water (Heinemann, 1987). This results in deterioration of the inhibitory surround, slow ephaptic and local synaptic spread of the ictal discharge with recruitment of adjacent neurons, and ultimately propagation along fiber tracts to contralateral and subcortical structures (Collins, 1978) (Fig. 4–4).

The behavioral characteristics of the seizure depend on the location of the initial focus and subsequent spread of epileptic discharges. Single clonic muscle twitches can appear with each interictal EEG spike when an acute experimental epileptic focus is placed in somatomotor cortex. With transition to the

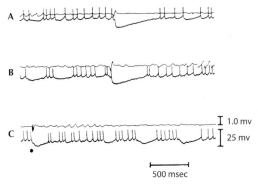

Figure 4–2. Three segments of intracellular recording from a neuron in a cortical inhibitory surround (lower trace) and simultaneous EEG (upper trace). **A, B.** Spontaneous surface paroxysmal discharges are associated with small EPSPs and long IPSPs (500 msec in **A**). **C.** IPSPs occurring spontaneously or following stimulation of ventrolateral nucleus (*dot*) are smaller in amplitude and duration than those associated with surface paroxysmal discharges. (From Prince and Wilder, 1967, with permission.)

ictal phase, focal tonic muscle contraction can occur, followed by slow spread to other muscle groups. A secondarily generalized tonic-clonic seizure results from axonal propagation of ictal discharge to contralateral cortex and subcortical structures (Fromm, 1987; Fromm et al., 1987).

Focal electrical stimulation and local application of convulsant drugs to limbic structures, particularly hippocampus and amygdala, as well as systemic administration of excitotoxic drugs that selectively activate hippocampus, such as *kainic acid* and *pilocarpine*, cause acute focal seizures with arrest reactions, chewing, and other oroalimentary symptoms, as originally described with *amygdala kindling* (Racine, 1972b), which will be discussed later. These ictal events are similar to limbic seizures seen in humans (Chapter 6). Secondarily generalized seizures develop less rapidly with limbic than with frontal neocortical experimental epileptic foci (Wada et al., 1978). The 6-Hz mouse model, believed to mimic pharmacoresistant limbic seizures in humans, is commonly used for screening of potential antiseizure drugs. These seizures are induced by 3 seconds of low-voltage 6-Hz stimulation via corneal electrodes (Barton et al., 2001).

Some parts of the brain have greater susceptibility to the induction of epileptic seizures than others. In general, hippocampus and amygdala have a lower threshold for electrically induced

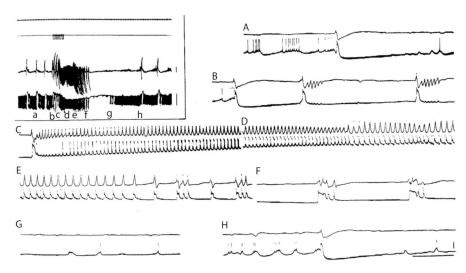

Figure 4–3. An ictal episode in a penicillin focus induced in the postsigmoid gyrus of a cat. The entire episode (including the preceding interictal pattern, the postictal stage, and its recovery) is shown in the inset, consisting of an ink-writing trace of the gross surface (*above*) and intracellular (*below*) activities. The ictal episode here is "facilitated" by a brief train of shocks at 1.5 Hz applied to the contralateral homologous region. Calibrations: 1 second, 2 mV for surface record, and 20 mV for intracellular record. Portions *a–h* are displayed for greater detail in oscilloscope tracings identified by the corresponding letters (*A–H*). The first three stimuli are shown in *B*. Note, in the postictal phase, the late recovery of PDS in comparison with that of "normal" action potentials *G* and *H*. Calibrations for intracellular record only: 500 msec and 10 mV. (From Ajmone-Marsan, 1969, with permission.)

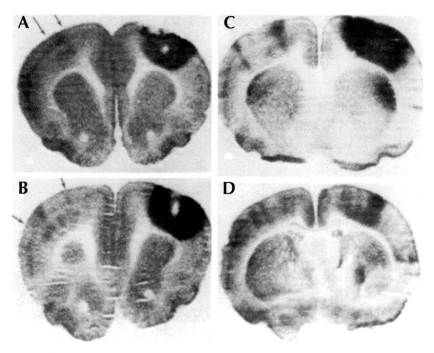

Figure 4–4. Deoxyglucose autoradiographs of an epileptogenic zone during repeated local application of penicillin. **A**. First injection of 25 units. The cortical focus is small and tightly contained on each side. The projection site contralateral to the focus is limited to a small patch of activity in layers III and V between the *arrows*. **B**. Tenth injection of 25 units. The focus is slightly larger and relatively more intense. The projection site in the contralateral cortex is considerably larger but still shows activity predominantly in the fifth lamina, with columnar extensions above this from layer III to the surface. **C**. After 100 units of penicillin the contralateral cortex shows prominent columnar activity. Columns run full thickness, with particular accentuation in layers III and V. There is increased activity in the dorsolateral aspect of both caudates, with a laminar pattern seen on the *left*. **D**. This section just posterior to the focus at the level of the anterior commissure shows columns in both hemispheres. The relative pallor lateral to the focus and absence of layer IV can be appreciated, reflecting decreased input from the inhibitory surround, which is contained within the area of hypermetabolism (Adapted from Collins, 1978, with permission.)

afterdischarge than neocortex (Seki and Wada, 1986). Even within relatively small structures such as the amygdala, regional differences in afterdischarge thresholds can be demonstrated (le Gal la Salle, 1981). An area in the *deep prepiriform cortex* of rats, *area tempestas*, has an extremely low threshold for seizures induced by local application of bicuculline, kainic acid, and carbachol (Gale, 1984; Gale et al., 2008). It is unknown what features of this area or its connections underlie its unique epileptogenicity. As with phylogenetic (Wada, 1978; Wilder et al., 1968) and ontogenetic (Holmes, 1986; Moshé, 1987; Schwartzkroin, 1984) differences in seizure susceptibility, these observations on regional anatomical differences could help to identify aspects of normal neuronal organization (Chapter 3) that predispose to the appearance of specific epileptiform phenomena.

IN VIVO MODELS OF GENERALIZED SEIZURES

Generalized seizures are commonly produced in mice by *electroconvulsive shock (ECS)*, administered to both ears or both eyes (Swinyard, 1972; Mares and Kubová, 2006). Systemic or *intracerebroventricular (ICV)* injection of most of the epileptogenic agents listed in Table 4–2, as well as inhalation of substances such as *flurothyl*, will give rise to generalized seizures (Velísek, 2006; Cortez and Snead, 2006). Phenomenological and pharmacological criteria have been used in classifying these generalized seizures as models of either human typical absences or generalized tonic-clonic seizures (see Table 4–1). Seizures that are commonly considered forms of experimental absence seizures consist largely of behavioral arrest and occasional twitching in association with bilaterally synchronous spike-and-wave EEG discharges (Cortez and Snead, 2006). Examples are the *subcutaneous pentylenetetrazol (PTZ) model* (Woodbury, 1972), the *feline generalized penicillin model* (induced by a large dose of intramuscular penicillin) (Gloor et al., 1977), the rat ICV enkephalin model (Urca et al., 1977), the α-*hydroxybutyrate model* (Snead, 1978), and the *tetrahydroxyisoxozolopyridine model* (Fariello and Golden, 1987). The mouse and rat *maximal electroshock seizure (MES)* is the classical animal model of a generalized tonic-clonic seizure (Swinyard, 1972; Mares and Kubová, 2006).

Experimental seizures blocked by drugs used clinically to treat typical absences (such as *ethosuximide* and *valproic acid*) are presumed to be generated by mechanisms similar to those that underlie these events in patients, whereas those blocked by drugs that are clinically effective against generalized tonic-clonic, but not absence, seizures (such as *phenytoin* and *carbamazepine*) are presumed to be generated by mechanisms similar to those underlying human generalized tonic-clonic seizures. Other drugs that have a broad spectrum of action against most types of experimental epilepsy do not elucidate the clinical relevance of specific experimental epileptic phenomena.

Several experimental models of generalized epileptic seizures are useful for screening potential anticonvulsant and antiabsence medications (Loscher and Schmidt, 1988; White et al., 2006). Maximal seizures induced by ECS, PTZ, and flurothyl are commonly used to identify drugs with possible anticonvulsant properties. The ability of pharmacological agents to reduce *posttetanic potentiation* in the spinal cord of cats also predicts their efficacy against generalized tonic-clonic seizures in humans (Woodbury, 1972). The subcutaneous PTZ-induced mouse seizure is the classical experimental model for screening potential antiabsence drugs; subcortical lesions and stimulation, as well as repetitive stimulation of the spinal cord of cats, have also been used for this purpose (Woodbury, 1972). The relative ineffectiveness of pharmacotherapy for limbic seizures probably reflects the failure, until recently, to include an animal model of these ictal events (e.g., *amygdala-kindled seizures*) during routine screening of drugs for antiseizure properties.

Some agents can produce both generalized tonic-clonic and absence-like seizures. Experimental absence seizures induced by PTZ (Woodbury, 1972) and some opioids (Snead and Bearden, 1980) are effectively blocked by ethosuximide but can progress to become generalized tonic-clonic seizures blocked by phenytoin. The generalized tonic-clonic seizures prevented by phenytoin most likely result from the ability of high-dose PTZ and opioids to interfere with GABA-mediated inhibition (Woodbury, 1980). The mechanisms responsible for the absence-like forms of PTZ- and opioid-induced seizures are related to their effects on inhibition in the thalamus, while convulsive opioid-induced seizures can result from disinhibition of hippocampal neurons (Dingledine, 1981). The bilaterally symmetrical 3-Hz spike-and-wave EEG discharges of the feline generalized penicillin model of petit mal epilepsy are generated in neocortex but triggered by synchronizing afferent input from those thalamic nuclei that normally produce augmenting and recruiting responses (Gloor et al., 1977) (Fig. 4–5). These observations led to replacement of the term *centrencephalic epilepsy* with *corticoreticular epilepsy* for clinical petit mal absence-type phenomena (Gloor, 1968).

It has been argued that petit mal absences are predominantly inhibitory seizures, because the prominent EEG slow waves suggest inhibitory axosomatic membrane events and because ethosuximide acts by antagonizing the effects of thalamic inhibition (Engel, 1987; 1988a). Studies of the feline generalized penicillin model have demonstrated that the slow wave of the spike-and-wave discharge is associated with chloride-sensitive (and therefore GABA-mediated) IPSPs in neocortical neurons (Giaretta et al., 1987). Some GABA agonists can actually produce these absence-like seizures (Fariello and Golden, 1987; Cortez and Snead, 2006). The cortical spike-and-wave discharge results from pacemaking discharges of cortically projecting neurons in thalamic relay nuclei. The rhythmic firing of these cells is mediated by *low-voltage T-type Ca²⁺ currents* and *hyperpolarization-activated cyclic nucleotide-gated cation (HCN) channels* activated by hyperpolarizing inhibitory input from GABAergic neurons in the thalamic reticular formation (McCormick and Contreras, 2001; Blumenfeld and Coulter, 2008) (Fig. 4–6) (Chapter 3). These discharges can be provoked

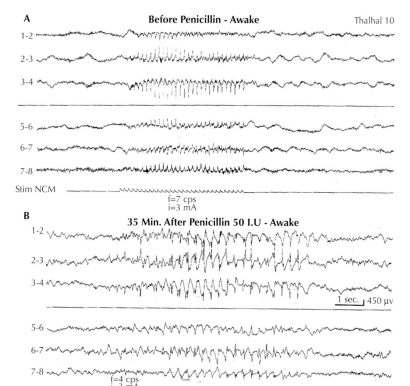

Figure 4–5. Cortical EEG recording from a cat. **A.** Before penicillin application, 7-Hz stimulation of nucleus centre median (*NCM*) elicits a recruiting response. **B.** After diffuse cortical penicillin application in the same animal, 4-Hz stimulation of nucleus centre median elicits bilaterally synchronous spike-and-wave activity. The letter *i* signifies intensity, and *f* frequency, of stimulation. (From Gloor et al., 1977, with permission.)

by thalamic stimulation when penicillin is selectively applied to the neocortex but not to the thalamus, which indicates that the abnormality can result from normal afferent input to abnormally epileptogenic neocortex.

Although generalized tonic-clonic seizures can be provoked by stimulation of subcortical structures, most evidence supports a view that these seizures are initiated in neocortex (Gloor, 1968; Velísek, 2006; Mares and Kubová, 2006). Minimal electroshock–induced seizures are likely models of myoclonic seizures, while MES models generalized tonic-clonic seizures. The mechanisms responsible for propagation of ictal discharge to spinal motor neurons are unknown but must involve the reticular core of the brain stem and spinal cord (Fromm et al., 1987). Lesion experiments suggest that structures in the pontine reticular formation mediate the tonic phase of generalized tonic-clonic seizures and the running, bouncing clonus of audiogenic seizures, but not the clonic phase of PTZ or flurothyl seizures (Browning, 1987). The use of 2-deoxyglucose (2DG) autoradiography clearly shows activation of *substantia*

nigra during generalized motor seizures (Engel et al., 1978), but whether this structure plays a facilitatory (Gale, 1984) or an inhibitory (Moshé et al., 1986) role remains controversial (Gale et al., 2008).

IN VITRO STUDIES OF ACUTE SEIZURES

Tissue-slice preparations and *dissociated cell cultures* are also used in the study of acute epileptic phenomena. Epileptiform electrographic discharges can be induced in tissue slices by a variety of manipulations, including bathing the medium in convulsant drugs, changing relative ionic concentrations, and applying specific electrical stimulation (Heinemann and Lambert, 1986; Schwartzkroin, 1986; Swartzwelder et al., 1987; Jefferys, 2008; see also Pitkänen et al., 2006b). These studies have helped researchers to define the local circuits involved in ictal discharges recorded from hippocampal and neocortical slices, to identify factors that lead to epileptiform excitability, and to construct models of neural networks that might explain hypersynchrony on the basis of

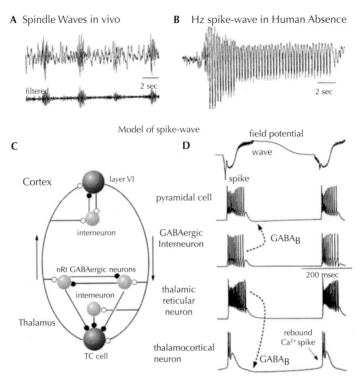

Figure 4–6. Possible cellular mechanisms of the generation of spike-wave seizures in human absence. A. Spindle waves during slow-wave sleep in the normal EEG are intermixed with delta waves and recur once every few seconds. **B.** Single EEG trace during an absence attack, illustrating the striking 3-Hz spike-wave activity that characterizes this state. This spike-wave activity is widely synchronized throughout the EEG (not shown). **C.** Simplified diagram of thalamocortical interactions proposed to underlie the generation of some forms of spike-wave activities. Cortical pyramidal cells (in layer VI) and thalamocortical cells (*TC cell*) form mutually excitatory connections (*open circles*) that are regulated through the activation of GABAergic interneurons within the thalamus, cortex, and thalamic reticular nucleus (*nRt*). (Inhibitory synaptic connections are denoted with *filled circles*.) **D.** Stimulation of one cycle of a spike-wave seizure in thalamocortical networks. A burst of spikes in a neuron activates the cortical network, which generates a strong burst of action potentials through intracortical recurrent excitatory connections. This activity strongly activates both local GABAergic neurons and thalamic reticular neurons. The buildup of K^+ currents, including the activation of $GABA_B$ receptors and the inactivation of depolarizing currents such as the low-threshold Ca^{2+} spike in thalamocortical cells, results in the cessation of activity in the network. The generation of a rebound Ca^{2+} spike in the thalamocortical cell 300 msec later initiates the next cycle of the oscillation. (From McCormick and Contreras, 2001, with permission.)

nonsynaptic as well as synaptic mechanisms (Knowles et al., 1985). Although inhibition promotes synchrony (Chapter 7), some studies have suggested that hypersynchronization may result in part from loss of inhibitory control over recurrent polysynaptic excitatory pathways (Miles and Wong, 1987) and that NMDA receptor–mediated mechanisms are responsible for stimulation-induced reductions in GABAergic inhibition (Stelzer et al., 1987). Dissociated cell cultures can be used to examine synaptic and nonsynaptic membrane responses to various convulsant agents and antiseizure drugs (McLean and Macdonald, 1986; Stewart et al., 2006; Dichter and Pollard, 2006), in some cases using recordings from single channels.

Although in vitro techniques are well suited for dissecting out specific mechanisms of excitability at the membrane and local circuit level, these preparations lack many important afferent and efferent synaptic connections that exist in the intact brain. Furthermore, electrotonic and field potential influences, which are important for regulating activity within a small population of neurons, may not be sufficient for synchronizing the larger, often widespread epileptogenic regions necessary for behavioral seizures to occur. Insights obtained from in vitro studies, therefore, must be coordinated with data obtained at the systems level from in vivo experimental models of seizures and epilepsy and, as with all animal research, must be validated in the human condition.

Chronic Models

Chronic models of epilepsy more faithfully reproduce the phenomenology of human epilepsy than acute models of seizures and allow investigation of interictal epileptogenic abnormalities and ictogenesis. However, chronic models are more expensive to prepare and maintain than acute models and are much more difficult in many respects to bring under adequate experimental control. Although the focal/generalized dichotomy no longer is used with respect to clinical epilepsy syndromes (Chapter 1), it is useful to divide chronic models into those that give rise to focal seizures and those that give rise to generalized seizures. It is important to note that animal models of chronic epilepsy are created by inducing an epileptogenic disturbance into an animal with a presumably normal brain, which is not necessarily the situation with human epilepsy. We now know that certain *susceptibility genes* and other predisposing factors may be necessary before a specific epileptogenic insult can cause the development of acquired epilepsy in some patients, the so-called *two-hit hypothesis* (Chapter 5). More accurate animal models of acquired human epilepsy conditions will require that the genetic substrates and predisposing factors of human acquired epilepsies be identified and that experimental epileptogenic insults be introduced in appropriately susceptible animals (Engel and Bertram, 2004).

IN VIVO MODELS OF EPILEPSY WITH FOCAL SEIZURES

Lesion and Insult Models

Perhaps the oldest experimental model of epilepsy is the *cortical freeze* model (Lewin, 1972, Luhmann, 2006), which was first produced 140 years ago by Openchowski (Openchowski, 1883). Brief exposure of a small area of cortex to dry ice, ethyl chloride spray, or a cold metal rod leads to the gradual appearance of focal interictal spikes. However, spontaneous seizures develop in only a minority of animals so treated. The interictal focal epileptiform abnormality can persist for many weeks, although it may be necessary to activate it with convulsant

drugs such as PTZ. Intracellular recordings have revealed PDS generation similar to that seen in the penicillin focus (Goldensohn, 1969). Freezing is believed to create structural changes in membranes that disrupt water and ion movement, but the exact mechanism of epileptogenicity in this model is unknown.

Undercutting and partially transecting an area of neocortex is another old technique for producing a chronic intermittent experimental epileptic focus (Echlin, 1959; Graber and Prince, 2006). Neurons within this *partially isolated cortical slab* show enhanced responsiveness to topically applied *acetylcholine (ACh)*, presumably as a result of denervation hypersensitivity (Echlin, 1959). Structural reorganization also occurs with growth of the severed axons back into the partially isolated slab, enhancing recurrent excitation (Purpura, 1961). The chronic epileptiform excitability can be prevented by repeated electrical stimulation of the cortical slab, which appears to reduce excitatory and increase inhibitory synaptic terminals within the reorganized cortical tissue (Rutledge et al., 1967). Studies of the neuronal reorganization that occurs after partial isolation could provide insights into the development of *posttraumatic epilepsy (PTE)* in patients (Graber and Prince, 2006).

Local application of toxic metals is commonly used for inducing focal epileptogenesis. Such epileptogenic agents include *alumina cream* or *aluminum hydroxide gel, cobalt, tungstic acid,* and *iron* or *ferric chloride* (Wilson et al., 1987; Ribak et al., 2006; Ueda et al., 2006). The last two are of theoretical interest because cortical hemosiderin deposits resulting from hemoglobin breakdown may be important in the development of PTE (Wilson et al., 1987; Ueda et al., 2006).

The *monkey alumina model* (Lockard et al., 1980; Ribak et al., 2006) was considered a useful model of human focal epilepsy in the past, but it has become unpopular because of the high cost of animal maintenance and limitations placed on primate research. Alumina lesions can generate spontaneous seizures that last for years. Monkeys can be observed continuously for alterations in seizure severity and frequency due to treatment with specific antiseizure drugs (Lockard and Levy, 1982) as well as to other manipulations and to physiological state changes such as diurnal cycles and pregnancy (Phillips and Lockard, 1985). Although the usual monkey alumina lesion is neocortical, limbic seizures can also be induced, by introduction of alumina into the amygdala and hippocampus. In this situation, bilateral lesions are necessary for the development of spontaneous recurrent limbic seizures (Soper et al., 1978).

Intracellular microelectrode recordings from alumina neocortical foci demonstrate large depolarization shifts followed by prolonged hyperpolarizations, similar to membrane events seen in the interictal penicillin focus (Prince and Futamachi, 1970). However, these are not as common or robust as in the penicillin focus, nor are burst firing events as synchronous (Wyler, 1986). One view is that a small population of pacemaker neurons initiate the interictal paroxysmal events and that passive neurons are then recruited into the process during the transition from the interictal to the ictal state (Wyler et al., 1975).

The dendrites of some pyramidal neurons within the neocortical alumina focus have decreased branching and are denuded of normal spinous processes (Westrum et al., 1964). There is also evidence for a decreased number of GABAergic inhibitory synapses (Ribak et al., 1979). Epileptogenicity in this situation could theoretically result from (1) enhanced excitatory influences due to the presence of excitatory synaptic terminals ending directly on the dendritic shaft and closer to the axon hillock, (2) reorganization of Ca^{2+} channel distribution, giving rise to large depolarization shifts closer to the axon hillock, and (3) a reduction in GABA-mediated inhibitory synaptic influences (Schwartzkroin and Wyler, 1980). Although there is no direct evidence that these structurally abnormal neurons in the monkey alumina model generate epileptiform membrane events, such events have been shown with similarly abnormal neurons in slice preparations from patients (Isokawa and Levesque, 1991), as will be discussed later.

Experimental *status-induced hippocampal sclerosis* with resultant spontaneous limbic seizures in rats and mice is now the model most commonly used for studying fundamental neuronal mechanisms of limbic epilepsy. Prolonged electrical stimulation of limbic structures, the *self-sustained status epilepticus (SSE)* model (Handforth and Ackermann, 1989; Lothman and Williamson, 1994; McIntyre et al., 1982; Mazarati et al., 2006), systemic application of *pilocarpine* (Cavalheiro et al., 2006), both local and systemic application of *kainic acid* (Ben-

Ari et al., 1981; Bragin et al., 1999c; 2005; Tanaka et al., 1982; Dudek et al., 2006), and, most recently, hyperthermia- and perinatal hypoxia-induced status epilepticus (Dubé and Baram, 2006; Sanchez and Jensen, 2006) lead to hippocampal cell loss and neuronal reorganization. These pathological changes resemble the *hippocampal sclerosis* commonly found in patients with limbic seizures (Babb and Brown, 1987; Margerison and Corsellis, 1966; Mathern et al., 2008) (Chapters 5 and 6). Because these *poststatus models* result in an enduring disturbance that generates spontaneous recurrent limbic seizures weeks or months later (Tanaka et al., 1982), they are regarded as models of human *mesial temporal lobe epilepsy (MTLE) with hippocampal sclerosis* (Chapter 7). The characteristic poststatus cell loss in the rat primarily involves pyramidal cells in area CA3 of hippocampus, inhibitory interneurons containing *somatostatin* and *neuropeptide Y (NPY)* as well as excitatory mossy cells in the hilus, and principal neurons of the subiculum. Loss of mossy cells results in degeneration of their axon projections back to the *inner molecular layer* of the dentate gyrus. Denuded postsynaptic membranes of proximal granule cell dendrites secrete trophic factors which induce the granule cell axons (*mossy fibers*) to sprout collaterals and reinnervate the inner molecular layer of the dentate (Fig. 4–7). *Mossy fiber sprouting* not only results in excitatory synapses on proximal granule cell dendrites, creating a monosynaptic recurrent excitatory circuit (Tauck et al., 1985; Engel et al., 2008a), but also in enhanced feedback inhibition due to increased excitatory collateral innervation of inhibitory interneurons in the inner molecular layer (Sloviter et al., 2006; Engel et al., 2008a). This mechanism reinforces dentate gate restriction on the flow of activity from entorhinal cortex to the hippocampus proper, providing a homeostatic protective mechanism. However, once epileptiform discharges break through, dentate inhibition also induces hypersynchronization, predisposing to the characteristic hypersynchronized EEG ictal onset pattern recorded from status models of MTLE as well as from patients with hippocampal sclerosis, as discussed later in this chapter (Engel et al., 2008a). Animals with hippocampal damage induced by status epilepticus also exhibit interictal behavioral changes (Engel et al., 1986a;b; Griffith et al., 1987), which could share common mechanisms with

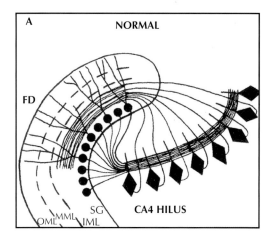

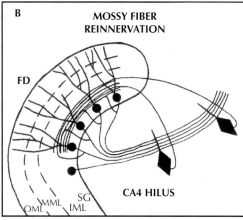

Hz (higher than that of normal ripples) termed *fast ripples* (Engel and Lopes da Silva, 2012; Le Van Quyen and Gotman, 2012; Staba and Bragin, 2011; Worrell and Gotman, 2011) (Figs. 4–8 and 4–9). These can be recorded from the sclerotic hippocampus of poststatus rat models as well as from patients with MTLE (Bragin et al., 1999a;b). Although HFOs in the 100- to 200-Hz range, termed *ripples*, are normal electrophysiological events (Chapter 3), it is now known that oscillation frequency does not distinguish between normal and pathological oscillations. Ripple-frequency oscillations can be recorded from

Figure 4–7. This schematic diagram illustrates the reorganization of neuronal integration observed in sclerotic hippocampus surgically removed from patients with temporal lobe epilepsy. **A.** Under normal conditions, dentate granule cells (*black circles*) located in fascia dentata (*FD*) send mossy fiber axons to excite dendrites of hilar cells (*black diamonds*) located in the CA4 region of hippocampus. These hilar cells send axons back into the inner molecular layer (*IML*) of the fascia dentata to excite proximal dendrites of granule cells. **B.** With hippocampal sclerosis some hilar cells die, afferent input of IML is lost, and mossy fibers sprout to occupy vacated postsynaptic membrane. Such reinnervation of granule cell dendrites by granule cell axons is believed to constitute monosynaptic recurrent excitatory circuits, which could contribute to the development of epileptiform activity. *SG, MML,* and *OML* refer to the stratum granulosum, middle molecular layer, and outer molecular layer divisions of the fascia dentata.

epilepsy-related behavioral disturbances seen in patients with limbic seizures (Chapter 11).

Of particular recent interest is the identification of *pathological high-frequency oscillations (pHFOs),* first defined as brief abnormal events with a frequency of 200–600

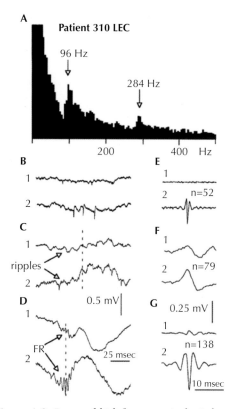

Figure 4–8. Low- and high-frequency ripples in human entorhinal cortex. **A.** Power spectrum of electrical activity recorded from microelectrode 2. Recording bandwidth: 0.1–10,000 Hz. Note peaks at 96 and 284 Hz. **B-D.** Examples of the unit activity, ripples, and fast ripples (*FR*) recorded from the same file with two electrodes within entorhinal cortex. **E-G.** Averages of events for electrodes 1 and 2; *n* is the number of events in each average. Because of similarities of amplitudes, the events were selected into different files by visual estimation. Single-unit activity was recorded only from microelectrode 2; note that ripples are in phase on both electrodes and the fast ripples are out of phase. (From Bragin et al., 1999a, with permission.)

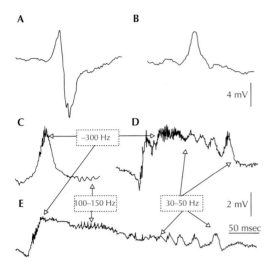

Figure 4–9. Examples of interictal spikes (**A**, **B**), fast ripples (**C**), and fast ripple-tail gamma complexes (**D**, **E**) recorded during the interictal state. Numbers within dashed boxes indicate the frequency of oscillations indicated by arrows. Upper amplitude calibration is for **A** and **B**, bottom for **C–E**. The time calibration is the same for all records. The large amplitude of the events in **A** and **B** identifies them as interictal spikes (IISs). (From Bragin et al., 1999b, with permission.)

epileptic dentate gyrus, which is not capable of generating normal ripples, indicating that these are pHFOs, while some normal neocortical areas can generate fast-ripple-frequency oscillations (Engel et al., 2009). It is, therefore, likely that at least some ripple-frequency oscillations in epileptic hippocampus and other limbic structures where normal ripples occur are actually pHFOs, while not all fast-ripple-frequency oscillations in neocortex are necessarily abnormal.

Pathophysiological oscillations can be distinguished from normal oscillations electrophysiologically. Whereas normal ripples occur diffusely over wide areas of tissue and reflect summated IPSPs (Buzsáki et al., 1992; Ylinen et al., 1995), pHFOs are localized to small neuronal clusters, are associated with decreased firing of interneurons, and reflect summated action potentials (*population spikes*), most likely from the synchronously bursting neurons that characterize the epileptogenic region (Engel et al., 2009; Staba and Bragin, 2011). Importantly, pHFOs appear to initiate ictal events (Bragin et al., 1999c) and to be uniquely

localized to brain tissue capable of generating spontaneous seizures, both in experimental animal models and in patients (Staba and Bragin, 2011; Jacobs et al., 2010; Worrell and Gotman, 2011), suggesting that they reflect the basic neuronal substrates of epilepsy. Pathological HFOs can also be recorded early after status and predict which animals will develop spontaneous seizures (Bragin et al., 2004). Therefore, pHFOs appear to be indicators of epileptogenic mechanisms and, interestingly, do not depend on mossy fiber sprouting, which occurs later (Bragin et al., 2004). Based on these findings, pHFOs are being considered as potential clinical biomarkers of epileptogenesis and epileptogenicity (Chapter 12).

Pathological HFOs are not widely distributed throughout epileptic hippocampus but are generated in small clusters of neurons embedded within more normal tissue (Bragin et al., 1999a;b). These clusters are spatially stable over time (Bragin et al., 2003) but increase in size with decreases in tonic inhibition (Bragin et al., 2002a) (Fig. 4–10). Evidence suggests that bursts of pHFOs, generated by principal neurons, are preceded by a reduction in firing of inhibitory neurons (Bragin et al., 2011). Therefore, a potential mechanism of ictogenesis is that naturally occurring alterations in the extracellular milieu that reduce inhibitory influences could cause these clusters to enlarge, coalesce, synchronize, and propagate (Engel et al., 2009) (Figs. 4–11 and 4–12).

The *lateral fluid percussion model* of *traumatic brain injury (TBI)* and PTE (Pitkänen et al., 2006a) are under intensive investigation, because of the increasing incidence of TBI and PTE as a result of the wars in Iraq and Afghanistan. There are several approaches to fluid percussion, but the most commonly used model induces a large area of lateral cortical encephalomalacia, hippocampal sclerosis, and chronic seizures; however, the exact site of ictal onset, hippocampal or neocortical, has not yet been established. Less severe percussion produces brief, subtle events that could reflect ictal mechanisms similar to those of human frontal lobe seizures (D'Ambrosio and Miller, 2010a;b), but this interpretation has been challenged (Dudek and Bertram, 2010).

Other acquired focal models of chronic epilepsy include manipulations such as infection (Stringer, 2006); *experimental brain tumors*

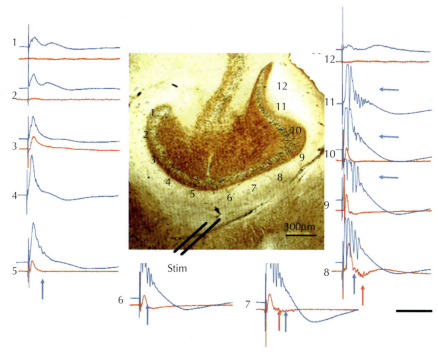

Figure 4–10. *1–12:* Fast-ripple-like responses from the in vitro dentate gyrus in normal ACSF *(thick lines)* and after the addition of 10 μm bicuculline to the perfusate *(thin lines)*. *Center:* Timm's-stained section demonstrating sprouting of mossy fibers in the inner molecular layer in relation to the positions of the recording sites that were stimulated to evoke the field potentials shown in *1–12*. (From Bragin et al., 2002a, with permission.)

(Gorji and Speckmann, 2006); focal application of *anti-GM1 ganglioside antibodies* (Karpiak et al., 1982); and cortical and hippocampal injections of *tetanus toxin*, which blocks GABA release and produces chronic focal seizures, though the primary cause of epileptogenesis in this case remains unclear (McIntyre and Goddard, 1973; Jefferys and Walker, 2006). A rat model of *Alzheimer disease (AD)* also exhibits spontaneous epileptic seizures (Palop et al., 2007), and there is increasing interest in possible mechanistic relationships between epilepsy and AD. The discovery of genetic mutations responsible for some human epilepsy conditions has made it at least theoretically possible to produce transgenic mice that can be used to study fundamental mechanisms of those disorders as well as to screen potential antiseizure drugs. An example of such a disorder is *autosomal dominant nocturnal frontal lobe epilepsy (ADNFLE)* (Klaassen et al., 2006; Mann and Mody, 2008) (Chapter 7).

Models in the Developing Brain

Epileptogenesis in the developing brain is not necessarily similar to epileptogenesis in the adult brain, and there is a great need for valid animal models of pediatric epilepsy syndromes (Auvin et al., 2012; Nehlig et al., 2012). The lesions and other insults described above are not models of pediatric epilepsy; not only is the immature brain relatively resistant to these epileptogenic mechanisms (Chapter 3), but when an epileptogenic insult introduced in the immature brain eventually results in spontaneous seizures, they begin in adulthood. Specific pediatric epilepsy conditions with focal seizures that have been reproduced in the animal laboratory include *perinatal hypoxia, complex febrile seizures* or *febrile status epilepticus, cortical dysplasia*, and *tuberous sclerosis*.

Perinatal hypoxia induces immediate and late-onset seizures in rodents and can be used to model neonatal hypoxic seizures, hypoxic encephalopathy, and resultant chronic, presumably focal seizures in humans (Sanchez

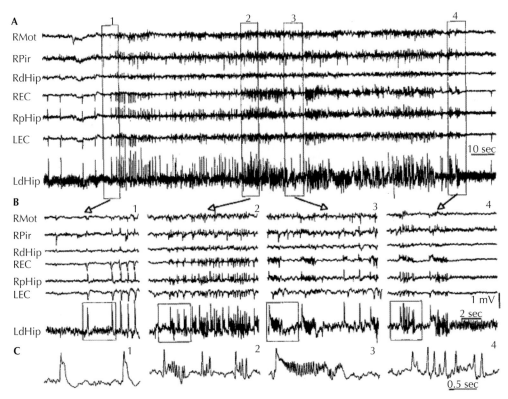

Figure 4–11. A. Example of a hypersynchronous-onset seizure in a rat. **B, C.** Expanded parts indicated by boxes. *B1, C1:* Seizure onset with a pattern similar to IIS in the period preceding the seizure. *B2, C2:* Transition period between IIS and fast ripple-tail gamma (FRTG) complex. *B3, C3:* Period of seizure dominated by FRTG complexes. *B4, C4:* Spike-burst pattern at the end of the seizure. (Fast ripples cannot be seen in this illustration because of low sampling rate of the recording.) (From Bragin et al., 1999b, with permission.)

and Jensen, 2006; Rakhade et al., 2011). *Hyperthermia-induced* generalized seizures in immature animals have been used as an experimental model of human febrile seizures (Millichap, 1968; Swann et al., 2008; Dubé and Baram, 2006). Susceptibility to hyperthermia-induced seizures is age-related. Newborn rats are less susceptible than adults to kainic acid–induced hippocampal cell damage (Albala et al., 1984; Nehlig et al., 2012), and a few seizures produced at an early age by this method have not affected the rate of subsequent kindling in adulthood (Okada et al., 1984). Repetitive seizures in neonatal rats can, however, alter the seizure threshold later in life and cause cognitive deficits that are worsened by maternal deprivation (Swann et al., 2008; Zhao and Holmes, 2006; Nehlig et al., 2012). A concern about the neonatal hypoxia (Rakhade et al., 2011) and hyperthermia (Dubé and Baram, 2006) models, as currently used, is that

they do not appear to cause neuronal structural brain damage; there remains controversy as to whether acquired epileptogenesis occurs without cell loss (Baram et al., 2011; Dudek et al., 2010).

Animal models of *cortical dysplasia* can be produced by *methylazoxymethanol acetate (MAM)* administration, *freezing, radiation,* and *ibotenate* injection in fetal and newborn rodents (Battaglia and Bassanini, 2006; Lin and Roper, 2006; Auvin et al., 2012; Nehlig et al., 2012). Although these interventions disrupt cortical development and produce seizures, they do not produce *balloon cells* or replicate histopathological features of *Taylor-type cortical dysplasia* (Chapter 5). Several rodent genetic models of cortical dysplasia are under investigation (Nehlig et al., 2012). Transgenic mice have also been developed to model *tuberous sclerosis,* which can be prevented by early inhibition of the *mammalian target of rapamycin*

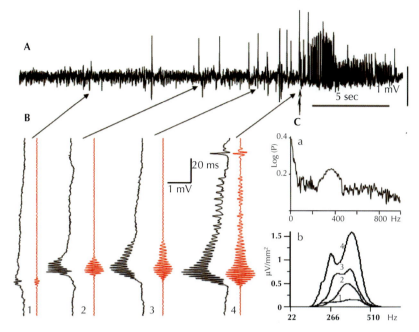

Figure 4–12. Evolution of EEG interictal spikes and fast ripple (FR)-frequency oscillations occurring at different times before seizure onset. **A.** EEG record of seizure. FR frequency, amplitude, and duration increase with proximity to seizure. Seizure onset indicated by *double-headed arrow*. **B.** Expanded examples of wideband recorded EEG spikes (*left*) and bandpass-filtered (80–500 Hz) oscillations (*right*). **C.** *a:* Power spectrogram of averaged HFO in wideband records shown in part **B.** *b:* Power spectrogram of bandpass-filtered HFOs shown in part **B.** (From Bragin et al., 2005, with permission.)

(mTOR) signaling pathway by treatment with *rapamycin* (Zheng et al., 2008) (Chapters 5 and 7). Whereas tuberous sclerosis is characterized clinically by multiple tubers, the brain of this mouse model consists essentially of one large tuber. The *Eker rat,* a model caused by a mutation in the *TSC2* gene, does not have tubers or spontaneous seizures but does have an increased response to chemical kindling (Tschuluun et al., 2007; Waltereit et al., 2006).

Secondary Epileptogenesis

Chronic focal epileptogenic lesions of all kinds can cause distant areas to become capable of generating epileptiform electrical discharges and, in some cases, spontaneous epileptic seizures. The best-defined example of this *secondary epileptogenesis* is the *mirror focus* (Morrell, 1959/60), an independent epileptogenic area of cortex that is contralateral and homotopic to a primary epileptogenic lesion. The independence of a mirror focus is proven by its persistence after ablation of the primary epileptogenic lesion (Engel, 1968; Morrell, 1959/60).

Secondary epileptic foci presumably develop as a result of continuous epileptiform bombardment along fiber tracts, which can cause downstream morphological changes (Engel and Morrell, 1970). Because the corpus callosum appears to be the most effective pathway for mediating this effect, mirror foci do not develop in cortical areas without strong callosal connections to the opposite hemisphere (Harris and Lockard, 1981). Nor do they develop when the corpus callosum has been sectioned (Morrell 1959/60), although temporal lobe lesions in split-brain primates have been reported as an exception (Nie et al., 1974). The time required for development of the mirror focus depends on the species and the length of the connecting fiber pathway. This period ranges from days in a rat, through weeks in a cat, to months or years, if at all, in primates (Wilder et al., 1968). Whether or not mirror foci develop in humans with focal epilepsy and, if so, under what conditions are issues that continue to be debated (Chapter 8).

The fundamental mechanisms of epileptogenesis have been a matter of increasing interest as a result of renewed efforts to develop antiepileptogenic interventions that could prevent epilepsy (Löscher and Brandt, 2010; Pitkänen, 2010). Although all of the models of acquired chronic epilepsy discussed previously involve a latent period during which epileptogenesis occurs, the epileptogenic process is inconsistent and often difficult to study. Secondary epileptogenesis was long ago brought under experimental control by the procedure known as *kindling* (Corcoran and Moshé, 2005; Wada, 1976;1981;1986; McIntyre, 2006), whereby focal electrical stimulation substitutes for seizures of the primary epileptogenic area. The mechanisms of kindled epileptogenesis, however, also appear to reproduce some of the mechanisms responsible for epileptogenesis at the primary focus after local synchronous burst firing has already begun, and the model has been primarily used for this purpose. Brief trains of weak electrical stimulation (usually 1 second at 60–100 Hz) are repeatedly delivered at appropriate intervals (usually 2 to 24 hours) to susceptible brain areas. Stimuli that initially produce EEG afterdischarges without associated behavioral symptoms subsequently give rise to more prolonged afterdischarges and a gradual progression of epileptic behavior, evolving through various stages to a secondarily generalized tonic-clonic seizure (Racine, 1972a;b). If stimulation is terminated at this stage, restimulation following a long rest period (periods of up to three years have been studied) will still produce the epileptic behavior (Wada et al., 1974). Although kindled epileptogenicity is enduring, kindling, as usually practiced, is not actually a complete model of epilepsy, because seizures need to be triggered by stimulation and do not occur spontaneously. Prolonged kindling, however, can result in the appearance of spontaneous seizures as a result of epileptogenic plastic changes downstream from the stimulating electrodes (Pinel and Rovner, 1978; Wada et al., 1974). The clinical relevance of kindling has been challenged, because human epileptogenesis does not demonstrate the stereotyped progression of ictal symptoms observed in kindled animals; however, this variability could reflect the increased complexity of the human brain and the confounding factors of medical intervention (Engel, 1998a; Engel and Cahan, 1986; Engel and Shewmon, 1991; Morrell et al., 1987) (Chapter 8).

Kindling is worth discussing in detail, because it allows the epileptogenic process to be viewed as a number of distinct pathophysiological phenomena, each of which appears to involve different neuronal mechanisms, and each of which may be relevant to different aspects of human epilepsy: (1) Initially there is increasing excitability at the site of stimulation, best demonstrated by the fact that repeated subthreshold stimulation eventually results in the appearance of an afterdischarge (Racine, 1972a). Progressive changes in the pattern and duration of afterdischarge also indicate increased excitability of local neurons as well as functional neuronal reorganization. (2) Transsynaptic changes then occur within distant structures to which the afterdischarge projects. This can be demonstrated by enhanced evoked potentials (Racine et al., 1975) and by the *transfer effect*, in which a *secondary site* (e.g., contralateral amygdala or ipsilateral hippocampus after completion of amygdala kindling) kindles at a much faster rate than the same structure would as a primary site (McIntyre, 1975; McIntyre and Goddard, 1973). A negative *interference effect* also occurs, in which secondary-site kindling reduces the epileptogenicity of the primary site (McIntyre, 1975; McIntyre and Goddard, 1973). (3) At some point, a generalized seizure-generating mechanism is engaged. The cerebral systems responsible for this predictable and stereotyped seizure stage are accessed by both limbic and nonlimbic kindling. Use of 2DG autoradiography indicates involvement of bilateral cerebral structures, including the thalamus, substantia nigra, and neocortex (Fig. 4–13) (Engel et al., 1978). The corpus callosum appears to be necessary for the development of bilateral synchrony (Wada and Komai, 1985). Bilateral frontal lesions can delay, but not prevent, the appearance of generalized seizures (Wada and Wake, 1977). Lesions of the mesencephalic reticular formation abolish fully kindled generalized seizures but have no effect on the development of kindled epileptogenesis (Wada and Sato, 1975). These last findings demonstrate that the neuronal mechanisms underlying the establishment of kindled epileptogenesis are different from those responsible for kindled ictogenesis (Albala et al., 1984). (4) Finally, additional enduring disturbances occur at a distance from the stimulation electrodes, accounting for the appearance of spontaneous

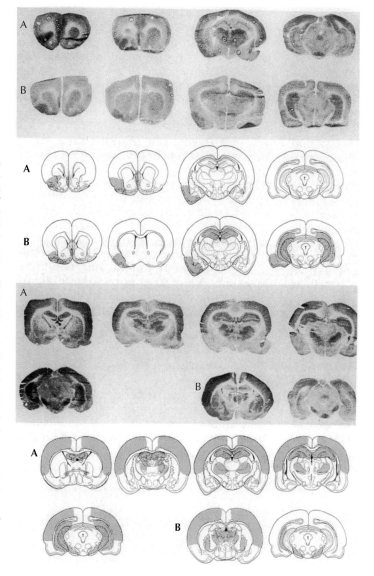

Figure 4–13. *Top:* Representative autoradiograms with line interpretations from two rats (*A* and *B*) with Stage 1 kindled seizures. Both show increased deoxyglucose (DG) uptake in the left anterior limbic field, medial septal area, and entorhinal and piriform cortices. Some uptake in ipsilateral or contralateral basolateral nucleus of the amygdala is also seen. One rat shows bilateral hippocampus uptake. *Bottom:* Representative autoradiograms, with line interpretations, from two rats (*A* and *B*) with Stage 5 and 4 kindled seizures, respectively. Note increased DG uptake bilaterally in the substantia nigra, specific and nonspecific thalamus, and neocortex in both animals. One rat also shows bilaterally increased uptake in a small area ventral to the anterior commissure and lateral to the bed nuclei of the stria terminalis as well as in the right basolateral amygdala, whereas the other demonstrates bilateral uptake in the globus pallidus. The hippocampus is bilaterally involved in one rat and unilaterally involved in the other. Stimulating electrodes for all rats were in the left amygdala. In the line interpretations, areas of increased DG uptake are indicated by dots. (From Engel et al., 1978, with permission.)

epileptic seizures in animals that have been kindled for prolonged periods.

The rate of kindling—that is, the number of afterdischarges required to achieve a generalized tonic-clonic seizure—depends on many factors, including the interval between stimulus trains, the site of stimulation, the age of the animal, and the species stimulated. Under most conditions, an interval of 24 hours between kindling stimuli is most effective. More afterdischarges are required as stimulus trains are given at shorter intervals, and kindling generally fails when stimulations are separated by minutes rather than hours (Goddard et al., 1969). *Rapid*

kindling, however, can be achieved with longer stimulus trains (10 seconds) given at 30-minute intervals (Lothman and Williamson, 1994).

Kindled epileptogenesis can be achieved in most forebrain gray matter structures but does not occur with stimulation of brain stem or cerebellum (Goddard et al., 1969). Of limbic structures, piriform and perirhinal cortex require the fewest daily afterdischarges, approximately 3 to 10 in the rat. Amygdala kindling requires about 14 days, and hippocampus twice as many (Goddard et al., 1969). Kindling of limbic structures produces a stereotyped progression of symptoms without regression. In the rat, these begin with an arrest reaction and clonic twitching of the ipsilateral eye, followed by chewing (Stage 1), head bobbing (Stage 2), forelimb clonus (Stage 3), rearing (Stage 4), and falling (Stage 5) (Racine, 1972b). Neocortical, thalamic, and caudate kindling result in few behavioral changes until the explosive appearance of generalized motor seizure activity. These latter seizures are initially unstable, with frequent regression on repeated stimulations (Seki and Wada, 1986).

Kindling in cats involves similar progressive ictal changes (Shouse, 2006). The number of afterdischarges required for completion of kindling, however, is greater than in the rat, and kindling in the primate takes even longer (Wada, 1978). Amygdala kindling in the rhesus monkey takes several hundred days, but kindling in the genetically photosensitive baboon, *Papio papio*, takes only about 70 days. The end point of kindling in *Papio papio* is a generalized seizure, which does not occur in the rhesus monkey (Wada and Osawa, 1976). This demonstrates the important contribution of genetic factors in the development of an acquired epilepsy condition (Chapter 5).

Morphological damage has been difficult to document in kindled animals. Mossy fiber sprouting similar to that described for kainic acid lesions (Sutula et al., 1988) and an increase in the ratio of perforated to nonperforated synapses in the middle molecular layer of the dentate gyrus (Geinisman et al., 1988) have been reported following perforant path kindling in the rat; these changes could reflect responses to repetitive epileptiform activity or perhaps to cell loss. Whether kindling requires cell loss, however, is still debated (McIntyre, 2006), and kindling can occur in the absence of mossy fiber sprouting (Sperber et al., 1991). Electrophysiological studies have demonstrated enhanced excitatory influences, as evidenced by bursting neurons (Racine et al., 1981), as well as enhanced inhibitory influences, as evidenced by perforant path hippocampal *paired-pulse suppression* (Tuff et al., 1983a), but pHFOs do not occur, presumably because the brain is not capable of generating spontaneous seizures (Bragin et al., 1999b). Perforant path hippocampal paired pulse suppression refers to the absence of normal *paired-pulse facilitation* (Chapter 3): the second of two pulses to entorhinal cortex, 40–100 msec after the first produces a reduced response, rather than a normal enhanced response, in the dentate gyrus of the hippocampus. Response decrement to the second stimulus can last many hundreds of milliseconds. This pronounced refractory period after the initial evoked potential is believed to reflect a chronic upregulation of recurrent GABAergic inhibitory mechanisms (Tuff et al., 1983b), although this interpretation has been challenged (Waldbaum and Dudek, 2009). Enhanced excitability, however, has been demonstrated by paired-pulse facilitation with stimulation of hippocampal association pathways (Wilson et al., 1998), indicating that inhibitory and excitatory pathways are both facilitated in the epileptogenic hippocampus.

The first studies to clearly demonstrate increased seizure susceptibility of the immature brain and to elucidate developmental aspects of epileptic excitability used kindling (Moshé, 1981). Kindled rat pups rarely exhibit Stage 5 seizures but do progress from focal to tonic seizures (Moshé and Albala, 1983). Postictal seizure suppression is markedly reduced compared with adults (Baram et al., 1998), and there is no negative interference effect with bilateral kindling (Haas et al., 1990), indicating that certain homeostatic inhibitory systems are absent early in life. The *substantia nigra pars reticulata* has been implicated in this maturational process (Moshé, 1987). Kindling does not cause cell loss or mossy fiber sprouting in rat pups, but these animals rekindle rapidly as adults with stimulation on either side, indicating that obvious structural changes are not necessary to retain enhanced epileptogenicity. Kindling has provided an ideal means to bring differences in the process of secondary epileptogenesis under laboratory control in order to elucidate fundamental mechanisms that promote and suppress epileptic excitability.

Investigations into the molecular basis of kindling (Morimoto et al., 2004) have been inconclusive. *Chemical kindling* occurs with repeated focal application of *muscarinic* drugs such as *carbachol*, which suggests a role for muscarinic receptors in kindled epileptogenesis (Wasterlain and Fairchild, 1985; Gilbert and Goodman, 2006). However, attempts to block electrical kindling with the muscarinic antagonist *atropine* have yielded conflicting data (Corcoran et al., 1976). The *biogenic amines* appear to suppress kindling, because stimulation of raphe nucleus serotonergic neurons retards the development of kindled seizures (Kovacs and Zoll, 1974) whereas depletion of forebrain noradrenaline facilitates it (Ehlers et al., 1980). Amygdala kindling has been reported to produce prolonged reduction in amygdala dopamine (Engel and Sharpless, 1977). Acetylcholine levels are decreased and benzodiazepine receptors are increased after amygdala-kindled seizures (Dashieff et al., 1981), and there is some evidence for more enduring changes in *benzodiazepine receptors* with kindling (Burnham et al., 1983; Tuff et al., 1983b). *Endogenous opioids* and other peptides are released during amygdala-kindled seizures (Vindrola et al., 1981). These substances may have a role in mediating postictal symptoms (Caldecott-Hazard and Engel, 1987; Engel et al., 1984a;b) but do not appear to be involved in seizure generation. GABA agonists retard the development of kindling (Burnham, 1985); these drugs act on nonspecific inhibitory influences, however, and there is continued controversy regarding the role of GABA-mediated synchronization in epileptogenesis (Engel et al., 2008a). Involvement of the NMDA–cation channel complex, similar to that proposed for *long-term potentiation* (LTP) (Collingridge and Bliss, 1987) (Chapter 3), is suspected (Mody and Heinemann, 1987). However, kindling and LTP are clearly quite different phenomena, because LTP dissipates with time.

The mechanisms underlying secondary epileptogenesis and kindling could contribute to a number of phenomena associated with clinical epilepsy. Similar pathophysiological processes might act in patients to (1) allow subclinical electrical discharges to manifest eventually as behavioral seizures, (2) extend the area of an epileptogenic zone, making seizures more severe and more resistant to treatment, (3) recruit distant structures into the epileptogenic process and produce new ictal symptoms, (4) establish distant epileptogenic zones with the capability of generating independent spontaneous seizures, and (5) give rise to enduring interictal behavioral disturbances (Engel and Cahan, 1986; Morrell et al., 1987). Because these phenomena presumably involve neuronal mechanisms available to the normal brain, they could indicate a relationship between aspects of clinical epilepsy and other, more general abnormal phenomena such as reverse tolerance to drugs (Post, 1981) as well as normal acquired behavior such as memory and learning.

Morimoto and colleagues (2004) have reviewed and synthesized several decades of research on kindling and status epilepticus models of epilepsy that implicate numerous mechanisms underlying the rewiring responsible for epileptogenesis and epileptogenicity. In the poststatus model, principal neurons are lost because of both necrosis and apoptosis, but interneurons are selectively preserved. This cell loss promotes synaptic reorganization. The initial responses to damage are presumably mediated by *inflammatory reactions* (Vezzani et al., 2008), which cause small numbers of neurons to burst synchronously; kindling stimulation produces this effect artificially. Once synchronous bursting is established in the status models, however, mechanisms similar to kindling can account for incorporation of local and distant structures into the epileptogenic process. These mechanisms include activation of *glutamate receptors*, *second messengers*, *immediate early genes*, *transcription factors*, *neurotropic factors*, *axon guidance molecules*, *neurogenesis*, and *synaptogenesis* (Scharfman and Schwarcz, 2008; Löscher and Brandt, 2010; Pitkänen, 2010). Kindling and status presumably increase glutamate and GABA release, with primary excitation mediated by AMPA receptors and compensatory inhibition by $GABA_A$ receptors. Prolonged depolarization secondarily activates NMDA receptors and voltage-dependent Ca^{2+} influx. Intracellular Ca^{2+} triggers intracellular cascades, resulting in morphological changes including *neurogenesis*, *axonal sprouting*, *synaptogenesis*, *gliosis*, and *angiogenesis* (Parent et al., 2008). *Nerve growth factor (NGF)* and axon guidance factors are important for mossy fiber sprouting, but *brain-derived neurotrophin factor (BDNF)* and *neurotrophin 3 (NP3)* mediate neurogenesis and morphological changes in interneurons. With amygdala kindling, bursting activity initially is most prominent in piriform and perirhinal cortex, but hyperexcitability also develops in CA1 and CA3. This activity is accompanied by increased inhibition in the dentate gyrus mediated by aberrant feedback on $GABA_A$ and benzodiazepine receptors. There is also increased activity by inhibitory neurons containing NPY, which has been shown to have both pro- and anticonvulsant effects. Increased excitation and inhibition via novel recurrent circuits, synaptogenesis, loss of presynaptic autoreceptors, and altered receptor subunit composition promote hypersynchronization.

Most epileptic seizures are followed by a *postictal refractory period,* when seizures cannot be induced. This seizure-suppressing effect can be revealed easily in kindled animals by the failure to respond to recycling stimuli (repeated stimulations at 2-minute intervals) (Engel and Ackermann, 1980). Postictal refractoriness to subsequent ictal generation can last weeks after a series of seizures (Mucha and Pinel, 1977). Differences exist among rats with respect to the length of postictal refractoriness (Engel and Ackermann, 1980), and this period is very short in the immature rat (Moshé et al., 1983), indicating the existence of genetic and maturation-dependent protective mechanisms. The postictal refractory period, in addition to other postictal characteristics (Chapter 9), appears to reflect continued action of those mechanisms that terminate ictus (Engel et al., 1981). This process is not due to neuronal exhaustion (Caspers and Speckmann, 1972). Although the specific mechanisms of ictal termination are unknown, active inhibition often appears to be responsible. Adenosine has been suggested as one possible transmitter involved (Dragunov et al., 1985), and endogenous opioid peptides released during seizures appear to mediate some postictal behaviors (Caldecott-Hazard and Engel, 1987; Engel et al., 1986b; Engel et al., 1984b) (Chapter 9).

IN VIVO MODELS OF EPILEPSY WITH GENERALIZED SEIZURES

A chronic generalized seizure disorder can be produced in animals by creating *multiple bilateral epileptogenic lesions* (Marcus, 1972) which are comparable, perhaps, to some forms of nongenetic generalized epilepsy (Chapter 7). A particularly pharmacoresistant form of acquired generalized seizures is *infantile spasms* (Chapter 6), seen in *West syndrome,* which is characterized by onset of epileptic spasms usually in the first year of life, a unique EEG pattern referred to as *hypsarrhythmia,* and cognitive impairment, which can be severe (Chapter 7). Investigations into basic mechanisms of this condition and screening for effective antiseizure drugs have been greatly hampered by the lack of an adequate experimental model. Four lesion-induced and three genetically engineered animal models incompletely replicate human infantile spasms (Auvin et al., 2012; Nehlig et al., 2012; Swann

and Moshé, 2012). Intrahippocampal infusion of *tetrodotoxin,* which blocks sodium channels (Galvan et al., 2003); systemic injection of *corticotropin-releasing hormone (CRH)* during the second week of life (Baram and Schultz, 1995); variations of systemic *NMDA* injection (Chachua et al., 2011); and the *triple-hit model,* which involves intracerebral injection of two toxins, *doxorubicin* in the brain stem and *lipopolysaccharide* in the cortex, followed by systemic p-*chlorophenylalanine* to deplete *serotonin* (Scantlebury et al., 2010) all cause epileptiform EEG changes and spasms and provide insights into the basic mechanisms underlying human infantile spasms. These animals are providing unique insights regarding age-related epileptic manifestations of spasms based on possible genetic, epigenetic, and structural etiologies. The stress theory is not fully supported, as spasms cannot be induced by intraventricular injection of CRH (Baram and Schultz, 1995). However, stress induced by intrauterine *betamethasone* injection primes the brain to NMDA-induced seizures (Velísek et al., 2007). In the latter model, pretreatment with *adrenocorticotropic hormone (ACTH)* decreases the number of spasms induced by NMDA (Velísek et al., 2007). In the triple-hit model, administration of ACTH after the onset of spasms does not control the spasms, while rapamycin does (Raffo et al., 2011). Thus this chronic model can be used to identify new treatments.

The *Ts65DN mouse* is a *Down syndrome model* that overexpresses *GABA$_B$ receptors* and exhibits spike-and-wave EEG discharges but does not have spontaneous seizures. Administration of *GABA$_B$* agonists in this model causes spasms that respond to *ACTH, valproic acid,* and *vigabatrin* (Cortez et al., 2001). The *Aristaless-related homeobox (ARX) model* (Marsh, 2009) and a *triplet repeat of the ARX gene* (Price et al., 2009) have impaired GABA inhibition and are X-linked; the former model is lethal. With the recognition of specific genetic disturbances underlying certain other severe pediatric syndromes, animal models can be genetically engineered. An example is the *SCN1A knockout mouse,* which reproduces some of the deficits of *Dravet syndrome* (Yu et al., 2006) (Chapter 7).

Several naturally occurring genetic generalized epilepsy conditions in animals can be exploited for research purposes, including those of a number of *mutant rat and mouse models* (Seyfried et al., 1986, Ramos and Loturco, 2006; Noebels, 2006), such as the *genetically epilepsy-prone rat (GEPR)* (Vergnes et al., 1982), the *genetic absence epilepsy rat from Strasbourg (GAERS)*, and the *WAG/Rij* rat from Rijswick (DePaulis and Van Luijtelaar, 2006); the *seizure-prone gerbil* (Loskata et al., 1974; Buckmaster, 2006); the epileptic beagle (Edmonds et al., 1979); *photosensitive baboon species*, the most sensitive and most studied being *Papio papio* (Killam et al., 1966; Jobe and Browning, 2006); and the photosensitive *epileptic fowl* (Johnson et al., 1979). In most of these animal models reflex seizures are induced by sensory stimulation, such as sound in the *audiogenic mouse mutant* and GEPR, somatosensory stimulation in the gerbil, and intermittent light stimulation in the baboon and fowl. A number of studies have implicated the frontal cortex as a major site of epileptic discharges in *Papio papio* (Naquet and Meldrum, 1972). In some rat strains, seizure susceptibility appears during a critical window in development and may persist for only a specific period, as is the case for age-dependent genetic human epilepsies (Chapters 5 and 7). Of considerable interest is the fact that early treatment of *WAG/Rij* rats with *ethosuximide* prevents the later appearance of seizures, presumably by blocking the expression of *HCN* channels responsible for epileptogenesis (Blumenfeld et al., 2008). This suggests that certain forms of genetic epilepsy can be prevented (Giblin and Blumenfeld, 2010). Epilepsy-like phenomena have also been modeled in lower species such as the *zebra fish* (Baraban, 2006), flies (Tempel et al., 1987), and the worm *C. elegans* (Williams et al., 2004).

None of the genetically determined animal epilepsy conditions faithfully reproduces, in toto, any of the human genetic generalized epilepsies. However, they all provide an opportunity to study mechanisms of neuronal excitability at the level of gene expression. Identification and localization of the genes and gene products responsible for specific epileptiform traits allow their role in brain development to be investigated (Noebels, 2006; Burgess, 2006). Given the possibility that the basic defects responsible for the development of most forms of animal and human epilepsy consist of subtle molecular or structural changes in relatively few, widely dispersed neurons,

some of which may no longer even exist by the time seizures manifest, tracing the evolution of defects from their genetic determinants allows the problem to be approached from a different direction. The diversity of human epilepsy phenotypes and the complexity of the human genome, however, offer a formidable challenge to molecular neurobiologists interested in basic mechanisms of human epilepsy.

IN VITRO STUDIES OF CHRONIC EPILEPSY

Chronic models of epilepsy have been studied in vitro largely by the hippocampal slice technique. No consistent changes in excitability have been demonstrated in the kindling model of epilepsy with this approach; however, paired pulse suppression, similar to that seen in vivo, has been demonstrated in the dentate gyrus (Oliver and Miller, 1985). On the other hand, NMDA receptors may be uncovered by kindling in this structure (Mody and Heinemann, 1987). Increased bursting of neurons in piriform cortex has also been described (McIntyre, 1986), confirming in vivo evidence of enduring transsynaptic enhancement of susceptibility to epileptiform activity. Hippocampal slice preparations from the GEPR, the hippocampal kainic acid model, and slices from cortical alumina foci of monkeys have yielded preliminary equivocal and inconsistent results (Schwartzkroin, 1986; Bernard, 2008). Although pHFOs have been recorded from hippocampal slices taken from rat models of MTLE (Foffani et al., 2007), because there is acute disconnection it is not clear which, if any, of these oscillations are normal and which represent pathological phenomena (Engel et al., 2009). Slices from the partially isolated cortical slab, however, have provided insights into the synaptic reorganization responsible for epileptogenicity (Graber and Prince, 2006).

The problems introduced by disconnection in the in vitro slice preparations have been largely overcome with the *isolated guinea pig brain* model, which can be maintained in vitro for detailed electrophysiological investigations (Gnatkovsky et al., 2008; DeCurtis and Gnatkovsky, 2009). Mirror focus formation in the neonatal brain has been investigated using a *three-compartment chamber*, one for each hippocampus and one for the connecting commissural fibers. After seizures are induced in one hippocampus with *kainate*, transmission is interrupted by application of tetrodotoxin to the commissural chamber, and epileptogenesis can be studied in the contralateral hippocampus. Results of this work confirm activation of NMDA receptors and conversion of the GABA effect of Cl⁻ channels from hyperpolarization to depolarization (Khalilov et al., 2003) (Chapter 3).

STUDIES OF HUMAN EPILEPSY

With advances in neuroimaging and neurosurgical treatment for seizures, it is becoming increasingly possible to carry out research on basic mechanisms of epilepsy with patients (Engel, 2001; Engel et al., 1987; 1989; 2008a). Relatively noninvasive early approaches used the EEG to examine electrophysiological abnormalities and body fluids to investigate biochemical disturbances. Coupled with EEG, functional imaging of the human brain with *positron emission tomography (PET)* and structural and functional *magnetic resonance imaging (MRI)* now provide unparalleled new noninvasive opportunities for identifying physiological, biochemical, and anatomical substrates of human epileptogenicity (Chapter 12). Centers that perform surgical treatment for epilepsy offer opportunities for invasive research directly on the human brain (Engel et al., 1987; Engel, 1990; 1998a). In these settings electrophysiological measurements can be made from the brain's surface, as well as within specific brain structures, using clinical macroelectrodes and microelectrodes to record field potentials and single cells (Engel et al., 2008a), and microdialysis probes can be used for simultaneous monitoring of release of neurotransmitters and other molecules into the extracellular fluid (Cavus and Wilson, 2008; Wilson et al., 1996; Fried et al., 1999). In addition, molecular, morphological, and electrophysiological disturbances can be defined by in vitro investigations of surgically resected epileptogenic tissue.

Electrophysiological Investigations

The various interictal and ictal EEG abnormalities associated with human epileptic seizure types (Commission on Classification, 1981) (Chapter 6) and human epilepsy syndromes (Commission on Classification, 1989; Berg et al., 2010) (Chapter 7) are well known (Engel and Pedley, 2008; Panayiotopoulos, 2010). Whereas prolonged EEG discharges are usually associated with a recognizable clinical seizure, behavioral changes can occur but go unrecognized during single spike-and-wave events that are considered to be interictal. This concept is generally accepted for absence epilepsy, but behavioral correlates of focal interictal spikes have also been described (Shewmon and Erwin, 1988a;b;c). If *interictal EEG spikes* are actually fragments of seizures, this term is an oxymoron in at least some patients with focal and generalized epilepsies, and a clear distinction between interictal and ictal states does not actually exist.

A more detailed definition of focal epileptiform EEG events and their relationship to ictal clinical behavior has been derived from EEG recordings with *stereotactically placed depth electrodes (stereotactic EEG – SEEG)*, which record directly from presumed epileptogenic areas and their projection fields (Engel et al., 1983a; Talairach et al., 1974; Wieser, 1983; Spencer et al., 2008). Such studies are carried out in candidates for resective surgical treatment of focal seizures (Engel, 1987a; 1993) (Chapter 16). Interictal spike discharges recorded from the scalp EEG can reflect events projected to cortex from mesial temporal structures, but spikes in the hippocampus, amygdala, and parahippocampal gyrus often have no scalp-EEG correlates (Fig. 4–14). Ictal discharges also commonly occur in the hippocampus and amygdala without associated changes on the scalp EEG (Fig. 4–15). Both chronic and acute (intraoperative) recordings from the surface of the human brain and from deep structures indicate that patients with focal seizure disorders usually have multiple cerebral sites capable of independently generating interictal epileptiform discharges. In most cases, however, only one region consistently gives rise to the patient's habitual seizures (Engel, 1987a;b; Lüders et al., 1993) (Chapter 16).

The site of ictal onset for human limbic seizures is most often the anterior hippocampus, although they can also begin in other limbic structures as well as in neocortical areas that preferentially project to limbic structures (Wieser, 1983; Engel and Williamson, 2008).

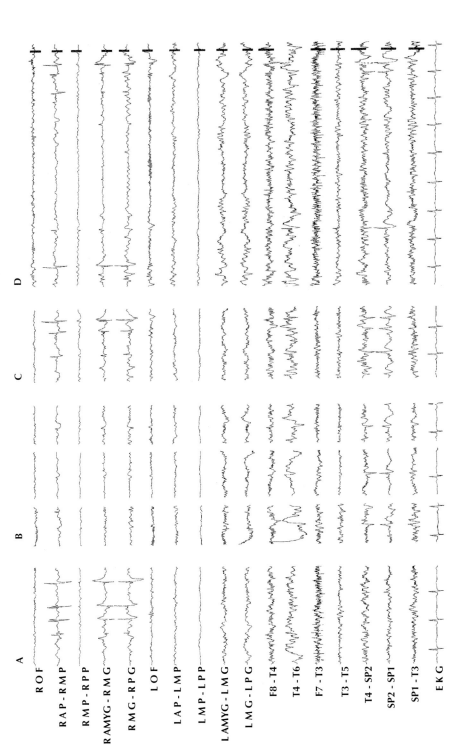

Figure 4–14. Interictal EEG recorded from stereotactically implanted depth electrodes as well as scalp (including sphenoidal [*SP1, SP2*]) electrodes. In segment *A*, interictal spikes are recorded from the right depth electrodes but not from the scalp. In segment *B*, interictal spikes are recorded from the right sphenoidal but not depth electrodes. In segment *C*, interictal spikes appear simultaneously in both depth and sphenoidal electrodes. In segment *D*, interictal spikes with all three topographical distributions occur within an 8-second period. Calibration: 100 μV. *ROF*, right orbital frontal cortex; *RAP*, right anterior hippocampal pes; *RMP*, right mid-hippocampal pes; *RPP*, right posterior hippocampal pes; *RAMYG*, right amygdala; *RMG*, right mid-hippocampal gyrus; *RPG*, right posterior hippocampal gyrus; *LOF*, left orbital frontal cortex; *LAP*, left anterior hippocampal pes; *LMP*, left mid-hippocampal pes; *LPP*, left posterior hippocampal pes; *LAMYG*, left amygdala; *LMG*, left mid-hippocampal gyrus; *LPG*, left posterior hippocampal gyrus.

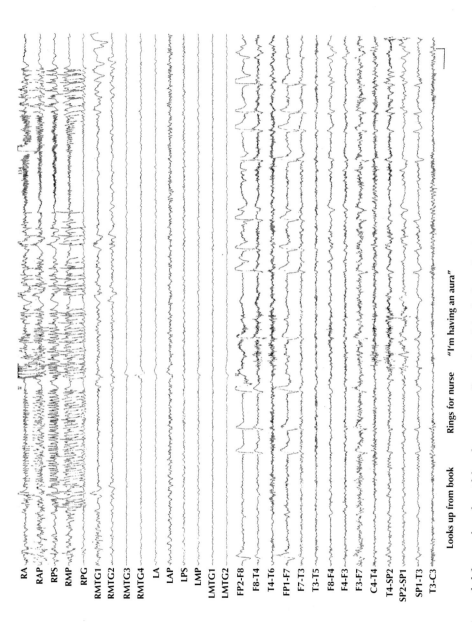

Figure 4–15. EEG recorded from scalp, sphenoidal, and stereotactically implanted depth electrodes during a focal seizure (aura) with no surface EEG correlates. Note the well-defined ictal discharge in right mesial temporal derivations reflected minimally at two of the four contacts in the right midtemporal gyrus and not at all at scalp and sphenoidal derivations. During the episode the patient rang for the nurse and indicated the occurrence of the aura. High-voltage transients during this time in the frontal areas represent eyeblinks. Calibration: 1 second. *RA*, right amygdala; *RAP*, right anterior hippocampal pes; *RPS*, right presubiculum; *RMP*, right mid-hippocampal pes; *RPG*, right posterior hippocampal pes; *RMTG*, right middle temporal gyrus (*1–4* represent anterior to posterior placements in neocortex); *LA*, left amygdala; *LAP*, left hippocampal pes; *LPS*, left presubiculum; *LMP*, left mid-hippocampal pes; *LMTG*, left middle temporal gyrus (*1* and *2* indicate more anterior and posterior placements in neocortex, respectively).

The electrophysiological patterns of hippocampal ictal onset are variable, but two discrete patterns have been described (Engel et al., 2008a; Engel et al., 1983a; Lieb et al., 1981a;b, Velasco et al., 2000) (Fig. 4–16). The most common pattern consists of repetitive high-amplitude spike or spike-and-wave discharges, referred to as the *hypersynchronous (HYP)* ictal onset pattern, resembling the rhythmic spike-and-wave ictal pattern of absence seizures. The other, referred to as the *low-voltage fast (LVF)* ictal onset pattern, is a buildup of low-voltage fast activity resembling the recruiting rhythm of a generalized tonic-clonic seizure or the pattern of ictal onset observed in the cat neocortical penicillin focus. Ictal discharges usually persist for long periods in mesiotemporal structures on one side before clinical symptoms appear. The HYP ictal onset pattern is well localized to a few electrodes and may be associated with an aura or no clinical signs or symptoms until it is transformed into an LVF pattern before propagation to the contralateral hemisphere (Fig. 4–17). Some hippocampal ictal events, however, consist entirely of HYP activity and terminate without propagating (Fig. 4–18). These may be associated with auras in isolation or have no clinical correlation. Ultraslow waves lasting 0.3 to 6 seconds also occur at the site of ictal onset (Vanhatalo, 2010) and are referred to as *initial slow waves (ISWs)* (Bragin et al., 2007; Bragin and Engel, 2008). These events may be generated by nonneuronal mechanisms, and their potential role in ictogenesis is unknown.

Relatively slow contralateral propagation occurs with hippocampal seizures (Lieb et al., 1986), which could be accounted for by poor or nonexistent hippocampal commissural connections (Wilson et al., 1987; 1991). However, similarly delayed propagation is also seen in the kainic acid and pilocarpine rat models of hippocampal sclerosis, and rats have extensive hippocampal commissures. Consequently, a more likely interpretation is that the hippocampus contains inherent homeostatic protective mechanisms that resist ictal propagation, perhaps involving enhancement of the dentate gate (Engel et al., 2008a). Neocortical ictal discharges, on the other hand, usually spread rapidly to the contralateral hemisphere, particularly from the frontal lobe (Bancaud et al., 1974). Bilateral mesial temporal involvement in the ictal discharge is associated with impaired consciousness; however, altered consciousness can occasionally be seen when the ictal discharges remain unilateral. Initial propagation of seizures with mesial temporal lobe onset is more often contralateral in women and ipsilateral in men (Savic and Engel, 1998), consistent with the known sexual dimorphism of callosal connections.

Application of penicillin to the human cortex produces EEG changes similar to those seen in the experimental penicillin focus of animals (Ralston and Papatheodoros, 1960), which indicates the existence of a similar neuronal substrate but does not imply a relationship to human epilepsy. Spontaneous epileptic phenomena in humans are considerably different from the effects of penicillin, which suggests that the penicillin model does not adequately reproduce human epileptiform pathophysiology. Human focal epilepsy very rarely results from a discrete focus, as in the penicillin model. Rather, large, irregular, and often multifocal brain regions demonstrate epileptogenic properties (Engel, 1987b; Wieser, 1983). Even if these widespread chronic disturbances are not all capable of generating spontaneous ictal activity, they (1) may be necessary for the

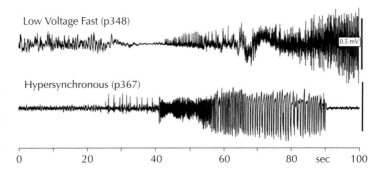

Figure 4–16. Single channels from depth electrode recordings of hippocampus, showing two different seizure onset patterns in two different patients with MTLE and hippocampal sclerosis. Top channel shows a typical low-voltage fast (LVF) ictal onset, and lower channel shows a typical hypersynchronous (HYP) ictal onset.

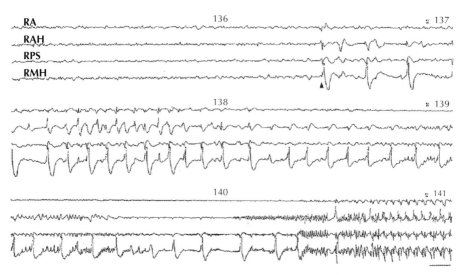

Figure 4–17. Telemetry recording showing EEG activity at selected depth electrodes (bipolar tips) during the onset of a complex partial seizure. Three continuous segments show a common ictal onset pattern, beginning with rhythmic high-amplitude sharp and slow transients (*arrowhead*), initially widely spaced but becoming faster and sharper. This eventually gives way to LVF discharge, which then evolves into higher-amplitude repetitive spikes or spike-and-wave discharges. Calibration: 1 second. *RA*, right amygdala; *RAH*, right anterior hippocampal pes; *RPS*, right presubiculum; *RMH*, right mid-hippocampal pes. (From Engel, 1988a, with permission.)

clinical manifestation of epileptic behavior, (2) certainly determine the pattern of ictal spread, if not the frequency and severity of epileptic seizures, and (3) perhaps mediate interictal behavioral disturbances (Engel et al., 1986; 2008b).

Both increased (Bernier et al., 1987) and decreased (Cherlow et al., 1977) afterdischarge thresholds have been reported with electrical stimulation of human epileptogenic brain areas. The reason for this discrepancy is unclear but may be related to stimulus parameters (Bernier et al., 1987). Connectivity between some cerebral structures is enhanced in the epileptic brain (Buser and Bancaud, 1983; Wilson et al., 1987), while in other areas on the side of the epileptogenic lesion, evoked potentials can be decreased or absent (Wilson et al., 1987). Paired-pulse suppression is often encountered in the human epileptogenic hippocampus (Wilson et al., 1987), resembling that demonstrated in the kindled rat (Tuff et al., 1983a). Chronic microelectrode recording reveals decreased unit firing rates (Babb and Crandall, 1976). Unit burst firing is encountered, but less often than in experimental animal models (Babb and Crandall, 1976; Wyler and Ward, 1986). As in animal models, unit burst firing

can correspond to the EEG spike and cessation of firing to the slow wave (Fig. 4–19); however, these events involve less than 5% of the total neuronal population (Babb and Crandall, 1976). Unit recordings reveal evidence of both excitatory and inhibitory influences at the time of seizure onset (Babb and Crandall, 1976; Babb et al., 1987).

Micro- and macroelectrode recordings from patients have defined the neuronal correlates of gamma- and normal ripple-frequency activity in the hippocampus (Le Van Quyen et al., 2008; 2010) and have confirmed that pHFOs recorded from humans, as in chronic rat models, are specifically localized to regions capable of generating spontaneous seizures (Bragin et al. 2002b; 2007; Staba et al., 2002a;b; 2004; 2012; Staba and Bragin, 2011; Worrell and Gotman, 2011). These studies established physiological properties of pHFOs and localized them to areas of cell loss where neuronal reorganization has taken place (Ogren et al. 2009b; Staba et al., 2007; 2012). The presence of pHFOs in human epileptic brain suggests the existence of small numbers of highly synchronized bursting neurons. This synchronization is likely to be dependent in part on pathological inhibitory influences. The more common HYP ictal onsets

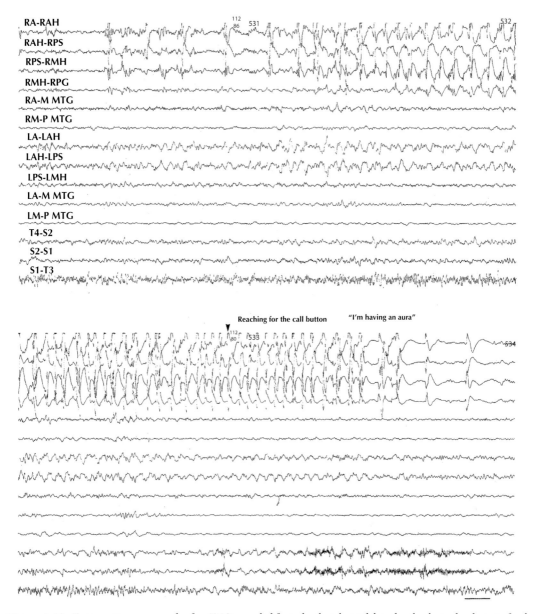

Figure 4–18. Forty continuous seconds of an EEG recorded from depth, sphenoidal, and scalp electrodes during a focal seizure (aura) involving the right temporal lobe. The ictal event begins in the left portion of the upper panel as an increase in interictal spike discharges maximal at the right anterior hippocampal pes electrode (*RAH*). After 8–9 seconds these spikes become regular, eventually developing into a 3-Hz spike-and-wave pattern involving all derivations from the right mesial temporal lobe before ending abruptly in the right portion of the lower panel. Note that no LVF ictal activity is seen, either initially or at any part of the ictal episode. Videotape analysis indicated that the patient reached for the call button at the *arrow*, at which point regular rhythmic slow activity is also seen in the left anterior hippocampus pes (*LAH*) and the right sphenoidal (S_2) electrode. The patient then indicated that she was having an aura, which consisted of a sensation of fear in her stomach. Calibration: 1 second. *RA*, right amygdala; *RPS*, right presubiculum; *RMH*, right mid-hippocampal pes; *RPG*, right posterior hippocampal gyrus; *RA-M MTG*, right anterior to mid-middle temporal gyrus; *RM-P MTG*, right mid- to posterior middle temporal gyrus; *LA*, left amygdala; *LPS*, left presubiculum; *LMH*, left mid-hippocampal pes; *LA-M MTG*, left anterior to mid-middle temporal gyrus; *LM-P MTG*, left mid- to posterior middle temporal gyrus. (From Engel, 1988a, with permission.)

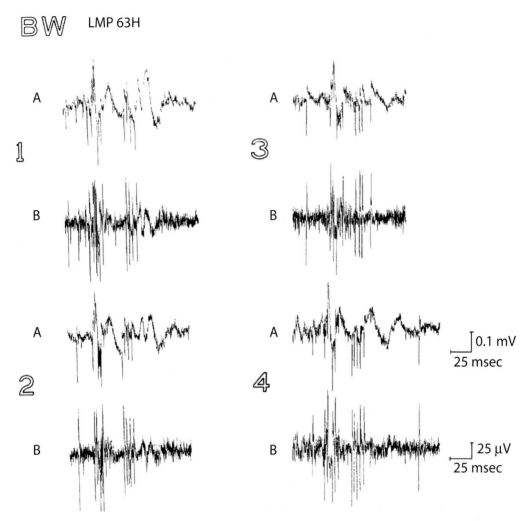

LMP 63H

Figure 4–19. EEG spikes (*A*) and action potentials (*B*) recorded from the same microelectrode in left mid-hippocampal pes (*LMP*) in a patient with clinical seizures originating in LMP. Tracings *1–4* were taken from the beginning to the end of the recording period, respectively, and were selected to have a similar EEG spike morphology, characterized by a fast rise time of the initial negative component. Tracing *A* is a wideband recording to show the EEG spike and slow wave superimposed on the unit discharges. For tracing *B*, additional high-pass filtering was used to enhance the neuronal discharges. Note increased unit firing during EEG spike and cessation of unit firing during EEG slow wave. (From Babb and Crandall, 1976, with permission.)

could be mediated by enhanced inhibitory and rebound excitatory mechanisms, perhaps similar to those responsible for the typical 3-Hz ictal EEG pattern of absence seizures (Engel et al., 2008a), whereas the LVF ictal onset pattern in hippocampus could reflect a disinhibitory mechanism similar to that seen in the penicillin focus (Matsumoto and Ajmone-Marsan, 1964b). However, recent data from the animal laboratory indicate that more pronounced continuous inhibitory mechanisms produce the beta gamma frequency and that firing of principal neurons actually ceases during this phase of ictal onset (Gnatkovsky et al., 2008; DeCurtis and Gnatkovsky, 2009). The LVF ictal onset is usually followed by high-amplitude ictal discharges, presumably representing a rebound excitatory effect, supporting the principle of synchronization through inhibition (Engel and Wilson, 1986; Klaassen et al., 2006). In vivo recordings of large ensembles of single neurons during seizure initiation and spread reveal highly heterogenous, not hypersynchronous, activity, which becomes more synchronous as the seizure progresses, followed by complete cessation of spiking at seizure termination (Truccolo et al., 2010). Changes in unit activity were also observed distant from the site of ictal onset minutes before the seizure, suggesting widespread complex interactions among neuronal networks before, during, and after the seizure.

The demonstration of increased inhibition within the human epileptic hippocampus (Wilson et al., 1987) could be explained by enhanced functions of the dentate gate as well as by observations in the human hippocampus that inhibitory interneurons are preferentially

spared (Babb et al., 1989a;b) and exhibit axonal sprouting (Davenport et al., 1990). Enhanced inhibitory mechanisms could be protective, but they could also play an important role in epileptiform hypersynchronization. Indeed, unit recordings from human epileptic hippocampus reveal that cells receiving strong inhibitory input are highly synchronized (Isokawa-Akesson et al., 1989; Staba et al., 2002a) (Fig. 4–20). Synchronized neuronal firing in epileptic tissue is best identified during sleep (Staba et al., 2002b).

Mossy fiber sprouting is also a prominent feature of human hippocampal sclerosis (Mathern et al., 2008). As in the monkey alumina focus, Golgi stains reveal that principal

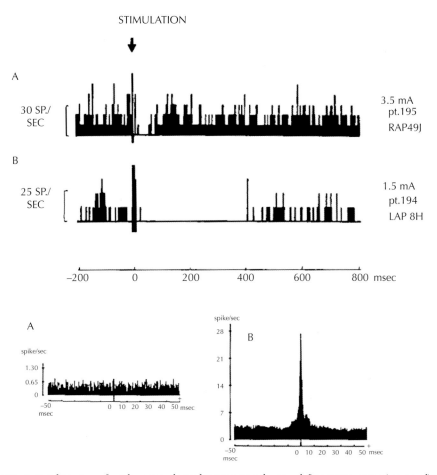

Figure 4–20. A: Unit histograms from human epileptic hippocampus show weak firing suppression (*top panel*) in neurons that were not firing synchronously as determined by cross-correlation histograms (*bottom left*). B: By contrast, strong firing suppression is evident (*bottom panel*) in neurons that were firing synchronously (*bottom right*). This provides indirect evidence for recurrent inhibitory circuits as a mechanism of hypersynchronization. (From Engel et al., 2008a, adapted from Isokawa-Akesson et al., 1989, with permission.)

neurons in the human epileptic hippocampus demonstrate varying degrees of degeneration, including loss of dendritic spines, dendritic beading, and eventual restriction of the dendritic domain (Scheibel et al., 1974) (Fig. 4–21). In vitro intracellular recordings from dentate granule cells of human epileptic hippocampus that exhibit degenerative changes indicate enhanced NMDA-mediated excitability, suggesting pathological uncovering of NMDA receptors (Isokawa and Levesque, 1991) similar to that described in the kindled rat (Mody and Heinemann, 1987). In vitro electrophysiological studies of human epileptogenic neocortex and hippocampus (Schwartzkroin, 1987) have also demonstrated bursting cells and, rarely, PDS-like membrane events. A major difficulty in such studies is the inability to reliably distinguish between epileptogenic and nonepileptogenic areas of the in vitro tissue. Until this can be done, it will not be possible to obtain adequate control data, if such is available at all, in brains of patients with epilepsy.

Investigations Using Brain Imaging Techniques

The use of PET with ^{18}F-*fluorodeoxyglucose* (*FDG*) in patients with focal epilepsy has revealed an *interictal zone of hypometabolism* involving the region of ictal onset (Engel et al., 1982a;b;c; Theodore et al., 1984) (Chapters 6 and 12). The degree of hypometabolism does not correlate with the frequency of interictal spikes, indicating that metabolic measures and electrophysiological measures assess different aspects of functional disturbance associated with epilepsy (Engel, 1988b; Engel et al., 1982). The interictal zone of hypometabolism is invariably larger than can be accounted for merely by cell loss or other structural lesions (Engel et al., 1982a). Furthermore, the hypometabolic zone becomes hypermetabolic during seizures (Engel et al., 1982d; 1983b; Theodore et al., 1984) and can disappear when seizures are controlled (Gur et al., 1982). At least some of these interictal metabolic disturbances, therefore, are believed to represent reversible functional abnormalities.

Ictal FDG scans obtained during focal seizures often contain large areas of hypometabolism in addition to localized regions of hypermetabolism (Fig. 4–22). The latter appear to correspond to the site of ictal onset and spread, whereas the former may reflect postictal changes associated with depressed metabolism (Engel et al., 1982d; 1983b). Similar changes have been demonstrated for oxygen metabolism and blood flow (Bernardi et al., 1983; Kuhl et al., 1980).

Children with absence epilepsy have normal interictal FDG scans and diffusely increased cerebral glucose metabolism during absences (Chapter 6). Ictal hypermetabolism with typical absences is greater than that seen with any other seizure type (Engel et al., 1985). This does not necessarily suggest that energy requirements for typical absences surpass those for focal or generalized tonic-clonic seizures. More likely, it reflects the fact that these absences are not associated with postictal depression, which would reduce the final weighted metabolic average measured by PET (Engel, 1984; 1983; Engel et al., 1985). Atypical absences, however, do not always produce hypermetabolic FDG scans (Ochs et al., 1987; Theodore et al., 1985). Consequently, generalized spike-and-wave EEG discharges do not represent a unitary pathophysiological process; these electrical events could result from several types of disturbances, each with different energy requirements.

Because GABA-mediated inhibitory synaptic activity requires as much or more energy than excitatory synaptic activity (Ackermann et al., 1984), ictal increases in FDG uptake could reflect enhanced synaptic excitation, enhanced synaptic inhibition, or probably both. Hypometabolism results from decreased neuronal activity, which could occur in projection fields of actively inhibited neurons, but also appears when excitatory inputs drive neurons at a rate slower than their random firing frequency (Ackermann et al., 1984). There is evidence for a relationship between temporal lobe hypometabolism and enhanced opiate receptor binding in the ipsilateral temporal neocortex (Chugani et al., 1984; Frost et al., 1988). If hypometabolism reflects abnormal opiate mechanisms, this would lend credence to the proposed role of endogenous opioids in postictal and interictal behavioral disturbances (Caldecott-Hazard and Engel, 1987; Engel et al., 1984b) (Chapters 9 and 11).

A variety of other PET tracers have been used to evaluate epilepsy (Henry and Chugani,

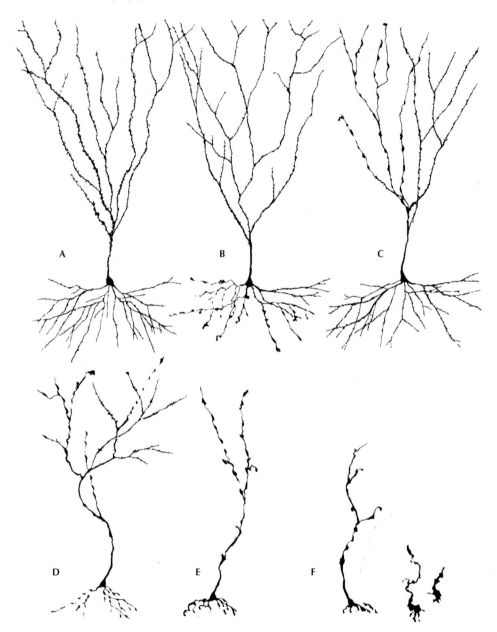

Figure 4–21. Drawing of human hippocampal pyramids from CA1 showing a series of changes of increasing severity leading to total cell destruction. Although all of these changes have been seen in many cells, it is not known that each cell in a pathological focus will follow this sequence of changes. **A.** Apparently normal pyramid. **B.** Loss of dendrite spines and development of nodulation ("string of beads" appearance) in approximately half of basilar dendrites. All other dendrite branches appear normal. **C.** Loss of dendrite spines and development of nodulation in approximately half the branches of the apical shaft. The rest of the dendrite system seems normal. The changes in cells **B** and **C** represent alternatives; the same neuron would obviously be unlikely to go through both changes. **D.** Some loss of branches and progressive distortion of the dendritic domain, patchy remaining areas of spines, and extensive areas of dendrite showing string-of-beads patterns. **E, F.** Terminal steps in cell death, with progressive loss of dendrite substance, increasing irregularity of the remaining shaft segments, angular distortion or curling of the dendrite branches, and swelling or shrinkage of the cell body (or both). Drawn from a number of sections stained by rapid Golgi variants; magnification × 100. (From Scheibel et al., 1974, with permission.)

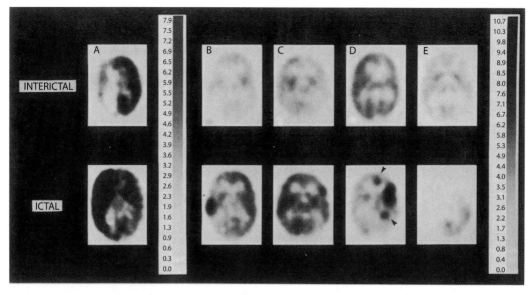

Figure 4–22. Representative planes of section of interictal (*top row*) and ictal (*bottom row*) FDG-PET scans from five patients with focal seizures. Scale indicates the calculated local cerebral metabolic rate for glucose in milligrams per 100 g per minute. Scans *B–E* are all displayed to the same scale, chosen to best illustrate values for maximal ictal activation. Scan *A* is scaled differently as a result of technical difficulties in displaying data. The number of ictal events occurring in the first half hour after FDG injection are described for each patient below. X-ray computed tomographic scans were abnormal for patient *A*, who had left hemisphere atrophy, and patient *E*, who had a small right occipital glioma. *A:* Ictal activation of the entire left hemisphere occurred with nine seizures that originated electrically in the left parietal area and spread to involve both sides of the body, the right side more than the left. *B:* Selective ictal activation of the left perisylvian area occurred within a larger zone of interictal hypometabolism during seven seizures that were confined electrographically to left temporal and central electrodes and behaviorally to the right arm and face. A second ictal scan in this patient demonstrated the same pattern. *C:* Hypermetabolism of the entire brain—prominent in the right precentral area, which was hypometabolic interictally—accompanied epilepsia partialis continua involving the left leg and arm. The ictal EEG contained no localizing abnormalities. *D:* Seven dyscognitive focal seizures with twitching of the left side of the mouth and head and eye turning to the left were associated with increased metabolic activity in right temporal and frontal structures, including discrete activation of hippocampus and cingulate cortex (*arrowheads*) and decreased metabolic activity elsewhere. *E:* Three seizures that originated in the right occiput and spread into the right temporal lobe began with formed visual auras in the left visual field, progressing to alteration of consciousness. This was associated with hypermetabolism of the right occipital and temporal lobes and hypometabolism elsewhere. (Note that older PET scans in this book are not reversed, right is on the right side and left is on the left side.) (From Engel et al., 1982d, with permission.)

2008). Two of particular interest are *flumazenil* (Henry et al., 1993; Savic et al., 1988) and α-*methyl-tryptophan* (*AMT*) (Kumar et al., 2011; Chugani, 2011). Uptake of flumazenil, a benzodiazepine receptor ligand, is selectively decreased in epileptogenic tissue, even in areas where FDG-PET is normal (Henry et al., 1993; Savic et al., 1988). This could reflect loss of inhibitory neurons, or it could indicate receptor downregulation as a result of enhanced presynaptic GABA release. AMT uptake is increased in epileptogenic tissue (Kumar et al., 2011), and although this tracer is involved in serotonin synthesis, it is not clear that these findings indicate a role for serotonin synthesis in epileptogenicity. Alternatively, it has been suggested that this increased AMT uptake reflects enhanced

activity in the *quisqualate* pathway, which has excitatory properties (Chugani, 2011).

MRI is able to demonstrate detailed cerebral anatomy and can reveal the location and extent of small structural lesions in many patients with epilepsy (Jackson et al., 1990; Sperling et al., 1986) (Chapter 12). MRI also provides an opportunity to define the precise anatomical boundaries of disturbances measured by PET and electrophysiological techniques, and correlative studies greatly enhance the anatomical specificity of these functional techniques (Salamon et al., 2008). *Voxel-based morphometry* of high-resolution MRI using *statistical parametric mapping (SPM)* now permits detailed reconstruction of epileptogenic tissue that is not clearly visualized on routine structural MRI, such as focal cortical dysplasia, other disturbances of neuronal migration, and hippocampal sclerosis. Such studies have revealed that the atrophy of hippocampal sclerosis is not homogeneous and diffuse but rather has a patchy distribution, which could be used to characterize different types of hippocampal sclerosis (Ogren et al., 2009a) (see Figs. 5–16 and 7–7). For instance, patterns of atrophy are different between patients with HYP and LVF ictal onsets, suggesting two different pathophysiological processes (Chapter 7) (Fig. 4–23). Such studies, coupled with *diffusion tensor imaging (DTI)*, which permits visualization of white matter tracts (Beaulieu, 2002; Gross, 2011), now allow noninvasive anatomical investigations with a degree of resolution approaching that of routine histology (Chapter 12). Whereas such anatomical studies were limited to surgically resected tissue in the past, EEG and behavioral findings can now also be correlated with the anatomy of the contralateral hippocampus and, when surgery is not performed, with the anatomy of the epileptogenic hippocampus.

Functional MRI (fMRI) takes advantage of differences in magnetic properties of oxygenated and deoxygenated hemoglobin using *blood oxygenation level-dependent (BOLD) signal* to identify areas of altered cerebral perfusion and define the anatomical substrates of complex behaviors (Cohen and Bookheimer, 2008). Functional MRI is a dynamic technique with a temporal resolution of seconds and has been used to image the onset and propagation of ictal activity (Jackson et al., 1994). More recently, simultaneous EEG-fMRI monitoring has been used to localize cerebral areas generating interictal EEG spikes and to define network abnormalities of the epileptic brain (Gotman and Pittau, 2011). Apart from the obvious clinical application of this technology (Chapter 12), it also greatly increases the ability to carry out detailed research on the structure-function relationships of epileptiform abnormalities noninvasively with high spatial and temporal resolution. Resting state *functional connectivity MRI (fcMRI)* (Chapters 3 and 12) is just beginning to be applied to research on human epilepsy, and this work will undoubtedly be

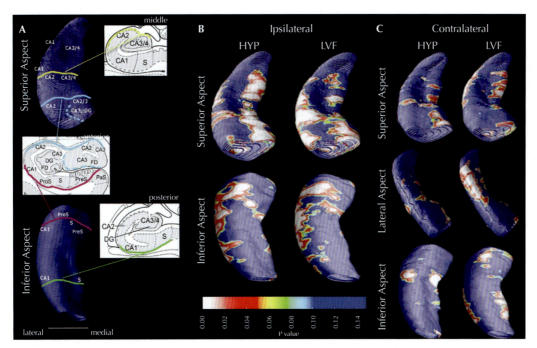

Figure 4–23. A. Three-dimensional contour map depicting location of dentate gyrus (*DG*), hippocampal subfields (*CA1–4*) and subicular cortex (*S*) within anterior, middle, and posterior regions of the hippocampal formation based on anatomical landmarks and atlas (Mai et al. 1997). **B, C.** Color-coded averaged contour maps comparing areas of significant atrophy (white and red) in hippocampus ipsilateral (**B**) and contralateral (**C**) to seizure onset between patients with hypersynchronous (HYP) and low-voltage fast (LVF) depth EEG ictal onset. (Modified from Ogren et al., 2009a, with permission.)

informed by ongoing basic research on neuronal connectivity using methodologies such as *optogenetics* and computer modeling of neuronal circuit organization, as discussed in Chapter 3.

Other clinical techniques that can be used for investigations into the fundamental mechanisms and anatomical substrates of human epileptic phenomena include *magnetic resonance spectroscopy (MRS)* (Petroff and Duncan, 2008), an application of MRI used to identify alterations in brain chemistry associated with epileptic seizures; *single photon emission computed tomography (SPECT)* (Kazemi et al., 2008); and the research tools of *optical imaging* (Haglund et al., 2008), which so far has only been clinically applied intraoperatively, and *cellular imaging* (Trevelyan and Yuste, 2008) (Chapter 12).

Microanatomical Investigations

Routine histopathological studies have demonstrated a characteristic pattern of hippocampal cell loss (hippocampal sclerosis) in most patients with limbic seizures (Babb and Brown, 1987; Mathern et al., 2008) (Chapter 5). Although surgical removal of a sclerotic hippocampus usually results in freedom from disabling seizures (Chapter 16), there remains debate over the degree to which this abnormality represents an epileptogenic lesion as opposed to the consequences of chronic recurrent epileptic seizures. Most likely it is both. The cell loss of human hippocampal sclerosis is similar to that already described for the post-status animal models. Synaptic reorganization, including mossy fiber and interneuron axonal sprouting, is also a feature of human hippocampal sclerosis (Maglóczky, 2010). These morphological disturbances appear to reflect the neuronal substrates of epileptogenicity, because chronic depth recordings in patients indicate that limbic seizures commonly originate within the sclerotic hippocampus and not from the more normal-appearing surrounding tissue (Babb et al., 1984). Pathological HFOs are more likely to be recorded from sclerotic hippocampus than hippocampus without evidence of atrophy on MRI (Staba et al., 2007). More detailed SPM MRI investigations reveal, as noted previously, that pHFOs are selectively generated within patches of atrophy (Ogren

et al., 2009b; Staba et al., 2012), suggesting that cell loss and subsequent synaptic reorganization is important for generation of synchronized burst discharges.

Biochemical and Molecular Investigations

Studies of neurotransmitters and their metabolites in blood and *cerebrospinal fluid (CSF)* of patients with epilepsy have yielded inconsistent and conflicting results. Reported alterations in GABA, biogenic amine metabolites, and ACh in the CSF cannot be directly related to the activities of these neurotransmitters in the brain. Pharmacological manipulation has also failed to define a single biochemical defect specifically responsible for a human chronic seizure disorder, with the exception of *pyridoxine-dependent seizures* (Swaiman and Millstein, 1970), which occur because pyridoxine is required for GABA synthesis. Such systemic studies are unlikely to be successful if specific biochemical defects are discretely localized within the brain, because drugs and endogenous neuroactive chemicals have diverse, and at times antagonistic, actions on different cerebral structures. PET holds more promise for identifying localized biochemical disturbances within the whole brain.

Genetic analysis, on the other hand, has identified gene products responsible for some epilepsy conditions (Chapter 5). Examples of such conditions include *GLUT1 deficiency* (DeVivo et al., 1991), the *CHRNA2* mutation that expresses an abnormal *nicotinic ACh receptor (nAChR)* in ADNFLE (Steinlein, 2008), and a variety of other ion channel and receptor mutations (Chapter 5) where the epileptogenic mechanisms can be reasonably assumed. However, for other gene products associated with epilepsy conditions, such as the product of the *leucine-rich glioma inactivated gene 1 (LGI1)* in *autosomal dominant lateral temporal lobe epilepsy* (Steinlein, 2008), the contribution of the molecular defect to the development of epileptogenicity is unknown (Chapter 5).

Epileptogenic tissue excised from patients undergoing surgical treatment may ultimately provide more direct opportunities to study the molecular abnormalities associated with chronic epilepsy. However, it is difficult to differentiate changes that could be responsible for the genesis of seizures from transient changes that are secondary to seizure occurrence and chronic interictal defects that represent homeostatic protective mechanisms. Increased glycine, decreased taurine, decreased glutamic acid, increased glutamic acid synthesis, decreased GABA synthesis, and increased catecholamine synthesis have been variously reported in excised epileptic human brain tissue. These findings provide a picture of altered energy, amino acid, and catecholamine metabolism (Sherwin and van Gelder, 1986; Sherwin et al., 1987). Hypotheses that implicate decreased GABA-mediated inhibition in epileptogenesis are not supported by immunocytochemical studies in human sclerotic hippocampus of the enzyme responsible for GABA synthesis, *glutamic acid decarboxylase (GAD)*, because surviving principal neurons are reported to have normal or increased GAD terminals (Fig. 4–24) and the ratio of GAD-containing neurons to principal neurons is also normal or increased (Babb, 1986; Babb and Brown, 1987).

MOLECULAR GENETIC INVESTIGATIONS

Tremendous advances in molecular genetics in recent years have provided unprecedented opportunities to identify disturbances at the molecular level in patients with epilepsy as well as in experimental animal models of epilepsy and have yielded an overwhelming amount of new data. A detailed discussion of potentially important findings is beyond the scope of this text, and the field is moving so rapidly that anything of a specific nature written today is almost certainly likely to be out of date by the time of publication. In any event, it is appropriate to discuss current approaches to molecular genetic research and present an overview of recent developments. The two broad types of molecular genetic investigations are *gene discovery*, or the identification of genetic mutations responsible for epilepsy conditions, and studies to elucidate *acquired genetic disturbances*, that is, alterations in gene expression associated with epilepsy both in humans and animal models.

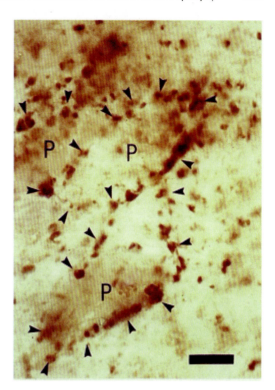

Figure 4–24. Hippocampal sclerosis. The inhibitory terminals (GAD puncta, *arrowheads*) that surround remnant pyramidal cells (*P*) in presubiculum extend around their somata and along their proximal dendrites. Hence, sclerotic epileptic tissue has intact inhibitory neurons and terminals on the remnant cells. (From Babb, 1986, with permission.)

Gene Discovery

Considerable progress has been made in identifying genetic abnormalities responsible for epilepsy disorders with *Mendelian modes of inheritance (autosomal dominant, autosomal recessive, and X-linked)* as well as *mitochondrial genetic defects* (Ottman and Winawer, 2008; Steinlein, 2008) (Chapter 5), but such disorders are rare. Complex modes of inheritance requiring more than one genetic defect or a genetic defect plus environmental factors are much more common, not only among the assumed genetic epilepsies, but also as *susceptibility genes*, for the acquired epilepsies. The genetic causes of epilepsy are discussed in detail in Chapter 5, but for the purposes of this chapter, it is important to note that identification of mutant genes that contribute to the development of human epilepsies greatly enhances the potential for research into basic mechanisms of epilepsy, and often of specific types of epilepsy. Understanding the function of proteins encoded by these genes provides insights into their role in epileptogenesis. Differences in genetic background also underlie individual variations in seizure threshold, reaction to neuronal injury, and response to antiseizure drugs. Not only can channel and other subcellular functions be studied by introduction of these genes into oocytes and other cells, but these genes can be deleted or inserted into mice and other animals to create *knockout* and *knock-in* models for in vivo investigations. *Viral vectors* are also now commonly used to determine the functional effects of genetic mutations of interest (Betley and Sternson, 2011).

Acquired Genetic Disturbances

Because most postmitotic neurons in the brain do not divide to form new neurons (neurogenesis), the function of DNA replication is to maintain the specific functions and structures of individual neurons (*phenotypic diversity*) and to mediate situation-induced alterations in function and structure (*phenotypic plasticity*). This is accomplished through *transcription* and *translation*. Transcription is the process whereby *RNA polymerase* copies the genetic code onto *messenger RNA (mRNA)*, and translation is the process by which mRNA forms the proteins responsible for the function and structure of cells. Current molecular genetic research is possible through the development of the *reverse transcription polymerase chain reaction (RT-PCR)*, which permits amplification of small DNA samples to produce *complementary DNA (cDNA)*; this in turn permits examination of altered expression of genes and gene profiles of selected brain tissues. *In situ hybridization* uses radiolabeled probes and autoradiography to localize the neurons and brain areas exhibiting specific alterations in gene expression.

Two experimental approaches are used to carry out molecular genetic investigations. The specific aims of *hypothesis-driven* approaches are to identify alterations in genes responsible for proteins that are known or highly suspected to be involved in mechanisms of epileptogenesis and epileptogenicity based on prior research. Alternatively, *discovery-driven* approaches use large microarrays consisting of tens of thousands of genes to identify clusters that are differentially upregulated or downregulated (or both) in association with specific aspects of epileptogenesis and epileptogenicity. Hypothesis-driven approaches have yielded important data confirming, for instance, involvement in epilepsy of ion channels, subunit composition of neurotransmitter receptors, neurotrophic factors, and active transport mechanisms but do not offer the same opportunities as the discovery-based approach to identify unanticipated novel alterations in gene expression that could result in a paradigm shift in understanding basic mechanisms of epileptic phenomena. Microarray research, however, has deficiencies that result in considerable inconsistencies among published research results. These discrepancies can be attributed to differences in technique, limited sensitivity of large microarrays, the fact that results can be diluted if relevant changes are limited to only a few cell types, and the need to distinguish among a variety of influences responsible for altered gene expression profiles in any given model or human disorder. Specifically, altered expression can reflect (1) transient normal responses to ictal activity, (2) early epileptogenic mechanisms that do not persist indefinitely after the epileptogenic insult, (3) transient or enduring responses to injury that are not epileptogenic, (4) enduring mechanisms that maintain epileptogenicity and promote progressive epileptogenesis, and (5) homeostatic protective mechanisms that develop in response to the epileptogenic process and act to maintain the interictal state.

Another confounding feature of microarray research is that a great many, often hundreds, of genes exhibit upregulation or downregulation in any given experiment. This difficulty has been overcome using bioinformatics to identify functional gene classes, or *gene ontology (GO)* terms (Lukasiuk et al., 2008), to elucidate the variety of mechanisms that might be represented by relatively large alterations in gene expression profiles. Results of these analyses can be confirmed in transgenic mutant mice and, in turn, lead to hypothesis-driven experimental designs.

Using GO terms, some of the more consistent findings can be summarized (Lukasiuk et al., 2008). Not surprisingly, immediately after status epilepticus in status rodent models of chronic epilepsy, there is upregulation of *immediate early genes (IEGs)* such as *c-fos*. These mediate transcription of other genes and can be used to localize brain structures involved in epileptic activity, much the same way that *2DG autoradiography* has been used. However, the exact function of these genes in terms of epileptogenic mechanisms is not known. Later, there is upregulation of genes involved in neurogenesis, and late in the development of epileptogenesis there are alterations in genes responsible for synaptic reorganization, plasticity, and neurotransmission.

It is important to recognize that some epilepsy-associated upregulation in gene expression must represent homeostatic protective mechanisms. For instance, increased expression of the vesicle-trafficking protein Sv2a, which is the target of the antiseizure drug levetiracetam (Lynch et al., 2004), occurs in regions adjacent to epileptogenic areas and could act to suppress the propagation of epileptiform discharges (Winden et al., 2011). Throughout all stages, there are alterations in genes responsible for cell motility, responses to stress and wounding, ion homeostasis, and cell death and survival; most consistently and most markedly, there is upregulation of genes responsible for immune reactions. From these studies, therefore, it is clear that immune reactions play an important role in initiating epileptogenesis and perhaps also in maintaining epileptogenicity, but exactly how is unknown.

Mechanisms by which inflammatory processes could mediate epileptogenesis involve innate reactions of neurons and glia, predominantly microglia, and adaptive mechanisms resulting from breakdown of the blood-brain barrier, permitting immune cells, antibodies, and antigens access to brain parenchyma (Vezzani et al., 2008; Vezzani and Ruegg, 2011a;b) (Fig. 4–25). Activation of innate inflammatory reactions results in the proliferation of *cytokines*, which reduce threshold to seizures, perhaps by inducing reactive gliosis, inhibiting neurogenesis, and upregulating ionotropic glutamate receptors. Cytokines also appear to have a protective effect, improving neuronal survival by stimulating production of NGF and other trophic molecules, by increasing calcium-binding proteins, which reduce intracellular Ca^{2+}, and by increasing antioxidant pathways. Molecules of interest in the cascade of chronic inflammatory events include *interleukin-1β and 6 (IL-1β, IL-6)*, *tumor necrosis factor-α (TNF-α)*, and inflammatory markers such as *prostaglandins*, *toll-like receptors*, *chemokines*, *nuclear factor-κB (NFκB)*, and *cyclooxygenase-2 (COX-2)*. Although the exact functions of these inflammatory molecules in the development of epileptogenesis have yet to be understood, they are potential targets of antiepileptogenic interventions. Other processes that appear to play a role in epileptogenesis, revealed in part by molecular genetic investigations, and that are potential targets of antiepileptogenic interventions, include reactive gliosis (Steinhauser et al., 2008), angiogenesis, and neurogenesis (Parent et al., 2008). New neurons are born throughout the adult life of the normal hippocampus, but neurogenesis is abnormally increased in the epileptic hippocampus, and seizures appear to induce that neurogenesis. However, the role of these newborn neurons in epileptogenesis and epileptogenicity is as yet unknown.

Research using molecular genetic approaches to define specific disturbances at the level of voltage- and ligand-gated channels and receptors (Chapter 3) and other important subcellular functions, as discussed here, is providing crucial insights into potential mechanisms of epileptogenesis and epileptogenicity. This work, however, is just the beginning of a long and difficult research process that will be necessary if we are to understand the possible function of these molecular aberrations. While some of the data suggest targets for novel approaches to antiepileptogenesis and antiseizure interventions, epilepsy is a disorder of neuronal interconnections as much as it is a disorder of individual neurons. Consequently, for each molecular defect identified, it becomes necessary to determine how it translates into the development of neuronal networks capable of generating spontaneous behavioral epileptic seizures. This will be possible only with exhaustive in vivo electrophysiological investigations at the systems level in experimental animal models and patients, perhaps greatly aided by advancing technologies in functional neuroimaging, such as PET and fMRI, capable of displaying localized biochemical alterations and interneuronal connections of the entire brain for comparison not

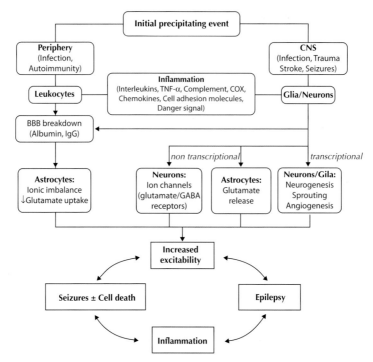

Figure 4–25. Simplified schema summarizing the interplay among inflammation, seizures, and epilepsy. *BBB*, blood brain barrier; *CNS*, central nervous system; *IgG*, immunoglobulin G. (From Vezzani and Ruegg, 2011b, with permission.)

only with controls but with the same animal and patient over time.

POSSIBLE MECHANISMS OF HUMAN EPILEPTIC PHENOMENA

The foregoing discussion of insights obtained from animal experiments and an increasing amount of data available from studies of patients allows speculation about the fundamental mechanisms of human epilepsy. Hypotheses, however, must take into account separately a number of individual epileptic phenomena: (1) *epileptogenesis*, or the mechanism by which an epileptic condition is acquired, (2) the disturbances that exist during the *interictal state* and predispose to the spontaneous recurrence of epileptic seizures, (3) the functional transition that leads to *ictal onset*, (4) the many manifestations of the *ictal state*, (5) *ictal termination*, (6) the unique features of the *postictal period*, and (7) the possible *consequences of epileptic seizures* for interictal brain function and structure and for behavior (Engel et al.,

2008b). Although molecular substrates of epilepsy are being rapidly identified, the manifestations of epileptic phenomena must ultimately be explained at the systems level, which will be the primary focus of the following discussion.

Epileptogenesis

The age-dependent appearance of spontaneous epileptic seizures in the genetic epilepsies presumably depends on a critical period during cerebral maturation when the genetically determined defect is expressed as a manifest change in behavior. Although it is likely that progressive epileptic changes must take place in the brain before a genetic epilepsy appears, it is most reasonable to discuss the concept of epileptogenesis as it might refer to acquired epilepsy disorders (Chapter 7).

In the acquired epilepsies, some structural lesion or metabolic disturbance is presumed to exist in the brain (Chapter 5) that renders individual neurons more excitable, reorganizes neuronal circuitry in a manner that enhances synchronization, or both. Inflammatory mechanisms induced by epileptogenic cerebral insults might (1) damage dendritic branching and abolish spinous processes, placing excitatory synapses closer to the axon hillock, (2) rearrange specific ion channel distributions, perhaps rendering Ca^{2+} and Na^+ channels more effective and Cl^- and K^+ channels less effective in influencing membrane events at the axon hillock; (3) destroy synaptic terminals, leading to sprouting of surviving axon fibers to increase synchronization, and create recurrent collateral excitation and inhibition, and (4) selectively attenuate and enhance different inhibitory influences, facilitating specific excitatory phenomena and also promoting synchronization (Fig. 4–26). Pathological disturbances in glial function mediate some of these inflammatory influences and also disrupt local neurotransmitter and ion concentrations by other mechanisms.

Structural or functional changes in afferent input might alter the availability of specific neurotransmitters and cause up- or down-regulation of receptors. At the molecular level, changes in the configuration of proteins, particularly those that regulate presynaptic and postsynaptic Ca^{2+}, would have profound effects on the efficacy of specific synaptic connections. Finally, chronic disturbances in the ionic microenvironment, water and pH balance, neuronal energy metabolism, and neurotransmitter deactivation could result from glial changes accompanying tissue damage or from alterations in neuronal firing patterns.

Such changes in the vicinity of a neocortical or hippocampal insult might give rise to intermittent synchronized burst discharges within neuronal aggregates. Repeated burst discharges resembling the stimulation-induced afterdischarges of the kindling model could then induce enduring reorganization of neuronal connections, locally and at a distance, mediated by mechanisms such as those proposed for the NMDA–cation channel complex (Chapter 3). This reorganization would result in extension of the epileptogenic zone, perhaps establishment of secondary epileptogenic areas, and eventual appearance of ictal clinical behavior.

Interictal State

The interictal state in most epileptic conditions is characterized by the appearance of interictal

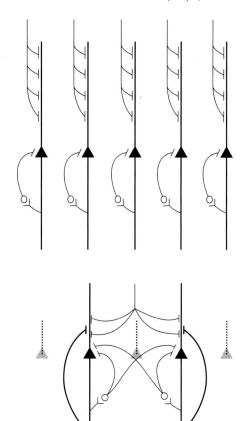

Figure 4–26. Reciprocal innervation of a hypothetical neuronal system. *Top:* Typical synaptic organization of neocortex and hippocampus. Excitatory afferent input terminates on the dendrites of principal neurons (*filled triangles*). Axon collaterals from these principal neurons terminate on inhibitory interneurons (*open circles*), which in turn make hyperpolarizing synapses on the somata of the same principal neurons as well as adjacent ones (not shown). *Bottom:* With cell loss, a number of synaptic reorganizations are likely to occur. Fewer afferent input fibers sprout, but they innervate more principal neurons, predisposing to hypersynchronization. Because the dendrites of principal neurons are shorter, these excitatory influences are closer to the axon hillock and more likely to induce neuronal firing. Neuronal excitability is further increased by the establishment of monosynaptic excitatory recurrent circuits (as also shown in Fig. 4–7). Inhibitory interneurons also sprout terminals to produce more powerful and/or more extensive recurrent inhibitory influences, further enhancing the potential for hypersynchronization. (From Engel, 1990, with permission.)

EEG spike-and-wave discharges, which are diffuse in the generalized epilepsies and localized in the focal epilepsies. In most cases it can be assumed that these events in humans reflect summated depolarizing and hyperpolarizing membrane events similar to those observed in acute animal models. The neurons contributing to the interictal EEG transients in human focal epilepsy represent only a small percentage of the neuronal aggregate, probably less than 5%, as opposed to over 90% in the penicillin focus.

Neurons in the human epileptogenic zone may have decreased afferent input. The interictal neuronal aggregate, therefore, may be hypersynchronous, but not necessarily hyperactive. This could explain the apparent discrepancy between metabolic measures of neuronal function determined by FDG-PET and electrophysiological measures with EEG. An interictal epileptogenic zone that demonstrates high-amplitude spike-and-wave discharges on the EEG is usually hypometabolic on FDG-PET. In this situation, only a small percentage of neurons are highly synchronized. In any event, metabolic measures such as PET and fMRI reflect energy-requiring synaptic and pump mechanisms that do not correlate directly with neuronal discharges. The reasons for hypometabolism of the epileptogenic region remain unknown.

In human focal epilepsy, strong inhibitory influences within the epileptogenic zone help to maintain the interictal state. These may include prolonged AHPs and perhaps some mechanism similar to that of the inhibitory surround. The latter, however, is likely to be admixed with, rather than encircling, a more diffuse epileptogenic region than seen in the experimental focus. While some inhibitory influences are homeostatic responses to epileptic excitability, others are important factors in the generation of hypersynchronized epileptiform discharges. Because normal synchronization in the central nervous system is achieved primarily through inhibitory mechanisms (Chapter 3), strong inhibition could predispose to the hypersynchronization that characterizes the interictal epileptiform discharge. Increased inhibitory function of the dentate gate blocks propagation of epileptiform discharges from entorhinal cortex to hippocampus proper and therefore suppresses the development of epileptic seizures, but when propagation does occur, this inhibitory mechanism could contribute to the hypersynchronized nature of the discharges that characterize hippocampal HYP ictal onsets. Enhanced inhibitory mechanisms also develop in distant structures and could play a role in the appearance of interictal behavioral disturbances (Chapter 11).

Pathological HFOs are recorded from the epileptogenic zone of human hippocampal and neocortical focal epilepsy and can be assumed to reflect summated action potentials of pathologically synchronized bursting neurons, as has been shown in rodents. These neurons are localized to small atrophic areas where cell death and reorganization have occurred, and they presumably form tightly interconnected clusters surrounded by more normal tissue. In animals, the size of these clusters can be increased by reducing inhibitory tone, indicating that surrounding inhibitory mechanisms serve to contain the spatial extent of bursting activity.

Although most interictal inhibition is GABAergic, other inhibitory mechanisms that reduce, rather than increase, energy requirements might contribute to the presence of interictal hypometabolism. Opioid peptide–mediated inhibition is one possible candidate.

Ictogenesis

A number of mechanisms undoubtedly account for transition to ictus in the human epilepsies; however, two predominant electrographic ictal onset patterns have been described. Generalized tonic-clonic seizures and some focal seizures begin with diffuse or focal LVF EEG rhythms, followed by evolution to slower, high-amplitude discharges. SEEG recordings of this type of ictal onset in patients with focal epilepsy reveal a morphological pattern and topographical distribution distinct from that of the interictal EEG spike, indicating in this case that different mechanisms underlie interictal and ictal electrographic events. As in the penicillin focus, this transition to ictus could involve a reversal of the AHP to a prolonged membrane depolarization, giving rise to continuous neuronal burst firing. However, more recent evidence indicates that the LVF activity represents enhanced inhibition, and that these seizures begin with desynchronization, perhaps followed by rebound synchronization. Gradual spread of focal discharges to adjacent brain tissue suggests ephaptic spread, followed by axonal propagation to distant ipsilateral and contralateral structures.

A second type of transition from interictal to ictal state, typified by absence seizures, consists of an abrupt onset of high-amplitude spike-and-wave or poly-spike-and-wave complexes with little or no morphological evolution. SEEG recordings reveal that most hippocampal and some neocortical seizures have similar but localized HYP ictal onset patterns. For this type of hypersynchronous seizure onset, the ictal EEG spike-and-wave complexes often appear to reflect the same enhanced excitation and inhibition that give rise to interictal EEG epileptiform transients.

Initiation of generalized hypersynchronous EEG discharges associated with absences in patients is likely precipitated by thalamic synchronizing afferent influences mediated by low-voltage T-type Ca^{2+} currents and HCN channels, which are in turn activated by GABAergic hyperpolarizing inhibitory input. Evidence suggests that focal hypersynchronous seizures such as those commonly seen in hippocampus could arise as a result of decreased tonic inhibition that causes the small pHFO-generating neuronal clusters to increase in size, coalesce, synchronize, and propagate. Whether hippocampal low-voltage T-type Ca^{2+} currents or HCN channels are also responsible for mediating the rhythmicity of these focal hypersynchronous discharges remains to be demonstrated. In any event, the neuronal mechanisms underlying both focal and generalized HYP onset seizures undoubtedly involve enhanced inhibitory as well as excitatory synaptic events, because inhibition is important for synchronization and is reflected in the wave of the spike-and-wave discharge. For focal seizures, however, decreased inhibition may also be an important precipitating factor causing expansion of pHFO-generating neuronal clusters. Consequently, simultaneous increases and decreases in specific inhibitory mechanisms may be important for ictogenesis.

Electrographic patterns of single focal seizure onsets recorded with depth electrodes can contain elements of both LVF and HYP ictal onsets. Focal seizures that begin with a HYP discharge will suddenly convert to an LVF pattern before propagation occurs. This could reflect recruitment of adjacent structures, engagement of a second ictal mechanism (perhaps involving breakdown of the dentate gate), or both. On the other hand, both focal and generalized seizures with an LVF onset pattern often evolve ultimately to high-amplitude hypersynchronous discharges that can reflect a rebound excitation, followed by phasing in of active inhibitory mechanisms that terminate the seizure.

Transition from the interictal to the ictal state appears to be the consequence of nonspecific influences acting on brain tissue that is abnormally susceptible to epileptiform excitation and synchronization. Available antiseizure medications presumably act by antagonizing these nonspecific precipitating influences rather than by correcting the specific pathophysiological disturbances responsible for individual chronic epilepsy conditions (Chapter 15). Recent advances in the molecular neurobiology of epileptogenesis and ictogenesis could lead to more specific pharmacological interventions.

Ictus

The neuronal bases of human *generalized seizures* are poorly understood, because invasive studies are rarely carried out on patients with these disorders. Animal research suggests a prominent inhibitory mechanism for absence seizures, generated by synchronizing thalamic input to abnormal cortex, but no comparable data exist for human absence epilepsies. Generalized tonic-clonic seizures presumably involve brain stem mechanisms for the tonic phase and require forebrain mechanisms for the clonic phase, although this also has never been directly demonstrated in humans. The thalamocortical mechanisms believed to underlie typical absences involve hyperpolarization-induced activity via T-type Ca^{2+} channels, but the pathophysiological basis of atypical absences is unknown; there appears to be a continuum between these events and certain frontal lobe seizures (Chapter 6). No electrophysiological features of secondary generalized epilepsy associated with slow EEG spike-and-wave patterns can definitively distinguish an interictal from an ictal state (Chapter 6).

In *focal seizures* it is presumed that containment of ictal discharge is mediated by synaptic inhibition; that local spread is a result, at least in part, of nonsynaptic ephaptic mechanisms similar to those in experimental epilepsy; and that intrahemispheric and interhemispheric propagation takes place along preferential fiber pathways. Hippocampal HYP ictal onset patterns transition to a LVF pattern before propagation, suggesting that the mechanisms that support HYP events also function to contain the ictal discharge, and perhaps involve the dentate gate. Patterns of distant propagation might be determined by several factors, including (1) the efferent projections of the structures involved in ictal onset, (2) transsynaptic alterations in excitability induced by mechanisms similar to those of kindling, and (3) genetic and acquired individual variations in preexisting functional neuronal networks. Propagation from hippocampus is typically delayed by many seconds and may not occur at all, resulting in auras in isolation. This was originally attributed to functional absence of the hippocampal commissure, but because this delay is also seen in rodents with well-developed interhippocampal connections, it appears to reflect intrinsic hippocampal mechanisms that resist propagation, perhaps related to the dentate gate. Mapping of the temporal sequence of ictal propagation by computer analysis of depth and scalp electrode EEG recordings and demonstration of anatomical substrates by PET and fMRI have revealed considerable variation from one patient to the next in the pattern of ictal spread, even when the sites of ictal onset are reasonably similar. Typical limbic seizures, however, ultimately involve first one and then both mesial temporal areas in a reasonably predictable fashion.

The progression to *secondarily generalized seizures* depends to a large extent on the ease of access from the site of seizure onset to the relevant brain stem and forebrain structures, as well as to the contralateral cortex. Differences in projection patterns, particularly the density of callosal connections, might explain why secondarily generalized tonic-clonic seizures are more common with frontal lobe lesions than with temporal lobe lesions. The receptivity of downstream structures to epileptiform input may be determined by genetic factors, acquired changes due to kindling-like effects, and a variety of exogenous and endogenous influences on excitability and synchronization (Chapter 3). Multiple mechanisms would account for interindividual variability, as well as variability in the same individual from one seizure to the next. Anticonvulsant medications appear to be more effective in preventing engagement of mechanisms that generate generalized tonic-clonic seizures than in preventing transition from the interictal to the ictal state.

Ictal Termination

Much less is known about the fundamental mechanisms of ictal termination than about mechanisms of ictal onset. Seizures do not cease as a result of neuronal exhaustion. Loss of synchrony, active inhibition, increased extracellular K^+, and depolarization block are the most common mechanisms. The clonic phase of a tonic-clonic seizure presumably reflects a phasing in of an active inhibitory mechanism, although not all generalized tonic-clonic seizures end with a clonic phase. Many generalized, and also focal, seizures have ictal EEG patterns that slowly deteriorate in a subtle fashion over many seconds, perhaps because of a gradual failure of synchronizing influences. Consequently, as with ictal onset, several mechanisms are likely to be responsible for the termination of ictal events.

Adenosine and a number of endogenous peptide neuromodulators are released during experimental epileptic seizures and may act to terminate ictus or prevent spread, but specific physiological or biochemical events that consistently end a seizure discharge have not been demonstrated in experimental animals, let alone in humans.

Status epilepticus (Chapter 10) results when mechanisms that ordinarily act to terminate epileptic seizures fail. The persistence of discretely localized *epilepsia partialis continua* for months or years indicates that ictal spread is limited by mechanisms different from those that terminate ictal events. That epilepsia partialis continua, *limbic status epilepticus*, and *absence status* rarely progress to generalized tonic-clonic seizures demonstrates the independence of influences that alter convulsive threshold from those that normally terminate nonconvulsive epileptic seizures. Such independent mechanisms would explain why anticonvulsant drugs that are used successfully to stop generalized tonic-clonic status epilepticus can be ineffective against focal and absence status.

Postictal Period

When active inhibitory influences or intrinsic membrane processes terminate the ictal event, they also appear to account for transient postictal seizure refractoriness. These inhibitory influences interfere with normal neuronal functions to cause transient behavioral and EEG depression, cognitive impairment, amnesia, reactive automatisms, and specific neurological deficits during the postictal period (Chapter 9). On the other hand, hypersynchronous absence seizures, as well as some focal auras associated with hypersynchronous ictal discharges, are not associated with postictal behavioral or EEG disturbances, suggesting that desynchronizing influences that act to terminate these events do not interfere with subsequent normal neuronal function. Although some postictal behaviors in experimental animals are mediated in part by endogenous opioid peptides and other substances released during epileptic seizures, this finding has not been verified in humans.

The classical *Todd's paralysis* following focal seizures in humans lasts 24–48 hours, but reversible focal neurological deficits occasionally last for many months (Chapter 9). Such enduring behavioral changes cannot be accounted for by transient biochemical disturbances induced by the seizure and must reflect more profound, perhaps structural changes that ultimately are compensated for by functional, if not structural, reorganization. It is possible, therefore, that events that are engaged to terminate the ictus and that subsequently give rise to postictal symptoms ultimately account for the appearance of more enduring interictal behavioral disturbances in some patients with chronic epilepsy (Chapter 11).

Possible Consequences of Epileptic Seizures

This chapter has been concerned with neuronal mechanisms of epileptogenesis, ictogenesis, and related disturbances in the immediate postictal period. Some of the most controversial issues in epileptology concern whether epileptic seizures can permanently alter the structure or function of the human brain. Epileptic encephalopathy is discussed in Chapter 7, the possibility that secondary epileptogenesis produces progressive changes in some patients with epilepsy is discussed in Chapter 8, brain damage caused by epileptic seizures is discussed in Chapter 10, and the neurobiological basis of interictal behavioral disorders is discussed in Chapter 11.

SUMMARY AND CONCLUSIONS

Although there are increasing opportunities to carry out basic research with patients, most of our understanding of the fundamental mechanisms of epilepsy derives from research with experimental animal models. A variety of animal models of epilepsy and epileptic phenomena are in use. Their relevance to the various types of human epilepsy has been presumed on the basis of EEG and behavioral similarities, as well as the responses of these models to anticonvulsant and anti-petit mal pharmacological agents. However, for reasons of cost and animal rights issues, the trend today is to use rodent models and even simpler systems and to move away from primates. In any event, such studies require validation of results in patients whenever possible. A precise animal model of an entire human epilepsy condition probably does not exist even in primates, but clinical epilepsy can be dissected into component parts, and certain similarities can be assumed between specific phenomena seen in experimental animals and clinical phenomena seen in patients.

Basic research carried out on patients using a variety of noninvasive and invasive techniques has confirmed that some of the findings in experimental animal models can be extrapolated to humans. However, the disturbances that give rise to human epilepsy appear to be much more complex than those implied by studies of experimental animal models. Multiple mechanisms underlie different epilepsy conditions, and multiple mechanisms also underlie the discrete epileptic phenomena encountered within each individual epileptic condition and within each single epileptic seizure.

Tremendous advances in genetic, genomic, and molecular biological research approaches have yielded voluminous insights into molecular neurobiology at the level of ion channels, receptors, active transport mechanisms, vesicle trafficking, and other subcellular processes that influence neuronal excitability and, to a certain extent, synchronization. Specific genetic defects have been identified for a few rare epilepsy diseases, but many other genetic defects and alterations in gene expression have been described in experimental animal models of epilepsy and in patients that could underlie epileptogenesis, ictogenesis, or increased susceptibility to epilepsy, as well as homeostatic protective mechanisms. Although a full understanding of how these molecular disturbances eventually manifest as clinical epilepsy ultimately requires elucidation at the systems level, these developments provide potential targets that could permit focused, more effective antiepileptogenic and anti-ictogenic therapeutic interventions with fewer side effects than systemic administration of currently available drugs and large surgical resections.

Because certain inhibitory mechanisms are enhanced in the interictal state, breakdown of these mechanisms appears to account for transition to some types of epileptic seizures. Other ictal phenomena, however, such as absences and some focal seizures, arise directly from interictal mechanisms and appear to depend on enhancement of some forms of inhibition to generate highly structured hypersynchronized spike-and-wave discharges, whereas decreases in certain types of inhibition could also play a role in initiating these events. Single-unit recordings in patients and animals indicate that neuronal firing is reduced and desynchronized prior to LVF ictal onsets, reinforcing the concept of rebound excitation. Only a small percentage of neurons are involved in the interictal EEG epileptiform events of chronic epilepsy, but epileptogenicity is more easily analyzed by recording pHFOs, which are field potentials of synchronously bursting neurons. These pHFOs are localized to the epileptogenic region, appear to be involved in initiation of many focal seizure types, and could reflect the basic epileptogenic abnormality of most acquired hippocampal and neocortical epilepsies. In addition to interest in HFOs, more attention needs to be paid to initial ultraslow waves seen at the onset of some seizures.

Epilepsy in humans is rarely, if ever, associated with a discrete epileptic focus. Epileptogenic zones are commonly diffuse and multiple. In some patients, widespread dysfunction suggests progressive changes similar to those encountered in experimental secondary epileptogenesis. Research at the molecular and systems levels is necessary to elucidate potential mechanisms by which recurrent epileptiform events induce widespread, enduring alterations in neuronal function and structure over time.

Attention in epilepsy research has focused primarily on abnormalities responsible for initiating ictal events and for mediating their spread. Prevention of epilepsy requires a better understanding of the neuronal basis of the development of epileptogenicity, before seizures ever occur, as well as of the homeostatic antiepileptogenic mechanisms that naturally oppose epileptogenesis. Very little is known about the mechanisms that suppress ictal events during the interictal state, limit their spread once they begin, and ultimately terminate them. Identification and characterization of these natural protective mechanisms would allow exploitation of endogenous neuronal processes for therapeutic purposes. Whether and how these mechanisms might contribute to the appearance of postictal and interictal behavioral disturbances are also unknown.

An important insight gained from genetic and molecular neurobiological investigations is that acquired epilepsies most likely develop preferentially in the context of molecular susceptibility. Identification of the factors contributing to this susceptibility will permit creation of more clinically relevant experimental animal models. The realization that seizures acutely induced in a normal brain are not the same as seizures that spontaneously occur in a chronically epileptogenic brain represented a paradigm shift for model development. Similarly, a second paradigm shift should result from the realization that chronic epileptogenicity induced in brains without regard for the underlying genetic substrate is not the same as chronic epileptogenicity induced in brains with specific genetic and molecular susceptibilities. It now remains to identify the susceptibility factors that predispose people to the various types of acquired as well as genetic epilepsies.

REFERENCES

Ackermann, RF, Finch, DM, Babb, TL, and Engel, J, Jr (1984). Increased glucose metabolism during long-duration recurrent inhibition of hippocampal pyramidal cells. J Neurosci 4:251–264.

Ajmone-Marsan, C (1969). Acute effects of topical epileptogenic agents. In Basic Mechanisms of the Epilepsies. Edited by HH Jaspers, AA Ward, Jr, and A Pope. Boston: Little, Brown & Co, pp. 299–319.

Ajmone-Marsan, C (1972). Focal electrical stimulation. In Experimental Models of Epilepsy—A Manual for the Laboratory Worker. Edited by DP Purpura, JK Penry, DB Tower, DM Woodbury, and R Walter. New York: Raven Press, pp. 147–172.

Albala, BJ, Moshé, SL, and Okada, R (1984). Kainic-acid-induced seizures: A developmental study. Dev Brain Res 13:139–148.

Andersen, P, and Sears, TA (1964). The role of inhibition in the phasing of spontaneous thalamo-cortical discharge. J Physiol 173:459–480.

Auvin, S, Pineda, E, Shin, D, Gressens, P, and Mazarati, A (2012). Novel animal models of pediatric epilepsy. Neurotherapeutics, 9:245–261.

Avanzini, GG, Treiman, DM, and Engel, J, Jr (2008). Animal models of acquired epilepsies and status epilepticus. In Epilepsy: A Comprehensive Textbook, 2nd ed. Edited by J Engel, Jr, and TA Pedley. Philadelphia: Lippincott Williams & Wilkins, pp. 415–444.

Babb, TL (1986). Metabolic, morphologic and electrophysiologic profiles of human temporal lobe: An attempt at correlation. In Excitatory Amino Acids and Epilepsy. Edited by R Schwarcz and Y Ben-Ari. New York: Plenum Press, pp. 115–125.

Babb, TL, and Brown, WJ (1987). Pathological findings in epilepsy. In Surgical Treatment of the Epilepsies. Edited by J Engel, Jr. New York: Raven Press, pp. 511–540.

Babb, TL, and Crandall, PH (1976). Epileptogenesis of human limbic neurons in psychomotor epileptics. Electroencephalogr Clin Neurophysiol 40:225–243.

Babb, TL, Lieb, JP, Brown, WJ, Pretorius, J, and Crandall, PH (1984). Distribution of pyramidal cell density and hyperexcitability in the epileptic human hippocampal formation. Epilepsia 25:721–728.

Babb, TL, Wilson, CL, and Isokawa-Akesson, M (1987). Firing patterns of human limbic neurons during stereoencephalography (SEEG) and clinical temporal lobe seizures. Electroencephalogr Clin Neurophysiol 66:467–482.

Babb, TL, Pretorius, JK, Kupfer, WR, et al. (1989a). Glutamate decarboxylase-immunoreactive neurons are preserved in human epileptic hippocampus. J Neurosci 9: 2562–2574.

Babb, TL, Pretorius, JK, Kupfer, WR, and Feldblum, S (1989b). Recovery of decreased glutamate decarboxylase immunoreactivity after rat hippocampal kindling. Epilepsy Res 3:18–30.

Bancaud, J, Talairach, J, Morel, P, Bresson, M, Bonis, A, Geier, S, Hemon, E, and Buser, P (1974). "Generalized" epileptic seizures elicited by electrical stimulation of the frontal lobe in man. Electroencephalogr Clin Neurophysiol 37:275–282.

Baraban SC (2006). Modeling epilepsy and seizures in developing zebrafish larvae. In Models of Seizures and Epilepsy. Edited by A Pitkänen, PA Schwartzkroin, and SL Moshé. Burlington, MA: Elsevier Academic Press, pp. 189–198.

Baram, TZ, and Schultz, L (1995). ACTH does not control neonatal seizures induced by administration of exogenous corticotropin-releasing hormone. Epilepsia 36:174–178.

Baram, TZ, Hirsch, E, Schultz, L, et al. (1998). Short interval electrical amygdala kindling in infant rats: The paradigm and its application to the study of age-specific convulsants. In Kindling 5. Edited by ME Corcoran, and SL Moshé. New York: Plenum Press, pp. 35–44.

Baram, TZ, Jensen, FE, and Brooks-Kayal, A (2011). Does acquired epileptogenesis in the immature brain require neuronal death? Epilepsy Curr 11:21–26.

Barton, ME, Klein, BD, Wolf, HH, and White, HS (2001). Pharmacological characterization of the 6 Hz psychomotor seizure model of partial epilepsy. Epilepsy Res 47:217–228.

Battaglia, G, and Bassanini, S (2006). MAM and other "lesion" models of developmental epilepsy. In Models of Seizures and Epilepsy. Edited by A Pitkänen, PA Schwartzkroin, and SL Moshé. Burlington, MA: Elsevier Academic Press, pp. 305–313.

Beaulieu, C (2002). The basis of anisotropic water diffusion in the nervous system—A technical review. NMR Biomed 15:435–455.

Ben-Ari, Y, Tremblay, E, Riche, D, Ghilini, G, and Naquet, R (1981). Electrographic, clinical and pathological alterations following systemic administration of kainic acid, bicuculline or pentetrazole: Metabolic mapping using the deoxyglucose method with special reference to the pathology of epilepsy. Neuroscience 6:1361–1391.

Berg, AT, Berkovic, SF, Brodie, MJ, et al. (2010). Revised terminology and concepts for organization of seizures and epilepsies: Report of the ILAE Commission on Classification and Terminology. Epilepsia 51:676–685.

Berkovic, S, Engel, J,Jr, Meldrum, BS, and Wasterlain, C (eds) (1996). Third Workshop on the Neurobiology of Epilepsy (WONOEP III): Mechanisms of Chronic Models of Epilepsy. Epilepsy Res 26(special issue):1–308.Bernard, C (2008). Synaptic plasticity. In Epilepsy: A Comprehensive Textbook, 2nd ed. Edited by J Engel, Jr, and TA Pedley. Philadelphia: Lippincott Williams & Wilkins, pp. 403–413.

Bernardi, S, Trimble, MR, Frackowiak, RSJ, Wise, RJS, and Jones, T (1983). An interictal study of partial epilepsy using positron emission tomography and the oxygen-15 inhalation technique. J Neurol Neurosurg Psychiatry 46:473–477.

Bernier, GP, Saint-Hilaire, J-M, Giard, N, Bouvier, G, and Mercier, M (1987). Commentary: Intracranial electrical stimulation. In Surgical Treatment of the Epilepsies. Edited by J Engel, Jr. New York: Raven Press, pp. 323–334.

Betley, JN, and Sternson, SM (2011). Adeno-associated viral vectors for mapping, monitoring, and manipulating neural circuits. Hum Gene Ther 22:669–677.

Blumenfeld, H, and Coulter, DA (2008). Thalamocortical anatomy and physiology. In Epilepsy: A Comprehensive Textbook, 2nd ed. Edited by J Engel, Jr, and TA Pedley. Philadelphia: Lippincott Williams & Wilkins, pp. 353–366.

Blumenfeld, H, Klein, JP, Schridde, U, Vestal, M, Rice, T, Khera, DS, Bashyal, C, Giblin, K, Paul-Laughinghouse, C, Wang, F, Phadke, A, Mission, J, Agarwal, RK, Englot, DJ, Motelow, J, Nersesyan, H, Waxman, SG, and Levin, AR (2008). Early treatment suppresses the development of spike-wave epilepsy in a rat model. Epilepsia 49:400–409.

Bragin, A, and Engel, J, Jr (2008). Slow waves associated with seizure activity. In Computational Neuroscience in Epilepsy. Edited by I Soltesz and K Staley. San Diego: Elsevier, pp. 440–453.

Bragin, A, Engel, J, Jr, Wilson, CL, Fried, I, and Buzsáki, G (1999a). High frequency oscillations in human brain. Hippocampus 9:137–142.

Bragin, A, Engel, J, Jr, Wilson, CL, Fried, I, and Mathern, GW (1999b). Hippocampal and entorhinal cortex high frequency oscillations (100–500 Hz) in kainic acid-treated rats with chronic seizures and human epileptic brain. Epilepsia 40:127–137.

Bragin, A, Engel, J,Jr, Wilson, CL, Vizentin, E, and Mathern, GW (1999c). Electrophysiologic analysis of a chronic seizure model after unilateral hippocampal KA injection. Epilepsia 40:1210–1221.

Bragin, A, Mody, I, Wilson, CL, and Engel, J, Jr (2002a). Local generation of fast ripples in epileptic brain. J Neurosci 22:2012–2021.

Bragin, A, Wilson, CL, Staba, RJ, Reddick, MS, Fried, I, and Engel, J, Jr (2002b). Interictal high frequency oscillations (80–500Hz) in the human epileptic brain: Entorhinal cortex. Ann Neurol 52:407–415.

Bragin, A, Wilson, CL, and Engel, J, Jr (2003). Spatial stability over time of brain areas generating fast ripples in the epileptic rat. Epilepsia 44:1233–1237.

Bragin, A, Wilson, CL, Almajano, J, Mody, I, and Engel, J, Jr (2004). High frequency oscillations after status epilepticus: Epileptogenesis and seizure genesis. Epilepsia 45:1017–1023.

Bragin, A, Azizyan, A, Almajano, J, Wilson, CL, and Engel, J, Jr (2005). Analysis of chronic seizure onsets after intrahippocampal kainic acid injection in freely moving rats. Epilepsia 46:1592–1598.

Bragin, A, Claeys, P, Vonck, K, Van Roost, D, Wilson, C, Boon, P, and Engel, J, Jr (2007). Analysis of initial slow waves (ISWs) at the seizure onset in patients with drug resistant temporal lobe epilepsy. Epilepsia 48:1883–1894.

Bragin, A, Benassi, SK, Kheiri, F, and Engel, J, Jr (2011). Further evidence that pathologic high-frequency oscillations are bursts of population spikes derived from recordings of identified cells in dentate gyrus. Epilepsia 52:45–52.

Browning, RA (1987). Effect of lesions on seizures in experimental animals. In Epilepsy and the Reticular Formation: The Role of the Reticular Core in Convulsive Seizures. Edited by GH Fromm, CL Faingold, RA Browning, and WM Burnham. New York: Alan R Liss, pp. 137–162.

Buckmaster, PS (2006). Inherited epilepsy in Mongolian gerbils. In Models of Seizures and Epilepsy. Edited by A Pitkänen, PA Schwartzkroin, and SL Moshé. Burlington, MA: Elsevier Academic Press, pp. 273–294.

Burgess, DL (2006). Transgenic and gene replacement models of epilepsy: Targeting ion channel and neurotransmission pathways in mice. In Models of Seizures and Epilepsy. Edited by A Pitkänen, PA Schwartzkroin, and SL Moshé. Burlington, MA: Elsevier Academic Press, pp. 199–222.

Burnham, WM (1985). Progabide and other GABA mimetics in the kindling model. In Epilepsy and GABA Receptor Antagonists: Basic and Therapeutic Research. Edited by G Bartholini, L Bossi, KG Lloyd, and PL Morselli. New York: Raven Press, pp. 121–127.

Burnham, WM, Nizik, HB, Okazaki, MM, and Kish, SJ (1983). Binding of ^{3}H-flunitrazepam and ^{3}H-RO5–4864 to crude homogenates of amygdala-kindled rat brain: Two months post-seizure. Brain Res 279:359–362.

Buser, P, and Bancaud, J (1983). Unilateral connections between amygdala and hippocampus in man: A study of epileptic patients with depth electrodes. Electroencephalogr Clin Neurophysiol 55:1–12.

Buzsáki, G, Horvath, Z, Urioste, R, Hetke, J, and Wise K (1992). High frequency network oscillation in the hippocampus. Science 256:1025–1027.

Caldecott-Hazard, S, and Engel, J, Jr (1987). Limbic postictal events: Anatomical substrates and opioid receptor involvement. Prog Neuropsychopharmacol Biol Psychiatry 11:389–418.

Caspers, H, and Speckmann, E-J (1972). Cerebral pO_2, pCO_2 and pH: Changes during convulsive activity and their significance for spontaneous arrest of seizures. Epilepsia 13:699–725.

Cavalheiro, EA, Naffah-Mazzacoratti, MG, Mello, LE, and Leite, JP (2006). The pilocarpine model of seizures. In Models of Seizures and Epilepsy. Edited by A Pitkänen, PA Schwartzkroin, and SL Moshé. Burlington, MA: Elsevier Academic Press, pp. 433–448.

Cavus, I, and Wilson, CL (2008). Microdialysis. In Epilepsy: A Comprehensive Textbook, 2nd ed. Edited by J Engel, Jr, and TA Pedley. Philadelphia: Lippincott Williams & Wilkins, pp. 1031–1039.

Chachua, T, Yum, M-S, Veliskova, J, and Velísek, L (2011). Validation of the rat model of cryptogenic infantile spasms. Epilepsia 52:1666–1677.

Cherlow, DG, Dymond, AM, Crandall, PH, Walter, RD, and Serafetinides, EA (1977). Evoked response and after-discharge thresholds to electrical stimulation in temporal lobe epileptics. Arch Neurol 34:527–531.

Chugani, DC (2011). α-Methyl-L-tryptophan: Mechanisms for tracer localization of epileptogenic brain regions. Biomarkers Med 5:567–575.

Chugani, HT, Ackermann, RF, Chugani, DC, and Engel, J, Jr (1984). Opioid-induced epileptogenic phenomena: Anatomical, behavioral, and electroencephalographic features. Ann Neurol 15:361–368.

Cohen, MS, and Bookheimer, SY (2008). Functional magnetic resonance imaging. In Epilepsy: A Comprehensive Textbook, 2nd ed. Edited by J Engel, Jr, and TA Pedley. Philadelphia: Lippincott Williams & Wilkins, pp. 989–998.

Collingridge, GL, and Bliss, TVP (1987). NMDA receptors—Theirrole in long-term potentiation. Trends Neurosci 10:288–293.

Collins, RC (1978). Kindling of neuroanatomic pathways during recurrent focal penicillin seizures. Brain Res 150: 503–517.

Commission on Classification and Terminology of the International League Against Epilepsy (1981). Proposal for revised clinical and electroencephalographic classification of epileptic seizures. Epilepsia 22:489–501.

Commission on Classification and Terminology of the International League Against Epilepsy (1989). Proposal for revised classification of epilepsies and epileptic syndromes. Epilepsia 30:389–399.

Corcoran, ME, and Moshé, SL (eds) (2005). Kindling 6. New York: Springer Science.

Corcoran, ME, Wada, JA, Wake, A, and Urstad, H (1976). Failure of atropine to retard amygdaloid kindling. Exp Neurol 51: 271–275.

Cortez, MA, and Snead, OC, III (2006). Pharmacologic models of generalized absence seizures in rodents. In Models of Seizures and Epilepsy. Edited by A Pitkänen, PA Schwartzkroin, and SL Moshé. Burlington, MA: Elsevier Academic Press, pp. 111–126.

Cortez, MA, McKerlie, C, and Snead, OC, 3rd (2001). A model of atypical absence seizures: EEG, pharmacology, and developmental characterization. Neurology 56:341–349.

D'Ambrosio, R, and Miller, JW (2010a) Point. Epilepsy Curr 10:90.

D'Ambrosio, R, and Miller, JW (2010b). What is an epileptic seizure? Unifying definitions in clinical practice and animal research to develop novel treatments. Epilepsy Curr 10:61–66.

Dashieff, RM, Byrne, MC, Patrone, V, and McNamara, JO (1981). Biochemical evidence of decreased muscarinic cholinergic neuronal communication following amygdalakindled seizures. Brain Res 206:233–238.

Davenport, CJ, Brown, WJ, and Babb, TL (1990). Sprouting of GABAergic and mossy fiber axons in dentate gyrus following intrahippocampal kainate in the rat. Exp Neurol 109:180–190.

deCurtis, M, and Gnatkovsky, V (2009). Reevaluating the mechanisms of focal ictogenesis: The role of low-voltage fast activity. Epilepsia 50:2514–2525.

DePaulis, A, and Van Luijtelaar, G (2006). Genetic models of absence epilepsy in the rat. In Models of Seizures and Epilepsy. Edited by A Pitkänen, PA Schwartzkroin, and SL Moshé. Burlington, MA: Elsevier Academic Press, pp. 233–248.

DeVivo, D, Trifiletti, RR, Jacobson, RI, Ronen, GM, Behmand, RA, and Harik, SI (1991). Defective glucose transient across the blood-brain barrier as a cause of persistent hypoglycorrhachia, seizures, and developmental delay. N Engl J Med 325:703–709.

Dichter, MA, and Pollard, J (2006). Cell culture models for studying epilepsy. In Models of Seizures and Epilepsy. Edited by A Pitkänen, PA Schwartzkroin, and SL Moshé. Burlington, MA: Elsevier Academic Press, pp. 23–34.

Dingledine, R (1981). Possible mechanisms of enkephalin action on hippocampal CA1 pyramidal neurons. J Neurosci 1:1022–1035.

Dragunov, M, Goddard, GV, and Laverty, R (1985). Is adenosine an endogenous anticonvulsant? Epilepsia 26:480–487.

Dubé, CM, and Baram, TZ (2006). Complex febrile seizures—An experimental model in immature rodents. In Models of Seizures and Epilepsy. Edited by A Pitkänen, PA Schwartzkroin, and SL Moshé. Burlington, MA: Elsevier Academic Press, pp. 333–340.

Dudek, FE, and Bertram, EH (2010). Counterpoint to "What is an epileptic seizure?" by D'Ambrosio and Miller. Epilepsy Curr 10:91–94.

Dudek, FE, Clark, S, Williams, PA, and Grabenstatter, HL (2006). Kainate-induced status epilepticus: A chronic model of acquired epilepsy. In Models of Seizures and Epilepsy. Edited by A Pitkänen, PA Schwartzkroin, and SL Moshé. Burlington, MA: Elsevier Academic Press, pp. 415–432.

Dudek, FE, Ekstrom, JJ, and Staley, KJ (2010). Is neuronal death necessary for acquired epileptogenesis in the immature brain? Epilepsy Curr 10:95–99.

Echlin, FA (1959). The supersensitivity of chronically "isolated" cerebral cortex as a mechanism in focal epilepsy. Electroencephalogr Clin Neurophysiol 11:697–722.

Edmonds, HL, Jr, Hegreberg, GA, van Gelder, NM, Sylvester, DM, Clemmons, RM, and Chatburn, CG (1979). Spontaneous convulsions in beagle dogs. Fed Proc 38:2424–2428.

Ehlers, CL, Clifton, DK, and Sawyer, CH (1980). Facilitation of amygdala kindling in the rat by transecting ascending noradrenergic pathways. Brain Res 189:274–278.

Elger, CE, and Speckmann, E-J (1983). Penicillin induced epileptic foci in the motor cortex: Vertical inhibition. Electroencephalogr Clin Neurophysiol 56:604–622.

Engel, J, Jr (1968). Secondary epileptogenesis in rats. Electroencephalogr Clin Neurophysiol 25:494–498.

Engel, J, Jr (1983). Metabolic patterns of human epilepsy: Clinical observations and possible physiological correlates. In Current Problems in Epilepsy 1: Cerebral Blood Flow, Metabolism and Epilepsy. Edited by M Baldy-Moulinier, DH Ingvar, and BS Meldrum. London: John Libbey, pp. 6–18.

Engel, J, Jr (1984). The use of positron emission tomographic scanning in epilepsy. Ann Neurol 15 (suppl 1): S190–S191.

Engel, J, Jr (ed) (1993). Surgical Treatment of the Epilepsies, 2nd ed. New York, Raven Press.

Engel, J, Jr (ed) (1987a). Surgical Treatment of the Epilepsies. New York: Raven Press.

Engel, J, Jr (1987b). New concepts of the epileptic focus. In The Epileptic Focus. Edited by HG Weiser, E-JSpeckmann, and J Engel, Jr. London: John Libbey, pp. 83–94.

Engel, J, Jr (1988a). Brain metabolism and pathophysiology of human epilepsy. In Mechanisms of Epileptogenesis: The Transition to Seizure. Edited by MA Dichter. New York: Plenum Press, pp. 1–15.

Engel, J, Jr (1988b). Comparison of positron emission tomography and electroencephalography as measures of cerebral function in epilepsy. In Functional Brain Imaging. Edited by G Pfurtscheller and FH Lopes da Silva. New York: Hans Huber, pp. 229–238.

Engel, J, Jr (1990). Functional explorations of the human epileptic brain and their therapeutic implications. Electroencephalogr Clin Neurophysiol 76:296–316.

Engel, J, Jr (1992). Experimental animal models of epilepsy: Classification and relevance to human epileptic phenomena. In Neurotransmitters and Epilepsy. Edited by G Avanzini, J Engel, Jr, R Fariello, and U Heinemann, Amsterdam: Elsevier, pp. 9–20.

Engel, J, Jr (1998a). Research on the human brain in an epilepsy surgery setting. Epilepsy Res 32:1–11.

Engel, J, Jr (1998b) The syndrome of mesial temporal lobe epilepsy: A role for kindling. In Kindling 5. Edited by M Corcoran and S Moshé. New York: Plenum Press, pp. 469–480.

Engel, J, Jr (2001). Mesial temporal lobe epilepsy: What have we learned? The Neuroscientist 7:340–352.

Engel, J, Jr, and Ackermann, RF (1980). Interictal EEG spikes correlate with decreased, rather than increased epileptogenicity in amygdaloid kindled rats. Brain Res 190:543–548.

Engel, J, Jr, and Bertram, EH (2004). The search for pharmacological and non-pharmacological targets for curing epilepsy: Chair summary. Epilepsy Res 60:125–131.

Engel, J, Jr, and Cahan, L (1986). Potential relevance of kindling to human partial epilepsy. In Kindling 3. Edited by J Wada. New York: Raven Press, pp. 37–51.

Engel, J, Jr, and Lopes daSilva, F (2012). High-frequency oscillations—Where we are and where we need to go. Prog Neurobiol 98:316–338.

Engel, J, Jr, and Morrell, F (1970). Turnover of RNA in normal and secondarily epileptogenic rabbit cortex. Exp Neurol 26:221–238.

Engel, J, Jr, and Pedley, TA (eds) (2008). Epilepsy: A Comprehensive Textbook, 2nd ed. Philadelphia: Lippincott Williams & Wilkins.

Engel, J, Jr, and Schwartzkroin, PA (2006). Who should be modeled? In Models of Seizures and Epilepsy.

Edited by A Pitkänen, PA Schwartzkroin, and SL Moshé. Burlington, MA: Elsevier Academic Press, pp. 1–14.

Engel, J, Jr, and Sharpless, NS (1977). Long-lasting depletion of dopamine in the rat amygdala induced by kindling stimulation. Brain Res 136:381–386.

Engel, J, Jr, and Shewmon, DA (1991). Impact of the kindling phenomenon on clinical epileptology. In Kindling and Synaptic Plasticity: The Legacy of Graham Goddard. Edited by F Morrell. Cambridge, MA: Birkhäuser Boston, pp. 195–210.

Engel, J, Jr, and Williamson, PD (2008). Limbic seizures. In Epilepsy: A Comprehensive Textbook, 2nd ed. Edited by J Engel, Jr, and TA Pedley. Philadelphia: Lippincott Williams & Wilkins, pp. 541–552.

Engel, J, Jr, and Wilson, CL (1986). Evidence for enhanced synaptic inhibition in epilepsy. In Neurotransmitters, Seizures, and Epilepsy III. Edited by G Nisticò, PL Morselli, KG Lloyd, RG Fariello, and J Engel, Jr. New York: Raven Press, pp. 1–13.

Engel, J, Jr, Wolfson, L, and Brown, L (1978). Anatomical correlates of electrical and behavioral events related to amygdaloid kindling. Ann Neurol 3:538–544.

Engel, J, Jr, Ackermann, RF, Caldecott-Hazard, S, and Kuhl, DE (1981). Epileptic activation of antagonistic systems may explain paradoxical features of experimental and human epilepsy: A review and hypothesis. In Kindling 2. Edited by JA Wada. New York: Raven Press, pp. 193–211.

Engel, J, Jr, Brown, WJ, Kuhl, DE, Phelps, ME, Mazziotta, JC, and Crandall, PH. (1982a). Pathological findings underlying focal temporal lobe hypometabolism in partial epilepsy. Ann Neurol 12:518–528.

Engel, J, Jr, Kuhl, DE, Phelps, ME, and Crandall, PH. (1982b).Comparative localization of epileptic foci in partial epilepsy by PCT and EEG. Ann Neurol 12:529–537.

Engel, J, Jr, Kuhl, DE, Phelps, ME, and Mazziotta, JC. (1982c). Interictal cerebral glucose metabolism in partial epilepsy and its relation to EEG changes. Ann Neurol 12:510–517.

Engel, J, Jr, Kuhl, DE, and Phelps, ME. (1982d). Patterns of human local cerebral glucose metabolism during epileptic seizures. Science 218:64–66.

Engel, J, Jr, Crandall, PH, and Rausch, R. (1983a). The partial epilepsies. In The Clinical Neurosciences, Vol 2. Edited by RN Rosenberg. New York: Churchill Livingstone, pp. 1349–1380.

Engel, J, Jr, Kuhl, DE, Phelps, ME, Rausch, R, and Nuwer, M. (1983b). Local cerebral metabolism during partial seizures. Neurology 33: 400–413.

Engel, J, Jr, Ackermann, RF, Caldecott-Hazard, S, and Chugani, HT. (1984a). Do altered opioid mechanisms play a role in human epilepsy? In Neurotransmitters, Seizures, and Epilepsy II. Edited by RG Fariello, PL Morselli, K Lloyd, LF Quesney, and J Engel, Jr. New York: Raven Press, pp. 263–274.

Engel, J, Jr, Caldecott-Hazard, S, Chugani, HT, and Ackermann, RF. (1984b). Neuropeptides, seizures and epilepsy. In Advances in Epileptology: XV Epilepsy International Symposium. Edited by RJ Porter, RH Mattson, AA Ward, and M Dam. New York: Raven Press, pp. 25–30.

Engel, J, Jr, Lubens, P, Kuhl, DE, and Phelps, M (1985). Local cerebral metabolic rate for glucose during petit mal absences. Ann Neurol 17:121–128.

Engel, J, Jr, Bandler, R, and Caldecott-Hazard, S. (1985–1986). Modification of emotional expression induced by clinical and experimental epileptic disturbances. Int J Neurol 19/20:30–39.

Engel, J, Jr, Caldecott-Hazard, S, and Bandler, R (1986). Neurobiology of behavior: Anatomic and physiologic implications related to epilepsy. Epilepsia 27(suppl 2): S3–S11.

Engel, J, Jr, Ojemann, G, Lüders, H, and Williamson, PD (eds) (1987). Fundamental Mechanisms of Human Brain Function: Opportunities for Direct Investigation in Association with the Surgical Treatment of Epilepsy. New York: Raven Press, p 288

Engel, J, Jr, Babb, TL and Crandall, PH (1989). Surgical treatment of epilepsy: Opportunities for research into basic mechanisms of human brain function. Acta Neurochir Suppl 46:3–8.

Engel, J, Jr, Wasterlain, C, Cavalheiro, E, Heinemann, U, and Avanzini, G (eds) (1992). Molecular Neurobiology of Epilepsy, Epilepsy Research (suppl 9). Amsterdam: Elsevier.

Engel, J, Jr, Dichter, MA, and Schwartzkroin, PA. (2008a). Basic mechanisms of human epilepsy. In Epilepsy: A Comprehensive Textbook, 2nd ed. Edited by J Engel, Jr, and TA Pedley. Philadelphia: Lippincott Williams & Wilkins, pp. 495–507.

Engel, J, Jr, Taylor, DC, and Trimble, MR. (2008b) Neurobiology of behavioral disorders. In Epilepsy: A Comprehensive Textbook, 2nd ed. Edited by J Engel, Jr, and TA Pedley. Philadelphia: Lippincott Williams & Wilkins, pp. 2077–2083.

Engel, J, Jr, Bragin A, Staba R, and Mody I (2009). High-frequency oscillations: What's normal and what is not? Epilepsia 50:598–604.

Fariello, RG, and Golden, GT (1987). The THIP-induced model of bilateral synchronous spike and wave in rodents. Neuropharmacology 26:161–165.

Fisher, RS, van Emde Boas, W, Blume, W, Elger, C, Engel, J, Jr, Genton, P, and Lee, P (2005). Epileptic seizures and epilepsy. Definitions proposed by the International League against Epilepsy (ILAE) and the International Bureau for Epilepsy (IBE). Epilepsia 46:470–472.

Foffani G, Uzcategui YG, Gal B, and Menendez de la Prida L (2007).Reduced spike-timing reliability correlates with the emergence of fast ripples in the rat epileptic hippocampus. Neuron 55:930–941.

Fried, I, Wilson, CL, Maidment, NT, Engel, J, Jr, Behnke, E, Fields, TA, MacDonald, KA, Morrow, JW, and Ackerson, L (1999).Cerebral microdialysis combined with single-neuron and electroencephalographic recording in neurosurgical patients. J Neurosurg 91:697–705.

Fromm, GH (1987). The brain-stem and seizures: Summary and synthesis. In Epilepsy and the Reticular Formation: The Role of the Reticular Core in Convulsive Seizures. Edited by GH Fromm, CL Faingold, RA Browning, and WM Burnham. New York: Alan R Liss, pp. 203–218.

Fromm, GH, Faingold, CL, Browning, RA, and Burnham, WM (eds) (1987). Epilepsy and the Reticular Formation: The Role of the Reticular Core in Convulsive Seizures. New York: Alan R Liss.

Frost, JJ, Mayberg, HS, Fisher, RS, Douglass, KH, Dannals, RF, Links, JM, Wilson, AA, Ravert, HT, Rosenbaum, AE, Synder, SH, and Wagner, HN (1988). Mu-opiate receptors measured by positron emission tomography are increased in temporal lobe epilepsy. Ann Neurol 23:231–237.

Galanopoulou, AS, Buckmaster, P, Staley, K, Moshé, SL, Perucca, E, Engel, J, Jr., Löscher, W, Noebels, JL, Pitkänen, A, Stables, J, White, SH, O'Brien, TJ, and Simonato, M (2012). Identification of new epilepsy treatments: issues in preclinical methodology. Epilepsia 53: 571–582.

Gale, K (1984). The role of the substantia nigra in the anticonvulsant actions of GABAergic drugs. In Neurotransmitters, Seizures, and Epilepsy II. Edited by RG Fariello, K Lloyd, PL Morselli, LF Quesney, and J Engel, Jr. New York: Raven Press, pp. 57–79.

Gale, K, Proctor, M, Velisková, J, and Nehlig, A (2008). Basal ganglia and brainstem anatomy and physiology. In Epilepsy: A Comprehensive Textbook, 2nd ed. Edited by J Engel, Jr, and TA Pedley. Philadelphia: Lippincott Williams & Wilkins, pp. 367–384.

Galvan, CD, Wenzel, JH, Dineley, KT, Lam, TT, Schwartzkroin, PA, Sweatt, JD, et al. (2003). Postsynaptic contributions to hippocampal network hyperexcitability induced by chronic activity blockade in vivo. Eur J Neurosci 18:1861–1872.

Geinisman, Y, Morrell, F, and deToledo Morrell, L (1988). Remodeling of synaptic architecture during hippocampal "kindling." Proc Natl Acad Sci USA 85:3260–3264.

Gerin, P (1960). Microelectrode investigations on the mechanisms of the electrically induced epileptiform seizure ("afterdischarge"). Arch Ital Biol 98:21–40.

Giaretta, A, Avoli, M, and Gloor, P (1987). Intracellular recordings in pericruciate neurons during spike and wave discharges of feline generalized penicillin epilepsy. Brain Res 405:68–79.

Giblin, KA, and Blumenfeld, H (2010). Is epilepsy a preventable disorder? New evidence from animal models. The Neuroscientist 16:253–275.

Gilbert, ME, and Goodman, JH (2006). Chemical kindling. In Models of Seizures and Epilepsy. Edited by A Pitkänen, PA Schwartzkroin, and SL Moshé. Burlington, MA: Elsevier Academic Press, pp. 379–393.

Gloor, P (1968). Generalized cortico-reticular epilepsies: Some considerations on the pathophysiology of generalized bilaterally synchronous spike and wave discharge. Epilepsia 9:249–263.

Gloor, P, Quesney, LF, and Zumstein, H (1977). Pathophysiology of generalized penicillin epilepsy in the cat: The role of cortical and subcortical structures. II. Topical applications of penicillin to the cerebral cortex and to subcortical structures. Electroencephalogr Clin Neurophysiol 43:79–94.

Gnatkovsky, V, Librizzi, L, Trombin, F, and deCurtis, M (2008). Fast activity at seizure onset is mediated by inhibitory circuits in the entorhinal cortex in vitro. Ann Neurol 64:674–686.

Goddard, GV, McIntyre, DC, and Leech, CK (1969). A permanent change in brain function resulting from daily electrical stimulation. Exp Neurol 25:295–330.

Goldensohn, ES (1969). Experimental seizure mechanisms (discussion). In Basic Mechanisms of the Epilepsies. Edited by HH Jasper, AA Ward, Jr, and A Pope. Boston: Little, Brown & Co, pp. 289–298.

Gorji, A, and Speckmann, E-J (2006). Brain tumour and epilepsy: A new neurophysiologic and neuropathologic ex vivo in vitro model. In Models of Seizures and Epilepsy. Edited by A Pitkänen, PA Schwartzkroin, and SL Moshé. Burlington, MA: Elsevier Academic Press, pp. 527–533.

Gotman, J, and Pittau, F (2011). Combining EEG and fMRI in the study of epileptic discharges. Epilepsia 52:38–42.

Graber, KD, and Prince, DA (2006). Chronic partial cortical isolation. In Models of Seizures and Epilepsy. Edited by A Pitkänen, PA Schwartzkroin, and SL Moshé. Burlington, MA: Elsevier Academic Press, pp. 477–493.

Griffith, N, Engel, J, Jr, and Bandler, R (1987). Ictal and enduring interictal disturbances in emotional behaviour in an animal model of temporal lobe epilepsy. Brain Res 400:360–364.

Gross, DW (2011). Diffusion tensor imaging in temporal lobe epilepsy. Epilepsia 52:32–34.

Gur, RC, Sussman, NM, Alavi, A, Gur, RE, Rosen, AD, O'Connor, M, Goldberg, HI, Greenberg, JH, and Reivich, M (1982). Positron emission tomography in two cases of childhood epileptic encephalopathy (Lennox-Gastaut syndrome). Neurology 32:1191–1194.

Haas, KZ, Sperber, EF, and Moshé, SL (1990). Kindling in developing animals: Expression of severe seizures and enhanced development of bilateral foci. Brain Res Dev Brain Res 56(2):275–280.

Haglund, MM, Hochman, D, and Toga, AW (2008). Optical imaging of seizure activity. In Epilepsy: A Comprehensive Textbook, 2nd ed. Edited by J Engel, Jr, and TA Pedley. Philadelphia: Lippincott Williams & Wilkins, pp. 1025–1030.

Handforth, A, and Ackermann, RF (1989). Electrically induced limbic status and kindled seizures. In Anatomy of Epileptogenesis. Edited by BS Meldrum, JA Ferendelli, and HG Wieser. London: John Libbey, pp. 71–87.

Harris, AB, and Lockard, JS (1981). Absence of seizures or mirror foci in experimental epilepsy after excision of alumina and astrogliotic scar. Epilepsia 22:107–122.

Heinemann, U (1987). Changes in the neuronal micro-environment and epileptiform activity. In Current Problems in Epilepsy 3: The Epileptic Focus. Edited by HG Wieser, E-J Speckmann, and J Engel, Jr. London: John Libbey, pp. 27–44.

Heinemann, U, and Lambert, JC (1986). Changes in extracellular calcium and magnesium concentration and their consequences for the development of seizure activity. In Neurotransmitters, Seizures, and Epilepsy III. Edited by G Nisticò, PL Morselli, KG Lloyd, RG Fariello, and J Engel, Jr. New York: Raven Press, pp. 65–74.

Heinemann, U, Engel, J, Jr, Meldrum, BS, Wasterlain, C, Avanzini, G and Mouritzen-Dam, A (eds) (1996). The Progressive Nature of Epilepsy, Epilepsy Research (suppl 12). Amsterdam: Elsevier.

Heinemann, U, Kann, O, and Schuchmann, S (2006). An overview of in vitro seizure models in acute and organotypic slices. In Models of Seizures and Epilepsy. Edited by A Pitkänen, PA Schwartzkroin, and SL Moshé. Burlington, MA: Elsevier Academic Press, pp. 35–44.

Henry, TR, and Chugani, HT (2008). Positron emission tomography. In Epilepsy: A Comprehensive Textbook, 2nd ed. Edited by J Engel, Jr, and TA Pedley. Philadelphia: Lippincott Williams & Wilkins, pp. 945–964.

Henry, TR, Frey, KA, Sackellares, JC, Gilman, S, Koeppe, RA, Buchtel, HA, Brunberg, JA, Ross, DA, Berent, S, Young, AB, and Kuhl, DE (1993). In vivo cerebral metabolism and central benzodiazepine receptor binding in temporal lobe epilepsy. Neurology 43:1998–2006.

Holmes, GL (1986).Morphological and physiological maturation of the brain in the neonate and young child. J Clin Neurophysiol 3:209–238.

Isokawa, M, and Levesque, MF (1991). Increased NMDA responses and dendritic degeneration in human epileptic hippocampal neurons in slices. Neurosci Lett 132:212–216.

Isokawa-Akesson, M, Wilson, CL, and Babb, TL (1989). Inhibition in synchronously firing human hippocampal neurons. Epilepsy Res 3:236–247.

Jackson, GD, Berkovic, SF, Tress, BM, Kalnins, RM, Fabinyi, G, and Bladin, PF (1990). Hippocampal sclerosis can be reliably detected by magnetic resonance imaging. Neurology 40:1869–1875.

Jackson, GD, Connelly, A, Cross, JH, Gordon, I, and Gadian, DG (1994). Functional magnetic resonance imaging of focal seizures. Neurology 44:850–856.

Jacobs, J, Zijlmans, M, Zelmann, R, Chatillon, CE, Hall, J, Olivier, A, Dubeau, F, and Gotman, J (2010). High-frequency electroencephalographic oscillations correlate with outcome of epilepsy surgery. Ann Neurol 67:209–220.

Jacobs, MP, Fischbach, GD, Davis, MR, Dichter, MA, Dingledine, R, and Lowenstein, DH (2001). Future directions for epilepsy research. Neurology 57:1536–1542.

Jefferys, JGR (2008). Epilepsy in vitro: Electrophysiology and computer modeling. In Epilepsy: A Comprehensive Textbook, 2nd ed. Edited by J Engel, Jr, and TA Pedley. Philadelphia: Lippincott Williams & Wilkins, pp. 457–468.

Jefferys JGR, and Walker MC (2006). Tetanus toxin model of focal epilepsy. In Models of Seizures and Epilepsy. Edited by A Pitkänen, PA Schwartzkroin, and SL Moshé. Burlington, MA: Elsevier Academic Press, pp. 407–414.

Jobe, PC, and Browning, RA (2006). Mammalian models of genetic epilepsy characterized by sensory-evoked seizures and generalized seizure susceptibility. In Models of Seizures and Epilepsy. Edited by A Pitkänen, PA Schwartzkroin, and SL Moshé. Burlington, MA: Elsevier Academic Press, pp. 261–271.

Johnson, DD, Jaju, AR, Ness, L, Richardson, JR, and Crawford, RD (1979). Brain norepinephrine, dopamine, and biochemical studies in epileptic fowl. Fed Proc 38:2417–2423.

Johnston, D, and Brown, TH (1981). Giant synaptic potential hypothesis for epileptiform activity. Science 211:294–297.

Karpiak, SE, Huang, YL, and Rapport, MM (1982). Immunological model of epilepsy: Epileptiform activity induced by fragments of antibody to GM1 ganglioside. J Neuroimmunol 3:15–21.

Kazemi, NJ, O'Brien, TJ, Cascino, GD, and So, EL (2008). Single photon emission computed tomography. In Epilepsy: A Comprehensive Textbook, 2nd ed. Edited by J Engel, Jr, and TA Pedley. Philadelphia: Lippincott Williams & Wilkins, pp. 965–973.

Kelly, MS, Jacobs, MP, and Lowenstein, DH (2009). The NINDS epilepsy research benchmarks. Epilepsia 50:579–582.

Khalilov, I, Holmes, GL, and Ben-Ari, Y (2003). In vitro formation of a secondary epileptogenic mirror focus by interhippocampal propagation of seizures. Nat Neurosci 6:1079–1085.

Killam, KF, Naquet, R, and Bert, J (1966). Paroxysmal responses to intermittent light stimulation in a population of baboons (Papio papio). Epilepsia 7:215–219.

Klaassen, A, Glykys, J, Maguire, J, Labarca, C, Mody, I, and Boulter, J (2006). Seizures and enhanced cortical GABAergic inhibition in two mouse models of human autosomal dominant nocturnal frontal lobe epilepsy. Proc Natl Acad Sci USA 103:19152–19157.

Knowles, WD, Traub, RD, Wong, RKS, and Miles, R (1985). Properties of neural networks: Experimentation and modeling of the epileptic hippocampal slice. Trends Neurosci 8:73–79.

Kovacs, DA, and Zoll, JG (1974). Seizure inhibition by median raphe nucleus stimulation in the rat. Brain Res 70:165–169.

Kuhl, DE, Engel, J, Jr, Phelps, ME, and Selin, C (1980). Epileptic patterns of local cerebral metabolism and perfusion in humans determined by emission computed tomography of ^{18}FDG and ^{13}NH$_3$. Ann Neurol 8:348–360.

Kumar, A, Asano, E, and Chugani, HT (2011). α-[^{11}C]-methyl-L-tryptophan PET: Clinical studies. Biomarkers Med 5:577–584.

Le Van Quyen, M, J (2012). High frequency oscillations. Prog Neurobiol 98:239–318.

Le Van Quyen, M, Bragin, A, Staba, R, Crépon, B, Wilson, CL, and Engel, J, Jr (2008). Cell type-specific firing during ripple oscillations in the hippocampal formation of humans. J Neurosci 28:6104–6110.

Le Van Quyen, M, Staba, R, Bragin, A, Dickson, C, Valderrama, M, Fried, I, and Engel, J, Jr (2010). Large-scale microelectrode recordings of high-frequency gamma oscillations in human cortex during sleep. J Neurosci 30:7770–7782.

Lewin, E (1972). The production of epileptogenic cortical foci in experimental animals by freezing. In Experimental Models of Epilepsy—A Manual for the Laboratory Worker. Edited by DP Purpura, JK Penry, DB Tower, and RD Walter. New York: Raven Press, pp. 37–49.

Lieb, JP, Engel, J, Jr, Gevins, AS, and Crandall, PH. (1981a). Surface and deep EEG correlates of surgical outcome in temporal lobe epilepsy. Epilepsia 22:515–538.

Lieb, JP, Engel, J, Jr, Brown, WJ, Gevins, AS, and Crandall, PH. (1981b) Neuropathological findings following temporal lobectomy related to surface and deep EEG patterns. Epilepsia 22:539–549.

Lieb, JP, Engel, J, Jr, and Babb, TL (1986). Interhemispheric propagation time of human hippocampal seizures. I. Relationship to surgical outcome. Epilepsia 27(3): 286–293.

Lin, DD, and Roper, SN (2006). In uteroirradiation as a model of cortical dysplasia. In Models of Seizures and Epilepsy. Edited by A Pitkänen, PA Schwartzkroin, and SL Moshé. Burlington, MA: Elsevier Academic Press, pp. 315–322.

Lockard, JS, and Levy, RH (1982). Experimental quantification and evaluation of anticonvulsant drugs in a primate model. In Antiepileptic Drugs, 2nd ed. Edited by DM Woodbury, JK Penry, and CE Pippenger. New York: Raven Press, pp. 127–140 .

Lockard, JS, Cangdon, WC, DuCharme, LL, and Finch, CA (1980). Slow-speed EEG for chronic monitoring of clinical seizures in monkey model. Epilepsia 21:325–334.

Löscher, W, and Brandt, C (2010). Prevention or modification of epileptogenesis after brain insults: Experimental approaches and translational research. Pharmacol Rev 62:668–700.

Löscher, W, and Schmidt, D (1988). Which animal models should be used in the search for new antiepileptic drugs? A proposal based on experimental and clinical considerations. Epilepsy Res 2:145–181.

Loskata, WJ, Lomax, P, and Rich, ST (1974). The gerbil as a model for the study of the epilepsies: Seizure patterns and ontogenesis. Epilepsia 15:109–119.

Lothman, EW, and Williamson, JM (1994). Closely spaced recurrent hippocampal seizures elicit two types of heightened epileptogenesis: a rapidly developing, transient kindling and a slowly developing, enduring kindling. Brain Res 649:71–84.

Lüders, HO, Engel, J, Jr, and Munari, C (1993). General principles. In Surgical Treatment of the Epilepsies, 2nd ed. Edited by J Engel, Jr. New York: Raven Press, pp. 137–153.

Luhmann, HJ (2006). The cortical freeze lesion model. In Models of Seizures and Epilepsy. Edited by A Pitkänen, PA Schwartzkroin, and SL Moshé. Burlington, MA: Elsevier Academic Press, pp. 295–303.

Lukasiuk, K, Dingledine, R, Lowenstein, DH, and Pitkänen, A (2008). Gene expression underlying changes in network excitability. In Epilepsy: A Comprehensive Textbook, 2nd ed. Edited by J Engel, Jr, and TA Pedley. Philadelphia: Lippincott Williams & Wilkins, pp. 307–322.

Lynch, BA, Lambeng, N, Mocka, K, Kensel-Hammes, P, Bajjalieh, SM, Matagne, A, and Fuks, B (2004). The synaptic vesicle protein SV2A is the binding site for the antiepileptic drug levetiracetam. Proc Natl Acad Sci USA 101:9861–9866.

Maglóczky, Z (2010). Sprouting in human temporal lobe epilepsy: Excitatory pathways and axons of interneurons. Epilepsy Res 89:52–59.

Mai, JK, Assheuer, J, and Paxinos, G (1997). Atlas of the Human Brain. San Diego: Academic Press.

Mann, EO, and Mody, I (2008). The multifaceted role of inhibition in epilepsy: Seizure-genesis through excessive GABAergic inhibition in autosomal dominant nocturnal frontal lobe epilepsy. Curr Opin Neurol 21:155–160.

Marcus, EM (1972). Experimental models of petit mal epilepsy. In Experimental Models of Epilepsy—A Manual for the Laboratory Worker. Edited by DP Purpura, JK Penry, DB Tower, DM Woodbury, and R Walter. New York: Raven Press, pp. 113–146.

Mares, P, and Kubová, H (2006). Electrical stimulation-induced models of seizures. In Models of Seizures and Epilepsy. Edited by A Pitkänen, PA Schwartzkroin, and SL Moshé. Burlington, MA: Elsevier Academic Press, pp. 153–159.

Margerison, JH, and Corsellis, JA (1966). Epilepsy and the temporal lobes: A clinical, electroencephalographic and neuropathological study of the brain in epilepsy, with particular reference to the temporal lobes. Brain 89:499–530.

Marsh, E, Fulp, C, Gomez, E, Nasrallah, I, Minarcik, J, Sudi, J, et al. (2009). Targeted loss of Arx results in a developmental epilepsy mouse model and recapitulates the human phenotype in heterozygous females. Brain 132: 1563–1576.

Mathern, GW, Wilson, CL, and Beck, H (2008). Hippocampal sclerosis. In Epilepsy: A Comprehensive Textbook, 2nd ed. Edited by J Engel, Jr, and TA Pedley. Philadelphia: Lippincott Williams & Wilkins, pp. 121–136.

Matsumoto, H, and Ajmone-Marsan, C (1964a). Cortical cellular phenomena in experimental epilepsy: Interictal manifestations. Exp Neurol 9:286–304.

Matsumoto, H, and Ajmone-Marsan, C (1964b). Cortical cellular phenomena in experimental epilepsy: Ictal manifestations. Exp Neurol 9:305–326.

Mazarati, AM, Thompson, KW, Lucie, S, Sankar, R, Shirasaka, Y, Nissinen, J, Pitkänen, A, Bertram, E, and Wasterlain, C (2006). Status epilepticus: Electrical stimulation models. In Models of Seizures and Epilepsy. Edited by A Pitkänen, PA Schwartzkroin, and SL Moshé. Burlington, MA: Elsevier Academic Press, pp. 449–464.

McCormick, DA, and Contreras, D (2001). On the cellular and network bases of epileptic seizures. Annu Rev Physiol 63:815–846.

McIntyre, DC (1975). Split brain rat: Transfer and interference of kindled amygdala convulsions. Can J Neurol Sci 2:429–437.

McIntyre, DC (1986). Kindling and the pyriform cortex. In Kindling 3. Edited by JA Wada. New York: Raven Press, pp. 249–262.

McIntyre, DC (2006). The kindling phenomenon. In Models of Seizures and Epilepsy. Edited by A Pitkänen, PA Schwartzkroin, and SL Moshé. Burlington, MA: Elsevier Academic Press, pp. 351–353.

McIntyre, DC, and Goddard, GV (1973). Transfer, interference and spontaneous recovery of convulsions kindled from the rat amygdala. Electroencephalogr Clin Neurophysiol 35:533–543.

McIntyre, DC, Nathanson, D, and Edson, N (1982). A new model of partial status epilepticus based on kindling. Brain Res 250:53–63.

McLean, MJ, and Macdonald, RL (1986). Limitation of sustained high frequency repetitive firing: A common anticonvulsant drug mechanism of action? In Neurotransmitters, Seizures, and Epilepsy III. Edited by G Nisticò, PL Morselli, KG Lloyd, RG Fariello, and J Engel, Jr. New York: Raven Press, pp. 23–41.

Miles, R, and Wong, RKS (1987). Inhibitory control of local excitatory circuits in the guinea-pig hippocampus. J Physiol 388:611–629.

Millichap, JG (1968). Febrile Convulsions. New York: Macmillan.

Mody, I, and Heinemann, U (1987). NMDA receptors of dentate gyrus granule cells participate in synaptic transmission following kindling. Nature 326: 701–704.

Morimoto, K, Fahnestock, M, and Racine, RJ (2004). Kindling and status epilepticus models of epilepsy: Rewiring the brain. Prog Neurol 73:1–60.

Morrell, F (1959/60). Secondary epileptogenic lesions. Epilepsia 1:538–560.

Morrell, F, Wada, JA, and Engel, J, Jr (1987). Potential relevance of kindling and secondary epileptogenesis to the consideration of surgical treatment for epilepsy. In Surgical Treatment of the Epilepsies. Edited by J Engel, Jr. New York: Raven Press, pp. 699–705.

Moshé, SL (1981). The effects of age on the kindling phenomenon. Dev Psychobiol 14(1):75–81.

Moshé, SL (1987). Epileptogenesis and the immature brain. Epilepsia 28(suppl 1):S3–S15.

Moshé, SL, and Albala, BJ (1983). Maturational changes in postictal refractoriness and seizure susceptibility in developing rats. Ann Neurol 13(5):552–557.

Moshé, SL, Albala, BJ, Ackermann, RF, and Engel, J, Jr (1983). Increased seizure susceptibility of the immature brain. Dev Brain Res 7:81–85.

Moshé SL, Ackermann, RF, Albala, BJ, and Okada, R (1986). The role of substantia nigra in seizures of developing animals. In Kindling 3. Edited by JA Wada. New York: Raven Press, pp. 91–106.

Moshé, SL, Engel, J, Jr, Mathern, GW, Nehlig, A, Pitkänen, A, and Vezzani, A (eds) (2000). Fifth Workshop on the Neurobiology of Epilepsy (WONOEP V):Brain Plasticity and Epilepsy. Epilepsia 41(special issue): S1–S205.

Mucha, RF, and Pinel, JPJ (1977). Postseizure inhibition of kindled seizures. Exp Neurol 54:266–282.

Naquet, R, and Meldrum, BS (1972). Photogenic seizures in baboon. In Experimental Models of Epilepsy—A Manual for the Laboratory Worker. Edited by DP Purpura, JK Penry, DB Tower, DM Woodbury, and RD Walter. New York: Raven Press, pp. 373–406.

Nehlig, A, Coppola, A, and Moshé, SL (2012). Syndromes and brain development. In Epileptic Syndromes in Infancy, Childhood and Adolescence. Edited by M Bureau, P Genton, C Dravet, A Delgado-Escueta, CA Tassinari, P Thomas, and P Wolf. Paris: John Libbey Eurotext (in press).

N'Gouemo, P, and Rogawski, MA (2006). Alcohol withdrawal seizures. In Models of Seizures and Epilepsy. Edited by A Pitkänen, PA Schwartzkroin, and SL Moshé. Burlington, MA: Elsevier Academic Press, pp. 161–177.

Nie, V, McCabe, JJ, Ettlinger, G, and Driver, MV (1974). The development of secondary epileptic discharges in the rhesus monkey after commissure section. Electroencephalogr Clin Neurophysiol 37:473–481.

Noebels, JL (2006). Spontaneous epileptic mutations in the mouse. In Models of Seizures and Epilepsy. Edited by A Pitkänen, PA Schwartzkroin, and SL Moshé. Burlington, MA: Elsevier Academic Press, pp. 223–232.

Ochs, RF, Gloor, P, Tyler, JL, Wolfson, T, Worsley, K, Andermann, F, Diksic, M, Meyer, E, and Evans, A (1987). Effect of generalized spike-and-wave discharge on glucose metabolism measured by positron emission tomography. Ann Neurol 21:458–464.

Ogren, JA, Bragin, A, Wilson, CL, Hoftman, GD, Lin, JJ, Dutton, RA, Fields, TA, Toga, AW, Thompson, PM, Engel, J, Jr, and Staba, RJ (2009a). Three-dimensional hippocampal atrophy maps distinguish two common temporal lobe seizure-onset patterns. Epilepsia 50:1361–1370.

Ogren, JA, Wilson, CL, Bragin, A, Lin, JJ, Salamon, N, Dutton, RA, Luders, E, Fields, TA, Fried, I, Toga, AW, Thompson, PM, Engel, J, Jr, and Staba, RJ (2009b). Three-dimensional surface maps link local atrophy and fast ripples in human epileptic hippocampus. Ann Neurol 66:783–791.

Okada, R, Moshé, SL, and Albala, BJ (1984). Infantile status epilepticus and future seizure susceptibility in the rat. Dev Brain Res 15:177–183.

Oliver, MW, and Miller, JJ (1985). Alterations of inhibitory processes in the dentate gyrus following kindling-induced epilepsy. Exp Brain Res 57:443–447.

Openchowski, P (1883). Sur l'action localisée du froid, appliquéà la surface de la région corticale du cerveau. C R Seances Memoires Soc Biol, 7th Ser, 4:38–43.

Ottman, R, and Winawer, MR (2008). Genetic epidemiology. In Epilepsy: A Comprehensive Textbook, 2nd ed. Edited by J Engel, Jr, and TA Pedley. Philadelphia: Lippincott Williams & Wilkins, pp. 161–170.

Palop, JJ, Chin, J, Roberson, ED, Wang, J, Thwin, MT, Bien-Ly, N, Yoo, J, Ho, KO, Yu, G-Q, Kreitzer, A, Finkbeiner, S, Noebels, JL, and Mucke, L (2007). Aberrant excitatory neuronal activity and compensatory remodeling of inhibitory hippocampal circuits in mouse models of Alzheimer's disease. Neuron 55:697–711.

Panayiotopoulos, CP (ed), Benbadis, SR, Beran, RG, Berg, AT, Engel, J, Jr, Galanopoulou, AS, Kaplan, PW, Koutroumanidis, M, Moshé, SL, Nordli, DR, Jr, Serratosa, JM, Sisodiya, SM, Tatum, WO, IV, Valeta, T, and Wilner, AN (section eds) (2010). Atlas of Epilepsies, Vols I–III. London: Springer,

Pappas, GD, and Purpura, DP (1972). Structure and Function of Synapses. New York: Raven Press.

Parent, JM, Coulter, DA, and Bertram, EH (2008). The effect of seizures on the brain. In Epilepsy: A Comprehensive Textbook, 2nd ed. Edited by J Engel, Jr, and TA Pedley. Philadelphia: Lippincott Williams & Wilkins, pp. 481–493.

Petroff, OAC, and Duncan, JS (2008). Magnetic resonance spectroscopy. In Epilepsy: A Comprehensive Textbook, 2nd ed. Edited by J Engel, Jr, and TA Pedley. Philadelphia: Lippincott Williams & Wilkins, pp. 975–988.

Phillips, NK, and Lockard, JS (1985). A gestational monkey model: Effects of phenytoin versus seizures on neonatal outcome. Epilepsia 26:697–703.

Pinel, JPJ, and Rovner, LI (1978). Experimental epileptogenesis: Kindling-induced epilepsy in rats. Exp Neurol 58:190–202.

Pitkänen, A (2010). Therapeutic approaches to epileptogenesis—Hope on the horizon. Epilepsia 51(suppl 3): 2–17.

Pitkänen, A, Kharatishvili, I, Nissinen, J, and McIntosh, TK (2006a). Posttraumatic epilepsy induced by lateral fluid-percussion brain injury in rats. InModels of Seizures and Epilepsy. Edited by A Pitkänen, PA Schwartzkroin, and SL Moshé. Burlington, MA: Elsevier Academic Press, pp. 465–476.

Pitkänen A, Schwartzkroin PA, and Moshé SL (eds) (2006b). Models of Seizures and Epilepsy. Burlington, MA: Elsevier Academic Press.

Pollen, DA (1964). Intracellular studies of cortical neurons during thalamic induced wave and spike. Electroencephalogr Clin Neurophysiol 17:398–404.

Post, RM (1981). Lidocaine-kindled limbic seizures: Behavioral implications. In Kindling 2. Edited by JA Wada. New York: Raven Press, pp. 149–157.

Price, MG, Yoo, JW, Burgess, DL, Deng, F, Hrachovy, RA, Frost, JD, Jr, et al. (2009). A triplet repeat expansion genetic mouse model of infantile spasms syndrome, Arx(GCG)10+7, with interneuropathy, spasms in infancy, persistent seizures, and adult cognitive and behavioral impairment. J Neurosci 29:8752–8763.

Prince, DA (1968). The depolarization shift in "epileptic" neurons. Exp Neurol 21:467–485.

Prince, DA, and Connors, BW (1986). Mechanisms of interictal epileptogenesis. Adv Neurol 44:275–299.

Prince, DA, and Futamachi, KJ (1970). Intracellular recordings from chronic epileptogenic foci in the monkey. Electroencephalogr Clin Neurophysiol 29:496–509.

Prince, DA, and Wilder, BJ (1967). Control mechanisms in cortical epileptogenic foci: "Surround" inhibition. Arch Neurol 16:194–202.

Purpura, DP (1961). Analysis of axodendritic synaptic organization in immature cerebral cortex. Ann NY Acad Sci 94:604–654.

Racine, RJ (1972a). Modification of seizure activity by electrical stimulation. I. After discharge threshold. Electroencephalogr Clin Neurophysiol 32:269–279.

Racine RJ (1972b). Modification of seizure activity by electrical stimulation: II. Motor seizure. Electroencephalogr Clin Neurophysiol 32:281–294.

Racine, R, Newberry, F, and Burnham, WM (1975). Post-activation potentiation and the kindling phenomenon. Electroencephalogr Clin Neurophysiol 39:261–271.

Racine, R, Kairiss, E, and Smith, G (1981). Kindling mechanisms: The evolution of the burst response versus enhancement. In Kindling 2. Edited by JA Wada. New York: Raven Press, pp. 15–27.

Raffo, E, Coppola, A, Ono, T, Briggs, SW, and Galanopoulou, AS (2011). A pulse rapamycin therapy for infantile spasms and associated cognitive decline. Neurobiol Dis 43:322–329.

Rakhade, SN, Klein, PM, Huynh, T, Hilario-Gomez, C, Kosaras, B, Rotenberg, A, and Jensen, FE (2011). Development of later life spontaneous seizures in a rodent model of hypoxia-induced neonatal seizures. Epilepsia 52:753–765.

Ralston, BL, and Papatheodoros, CA (1960). The mechanism of transition of interictal spiking foci into ictal seizure discharges. II. Observations in man. Electroencephalogr Clin Neurophysiol 12:297–304.

Ramos, RL, and Loturco, JJ (2006). Models with spontaneous seizures and developmental disruption of genetic etiology. In Models of Seizures and Epilepsy. Edited by A Pitkänen, PA Schwartzkroin, and SL Moshé. Burlington, MA: Elsevier Academic Press, pp. 249–259.

Ribak, CE, Harris, AB, Vaughn, JE, and Roberts, E (1979). Inhibitory GABAergic nerve terminals decrease at sites of focal epilepsy. Science 205:211–214.

Ribak, CE, Shapiro, LA, Seress, L, and Bakay, RA (2006). Alumina gel injection models of epilepsy in monkeys. In Models of Seizures and Epilepsy. Edited by A Pitkänen, PA Schwartzkroin, and SL Moshé. Burlington, MA: Elsevier Academic Press, pp. 179–187.

Rutledge, LT, Ranack, JB, Jr, and Duncan, JA (1967). Prevention of supersensitivity in partially isolated cerebral cortex. Electroencephalogr Clin Neurophysiol 23:256–262.

Salamon, N, Kung, J, Shaw, SJ, Koo, J, Koh, S, Wu, JY, Lerner, JT, Sankar, R, Shields, WD, Engel, J, Jr, Fried, I, Miyata, H, Yong, WH, Vinters, HV, and Mathern, GW (2008). FDG-PET/MRI coregistration improves detection of cortical dysplasia in patients with epilepsy. Neurology 71:1594–1601.

Sanchez, RM, and Jensen, FE (2006). Modeling hypoxia-induced seizures and hypoxic encephalopathy in the neonatal period. In Models of Seizures and Epilepsy. Edited by A Pitkänen, PA Schwartzkroin, and SL Moshé. Burlington, MA: Elsevier Academic Press, pp. 323–331.

Savic, I, and Engel, J, Jr (1998). Sex differences in patients with mesial temporal lobe epilepsy. J Neurol Neurosurg Psychiatry 65:910–912.

Savic, I, Persson, A, Roland, P, Pauli, S, Sedvall, G, and Widen, L (1988). In-vivo demonstration of reduced benzodiazepine receptor binding in human epileptic foci. Lancet 8616:863–866.

Scantlebury, MH, Galanopoulou, AS, Chudomelova, L, Raffo, E, Betancourth, D, and Moshé, SL (2010). A model of symptomatic infantile spasms syndrome. Neurobiol Dis 37:604–612.

Scharfman, HE, and Schwarcz, R (2008). Neuromodulation of seizures, epileptogenesis, and epilepsy. In Epilepsy: A Comprehensive Textbook, 2nd ed. Edited by J Engel, Jr, and TA Pedley. Philadelphia: Lippincott Williams & Wilkins, pp. 289–305.

Scheibel, ME, Crandall, PH, and Scheibel, AB (1974). The hippocampal-dentate complex in temporal lobe epilepsy. Epilepsia 15:55–80.

Schwartzkroin, PA (1984). Epileptogenesis in the immature central nervous system. In Electrophysiology of Epilepsy. Edited by PA Schwartzkroin and H Wheal. New York: Academic Press, pp. 389–412.

Schwartzkroin, PA (1986). Hippocampal slices in experimental and human epilepsy. Adv Neurol 44:991–1010.

Schwartzkroin, PA (1987). The electrophysiology of human brain slices resected from "epileptic" brain tissue. In Fundamental Mechanisms of Human Brain Function. Edited by J Engel, Jr, GA Ojemann, HO Lüders, and PD Williamson. New York: Raven Press, pp. 145–154.

Schwartzkroin, PA (ed) (2009). Encyclopedia of Basic Epilepsy Research. Amsterdam: Elsevier.

Schwartzkroin, PA, and Wyler, AR (1980). Mechanisms underlying epileptiform burst discharge. Ann Neurol 7:95–107.

Schwartzkroin, PA, Avanzini, G, Cavalheiro, EA, Engel, J, Jr, Heinemann, U, Meldrum, BS, Moshé, SL, Suzuki, J, and Wasterlain, CG (eds) (1998). Fourth Workshop on the Neurobiology of Epilepsy (WONOEP IV): Parallel Studies of Epileptogenesis in Human Tissue and Animal Models. Epilepsy Res 32(special issue):1–333.

Seki, K, and Wada, JA (1986). Kindling of cortical association area 5 in the cat. In Kindling 3. Edited by JA Wada. New York: Raven Press, pp. 429–446.

Seyfried, TN, Glaser, GH, Yu, RK, and Palayoor, ST (1986). Inherited convulsive disorders in mice. Adv Neurol 44:115–133.

Sherwin, AL, and van Gelder, NM (1986). Amino acid and catecholamine markers of metabolic abnormalities in human focal epilepsy. Adv Neurol 44:1011–1032.

Sherwin, A, Robitaille, Y, Quesney, L, Reader, T, Olivier, A, Briére, R, Andermann, E, Andermann, F, Feindel, W, Leblanc, R, Matthew, E, Ochs, R, Villemure, J, and Gloor, P (1987). Noradrenergic abnormalities in human cortical seizure foci. In Fundamental Mechanisms of Human Brain Function. Edited by J Engel, Jr, GA Ojemann, HO Lüders, and PD Williamson. New York: Raven Press, pp. 249–258.

Shewmon, DA, and Erwin, RJ (1988a). The effect of focal interictal spikes on perception and reaction time.

I. General considerations. Electroencephalogr Clin Neurophysiol 69:319–337.

Shewmon, DA and Erwin, RJ (1988b). The effect of focal interictal spikes on perception and reaction time. II. Neuroanatomic specificity. Electroencephalogr Clin Neurophysiol 69:338–352.

Shewmon, DA, and Erwin, RJ (1988c). Focal spike induced cerebral dysfunction is related to the after-coming slow wave. Ann Neurol 23:131–137.

Shouse, MN (2006). Kindling kittens and cats. In Models of Seizures and Epilepsy. Edited by A Pitkänen, PA Schwartzkroin, and SL Moshé. Burlington, MA: Elsevier Academic Press, pp. 365–369.

Sloviter, RS, Zappone, CA, Harvey, BD, et al. (2006). Kainic acid-induced recurrent mossy fiber innervations of dentate gyrus GABAergic interneurons; possible anatomical substrate of granule cell hyperinhibition in chronically epileptic rats. J Comp Neurol 494:944–960.

Snead, OC (1978). Gamma hydroxybutyrate in the monkey. III. Effects of intravenous anticonvulsant drugs. Neurology 28:1173–1178.

Snead, OC, and Bearden, LJ (1980). Naloxone overcomes the dopaminergic, EEG, and behavioral effects of γ-hydroxybutyrate. Neurology 30:832–838.

Soper, HV, Strain, GM, Babb, TL, Lieb, JP, and Crandall, PH (1978). Chronic alumina temporal lobe seizures in monkeys. Exp Neurol 62:99–121.

Spencer, SS, Sperling, MR, Shewmon, DA, and Kahane, P (2008). Intracranial electrodes. In Epilepsy: A Comprehensive Textbook, 2nd ed. Edited by J Engel, Jr, and TA Pedley. Philadelphia: Lippincott Williams & Wilkins, pp. 1791–1815.

Sperber, EF, Haas, KZ, Stanton, PK, and Moshé, SL (1991). Resistance of the immature hippocampus to seizure-induced synaptic reorganization. Dev Brain Res 60:88–93.

Sperling, MR, Wilson, G, Engel, J, Jr, Babb, TL, Phelps, ME, and Bradley, W (1986). Magnetic resonance imaging in intractable partial epilepsies: Correlative studies. Ann Neurol 20:57–62.

Staba, RJ, and Bragin, A (2011). High-frequency oscillations and other electrophysiological biomarkers of epilepsy: Underlying mechanisms. Biomarkers Med 5:545–556.

Staba, RJ, Wilson, CL, Bragin, A, Fried, I, and Engel, J, Jr (2002a). Quantitative analysis of high frequency oscillations (80–500 Hz) recorded in human epileptic hippocampus and entorhinal cortex. J Neurophysiol 88:1743–1752.

Staba, RJ, Wilson, CL, Bragin, A, Fried, I, and Engel, J, Jr (2002b). Sleep states differentiate single neuron activity recorded from human epileptic hippocampus, entorhinal cortex and subiculum. J Neurosci 22:5694–5704.

Staba, RJ, Wilson, CL, Bragin, A, Fried, I, and Engel, J, Jr (2004). High frequency oscillations recorded in human medial temporal lobe during sleep. Ann Neurol 56:108–115.

Staba, RJ, Frighetto, L, Behnke, EJ, Mathern, GW, Fields, T, Bragin, A, Ogren, J, Fried, I, Wilson, CL, and Engel, J, Jr (2007). Increased fast ripple to ripple ratios correlate with reduced hippocampal volumes and neuron loss in temporal lobe epilepsy patients. Epilepsia 48:2130–2138.

Staba, RJ, Ekstrom, AD, Suthana, NA, Burggren, A, Fried, I, Engel, J, Jr, and Bookheimer, SY (2012). Gray matter loss correlates with mesial temporal lobe neuronal hyperexcitability inside the human seizure-onset zone. Epilepsia 53:25–34.

Steinauser, C, Haydon, PG, and De Lanerolle, NC (2008). Astroglial mechanisms in epilepsy. In Epilepsy: A Comprehensive Textbook, 2nd ed. Edited by J Engel, Jr, and TA Pedley. Philadelphia: Lippincott Williams & Wilkins, pp. 277–288.

Steinlein, OK (2008). Genetics of epilepsy syndromes. In Epilepsy: A Comprehensive Textbook, 2nd ed. Edited by J Engel, Jr, and TA Pedley. Philadelphia: Lippincott Williams & Wilkins, pp. 195–210.

Stelzer, A, Slater, NT, and ten Bruggencate, G (1987). Activation of NMDA receptors blocks GABAergic inhibition in an in vitromodel of epilepsy. Nature 326:698–701.

Stewart, M, Chen, W-P, and Wong, RKS (2006). Single nerve cells acutely dissociated from animal and human brains for studies of epilepsy. In Models of Seizures and Epilepsy. Edited by A Pitkänen, PA Schwartzkroin, and SL Moshé. Burlington, MA: Elsevier Academic Press, pp. 15–22.

Stringer JL (2006). Models available for infection-induced seizures. InModels of Seizures and Epilepsy. Edited by A Pitkänen, PA Schwartzkroin, and SL Moshé. Burlington, MA: Elsevier Academic Press, pp. 521–526.

Sutula, T, He, X-X, Cavazos, J, and Scott, G (1988). Synaptic reorganization in the hippocampus induced by abnormal functional activity. Science 239:1147–1150.

Swaiman, KF, and Millstein, TM (1970). Pyridoxine-dependency and penicillin. Neurology 20:78–81.

Swann, JW, and Moshé, SL (in press). On the basic mechanisms of infantile spasms. In Jaspers's Basic Mechanisms of the Epilepsies, 4th ed. Edited by J Noebels, M Avoli, M Rogawski, R Olsen, and A Delgado-Escueta. Oxford: Oxford University Press.

Swann, JW, Baram, TZ, Jensen, FE, and Moshé, SL (2008). Seizure mechanisms and vulnerability in the developing brain. In Epilepsy: A Comprehensive Textbook, 2nd ed. Edited by J Engel, Jr, and TA Pedley. Philadelphia: Lippincott Williams & Wilkins, pp. 469–479.

Swartzwelder, HS, Lewis, DV, Anderson, WW, and Wilson, WA (1987). Seizure-like events in brain slices: Suppression by interictal activity. Brain Res 410:362–366.

Swinyard, EA (1972). Electrically induced convulsions. In Experimental Models of Epilepsy—A Manual for the Laboratory Worker. Edited by DP Purpura, JK Penry, DB Tower, and RD Walter. New York: Raven Press, pp. 433–458.

Talairach, J, Bancaud, J, Szikla, G, Bonis, A, Geier, S, and Vedrenne, C (1974). Approche nouvelle de la neurochirurgie de l'épilepsie: Méthodologie stéréotaxique et résultats thérapeutiques. Neurochirurgie 20(supp 1).

Tanaka, T, Kaijima, M, Daita, G, Oghami, S, Yonemasu, Y, and Riche, D (1982). Electroclinical features of kainic acid-induced status epilepticus in freely moving cats: Microinjection into the dorsal hippocampus. Electroencephalogr Clin Neurophysiol 54:288–300.

Tauck, DL, and Nadler, JV (1985). Evidence of functional mossy fiber sprouting in hippocampal formation of kainic acid-treated rats. J Neurosci 4:1016–1022.

Tempel, BL, Papazian, DM, Schwarz, TL, Jan, YN, and Jan, LY (1987). Sequence of a probable potassium channel component encoded at Shaker locus of Drosophila. Science 237:770–775.

Theodore, WH, Newmark, ME, Sato, S, De LaPaz, R, DiChiro, G, Brooks, R, Patronas, N, Kessler, RM, Manning, R, Margolin, R, Channing, M, and Porter, RJ (1984). ^{18}F-fluorodeoxyglucose positron emission tomography in refractory complex partial seizures. Ann Neurol 14:429–437.

Theodore, WH, Brooks, R, Margolin, R, Patronas, N, Sato, S, Porter, RJ, Mansi, L, Bairamian, D, and DiChiro, G (1985). Positron emission tomography in generalized seizures. Neurology 35:684–690.

Trevelyan, AJ, and Yuste, RM (2008). Cellular imaging of epilepsy. In Epilepsy: A Comprehensive Textbook, 2nd ed. Edited by J Engel, Jr, and TA Pedley. Philadelphia: Lippincott Williams & Wilkins, pp. 1051–1056.

Truccolo, W, Donoghue, JA, Hochberg, LR, Eskandar, EN, Madsen, JR, Anderson, WS, Brown, EN, Halgren, E, and Cash, SS (2010). Single-neuron dynamics in human focal epilepsy. Nat Neurosci 14:635–641.

Tschuluun, N, Wenzel, HJ, and Schwartzkroin, PA (2007). Irradiation exacerbates cortical cytopathology in the Eker rat model of tuberous sclerosis complex, but does not induce hyperexcitability. Epilepsy Res 73:53–64.

Tuff, LP, Racine, RJ, and Adamec, R (1983a). The effects of kindling on GABA-mediated inhibition in the dentate gyrus of the rat. I. Paired-pulse depression. Brain Res 277:79–90.

Tuff, LP, Racine, RJ, and Mishra, RK (1983b). The effects of kindling on GABA-mediated inhibition in the dentate gyrus of the rat. II. Receptor binding. Brain Res 277:91–98.

Ueda, Y, Triggs, WJ, and Willmore, LJ (2006). Head trauma: Hemorrhage-iron deposition. In Models of Seizures and Epilepsy. Edited by A Pitkänen, PA Schwartzkroin, and SL Moshé. Burlington, MA: Elsevier Academic Press, pp. 495–500.

Urca, G, Frenk, H, Liebeskind, JC, and Taylor, AN (1977). Morphine and enkephalin: Analgesic and epileptic properties. Science 197:83–86.

Vanhatalo S, Voipios, Kaila K (2010). Infraslow EE6 activity. In Niedermeyer's Electroncephalography: Basu Principles, clinical application, and related fieldo. 6th ed. Edited by D. Schomer, F. Lopesda silva. Philabelphia: Lippencott Williams & Wilkins, pp. 741–747.

Velasco, AL, Wilson, CL, Babb, TL and Engel, J, Jr (2000). Functional and anatomic correlates of two frequently observed temporal lobe seizure-onset patterns. Neural Plast 7, 49–63.

Velísek, L (2006). Models of chemically-induced acute seizures. In Models of Seizures and Epilepsy. Edited by A Pitkänen, PA Schwartzkroin, and SL Moshé. Burlington, MA: Elsevier Academic Press, pp. 127–152.

Velísek, L, Jehle, K, Asche, S, and Velisková, J (2007). Model of infantile spasms induced by N-methyl-D-aspartic acid in prenatally impaired brain. Ann Neurol 61:109–119.

Vergnes, M, Marescaux, C, Micheletti, G, Reis, J, Depaulis, A, Rumbach, L, and Warter, JM (1982). Spontaneous paroxysmal electroclinical patterns in rat: A model of generalized non-convulsive epilepsy. Neurosci Lett 33:97–101.

Vezzani, A, and Rüegg, S (eds) (2011a). Proceedings of the First Meeting on Immunity and Inflammation in Epilepsy: Mechanistic Insights and Therapeutic Perspectives. Epilepsia 52(suppl 3):1–53.

Vezzani, A, and Rüegg, S (2011b). Introduction. In Proceedings of the First Meeting on Immunity and Inflammation in Epilepsy: Mechanistic Insights and Therapeutic Perspectives. Edited by A Vezzani and S Rüegg. Epilepsia 52(suppl 3):1–4.

Vezzani, A, Peltola, J, and Janigro, D (2008). Inflammation. In Epilepsy: A Comprehensive Textbook, 2nd ed. Edited by J Engel, Jr, and TA Pedley. Philadelphia: Lippincott Williams & Wilkins, pp. 267–276.

Vindrola, O, Briones, R, Asai, M, and Fernandez-Guardiola, A (1981). Brain content of Leu^5- and Met^5-enkephalin changes independently during the development of kindling in the rat. Neurosci Lett 26:125–130.

Wada, JA (ed) (1976). Kindling. New York: Raven Press.

Wada, JA (1978). The clinical relevance of kindling: Species, brain sites and seizure susceptibility. In Limbic Mechanisms. Edited by KE Livingston and O Hornykiewicz. New York: Plenum Press, pp. 369–388.

Wada, JA (ed) (1981). Kindling 2. New York: Raven Press.

Wada, JA (ed) (1986). Kindling 3. New York: Raven Press.

Wada, JA, and Komai, S (1985). Effect of anterior two-thirds callosal bisection upon bisymmetrical and bisynchronous generalized convulsions kindled from amygdala in epileptic baboon, Papio papio. In Epilepsy and the Corpus Callosum. Edited by AG Reeves. New York: Plenum Press, pp. 75–97.

Wada, JA, and Osawa, T (1976). Spontaneous recurrent seizure state induced by daily electrical amygdaloid stimulation in Senegalese baboons, Papio papio. Neurology 26:273–286.

Wada, JA, and Sato, M (1975). Effects of the unilateral lesion in the midbrain reticular formation on kindled amygdaloid convulsion in cats. Epilepsia 16:693–697.

Wada, JA, and Wake, A (1977). Dorsal frontal, orbital and mesial frontal cortical lesion and amygdaloid kindling in cats. Can J Neurol Sci 4:107–115.

Wada, JA, Sato, M, and Corcoran, ME (1974). Persistent seizure susceptibility and recurrent spontaneous seizures in kindled cats. Epilepsia 15 (1978). 465–478.

Wada, JA, Mizoguchi, T, and Osawa, T (2009). Secondarily generalized convulsive seizures induced by daily amygdaloid stimulation in rhesus monkeys. Neurology 28:1026–1036.

Waldbaum, S, and Dudek, FE: Single and repetitive paired-pulse suppression: A parametric analysis and assessment of usefulness in epilepsy research. Epilepsia 50:904–916.

Waltereit, R, Welzl, H, Dichgans, J, Lipp, HP, Schmidt, WJ, and Weller, M (2006). Enhanced episodic-like memory and working epilepsy in a rat model of tuberous sclerosis. J Neurochem 96:407–413.

Wasterlain, CG, and Fairchild, MD (1985). Transfer between chemical and electrical kindling in the septal-hippocampal system. Brain Res 331:261–266.

Westrum, LE, White, LE, Jr, and Ward, AA, Jr (1964). Morphology of the experimental epileptic focus. J Neurosurg 21:1033–1046.

White, HS, Smith-Yockman, M, Srivastava, A, and Wilcox, KS (2006). Therapeutic assays for the identification and characterization of antiepileptic and antiepileptogenic drugs. In Models of Seizures and Epilepsy. Edited by A Pitkänen, PA Schwartzkroin, and SL Moshé. Burlington, MA: Elsevier Academic Press, pp. 539–549.

Wieser, HG (1983). Electroclinical Features of Psychomotor Seizure: A Stereoelectroencephalographic Study of Ictal Symptoms and Chromatographical Seizure Patterns Including Clinical Effects of Intracerebral Stimulation. London: Butterworths.

Wilder, BJ, King, RL, and Schmidt, RP (1968). Comparative study of secondary epileptogenesis. Epilepsia 9:275–289.

Williams, SN, Locke, CJ, Braden, AL, Caldwell, KA, and Caldwell, GA (2004). Epileptic-like convulsions associated with LIS-1 in the cytoskeletal control of neurotransmitter signaling in Caenorhabditis elegans. Hum Mol Genet 13:2043–2059.

Wilson, CL, Isokawa-Akesson, M, Babb, TL, Engel, J, Jr, Cahan, LD, and Crandall, PH (1987). A comparative view of local and interhemispheric limbic pathways in humans: An evoked potential analysis. In Fundamental Mechanisms of Human Brain Function. Edited by J Engel, Jr, GA Ojemann, HO Lüders, and PD Williamson. New York: Raven Press, pp. 27–38.

Wilson, CL, Isokawa, M, Babb, TL, Crandall, PH, Levesque, MF and Engel, J, Jr (1991). Functional connections in the human temporal lobe: II. Evidence for a loss of functional linkage between contralateral limbic structures. Exp Brain Res 85:174–187.

Wilson, CL, Maidment, NT, Shomer, MH, Behnke, EJ, Ackerson, L, Fried, I, and Engel, J, Jr (1996). Comparison of seizure related amino acid release in human epileptic hippocampus versus a chronic, kainate rat model of hippocampal epilepsy. Epilepsy Res 26:245–254.

Wilson, CL, Khan, SU, Engel, J, Jr, Isokawa, M, Babb, TL, and Behnke, EJ (1998). Paired pulse suppression and facilitation in human epileptogenic hippocampal formation. Epilepsy Res 31:211–230.

Winden, KD, Karsten, S, Bragin, A, Kudo, L, Gehman, L, Ruidera, J, Engel, J, Jr, and Geschwind, DH (2011). A systems level, functional genomics analysis of chronic epilepsy. PLoS One 6:e2063.

Withrow, CD (1972). Systemic carbon dioxide derangements. In Experimental Models of Epilepsy—A Manual for the Laboratory Worker. Edited by DP Purpura, JK Penry, DB Tower, and RD Walter. New York: Raven Press, pp. 477–494.

Woodbury, DM (1972). Applications to drug evaluations. In Experimental Models of Epilepsy—A Manual for the Laboratory Worker. Edited by DP Purpura, JK Penry, DB Tower, and RD Walter. New York: Raven Press, pp. 557–583.

Woodbury, DM (1980). Convulsant drugs: Mechanisms of action. Adv Neurol 27:249–303.

Worrell, G, and Gotman, J (2011). High-frequency oscillations and other electrophysiological biomarkers: Clinical studies. Biomarkers Med 5:557–566.

Wyler, AR (1986). Synchrony between cortical neurons in normal and epileptogenic cortex of monkey. Epilepsia 27:171–176.

Wyler, AR, and Ward, AA, Jr (1986). Neuronal firing patterns from epileptogenic foci of monkey and human. Adv Neurol 44:967–989.

Wyler, AR, Fetz, EE, and Ward, AA, Jr (1975). Firing patterns of epileptic and normal neurons in the chronic alumina focus in undrugged monkeys during different behavioral states. Brain Res 98:1–20.

Ylinen, A, Bragin, A, Nádasdy, Z, Jando, G, Szabo, I, Sik, A, and Buzsáki, G (1995). Sharp wave-associated high-frequency oscillation (200 Hz) in the intact hippocampus: Network and intracellular mechanisms. J Neurosci 15:30–46.

Yu, FH, Mantegazza, M, Westerbroek, RE, Robbins, CA, Kalume, F, Burton, KA, Spain, WJ, McKnight, GS, Scheuer, T, and Caterall, WA (2006). Reduced sodium current in GABAergic interneurons in a mouse model of severe myoclonic epilepsy in infancy. Nat Neurosci 9:1142–1149.

Zhao, Q, and Holmes, GL (2006). Repetitive seizures in the immature brain. In Models of Seizures and Epilepsy. Edited by A Pitkänen, PA Schwartzkroin, and SL Moshé. Burlington, MA: Elsevier Academic Press, pp. 341–350.

Zheng, LH, Xu, L, Gutmann, DH, and Wong, M (2008). Rapamycin prevents epilepsy in a mouse model of tuberous sclerosis complex. Ann Neurol 63:444–453.

Chapter 5

Causes of Human Epilepsy

NONSPECIFIC PREDISPOSING FACTORS
Genetic Factors
Environmental Factors
Dynamic Aspects of Threshold

SPECIFIC EPILEPTOGENIC DISTURBANCES
Genetic Causes of Epilepsy Disorders

Acquired Causes of Epilepsy Disorders

PRECIPITATING FACTORS
Nonspecific Precipitating Factors
Specific Precipitating Factors

SUMMARY AND CONCLUSIONS

In the past, epilepsy disorders were considered to be either *idiopathic* (*essential, primary*) or *symptomatic* (*acquired, secondary*) (Chapter 1). Today, we recognize that a variety of genetic, environmental, and physiological factors influence the appearance of epilepsy (see Table 1–10). Thus a *multifactorial approach* is needed to fully understand the causes of human epilepsy (Andermann, 1982; Anderson et al., 1991; Engel, 1984; Engel and Pedley, 2008; Gloor, 1977; Lennox, 1960; Shorvon et al., 2011).

The causes of epileptic seizures and epilepsy can be viewed as belonging to three categories: (1) *nonspecific predisposing factors*, which determine differences in individual susceptibility to generating epileptic seizures and developing chronic epilepsy, (2) *specific epileptogenic*

disturbances, which account for chronic epilepsy disorder disorders in susceptible individuals, and (3) *precipitating factors*, which are endogenous or exogenous perturbations capable of acutely evoking epileptic seizures in persons with chronic epilepsy and, in some cases, reactive seizures in nonepileptic individuals.

Predisposing factors determine the *threshold* for seizure occurrence and susceptibility to epileptogenesis. Specific epileptogenic disturbances that chronically enhance neuronal excitation and synchronization will not cause chronic recurrent epileptic seizures when the seizure threshold is high (Fig. 5–1). In the presence of an intermediate threshold for seizure generation, specific epileptogenic disturbances can lead to chronic recurrent seizures when precipitating factors provide sufficient

157

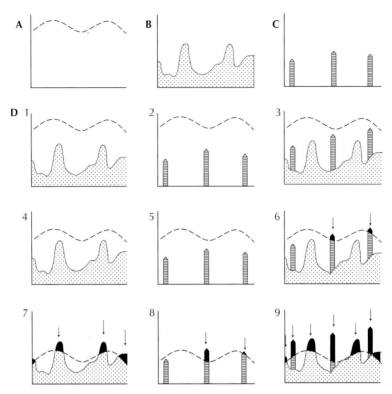

Figure 5–1. Schematic diagram illustrating interactions of the fluctuating threshold for seizures determined by nonspecific predisposing factors (**A**); independent fluctuations of a specific epileptogenic disturbance (**B**); and intermittent precipitating factors (**C**). **D.** With a high threshold, epileptogenic disturbances and precipitating factors alone (*1, 2*) and combined (*3*) fail to generate seizures. With an intermediate threshold, epileptogenic disturbances and precipitating factors alone (*4, 5*) fail to generate seizures, but seizures (*arrows*) occur when these factors are combined (*6*). With a low threshold, epileptogenic disturbances and precipitating factors alone (*7, 8*) are each capable of generating seizures and combined (*9*) generate even more seizures, perhaps constituting status epilepticus.

additional excitatory or synchronizing influences (or both) to initiate epileptiform activity. If the seizure threshold is low, specific epileptogenic disturbances might induce spontaneous ictal events even in the absence of identifiable precipitating factors, or precipitating factors might induce reactive seizures in patients without chronic epilepsy.

With respect to the simplified concepts illustrated in Figure 5–1, the primary approach to the treatment of epilepsy is to alter the seizure threshold with antiseizure drugs. Specific epileptogenic disturbances in some cases can be surgically resected, but primary prevention involves public health efforts that could reduce the incidence of epileptogenic insults that lead to acquired epilepsies, such as the use of seat belts, appropriate prenatal and perinatal care, and adequate standards for nutrition and hygiene. Understanding the basic mechanisms

of epileptogenesis in acquired epilepsies, as well as in the genetic epilepsies, will ultimately lead to the development of secondary preventive interventions. Recognition of precipitating factors is important when these can be reasonably avoided.

The distinctions among nonspecific predisposing factors, specific epileptogenic disturbances, and precipitating factors are actually artificial, and the categories overlap considerably. Some factors that can be specifically epileptogenic in one situation can act as predisposing factors in another or as precipitating factors in a third. For example, acute hypoxia can act as a precipitating factor and cause a reactive seizure, whereas more prolonged or severe hypoxia can induce cerebral damage that might lower the seizure threshold and act as a predisposing factor or that might give rise to an epilepsy disorder and constitute a specific epileptogenic disturbance. It is nevertheless useful to investigate patients with a view toward identifying reversible nonspecific predisposing factors, treatable specific epileptogenic disturbances, and avoidable precipitating factors.

NONSPECIFIC PREDISPOSING FACTORS

An epileptic seizure can be provoked in anyone, given the right combination of circumstances. The ease with which seizures can be induced varies considerably, owing to individual differences in threshold. Although threshold is commonly viewed as a *level* that might be raised or lowered, depending on various factors, threshold effects are actually determined by the resting state of neuronal excitability and synchronization and the ease or rapidity with which this level can be brought to the point of a seizure. A lower threshold for epileptic seizures, therefore, can result from a combination of an increased resting state of neuronal excitability and synchronization, an increased potential for further enhancing neuronal excitation and synchronization, and a decreased degree of excitation and synchronization required for this neuronal activity to develop into epileptiform discharges. Threshold is a dynamic concept; it can be influenced by a variety of nonspecific predisposing factors that vary over time and space (Chapter 9). The relationship between threshold for ictogenesis and susceptibility to epileptogenesis is complex and poorly understood.

Genetic Factors

Genetic factors influence epileptogenicity and epileptogenesis in three major ways: (1) In the genetic epilepsies, approximating what were formerly called idiopathic epilepsies, genetic factors are paramount. A minority of these are monogenic disorders, and the rest are polygenic. Most mutations discovered to date disrupt ligand- and voltage-gated ion channels (*channelopathies*) (Guerrini et al., 2011; Helbig et al., 2008; Steinlein, 2008). (2) Genetic mutations also give rise to diseases, such as *tuberous sclerosis complex (TSC)* or certain *malformations of cortical development,*

that are associated with variable clinical signs and symptoms among which epilepsy may be more or less common, but not inevitable (Bonkowsky et al., 2008; Guerrini et al., 2011; Helbig et al., 2008). (3) Perhaps most important, yet most difficult to define, are genetic disturbances that alter the predisposition for seizures and epilepsy in a nonspecific fashion. Such *susceptibility genes* can influence the appearance and manifestations of genetic as well as acquired epilepsies. These nonspecific genetic influences could increase the risk for all or most epilepsies globally or could have more selective effects, perhaps constituting essential cofactors for the development of specific epilepsy syndromes (Ottman and Winawer, 2008). At present, sufficiently large *genome-wide association studies (GWAS)* have not been performed to detect these genes (Klassen et al., 2011). Genetic factors can alter susceptibility or cause epilepsy directly throughout life, be age-specific in their effects, or exert their influences during fetal or postnatal development, in which case all traces of the direct genetic effect might be gone by the time the epilepsy condition manifests (Fig. 5–2).

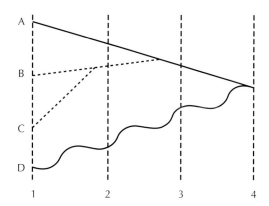

Figure 5–2. Potential developmental influence of four etiologies producing the same phenotype. Several separate etiologies (e.g., four sodium channel gene mutations, *A*, *B*, *C*, and *D*) could ultimately give rise to the same ictal generation directly (*solid straight line*), by altering developmental patterns (*dotted lines*), or by some circuitous unknown mechanism (*wavy line*). In this example, examining the etiology too early (*dashed line 1*) could falsely increase the number of pathophysiological mechanisms and anatomical substrates, while observing the end point (*dashed line 4*) would give the mistaken impression that there was only one mechanism. Where along the causal pathway (*dashed line 2 or 3*) the correct determination of the mechanisms should be made, however, remains unclear. (From Engel, 2006, with permission.)

There is an increasing tendency to refer to the genetic disturbances underlying the epilepsies when these conditions are discussed among professionals and with the lay public and patients. This association can have adverse consequences in cultures where not only is it difficult for people with epilepsy to marry but the stigma can extend to the entire family for fear that other members might possess an "epilepsy gene." It is important to recognize, therefore, that *genetic* is not the same as *inherited*. Sporadic gene mutations often cause epilepsy syndromes, diseases associated with epilepsy, and increased susceptibility to epilepsy without there being any genetic disturbances in other family members. Even with inherited epilepsies, there usually is a relatively low risk that genetic abnormalities in a parent will manifest as a clinically significant phenotype in their children.

Regulation of cortical excitability in the normal brain depends on ionic fluxes across membranes, neuronal morphology, neurotransmitter-receptor interactions, neuronal circuitry, and extracerebral systems that influence cerebral function (Chapter 3). Although these molecular and structural features all represent the expression of genetic information, when a single phenotype has many causes, it becomes difficult to determine patterns of genetic transmission. Classical approaches to gene identification derive from analyses of families with single-gene-locus (*Mendelian*) modes of inheritance, which include *autosomal dominant*, *autosomal recessive*, and *X-linked* forms. In addition, *mitochondrial* inheritance is selectively transmitted maternally. Studies of genetic mutations with Mendelian and mitochondrial inheritance patterns have identified specific epileptogenic disturbances in rare instances, as discussed later in this chapter, but nonspecific predisposing genetic factors are more likely to be mediated by *complex disease genes*, or *susceptibility genes*, which often require polygenic mutations, as well as by environmental factors, which additively increase the risk for epilepsy (Ottman and Winawer, 2008).

The increased susceptibility for epileptiform EEG patterns and epileptic seizures among first-degree relatives of individuals with epilepsy is in agreement with the shift in normal Gaussian distribution expected for a multifactorial inheritance pattern (Andermann, 1982) (Fig. 5–3). Large family studies indicate that

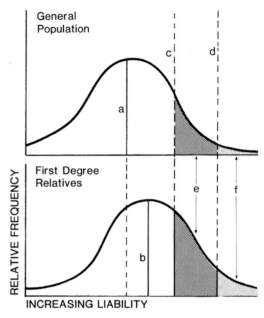

Figure 5–3. Diagrammatic representation of multifactorial inheritance, adapted for EEG abnormalities and epilepsy. Distribution of seizure susceptibility is Gaussian, but the curve is shifted toward increased susceptibility for first-degree relatives of patients with epilepsy. The mean susceptibility for relatives (*b*) is greater than for the greater population (*a*); and given the same threshold for expression of EEG abnormalities (*c*) and seizures (*d*), a larger percentage of the relatives exhibit these epileptiform or epileptic phenomena (*e*, EEG abnormalities; *f*, seizures). (Redrawn from Andermann, 1982, with permission.)

15% of patients with a diagnosis of an idiopathic generalized epilepsy have a positive family history of epilepsy, but it has been difficult to demonstrate increased risk of epilepsy in relatives of patients with acquired epilepsies (Ottman and Winawer, 2008). Nevertheless, a genetic basis for nonspecific seizure susceptibility has been generally accepted for some time (Andermann, 1982; Anderson et al., 1991; Newmark and Penry, 1980; Ottman and Winawer, 2008). However, the manifestation of epileptiform EEG abnormalities and epileptic seizures presumably requires the interplay of additional specific genetic or environmental factors (or both), making more precise genetic modeling impossible at present. Genetic traits that underlie specific epileptogenic EEG traits (e.g., the 3-Hz spike-and-wave or photosensitivity) have better-understood inheritance patterns (Pedley, 2008).

Genetic factors must also account for the naturally occurring differences among cerebral structures in their predisposition to the development of epileptiform discharges and epileptogenesis. The hippocampus is naturally highly susceptible to epileptiform activity (Chapter 3), and the epileptogenicity of neocortex varies somewhat from one cortical region to another (Chapter 8). As with other aspects of threshold, the anatomical distribution of seizure susceptibility differs depending on specific epileptogenic features. Thus the unique input to visual cortex renders it selectively susceptible to disturbances that produce photosensitive seizures, the local physiology of perirolandic cortex may predispose it to the disturbances that cause benign centrotemporal spikes and seizures in children, and the outflow patterns of frontal cortex increase the likelihood that disturbances in this area will result in generalized tonic-clonic seizures.

Environmental Factors

Superimposed on the naturally occurring, genetically determined factors that influence epileptogenicity are environmental factors that alter the capacity of cerebral neurons to be excited or synchronized. Environmental factors presumably increase or decrease not only seizure susceptibility but also susceptibility to epileptogenesis and chronic epilepsy, therefore contributing to the Gaussian distribution shown in Fig. 5–3. Seizure susceptibility can be profoundly and permanently affected by in utero insults that diffusely disrupt the development of neuronal circuitry or neurotransmitter systems. Such disturbances increase the risk of seizures and epilepsy in the presence of specific epileptogenic factors, but on their own would not give rise to either. Common examples of environmental factors that nonspecifically lower the seizure threshold throughout life are systemic illness, psychological stress, sleep deprivation, alcohol or sedative drug withdrawal, and fever (Chapter 9). In certain situations, these influences can also act as precipitating factors.

Risk factors are variables associated with an increased probability of a disease process for any reason and do not always have a defined pathophysiological basis. Therefore, risk factors for epilepsy can include more than predisposing factors that influence the threshold for seizure occurrence. Apart from influences that alter seizure threshold per se, risk factors for epileptogenesis are somewhat different for children than adults (Hesdorffer, 2008). Whereas head trauma, central nervous system (CNS) infections, and family history, which are usually risk factors for specific epileptogenic disturbances, are common to children and adults, important risk factors for children include febrile seizures, mental retardation, cerebral palsy, and *attention deficit hyperactivity disorder*, while important risk factors for adults include CNS malignancies, cardiovascular disease, Alzheimer's disease and other dementias, multiple sclerosis, hypertension, stroke risk, major depression, alcohol abuse, use of certain illicit drugs, and low socioeconomic status. Many of these conditions are associated with basic neuronal disturbances that constitute nonspecific predisposing factors, but more research is necessary before we can understand how some of these, for instance major depression, reflect brain function that is disturbed in a way that increases susceptibility to epileptic seizures (Kanner and Blumer, 2008) (Chapter 11).

In contrast to the risk factors and predisposing factors that increase susceptibility to epileptogenesis and ictogenesis, there are undoubtedly naturally occurring environmental factors that reduce susceptibility to these epileptogenic phenomena. Mechanisms that explain why specific epileptogenic disturbances cause epileptic seizures in some persons and not others and why some persons with chronic epilepsy experience spontaneous seizure-free periods are neglected and potentially fruitful areas of investigation.

Pharmacological agents nonspecifically alter the threshold for epileptic seizures. Certain drugs, such as the neuroleptics and antidepressants, are not likely to cause epileptic seizures in people without epilepsy but may increase the risk of seizures in those in whom specific epileptogenic factors exist (Messing et al., 1984; Elliott et al., 2009). The risk of seizures from psychotropic drugs is dose dependent; *maprotiline, clomipramine, chlorpromazine,* and *clozapine* have a relatively high ictogenic potential, while *phenelzine, tranylcypromine, fluoxetine, paroxetine, sertraline, venlafaxine, trazodone, fluphenazine, haloperidol, pimozide,* and *risperidone* have a relatively low risk (Pisani et al., 2002). Despite attempts to design pharmacological interventions that act on specific mechanisms of epilepsy, current anti-seizure medications appear to work primarily by raising the seizure threshold nonspecifically (Chapters 3 and 15).

Acquired brain lesions can alter the anatomical pattern of epileptic susceptibility by selectively lowering or raising seizure threshold in specific cerebral areas. Reactive seizures induced by nonspecific precipitating factors can have focal features when such lesions exist. For instance, cortical scars are common in alcoholics who have experienced multiple episodes of head trauma. When these scars are not sufficiently epileptogenic to cause spontaneous ictal events, they can generate focal seizures during alcohol withdrawal. These are reactive seizures and should not be considered evidence for a chronic focal epilepsy disorder (Chapter 12). Another common example is the elderly stroke patient with hemiparesis and a systemic toxic or metabolic insult. If the damaged brain has an elevated threshold for seizure generation or perhaps a decreased ability to generate motor manifestations of the seizure, ictal symptoms of a generalized reactive epileptic event can be limited to the side contralateral to the hemiparesis.

Dynamic Aspects of Threshold

Susceptibility to ictogenesis is not a stable phenomenon. For instance, seizure thresholds change constantly over time as a result of *maturational factors*. Studies of experimental models of epilepsy have shown that the threshold for epileptic seizures is decreased in immature animals compared to young adults (Holmes, 1986; Nelson and Ellenberg, 1978; Galanopoulou and Moshé, 2009) and increased in aged animals (DeToledo-Morrell et al., 1984) (Chapter 4). Susceptibility to the development of chronic seizures, however, is increased in the immature compared to young adults, as well as in the aged brain (Chapter 4), yet there is an increased incidence of epilepsy at the extremes of age (Hauser and Kurland, 1975; Banerjee and Hauser, 2008). This age-related increased incidence, which appears paradoxical, can be due to many factors, including (1) genetically determined nonspecific predisposing factors, (2) specific genetic factors with age-dependent penetrance, such as those that underlie *febrile seizures* (Tsuboi,

1982), *childhood absence epilepsy* (*petit mal*) (Metrakos and Metrakos, 1966), and *benign childhood epilepsy with centrotemporal spikes* (Bray and Wiser, 1964), and (3) the greater risk of certain environmental epileptogenic influences in infancy and early childhood, such as trauma and infection, and in the elderly, such as stroke and neoplasms. Presumably, all of these factors interact to explain the age-related expression of specific epileptogenic processes. Furthermore, maturational factors appear to affect thresholds differently for different epileptic phenomena. Consequently, some types of seizures are more likely to occur in infancy; others, in childhood or adolescence (Chapter 6).

Fluctuations in the threshold for epileptic seizures also result from normal *biorhythms*, which may be genetically determined. *Circadian rhythms* are related to *diurnal cycles* in hormone levels or to alterations in neuronal activity accompanying *sleep* and *wakefulness* (Chapters 3 and 9). Thresholds can change in different directions for different types of epileptic phenomena, so that some individuals will have seizures predominantly during wakefulness and others predominantly during sleep, while still others demonstrate no specific circadian pattern. Shorter, *ultradian* (Kellaway, 1985; Stevens et al., 1971) and longer cyclical fluctuations in threshold also occur. A common example of the latter is *catamenial epilepsy*: increased seizure occurrence in women around the time of menses and ovulation due largely to changes in estrogen and progesterone levels (Chapters 3 and 9).

SPECIFIC EPILEPTOGENIC DISTURBANCES

Specific disturbances that give rise to epileptic seizures (Chapter 6) or epilepsy syndromes (Chapter 7) have been identified, but their mechanisms of action are often incompletely understood (Shorvon et al., 2011). They can be genetic or acquired and are presumed to be primarily responsible for the initiation of epileptiform activity in the brain. As with seizure threshold, specific epileptogenic influences can be viewed as dynamic, with certain spatial distributions and temporal fluctuations. The appearance of epileptic seizures is determined, in fact, by the interaction of these specific epileptogenic processes with threshold at a given time and a given place within the brain.

In a study of siblings and children of persons with focal seizures, presumably due to acquired cerebral lesions, 20% demonstrated EEG abnormalities, 7% had had one or more seizures, and 4% had chronic epilepsy conditions (Andermann, 1982). Although the incidence of chronic recurrent seizures in close relatives of persons with acquired focal epilepsy was greater than in the general population, the difference was not significant, as noted in many subsequent studies (Ottman and Winawer, 2008). However, there is a significantly greater incidence of EEG abnormalities in those relatives, consistent with the view that inherited nonspecific predisposing factors increase the probability that acquired specific epileptogenic disturbances will produce seizures in this population. In the aforementioned study, the patients with focal seizures were part of a population treated surgically. Postoperative outcome was significantly better in those whose relatives showed epileptiform EEG abnormalities than in those whose relatives did not (Andermann, 1982). This seemingly paradoxical finding has a reasonable explanation: because a low seizure threshold might allow a relatively small cerebral lesion to cause a chronic epilepsy condition, patients with a familial predisposition to epilepsy would be more likely to have discrete structural abnormalities amenable to complete surgical resection (Engel et al., 1983).

Genetic Causes of Epilepsy Disorders

Specific genetic epileptogenic disturbances are of two types: (1) genetic epilepsies, or epilepsies in which epileptic seizures are the principal or only phenotypic expression of the genetic defect (Chapter 7), and (2) genetic disorders associated with epilepsy, or epilepsies in which the phenotypic expression is a neurological or systemic disorder that is incidentally but not always associated with cerebral disturbances causing epileptic seizures (Berg et al., 2010; Guerrini et al., 2011).

Based on clinical genetic studies, 30–40% of all epilepsies are believed to be inherited genetic epilepsies, formerly referred to as idiopathic epilepsies (Steinlein, 2008). These are age-dependent disturbances and most but not all are generalized. Very few are *monogenic*, the majority being *polygenic (oligogenic)* forms, all with variable penetrance, indicating the importance of predisposing factors, either susceptibility genes or environmental influences, for phenotypic expression. Mendelian and mitochondrial modes of inheritance have been identified for genetic disturbances associated with epilepsy.

Genetic analysis begins with accurate phenotypic description, which is hampered by the fact that there are many types of epilepsy and that the clinical manifestation of epilepsy disorders is extremely variable. Consequently, genetic studies have been possible only for relatively well-defined epilepsy syndromes that represent reasonably homogeneous conditions. The genetic epilepsy syndromes are initially recognized by *family aggregation*, that is, identification of families with many members who display similar clinical features. *Twin studies* help to determine that the clinical features result from shared genes rather than shared environment. Elucidation of molecular mechanisms underlying these disorders then requires identification of specific genes, beginning with *linkage analysis*, followed by *positional cloning* and *allelic association* studies (Ottman and Winawer, 2008).

In genetic studies, the affected individual of interest is referred to as the *proband*. Linkage analysis is carried out in families where the proband has multiple affected relatives and is based on the fact that the closer two markers are on a chromosome, the more likely they are to be inherited together. The likelihood of linkage is expressed as the *log of the odds ratio (lod) score*; in a genome-wide analysis, a lod score of 3.0 is considered significant evidence for linkage (Ottman and Winawer, 2008). Linkage analysis helps to identify the location of a putative epileptogenic gene mutation on a specific chromosome, and sequencing of genes in the region then allows identification of the causative variant, particularly in monogenic disorders. In polygenic disorders, *allelic association* studies are used to identify putative variants, and it is becoming increasingly feasible to carry out genome-wide allelic investigations without first performing linkage analysis. Multiple variants of a gene are referred to as *polymorphisms*, and most genetic variants investigated in epilepsy are *single-nucleotide polymorphisms (SNPs)*, where one of the four nucleotides that represent the DNA code is substituted for another. Such *point mutations* can result in *missense*, in which the sequence now codes for a different amino acid, or *nonsense*, in which the sequence now codes for a stop, resulting in a truncated protein. *Copy number variants (CNVs)* are also under investigation, as are other abnormal deletions and insertions that might influence epileptogenicity. As noted in Chapter 3, research on genomic sequencing is advancing so quickly that any further discussion here will be outdated by the time this text is published.

A family history of epilepsy is not present with *de novo mutations,* which are now known to cause a number of sporadic epilepsy syndromes due to a variety of defects to specific genes, such as *SCN1A* for most cases of *Dravet syndrome*, *STXBP1* for some cases of *Ohtahara syndrome* (Chapter 7), and an increasing number of rare conditions that have not yet been listed among the syndromes recognized by the International League Against Epilepsy (ILAE).

GENETIC EPILEPSIES

Genes have now been identified for a number of epilepsy syndromes, as shown in Table 5–1

(see also Chapter 7). This table demonstrates *locus heterogeneity*, meaning that a single phenotype can be caused by more than one gene mutation, and *variable expressivity*, meaning that a single gene can produce more than one phenotype, as evidenced, for instance, by the condition known as *Genetic epilepsy with febrile seizures plus (GEFS+)*, where members of the same family exhibit different epilepsy conditions (Chapter 7). The same can be said for the so-called *idiopathic generalized epilepsies*, where absence and myoclonic forms of the disorder occur in different members of the same family (Ottman and Winawer, 2008) (Chapter 7).

Penetrance for genetic defects is influenced by sex and maturation. Consequently, most of the genetic epilepsies are age dependent, and some are represented unequally between males and females. These facts are useful for diagnostic purposes and also for genetic counseling. When attempting to elicit a history of a specific genetic epilepsy in family members, it is important to inquire about seizures during the appropriate period of childhood and not just around the time of interview.

Whereas in the past the genetic epilepsies, formerly called idiopathic epilepsies, were believed to be benign, often age-limited

Table 5–1 **Mendelian Idiopathic Epilepsy Syndromes with Genes Identified by Postictal Cloning (as of December 2005)**

Epilepsy Syndrome	Gene	Chromosomal Location
Benign familial neonatal seizures	KCNQ2	20q13
	KCNQ3	8q24
Generalized epilepsy with febrile seizures plus (GEFS+)	SCN1B	19q13
	SCN1A°°	2q24
	SCN2A°	2q24
	GABRG2°	5q31
Benign familial neonatal-infantile seizures	SCN2A°	2q24
Childhood absence epilepsy with febrile seizures	GABRG2°	5q31
Autosomal dominant juvenile myoclonic epilepsy	GABRA1	5q34
	EFHC1	6p12
Autosomal dominant nocturnal frontal lobe epilepsy	CHRNA4	20q13
	CHRNB2	1q21
Autosomal dominant focal epilepsy with auditory features	LGI1	10q24

°Mutations identified in more than one epilepsy syndrome.
°°Mutations (many of which are de novo) also identified in severe myoclonic epilepsy of infancy.
Adapted from Ottman and Winawer, 2008, with permission.

conditions, modern genetic analysis has revealed that these genetic epilepsies have much more variable manifestations, which are difficult to understand from the underlying genetic mutation. For instance, mutations in the *SCN1A gene* have been identified as the causative factor in most patients with Dravet syndrome, a severe progressive epilepsy disorder of infancy which actually belongs to this category of conditions. Also, it is difficult to understand why a seemingly diffuse mutation of the gene expressing the *nicotinic acetylcholine receptor* would give rise to the focal seizures of *autosomal dominant nocturnal frontal lobe epilepsy (ADNFLE)* and why mutations in the *leucine-rich repeat protein (LGI1)* gene, which influences K^+ currents, causes the focal seizures of *autosomal dominant focal epilepsy with auditory features*. The genetic heterogeneity of GEFS+ identifies it as a family of epilepsy conditions rather than a single syndrome. It may be that familial, and possibly even sporadic, forms of *mesial temporal lobe epilepsy (MTLE) with hippocampal sclerosis*, which is often associated with febrile seizures, as well as the sporadic Dravet syndrome, also belong to the GEFS+ family.

Other rare single-gene epilepsies have been identified (Guerrini et al., 2011). Mutations of the *protocadherin 19 (PCDH19) gene* have been associated with an X-linked disorder, *epilepsy and mental retardation limited to females (EFMR)*, and have also been seen in some cases of Dravet syndrome (Chapter 7). Mutations of the *Aristaless-related homeobox (ARX)* and *syntaxin binding protein 1 (STXBP1) genes* can cause the devastating *early infantile epileptic encephalopathy* and Ohtahara syndrome. The role of these genes in the manifestation of these conditions is not understood, because mutations of the same genes are implicated in other disorders, and these syndromes also have other causes.

Genetic bases have also been demonstrated for three other specific epileptic or epilepsy-related phenomena that do not in themselves constitute chronic epilepsy conditions (Table 5–2). The most common inherited epilepsy condition is *febrile seizures* (Chapter 7). The inheritance pattern for febrile seizures is complicated and is usually polygenic rather than autosomal dominant (Tsuboi, 1982). Other than in the well-defined conditions of GEFS+ and Dravet syndrome, there is a complex relationship between the genetic predisposition for febrile seizures and the genetic predisposition for epilepsy (Chapter 7). Although the incidence of febrile seizures is not increased among offspring of patients with chronic epilepsy conditions (Beck-Mannagetta and Janz, 1982), a presumed genetic association exists between the occurrence of benign febrile seizures and the development of *benign epilepsy of childhood with centrotemporal spikes* (Lüders et al., 1987). There is also a high incidence of prolonged febrile seizures among patients with acquired limbic seizures (Falconer, 1971). This may represent the ease with which a precipitating factor (fever), on the one hand, and a specific epileptogenic disturbance (focal brain lesion), on the other, can independently give rise to epileptic seizures in a person with an inherited predisposing factor that nonspecifically lowers seizure threshold. Although older prospective studies of patients with febrile seizures have failed to relate this genetic predisposition per se to a significant incidence of subsequent limbic seizures (Hauser and Annegers, 1987; Nelson and Ellenberg, 1981; Nelson and Ellenberg, 1978) (Chapter 7), investigations using *magnetic resonance imaging (MRI)* indicate that after complex and prolonged febrile seizures some children develop enduring hippocampal abnormalities that may eventually lead to MTLE with hippocampal sclerosis (Gomes and Shinnar et al., 2011). In these situations,

Table 5–2 **Genetic Characteristics of Some Epileptic and Epileptiform Phenomena**

Phenomenon	Likely Mode of Inheritance	Sex Ratio	Age Incidence
Febrile convulsions	Polygenic	Equal	1–5 years
Photosensitivity	Polygenic	Female > male	4–16 years
4- to 7-Hz EEG	Polygenic	Equal	2–6 years

febrile seizures could be predisposing factors themselves, could indicate the occurrence of specific epileptogenic inflammatory insults such as viral infections, or could reflect a pre-existing epileptogenic abnormality.

Photosensitivity (epileptiform EEG discharges in response to intermittent photic stimulation) has been reported to occur in up to 9% of children without epileptic seizures (Petersen et al., 1976) and can be seen in a high percentage of children with genetic generalized epilepsies as well as in those who have a relatively rare epileptic condition with seizures that occur only in response to intermittent-light stimulation (Doose, 1982; Newmark and Penry, 1980; Newmark and Penry, 1979) (Chapter 9). The Japanese *Pocket Monster* (*Pokémon*) video cartoon experience in 1997 highlighted the prevalence of photosensitivity in school-age children (Ishida et al., 1998) (Chapter 9). Undoubtedly, many types of photosensitivity exist, and none appear to have an inheritance pattern consistent with a single-gene disorder (Pedley, 2008).

A bilaterally synchronous, monomorphic *4- to 7-Hz interictal EEG rhythm* can be seen in children with various forms of epilepsy, particularly genetic epilepsies (Baier and Doose, 1987). It has been reported to occur in 50% of children with febrile seizures and in up to 30% of siblings of children with epilepsy (Doose and Gundel, 1982). This EEG pattern may reflect a specific epileptogenic susceptibility or a nonspecific predisposing factor, and it does not have a single-gene pattern of inheritance.

GENETIC DISORDERS ASSOCIATED WITH EPILEPSY

Genetic disorders associated with cerebral lesions that give rise to epileptic seizures are not considered to be genetic epilepsy disorders, even though they are genetically determined. The reasons for this are that (1) the seizures are an incidental consequence of a genetically determined cerebral disturbance and not the direct result of a primary genetic defect, (2) epileptic seizures do not necessarily occur in every person with these conditions, and (3) individuals with these conditions have other important neurological disturbances. Table 5–3 shows the risks for seizures and epilepsy in a number of genetic disorders (Bonkowsky et al., 2008). A complete discussion of all the genetic disorders

associated with epilepsy is beyond the scope of this text, but a few with relatively well-understood mechanisms of action can be mentioned (see also Shorvon et al., 2011).

Disorders of *amino acid* and *protein metabolism* (such as *phenylketonuria* and *porphyria*) disrupt synthesis of proteins important to neural function and cause toxic substances to accumulate. Some of these disorders may be treated by dietary restriction.

Many *lysosomal storage diseases*, including the *gangliosidoses*, *neuronal ceroid lipofuscinoses*, *mucolipidoses*, and *neuraminidase deficiencies* cause intracellular accumulation of toxic molecules and structural disturbances in the brain that influence neuronal excitability.

Myelin disorders (such as *Krabbe's disease* and *adrenoleukodystrophy*) can be associated with lesions of the immediate subcortical white matter, which presumably affect adjacent cell bodies and occasionally induce epileptic seizures.

Disorders of *vitamin*, *electrolyte*, and *endocrine metabolism* (such as *pyridoxine dependency*, *hyperparathyroidism*, *hypoparathyroidism*, and *hypomagnesemia*) disrupt neuronal excitability by influencing neurotransmitter function and the ionic microenvironment.

A number of disorders classified as genetic malformations may be inherited (such as *Aicardi's syndrome*, *lissencephaly*, *holoprosencephaly*, *double cortex syndrome*, and the *X-linked periventricular nodular heterotopia*) (Fig. 5–4). *Microdysgenesis* has been reported in patients with genetic epilepsy disorders (Meencke and Janz, 1984) but appears to be more significant as a marker than as a cause of epileptogenesis. Abnormal neuronal circuitry may be responsible for epileptogenesis in patients with these disorders.

The *progressive myoclonus epilepsies* consist of many types, including *Unverricht-Lundborg*, *Lafora*, *myoclonus epilepsy with ragged red fibers* (*MERRF*), and some *lipid storage disorders* (Chapter 7). Lesions in the cerebellum, brain stem, and diencephalon appear to be responsible for myoclonic symptoms, whereas lesions in the cerebral cortex cause epileptic seizures and dementia.

Some disorders (such as TSC and *neurofibromatosis*) are associated with abnormal growth, development, maturation, and cellular organization within brain tissues, which disrupt

Table 5–3 **Risk for Epilepsy and Other Seizure Associations in Genetic Disorders**

Risk for Epilepsy		Seizure Association
>75%	*<30%*	*Burst suppression*
Angelman syndrome	Acute intermittent porphyria	Nonketotic hyperglycemia
Fukuyama congenital muscular	Adrenoleukodystrophy	*Hypsarrhythmia*
dystrophy	Alzheimer's disease	Menkes disease
Hemimegencephaly	Autism	Nonketotic hyperglycemia
Lissencephaly	Börjeson-Forssman-Lehmann	*Infantile spasms*
MELAS syndrome	syndrome	Hypomelanosis of Ito
Periventricular nodular heterotopia	Brachmann-de Lange syndrome	Lissencephaly
Sturge-Weber syndrome	Cardiofaciocutaneous syndrome	Tuberous sclerosis
Tuberous sclerosis	Cohen syndrome	Wolf-Hirschhorn syndrome
Zellweger spectrum disorders	Crouzon syndrome	*Other nonepileptic events*
50%–75%	Fragile X syndrome	Alzheimer's disease (myoclonus)
Biotinidase deficiency	Huntington's disease	Angelman syndrome (myoclonus)
Christian syndrome	Homocystinuria	Coffin-Lowry syndrome
Landau-Kleffner syndrome	Leigh syndrome	(stimulus-induced drop attacks)
Linear nevus sebaceous syndrome	Neurofibromatosis, Types 1	Niemann-Pick disease, Type C
Rett syndrome	and 2	(gelastic cataplexy)
Wolf-Hirschhorn syndrome	Parry-Romberg syndrome	Trisomy 13 (apneic spells)
30–50%	Prader-Willi syndrome	
Congenital disorders of	Trisomy 13	
glycosylation	Trisomy 21	
Glycogen storage disease I and III	Velocardiofacial syndrome	
Hypomelanosis of Ito	Wilson's disease	
McLeod neuroacanthocytosis	*No increased risk*	
syndrome	Cri-du-chat syndrome	
Metachromatic leukodystrophy	Sex chromosome aneuploidies	
Niemann-Pick disease, Type C	Subtelomeric deletions	
Saethre-Chotzen syndrome	Williams syndrome	
Schizencephaly	Smith-Magenis syndrome	
	Lesch-Nyhan syndrome	
	Mucopolysaccharidoses	

MELAS = mitochondrial encephalomyopathy with lactic acidosis and stroke-like episodes.
From Bonkowsky et al., 2008, with permission.

adjacent neuronal function, structure, or both to produce focal cortical epileptogenic zones. TSC (Fig. 5–5) results from mutations in the *TSC1* and *TSC2* genes, which code for *hamartin* and *tuberin* (Chu-Shore and Thiele, 2011). These two proteins form a heterodimer that inhibits the *mammalian target of rapamycin (mTOR)*, a serine/threonine kinase involved in cell growth and proliferation. The genetic mutation causes hyperactivation of this signaling pathway. Epilepsy and death in a mouse model of TSC was prevented by treatment with rapamycin, which antagonizes the effect of mTOR (Zheng et al., 2008), an approach that is gaining interest for treatment of other causes of epilepsy (Chapters 3 and 4).

Disorders of *carbohydrate metabolism*, such as *von Gierke's disease, leucine-induced hypoglycemia*, and *glucose-transporter-1 (GLUT1) deficiency*, enhance neuronal excitability by disrupting energy supplies. GLUT1 deficiency results from mutations in the *SLC2A1* gene and can manifest as a variety of severe and benign epilepsy syndromes (Chapter 7). Recognition of these conditions is important because they respond to treatment with the *ketogenic diet* (Chapter 16).

Rett syndrome is an X-linked progressive condition that occurs only in girls and is caused by a mutation of the *MECP2* gene, whose expression is important for normal neuronal maturation and synaptogenesis (Bonkowsky et al., 2008). Symptoms begin at 4–18 months of age, and minor motor seizures, which are easily controlled by *valproic acid*, appear at 3–6 years of age.

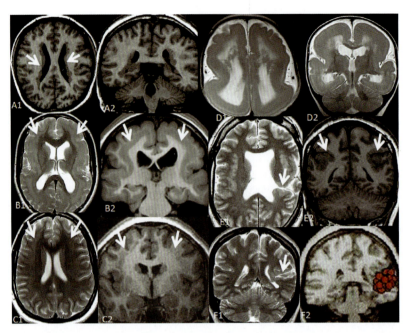

Figure 5–4. Malformations of cortical development. **A1, A2.** Axial T1-weighted (**A1**) and coronal T1- weighted (**A2**) MRI images show diffuse periventricular heterotopias (*arrows* in **A1**). **B1.** Axial T2-weighted image demonstrates gray matter signal intensity bands (*arrows*) in the subcortical white matter, consistent with band heterotopia. **B2.** Coronal T1-weighted image demonstrates band heterotopia seen as low T1-weighted signal (arrows). **C1.** Axial T2-weighted image shows subtle gray matter heterotopia (arrows). **C2.** Coronal T1-weighted image shows low T1 signal band in the subcortical white matter. Heterotopia is better seen in T1-weighted image (arrows). **D1, D2.** Axial T2-weighted (**D1**) and coronal T2-weighted (**D2**) images show smooth cortical surface with very thick cortex, consistent with lissencephaly. **E1.** Axial T2-weighted image shows open lip schizencephaly (*arrow*). **E2:** Coronal T1-weighted image shows bilateral posterior sylvian polymicrogyria (arrows). **F1:** Coronal T2-weighted image shows closed lip schizencephaly (*arrow*). **F2:** Magnetic source image (MSI) shows clustered spikes (*red*) in the area of schizencephaly shown in **F1**. (Courtesy of Dr. Noriko Salamon.)

Among the few chromosome disorders that are consistently associated with epileptic seizures are *terminal deletion chromosome 1p36, Wolf-Hirschhorn syndrome (4p⁻), Angelman syndrome, inversion duplication 15 syndrome (IDIC 15), Miller-Dieker syndrome, Ring 14 syndrome (r14)* and *Ring 20 syndrome (r20)* (Zuberi, 2010). Whereas early onset of seizures, dysmorphic features, and mental retardation are characteristic of most of these rare conditions, as well as *early infantile epileptic encephalopathy* in some, r20 is an exception. In r20, there are no dysmorphic features, seizures begin in childhood or even adolescence,

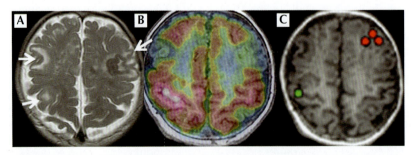

Figure 5–5. Tuberous sclerosis complex. **A.** Axial T2-weighted image shows multiple foci of high T2 signal (*arrows*) consistent with cortical tubers. **B.** Fusion of positron emission tomography (PET) and MRI images shows areas of hypometabolism in the corresponding tubers. **C.** Magnetoencephalography shows spikes (*red*) in the epileptogenic tuber. Sensory stimulation response is noted (*green*) in the right sensory cortex in the postcentral gyrus. (Courtesy of Dr. Noriko Salamon.)

and cognitive decline appears only after onset of seizures (Bernard and Andermann, 2011). In these conditions, there is a peculiar theta-delta EEG pattern, focal dyscognitive status epilepticus is common, and it is important to recognize that these children are not candidates for surgical therapy.

Of the mitochondrial disorders, MERRF is considered by some to be a primary genetic epilepsy, as seizures are a defining clinical feature; however, the mutation also causes hearing loss, dementia, peripheral neuropathy, short stature, exercise intolerance, lipomas, and lactic acidosis. The seizures in *mitochondrial encephalomyopathy, lactic acidosis, and stroke-like episodes (MELAS)* are initially caused by lactic acidosis but are also secondary to infarcts (Hirano et al., 2008). Drugs affecting the respiratory chain, including valproic acid, should be used with caution in mitochondrial disorders, and valproic acid is absolutely contraindicated in mitochondrial DNA *polymerase γ (POLG) gene* mutations (Stewart et al., 2010) (Chapter 15).

Many of the genetic disorders shown in Table 5–3 can be epileptogenic by more than one mechanism, and often the exact mechanisms of epileptogenesis are unknown.

Acquired Causes of Epilepsy Disorders

Acquired epilepsy disorders characterized by generalized onset seizures result from diffuse lesions of the brain, usually following devastating prenatal or perinatal brain injuries resulting from events such as *hypoxia, physical trauma*, and *infections*. Localized *congenital cerebral malformations* result from less severe disturbances of many types in utero and can cause focal seizures later in life. Widespread cerebral damage occurs uncommonly in the mature brain and when it does more often results in focal seizures or myoclonic phenomena than in generalized onset seizures (Shorvon et al., 2011). Well-defined localized pathophysiological processes such as neoplasms, infections, scars, and vascular malformations are easily identified causes of focal seizures on MRI; however, small focal lesions can still be unexpectedly encountered at autopsy or after surgical resection (Armstrong and Bruton, 1987; Babb and Brown, 1987).

Many of the latter are presumed to be congenital lesions. A partial list of systemic diseases associated with epileptic seizures appears in Table 5–4, but most of these disorders cause reactive seizures rather than epilepsy. Insults provoking reactive seizures should be considered precipitating factors unless they also cause brain damage and a chronic epilepsy condition.

A well-documented study of 516 patients treated for epilepsy between 1935 and 1967 in Rochester, Minnesota, identified specific causes in only 23.3% of cases (Hauser and Kurland, 1975). Although these data are pre-MRI, when autopsies were carried out the resulting data did not significantly increase the incidence of identifiable causes. Prior to MRI, however, unsuspected specific structural lesions were demonstrated with careful pathological evaluation of most temporal lobes removed surgically as treatment for MTLE (Armstrong and Bruton, 1987; Babb and Brown, 1987; Engel et al., 1987). The incidences of various identified causes of epilepsy in the Rochester study appear in Table 5–5. This is an example of the distribution of common causes and not a definitive statement of their rates of occurrence, because even though the study was large the number of patients with identifiable causes was relatively small. Furthermore, the distribution of etiologies differs from one demographic area to another. Data from more recent studies also appear in Table 5–5, indicating only relatively minor differences. The usual causes of neonatal seizures are somewhat different from those of seizures later in life (Lombroso, 1983; Rose and Lombroso, 1970; Volpe, 1987) and have changed over the past 20 years (Table 5–6).

ANOXIA AND TRAUMA

Anoxia and physical trauma that occur in utero, during delivery, or in the neonatal period, can cause extensive damage to the CNS that can lead to chronic epileptic seizures (Shorvon et al., 2011). The resultant disorder is usually characterized by generalized onset seizures of one or more types associated with mental retardation and other severe neurological impairments. Although hypoxia and brain distortion occurring during delivery were once thought to cause hippocampal sclerosis and temporal lobe seizures (Earle et al., 1953). this is no longer

Table 5–4 Systemic Diseases Associated with Epileptic Seizures

Cardiovascular diseases
Congenital heart disease
Acquired heart disease
    Mitral stenosis
    Aortic stenosis
    Myocardial infarction
Hypertensive encephalopathy
Hypotension
Obstruction of superior vena cava

Endocrine disorders
Hyperinsulinism
Diabetes mellitus
Hyperthyroidism
Hypothyroidism
Hyperparathyroidism
Hypoparathyroidism
Cushing's syndrome
Addison's disease
Adrenogenital syndrome
Hypopituitarism
Pheochromocytoma

Connective tissue and inflammatory diseases
Systemic lupus erythematosus
Vasculitis
Rheumatic fever
Behçet's disease

Gastrointestinal disorders
Celiac disease
Inflammatory bowel disease
Whipple's disease

Neoplastic diseases
Metastatic carcinoma
Hodgkin's disease

Water, electrolyte and acid-base imbalances
Water intoxication
Dehydration
Hyponatremia
Hypernatremia
Acidosis
Hypocalcemia
Hypomagnesemia

Metabolic disorders
Uremia
Hepatic insufficiency
Xanthomatosis
Hypoglycemia
Inherited metabolic disorder

Hematological disorders
Sickle cell anemia
Leukemia
Polycythemia
Purpura
    Thrombotic thrombocytopenia
    Henoch-Schönlein syndrome

Allergic disorders
Postvaccinal
Anaphylactic shock

Nutritional deficiencies
Beriberi
Rickets
Pyridoxine deficiency

Pregnancy
Eclampsia
Cerebral venous thrombosis

Infections
Viral
Richettsial
Bacterial
Spirochetal
Fungal
Protozoan (especially malaria toxoplasmosis)
Metazoan (especially *Ascaridia, Toxocara, Trichinella, Schistosoma, Paragonimus, Cysticercus, Echinococcus*)

Osteogenic diseases
Oral-facial-digital syndrome
Cleidocranial dysostosis
Paget's disease

Dermatological conditions
Tuberous sclerosis
Sturge-Weber syndrome
Lipoid proteinosis
Pseudoxanthoma
Ichthyosis
Keratosis palmoplantaris
Xeroderma pigmentosum
Incontinentia pigmentosum
Ectodermal dysplasia
Ehlers-Danlos syndrome
Cutaneous melanosis
Congenital lymphedema
Acanthosis nigricans

Adapted from Alia, 1964, and Riggs, 1991, with permission.

Table 5–5 **Causes of Epilepsy, 1935–2008**

Cause	Rochester 1935–1967 (%)	Iceland 1995–1999 (%)	Hauser, 2008 (%)
Trauma	5.2	4.6	8.8
Vascular	5.2	9.0	9.3
Neoplastic	4.1	5.8	2.7
Congenital	3.9	4.2	3.5
Infection	2.9	1.4	2.2
Birth anoxia	1.4		
Degenerative	0.6	6.6	4.0
Unknown (other)	76.7	68.5	63.7

Adapted from Banerjee and Hauser, 2008, with permission.

believed to be the case. The pattern of hippocampal cell loss associated with hypoxia is different from that seen in hippocampal sclerosis (Babb and Brown, 1987), as discussed later in this chapter.

Hypoxic insults in older persons preferentially cause chronic nonepileptic myoclonus (Lance and Adams, 1963), perhaps related to the fact that maturation increases the relative susceptibility of subcortical structures, particularly the cerebellum, to anoxic brain damage (Schneck, 1985). Acute postanoxic coma, often seen in older persons after cardiac and respiratory arrest, can be accompanied by *pseudoperiodic lateralized epileptiform EEG discharges (PLEDs)* (Chatrian et al., 1964) inconsistently associated with focal motor seizures. This condition usually has characteristics more like those of myoclonus than of epilepsy (Chapters 6 and 10).

In all age groups, *traumatic brain injury (TBI)* can produce acute epileptic seizures,

Table 5–6 **Trends in Etiological Factors of Neonatal Seizures at Texas Children's Hospital, 1962–1995**

	1971 n = 228 (%)	1977 n = 80 (%)	1987 n = 95 (%)	1995 n = 100 (%)
Etiologies in initial series				
Hypoxic-ischemic encephalopathy	36	36	42	32
Hypocalcemia	31	12	1	4
Hypoglycemia	5	4	3	2
Congenital brain malformation	6	5	5	3
CNS infection	4	12	17	14
Unknown	23	30	5	9
Additional etiologies identified in 1987 series				
Infarction			6	7
Intracerebral hemorrhage			8	15
Intraventricular hemorrhage			4	1
Inborn errors of metabolism			4	3
Subarachnoid hemorrhage			3	1
Additional etiologies identified in 1995 series				
Chromosomal abnormalities				4
Neurodegenerative disorders				3
Multiple congenital abnormalities				1
Benign familial neonatal convulsions				1
Benign neonatal convulsions				1

From Mizrahi and Kellaway, 1998, with permission.

occurring within the first few days after con-cussion. These seizures do not necessarily pre-dict the development of *posttraumatic epilepsy (PTE)* (Jennett, 1975) (Chapter 8). Such acute events should be considered reactive seizures and the head trauma a precipitating factor. Closed head injury that causes cerebral contu-sion, laceration, and hematoma formation, as well as open head injuries such as bullet wounds and depressed skull fractures, can also produce acute epileptic seizures, but these conditions are associated with a much higher incidence of chronic recurrent seizures (Jennett, 1975) (Chapter 8). The traumatic epileptogenic lesion is encephalomalacia or a cicatrix, with cell loss, gliosis, and sometimes variable degrees of cystic cavitation. Hemosiderin deposits as a result of extravasated blood constitute an epileptogenic factor (Wilmore et al., 1978). The latency of months to more than 10 years between TBI and onset of recurrent epileptic seizures (Raymont et al., 2010), referred to as the *latent period* or *ripening of the scar* (Glaser, 1987; Penfield and Jasper, 1954), reflects a variable time course of epileptogenesis from one person to another. The incidences of TBI and PTE have increased in recent years as a result of casualties from the wars in Iraq and Afghanistan and improved survival after battle-field injuries. This has sparked an increase in interest in basic research on experimental ani-mal models of TBI (Chapter 4). Investigations into the fundamental neuronal disturbances that occur during the latent period are provid-ing important insights into the mechanisms of epileptogenesis that will suggest approaches to prevention.

Two iatrogenic traumatic causes of epi-lepsy were noted in the Rochester series: *intracranial surgery* and *electroshock ther-apy* (Hauser and Kurland, 1975). For three of the four patients with postsurgical seizures in this series, the surgical intervention was prefrontal lobotomy. The risk of epileptic seizures following other types of intracra-nial surgery remains an important and con-troversial clinical issue (North et al., 1983) (Chapter 8). The possibility that repeated trials of electroshock therapy can lead to chronic recurrent epileptic seizures, pre-sumably by a mechanism similar to that of kindling in animals (Chapter 4), is also con-troversial (Devinsky and Duchowny, 1983; Small et al., 1981) (Chapter 8).

CEREBROVASCULAR DISORDERS

All forms of cerebral vascular disease can cause acute reactive seizures or chronic epilepsy, including cerebral hemorrhage; infarction; vascular malformations such as arteriovenous malformations, aneurysms, and cavernous angiomas (Shorvon et al., 2011); and vascular complications of entities such as *Moyamoya syndrome, cerebral autosomal dominant arte-riopathy with subcortical infarcts and leuko-encephalopathy (CADASIL), cerebral venous thrombosis,* the *antiphospholipid syndrome, cerebral amyloid angiopathy, Ehler-Danlos syndrome, Marfan syndrome, cerebral angiitis,* and *Takayasu arteritis* (Gjerstad and Tauboll, 2011).

Strokes cause acute reactive seizures in 10–15% of patients and recurrent seizures in 15% (Hauser et al., 1984). When acute seizures are encountered, they are generally assumed to indicate a carotid occlusion (Cocito et al., 1982) or an embolic or hemorrhagic event (Lesser, 1985), but this specificity has been questioned (Hauser et al., 1984). Glial scars, sometimes associated with hemosiderin deposits, which are hemorrhagic residua, are responsible for the late development of focal and generalized onset seizures. As with trauma, acute reactive seizures associated with strokes do not neces-sarily predict the onset of a chronic recurrent epileptic condition (Chapter 8) (Lesser, 1985). Because *silent strokes* are relatively common among the elderly, and such small lesions often are detected at the time epileptic symptoms appear, these are generally assumed to be the cause of most seizure disorders in older patients whose conditions have no other apparent etio-logical diagnosis.

Vascular lesions in utero can result in forma-tion of *porencephalic cysts* (Fig. 5–6), which is a common congenital cause of epilepsy (Friede, 1975), as well as *cystic-gliotic enceph-alopathy (ulegyria).* Prenatal and perinatal arterial occlusion leads to *infantile hemiplegia* (Solomon et al., 1970) associated with epileptic seizures. Similar insults on a smaller scale dur-ing the prenatal or perinatal period can cause chronic focal seizures later in life (Remillard et al., 1974).

Vascular malformations, including *aneu-rysms,* cause chronic seizures by leaking blood into surrounding cortex and by producing irri-tation through mass effect or pulsations. Large

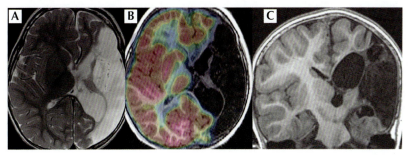

Figure 5–6. Porencephalic cyst secondary to a perinatal infarction. **A.** Axial T2-weighted image shows large stroke in the left middle cerebral artery territory with encephalomalacia and atrophy of the left hemisphere. The left lateral ventricles are larger than those on the right (ex vacuo dilatation). **B.** Coregistration of images obtained using PET with ^{18}F-fluorodeoxyglucose (FDG-PET) and MRI shows loss of normal metabolism in the area of left middle cerebral artery territory stroke. The left anterior and posterior cerebral artery territories show normal metabolism. **C.** Coronal T1-weighted image demonstrates fluid-like intensity in the infarcted tissue of the left middle cerebral artery territory with marked enlargement of the left lateral ventricle and atrophy of the left thalamus. (Courtesy of Dr. Noriko Salamon.)

arteriovenous malformations can also create a steal phenomenon, rendering nearby regions of the brain ischemic. *Venous angiomas,* however, are not generally epileptogenic. *Sturge-Weber syndrome* involves a specific congenital vascular malformation commonly associated with epilepsy in children. *Cavernous angiomas* also cause seizures as a result of bleeding, which produces a characteristic hemosiderin ring on MRI and *computed tomography (CT)* (Fig. 5–7), and when such angiomas are in the temporal lobe, adjacent mesial temporal structures often become epileptogenic (Upchurch et al., 2010). Not all cavernomas necessarily cause seizures, however, so it is important to be aware that the appearance of a cavernoma on the MRI of a person with epilepsy can

be an incidental finding. *Multiple cavernous angiomas,* a condition resulting from mutations in any one of several genes, is associated with as many as 20 or more cavernomas, but only one might be responsible for the patient's seizures. Seizures are acutely induced by *subarachnoid hemorrhage, vasospasm, venous thrombosis,* and *hypertensive encephalopathy,* the cause of seizures in *toxemia of pregnancy* and *posterior reversible encephalopathy syndrome (PRES),* and residual pathological changes can act as a focus for chronic epilepsy. Seizures can also occur from small cerebral hemorrhages associated with *sickle cell anemia* and *coagulopathies*; perivascular infiltrates due to *leukemia*; and cerebral disturbances induced by *collagen vascular diseases.*

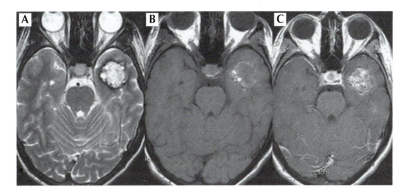

Figure 5–7. Cavernous angioma. **A.** Axial T2-weighted image demonstrates a high signal focus with surrounding low-signal rim within the left anterior temporal lobe, consistent with cavernous malformation and surrounding hemosiderin. **B.** Precontrast T1-weighted image shows foci of mixed signal intensity in the left anterior temporal lesion. **C.** Postcontrast T1-weighted image shows heterogeneous enhancement, often seen with cavernous malformation. No associated developmental venous anomaly is seen. (Courtesy of Dr. Noriko Salamon.)

BRAIN TUMORS

Epileptic seizures occur in 20–70% of patients with various types of intracranial tumors (Hoefer et al., 1947; Farrell et al., 2008; Shorvon et al., 2011) (Table 5–7). Although high-resolution MRI can identify most brain tumors, small epileptogenic neoplasms still escape detection in some patients, in which case serial scans are necessary to reveal the progressive lesion.

Small *meningiomas* and *arachnoid cysts* are usually incidental findings, but large meningiomas and some cysts presumably produce seizures by irritation and compression, rather than destruction, of adjacent cortex. *Gliomas* and *gangliogliomas* (mixed neoplastic neuronal and glial tissue) are the most commonly encountered neoplasms in epilepsy surgical specimens (Spencer et al., 1984). These small lesions are not particularly invasive or aggressive; often they are associated with a long history of seizures and have a low incidence of recurrence (Armstrong and Bruton, 1987; Babb and Brown, 1987). *Hamartomas*, nonneoplastic masses consisting of abnormal mixtures of vascular, glial, and neuronal tissue, are also encountered in temporal lobe tissue removed from patients with limbic seizures (Armstrong and Bruton, 1987; Babb and Brown, 1987). The term *hamartoma* has been variously used to indicate vascular malformations, tubers, and forms of ectodermal dysplasia (Armstrong and Bruton, 1987). *Tubers* consist of disorganized collections of large pleomorphic astrocytes resembling *gemistocytic astrocytes*, often with calcification, and neurons showing cytoskeletal abnormalities. It is not clear whether these represent a forme fruste of TSC or an acquired lesion. Ectopic tissue such as *epidermoids* and *dermoids*, particularly in mesial temporal structures, can give rise to epileptic seizures. Many tumors previously diagnosed as hamartomas, tubers, epidermoids, and dermoids are now classified as *dysembryoplastic neuroepithelial tumors (DNETs)*, which are extremely indolent but have a strong association with epilepsy (Farrell et al., 2008) (Fig. 5–8). Although DNETs represent only about 1% of neuroepithelial tumors, they are disproportionately represented in patients with pharmacoresistant focal seizures who are candidates for surgical treatment. Seizures from DNETs almost always begin before the age of 20, and successful surgical removal offers an excellent prognosis for a seizure-free outcome. A particular form of hamartoma, *hypothalamic hamartoma*, gives rise to a specific syndrome associated with *gelastic seizures* (Harvey et al., 2008; Kerrigan, 2011) (Chapter 7).

Hemimegalencephaly, a rare congenital disorder invariably associated with severe seizures, has been considered a form of brain tumor (Townsend et al., 1975a) but now is regarded as a malformation of cortical development (Kuzniecky and Jackson, 2008) (Fig. 5–9). Bony skull growths encroaching on the intracranial vault that occur with malformations such as *cleidocranial dysostosis* and *Paget's disease* can also mechanically irritate cortex and cause epileptic seizures (Aita, 1964).

INFECTIOUS DISEASES

Prenatal and perinatal infections (such as *toxoplasmosis, cytomegalic inclusion disease,*

Table 5–7 **Relative Frequency of Convulsive Seizures in Various Types of Tumors of the Cerebral Hemispheres**

Type of Tumor	Number of Cases	% with Seizures
Hemangioma and blastoma	13	69
Cysts	5	60
Astrocytoma	85	55
Abscess	12	50
Meningiomas	84	41
Metastatic tumors	34	35
Glioblastomas	149	31
Other gliomas	34	26
Subdural hematoma	17	23

From Hoefer et al., 1947, with permission.

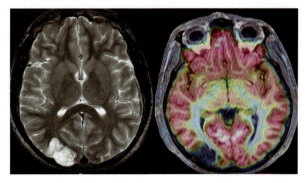

Figure 5–8. Dysembrioplastic neuroepithelial tumor (DNET). *Left:* Axial T2-weighted image of 16-year-old patient with a right occipital DNET. There is a well-defined cystic lesion with internal septation in the right occipital lobe. Adjacent bone erosion is seen, suggesting a slow-growing process. *Right:* Coregistration of FDG-PET and MRI images demonstrates hypometabolism in the lesion. Adjacent gray matter demonstrates normal metabolism. (Courtesy of Dr. Noriko Salamon.)

rubella, *herpes*, and *syphilis*) produce diffuse static neocortical and hippocampal damage. This results in chronic epileptic conditions, usually associated with generalized onset seizures and developmental delay. A late *progressive encephalitis* associated with epileptic seizures has been reported to occur in the second decade of life in children with congenital rubella (Townsend et al., 1975b; Weil et al., 1975), and rubella virus is believed to be responsible (Falconer, 1971). *Cerebral malaria* in young children is a cause of refractory epilepsy later in life and can now be readily diagnosed in endemic countries (which usually have limited resources) by identification of a characteristic malaria retinopathy (Birbeck et al., 2010). *Meningitis, encephalitis, abscesses,* and *granulomas* commonly induce acute epileptic seizures. After effective treatment, residual structural changes can continue to act as

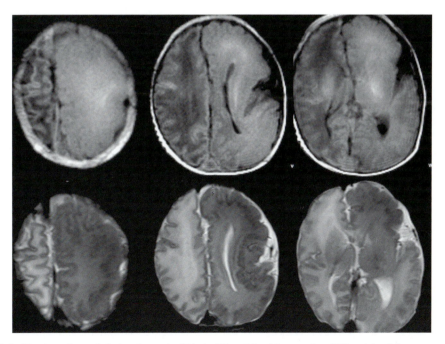

Figure 5–9. Hemimegalencephaly in a 3-month-old baby. T1-weighted (*top row*) and T2-weighted (*bottom row*) images demonstrate large left hemisphere and thickened cortex with increased T1- and decreased T2-weighted signal in the left hemispheric white matter, suggesting accelerated myelination. (Courtesy of Dr. Noriko Salamon.)

chronic epileptogenic lesions. Parasitic infections can also cause epileptic seizures. (See also Shorvon et al., 2011.)

Cysticercosis is the most common cause of focal seizures in Latin America, is a major health problem in Asia and Africa, and is increasingly encountered elsewhere among immigrants from endemic areas (Miller et al., 1983; Del Brutto, 2008). The residual cyst can cause recurrent seizures, but it remains uncertain how often this infection is responsible for chronic epilepsy. Cysts on CT-MRI scans in patients with focal epilepsy from endemic areas can be incidental findings. Recent evidence indicates that many patients with neurocysticercosis and epilepsy actually have MTLE with hippocampal sclerosis, suggesting that the cysts per se are not the cause of chronic epilepsy but somehow predispose to hippocampal atrophy and epileptogenesis (da Gama et al., 2005).

The *acquired immunodeficiency syndrome (AIDS)* is an important cause of neurological symptoms in adults and children. Cerebral dysfunction in AIDS results from *opportunistic infections*, especially *cytomegalovirus, cryptococcus*, and *progressive multifocal leukoencephalopathy (PML)*, associated CNS *lymphomas*, and encephalopathy due directly to the *human immunodeficiency virus (HIV)*, all of which can manifest with epileptic seizures (Rosenblum et al., 1988a; Sever and Gibbs, 1988). Seizures were reported in 18% of children with HIV infections (Epstein et al., 1988) and in 14% of adults with CNS lymphomas and AIDS (Rosenblum et al., 1988b).

INFLAMMATION AND IMMUNE-MEDIATED DISORDERS

Research on basic mechanisms of epileptogenesis is demonstrating an increasingly important role for immunity and inflammatory processes (Vezzani and Rüegg, 2011) (Chapter 4). Brain insults such as infection, trauma, and stroke, as well as seizures themselves, induce inflammatory changes in the brain (*innate immunity*). Breakdown in the blood-brain barrier permits peripheral immune responses as well as specific antibody production to affect the brain (*adaptive immunity*). *Rasmussen's encephalitis*, the first epilepsy disorder to be recognized as inflammatory, is usually unilateral, progressive, and associated with focal status epilepticus (Aguilar and Rasmussen, 1960; Rasmussen, 1978; Farrell et al., 1995; Del Brutto, 2008) (Chapter 7).

Other epilepsy syndromes that could involve similar immune-mediated processes include *West syndrome, Landau-Kleffner syndrome, hemiconvulsion-hemiplegia syndrome, Batten disease*, and *limbic encephalitis* (Granata et al., 2011) (Chapter 7). Limbic encephalitis may or may not be *paraneoplastic*. Seizures in these conditions are often associated with specific antibodies to the N-*methyl-*D-*aspartate (NMDA)* receptor, γ-*aminobutyric acid B (GABA$_B$)* receptor, α-*amino-3-dehydroxy-5-methyl-4-isoxazole proprionic acid (AMPA)* receptor, and, most recently, molecules associated with the *voltage-gated potassium channel (VGKC)* complex, all located on the surface of neurons. Antibodies to VGKC can produce frequent faciobrachial clonic seizures (Irani et al., 2011) and in 90% of cases targets the LGI1 protein, which is curious not only because of the focal nature of the phenotype, given the general distribution of this protein, but also because mutation of the gene that encodes this protein is responsible for *temporal lobe epilepsy with auditory features* (Chapter 7). It is important to recognize these conditions, because they can be responsive to anti-immune therapy, including steroids, *intravenous immunoglobulin (IVIG)*, and *plasmapheresis* (Ozkara and Vigevano, 2011). Inflammatory mechanisms may also be involved in seizures associated with known autoimmune disorders such as *multiple sclerosis, systemic lupus erythematosus, type 1 diabetes mellitus, Hashimoto's encephalopathy*, and *celiac disease*, which is associated with occipital calcifications and seizures (Vincent and Crino, 2011). Individuals with *Alzheimer's disease* have a 10-fold increase in the incidence of epileptic seizures (Hauser et al., 1986), which could conceivably be related to some inflammatory processes, including microglial activation as the result of brain amyloid deposition.

There is no evidence to support the persistent fear that vaccinations cause encephalopathy that leads to chronic epilepsy and other neurological disturbances (Cendes and Sankar, 2011). Epileptic seizures that occur during the first 72 hours following immunization with whole cell killed bacteria containing endotoxins, such as the *pertussis* vaccine, and 7–10 days following live attenuated virus immunizations, such as the *measles* vaccine, indicate benign febrile seizures due to the immunization-induced fever and not allergic encephalopathy caused by the immunizing agent (Hirtz et al., 1983). Whereas immunization is not recommended in children who have had epileptic seizures (to avoid precipitating a seizure, not for fear of producing an allergic encephalopathy), a family history of epilepsy is not considered a contraindication (Committee on Infectious Diseases, 1987). When routine vaccination causes a febrile seizure that is followed by an encephalopathy, this reflects induction of an ictal event in a child with a preexistent epileptogenic abnormality, a common scenario for Dravet syndrome, which can be diagnosed by genetic testing (Ottman et al., 2010).

MALFORMATIONS OF CORTICAL DEVELOPMENT

With the advent of high-resolution MRI, a large variety of *malformations of cortical development (MCDs)* can now be visualized and are recognized as a major cause of epilepsy (Kuzniecky and Jackson, 2008; Vinters et al., 2008; Shorvon et al., 2011). MCDs, both genetic and acquired, range from widespread disturbances associated with developmental delay, skin lesions, and organ malformations, to small, isolated focal lesions that are not readily apparent on MRI and require specialized imaging when surgical treatment is considered or that may be revealed only by pathological evaluation of the postoperative surgical resection. MCDs are increasingly recognized as a major cause of pharmacoresistant, often surgically remediable epilepsy. Table 5–8 shows the classification scheme for these disorders (Kuzniecky and Jackson, 2008). Large areas of *cortical dysplasia, polymicrogyria,* and *hemimegalencephaly* usually manifest as severe seizures very early in life, often as West syndrome in infancy. Many infants with these conditions can be treated by large multilobar resections or hemispherectomy (Chapter 16). *Schizencephaly* is of particular interest, because these large developmental defects can cause few or no obvious clinical signs or symptoms. Seizures, when they occur, are usually focal and can develop late. The epileptogenic regions in these patients are often limited to a small area of the cleft that can be surgically removed with beneficial effects (Landy et al., 1992).

Focal cortical dysplasia (FCD) is a common cause of focal seizures beginning in adolescence or later that often become pharmacoresistant but can be treated surgically. Originally described by Taylor et al. (1971) on pathological examination of surgically resected specimens from patients with intractable epilepsy, this lesion can now frequently be identified by MRI in patients with focal seizures who in the past would have been diagnosed as having a cryptogenic epilepsy condition. Considerable attention is now being paid to the pathological characteristics of different types of FCD (Blümcke et al., 2011) (Table 5–9; Fig. 5–10), which are now the most common surgically remediable epileptogenic lesions in children (Lerner et al., 2009). *FCD Types I* (Fig. 5–11) and *II* are isolated lesions often associated with frequent pharmacoresistant seizures. A characteristic feature of FCD Type IIa is the presence of enlarged, dysmorphic, and disorganized neurons (Fig. 5–12), while Type IIb also has gemistocyte-like large *balloon cells* (Fig. 5–13). Microscopically, FCD Type IIb is almost indistinguishable from a tuber of TSC. *FCD Type III* is a variant associated with other lesions such as hippocampal sclerosis, neoplasms, vascular malformations, and trauma. Examples of neuropathological features of these different conditions can be found on the ILAE Brain Bank web site (www.epicurebank.org).

TOXIC AND METABOLIC DISTURBANCES

Common seizure-inducing exogenous toxic substances include *heavy metals* (particularly *lead* in children), *organic* and *inorganic compounds,* and *proconvulsant drugs.* Common seizure-inducing endogenous toxic-metabolic processes are *uremia* and *hyperammonemia* as well as disruption of *electrolyte* and *water balance, pH,* and *carbohydrate metabolism.* All of these insults should be considered precipitating factors rather than specific epileptogenic disturbances. However, prolonged exposure to toxins and metabolic abnormalities can lead to structural damage and recurrent epileptic seizures. Alcohol and drug abuse have a strong association with epilepsy, for a variety of reasons ranging from direct effects to secondary brain damage from trauma and intravenous injections (Brust, 2008).

HIPPOCAMPAL SCLEROSIS

Hippocampal sclerosis is the most common lesion encountered in patients with limbic seizures (Chapter 6) and MTLE (Chapter 7) (Babb and Brown, 1987; Cendes and Morita,

Table 5–8 Classification Scheme of Malformations of Cortical Development

I. Malformations due to abnormal neuronal and glial proliferation or apoptosis
   A. Decreased proliferation/increased apoptosis or increased proliferation/decreased apoptosis—abnormalities of brain size
      1. Microcephaly with normal to thin cortex
      2. Microlissencephaly (extreme microcephaly with thick cortex)
      3. Microcephaly with extensive polymicrogyria
      4. Macrocephalies
   B. Abnormal proliferation (abnormal cell types)
      1. Nonneoplastic
         a. Cortical hamartomas of tuberous sclerosis
         b. Cortical dysplasia with balloon cells
         c. Hemimegalencephaly
      2. Neoplastic (associated with disordered cortex)
         a. Dysembryoplastic neuroepithelial tumor
         b. Ganglioglioma
         c. Gangliocytoma
II. Malformations due to abnormal neuronal migration
   A. Lissencephaly/subcortical band heterotopia spectrum
   B. Cobblestone complex/congenital muscular dystrophy syndromes
   C. Heterotopia
      1. Subependymal (periventricular)
      2. Subcortical (other than band heterotopia)
      3. Marginal glioneuronal
III. Malformations due to abnormal cortical organization (including later neuronal migration)
   A. Polymicrogyria and schizencephaly
      1. Bilateral polymicrogyria syndromes
      2. Schizencephaly (polymicrogyria with clefts)
      3. Polymicrogyria or schizencephaly as part of multiple congenital anomaly/mental retardation syndromes
   B. Cortical dysplasia without balloon cells
   C. Microdysgenesis
IV. Malformations of cortical development, not otherwise classified
   A. Malformations secondary to inborn errors of metabolism
      1. Mitochondrial and pyruvate metabolic disorders
      2. Peroxisomal disorders
   B. Other unclassified malformations
      1. Sublobar dysplasia
      2. Others

From Kuzniecky and Jackson, 2008, with permission.

2011; Margerison and Corsellis, 1966; Mathern et al., 2008). This lesion was first identified grossly by Bouchet and Cazauvieilh in 1825 (Bouchet and Cazauvieilh, 1825) and studied microscopically by Sommer in 1880 (Sommer, 1880) and Bratz in 1899 (Bratz, 1899) (Fig. 5–14). Subsequently, terms such as *Ammon's horn sclerosis, mesial temporal sclerosis, incisural sclerosis, pararhinal sclerosis,* and *mesial sclerotic temporal atrophy* have been applied to mesial temporal lesions with various patterns of cell loss and gliosis. The cell loss can range from involvement of the end folium or hilus of the dentate gyrus only (although this *end folium sclerosis* is a dubious entity) to widespread cell loss of most or all of the hippocampus as well as parts of amygdala and parahippocampal gyrus (Armstrong and Bruton, 1987; Babb and Brown, 1987; Mathern et al., 2008). Hippocampal atrophy resembling hippocampal sclerosis can also be seen in the absence of epilepsy, for instance in dementia and depression (Chapter 11). Hippocampal sclerosis can be bilateral and is not the only pathological finding in classical MTLE; thalamus, basal ganglia, and wide areas of neocortex, ipsilaterally and contralaterally, can be involved (Engel and Thompson, 2012) (Chapter 7).

Table 5–9 **Three-Tiered ILAE Classification System of Focal Cortical Dysplasia (FCD), Distinguishing Isolated Forms (Types I and II) from Those Associated with Another Principal Lesion (Type III)**

FCD Type I (isolated)	Focal cortical dysplasia with abnormal radial cortical lamination (FCD Type Ia)	Focal cortical dysplasia with abnormal tangential cortical lamination (FCD Type Ib)	Focal cortical dysplasia with abnormal radial and tangential cortical lamination (FCD Type Ic)	
FCD Type II (isolated)	Focal cortical dysplasia with dysmorphic neurons (FCD Type IIa)		Focal cortical dysplasia with dysmorphic neurons and balloon cells (FCD Type IIb)	
FCD Type III (associated with principal lesion)	Cortical lamination abnormalities in the temporal lobe associated with hippocampal sclerosis (FCD Type IIIa)	Cortical lamination abnormalities adjacent to a glial or glioneuronal tumor (FCD Type IIIb)	Cortical lamination abnormalities adjacent to vascular malformation (FCD Type IIIc)	Cortical lamination abnormalities adjacent to any other lesion acquired during early life, e.g., trauma, ischemic injury, encephalitis (FCD Type IIId)

FCD Type III (not otherwise specified, NOS): if clinically/radiologically suspected principal lesion is not available for microscopic inspection.

Please note that the rare association between FCD Types IIa and IIb with hippocampal sclerosis, tumors, or vascular malformations should not be classified as FCD Type III variant.

From Blümcke et al., 2011, with permission.

For many years, there was considerable debate over whether hippocampal sclerosis results from epileptic activity (Meldrum et al., 1974) or whether the lesion precedes the epileptic condition and is the cause of seizures (Earle et al., 1953). A unifying hypothesis was initially proposed by Falconer (Falconer, 1971): Prolonged febrile seizures, which are commonly reported in the history of patients with limbic seizures, produce hippocampal damage. Later in life, this structural abnormality itself becomes an epileptogenic lesion. In this situation, a genetic predisposition for epilepsy could underlie both the appearance of febrile seizures and the epileptogenic potential of hippocampal sclerosis. Although there is increasing evidence that prolonged febrile seizures can cause hippocampal changes associated in some cases with later seizures (Gomes and Shinnar, 2011), Falconer's hypothesis remains controversial: patients with simple febrile seizures do not appear to be at great risk for subsequent chronic seizures (Hauser and Annegers, 1987; Nelson and Ellenberg, 1981; Nelson and Ellenberg, 1978) (Chapter 7), and primates with hippocampal sclerosis induced by prolonged generalized tonic-clonic seizures have not demonstrated spontaneous epileptogenic properties (Meldrum, 1988). In rodents and other mammals, status epilepticus produces hippocampal damage similar to hippocampal sclerosis that results in spontaneous seizures, and this has become a popular experimental model of MTLE with hippocampal sclerosis; however, prolonged heat-induced seizures in rodents do not cause cell death but may cause subsequent seizures (Chapter 4). A finding of hippocampal sclerosis in temporal lobe tissue resected from patients with medically intractable focal seizures usually predicts a good surgical outcome (Armstrong and Bruton, 1987; Babb and Brown, 1987; Falconer and Serafetinides, 1963; Falconer and Taylor, 1968), and ictal depth electrode

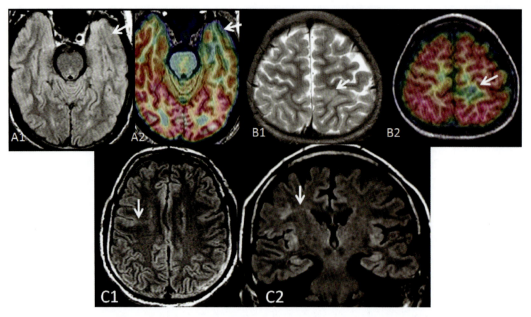

Figure 5–10. Focal cortical dysplasia (FCD). **A.** Type I FCD. *A1*: Axial fluid attenuated inversion recovery (FLAIR) image shows high signal intensity in the left temporal pole (*arrow*). Asymmetry of the temporal lobe is present. *A2*: Coregistration of FDG-PET-and MRI images demonstrates subtle hypometabolism (*arrow*) in the left anterior temporal lobe. **B.** Type IIa FCD. *B1*: Axial T2-weighted image shows thickening of the gray matter of the left paracentral lobule (*arrow*). *B2*: FDG-PET and MRI coregistration demonstrates clear hypometabolism (*arrow*) in the left paracentral lobule. **C.** Type IIb FCD. Axial FLAIR (*C1*) and coronal FLAIR (*C2*) images show right frontal gray-white matter blurring with transmantle tail (*arrow*) toward the right lateral ventricle. (Courtesy of Dr. Noriko Salamon.)

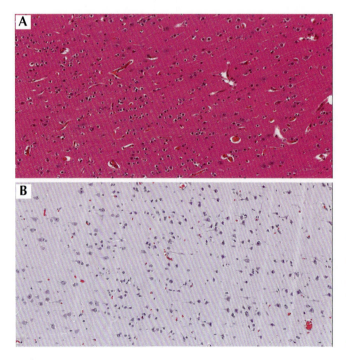

Figure 5–11. Type I FCD. The two panels show micrographs photographed at the same original magnification (X 10). **A.** Image from relatively normal cortex, with well-organized cortical neurons. **B.** Image from a subject with Type I FCD. Note disorganization and clustering of neurons, with frequently abnormal polarity. Difference in staining intensity reflects interday laboratory variation. (Courtesy of Dr. Harry Vinters.)

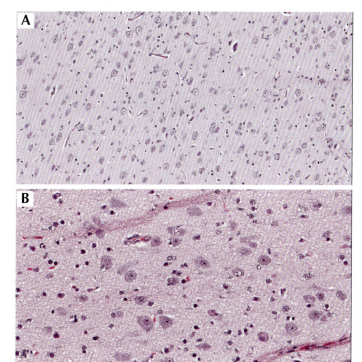

Figure 5–12. Type IIa FCD. **A.** Micrograph photographed at magnification identical to that for Figure 5–11. Note abnormal organization and crowding of neurons, with neuronal enlargement and dysmorphism. **B.** The same features shown at higher magnification (original × 20) (Courtesy of Dr. Harry Vinters.)

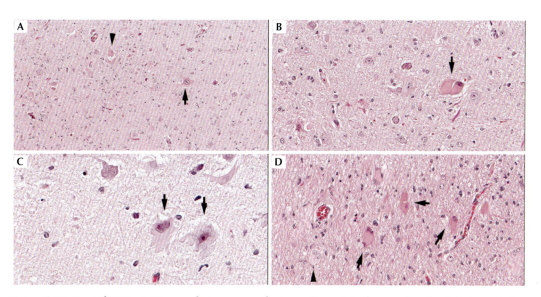

Figure 5–13. Type IIb FCD. **A.** Micrograph at same magnification as Figure 5–11 shows profound cortical disorganization and dyslamination, as well as dysmorphic neurons (*arrow*) and balloon cells (*arrowhead*). **B, D.** Image at original magnification × 20 shows detail of gemistocyte-like balloon cells (*arrows*); *arrowhead* in **D** indicates a binucleated balloon cell. **C.** Image at original magnification × 20 shows markedly dysmorphic neurons with pale eosinophilic cytoplasm (lacking Nissl substance). (Courtesy of Dr. Harry Vinters.)

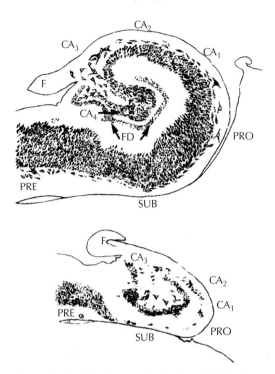

Figure 5–14. Wood-carved plate by Bratz (1899) of cells in normal (*top*) and atrophied epileptic (*bottom*) hippocampus. Although the numbers of pyramidal cells are overrepresented at the top, the Ammon's horn (*CA*), fascia dentata (*FD*), and subicular complex are identifiable in both normal and sclerotic hippocampus. The important subfields are labeled, and one can note in the normal hippocampus (*top*) large CA3 pyramids, properly oriented pyramids around Ammon's horn to the presubiculum (*PRE*), smaller granule cells of the fascia dentata, and the white matter of the fimbria-fornix (*F*). In the epileptic hippocampus, granule cells of the fascia dentata and CA4 pyramids are less damaged than in CA3, CA1, and prosubiculum (*PRO*). Most notable is the preservation of CA2 and the relatively intact presubiculum adjacent to the damaged subiculum (*SUB*). This epileptic pattern is found in temporal lobe resections and autopsies of patients who have suffered from temporal lobe epilepsies.

recordings from these patients prior to surgery show that the habitual seizures begin within the sclerotic hippocampus (Babb et al., 1984). It seems clear, therefore, that the structural hippocampal abnormality does play a role in epileptogenesis in this situation, even though the cause of the sclerosis remains unknown (Chapter 4).

Careful quantitative analysis of hippocampal cell densities in tissue removed from patients with temporal lobe epilepsy has revealed a characteristic pattern of cell loss. Although the loss is widespread in hippocampus, it

is most marked in CA1 and CA3 and tends to spare CA2 (Babb and Brown, 1987; Mouritzen-Dam, 1982). It has been proposed that this specific pattern is peculiar to the form of hippocampal sclerosis that generates epileptic seizures, because the more diffuse hippocampal lesions due to anoxia and other systemic injuries are not particularly epileptogenic (Babb and Brown, 1987) (Fig. 5–15). More detailed clinical pathological correlations have now suggested that there most likely is more than one type of hippocampal sclerosis leading to epilepsy and that MTLE with hippocampal sclerosis is not a single syndrome (Wieser et al., 2004). Statistical parametric mapping of high-resolution MRI scans reveals that atrophy is not diffusely distributed but occurs in a patchy pattern. (see Fig. 4–23). Different patterns of atrophy can be identified that correlate, for instance, with the occurrence of *fast ripples* (Ogren et al., 2009a;b) (Fig. 5–16). It is clear now that this disorder is not limited to the hippocampus; there are also large areas of neocortical atrophy, often bilateral, as well as involvement of subcortical structures, including basal ganglia and thalamus (Mathern et al., 2008; Lin et al. 2005; 2007). Work is under way to create an international classification for hippocampal sclerosis, and pathological specimens can be viewed on the ILAE Brain Bank web site (www.epicure-bank.org).

PRECIPITATING FACTORS

Precipitating factors determine the time of occurrence of epileptic seizures in persons with chronic epilepsy. In susceptible persons with low thresholds for epileptic seizure generation, some precipitating factors can also provoke reactive seizures in the absence of a specific epileptogenic disturbance (see Fig. 5–1). In that situation, seizures can often be controlled by limiting exposure to the precipitating factors, obviating the need for antiseizure medication.

Precipitating factors can be nonspecific events that enhance neuronal excitation and synchronization in a general fashion or specific events that enhance excitation and synchronization in discrete regions of the brain uniquely receptive to these influences (Jallon and Zifkin, 2008; Shorvon et al., 2011) (Chapter 9).

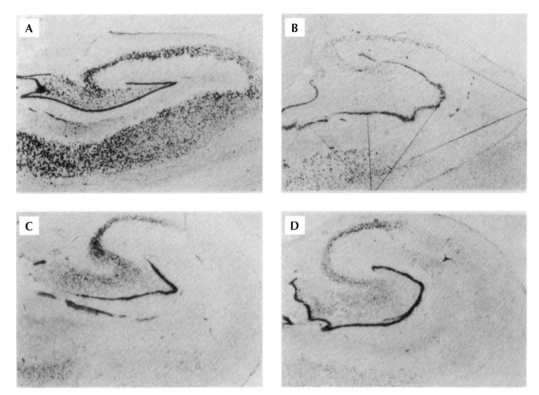

Figure 5–15. Four photomicrographs used by Spielmeyer (1927) to illustrate normal hippocampus (**A**) and hippocampal cell loss with epileptic seizures (**B**), opium poisoning fatality (**C**), and fatal tuberculin meningitis (**D**). Hippocampal damage has different patterns depending on cause. **B.** Epileptic seizures are associated here with the most hippocampal cell loss, but presubiculum is spared (typical hippocampal sclerosis). **C.** More uniform loss extending past the subiculum is seen with opium death. **D.** Severe loss of neurons from CA1 through subiculum proper occurs with meningitis.

Nonspecific Precipitating Factors

Nonspecific influences that can provoke epileptic seizures under appropriate conditions include stress, sleep deprivation, convulsant drugs, withdrawal of alcohol and sedative (often antiseizure) drugs, fever, infectious processes, head trauma, and various toxic and metabolic conditions (such as *hyponatremia*, *hypocalcemia*, *hypoglycemia*, *hepatic encephalopathy*, and *hypoxia*) that disrupt water, pH, and electrolyte balance and energy metabolism (Chapter 3). Importantly, metabolic encephalopathies can occasionally cause focal as well as generalized seizures, and focal ictal events are commonly encountered with *nonketotic hyperglycemia* and *uremia* (Berkovic et al., 1982; Singh and Strobos, 1980). The former often responds to insulin but not antiseizure medications. Particularly pharmacoresistant focal seizures occur in hyperosmolar conditions when

shrinkage of brain tissue tears small bridging vessels.

Table 5–10 shows drugs reported to precipitate generalized tonic-clonic seizures. Of particular interest to neurologists are the *aqueous iodinated contrast agents* (such as *metrizamide*), which are used in myelography and may cause nonconvulsive status epilepticus as well as generalized tonic-clonic seizures (Levin and Lee, 1985), and several other agents that might be prescribed for patients with epilepsy (such as the *antidepressants* and *antipsychotics* mentioned earlier and *general anesthetics*). Although these latter agents should be used with caution in patients with known epileptogenic disorders, there is no reason to withhold their use when appropriate antiseizure drugs are also administered (Chapter 14). The antiseizure drugs *phenobarbital* and *phenytoin* are on this list because of the paradoxical effects sometimes seen with high doses of these medications

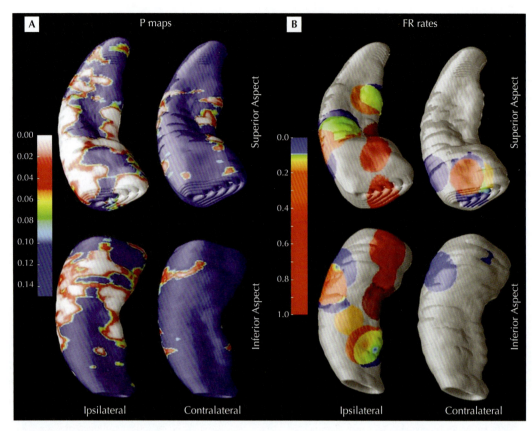

Figure 5–16. Statistical parametric mapping of high-resolution MRI images of patients with unilateral mesial temporal lobe epilepsy. **A.** Three-dimensional averaged contour map depicts areas of significant atrophy (*white and red*) on superior and inferior surfaces of hippocampus ipsilateral and contralateral to seizure onset. **B.** Maps from same patients indicating averaged fast ripple (FR) rates within a 5-mm radius of the tip of microelectrode position in hippocampus. Higher FR rates correlated with local areas of atrophy shown in **A.** Colors represent rates of FR occurrence: blue, purple and yellow are slower (< 0.2/min.), and orange and red are faster (0.2–1.0/min). (Modified from Ogren et al., 2009b, with permission.)

as well as other antiseizure drugs (Chapter 14). Alcohol and drug abuse are particularly problematic for people with epilepsy (Brust, 2008). *Lindane*, an ingredient in some antidandruff shampoos, has been reported to be proconvulsant (Stark et al., 1987), and a number of environmental toxins, particularly pesticides, have epileptogenic potential (Table 5–11).

Specific Precipitating Factors

Certain individuals are particularly sensitive to specific seizure-precipitating factors (Jallon and Zifkin, 2008). Photosensitivity and susceptibility to febrile seizures are two inherited conditions in which reactive epileptic seizures can occur in response to specific precipitating influences. Chronic epilepsy conditions known

as *reflex epilepsies* (Forster, 1977) (Chapters 7 and 9) can be inherited or acquired. In these disorders, generalized or focal seizures can be provoked by exquisitely specific sensory stimulation. The selectively precipitated effect varies in severity; for instance, photosensitivity can manifest merely as a paroxysmal EEG response to intermittent photic stimulation or, in more susceptible individuals, as clinical seizures (Newmark and Penry, 1979). The effectiveness of the photic stimulation depends on its frequency, which suggests hypersynchronization as a mechanism of action. Hypersynchronization could also account for seizures caused by sudden startling stimuli (Chapter 9). It is not clear, however, how the discrete sensitivity develops and by what mechanism the stimulus itself acts in individuals with reflex epilepsies induced only by extremely specific precipitating

Table 5–10 Drugs Reported to Cause Convulsions

Anticholinergics
Anticholinesterase agents (organophosphates, physostigmine)
Antidepressants
Antihistamines
Antipsychotics
Aqueous iodinated contrast agents
Baclofen
Beta-blockers (propranolol, oxprenolol)
Bronchodilators
Camphor
Chlorambucil
Cocaine
Cycloserine
Cyclosporin A
Ergonovine
Folic acid
General anesthetics (ketamine, halothane, Althesin, enflurane, propanidid)
Hyperbaric oxygen
Hypoglycemic agents
Hyposmolar parenteral solutions
Insulin
Isoniazid
Local anesthetics (bupivacaine, lidocaine, procaine, etidocaine)
Mefenamic acid
Methylxanthines
Metronidazole
Misonidazole
Nalidixic acid
Narcotic analgesics (fentanyl, merperidine, pentazocine, propoxyphene)
Oxytocin (secondary to water intoxication)
Penicillins
Phencyclidine
Phenobarbital
Phenytoin
Prednisone (with hypocalcemia)
Sympathomimetics (amphetamines, ephedrine, phenylpropanolamine, terbutaline)
Vitamin K oxide

From Messing et al., 1984, with permission.

factors such as certain strains of music or eating (Chapter 9).

SUMMARY AND CONCLUSIONS

Patients with epilepsy benefit when approaches to management take into account the multifactorial causes of human epilepsy conditions.

Table 5–11 Potentially Proconvulsant Environmental Toxins

DDT
Lindane
Chlordane
Dieldrin
DDE
Endrin
Aldrin
Heptachlor
Hexachorocyclohexane
Toxaphene
Endosulfan
Methoxychlor
Heptachlor epoxide

Courtesy of Dr. Larry G. Stark, Department of Pharmacology, University of California, Davis.

Although identification of one or more specific epileptogenic disturbances is a major goal in diagnosis, such disturbances often cannot be found, and many of those that are revealed have no definitive treatment. Diagnostic evaluation, therefore, must also take into account nonspecific predisposing factors and precipitating factors that might be amenable to therapeutic manipulation.

Genetic investigations are greatly advancing our understanding of the causes of the epilepsies and rapidly identifying mutations responsible for epilepsy syndromes, diseases associated with epilepsy, and susceptibility factors that enhance the risks of acquired epilepsy. Genetic disturbances, however, are not necessarily inherited. Many of these mutations are sporadic. Furthermore, the risk of inheritance of most epileptogenic genetic disturbances is relatively low.

Improved understanding of structural abnormalities that act as specific epileptogenic disturbances increases the opportunity for devising effective treatment for individual patients. At present such treatment consists particularly of surgical resection of small tumors, hippocampal sclerosis, MCDs, and other focal cerebral lesions (Chapter 16). High-resolution MRI has contributed greatly to our ability to diagnose such defects, and other diagnostic tools have been useful for inferring their presence even when they are not visualized (Chapters 12 and 16). Characterization of particular aspects of cerebral insults that lead to the development of epileptic seizures might suggest selective interventions to block the epileptogenic process (Chapters 4 and 8). At the social level, primary preventive measures, such as the use of seat belts, attention to appropriate prenatal care, and improved standards for nutrition and hygiene, would contribute greatly to reducing the incidence of epilepsy due to avoidable epileptogenic lesions.

Nonspecific predisposing factors determine seizure threshold, a dynamic concept with spatial and temporal dimensions. Understanding genetic predisposing factors has relevance for genetic counseling, provides prognostic information, and can help basic scientists to elucidate fundamental mechanisms of epileptogenesis. Understanding environmental factors that alter the epileptic seizure threshold aids identification of reversible exogenous and endogenous processes that could be manipulated in individual patients. Examples include control of metabolic and endocrine influences by regulation of eating and sleeping habits, judicious use of proseizure and antiseizure pharmacological agents, and restructure of stressful behavioral patterns. Antiseizure medication regimens can also be arranged to provide higher drug levels at times of maximum risk, for instance, around the time of menses. Research is needed to identify factors that naturally raise seizure threshold and account for the fact that epilepsy does not develop in some victims of epileptogenic insults. Factors that influence thresholds for ictogenesis are not necessarily the same as those that influence thresholds for epileptogenesis. Much less is known about the latter, and this is an area of intensive investigation.

Precipitating factors determine the time of occurrence of individual epileptic seizures in patients with chronic epilepsy and can also provoke isolated reactive epileptic seizures in susceptible individuals who do not have a chronic epilepsy condition. In both cases, precipitating factors can be specific, such as selective sensory stimulation, or nonspecific, such as fever, sleep deprivation, alcohol withdrawal, or emotional stress. For some individuals, identifying precipitating factors may permit reorganizing the environment to reduce the risk of the occurrence of seizures.

It has been the nature of basic research on mechanisms of epilepsy, as perhaps it is with all medical disorders, that certain concepts and hypotheses become popular for a time and then lose their appeal. Clinical practitioners should be aware of current trends in basic research and should contribute their clinical experience to the evidence for and against the relevance of specific research observations. Clearly, the controversies engendered by various mechanisms proposed to underlie epilepsy and epileptic phenomena as well as the potential clinical relevance of these mechanisms, must ultimately be resolved by identification and characterization of the specific causes of human epilepsy.

REFERENCES

Aguilar, MJ, and Rasmussen, T (1960). Role of encephalitis in pathogenesis of epilepsy. Arch Neurol 2:663–676.

Aita, JA (1964). Neurologic Manifestations of General Diseases. Springfield, IL: Charles C Thomas.

Andermann, E (1982). Multifactorial inheritance of generalized and focal epilepsy. In Genetic Basis of the Epilepsies. Edited by VE Anderson, WA Hauser, JK Penry, and CF Sing. New York: Raven Press, pp. 355–374.

Armstrong, DD, and Bruton, CJ (1987). Postscript: What terminology is appropriate for tissue pathology? How does it predict outcome? In Surgical Treatment of the Epilepsies. Edited by J Engel, Jr. New York: Raven Press, pp. 541–552.

Anderson, VE, Hauser, WA, Penry, JK, and Sing, CF (Eds) (1982). Genetic Basis of the Epilepsies. New York (1991). Raven Press. See also Anderson, VE, Hauser, WA, Leppik, IE, Noebels, JL, and Rich, SS (Eds): Genetic Strategies in Epilepsy Research. Amsterdam: Elsevier.

Babb, TL, and Brown, WJ (1987). Pathological findings in epilepsy. In Surgical Treatment of the Epilepsies. Edited by J Engel, Jr. New York: Raven Press, pp. 511–540.

Babb, TL, Lieb, JP, Brown, WJ, Pretorius, J, and Crandall, PH (1984). Distribution of pyramidal cell density and hyperexcitability in the epileptic human hippocampal formation. Epilepsia 25:721–728.

Baier, WJ, and Doose, H (1987). Interdependence of different genetic EEG patterns in siblings of epileptic patients. Electroencephalogr Clin Neurophysiol 66:483–488.

Banerjee, PN, and Hauser, WA (2008). Incidence and prevalence. In Epilepsy: A Comprehensive Textbook, 2nd ed. Edited by J Engel, Jr, and TA Pedley. Philadelphia: Lippincott Williams & Wilkins, pp. 45–56.

Beck-Mannagetta, G, and Janz, D (1982). Febrile convulsions in offspring of epileptic probands. In Genetic Basis of the Epilepsies. Edited by VE Anderson, WA Hauser, JK Penry, and CF Sing. New York: Raven Press, pp. 145–150.

Berg, AT, Berkovic, SF, Brodie, MJ, Buchhalter, J, Cross, JH, van Emde Boas, W, Engel, J, Jr, French, J, Glauser, TA, Mathern, GW, Moshé, SL, Nordli, D, Jr, Plouin, P, and Scheffer, IE (2010). Revised terminology and concepts for organization of seizures and epilepsies: Report of the ILAE Commission on Classification and Terminology, 2005–2009. Epilepsia 51:676–685.

Berkovic, SF, Johns, JA, and Bladin, PF (1982). Focal seizures and systemic metabolic disorders. Aust N Z J Med 12:620–623.

Bernard, G, and Andermann, F (2011). Ring chromosome 20. In The Causes of Epilepsy: Common and Uncommon Causes in Adults and Children. Edited by SD Shorvon, F Andermann, and R Guerrini. Cambridge, UK: Cambridge University Press, pp. 285–287.

Birbeck, GL, Molyneux, ME, Kaplan, PW, Seydel, KB, Chimalizeni, YF, Kazawa, K, and Taylor, TE (2010). Blantyre Malaria Project Epilepsy Study (BMPES) of neurological outcomes in retinopathy-positive paediatric cerebral malaria survivors: A prospective cohort study. Lancet Neurology 9:1173–1181.

Blümcke, I, Thom, M, Aronica, E, et al. (2011). The clinicopathologic spectrum of focal cortical dysplasias: A consensus classification proposed by an ad hoc task force of the ILAE Diagnostic Methods Commission. Epilepsia 52:158–174.

Bonkowsky, JL, Nance, MA, Hauser, WA, and Anderson, VE (2008). Genetic diseases associated with epilepsy. In Epilepsy: A Comprehensive Textbook, 2nd ed. Edited by J Engel, Jr, and TA Pedley. Philadelphia: Lippincott Williams & Wilkins, pp. 183–193.

Bouchet, C, and Cazauvieilh, JB (1825). De l'epilepsie consideree dans ses rapports avec l'alienation mentale. Arch Gen Med 9:510–542.

Bratz, E (1899). Ammonshornbefunde der Epileptischen. Arch Psychiatr Nervenkr 31:820–836.

Bray, PF, and Wiser, WC (1964). Evidence for a genetic etiology of temporal-central abnormalities in focal epilepsy. N Engl J Med 271:926–933.

Brust, JCM (2008). Alcohol and drug abuse. In Epilepsy: A Comprehensive Textbook, 2nd ed. Edited by J Engel, Jr, and TA Pedley. Philadelphia: Lippincott Williams & Wilkins, pp. 2683–2687.

Cendes, F, and Morita, ME (2011). Hippocampal sclerosis. In The Causes of Epilepsy: Common and Uncommon Causes in Adults and Children. Edited by SD Shorvon, F Andermann, and R Guerrini. Cambridge, UK: Cambridge University Press, pp. 363–372.

Cendes, F, and Sankar, R (2011). Vaccinations and febrile seizures. Epilepsia 52(suppl 3):23–25.

Chatrian, GE, Shaw, CM, and Leffman, H (1964). The significance of periodic lateralized epileptiform discharges in EEG: An electrographic clinical and pathological study. Electroencephalogr Clin Neurophysiol 17:177–193.

Chu-Shore, CJ, and Thiele, EA (2011). Tuberous sclerosis complex. In Shorvon, SD, Andermann, F, and Guerrini, R (Eds). The Causes of Epilepsy: Common and Uncommon Causes in Adults and Children. Cambridge, UK: Cambridge University Press, pp. 177–182.

Cocito, L, Favale, E, and Reni, L (1982). Epileptic seizures in cerebral arterial occlusive disease. Stroke 13:189–195.

Committee on Infectious Diseases (1987). Family history of convulsions in candidates for immunization with pertussis-containing vaccines (diphtheria, tetanus, pertussis). Pediatrics 80:743–744.

da Gama, CN, Kobayashi, E, Li, LM, and Cendes, F (2005). Hippocampal atrophy and neurocysticercosis calcifications. Seizure 14:85–88.

Del Brutto, OH (2008). Infection and inflammatory diseases. In Epilepsy: A Comprehensive Textbook, 2nd ed. Edited by J Engel, Jr, and TA Pedley. Philadelphia: Lippincott Williams & Wilkins, pp. 2643–2652.

DeToledo-Morrell, L, Morrell, F, and Fleming, S (1984). Age-dependent deficits in spatial memory are related to impaired hippocampal kindling. Behav Neurosci 98:902–907.

Devinsky, O, and Duchowny, MS (1983). Seizures after convulsive therapy: A retrospective case survey. Neurology 33:921–925.

Doose, H (1982). Photosensitivity: Genetics and significance in the pathogenesis of epilepsy. In Genetic Basis of the Epilepsies. Edited by VE Anderson, WA Hauser, JK Penry, and CF Sing. New York: Raven Press, pp. 113–121.

Doose, H, and Gundel, A (1982). Four to 7 CPS rhythms in the childhood EEG. In Genetic Basis of the Epilepsies. Edited by VE Anderson, WA Hauser, JK Penry, and CF Sing. New York: Raven Press, pp. 83–93.

Earle, KM, Baldwin, M, and Penfield, W (1953). Incisural sclerosis and temporal lobe seizures produced by hippocampal herniation at birth. Arch Neurol Psychiatry 69:27–42.

Elliott, B, Amarouche, M, and Shorvon, SD (2009). Psychiatric features of epilepsy and their management. In The Treatment of Epilepsy, 3rd ed. Edited by S Shorvon, E Perucca, and J Engel, Jr. West Sussex, UK: Wiley-Blackwell, pp. 273–287.

Engel, J, Jr (1984). A practical guide for routine EEG studies in epilepsy. J Clin Neurophysiol 1:109–142.

Engel, J, Jr (2006). Report of the ILAE Classification Core Group. Epilepsia 47:1558–1568.

Engel, J, Jr, and Pedley, TA (2008). Introduction: What is epilepsy? In Epilepsy: A Comprehensive Textbook, 2nd ed. Edited by J Engel, Jr, and TA Pedley. Philadelphia: Lippincott Williams & Wilkins, pp. 1–7.

Engel, J, Jr, and Thompson, PM (2012). Going beyond hippocampocentricity in the concept of mesial temporal lobe epilepsy. Epilepsia 53:220–223.

Engel, J, Jr, Crandall, PH, and Rausch, R (1983). The partial epilepsies. In The Clinical Neurosciences, Vol 2. Edited by RN Rosenberg. New York: Churchill Livingstone, pp. 1349–1380.

Engel, J, Jr, Babb, TL, and Phelps, ME (1987). Contribution of positron emission tomography to understanding mechanisms of epilepsy. In Fundamental Mechanisms of Human Brain Function. Edited by J Engel, Jr, GA Ojemann, HO Lüders, and PD Williamson. New York: Raven Press, pp. 209–218.

Epstein, LG, Sharer, LR, and Goudsmit, J (1988). Neurological and neuropathological features of human immunodeficiency virus infection in children. Ann Neurol 23(suppl):S19–S23.

Falconer, MA (1971). Genetic and related aetiologiscal factors in temporal lobe epilepsy: A review. Epilepsia 12:13–31.

Falconer, MA, and Serafetinides, EA (1963). A follow-up study of surgery in temporal lobe epilepsy. J Neurol Neurosurg Psychiatry 26:154–165.

Falconer, MA, and Taylor, DC (1968). Surgical treatment of drug-resistant epilepsy due to mesial temporal sclerosis: Etiology and significance. Arch Neurol 19:353–361.

Farrell, MA, Droogan, O, Secor, DL, Poukens, V, Quinn, B, and Vinters, HV (1995). Chronic encephalitis associated with epilepsy: Immunohistochemical and ultrastructural studies. Acta Neuropathol 89:313–321.

Farrell, MA, Blümcke, I, Khanlou, N, and Vinters, HV (2008). General neuropathology of epilepsy. In Epilepsy: A Comprehensive Textbook, 2nd ed. Edited by J Engel, Jr, and TA Pedley. Philadelphia: Lippincott Williams & Wilkins, pp. 103–120.

Forster, FM (1977). Reflex Epilepsy, Behavioral Therapy and Conditional Reflexes. Springfield, IL: Charles C Thomas.

Friede, RL (1975). Developmental Neuropathology. New York: Springer-Verlag.

Galanopoulou, AS, and Moshé, SL (2009). Age-specific responses to antiepileptic drugs. In Encyclopedia of Basic Epilepsy Research. Edited by PA Schwartzkroin. Amsterdam: Elsevier, pp. 1025–1033.

Gjerstad, L, and Tauboll, E (2011). Other vascular disorders. In The Causes of Epilepsy: Common and Uncommon Causes in Adults and Children. Edited by SD Shorvon, F Andermann, and R Guerrini. Cambridge, UK: Cambridge University Press, pp. 565–571.

Glaser, GH (1987). Natural history of temporal lobe-limbic epilepsy. In Surgical Treatment of the Epilepsies. Edited by J Engel, Jr. New York: Raven Press, pp. 13–30.

Gloor, P (1977). The EEG and differential diagnosis of epilepsy. In Current Concepts in Clinical Neurophysiology. Edited by H van Duijn, DNJ Donker, and AC van Huffelen. The Hague: NV Drukkerij Trio, pp. 9–21.

Gomes, WA, and Shinnar, S (2011). Prospects for imaging-related biomarkers of human epileptogenesis: A critical review. Biomarkers Med 5:599–606.

Granata, T, Cross, H, Theodore, W, and Avanzini, G (2011). Immune-mediated epilepsies. Epilepsia 52(suppl 3):1–53.

Guerrini, R, Shorvon, SD, Andermann, F, and Andermann, E (2011). Introduction to the concept of genetic epilepsy. In The Causes of Epilepsy: Common and Uncommon Causes in Adults and Children. Edited by SD Shorvon, F Andermann, and R Guerrini. Cambridge, UK: Cambridge University Press, pp. 43–61.

Harvey, AS, Eeg-Olofsson, O, and Freeman, JL (2008). Hypothalamic hamartoma with gelastic seizures. In Epilepsy: A Comprehensive Textbook, 2nd ed. Edited by J Engel, Jr, and TA Pedley. Philadelphia: Lippincott Williams & Wilkins, pp. 2503–2509.

Hauser, WA, and Annegers, JF (1987). Prognosis of children with febrile seizures. In Advances in Epileptology, Vol 16. Edited by P Wolf, M Dam, D Janz, and FE Dreifuss. New York: Raven Press, pp. 155–161.

Hauser, WA, and Kurland, LT (1975). The epidemiology of epilepsy in Rochester, Minnesota, 1935 through 1967. Epilepsia 16:1–66.

Hauser, WA, Ramirez-Lassepas, M, and Rosenstein, R (1984). Risks for seizures and epilepsy following cerebrovascular insults. Epilepsia 25:666.

Hauser, WA, Morris, ML, Heston, LL, and Anderson, VE (1986). Seizures and myoclonus in patients with Alzheimer's disease. Neurology 36:1226–1230.

Helbig, I, Scheffer, IE, Mulley, JC, and Berkovic, SF (2008). Navigating the channels and beyond: Unravelling the genetics of the epilepsies. Lancet Neurol 7:231–245.

Hesdorffer, DC (2008). Risk factors. In Epilepsy: A Comprehensive Textbook, 2nd ed. Edited by

J Engel, Jr, and TA Pedley. Philadelphia: Lippincott Williams & Wilkins, pp. 57–63.

Hirano, M, Kunz, WS, and DiMauro, S (2008). Mitochondrial diseases. In Epilepsy: A Comprehensive Textbook, 2nd ed. Edited by J Engel, Jr, and TA Pedley. Philadelphia: Lippincott Williams & Wilkins, pp. 2621–2630.

Hirtz, DG, Nelson, KB, and Ellenberg, JH (1983). Seizures following childhood immunizations. J Pediatr 102:14–18.

Hoefer, PFA, Schlesinger, EB, and Pennes, HH (1947). Seizures in patients with brain tumors. Res Nerv Ment Dis Proc 26:50–58.

Holmes, GL (1986). Morphological and physiological maturation of the brain in the neonate and young child. J Clin Neurophysiol 3:209–238.

Irani, SR, Michell, AW, Lang, B, et al. (2011). Faciobrachial dystonic seizures precede Lgi1 antibody limbic encephalitis. Ann Neurol 69:892–900.

Ishida, S, Yamashita, Y, Matsuishi, T, Ohshima, M, Ohshima, H, Kato, H, and Maeda, H (1998). Photosensitive seizures provoked while viewing "Pocket Monsters," a made-for-television animation program in Japan. Epilepsia 39:1340–1344.

Jallon, P, and Zifkin, BG (2008). Seizure precipitants. In Epilepsy: A Comprehensive Textbook, 2nd ed. Edited by J Engel, Jr, and TA Pedley. Philadelphia: Lippincott Williams & Wilkins, pp. 77–80.

Jennett, B (1975). Epilepsy After Non-missile Head Injuries, 2nd ed. Chicago: William Heinemann.

Kanner, AM, and Blumer, D (2008). Affective disorders. In Epilepsy: A Comprehensive Textbook, 2nd ed. Edited by J Engel, Jr, and TA Pedley. Philadelphia: Lippincott Williams & Wilkins, pp. 2123–2138.

Kellaway, P (1985). Sleep and epilepsy. Epilepsia 26(suppl 1):S15–S30.

Kerrigan, JF (2011). Hypothalamic hamartoma and gelastic epilepsy. In The Causes of Epilepsy: Common and Uncommon Causes in Adults and Children. Edited by SD Shorvon, F Andermann, and R Guerrini. Cambridge, UK: Cambridge University Press, pp. 449–453.

Klassen, T, Davis, C, Goldman, A, Burgess, D, Chen, T, Wheeler, D, McPherson, J, Bourquin, T, Lewis, L, Villasana, D, Morgan, M, Muzny, D, Gibbs, R, and Noebels, J (2011). Exome sequencing of ion channel genes reveals complex profiles confounding personal risk assessment in epilepsy. Cell 145:1036–1048.

Kuzniecky, RI, and Jackson, GD (2008). Malformations of cortical development. In Epilepsy: A Comprehensive Textbook, 2nd ed. Edited by J Engel, Jr, and TA Pedley. Philadelphia: Lippincott Williams & Wilkins, pp. 2575–2588.

Lance, JW, and Adams, RD (1963). The syndrome of intention or action myoclonus as a sequel to hypoxic encephalopathy. Brain 86:111–136.

Landy, HJ, Ramsay, RE, Ajmone-Marsan, C, Levin, BE, Brown, J, Pasarin, G, and Quencer, RM (1992). Temporal lobectomy for seizures associated with unilateral schizencephaly. Surg Neurol 37:477–481.

Lennox, WG (1960). Epilepsy and Related Disorders, Vols 1–2. Boston: Little, Brown & Co.

Lerner, JT, Salamon, N, Hauptman, JS, Velasco, TR, Hemb, M, Wu, JY, Sankar, R, Shields, WD, Engel, J, Jr, Fried, I, Cepeda, C, Andre, VM, Levine, MS, Miyata, H,

Yong, WH, Vinters, HV, and Mathern, GW (2009). Assessment and surgical outcomes for mild type I and severe type II cortical dysplasia: A critical review and the UCLA experience. Epilepsia 50:1310–1335.

Lesser, RP, Lüders, H, Dinner, DS, and Morris, HH (1985). Epileptic seizures due to thrombotic and embolic cerebrovascular disease in older patients. Epilepsia 26:622–630.

Levin, R, and Lee, SI (1985). Nonconvulsive status epilepticus following metrizamide myelogram [letter]. Ann Neurol 17(5):518–519.

Lin, JJ, Salamon, N, Dutton, RA, Lee, AD, Geaga, JA, Hayashi, KM, Toga, AW, Engel, J, Jr, and Thompson, PM (2005). Three-dimensional preoperative maps of hippocampal atrophy predict surgical outcomes in temporal lobe epilepsy. Neurology 65:1094–1097.

Lin, JJ, Salamon, N, Lee, AD, Dutton, RA, Geaga, JA, Hayashi, KM, Luders, E, Toga, AW, Engel, J, Jr, and Thompson, PM (2007). Reduced neocortical thickness and complexity mapped in mesial temporal lobe epilepsy with hippocampal sclerosis. Cereb Cortex 17:2007–2018.

Lombroso, CT (1983). Neonatal seizures. In Epilepsy Diagnosis and Management. Edited by TR Browne and RG Feldman. Boston: Little, Brown & Co, pp. 297–313.

Lüders, H, Lesser, RP, Dinner, DS, and Morris, HH, III (1987). Benign focal epilepsy of childhood. Epilepsy: Electroclinical Syndrome. Edited by H Lüders and RP Lesser. London: Springer-Verlag, pp. 303–346.

Margerison, JH, and Corsellis, JA (1966). Epilepsy and the temporal lobes: A clinical, electroencephalographic and neuropathological study of the brain in epilepsy, with particular reference to the temporal lobes. Brain 89:499–530.

Mathern, GW, Wilson, CL, and Beck, H (2008). Hippocampal sclerosis. In Epilepsy: A Comprehensive Textbook, 2nd ed. Edited by J Engel, Jr, and TA Pedley. Philadelphia: Lippincott Williams & Wilkins, pp. 121–136.

Meencke, HJ, and Janz, D (1984). Neuropathological findings in primary generalized epilepsy: A study of eight cases. Epilepsia 25:8–21.

Meldrum, BS (1988). Personal communication.

Meldrum, BS, Horton, RW, and Brierley, JB (1974). Epileptic brain damage in adolescent baboons following seizures induced by allylglycine. Brain 97:407–418.

Metrakos, JD, and Metrakos, K (1966). Childhood epilepsy of subcortical ("centrencephalic") origin: Some questions and answers for the pediatrician. Clin Pediatr 5:537–542.

Miller, BL, Goldberg, MA, Heiner, D, and Myers, A (1983). Cerebral cysticercosis: An overview. Bull Clin Neurosci 48:2–5.

Mizrahi EM, Kellaway P (1998). Diagnosis and Management of Neonatal Seizures. Philadelphia: Lippincott-Raven.

Mouritzen-Dam, A (1982). Hippocampal neuron loss in epilepsy and after experimental seizures. Acta Neurol Scand 66:601–642.

Nelson, KB, and Ellenberg, JH (1978). Prognosis in children with febrile seizures. Pediatrics 61:720–727.

Nelson, KB, and Ellenberg, JH (Eds) (1981). Febrile Seizures. New York: Raven Press.

Newmark, ME, and Penry, JK (1979). Photosensitivity and Epilepsy: A Review. New York: Raven Press.

Newmark, ME, and Penry, JK (1980). Genetics of Epilepsy: A Review. New York: Raven Press.

North, JB, Penhall, RK, Hanieh, A, Frewin, DB, and Taylor, WB (1983). Phenytoin and postoperative epilepsy. J Neurosurg 58:672–677.

Ogren, JA, Bragin, A, Wilson, CL, Hoftman, GD, Lin, JJ, Dutton, RA, Fields, TA, Toga, AW, Thompson, PM, Engel, J, Jr, and Staba, RJ (2009a). Three-dimensional hippocampal atrophy maps distinguish two common temporal lobe seizure-onset patterns. Epilepsia 50:1361–1370.

Ogren JA, Wilson CL, Bragin A, Lin JJ, Salamon N, Dutton RA, Luders E, Fields TA, Fried I, Toga AW, Thompson PM, Engel, J, Jr, and Staba RJ (2009b). Three dimensional surface maps link local atrophy and fast ripples in human epileptic hippocampus. Ann Neurol 66:783–791.

Ottman R, and Winawer, MR (2008). Genetic epidemiology. In Epilepsy: A Comprehensive Textbook, 2nd ed. Edited by J Engel, Jr, and TA Pedley. Philadelphia: Lippincott Williams & Wilkins, pp. 161–170.

Ottman, R, Hirose, S, Jain, S, Lerche, H, Lopes-Cendes, I, Noebels, JL, Serratosa, J, Zara, F, and Scheffer, IE (2010). Genetic testing in the epilepsies—Report of the ILAE Genetics Commission. Epilepsia 51:655–670.

Ozkara, C, and Vigevano, F (2011). Immuno- and antiinflammatory therapies in epileptic disorders. Epilepsia 52(suppl 3):45–51.

Pedley, TA (2008). EEG traits. In Epilepsy: A Comprehensive Textbook, 2nd ed. Edited by J Engel, Jr, and TA Pedley. Philadelphia: Lippincott Williams & Wilkins, pp. 171–181.

Penfield, W, and Jasper, H (1954). Epilepsy and the Functional Anatomy of the Human Brain. Boston: Little, Brown & Co.

Petersen, I, Sellden, U, and Eeg-Olofsson, O (1976). The evolution of the EEG in normal children and adolescents from 1 to 21 years. In Handbook of Electroencephalography and Clinical Neurophysiology. Edited by A Remord. Amsterdam: Elsevier, pp. 6B31–6B68.

Pisani, F, Oteri, G, Costa, C, Di Raimondo, G, and Di Perri, R (2002). Effects of psychotropic drugs on seizure threshold. Drug Saf 25:91–110.

Rasmussen, T (1978). Further observations on the syndrome of chronic encephalitis and epilepsy. Applied Neurophysiol 41:1–12.

Raymont, V, Salazar, AM, Lipsky, R, Goldman, D, Tasick, G, and Grafman, J (2010). Correlates of posttraumatic epilepsy 35 years following combat brain surgery. Neurology 75:224–229.

Remillard, GM, Ethier, R, and Andermann, F (1974). Temporal lobe epilepsy and perinatal occlusion of the posterior cerebral artery: A syndrome analogous to infantile hemiplegia and a demonstrable etiology in some patients with temporal lobe epilepsy. Neurology 24:1001–1009.

Riggs, JE (1991). Systemic disease. In Neurology in Clinical Practice. Edited by WG Bradley, RB Daroff, GM Fenichel, and CD Marsden. Boston: Butterworth-Heinemann, pp. 841–860.

Rose, AL, and Lombroso, CT (1970). Neonatal seizure states: A study of clinical, pathological and electroencephalographic features in 137 full-term babies with a long-term follow-up. Pediatrics 45:404–425.

Rosenblum, ML, Levy, RM, and Bredesen, DE (Eds) (1988a). AIDS and the Nervous System. New York: Raven Press.

Rosenblum, ML, Levy, RM, Bredesen, DE, So, YT, Wara, W, and Ziegler, JL (1988b). Primary central nervous system lymphomas in patients with AIDS. Ann Neurol (suppl 23):S13–S16.

Schneck, SA (1985). Cerebral anoxia. In Clinical Neurology, Vol 2. Edited by AB Baker and RJ Joynt. Philadelphia: Harper & Row, pp. 1–25.

Sever, JL, and Gibbs, CJ, Jr (Eds) (1988). Retroviruses in the nervous system. Ann Neurol (suppl 23):S1–S217.

Shorvon, SD, Andermann, F, and Guerrini, R (Eds) (2011). The Causes of Epilepsy: Common and Uncommon Causes in Adults and Children. Cambridge, UK: Cambridge University Press.

Singh, BM, and Strobos, RJ (1980). Epilepsia partialis continua associated with non-ketotic hyperglycemia: Clinical and biochemical profile of 21 patients. Ann Neurol 8:155–160.

Small, J, Milstein, V, Small, IF, and Sharpley, PH (1981). Does ECT produce kindling? Biol Psychiatry 16:773–778.

Solomon, GE, Hilal, SK, Gold, AP, and Carter, S (1970). Natural history of acute hemiplegia of childhood. Brain 93:107–120.

Sommer, W (1880). Erkrankung des Ammonshorns als aetiologisches Moment der Epilepsie. Arch Pyschiatr Nervenkr 10:631–675.

Spencer, DD, Spencer, SS, Mattson, RH, and Williamson, PD (1984). Intracerebral masses in patients with intractable partial epilepsy. Neurology 34:432–436.

Spielmeyer, W (1927). Die Pathogenese des epileptischen Krampfes. Z Gesamte Neurol Psychiatr 109:501–520.

Stark, LG, Chuang, RY, and Joy, RM (1987). Biochemical markers of exposure to proconvulsant and anticonvulsant chlorinated hydrocarbons [abstract]. Epilepsia 28:584.

Steinlein, OK (2008). Genetics of epilepsy syndromes. In Epilepsy: A Comprehensive Textbook, 2nd ed. Edited by J Engel, Jr, and TA Pedley. Philadelphia: Lippincott Williams & Wilkins, pp. 195–210.

Stevens, JR, Kodama, H, Lonsbury, B, and Mills, L (1971). Ultradian characteristics of spontaneous seizure discharges recorded by radio telemetry in man. Electroencephalogr Clin Neurophysiol 31:313–325.

Stewart, JD, Horvath, R, Baruffini, E, Ferrero, I, Bulst, S, Watkins, PB, Fontana, RJ, Day, CP, and Chinnery, PF (2010). Polymerase γ gene POLG determines the risk of sodium valproate-induced liver toxicity. Hepatology 52:1791–1796.

Taylor, DC, Falconer, MA, Bruton, CJ, and Corsellis, JAN (1971). Focal dysplasia of the cerebral cortex in epilepsy. J Neurol Neurosurg Psychiatry 34:369–387.

Townsend, JJ, Nielsen, SL, and Malamud, N (1975a). Unilateral megalencephaly: Hamartoma or neoplasm? Neurology 25:448–453.

Townsend, JJ, Baringer, JR, Wolinsky, JS, Malamud, N, Mednick, JP, Panitch, HS, Scott, RAT, Oshiro, LS, and Cremer, NE (1975b). Progressive rubella panencephalitis: Late onset after congenital rubella. N Engl J Med 292:990–993.

Tsuboi, T (1982). Febrile convulsions. In Genetic Basis of the Epilepsies. Edited by VE Anderson, WA Hauser, PK Penry, and CF Sing. New York: Raven Press, pp. 123–134.

Upchurch, K, Stern, JM, Salamon, N, Dewar, S, Engel, J, Jr, Vinters, HV, and Fried, I (2010). Epileptogenic temporal cavernous malformations: Operative strategies and postoperative seizure outcomes. Seizure 19:120–128.

Vezzani, A, and Rüegg, S (Eds) (2011). Proceedings of the First Meeting on Immunity and Inflammation in Epilepsy: Mechanistic Insights and Therapeutic Perspectives. Epilepsia 52(suppl 3):1–53.

Vincent, A, and Crino, PB (2011). Systemic and neurologic autoimmune disorders associated with seizures or epilepsy. Epilepsia 52(suppl 3):12–17.

Vinters, HV, Salamon, N, Miyata, H, Khanlou, N, and Mathern, GW (2008). Neuropathology of developmental disorders associated with epilepsy. In Epilepsy: A Comprehensive Textbook, 2nd ed. Edited by J Engel, Jr, and TA Pedley. Philadelphia: Lippincott Williams & Wilkins, pp. 137–160.

Volpe, JJ (1987). Neurology of the Newborn, 2nd ed. Philadelphia: WB Saunders.

Weil, ML, Habashi, HH, Cremer, NE, Oshiro, LS, Lennette, EH, and Carnay, L (1975). Chronic progressive panencephalitis due to rubella virus simulating subacute sclerosing panencephalitis. N Engl J Med 292:994–998.

Wieser, H-G, Özkara, Ç, Engel, J, Jr, Hauser, AW, Moshé, SL, Avanzini, G, Helmstaedter, C, Henry, TR, and Sperling, MR (2004). Mesial temporal lobe epilepsy with hippocampal sclerosis: Report of the ILAE Commission on Neurosurgery of Epilepsy. Epilepsia 45:695–714.

Wilmore, LS, Sypert, GW, and Munson, JB (1978). Recurrent seizures induced by cortical iron injection: A model of post-traumatic epilepsy. Ann Neurol 4:329–336.

Wolf, P (1985). Juvenile absence epilepsy. In Epileptic Syndromes in Infancy, Childhood and Adolescence. Edited by J Roger, C Dravet, M Bureau, FE Dreifuss, and P Wolf. London: John Libbey, pp. 242–246.

Zheng, LH, Xu, L, Gutmann, DH, and Wong, M (2008). Rapamycin prevents epilepsy in a mouse model of tuberous sclerosis complex. Ann Neurol 63:444–453.

Zuberi, SM (2010). Chromosome disorders associated with epileptic seizures. In Atlas of Epilepsies. Edited by CP Panayiotopoulos. London: Springer-Verlag, pp. 121–128.

PART 3

Phenomenology

Chapter 6

Epileptic Seizures

NEUROBIOLOGICAL CONSIDERATIONS FOR THE DIAGNOSIS OF EPILEPTIC SEIZURE TYPES
Anatomical Substrates
Pathophysiological Mechanisms
Pharmacological Considerations

TYPES OF EPILEPTIC SEIZURES

FOCAL SEIZURES
Neocortical Seizures
Limbic Seizures
Focal Seizures Evolving into Secondarily Generalized Seizures

GENERALIZED SEIZURES
Tonic-Clonic Seizures
Typical Absence Seizures

Atypical Absence Seizures
Myoclonic Absences
Eyelid Myoclonia
Myoclonic Seizures
Myoclonic Atonic Seizures
Myoclonic Tonic Seizures
Clonic Seizures
Tonic Seizures
Atonic Seizures

UNCLASSIFIED SEIZURES
Epileptic Spasms
Reflex Seizures
Neonatal Seizures

MYOCLONUS

SUMMARY AND CONCLUSIONS

The 1981 *International Classification of Epileptic Seizures* (Chapter 1) was based entirely on signs, symptoms, and EEG findings that could be easily observed and generally agreed upon, because there was insufficient information about pathophysiological mechanisms and anatomical substrates to warrant construction of a more specific neurobiological classification. Although this remains true today, there is greater understanding about similarities and differences among the many forms of ictal events, justifying construction of a list of seizures based on the likelihood that each represents a unique diagnostic entity. As such, a diagnosis of a specific epileptic seizure type has etiological, therapeutic, and prognostic implications when a diagnosis of an epilepsy syndrome cannot be made (Engel, 2001, 2006; Berg et al., 2010). Primary considerations for concluding that a given epileptic seizure type is likely to be a unique diagnostic entity derives from understanding anatomical substrates, pathophysiological mechanisms, and responses to antiseizure drugs.

NEUROBIOLOGICAL CONSIDERATIONS FOR THE DIAGNOSIS OF EPILEPTIC SEIZURE TYPES

Anatomical Substrates

John Hughlings Jackson first called attention to the correlation between ictal behavioral manifestations and the location of the structural abnormalities seen on postmortem studies of the brain (Chapter 1). The demonstration that electrical stimulation of specific brain regions reliably induced habitual ictal behaviors further indicated that some epileptic seizures could be classified according to anatomical substrates (Penfield and Jasper, 1954). Electroclinical correlations derived from film, and later video, monitoring of spontaneous or induced ictal behaviors during scalp and intracranial EEG recording have resulted in more refined concepts of the anatomical basis of specific ictal behaviors (Ajmone-Marsan and Ralston, 1957; Wieser, 1983).

Most epilepsy surgery centers now perform long-term intracranial EEG recording in association with video monitoring as part of the presurgical evaluation in a subset of patients with epilepsy who are candidates for resective surgical treatment (Chapters 12 and 16). This technique allows detailed correlation between the spatial distribution of ictal discharges and the behavioral characteristics of clinical seizures. The site of ictal onset can then be substantiated in many patients when habitual seizures no longer occur after surgical resection of the suspected epileptogenic area. Based on this experience, Appendix I of the 1985 *Classification of the Epilepsies and Epileptic Syndromes* (Commission on Classification and Terminology, 1985) included a summary of impressions from several epilepsy surgery

centers concerning behavioral correlates of seizures originating in specific brain regions. These impressions, however, were preliminary, because experience between centers varied, ictal features of some anatomical substrates were derived from only a few patients, and electroclinical correlations do not necessarily differentiate between clinical signs and symptoms reflecting ictal onset and those reflecting ictal spread. Suggestions for revision were made by the Commission on Classification and Terminology of the International League Against Epilepsy (ILAE) in 1987 (Roger, 1987). Table 6–1 was derived from this revised version, which remains a reasonably valid approach for using ictal behavior to infer anatomical substrates, with the understanding that virtually no symptoms can be considered pathognomonic of involvement of a specific region of cerebral cortex (Ajmone-Marsan, 1978; Lesser et al., 1987) (Figs. 6–1 and 6–2). In general, the more sophisticated the analyses, the more variability has been found and the more exceptions to classical concepts have arisen (Penfield and Jasper, 1954; Halgren et al., 1978; Gloor et al., 1982; Ochs et al., 1984; McLachlan, 1987; Williamson et al., 1987). Therefore, in any given patient, the information listed in Table 6–1 can only provide clues to anatomical substrates and is not sufficient for localizing a specific site of ictal origin. It is noteworthy that large multilobar areas of the brain can produce similar signs and symptoms. Thus motor and sensory phenomena occur with epileptiform discharges in both pre- and postrolandic cortex, and other ictal features characterize the temporoparietal occipital junction and the frontal-parietal-temporal operculum (Table 6–1).

As discussed in more detail in Chapter 4, discrete, well-circumscribed epileptogenic regions are rarely encountered in the human brain. Intracranial EEG recordings from patients with focal seizures usually reveal diffuse or multiple areas capable of generating interictal and even ictal discharges (Engel and Crandall, 1983; Bancaud and Chauvel, 1987; Engel, 1987a, 1987b;). When a discrete structural lesion can be identified, the functionally abnormal brain is by no means limited to the site of this lesion (Engel et al., 1981a). Furthermore, habitual seizures can occasionally take on EEG and behavioral manifestations of ictal events originating at a distance from the

Table 6–1 Behavioral Signs and Symptoms Associated with Electrographic Ictal Discharges Recorded from Specific Cerebral Areas*

I. Features suggestive of seizures arising from the temporal lobe.

Simple partial seizures have autonomic signs or symptoms, psychic symptoms, and/or certain sensory symptoms. Seizures of hippocampal-amygdaloid (mesiobasal limbic or primary rhinencephalic psychomotor) origin often begin with an indescribable strange sensation, rising epigastric discomfort, or nausea. Other common initial signs and symptoms include fear, panic, and/or marked autonomic phenomena such as borborygmi, belching, pallor, fullness of the face, flushing of the face, arrest of respiration, and pupillary dilatation. Seizures of lateral temporal origin often begin with auditory or visual perceptual hallucinations, illusions, dreamy states, and/or vertiginous symptoms. Language disorders indicate involvement of the language-dominant hemisphere. Gustatory hallucinations may indicate involvement of parietal or rolandic operculum, and olfactory hallucinations may indicate involvement of orbital frontal cortex. Complex partial seizures often, but not always, begin with motor arrest, followed by oroalimentary automatisms. There must be amnesia for the ictal event. Common features include reactive automatisms, duration more than one minute, postictal confusion, and gradual recovery. Secondary generalization occurs occasionally.

II. Features suggestive of seizures arising from the frontal lobe.

Simple or complex partial seizures often have prominent motor manifestations, can include drop attacks, and may be mistaken for psychogenic seizures. Some seizure types are frequently associated with rapid secondary generalization or status epilepticus. Complex partial seizures are often brief, frequent, and with minimal or no postictal confusion and can be associated with urinary incontinence. Seizures involving supplementary motor cortex may have postural (including fencing postures) or focal tonic motor signs, vocalization, or speech arrest (M2e seizures of Ajmone-Marsan and Ralston, 1957). Seizures involving cingulate cortex may be associated with changes in mood and affect, vegetative signs, and elaborate motor gestural automatisms at onset. Seizures involving orbital frontal cortex may be associated with olfactory hallucinations and illusions; early motor signs, including gestural automatisms; and autonomic signs and symptoms. Dorsolateral frontal lobe involvement may give rise to simple partial seizures with tonic or, less commonly, clonic signs and versive eye and head movements. The signs and symptoms of seizures involving frontal operculum and prerolandic cortex are described below under "Features suggestive of seizures arising from multilobar regions."

III. Features suggestive of seizures arising from the parietal lobe.

Simple partial seizures consist of positive somatosensory signs and symptoms as described for the perirolandic area, an intra-abdominal sensation of sinking, choking, or nausea (particularly with inferior and lateral parietal lobe involvement), or, rarely, pain (either as superficial burning dysesthesia or as vague but severe episodic painful sensations); or of negative somatosensory symptoms, including numbness, feeling as if a body part were absent, loss of awareness of part or half of the body (asomatognosia, particularly seen with nondominant hemisphere involvement), and/or severe vertigo or disorientation in space (suggesting inferior parietal lobe involvement); and/or of receptive or conductive language disturbances (suggesting dominant parietal lobe involvement): and/or rotary or postural movements; and/or visual symptoms as described for the temporal-parietal-occipital junction.

IV. Features suggestive of seizures arising from the occipital lobe.

Simple partial seizures usually, but not exclusively, include visual phenomena. Visual symptoms consist of fleeting visual perceptions, which may be either negative (scotoma, hemianopsia, amaurosis) or, more commonly, positive (sparks or flashes, phosphenes), originating in the visual field contralateral to occipital cortical involvement, or of visual perceptual illusions or hallucinations as described for temporal-parietal-occipital junction. Motor signs include clonic and/or tonic controversion (or occasionally ipsiversion) of eyes and head or eyes only (oculoclonic or oculogyric deviation), palpebral jerks, or forced closure of the eyelids. Nonvisual sensory symptoms include sensations of ocular oscillation, whole-body oscillation, or headache (including migraine). Ictal discharges may spread to produce seizure manifestations of temporal lobe, parietal lobe, or frontal motor seizures. There is an occasional tendency to become secondarily generalized.

(continued)

Table 6–1 (Continued)

V. Features suggestive of seizures arising from multilobar regions. (Some seizure patterns are characteristic of more than one anatomically defined lobe of the brain.)

A. Features suggestive of seizures arising from the perirolandic (sensory motor) area can originate in either the precentral (frontal) or postcentral (parietal) gyrus. Simple partial seizures with motor signs and/or sensory symptoms involve body parts in proportion to their representation on the precentral and postcentral gyrus. Thus involvement of face, tongue, hand, and arm occur most often. Common signs and symptoms, which may occasionally spread in a jacksonian manner, include tonic or clonic movements, tingling, a feeling of electricity, a desire to move a body part, a sensation of a part being moved, and/or loss of muscle tone. Lower perirolandic involvement may be associated with speech arrest, vocalization, or dysphasia; movements of the face on the contralateral side: swallowing, tongue sensations of crawling, stiffness, or coldness; and/or facial sensory phenomena, which can occur bilaterally. Movements and sensory symptoms of the contralateral upper extremities occur with involvement of the middle and upper perirolandic area. Sensory symptoms and/or motor signs of the contralateral lower extremity, well-lateralized genital sensations, and/or tonic movements of the ipsilateral foot occur with involvement of the pericentral lobule. Postictal Todd's paralysis and secondary generalization occur frequently with seizures of perirolandic origin.

B. Features suggestive of seizures arising from the opercular (perisylvian, insular) area can originate in frontal, parietal, or temporal operculum. Mastication, salivation, swallowing, laryngeal symptoms, epigastric sensations with fear and/or vegetative phenomena are characteristic of opercular involvement. Simple partial seizures, particularly with clonic facial movements, are common. Secondary sensory symptoms include numbness, particularly in the hands. Bilateral movement of the upper extremities may be seen.

C. Features suggestive of seizures arising from the temporal-parietal-occipital junction commonly derive from epileptic discharges involving cortex of more than one lobe. Simple partial seizures often consist of visual perceptual illusions or formed hallucinations. Visual illusions include a change in size (macropsia or micropsia), a change in distance, an inclination of objects in a given plane of space, distortion of objects, or a sudden change of shape (metamorphopsia), which is more common with nondominant hemisphere involvement. Formed visual hallucinations may include complex visual perception, e.g., colorful scenes varying in complexity; in some cases the scene is distorted or made smaller, and in rare instances the subject sees his or her own image (autoscopy). Multimodality-formed hallucinations may include auditory and occasionally olfactory or gustatory symptoms and autonomic signs and symptoms appropriate to the visual perceptions. Vertiginous symptoms also arise from this region. Language deficits suggest dominant hemisphere involvement. Complex partial seizures often ensue, presumably due to mesial temporal spread.

* Signs and symptoms may be determined by functions of the cerebral structures indicated or their preferential propagation patterns. The information contained in this table was adapted in part from deliberations of the Commission on Classification and Terminology of the International League Against Epilepsy, chaired by Dr. J. Roger, and in part from the experiences of Dr. J. Bancaud and his group at Hôpital Sainte-Anne in Paris. The table is published with the permission of Drs. Roger and Bancaud, with the understanding that it often reflects an oversimplification of complicated anatomical interactions that are as yet incompletely identified. Although ictal behavioral signs and symptoms are useful in postulating possible anatomical substrates of epileptogenic dysfunction, such clinical information alone never definitively indicates the site of seizure origin.

actual structural abnormality (Falconer et al., 1962). A more realistic approach recognizes an *irritative zone* as the area demonstrating epileptiform EEG abnormalities, an *epileptogenic lesion* as the structural disturbance presumed responsible for the epilepsy condition, and an *epileptogenic zone*, which remains a theoretical concept derived from a complete battery of diagnostic testing, operationally defined as the area necessary and sufficient for spontaneous seizures to occur (Bancaud and Chauvel,

1987; Engel, 1987a;b; Lüders et al., 1993). For practical purposes, when surgery is being considered, the epileptogenic zone represents the minimum tissue that must be resected to render the patient seizure-free (Chapter 16).

Some epilepsy centers use a classification system devised at the Cleveland Clinic that consists of highly specific descriptions of the ictal behavior derived from long-term video-EEG monitoring (Lüders et al., 1998). This is not, strictly speaking, a classification, but

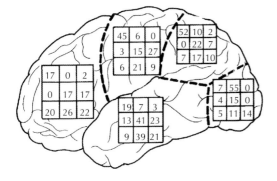

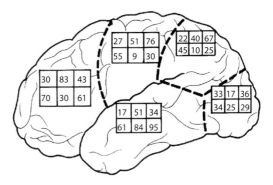

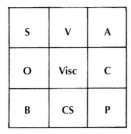

S	V	A
O	Visc	C
B	CS	P

Figure 6–1. Characteristics of auras associated with epileptiform EEG abnormalities in various regions of the brain. The numbers in each grid represent the percentages of patients with seizures characterized by the features noted in the large grid. The numbers in each grid may add up to more than 100 because seizures can have more than one feature. Note the relative lack of anatomical specificity for most phenomena. S, somatosensory; V, visual; A, auditory; O, olfactory and gustatory; Visc, visceral; C, cephalic; B, body; CS, complex subjective (emotional, feelings of unreality, discomfort); P, psychic. (Adapted from Ajmone-Marsan, 1978, with permission.)

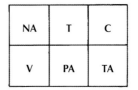

NA	T	C
V	PA	TA

Figure 6–2. Characteristics of focal seizures with motor signs associated with epileptiform EEG abnormalities in various regions of the brain. The numbers in each grid represent the percentages of patients with seizures characterized by the features noted in the large grid. The numbers in each grid may add up to more than 100 because seizures can have more than one feature. As in Figure 6–1, there is a relative lack of anatomical specificity for most of these phenomena. NA, no aura; T, tonic motor; C, clonic motor; V, versive posture; PA, pure automatisms (no other features); TA, total automatisms. (Adapted from Ajmone-Marsan, 1978, with permission.)

rather a descriptive diagnostic approach that can be applied to individual patients. For this reason, it has been incorporated into the diagnostic scheme recommended by the ILAE for descriptions of individual patients (Engel, 2001) (Chapter 1), and the ILAE has published an accompanying glossary of descriptive terminology to foster consistency in medical recording (Blume et al., 2001). This is, however, an optional axis for the diagnostic scheme, not only because detailed descriptions of ictal behavior are difficult to obtain in most patients but also because it has limited value with respect to diagnosis and treatment when surgery is not a consideration. The major purpose of careful observation of ictal phenomena is to provide clues to the anatomical localization of ictal onset, which is important only in candidates for resective surgical therapy (Chapter 16).

Because delineation of the epileptogenic zone based on clinical ictal behavior can be misleading, localization always requires correlative diagnostic information from electrophysiological and imaging studies as well as from a variety of other diagnostic tests usually performed at epilepsy surgery centers (Chapter 16). Even the grossest anatomical distinction, discriminating focal from generalized seizures, can be problematic, as discussed in Chapter 1. Nevertheless, the ILAE has considered it useful to continue the practice of dividing seizure types into focal and generalized, acknowledging that this is not an absolute dichotomy.

Pathophysiological Mechanisms

Different electrographic ictal onset patterns have been identified that appear to reflect different pathophysiological mechanisms. Of the two most common types recorded with depth electrodes from hippocampus, one consists of EEG suppression or low-voltage fast activity, while the other consists of repetitive spike-and-wave discharges reflecting abnormal hypersynchronization, which presumably requires enhanced excitation and inhibition (Gloor, 1979; Engel et al., 1981a; Engel and Wilson, 1986; Engel, 1987a; Gloor and Fariello, 1988; Spencer et al., 1992; Velasco et al., 2000; Ogren et al., 2009) (Chapter 4). Both patterns can be seen during a single epileptic seizure. One can evolve into the other, or one can occur at the site of seizure initiation while the other appears at propagation sites. Most epileptic seizures consist of a progression of signs and symptoms reflecting a series of anatomically and pathophysiologically discrete events (Chapter 4).

Pathophysiological mechanisms appear to cut across accepted categories of epileptic seizures. For instance, some focal seizures result from underlying mechanisms more similar to the mechanisms of certain types of generalized seizures than to those of other focal seizures. Focal and generalized ictal events are not clearly separate entities but represent a spectrum of symptoms lying along a continuum (Chapters 1 and 4). Whether a seizure remains in one part of the brain, spreads, or is generalized from the start depends less on the nature of the pathophysiological disturbance than on the size and location of the epileptogenic zone and the predisposition of the brain to manifest epileptic symptoms (Chapter 4).

A small, discrete lesion is likely to give rise to focal epileptic symptoms, whereas bilateral or diffuse lesions are more likely to rapidly recruit larger brain areas and give rise to generalized symptoms from the start. The potential for generalization is relatively low for lesions in primary cortical areas such as the motor strip and relatively high in certain association areas, particularly frontal cortex (Bancaud et al., 1974). This presumably reflects regional differences in neuronal connectivity and excitability (Chapter 8).

A lesion large enough to produce generalized seizures in a patient with a low threshold for epilepsy might produce only focal seizures in a patient with a higher threshold. The mechanisms that determine this threshold depend on inherited and acquired characteristics of neuronal function (Chapter 5). Focal seizures can manifest as generalized ictal events when the threshold is lowered, for instance, with sleep and drowsiness, fever, psychological stress, or withdrawal from sedative and antiseizure medications. On the other hand, institution of antiseizure medication to increase the seizure threshold in patients with apparent generalized epilepsy can occasionally unmask auras or other focal seizures.

The ILAE has emphasized the primary importance of pathophysiological mechanisms, which include an understanding of the etiological disturbance, over clinical ictal behavior in future classifications of epileptic seizures and epilepsy syndromes (Engel, 2001, 2006; Berg et al., 2010). Clearly the fundamental neuronal mechanisms underlying typical absence seizures are completely different from those of limbic seizures consisting solely of brief lapses of consciousness (Chapter 4), even though the clinical manifestations can be identical. On the other hand, a specific epileptogenic disturbance, such as focal cortical dysplasia, in the motor cortex will give rise to ictal behaviors entirely different from those due to the same lesion and the same pathophysiological mechanisms in the occipital lobe. Here, it is the underlying pathophysiology, and not the clinical manifestations or the anatomical location, that will ultimately determine specific nonsurgical therapeutic interventions. Furthermore, the pathophysiological mechanisms leading to epileptogenesis and epileptogenicity will likely differ considerably depending on the etiological agent. For instance, the fundamental neuronal mechanisms underlying the development of and ictogenesis in limbic seizures due to hippocampal sclerosis could be entirely different from those due to a neoplasm or a malformation of cortical development. Although these distinctions may have little practical value at present, elucidating the varieties of disturbed neurobiological mechanisms that lead to similar ictal phenomena could inform future approaches to more specific therapeutic interventions as well as more appropriately designed clinical trials for such interventions.

Pharmacological Considerations

Antiseizure drugs have different spectra of action (e.g., anticonvulsant or antiabsence), which can be used to classify epileptic phenomena (Chapter 1) and perhaps provide clues to underlying mechanisms (Chapters 3, 14, and 15). *Phenytoin* and *carbamazepine* are common *anticonvulsant* drugs with selective efficacy against both generalized tonic-clonic and focal seizures, whereas *ethosuximide* is an *antiabsence* drug with selective efficacy against petit mal absences and some atypical absences (Chapters 14 and 15). Certain *benzodiazepines*, *valproic acid*, and many of the new drugs have a broad spectrum of action and can be used to treat all forms of ictal behavior. Myoclonic jerks can be treated by most of these broad-spectrum drugs, but they do not respond to selective anticonvulsant or antiabsence medication. Atonic seizures are particularly pharmacoresistant, but *felbamate* and *rufinamide* are more effective treatment than other antiseizure drugs.

These selective effects of pharmacological agents suggest that some focal and generalized tonic-clonic seizures share common mechanisms distinct from those giving rise to absences, whereas myoclonic phenomena reflect yet other, most likely more than one, pathophysiological processes. For pharmacotherapeutic purposes, these three categories might be considered sufficient (Chapter 14). Further differences can be found within these three groups. For instance, focal seizures are more refractory to anticonvulsants than generalized tonic-clonic seizures, and limbic seizures appear to be the most difficult to control (Schmidt et al., 1986; Semah et al., 1998). Similarly, atypical absences are more refractory to antiabsence medication than typical absences and are occasionally responsive to anticonvulsant medications. This suggests that atypical absences reflect more complex or inconsistent pathophysiological mechanisms than typical absences. Therefore, responses to pharmacological treatment could allow further identification of certain epileptic seizure subtypes.

TYPES OF EPILEPTIC SEIZURES

Table 6–2 shows clinical and EEG features of the seizure types recognized by the 1981 International Classification of Epileptic Seizures (Commission on Classification and Terminology, 1981). This chapter, however, will consider the generalized seizure types

recognized by the 2010 ILAE report (Berg et al., 2010), which is slightly different from the 1981 classification. Following recent ILAE recommendations (Engel, 2001, 2006; Berg et al., 2010), this discussion will not divide focal seizures into simple and complex based on impairment of consciousness but will consider neocortical and limbic seizures separately. Specific ictal manifestations have been described in detail by many authors (see Lüders et al., 1998; Blume et al., 2001; Engel and Pedley, 2008; Panayiotopoulos, 2010; see also the electronic textbook MedLink [www.medlink.com] and videos of ictal and other related phenomena available on www.epilepticdisorders.com).

Focal seizures are now described by the ILAE as originating within networks limited to one hemisphere, which may be discretely localized or more widely distributed; thus they are not really *focal*. Focal seizures may originate in subcortical structures. Each seizure type shows a consistent ictal onset from one seizure to another and exhibits preferential propagation patterns, which can involve the contralateral hemisphere. In some patients, however, there is more than one epileptogenic network, and these can be bilateral but independent. Multiple epileptogenic networks can give rise to more than one seizure type in the same patient, but each seizure type has a consistent site of onset. Focal seizures do not fit easily into any recognized set of natural classes based on our current understanding of the mechanisms involved (Berg et al., 2010).

Generalized seizures are now defined by the ILAE as originating at some point within and rapidly engaging bilaterally distributed networks. Such bilateral networks can include cortical and subcortical structures, but do not necessarily include the entire cortex; thus they are not really *generalized*. Although individual seizure onsets can appear localized, their location and lateralization are not consistent from one seizure to another. Generalized seizures can be asymmetric (Berg et al., 2010).

These definitions attempt to overcome the false focal/generalized dichotomy by invoking the concept of ictal onsets within specific networks that are more or less localized. In focal seizures, the network responsible for seizure initiation is limited to one hemisphere, but a given patient could have bilateral independent networks giving rise to bilateral but

Table 6–2 **1981 Seizure Classification**

I. PARTIAL (FOCAL, LOCAL) SEIZURES

Partial seizures are those in which, in general, the first clinical and electroencephalographic changes indicate initial activation of a system of neurons limited to part of one cerebral hemisphere. A partial seizure is classified primarily on the basis of whether or not consciousness is impaired during the attack. When consciousness is not impaired, the seizure is classified as a simple partial seizure. When consciousness is impaired, the seizure is classified as a complex partial seizure. Impairment of consciousness may be the first clinical sign, or simple partial seizures may evolve into complex partial seizures. In patients with impaired consciousness, aberrations of behavior (automatisms) may occur. A partial seizure may not terminate, but instead progress to a generalized motor seizure. Impaired consciousness is defined as the inability to respond normally to exogenous stimuli by virtue of altered awareness and/or responsiveness.

There is considerable evidence that simple partial seizures usually have unilateral hemispheric involvement and only rarely have bilateral hemispheric involvement; complex partial seizures, however, frequently have bilateral hemispheric involvement.

Partial seizures can be classified into one of the following three fundamental groups:

A. Simple partial seizures
B. Complex partial seizures
    1. With impairment of consciousness at onset
    2. Simple partial onset followed by impairment of consciousness
C. Partial seizures evolving to generalized tonic-clonic convulsions (GTC)
    1. Simple evolving to GTC
    2. Complex evolving to GTC (including those with simple partial onset)

Clinical Seizure Type	EEG Seizure Type	EEG Interictal Expression
A. *Simple partial seizures* (consciousness not impaired)	Local contralateral discharge starting over the corresponding area of cortical representation (not always recorded on the scalp)	Local contralateral discharge

    1. With motor signs
        (a) Focal motor without march
        (b) Focal motor with march (Jacksonian)
        (c) Versive
        (d) Postural
        (e) Phonatory (vocalization or arrest of speech)
    2. With somatosensory or special sensory symptoms (simple hallucinations, e.g., tingling, light flashes, buzzing)
        (a) Somatosensory
        (b) Visual
        (c) Auditory
        (d) Olfactory
        (e) Gustatory
        (f) Vertiginous
    3. With autonomic symptoms or signs (including epigastric sensation, pallor, sweating, flushing, piloerection, and pupillary dilatation)
    4. With psychic symptoms (disturbances of higher cerebral function). These symptoms rarely occur without impairment of consciousness and are much more commonly experienced as complex partial seizures.
        (a) Dysphasic
        (b) Dysmnesic (e.g., déjà vu)
        (c) Cognitive (e.g., dreamy states, distortions of time sense)
        (d) Affective (fear, anger, etc.)
        (e) Illusions (e.g., macropsia)
        (f) Structured hallucinations (e.g., music, scenes)

(continued)

Table 6–2 (Continued)

Clinical Seizure Type	EEG Seizure Type	EEG Interictal Expression
B. *Complex partial seizures*		
(with impairment of consciousness; may sometimes began with simple symptomatology)	Unilateral or frequently bilateral discharge, diffuse or focal in temporal or frontotemporal regions	Unilateral or bilateral generally asynchronous focus; usually in the temporal or frontal regions

1. Simple partial onset followed by impairment of consciousness
    (a) With simple partial features (A.1.–A.4) followed by impaired consciousness
    (b) With automatisms
  2. With impairment of consciousness at onset
    (a) With impairment of consciousness only
    (b) With automatisms		

C. *Partial seizures evolving to* secondarily *generalized* seizures (this may be generalized tonic-clonic, tonic, or clonic)
  1. Simple partial seizures (A) evolving to generalized seizures
  2. Complex partial seizures (B) evolving to generalized seizures
  3. Simple partial seizures evolving to complex partial seizures evolving to generalized seizures
	Above discharges become secondarily and rapidly generalized	

II. GENERALIZED SEIZURES (CONVULSIVE OR NONCONVULSIVE)

Generalized seizures are those in which the first clinical changes indicate initial involvement of both hemispheres. Consciousness may be impaired, and this impairment may be the initial manifestation. Motor manifestations are bilateral. The ictal electroencephalographic patterns initially are bilateral and presumably reflect neuronal discharge, which is widespread in both hemispheres.

Clinical Seizure Type	EEG Seizure Type	EEG Interictal Expression
A. 1. *Absence seizures*	Usually regular and symmetrical 3-Hz but may be 2- to 4-Hz spike-and-slow-wave complexes and may have multiple spike-and-slow-wave complexes. Abnormalities are bilateral.	Background activity usually normal, although paroxysmal activity (such as spikes or spike-and-slow-wave complexes) may occur. This activity is usually regular and symmetrical.

(a) Impairment of consciousness only
  (b) With mild clonic components
  (c) With atonic components		

(continued)

Table 6–2 (Continued)

Clinical Seizure Type	EEG Seizure Type	EEG Interictal Expression
(d) With tonic components (e) With automatisms (f) With autonomic components (b through f may be used alone or in combination)		
2. *Atypical absence*	EEG more heterogeneous; may include irregular spike-and-slow-wave complexes, fast activity or other paroxysmal activity. Abnormalities are bilateral but often irregular and asymmetrical and asymmetrical	Background usually abnormal; paroxysmal activity (such as spikes or spike-and-slow-wave complexes) frequently irregular and asymmetrical
May have; (a) Changes in tone that are more pronounced than in A.1 (b) Onset and/or cessation that is not abrupt		
B. *Myoclonic* seizures Myoclonic jerks (single or multiple)	Polyspike and wave, or sometimes spike and wave or sharp and slow waves	Same as ictal
C. *Clonic* seizures	Fast activity (10 c/sec or more) and slow waves; occasional spike-and-wave patterns	Spike-and-wave or polyspike-and-wave discharges
D. *Tonic seizures*	Low voltage fast activity or a fast rhythm of 9–10 c/sec or more decreasing in frequency and increasing in amplitude	More or less rhythmic discharges of sharp and slow waves, sometimes asymmetrical. Background is often abnormal for age.
E. *Tonic-clonic seizures*	Rhythm at 10 or more c/sec decreasing in frequency and increasing in amplitude during tonic phase, interrupted by slow waves during clonic phase	Polyspike and waves, spike and wave, or, sometimes, sharp- and slow-wave discharges
F. *Atonic seizures* (astatic) (combinations of the above may occur, e.g., B and F, B and D)	Polyspikes and wave or flattening or low-voltage fast activity	Polyspikes and slow wave

III. UNCLASSIFIED EPILEPTIC SEIZURES

Includes all seizures that cannot be classified because of inadequate or incomplete data and some that defy classification in hitherto described categories. This includes some neonatal seizures, e.g., rhythmic eye movements, chewing, and swimming movements.

IV. ADDENDUM

Repeated epileptic seizures occur under a variety of circumstances: (1) as fortuitous attacks, coming unexpectedly and without any apparent provocation; (2) as cyclic attacks, attacks at more or less regular intervals (e.g., in relation to the menstrual cycle or the sleep-waking cycle); (3) as attacks provoked by (a) nonsensory factors (fatigue, alcohol, emotion, etc.) or (b) sensory factors, sometimes referred to as "reflex seizures."
Prolonged or repetitive seizures (status epilepticus). The term "status epilepticus" is used whenever a seizure persists for a sufficient length of time or is repeated frequently enough that recovery between attacks does not occur. Status epilepticus may be divided into partial (e.g., Jacksonian) or generalized (e.g., absence status or tonic-clonic status). When very localized motor status occurs, it is referred to as epilepsia partialis continua.

From Commission on Classification, 1981, with permission.

independent focal ictal onsets. This definition also accounts for a rapid spread from a unilateral network to produce an apparent generalized seizure, even though the ictal onset is consistently focal. For generalized seizures, the ILAE concept acknowledges that ictal onsets can be focal and unilateral but that the epileptogenic network is diffuse and bilateral, so that ictal onset does not originate at a fixed location, as it would for focal epilepsy, but rather can originate in either hemisphere and at times from multiple areas of each hemisphere (Hirsch et al., 2006).

Because the 1981 International Classification of Epileptic Seizures placed considerable emphasis on consciousness by dividing focal seizures into *simple partial*, without impairment of consciousness, and *complex partial*, with impairment of consciousness, and because this terminology is still commonly used, it is worth reviewing the original definitions. *Consciousness* was operationally defined as awareness of or responsiveness to externally applied stimuli (Commission on Classification and Terminology, 1981). A responsive patient can carry out simple commands or willed movements, and an aware patient has full contact with the environment. A patient with simple partial seizures might be unresponsive because of motor paralysis or aphasia but still be aware and able to recount the events that occurred after return of responsiveness. On the other hand, during a complex partial seizure a patient might appear to be appropriately responsive to stimuli, although in an automatic fashion, but unable to recall events that occurred during the ictal episode. Consequently, *amnesia for the ictal event* is a hallmark of the complex partial seizure.

Although it can be difficult to determine whether consciousness is impaired during habitual seizures, particularly when depending on historical information, and consciousness is no longer a criterion for defining a specific type of focal seizure, this remains an important descriptive factor for individual patients, because seizures with impairment of consciousness represent a much greater disability than seizures without impairment of consciousness (Berg et al., 2010). The term *focal dyscognitive seizure* is now preferred (Blume et al., 2001) when describing ictal events in individual patients.

Focal seizures without impairment of consciousness and symptoms apparent only to the patient, that evolve into ictal motor manifestations, impaired consciousness, or both are commonly referred to as *auras*. In this situation, the aura is assumed to be the beginning of the seizure. Occasionally, however, nonspecific sensations that occur preictally and may persist for prolonged periods of time reflect prodromal events that predispose to ictogenesis and are distinct from specific ictal events (Chapter 4). For some patients, auras invariably evolve into more apparent ictal events with motor features or impaired consciousness, whereas in others auras can also occur in isolation. Ictal events are dynamic phenomena, so not only do auras evolve into more severe focal seizures, but focal seizures can become secondarily generalized.

The term *convulsion* has been variably used to describe (1) all motor ictal phenomena, focal and generalized, (2) only generalized motor phenomena, or (3) only specific generalized motor phenomena. Most commonly, generalized tonic-clonic, clonic, and some tonic motor seizures are referred to as *convulsive generalized seizures*, while absences and atonic, brief tonic, and myoclonic seizures are commonly referred to as *nonconvulsive generalized seizures*.

Drop attacks are highly disabling ictal events occurring most often in patients with diffuse brain damage, who usually have multiple seizure types. The ILAE recognizes *atonic seizures* as a distinct seizure type, characterized by loss of tone, but the term *astatic seizure* is used to refer to drop attacks in general. Myoclonic, myoclonic atonic, myoclonic tonic, clonic, and brief tonic seizures all can cause patients to fall suddenly and are included in the concept of astatic seizures. Focal motor seizures, particularly those originating in frontal cortex, can also occasionally manifest as a drop attack.

Myoclonus refers to a wide variety of motor phenomena that have been extremely difficult to define and classify. Hallett and Shibasaki (2008) state:

> Myoclonus is characterized by quick muscle jerks, either irregular or rhythmic. Myoclonic movements are always simple in nature, and this is often a critical feature separating myoclonus from other types of involuntary movements. Myoclonus can be focal, involving only a few adjacent muscles; generalized, involving many or most of the muscles in the body; or multifocal, involving many muscles but in different jerks. Myoclonus can be spontaneous, can be activated or accentuated by voluntary movement

(action myoclonus), and can be activated or accentuated by sensory stimulation (reflex myoclonus).

Considerable debate persists regarding which myoclonic phenomena are epileptic and which are nonepileptic. Although myoclonic phenomena have been classified according to electrophysiological and to etiological features, this classification has not seemed to help in distinguishing epileptic from nonepileptic events. At present, it seems simpler to conclude that myoclonic jerks occurring in epilepsy conditions are epileptic and those not associated with epilepsy conditions are nonepileptic. This is still unsatisfactory, however, because an argument can be made that the myoclonic jerks in the *progressive myoclonus epilepsies* are nonepileptic and not fragments of the epileptic seizures that also occur in these conditions. In the following discussion, bilateral massive myoclonus, as seen in *juvenile myoclonic epilepsy* and some infantile genetic epilepsies, as well as focal myoclonus, most commonly encountered in *epilepsia partialis continua*, will be considered under discussions of generalized and focal epilepsies. The broader topic of myoclonus will be discussed separately.

FOCAL SEIZURES

Focal seizures are divided here into *neocortical* and *limbic*; however, ictal phenomenology does not always reflect the site of ictal onset but rather the site of propagation. The brain area giving rise to ictal clinical behavior has been referred to as the *symptomatogenic zone* (Lüders et al., 1993) and can be some distance from the epileptogenic zone, where seizures originate. Symptoms of focal seizures, therefore, often reflect where epileptiform activity is occurring but not necessarily where it originated. Likewise, postictal focal dysfunction has localizing value but does not reliably identify the site of ictal onset (Lesser et al., 1987).

Neocortical onset seizures can preferentially propagate to hippocampus and other limbic areas, giving rise to limbic seizures. Ictal onsets in temporal neocortex, as well as in the occipital lobe below the calcarine fissure, propagate preferentially to hippocampus, whereas ictal onsets in the occipital lobe superior to the calcarine fissure and in the parietal lobe preferentially propagate to frontal lobe. Ictal electrographic discharges originating in hippocampus typically are not associated with clinical signs or symptoms until they propagate. Consequently, although this propagation is usually within the limbic system, giving rise to typical limbic seizures, it can also be to other neocortical areas, in which case the ictal manifestations might be more characteristic of neocortical seizures. Ictal behavioral manifestations are more likely to reflect the epileptogenic zone when it is in primary cortical areas such as motor and sensory neocortex than when it is in association cortical areas, but in general the following discussion of seizure semiology will be in reference to the symptomatogenic zone, regardless of where the seizures actually begin. Epileptic seizures are dynamic events; thus limbic seizures that begin with typical limbic ictal symptoms and signs can propagate to neocortex, with evolution to neocortical signs and symptoms. Similarly, neocortical seizures can begin with typical neocortical signs and symptoms and propagate to mesial temporal structures, evolving into limbic seizures (*secondary temporalization*).

Neocortical Seizures

MECHANISMS

Uncomplicated motor and sensory symptoms usually indicate discrete lesions in or near the appropriate primary neocortical area, although this relationship is not absolute (Ajmone-Marsan, 1978; Lesser et al., 1987) (see Fig. 6–1). Although focal neocortical seizures most often are due to unilateral, relatively well-localized epileptogenic lesions, this is not always the case. Two prominent exceptions are (1) the seizures that occur in the focal genetic childhood epilepsies and (2) the childhood form of epilepsia partialis continua (Chapter 10). In the first group of disorders, there is no evidence for a structural lesion, and symptoms can shift from side to side. The second disorder is often associated with diffuse, usually unilateral, neocortical disturbances.

PHENOMENOLOGY

The phenomenology of focal neocortical seizures has been reviewed in detail by many authors (see Lüders et al., 1998; Engel and

Pedley, 2008; Panayiotopoulos, 2010; and the electronic textbook MedLink [www.medlink. com]). Signs and symptoms are described here individually, but focal neocortical seizures frequently consist of a combination of two or more of these phenomena, often changing over time and reflecting functional properties of adjacent cortical areas.

Motor Signs

Motor seizures can be clonic or tonic, involving any body part (Kotagal and Lüders, 2008). *Clonic motor seizures* affect specific body parts in direct relation to the size of the representation of the particular body part in the motor homunculus (Kotagal and Lüders, 2008; Sperling, 2010a). Consequently, focal clonic seizures most often involve the face and hands. Focal clonic seizures can occur with ictal discharges on either side of the Rolandic fissure (see Fig. 6–1), and some clonic motor symptoms are typical of activity outside the primary sensorimotor cortex. For instance, occipital lesions can produce eye movements, blinking, and twitching of periocular muscles, and temporal lobe lesions produce oral, buccal, lingual, and pharyngeal movements.

Rarely, clonic focal motor seizures begin in one part of the body and slowly spread to adjacent muscle groups, corresponding to slow, nonsynaptic spread (Chapter 4) of epileptic discharge along the motor cortex. This is the classical *Jacksonian march*, which is most easily recognized with focal lesions in the precentral gyrus.

Tonic motor seizures (Kotagal and Lüders, 2008; Jobst, 2010a) are less anatomically specific than clonic ones. Movements are most often *versive*; they consist of slow head and eye movements to one side and are occasionally associated with twisting of the entire body. *Asymmetrical dystonic posturing* of the limbs also occurs. Classical manifestations of *supplementary motor seizures* are *adversive* head turning with flexion of one arm and extension of the other. These are occasionally associated with leg posturing, vocalizations or speech arrest, and incontinence. This structure-function relationship, however, is not absolute (Williamson et al., 1987). Version is almost always contralateral to the site of ictal onset with frontal lobe seizures, but not reliably lateralizing when seizures begin in the temporal lobe.

Focal *hyperkinetic seizures* consist of complex, often directed, excessive bilateral motor activity resulting from epileptiform discharges usually originating in prefrontal cortex (Jobst, 2010b). Motor behaviors can be bizarre, including bicycling leg movements, flailing arm movements, sexual automatisms, and vocalizations. Consciousness may not be lost during these events.

Aphasic seizures can be negative ictal motor symptoms (Stern, 2010d). Brief episodes of *speech arrest* can result from ictal disturbances of motor areas in the language-dominant hemisphere. Rarely, weakness, paralysis, or a sensation of an inability to move other body parts or the whole body occur as *negative motor seizures* from epileptogenic lesions in the anterior supplementary motor cortex (Lesser et al., 1987; Skidmore, 2010b).

Focal motor seizures arising in or near the motor strip, with or without a march, can be followed by postictal localized paralysis of muscles involved in the seizure (*Todd's paralysis*) (Efron, 1961) (Chapter 9). Versive and postural seizures, however, are not associated with postictal paralysis.

Focal myoclonic seizures presumably occur as epileptic phenomena (Skidmore, 2010a). They are most commonly encountered in *epilepsia partialis continua*, a form of focal status epilepticus that can persist for days, weeks, or years (Chapter 10). Otherwise, brief focal jerks that appear to be fragments of focal motor seizures in patients who also demonstrate the latter epileptic phenomena would generally be considered epileptic. *Focal negative myoclonus*, brief cessation of tone, is also believed to be epileptic in some situations, but the most common manifestation of this phenomenon is *asterixis*, which is nonepileptic.

Gelastic seizures are a unique ictal phenomenon consisting of stereotyped recurrence of pathological laughter in the absence of external precipitants (Freeman and Eeg-Olofsson, 2008; Freeman, 2010). Associated tonic and clonic movements, impaired consciousness, and automatisms can occur. Gelastic seizures are the characteristic seizure type of the epilepsy syndrome of *hypothalamic hamartoma with gelastic seizures* (Chapter 7). In patients with hypothalamic hamartoma with gelastic seizures, the laughter is often said to be mirthless, although this remains a matter of debate. Ictal laughter can also occur with seizures originating in temporal and frontal lobe structures, in which case it can be mirthful. Gelastic seizures are associated with epileptiform EEG abnormalities, which vary depending on the etiology. In hypothalamic hamartoma with gelastic seizures, the gelastic seizures appear to originate within the hamartoma itself (Munari et al., 1995). Ictal crying, *dacrystic seizures*, is a related seizure type.

Sensory Symptoms

Ictal sensory symptoms can be negative or positive and generally indicate an epileptogenic lesion in or near the appropriate primary sensory cortex (Van Ness et al., 2008) (see Fig. 6–1). When these sensations occur de novo, they are called ictal *hallucinations*, whereas distortions of normal sensory perception are called ictal *illusions*. Complex illusions and formed hallucinations are also discussed later under "Psychic Symptoms."

Somatosensory seizures usually originate in the postcentral or precentral area (Van Ness et al., 2008; Zangaladze, 2010). Most consist of localized paresthesias or numbness, with the incidence of body part involvement related to the size of the representation of that part on the somatosensory homunculus. Positive symptoms often take the form of bizarre, disturbing sensations, and pain occasionally occurs (Young and Blume, 1983). A rare negative symptom is loss of awareness of a body part (*asomatognosia*), usually due to right parietal involvement. Sensory seizures can exhibit a Jacksonian march, and paresthesias can be followed by postictal numbness corresponding to a sensory Todd's phenomenon.

Ictal *visual symptoms* usually consist of white or colored luminous spots or patterns (*phosphenes*) in one visual field, which can be static or moving (*paropsia*) (Van Ness et al., 2008; Jobst, 2010d). Negative symptoms such as small scotomata, complete hemifield defects, and blindness in full consciousness occur ictally but are more common during the postictal period. Both positive and negative unformed visual symptoms correlate highly with an epileptogenic lesion in the contralateral occipital lobe but not necessarily in the calcarine cortex.

Ictal *auditory symptoms* occur most often with lesions in the lateral temporal lobe (Van Ness et al., 2008; Jobst, 2010c). Positive symptoms (*paracusis*) can take the form of perceived sounds, such as hissing, ringing, and buzzing, or distorted sounds, including increased (*hyperacusis*) or decreased (*hypoacusis*) sensitivity to sound. Deafness is a rare ictal or postictal symptom.

Ictal *vertiginous symptoms* occur most commonly with epileptogenic lesions of the lateral temporal and parietal lobes (Van Ness et al., 2008; Stern, 2010c). Patients may complain of vague dizziness or a specific sensation of vertigo, although symptoms often lack a well-defined directional component.

Complex ictal *illusions* and formed *hallucinations* have been attributed to association neocortex of the temporal-parietal-occipital junction (Van Ness et al., 2008; Jobst, 2010d). Evidence suggests, however, that some of these *experiential* phenomena can occur with mesial temporal discharges (Gloor et al., 1982). Symptoms most often have visual features. During visual illusions objects can appear smaller (*micropsia*) or larger (*macropsia*), can be increased in number (*polyoptic seizures*), as in *monocular diplopia*, can appear to move closer or farther away (*microteleopsia*), or can change in form (*metamorphopsia*). Similarly, complex somesthetic, auditory, olfactory, and gustatory illusions occur. Ictal formed hallucinations are stereotyped and may be extremely detailed, for instance, an elaborate scene with many people each of whom has distinguishing features or a completely recreated episode from the past (*panoramic vision*). Multimodal hallucinations are common: faces can speak, and familiar places can have their characteristic odors. These ictal experiences are also often associated with affective symptoms, usually fear or other emotional states appropriate to the hallucination.

EEG

The *interictal EEG* in patients with focal neocortical seizures most often reveals focal spike-and-wave discharges over the appropriate neocortical region. Because interictal spikes often are inconsistently present, they may not be detected on a single routine EEG and in some patients do not appear even in serial EEGs or during long-term EEG monitoring. Interictal spike frequency does not correlate with degree of seizure control (Chapter 14). Runs of rhythmic focal slowing in the area of the epileptogenic zone can represent epileptiform activity, especially if the slow waves are notched in appearance. Continuous focal slowing, however, is often postictal and transient. Consequently, when serial EEGs reveal a new slow-wave focus in a patient with long-standing epilepsy, inquiry concerning the last seizure and a repeat EEG in several days are usually more appropriate than a structural imaging study.

Ictal EEG changes include suppression of ongoing EEG activity, a buildup of low-voltage fast activity, or polyspike-and-wave discharges exhibiting temporal and spatial evolution (Chapter 13). These patterns are usually localized to the appropriate neocortical area but can be diffusely distributed over one hemisphere; occasionally, however, they have no focal or lateralizing features. Diffuse or nonlocalizing ictal changes are characteristic of one form of epilepsia partialis continua (Chapter 10). Auras typically are not associated with ictal EEG changes unless or until the ictal event progresses to include pronounced motor or cognitive signs, although interictal spikes cease during this time.

Figure 6–3 shows an EEG recording from the scalp during a focal seizure of lateral temporal origin, and Figure 6–4 shows the image simultaneously obtained with positron emission

tomography with ^{18}F-fluorodeoxyglucose (FDG-PET), which confirmed that the ictal event was limited to the temporal lobe. For further discussion of the use of EEG in diagnosis of focal seizures, see Chapters 12 and 13.

CLINICAL CONSIDERATIONS

Focal neocortical seizures are the primary complaint of about 10% of patients with epilepsy (Gastaut et al., 1975). Auras can occur frequently with little consequent disability and are usually recognized as ictal events only if they also appear preceding clinically apparent seizures.

Diagnosis of focal neocortical seizures indicates a need to look for an underlying cause and to rule out a progressive lesion. Relatively brief and intermittent seizures that occur without progression to impaired consciousness or secondary generalization can usually be distinguished from more persistent signs and symptoms of other neurological or psychiatric disorders. Differential diagnosis can be a problem, however, when the seizures are prolonged for days and weeks (Wieser et al., 1985) (Chapters 10, 11, and 13). Recurrent epileptic hallucinations can be confused with psychotic hallucinations, particularly when the character

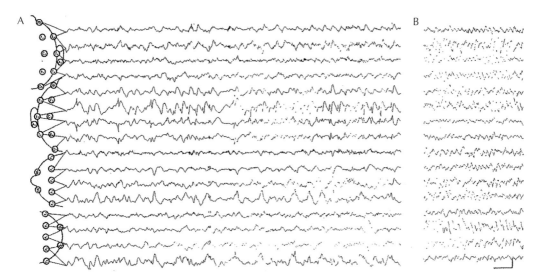

Figure 6–3. A. EEG recording of the onset of a typical focal motor seizure that occurred during the ictal FDG-PET study shown in Figure 6–4C. Seizures in this child consisted of twitching of the right face and arm associated with aphasia but no alteration of consciousness. Ictal discharges began with irregular spikes at T_3, which increased in frequency but remained localized to this area. **B.** EEG recorded in the same patient one year later, during the interictal FDG-PET study shown in Figure 6–4D, shows diffuse slowing and depression in the left temporal area. This child had epilepsia partialis continua and was eventually diagnosed with Rasmussen's encephalitis. (From Engel et al., 1983a, with permission.)

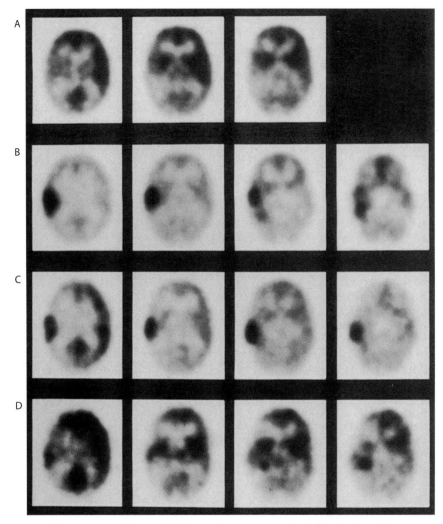

Figure 6–4. Representative sections from one interictal (**A**) and two ictal (**B, C**) FDG-PET scans obtained from the patient whose EEG is shown in Figure 6–3 during his first hospitalization and another interictal scan (**D**) obtained from the same patient one year later. Scans are scaled to best display abnormalities and not according to an absolute standard. The first interictal scan demonstrates a large zone of hypometabolism involving the left frontal and temporal lobes. Both ictal scans demonstrate a discrete zone of hypermetabolism in the left temporal region. The patterns on both ictal scans are similar, although the first suggests that the temporal hypermetabolism may be broken into two zones, one perhaps conforming to posterior hippocampus. The second interictal scan shows a small zone of hypermetabolism in the left perisylvian area and left hippocampus, although EEG and behavioral observation indicated that no seizure occurred during the study. EEGs obtained during scans 4C and 4D are shown in Figure 6–3. (Note that older PET scans in this look are not reversed, right is in the right side and left is in the left side.) (From Engel et al., 1983a, with permission.)

of the ictal events has been influenced by personal experiences and lends itself to psychodynamic interpretation. Major features of an epileptic, as opposed to a schizophrenic, hallucination are the stereotyped nature of the event and the propensity for visual and mixed-modality perceptions. Schizophrenic hallucinations are more often auditory, usually consisting of voices in isolation. Also, the patient with epilepsy is commonly aware that the hallucinations are not real, whereas the acutely psychotic patient is not.

Focal neocortical seizures are often resistant to pharmacotherapy, but if a discrete structural lesion is present, surgical resection offers an excellent prognosis. Natural history depends on the underlying cause. If focal neocortical seizures are unassociated with impairment of consciousness, do not progress to more severe ictal events, and do not interfere with quality of life, they may not need to be treated. There is no clinical evidence that such seizures cause progressive changes in brain function or influence the later development of more severe seizures (Chapter 8).

Limbic Seizures

MECHANISMS

Limbic seizures most commonly begin in hippocampus but can also originate in parahippocampal structures or in distant limbic areas such as cingulate and orbital frontal cortex (Engel and Williamson, 2008). Typical limbic seizures can also arise from silent association areas of neocortex that preferentially project to mesial temporal structures. There is reason to believe that fundamental mechanisms of limbic seizures originating in hippocampus and parahippocampal structures are different from those of seizures originating in neocortex (Chapter 4), but this chapter is more concerned with structures generating ictal clinical behavior. The symptomatogenic zone for typical limbic auras and automatisms is not the hippocampus but propagation areas including insula, amygdala, hypothalamus, and limbic neocortex.

Depth electrode recordings from patients under evaluation for resective surgery indicate that the most common electrophysiological correlate of impaired consciousness during dyscognitive limbic seizures is bilateral mesial temporal ictal activity. Although it is generally assumed that bilateral hippocampal involvement is necessary for the manifestation of dyscognitive signs and symptoms, impaired consciousness and postictal amnesia can occasionally occur when ictal discharges are seen in only one hippocampus. In this situation, there may be many ways that epileptiform activity could affect structures outside the hippocampus to alter consciousness (Blumenfeld, 2011). Consciousness can also be impaired when ictal discharges involve one hippocampus and the other is structurally damaged. Although it is reasonable to account for postictal amnesia by invoking involvement of both hippocampi in the ictal event, the actual structures involved in various types of impaired consciousness and dyscognitive signs and symptoms during

limbic seizures are unknown. Similar signs and symptoms can occur with neocortical seizures without involving mesial temporal structures, and limbic status epilepticus with epileptiform discharges recorded from depth electrodes in frontal cortex but not hippocampus has been reported (Williamson et al., 1985) (Chapter 10).

Limbic seizures are perhaps the most pharmacoresistant seizure type (Semah et al., 1998) but are the most commonly treated surgically, usually with excellent results (Chapter 16). There is evidence that repeated limbic seizures can produce progressive functional and structural disturbances (Chapters 8 and 10).

PHENOMENOLOGY

Limbic seizures usually begin with autonomic, psychic, or certain sensory auras, which can also occur in isolation. The latter can be olfactory, gustatory, or nonspecific somatosensory such as bilateral tingling of the face or hands, but specific sensory auras indicate a neocortical onset that preferentially projects to limbic structures. Although limbic seizures can consist only of impairment of consciousness, they usually include *automatisms*. A common initial feature of typical limbic seizures is an *arrest reaction* or *motionless stare* (Wieser, 1983; Engel and Williamson, 2008). The only evidence of impaired consciousness at this time may be amnesia for the ictal event. Automatisms usually follow impairment of consciousness but rarely occur during the aura, in which case they are recalled by the patients. Automatisms can also occur during the postictal period (Chapter 9). Some patients experience a loss of tone during focal dyscognitive seizures and slump slowly to the ground. A sudden drop (*temporal lobe syncope*) (Caffi, 1973), however, is rare and usually suggests a frontal lobe origin.

Limbic Sensory Symptoms

Ictal *olfactory symptoms* are commonly identified with lesions in anterior mesial temporal and orbital frontal structures (Engel and Williamson, 2008; Stern, 2010b). Ictal smells (*parosmia*), which are usually disagreeable, are referred to as *uncinate fits* and are said to have a higher correlation with neoplasms than other forms of focal epilepsy (Penfield and Jasper, 1954), although this has been disputed

(Howe and Gibson, 1982). *Anosmia* is rarely noted as an ictal or postictal symptom, but its occurrence is likely to be missed.

Ictal *gustatory symptoms* have been associated with mesial temporal lesions, particularly in the insular and peri-insular regions, although there is evidence to implicate the parietal operculum (Hausser-Hauw and Bancaud, 1987; Engel and Williamson, 2008; Stern, 2010a). They consist of taste sensations (*parageusia*), which are also usually disagreeable.

Autonomic Symptoms and Signs

Ictal autonomic symptoms are most often associated with epileptiform discharges in limbic portions of the temporal and frontal lobes (Engel and Williamson, 2008; Sperling, 2010b). They can occur in isolation and can be difficult to diagnose as epileptic unless followed by more obvious symptoms, usually dyscognitive focal seizures. The most common ictal autonomic symptoms are *gastrointestinal*, consisting of abdominal discomfort or nausea, often ascending to the throat (*epigastric rising*); stomach pain; borborygmi; belching; flatulence; and even vomiting (Van Buren, 1963). The last has been reported to be more frequent with right than left mesial temporal ictal discharge. These ictal symptoms in isolation have been referred to as *abdominal epilepsy*; however, this diagnosis has been greatly abused and only rarely is justified. Other autonomic symptoms, such as pallor, flushing, sweating, piloerection, pupil dilatation, alterations in heart rate and respiration, and urination, also occur. Sexual arousal, penile erection, and orgasm have been reported occasionally (Lesser et al., 1987). Autonomic signs and symptoms might also reflect a reaction to the occurrence of an epileptic seizure.

Psychic Symptoms

Ictal psychic symptoms usually indicate epileptic activity in mesial temporal or other limbic structures and often evolve into typical limbic seizures (Engel and Williamson, 2008; Stern, 2010e). Psychic, autonomic, olfactory, and gustatory ictal symptoms without impairment of consciousness are still considered to be *limbic*, *temporal lobe*, or *psychomotor seizures*, but they were called simple partial seizures according to the 1981 International Classification.

Ictal *dysphasic symptoms* usually indicate a lesion in the language-dominant hemisphere (Engel and Williamson, 2008; Stern, 2010d). These psychic phenomena are not always clearly distinguishable from negative motor symptoms. The former refer to more complex disturbances with various forms of aphasic speech as opposed to simple speech arrest. Receptive aphasias can also occur.

Ictal *dysmnesic symptoms* are distorted memory experiences, such as inappropriate feelings of familiarity (*déjà vu*, *déjà entendu*, and *déjà vécu*) or strangeness (*jamais vu*, *jamais entendu*, and *jamais vécu*), flashbacks, forced thinking, and rapid recollection of episodes from the past (Engel and Williamson, 2008; Stern, 2010e). Although memory experiences are disturbed, registration of new memory traces during these seizures is not, because the patient is not amnesic with regard to these events.

Ictal *cognitive disturbances* include dream states, distortion of time sense, sensations of unreality, and depersonalization, but any specific cognitive dysfunction can occur (Engel and Williamson, 2008; Stern, 2010e).

The most common ictal *affective symptom* is fear, often associated with appropriate autonomic changes (Engel and Williamson, 2008; Stern, 2010e). Patients also occasionally experience anger, depression, or embarrassment. Gelastic seizures (ictal inappropriate sudden laughter), as discussed above, can express an emotion, particularly when of limbic origin, or may be confined to the motor manifestations of laughter.

Automatisms

Automatisms consist of involuntary, automatic motor behaviors usually occurring when consciousness is impaired (Engel and Williamson, 2008; Stern, 2010e). They can be ictal or postictal and are of two forms, spontaneous and reactive. *Spontaneous automatisms* tend to be stereotyped and are a constant feature of the patient's habitual seizure. The most common examples of these behaviors are *oroalimentary automatisms*, such as lip smacking, chewing, and swallowing. Involvement of the amygdala is implied, but this is not necessarily the site of ictal origin. Some investigators believe swallowing indicates ictal activity in frontal operculum (Munari et al., 1980). *Mimetic automatisms* consist of facial expressions indicating emotion; *gestural automatisms* include picking at clothes, scratching, dressing and undressing, or rearranging objects; *ambulatory automatisms* involve walking or running (*cursive epilepsy*), usually in a particular pattern while easily avoiding obstacles; *verbal automatisms*, which have no lateralizing significance, are stereotyped and consist of simple phrases such as "Help me," "Oh, no, here it comes again," or calling someone's name. *Sexual automatisms*, such as pelvic thrusting and masturbation, are rare and can indicate frontal lobe involvement (Spencer et al., 1983). Other spontaneous automatisms are less well defined, such as chaotic flailing of the limbs and bicycle movements of the legs, referred to as *hyperkinetic automatisms*; humming; screaming; and spitting. These also can indicate a neocortical disturbance, which is usually in the frontal lobe. Unilateral dystonic posturing contralateral to the side of ictal onset is commonly encountered during limbic seizures. Consequently, when movements, such as gestural automatisms, are unilateral, they are usually ipsilateral to the epileptogenic zone, because the contralateral side is dystonic.

Occasionally, stereotyped automatisms, particularly verbal and gestural automatisms, are influenced by situations that were present when the first seizure occurred or by other important factors in the patient's life at that time. An example of the former is a patient who was playing basketball when he experienced his first seizure and whose repeated verbal automatism is "over here." An example of the latter is a priest whose gestural automatisms consist of crossing himself and putting his hands together in prayer. How such ictal events develop is unknown, and investigations might inform our understanding of the mechanisms of epileptogenesis.

Reactive automatisms are not stereotyped, because they are determined by environmental stimuli at the time of the seizure. Commonly, simple activities in progress at the time of seizure onset can be continued with sufficient skill that a naive observer might not realize a seizure is occurring. Consequently, a patient can continue to wash dishes or write (although the writing is unintelligible) but have no memory of the event afterward. Patients can often answer questions, follow simple commands, or respond correctly to new situations, such as avoiding cars while crossing the street. Such responses can occasionally lead to the erroneous assumption that consciousness is not impaired. More often, however, reactive automatisms are inappropriate and can be disturbing to others who do not understand the disorder. For instance, when handed paperwork to do, the patient may proceed to tear the paper into small pieces or crumple it into a ball. A more troublesome example is the violent reaction to perceived threat, which is why it is unwise to attempt to restrain a patient during or after a limbic seizure (Chapter 9). Reactive automatisms have no specific anatomical substrate and can be ictal or postictal. They can also be seen, to some extent, during absences as well as following generalized convulsions. Consequently, these behaviors appear to be nonspecific *release* activities resulting from functional ablation of conscious control mechanisms.

Other motor symptoms besides automatisms can occur with limbic seizures. Most commonly these are tonic postural or versive behaviors. Movements that are *contraversive* (away from the lesion) as well as those that are *ipsiversive* (toward the lesion) are seen. Thus, initial head and body turning has no specific lateralizing or localizing value for limbic seizures (Ochs et al., 1984). However, definite forced (involuntary) versive movements that involve the eyes and head just prior to a secondarily generalized seizure correlate highly with ictal onset in the contralateral hemisphere (Wyllie et al., 1986; McLachlan, 1987). Initial postural changes of temporal lobe origin tend to be slow and deliberate during impairment of consciousness. Tonic motor symptoms of frontal lobe origin, on the other hand, are more rapid, brief, and repeated. They are inconsistently associated with impaired consciousness (McLachlan, 1987) and may be sufficiently bizarre to suggest psychogenic nonepileptic seizures (Ajmone-Marsan and Ralston, 1957; Williamson et al., 1987). Clonic movements during limbic seizures most often involve muscles of the face or oroalimentary muscles. Interestingly, unilateral blinking can rarely occur ipsilateral to mesial temporal ictal discharge (Wada, 1980), similar to the early ictal response to amygdala stimulation in kindling (Racine, 1972).

Limbic seizures are almost invariably followed by a period of confusion, although the transition from the ictal to the postictal state is not always clear. Rarely, the change is abrupt, with apparent immediate return of awareness and responsiveness. In these situations, a brief period of postictal cognitive disturbance can usually be found if the patient is examined properly. The most commonly encountered postictal symptoms are anterograde amnesia and, if the language-dominant hemisphere is primarily involved, receptive or expressive aphasia. In some patients, specific behaviors such as a cough or rubbing the nose may reliably indicate the end of the ictal discharge, even when impaired consciousness or confusion persists for some time afterward. A postictal nose wipe is usually made with the hand ipsilateral to seizure onset. During the postictal period of confusion, patients can occasionally react violently to a perceived threat or attempts at restraint, as noted previously. This is a nonspecific response and not evidence of ictal or postictal directed aggression (Chapter 9). Reactive automatisms can continue or initially appear during the postictal period. Disability due to disorientation, fatigue, and occasionally headache can dissipate in minutes after the seizure terminates or can last for hours. Anterograde amnesia can sometimes persist for weeks after repeated limbic seizures (Engel et al., 1978).

Limbic dyscognitive seizures involving frontal areas can be difficult to distinguish behaviorally from those involving mesial temporal structures, but a characteristic feature of some frontal lobe dyscognitive seizures is brief, frequent events involving more pronounced motor activity initially and a short period of postictal confusion. Urinary incontinence and drop attacks during dyscognitive seizures and nocturnal ictal events also suggest frontal lobe involvement. Auras in isolation are a characteristic feature of limbic seizures originating in mesial temporal structures but not of those originating in frontal lobe structures or other neocortical areas (Chapter 4).

EEG

Interictal EEGs in patients with limbic seizures usually demonstrate unilateral or independent bilateral anterior temporal spike foci. These transients are best seen with basal electrodes (Fig. 6–5) (Chapters 12 and 13). Sleep characteristically activates anterior temporal spike foci, although spikes that occur during slow-wave sleep have less lateralizing or localizing value than those that occur during wakefulness

(Lieb et al., 1980). Intermittent interictal temporal theta or delta rhythms (*temporal intermittent rhythmic delta activity*, or *TIRDA*) usually reflect spike-and-wave discharges in deep mesial temporal or orbital frontal regions when the more rapid transients are not recorded at the surface.

Limbic auras in isolation usually have no EEG correlate, and when these events occur as auras for dyscognitive seizures, the ictal EEG abnormalities typically do not appear until consciousness becomes impaired. *Ictal EEGs* are almost always abnormal during hippocampal onset limbic seizures after consciousness becomes impaired, although the abnormality can range from mild focal or diffuse slowing to well-defined ictal discharges localized initially to one temporal lobe. The latter, when present, usually take the form of a variable suppression of baseline rhythms evolving into a higher-amplitude 5- to 7-Hz rhythm, which spreads ipsilaterally and then contralaterally. In patients with mesial temporal lesions, this ictal pattern is often seen in one basal electrode before it spreads to lateral temporal derivations (*initial focal onset*), or it may appear predominantly in one basal electrode many seconds after a nonlocalizing ipsilateral or bilateral onset (*delayed focal onset*) (Risinger et al., 1989) (Fig. 6–6). Depth electrode recordings demonstrate both low-voltage fast and high-amplitude spike-and-wave (hypersynchronous) patterns of ictal onset, but the latter is more common with hippocampal onset (Velasco et al., 2000) (Chapter 4). Depth-recorded hypersynchronous discharges usually are not reflected in the scalp EEG and can be associated with an aura or no symptoms at all. Figure 4–18 shows a depth electrode recording of a focal seizure of hippocampal origin that had no scalp EEG changes. Hypersynchronous discharges characteristically remain for many seconds or even minutes in one hippocampus before spreading to the contralateral side, at which point consciousness becomes impaired (Lieb et al., 1986). This delay is characteristic of hippocampal, as opposed to neocortical, seizures and is believed to be an intrinsic property of hippocampus that resists propagation rather than reflecting the functional absence of a hippocampal commissure (Wilson et al., 1987) (Chapter 4). FDG-PET scans during limbic seizures can reveal regions of ictal propagation (Fig. 6–7). Postictal EEG depression,

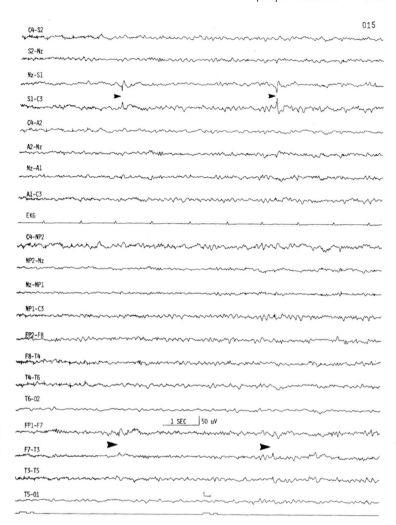

Figure 6–5. EEG showing mesial spikes at the left sphenoidal electrode (S$_1$), reflected at F$_7$ (*arrowheads*). Note that this spike is not seen by nasopharyngeal (NP$_1$) or ear (A$_1$) electrodes. (From Sperling et al., 1986, with permission.)

a common feature of limbic seizures, is also reflected in the FDG-PET scan as diffuse hypometabolism superimposed on the focal hypermetabolism of the area of ictal onset and spread (Fig. 6–7). Dyscognitive seizures of frontal lobe onset have variable, often poorly localized and lateralized ictal onset patterns, even with invasive recording.

CLINICAL CONSIDERATIONS

Studies of incidence and prognosis have not distinguished between limbic dyscognitive seizures with mesial temporal and neocortical onset, but the differential diagnosis is important when surgical resection is considered (Chapter 16). Limbic dyscognitive seizures are the predominant seizure type in approximately 40% of patients with epilepsy (Gastaut et al., 1975). They tend to be more refractory to medical treatment than most other types of seizures (Schmidt et al., 1986; Semah et al., 1998) (Chapter 7). Risk of relapse after remission is great. The ictal events that have been called *complex partial seizures in infancy* are almost always indicative of extensive cerebral rather than specifically limbic dysfunction and have a poor prognosis (Duchowny, 1987).

In contrast to their relatively high incidence of medical intractability, limbic seizures are more likely than other seizure types to be amenable to resective surgical therapy (Chapter 16). Limbic seizures usually indicate an epileptogenic lesion in mesial temporal structures, but they also occur with lateral temporal, frontal limbic, and other neocortical

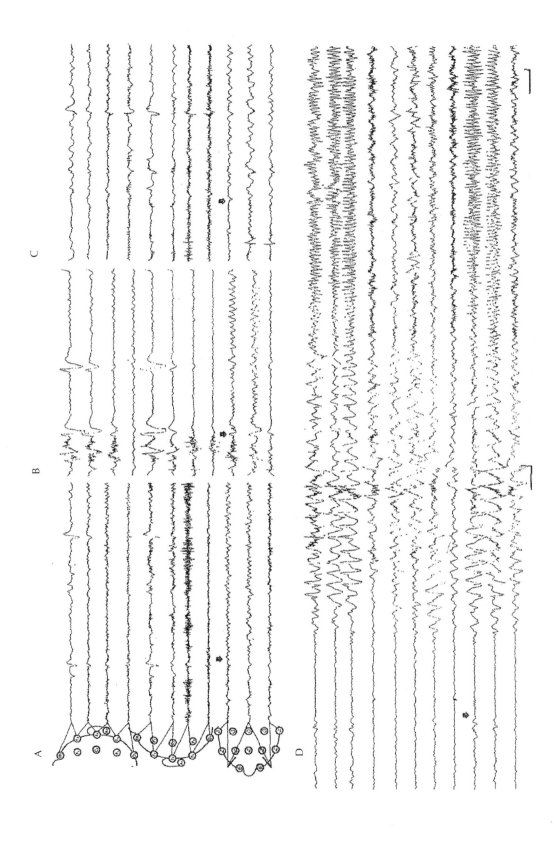

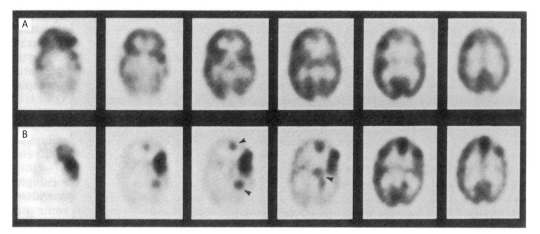

Figure 6–7. A. Interictal FDG-PET scan revealing a wide area of hypometabolism in the right frontal and temporal lobes. **B.** Scan obtained when FDG was injected just prior to several dyscognitive focal seizures. The most marked zone of hypermetabolism involves the right posterior frontal and anterior temporal lobes, but discrete smaller areas of increased metabolic activity can be seen in the right cingulate cortex (*top arrowhead*), posterior hippocampus (*bottom arrowhead*), and thalamus (*middle arrowhead*). (Note that older PET scans in this look are not reversed, right is in the right side and left is in the left side.) (From Engel et al., 1983a, with permission).

epileptogenic lesions when ictal discharges propagate to the mesial temporal lobe. There are no data to suggest that the prognosis and medical management of limbic seizures would differ among the forms of limbic epilepsy, but accurate localization of the site of ictal onset is essential when patients are candidates for resective surgical treatment (Chapters 12 and 16). Limbic status epilepticus, however, may occur more often with frontal lobe than with mesial temporal disturbances (Williamson et al., 1985) (Chapter 10). Lateralization of ictal onset also has no prognostic or therapeutic value unless surgery is contemplated. In this situation, particularly when neuroimaging is negative, lateralization depends on EEG and ictal semiology. Some useful lateralizing ictal and postictal signs and symptoms are shown in Table 6–3.

Focal Seizures Evolving into Secondarily Generalized Seizures

MECHANISMS

When focal seizures evolve into generalized seizures, it is assumed that some generalized seizure–generating mechanism is responsible for the characteristic tonic and clonic motor manifestations. The mechanisms and anatomical substrates for these events are not known; however, brain stem structures appear to be essential for generation of the tonic components, whereas the cortex probably mediates the clonic components (Chapter 4). Secondarily generalized seizures are most common with epileptogenic lesions in the frontal lobe and can occasionally be the only ictal manifestation of a frontal lobe lesion.

Figure 6–6. Examples of EEG telemetry-recorded ictal onsets from four patients with temporal lobe seizures. **A.** Low-voltage 6- to 7-Hz rhythmic activity appears at the right sphenoidal electrode (*arrow*) 5 seconds before it is seen over the right temporal convexity. **B.** After a diffuse burst of muscle and eye movement artifact, low-voltage fast activity is recorded by the right sphenoidal electrode (*arrow*). This becomes progressively slower, and the amplitude increases; 5 seconds later it is seen diffusely over the right hemisphere. **C.** Irregular, sharply contoured slow waves demonstrate phase reversal at the right sphenoidal electrode (*arrow*) and are reflected as low-amplitude delta waves, without phase reversal, over the right hemisphere. **D.** In this lateralized but not localized ictal onset, voltage suppression and low-voltage fast activity occur over the right frontotemporal area and are best seen at the right sphenoidal electrode (*arrow*). This precedes by 3 seconds the appearance of diffuse 3-Hz spike-and-wave discharges, which are prominent from the right frontotemporal and sphenoidal derivations. After 10 seconds this latter activity evolves into high-voltage 7-Hz rhythmic activity, which phase reverses at the right sphenoidal electrode and laterally at the right anterior to midtemporal region. Patterns shown in **A** and **B** (initial focal onsets) and **D** (delayed focal onset) have more reliable localizing significance than the irregular delta pattern shown in **C**. (From Engel et al., 1983b, with permission.)

Table 6–3 Ictal and Postictal Lateralizing Signs and Symptoms

Primary sensory symptoms—contralateral
Clonic motor, especially Jacksonian
  march—contralateral
Versive head and eye turning before a secondarily
  generalized seizure, and with frontal (but not
  necessarily temporal) onset—contralateral
Dystonic posturing—contralateral
Unilateral automatism—ipsilateral
Postictal nose wipe—ipsilateral
Retching—right hemisphere
Aphasic features—language-dominant hemisphere

PHENOMENOLOGY

When focal seizures generalize, they do not have the features typical of generalized tonic-clonic seizure onsets but rather begin with irregular, usually asymmetrical clonic movements. Occasionally there is no tonic phase, suggesting that propagation from the limbic system can preferentially avoid brain stem structures that produce tonic events (Chapter 4). Secondarily generalized seizures often begin with contralateral tonic version of the head and eyes and sometimes the whole body. Typically, there is brief flexion of the body and extremities, which can be followed by extension of one upper extremity, usually contralateral to the site of ictal onset, while the ipsilateral limb remains flexed—referred to as the *figure 4 sign*—before the period of bilateral upper extremity tonic extension (Kotagal et al., 2000) (Fig. 6–8). Most secondarily generalized seizures eventually evolve into tonic-clonic events that have behavioral and EEG features similar to those

described for generalized tonic-clonic seizures in the next section. However, clonic-tonic-clonic seizures, tonic seizures, clonic seizures, unilateral or incomplete tonic or clonic seizures, and other, less organized generalized motor manifestations can be seen.

CLINICAL CONSIDERATIONS

Although secondarily generalized seizures occur at some time in most patients with focal seizures, they are infrequent and are usually easily controlled by antiseizure medication. Secondarily generalized seizures occur more often in children than in adults and are the predominant seizure type in 16% of the former and 9% of the latter (Gastaut et al., 1975). They can occasionally begin so rapidly that the initial focal symptomatology is not noted. In this situation, ictal EEG recordings or other tests are necessary to identify the focal onset and differentiate the seizure from one that is generalized from the start. When neuroimaging is negative, this distinction often cannot be made with certainty. The prognosis for focal seizures is worse if secondarily generalized seizures occur frequently (Schmidt et al., 1983).

GENERALIZED SEIZURES

Tonic-Clonic Seizures

MECHANISMS

Generalized tonic-clonic seizures (*GTS*), also referred to as *generalized tonic-clonic convulsions*, *major motor seizures*, and *grand mal*

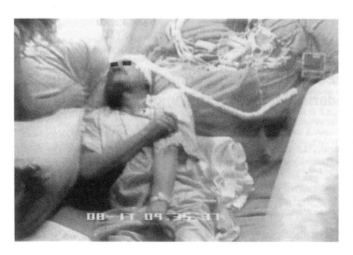

Figure 6–8. Asymmetric limb posturing during a secondarily generalized tonic-clonic seizure that began in the right occipital region. After version of the head and eyes to the left, the head returns to the midline, and the left arm is tonically extended while the right arm is flexed at the elbow. This posture resembles the figure 4. Thereafter both arms became tonically extended, followed by clonic jerking of the extremities and facial muscles. (From Kotagal at el., 2000, with permission.)

seizures, are the typical ictal expression of reactive seizures occurring in patients without a chronic epileptic condition (Zifkin and Dravet, 2008; Zifkin and Andermann, 2010). They also are considered to be the usual form taken by focal seizures that secondarily generalize (although that often does not happen, as noted previously). Consequently, the neuronal substrates required for this particular ictal expression appear to exist in the normal brain and can be engaged through a variety of initial mechanisms. Classical animal experiments indicate that the clonic component requires neocortex, whereas the tonic component is mediated through brain stem structures (Browning, 1985; Burnham, 1985; Browning, 1994; Morales et al., 2005) (Chapter 4). Why generalized motor seizures sometimes have only tonic or clonic, rather than tonic-clonic, components is not known. Generalized tonic-clonic seizures occur in both genetic epilepsies and epilepsy conditions associated with diffuse brain damage. In the former, the basic defects involve various global molecular disturbances, often consisting of channelopathies or neurotransmitter dysfunction (Chapters 4 and 5), but remain for the most part undetermined, whereas in the latter the structural or metabolic cortical disturbance is presumably so diffuse or widespread and multifocal that epileptic seizures appear to begin in a generalized fashion. Some localized epileptogenic lesions, particularly those in the frontal lobe, have preferential projections to structures responsible for generalized tonic-clonic seizures. Lesions in these areas can give rise to seizures that generalize so rapidly they appear to be generalized from the start (Bancaud et al., 1974).

PHENOMENOLOGY

Generalized tonic-clonic seizures are the most common seizure type, because they are the characteristic manifestation of reactive seizures. Rarely, in patients with chronic generalized tonic-clonic seizures, there may be a nonspecific prodrome beginning hours before seizure onset. This is not an aura in the usual sense; it probably reflects a state change that predisposes to seizures rather than an ictal phenomenon (Chapter 9). Much more often, however, the seizures begin suddenly, without warning, and follow a stereotyped pattern (Fig. 6–9). Occasionally, the tonic phase is immediately preceded by one or more brief myoclonic jerks,

giving rise to a clonic-tonic-clonic ictal pattern. There is initial brief flexor spasm involving axial and then extremity muscles, associated with loss of consciousness, but this rapidly becomes extensor spasm. Typically, there is a cry resulting from tonic spasm of truncal muscles; upward deviation of the eyes, which usually remain open; pupillary dilatation; and rigidity of the jaw, which forcefully closes, often causing trauma to the sides of the tongue and the inside of the cheek. The resultant rigidity is eventually interrupted by brief, intermittent muscle relaxation, which creates the clonic phase. The periods of relaxation become longer and closer together, causing the clonic movements to decrease in frequency and duration until they cease completely. The tonic and clonic phases are associated with large increases in heart rate and blood pressure, glandular hypersecretion, and prolonged apnea leading to cyanosis. Incontinence commonly occurs at the beginning of the postictal period. Respiration returns postictally, but excessive salivation and flaccid pharyngeal musculature can lead to airway obstruction. Rarely, the motor manifestations can be so violent that they cause joint (usually shoulder) dislocation or spinal fractures. The ictal episode usually lasts for a minute or less, and a second tonic phase occasionally occurs. Postictal muscular flaccidity and coma lasts for a variable period of time. The patient is disoriented as consciousness is regained and frequently experiences a headache and fatigue. After a generalized tonic-clonic seizure, patients often fall into a deep sleep and can awaken minutes or hours later, at times with minimal symptoms.

EEG

The EEG correlate of the tonic phase consists of a buildup of generalized low-voltage fast activity, also called a *recruiting rhythm*. This typically evolves into a high-amplitude generalized polyspike or polyspike-and-wave discharge. The brief periods of muscular relaxation responsible for the jerking of the clonic phase of the seizure are associated with generalized EEG suppression, creating a pattern of high-amplitude polyspike or polyspike-and-wave discharges during muscular contraction alternating with low-amplitude slowing or EEG silence. Usually the clonic phase ends abruptly, referred to as *fit switch*, but gradual dissipation can also occur. Postictally, the EEG shows diffuse slowing (Fig. 6–10). PET scans carried

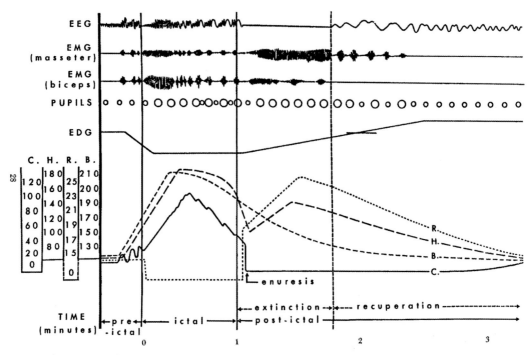

Figure 6–9. Schematic representation of a generalized tonic-clonic seizure. The immediate *preictal* period is often characterized by massive bilateral myoclonus (electromyogram [*EMG*]), and generalized polyspike discharges (*EEG*), a sudden fall in skin resistance (electrodermogram [*EDG*]), increases in systolic and diastolic blood pressure (*B*, blood pressure) and intravascular pressure (*C*, cystogram), and tachycardia (*H*, heart rate). The *seizure* proper lasts an average of a little less than a minute and is expressed in the EEG and EMG by sustained and then rhythmic discharges accompanied by marked vegetative phenomena: apnea (*R*, respiration), arterial hypertension (120 increasing to about 210 mm Hg, systolic), intravesicular hypertension (20 up to 100 cm H_2O), tachycardia (75 to 190 beats per minute [bpm]), drop in skin resistance, and mydriasis, which disappears rhythmically with each muscle relaxation of the clonic phase, producing hippus. Except for the apnea, which persists during the entire seizure, all autonomic changes attain their maxima, as indicated, at the end of the tonic phase and then progressively attenuate during the clonic phase. The immediate *postictal* period consists of complete electroencephalographic silence, a second phase of tonic muscular contraction of variable intensity and predominating in axial and head muscles (see masseter versus biceps EMG), recurrence of mydriasis, and intense tachycardia (140 bpm) with tachypnea (27 respirations per minute), respiration having returned after the last myoclonus. Only during the brief period (several seconds) between this final jerk and the reappearance of tonic spasm is the subject in complete muscular relaxation. Urinary incontinence may occur at this time because of the loss of sphincter muscle tone and be associated (as shown) with a drop of intravesicular pressure to zero. The recuperative phase contains a return to normal of all of the previously disturbed vegetative phenomena. Note the new episode of hippus, corresponding to rhythmic interruptions of mydriasis during each interval of muscle relaxation that interrupts the postictal hypertonic spasm. This spasm lasts longer in the masticatory muscles than in the limbs, where it is also less intense. The EEG exhibits slow-wave activity that later progressively accelerates until the normal cerebral rhythms return. (From Gastaut and Broughton, 1972, with permission.)

Figure 6–10. EEG correlate of a generalized convulsion. In this patient, electroconvulsive shock treatment (ECT) was administered under light methohexital anesthesia and mild succinylcholine paralysis. Consequently, muscle artifact is negligible. The EEG tracing begins immediately after the application of electroshock (*upper left*) and demonstrates a generalized recruiting rhythm, which gradually evolves into a bilaterally synchronous, 4-Hz polyspike-and-wave pattern. The generalized polyspikes and waves first increase and then decrease in amplitude, while decreasing in frequency, and ultimately stop suddenly (*bottom right*), to be replaced by postictal EEG depression. The clonic phase is not particularly marked in this example, in part because of the absence of muscle artifact. Three seconds are missing between the top and bottom panels. Calibration: 1 second, 100 μV.

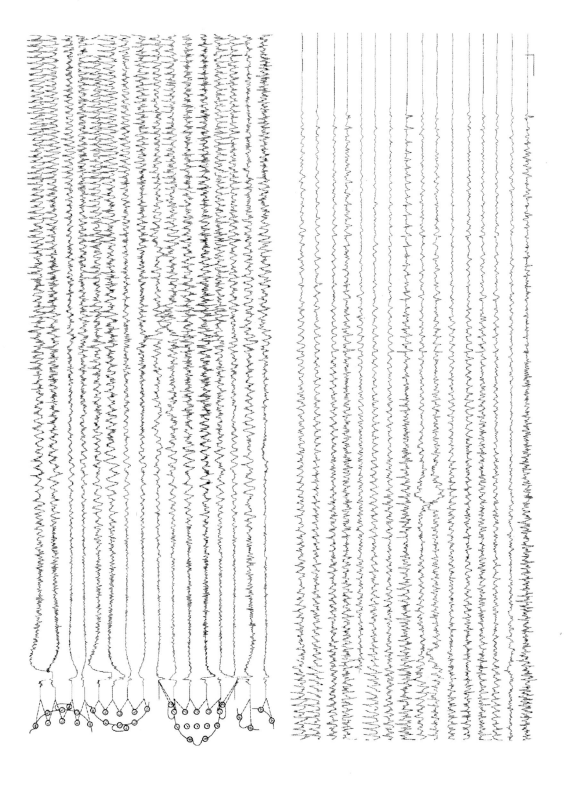

out during generalized tonic-clonic seizures induced by electroconvulsive shock treatment confirm diffuse brain involvement in both the ictal and postictal phases (Ackermann et al., 1986; Engel et al., 1982) (Fig. 6–11).

CLINICAL CONSIDERATIONS

Generalized tonic-clonic seizures are the predominant seizure type in approximately 10% of persons with chronic epilepsy (Gastaut et al., 1975) and in most persons who experience reactive seizures. Focal behavioral or EEG features seen at onset or postictally that are consistently lateralized indicate a focal seizure that has secondarily generalized. Initial focal features that are inconsistently lateralized and occur with equal frequency on both sides are not unusual with generalized tonic-clonic seizures. Generalized tonic-clonic seizures are controlled by anticonvulsant drugs in 60–80% of patients (Chadwick, 1985).

Typical Absence Seizures

MECHANISMS

Typical absence seizures, previously referred to as *petit mal seizures*, result from inherited diffuse epileptogenic disturbances of the brain and cannot be accounted for by observable structural lesions (Stefan et al., 2008; Camfield and Camfield, 2010). These seizures begin early in life and often resolve with time, presumably reflecting biochemical or microstructural abnormalities that disappear or are compensated for during development. The relevance of mechanisms elucidated in several animal models with absence-like seizures to the clinical condition has not been definitively demonstrated (Chapter 4). On the basis of these animal studies, however, most workers now regard absence seizures as responses of abnormal neocortex to synchronizing input from thalamus and brain stem (*corticoreticular epilepsy*) (Gloor et al., 1977; Quesney et al., 1977) and

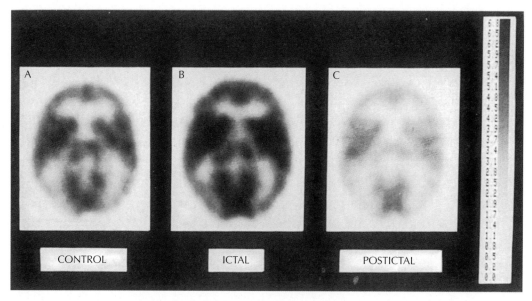

Figure 6–11. Representative sections from three FDG-PET scans of a patient undergoing ECT for depression. The control scan (**A**) was obtained when the patient was not undergoing ECT. The ictal scan (**B**), obtained when FDG was injected just before the seizure, shows a diffuse increase in the local cerebral metabolic rate for glucose, whereas the postictal scan (**C**), obtained when FDG was injected immediately after the electrographic seizure, at the beginning of postictal electroencephalographic depression, shows a diffuse decrease in local cerebral metabolic rate for glucose. The scale for the metabolic rate is in milligrams per minute per 100 g tissue. (From Engel et al., 1982, with permission.)

consider inhibitory events to play a prominent role in ictal manifestation (Gloor, 1979; Engel et al., 1981b; Fromm, 1986; Gloor and Fariello, 1988; McCormick and Contreras, 2001; Blumenfeld and Coulter, 2008) (Chapter 4). Typical petit mal absences are associated with diffuse increased metabolism on FDG-PET scans (Engel et al., 1985) (Fig. 6–12), which could indicate enhanced excitatory or inhibitory neuronal activity or both.

PHENOMENOLOGY

Typical absence seizures are characterized by lapses of consciousness that are sudden in onset and offset and rarely last longer than 10 seconds (Stefan et al., 2008). Absences associated with only impairment of consciousness constitute less than 10% of all absence seizures (Penry et al., 1975). Absences of this sort consist of sudden and complete cessation of all ongoing activities and a brief motionless stare. The eyes may rotate upward, and the eyelids may droop, but there are no other motor manifestations. The episode ends as suddenly as it begins. Afterward, the patient frequently is unaware that an absence has occurred and continues pre-ictal activities as though nothing had happened. Absences are much more often associated with a variety of additional signs and symptoms: clonic movements, increased or decreased postural tone, automatisms, and autonomic phenomena (Penry et al., 1975; Stefan et al., 2008).

Clonic manifestations of absences are bilaterally symmetrical. They most commonly involve the eyelids, producing rapid blinking, but can also involve other facial muscles, upper more than lower extremities, and at times even truncal muscles. In their most severe form, the clonic movements cause the patient to drop or fling objects held in the hand.

Increased tone can be asymmetrical, resulting in truncal arching and retropulsion, propulsion, and versive movements. Decrease in tone is most often manifested as head drop, although relaxation of the limbs and trunk also occur, on rare occasions causing patients to fall. Such absences may be mistaken for atonic (drop) attacks.

Automatisms during absences are not as rich in ictal symptomatology as those during limbic seizures but when present can have specific features that are identical to the latter, including oroalimentary and facial movements, fumbling, and humming. A variety of reactive automatisms can take the form of a continuation of ongoing behavior such as scratching or rocking; the patient might push a noxious stimulus away or take a stick of gum that is offered and chew it. Automatisms rarely begin at the onset of an absence and are more common when absences are prolonged.

Autonomic phenomena associated with absences include pallor, pupil dilatation, flushing, piloerection, tachycardia, salivation, and occasionally urinary incontinence.

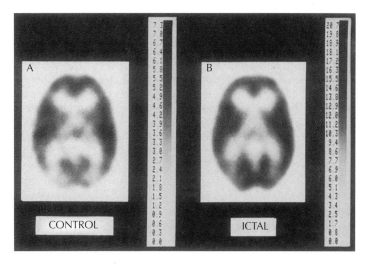

Figure 6–12. Representative sections from two FDG-PET scans of a child with petit mal absences. **A.** Control study, obtained several months after successful treatment, during 10 minutes of hyperventilation when no absences occurred. **B.** Ictal study, obtained before treatment, was instituted during 10 minutes of hyperventilation when absences were frequent. Note that the gray scales are different for the two studies and that although the patterns are identical, the ictal study shows a global threefold increase in estimated metabolic rate for glucose, indicated in milligrams per minute per 100 g tissue. (From Engel et al., 1982, with permission.)

EEG

Typical absence seizures are classically associated with regular, bilaterally synchronous, frontally predominant but generalized *3-Hz spike-and-wave discharges* (Fig. 6–13) that begin suddenly from normal background and end abruptly without postictal slowing or other EEG disturbances. These spike-and-wave discharges can be activated by hyperventilation and, in some patients, by eye closure and photic stimulation (Newmark and Penry, 1979) (Chapter 9). The relationship between the EEG discharge and the lapse of consciousness is inexact. Inattention may begin after onset of the EEG abnormality (Porter et al., 1973). Isolated spike-and-wave discharges or brief runs identical to ictal events are unassociated with a perceptible lapse of consciousness and occur at varying intervals as the only abnormality in the interictal EEG tracing. Distinction between ictal and interictal events in this situation, however, is unclear (Chapter 4). Whether detectable behavioral manifestations occur depends on the duration of the discharge (and on the sophistication of testing techniques).

Considerable variance from the classical bilaterally synchronous 3-Hz spike-and-wave EEG discharge is acceptable when clinical features otherwise suggest a diagnosis of a genetic absence epilepsy (Chapter 7). Patients can show some change in frequency during a prolonged burst, and a few high-amplitude slow waves without spikes can occur at the termination of an ictal episode. Spike-and-wave frequency can be 6–12 Hz in some patients, but frequencies that dip down below the 2.5-Hz range, characteristic of the *Lennox-Gastaut syndrome* (Chapter 7), rarely occur with typical absences. Slight asymmetries in time of onset or amplitude of spike-and-wave discharges are encountered with typical absence seizures, usually shifting from side to side. Bilaterally independent frontopolar spikes are not uncommon interictally in patients with typical absences. Spike-and-wave discharges become more irregular during sleep and commonly take on atypical patterns if the condition persists into adulthood. Such variant patterns can be referred to as *atypical spike-and-wave* but do not necessarily alter a diagnosis of typical absence if other features are consistent with a genetic absence syndrome (Chapter 7).

CLINICAL CONSIDERATIONS

Typical absences are the predominant seizure type in 15–20% of children with epilepsy (Gastaut et al., 1975) (Chapter 7). They are the principal symptoms of *childhood* and *juvenile absence (petit mal) epilepsy* and occur in 15% of patients with *juvenile myoclonic epilepsy*. Response to antiabsence drugs is usually excellent. Distinction between the typical absences described here and other absences described in the following sections is an important aspect of the differential diagnosis of genetic epilepsies with a relatively good prognosis and other epilepsies with a relatively poor prognosis (Chapter 7). Typical absences can be evoked in the examining room by hyperventilation and occasionally by photic stimulation; atypical absences are usually not induced in this manner. The remission rate has been reported to be as high as 80% for absences associated with impaired consciousness only and as low as 35% for absences with other features (Chadwick, 1985). Because the latter probably include atypical absences as well, absence type may not influence remission rate if only typical absences are considered (Sato et al., 1976).

Atypical Absence Seizures

MECHANISMS

Atypical absences usually occur in patients with diffuse or multifocal structural lesions of the brain (Stefan et al., 2008). Presumably, extensive cortical disruption is responsible for epileptic seizures being generalized rather than focal at onset. It is not known why these seizures manifest as absences with EEG spike-and-wave discharges rather than as tonic-clonic events. The neuronal mechanisms underlying atypical absences are not identical to those underlying typical absences and appear to involve limbic as well as thalamocortical circuits. Unique mechanisms are implied by the fact that antiabsence medications are not necessarily effective against atypical absences (Chapter 14). Atypical absences have a much greater tendency than typical absences to develop into absence status, and there could be a relationship between atypical absence status and frontal lobe limbic status (Chapter 10).

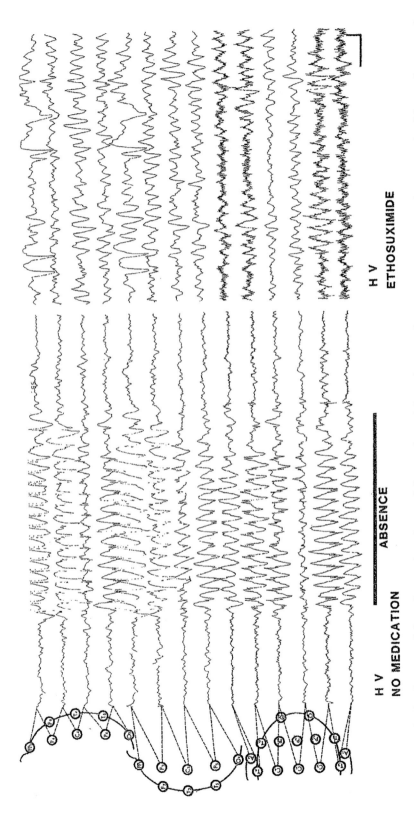

Figure 6–13. *Left*: The electroencephalographic correlate of a typical absence observed during hyperventilation prior to treatment. *Right*: An example of slowing that occurred during hyperventilation in the same patient several months after successful treatment with ethosuximide. These EEGs were obtained during the FDG-PET scans shown in Figure 6–12. Calibration: 1 second, 100 μV. (From Engel et al., 1985, with permission.)

PHENOMENOLOGY

Behaviorally, atypical absences are almost always associated with motor signs, particularly changes in tone, which can be more pronounced than those occurring with typical absences. Atypical absences can have minor focal or lateralizing features. They often last longer than 10 seconds, onset and cessation are usually not as abrupt as with typical absences, and there commonly is some degree of postictal confusion. Consciousness is variably impaired during atypical absences. Both brief events and prolonged absence status can range from complete unresponsiveness to a barely recognizable dulling of mental capacity. Atypical absences are most likely to occur during drowsiness and on awakening but are not usually activated by hyperventilation or photic stimulation.

EEG

EEGs of patients with atypical absences characteristically show a generalized *slow spike-and-wave pattern* (Blume et al., 1973) at 2.5 Hz or less (Fig. 6–14). Other epileptiform transients can occur, such as diffuse polyspikes and polyspike-and-wave discharges, occasionally with focal features. The appearance of the slow spike-and-wave EEG pattern is not clearly associated with a change in clinical behavior, and it can be impossible to determine from the EEG alone whether an atypical absence has occurred. Interictal EEGs also usually show excessive slowing of baseline rhythms, often with a degree of focal or lateralized predominance.

CLINICAL CONSIDERATIONS

Atypical absences are characteristic of the *Lennox-Gastaut syndrome* and other epilepsies associated with diffuse brain disturbances and seizures beginning in childhood or adolescence. Recognizing atypical absences is important in differentiating these disorders from the more benign genetic epilepsies of childhood and adolescence (Chapter 7).

Myoclonic Absences

The term *myoclonic absences* refers to a specific type of absence associated with the syndrome of the same name (Stefan et al., 2008) (Chapter 7). These seizures are characterized by variable impairment of consciousness during which patients can continue to carry out simple normal activities. There are rhythmic myoclonic jerks lasting between 10 and 60 seconds, primarily involving shoulders, arms, and occasionally legs, as well as jerks of the head. Perioral myoclonias can be frequent, but eyelid twitching is rare. Tonic contractions can cause the arms to be slightly elevated. The motor manifestations are more pronounced than in typical and atypical absences and can be asymmetric

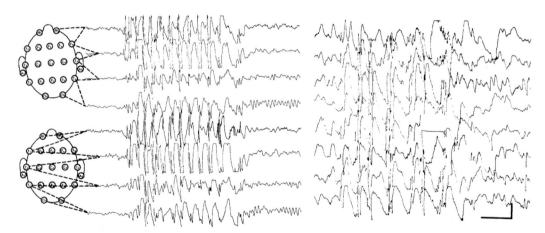

Figure 6–14. Segments from EEG recordings of two patients with absence seizures. *Left:* A well-organized, regular, symmetrical, and synchronous 3-Hz spike-and-wave discharge that begins and ends abruptly, characteristic of petit mal epilepsy. *Right:* A slower, poorly organized, and irregular spike-and-wave discharge characteristic of patients with atypical absences such as those seen with the Lennox-Gastaut syndrome. Calibration: 1 second, 100 µV.

or unilateral. Myoclonic absences are associated with bilateral, frontal-predominant 3-Hz spike-and-wave or polyspike-and-wave discharges on EEG. Response to medication is not as good as for typical absences but is better than for atypical absences.

Eyelid Myoclonia

Eyelid myoclonia characterize the condition of *eyelid myoclonus with absences*, or *Jeavons syndrome* (Jeavons, 1977; Duncan and Panayiotopoulos, 1996; Stefan et al., 2008) (Chapter 7). Because eyelid myoclonia are not always associated with absences, however, there is disagreement as to whether the seizures should be classified as absences or as myoclonic seizures. Eyelid myoclonia consists of brief episodes of marked jerks of the eyelids, often associated with upward deviation of the eyeballs and occasionally with retropulsion of the head. They typically occur after eye closure. Alteration of consciousness is not a consistent feature. Associated EEG abnormalities consist of generalized spike-and-wave discharges that are inhibited by total darkness. Studies with combined EEG and functional magnetic resonance imaging (fMRI) implicate involvement of the thalamus; mesial temporal, frontal, and parietal cortices; and cerebellum (Liu et al., 2008).

Myoclonic Seizures

The term *myoclonus* is applied to a class of motor symptoms characterized by quick muscle jerks due to both epileptic and nonepileptic mechanisms (Inoue et al., 2008; Nordli, 2010a). Myoclonus is discussed in more detail later in this chapter, but some specific myoclonic phenomena, referred to as *myoclonic seizures*, are considered to be forms of epileptic myoclonus, and three forms are included in the most recent list of ILAE-accepted seizure types (Berg et al., 2010). The most common are the massive myoclonic events of *myoclonic seizures per se*; the other two variant forms, *myoclonic atonic seizures* and *myoclonic tonic seizures*, are discussed in later sections. There continues to be debate concerning which myoclonic phenomena are epileptic and which are not.

MECHANISMS

Simultaneous EEG and *electromyography (EMG)*, *somatosensory evoked potentials (SEPs)*, C-reflex, and jerk-locked back averaging have been used to characterize three types of myoclonus: *cortical myoclonus*, *primary generalized epileptic myoclonus*, and *reticular myoclonus* (Guerrini et al., 2002; Inoue et al., 2008). Cortical myoclonus can be a fragment of focal epilepsy and includes the myoclonic phenomena of *epilepsia partialis continua* as well as other spontaneous focal myoclonic jerks such as *multifocal reflex* and *action myoclonus*. Primary generalized epileptic myoclonus and reticular myoclonus can be fragments of epileptic events associated with generalized epilepsies and in this situation are believed to reflect thalamocortical mechanisms similar to those seen with the absence epilepsies; however, consciousness is usually not impaired during the myoclonic jerks. Massive bilaterally synchronous epileptic myoclonus characterizes *juvenile myoclonic epilepsy*, *benign myoclonic epilepsy of infancy*, and *Dravet syndrome* but can occur with diffuse structural or metabolic disorders such as the *progressive myoclonus epilepsies* (Chapter 7). Nonepileptic myoclonus is discussed in the section on myoclonus later in this chapter.

Massive bilateral myoclonic jerks can occur repetitively without alteration in consciousness, which indicates that the pathophysiological process, anatomical substrate, or both cannot be identical to those of other generalized epileptic seizures. Some myoclonic seizures resemble a normal startle reflex (Eaton, 1984), although careful evaluation reveals physiological differences (Wilkins et al., 1986) (Chapter 13). Mechanisms similar to those that give rise to certain forms of nonepileptic myoclonus (as discussed later in this chapter) could also play a role in some phenomena currently considered to be epileptic myoclonus. Consequently, enhanced subcortical excitability may be necessary in addition to epileptiform cortical disturbances for manifestation of myoclonic seizures.

PHENOMENOLOGY

Generalized myoclonic seizures are bilaterally synchronous jerks that can be single or repeated in trains (Gastaut, 1968). Muscle masses involved can be restricted, usually to periocular or facial muscles, or extensive, involving arms and legs, with falling or retropulsion. Myoclonic seizures are often provoked by simple sensory stimulation (Chapter 9), particularly photic stimulation. They typically occur in clear consciousness, although repeated events at one to five per second that last minutes or hours (*myoclonic status, myoclonic storm*) can be associated with some mental impairment.

Myoclonus and myoclonic phenomena remain poorly categorized with respect to which are epileptic phenomena and which are not (Shibasaki and Hallett, 2005). Massive bilaterally synchronous myoclonus, as seen with juvenile myoclonic epilepsy, is definitely classified as epileptic, as discussed later, but focal or multifocal myoclonic seizures also exist, and some of these might be considered epileptic. For instance, the motor manifestations of epilepsia partialis continua have been considered focal myoclonic seizures (Chapter 10). Focal *negative myoclonus* refers to brief lapses of postural control, similar to asterixis; however, these events can occur in association with EEG spike-and-wave discharges in certain epileptic conditions and could represent epileptic phenomena.

EEG

EEG shows bilaterally synchronous spike-and-wave discharges during myoclonic seizures, but the temporal relationship between EEG paroxysms and muscle jerks is not always fixed. Polyspikes can occur at double or triple the frequency of myoclonic jerks, usually at the beginning of a repeated train.

CLINICAL CONSIDERATIONS

Myoclonic seizures are the predominant seizure type in about 4% of patients with epilepsy (Gastaut et al., 1975). They typically occur in genetic generalized epilepsies but occasionally are seen in epilepsies caused by diffuse brain disturbances. They may be associated features of absences or atonic seizures and are the principal disturbance of juvenile myoclonic epilepsy (Chapter 7). Myoclonic seizures must be distinguished from other forms of nonepileptic myoclonus, which are more likely to be sporadic and multifocal, are often activated by movement, and are seen in a variety of disorders (see below and Chapter 7).

Myoclonic Atonic Seizures

Myoclonic atonic seizures, also called *myoclonic-astatic seizures*, occur in the syndrome of the same name (Chapter 7) and are also bilaterally synchronous events (Inoue et al., 2008). They differ from massive bilaterally synchronous myoclonic seizures in that the brief jerks involve more proximal muscles with head nodding and in that the jerks can include abrupt loss of muscle tone, causing falls. Injuries can be severe because the atonia prevents protective movements. Jerks typically last less than 100 msec and are associated with brief paroxysms of bilaterally synchronous spike-and-wave and polyspike-and-wave discharges on EEG. The jerk occurs during the spike and the atonia during the slow wave. These events can occur repetitively at approximately 3-Hz. It is unclear whether myoclonic atonic seizures represent a thalamocortical or a cortical form of myoclonus.

Myoclonic Tonic Seizures

Myoclonic tonic seizures are recently described ictal events noted in a few infants that begin after the first year of life. Several features distinguish them from *infantile spasms* of *West syndrome*: brief tonic or myoclonic onset is followed by behavioral arrest and slight decrease in body tone lasting less than 10 seconds associated with an electrodecremental response on EEG, sometimes with 20- to 25-Hz activity. There are interictal posterior epileptiform discharges but no *hypsarrhythmia* or *slow spike-and-wave activity*. Seizures tend to cluster with an irregular pattern. Patients have probable or known structural etiologies (Nordli et al., 2007).

Clonic Seizures

MECHANISMS

Mechanisms of *clonic seizures* are poorly understood (Dravet and Seino, 2008; Nordli, 2010d). These events resemble myoclonic seizures, but contractions are repeated at a regular rate of 0.2–5 per second. *Hemiclonic seizures*, involving one side of the body, also occur. In this situation, the underlying mechanisms are assumed to be similar to those of generalized epilepsies but limited to one hemisphere, as opposed to a focal mechanism.

PHENOMENOLOGY

Generalized clonic seizures are predominantly observed in infants and young children and are characterized by loss of consciousness, massive autonomic discharge, and rhythmically repeated bilateral clonic contractions (Dravet and Seino, 2008). The generalized clonic movements are often asymmetrical and can be unilateral (hemiclonic). Attacks can begin with sudden hypotonia or tonic spasm with falling. Motor manifestations can at times be chaotic, demonstrating extreme variability of amplitude, frequency, and spatial distribution. The ictal episode can be prolonged, causing bronchial secretions and respiratory distress. Consciousness during hemiclonic seizures is difficult to assess, and variations on this condition involve seizures that move from one side of the body to the other or that involve upper limbs on one side and lower limbs on the other. Hemiclonic seizures are usually followed by flaccid hemiplegia, and if prolonged they can evolve into a spastic hemiplegia, resulting in the *hemiconvulsion-hemiplegia-epilepsy (HHE)* syndrome (Chapter 7).

EEG

Ictal EEG patterns in clonic seizures are extremely variable, usually consisting of irregular spike-and-wave discharges. The EEG during hemiclonic seizures usually consists of bilateral slow waves with higher amplitude contralateral to the clonic movements.

CLINICAL CONSIDERATIONS

Generalized clonic seizures are a manifestation of a wide variety of conditions occurring in early childhood, ranging from relatively benign disorders such as febrile seizures to severe epilepsies due to toxic and metabolic encephalopathies. Hemiclonic seizures can be seen in the genetic focal epilepsies such as *benign epilepsy with centrotemporal spikes* and *Panayiotopoulos syndrome* (Chapter 7). Both

generalized clonic and hemiclonic seizures are often prolonged and can evolve into status epilepticus. Consequently, aggressive treatment is required. They respond well to intravenous benzodiazepines. Response to antiseizure medication in general depends on etiology.

Tonic Seizures

MECHANISMS

As with tonic-clonic seizures, most tonic seizures are believed to originate in brain stem structures (Fusco et al., 2008; Nordli, 2010c). Whereas a brain stem origin is accepted for tonic seizures in *early infantile epileptic encephalopathy, early myoclonic encephalopathy,* and the *Lennox-Gastaut syndrome,* a cortical mechanism is suspected for reflex tonic seizures, such as those seen in startle-induced epilepsy (Fusco et al., 2008). Corpus callosotomy can be effective in treating refractory tonic seizures of presumed brain stem origin, suggesting that their manifestation requires interhemispheric synchronization above the brain stem level.

PHENOMENOLOGY

Tonic seizures are brief events involving flexor contractions of axial and limb muscles, with a duration of 5–20 seconds, somewhat longer than that of myoclonic seizures and epileptic spasms. They typically occur early during non–rapid eye movement (non-REM) sleep, and when they occur during wakefulness, patients lose consciousness and can fall. Autonomic features include alterations in respiration with apnea, alterations in heart rate, pupillary dilatation, and facial flushing. Frequency and intensity vary greatly and more violent events can be followed by postictal drowsiness and sleep. Startle-induced tonic seizures involve predominantly postural muscles asymmetrically, causing the patient to assume particular postures.

EEG

In infants, tonic spasms are associated with a burst suppression EEG pattern, and the tonic seizure is associated with the burst. In older patients, the EEG correlate of tonic seizures is variable, usually consisting of rhythmic spiking or a desynchronized rhythm.

CLINICAL CONSIDERATIONS

Tonic seizures are the characteristic seizure type of severe epilepsies in infancy, particularly early infantile epileptic encephalopathy and early myoclonic encephalopathy associated with burst suppression EEG patterns, and also in older patients with Lennox-Gastaut syndrome and *startle-reflex epilepsy*. These are all severe epilepsy conditions associated with diffuse brain disturbances, developmental delay, and cognitive and neurological deficits. Seizures are often pharmacoresistant.

Atonic Seizures

MECHANISMS

There are no experimental animal models of atonic seizures, and the neuronal substrates of this sudden loss of tone are unknown (Tassinari et al., 2008; Nordli, 2010b; Oguni, 2010). Pathophysiological mechanisms similar to those that intersperse with muscular contraction during clonic seizures may be involved. Interhemispheric synchronization of discharges via the corpus callosum appears to be important, because section of this commissure has been relatively successful in abolishing atonic seizures clinically (Reeves, 1985; Spencer et al., 1987).

PHENOMENOLOGY

Atonic seizures consist of a sudden loss of tone in postural muscles (Tassinari et al., 2008). In some patients this can be preceded by one or more generalized clonic jerks (*myoclonic atonic seizures*), as discussed above. When atonic seizures are mild, the head drops, but in their more severe form, the patient suddenly collapses to the floor. The attack usually lasts only a few seconds and can be associated with briefly impaired consciousness but shows no noticeable postictal symptoms. Less commonly, atonic seizures can be prolonged; the patient suddenly falls to the floor and remains unconscious and flaccid for one or more minutes.

EEG

The ictal EEG can show polyspike-and-wave discharges or a suppression of electrical activity (*electrodecremental response*) at the time of the atonic seizure (see Fig. 6–16).

CLINICAL CONSIDERATIONS

Atonic seizures occur with generalized epilepsies due to diffuse brain disturbances and are a major cause of disability in the Lennox-Gastaut syndrome (Chapter 7). Frequent falls often result in injury. Drop attacks can be extremely difficult to treat medically but respond better than any other seizure type to *corpus callosum section* (Reeves, 1985; Spencer et al., 1987) (Chapter 16). *Felbamate* and *rufinamide* appear to be more effective against drop attacks than other antiseizure drugs (Chapter 15), and *vagus nerve stimulation* may be as effective as corpus callosotomy (Chapter 16).

UNCLASSIFIED SEIZURES

Epileptic Spasms

Infantile spasms were not included in the 1981 classification of epileptic seizures, because this condition was believed to be a syndrome rather than a seizure type (Chapter 4). The syndrome is now called *West syndrome*, and *epileptic spasms* are now recognized as an epileptic seizure type that is a characteristic of West syndrome but not necessarily limited to infancy (Engel, 2001, 2006; Berg et al., 2010). Because epileptic spasms can be both focal and generalized, the most recent ILAE report lists them separately as unclassified (Berg et al., 2010). The basic mechanisms of epileptic spasms are unknown, but in the infant they reflect an age-specific response to multiple pathological conditions, acquired and genetic, most likely involving more than one mechanism. It has also been suggested that the primary generators of these ictal phenomena are nonepileptic (Kellaway et al., 1983).

Although epileptic spasms as a recognized seizure type can occur in older children and even occasionally in adults (Tinuper et al., 2003), the classical form, which has been extensively studied, is the infantile form (Holmes et al., 2008; Nordli, 2010e). Consequently, this section is limited to a discussion of infantile spasms, which are also known as *tics de salaam* in French and *Blitz-Nick-Salaam Krampfe* in German. Infantile spasms have been electro-clinically characterized (Kellaway et al., 1979). They are almost always bilateral and sym-metrical and consist of a brief (less than 2 sec-ond) phasic event usually followed by a slower (2–10 second) tonic event. Akinesia (arrest) lasting up to 90 seconds may be seen after the spasm and sometimes appears in isolation. Mixed flexor-extensor spasms are more com-mon than flexor spasms, and extensor spasms occur least often. Most babies with infantile spasms experience more than one type of sei-zure. The classical *salaam*, or *jackknife, seizure* consists of flexion at the neck, waist, arms, and legs with abduction or adduction of the arms. Barely perceptible spasms can affect only selected areas such as face, neck, or abdomen. Spasms can be repetitive and occur hundreds of times a day, can cluster, or can occasionally, though rarely, appear as infrequently as once every several days. Infantile spasms occur more frequently on awakening from sleep and occasionally can be exacerbated by other forms of stimulation, such as sudden noise or feeding.

The baseline EEG in this disorder classi-cally shows *hypsarrhythmia* (Gibbs and Gibbs, 1952), continuous high-amplitude, irregular, and asynchronous sharp and slow waves occur-ring in a chaotic fashion (Fig. 6–15). The elec-trographic correlate of the spasm is usually a high-amplitude, frontally predominant delta wave followed by a brief cessation of activity, the electrodecremental response (Fig. 6–16). Generalized attenuation, fast activity, slow waves, and sharp and slow complexes, in com-bination or alone, can also occur during spasms, and electrodecremental responses can be seen without behavioral correlates (Kellaway et al., 1979). Hypsarrhythmia can be quite variable and can disappear at times, particularly dur-ing REM sleep. Hypsarrhythmia patterns that include some degree of organization have been referred to as *modified hypsarrhythmia* and have the same diagnostic and prognostic sig-nificance as hypsarrhythmia (Hrachovy et al., 1984). In some patients a burst suppression EEG pattern can indicate a poorer prognosis (Lombroso, 1983), whereas in others, particu-larly those with the so-called cryptogenic form of infantile spasms, the EEG may be more

normal, indicating a better prognosis (Lacy and Penry, 1976) (Chapter 7).

Reflex Seizures

Seizures that are objectively and consistently demonstrated to be evoked by a specific affer-ent stimulus or by activity of the patient are referred to as reflex seizures (Blume et al., 2001; Zifkin, 2010). The term *reflex seizures* denotes a precipitating factor, and the seizure type is defined according to the ictal manifesta-tions. Provocative stimuli can be simple sensory, such as flashing light or a startling event, or can be elaborate and structured, such as reading (Chapter 9). Reflex seizures occur in many epi-lepsy syndromes in which spontaneous seizures also occur, but reflex epilepsies also are recog-nized where virtually all seizures are precipi-tated by specific stimuli (Chapter 7).

Neonatal Seizures

In the past, seizures that occur during the neonatal period were considered to be phe-nomenologically distinct from epileptic events in older children and adults. However, neonatal seizures were not included in the 1981 International Classification of Epileptic Seizures (Commission on Classification and Terminology, 1981). The most recent report of the ILAE Commission on Classification and Terminology (Berg et al., 2010) states: "neonatal seizures are no longer regarded as a separate entity. Seizures in neonates can be classified within the proposed scheme." Nonetheless, many decades of work have been devoted to establishing approaches to defining and classi-fying what may be unique neonatal ictal phe-nomena (Mizrahi and Kellaway, 1987; Volpe, 1987; Mizrahi, 2010). In any event, the general neurological condition (Holmes, 1987; Volpe, 1987) and interictal EEG (Tharp, 1980; Tharp et al., 1981) are important for determining eti-ology and prognosis of seizures in the newborn (Chapter 7), and certain behavioral and EEG characteristics can be correlated with outcome (Mizrahi et al., 2008; Mizrahi, 2010).

According to Volpe's (1987) proposal for a classification of neonatal seizures (Table 6–4), *subtle seizures* are by far the most common ictal patterns. Outcome appears to be generally

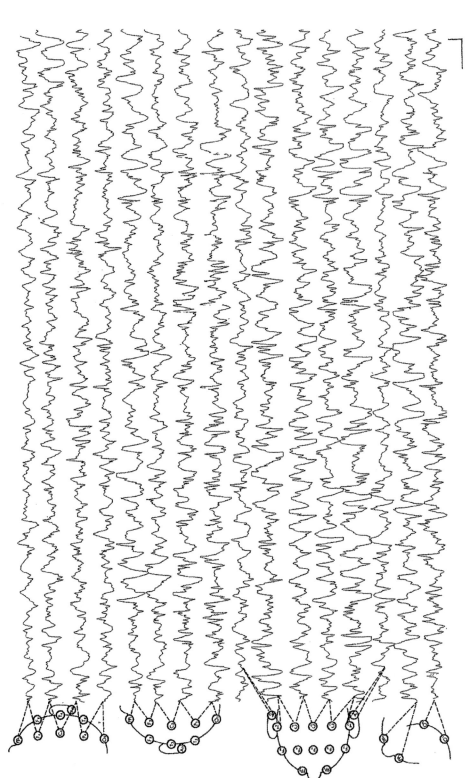

Figure 6–15. Hypsarrhythmic EEG with a chaotic high-amplitude, sharp- and slow-wave pattern. Note that the gain is approximately one-third that of the usual EEG setting. Calibration: 1 second, 300 μV.

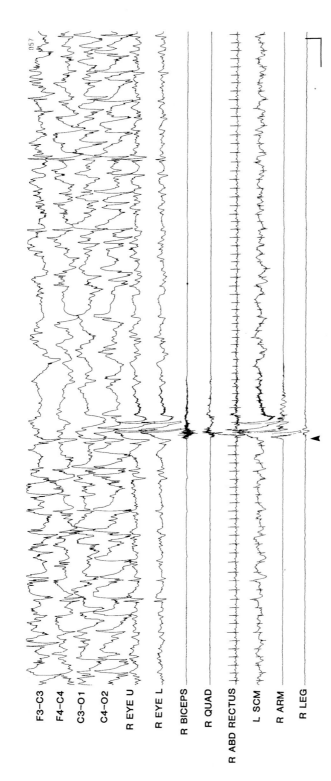

Figure 6–16. Hypsarrhythmic EEG with an electrodecremental response at the time of an infantile spasm beginning at the *arrowhead*. As with the previous figure, the gain is one-third that of the usual EEG setting, but paper speed is also slowed to 15 mm/sec. For eye movement channels, *U* indicates the upper canthus and *L* the lower canthus. EMG channels include right biceps, right quadriceps (*R QUAD*), right rectus abdominis (*R ABD RECTUS*), and left sternocleidomastoid (*L SCM*). Accelerometers record right arm and right leg movement. Calibration: 2 seconds and, for EEG only, 300 μV. (Recording courtesy of Dr. Alan Shewmon, University of California, Los Angeles.)

Table 6–4 Classification of Neonatal Seizures

Subtle seizures
  Premature and full-term infants
  Ocular-tonic horizontal deviation of the eyes with or without jerking; sustained eye opening with ocular fixation
  Eyelid blinking or fluttering
  Sucking, smacking, drooling, and other oral-buccal-lingual movements
  Swimming, rowing, and pedaling movements
  Apneic spells
Generalized tonic seizures
  Primarily premature infants
  Tonic extension of upper and lower limbs (mimics decerebrate posturing)
  Tonic flexion of upper limb and extension of lower limb (mimics decorticate posturing)
Multifocal clonic seizures
  Primarily full-term infants
  Multifocal clonic movements: simultaneous or in sequence
  Nonordered (non-Jacksonian) migration
Focal clonic seizures
  Full > premature infants
  Well-localized clonic jerking
  Infant usually not unconscious
Myoclonic seizures
  Premature and full-term infants
  Single or several synchronous jerks of flexion of upper > lower limb
  May presage hypsarrhythmia

From Volpe (1987), with permission.

Table 6–5 Classification of Neonatal Seizures Based on Electroclinical Findings

Clinical seizures with a consistent electrocortical signature (pathophysiology: Epileptic)
  Focal clonic
    Unifocal
    Multifocal
    Hemiconvulsive
    Axial
  Focal tonic
    Asymmetrical truncal posturing
    Limb posturing
    Sustained eye derivation
  Myoclonic
    Generalized
    Focal
  Spasms
    Flexor
    Extensor
    Mixed extensor/flexor
Clinical seizures without a consistent electrocortical signature (pathophysiology: Presumed nonepileptic)
  Myoclonic
    Generalized
    Focal
    Fragmentary
  Generalized tonic
    Flexor
    Extensor
    Mixed extensor/flexor
  Motor automatisms
    Oral-buccal-lingual movements
    Ocular signs (aside from sustained eye derivation)
    Progression movements
    Complex purposeless movements
Electrical seizures without clinical seizure activity

From Mizrahi and Kellaway, 1998, with permission.

worse for subtle, *generalized tonic*, and *myoclonic seizures* and generally better for *focal clonic seizures*.

Marked ictal EEG changes can occur in the absence of clinical alterations, and newborns who clinically appear to be having seizures may show no clear epileptiform abnormalities on the EEG (Tharp, 1980; Mizrahi and Kellaway, 1987). Mizrahi and Kellaway (1987, 1998) have proposed a classification based on the relationship between EEG seizure discharges and clinical behavior (Table 6–5). Seizures with closely correlated ictal EEG discharges, particularly clonic focal, tonic focal, and some myoclonic seizures, are associated with well-circumscribed pathological lesions and a favorable short-term outcome. Seizures with no or poorly correlated ictal EEG events, particularly so-called motor automatisms (*subtle seizures*), generalized tonic seizures, and some myoclonic seizures, are associated with diffuse encephalopathic processes and a poor short-term outcome. It has been suggested that seizures in this latter group may not reflect epileptic mechanisms, because their additional clinical features resemble brain stem release phenomena (Kellaway and Mizrahi, 1987; Mizrahi and Kellaway, 1987, 1998). These issues define an increasing role for EEG telemetry and video monitoring (Chapter 12) in the newborn nursery.

Differential diagnosis to exclude nonepileptic phenomena is important. The opisthotonic posturing associated with intraventricular hemorrhage (Mellits et al., 1981) and a poor prognosis is not considered to be a neonatal seizure. *Jitteriness*, a benign phenomenon commonly confused with seizures in the newborn (Chapter 13), is more likely to be stimulus-sensitive than are epileptic seizures and can be abolished by limb flexion or restraint.

Many normal and nonepileptic abnormal EEG phenomena in the newborn have sharp or spike-like configurations and are not interpreted as interictal epileptiform discharges. Consequently, the contribution of the EEG to a diagnosis of epilepsy at this age depends almost entirely on identification of clearly epileptiform *ictal* events (Fig. 6–17). The diagnostic and prognostic value of interictal EEG is based on interpretation of nonepileptiform abnormalities (Chapter 7). The field of neonatal EEG continues to evolve, and interpretation of recordings requires specialized training.

MYOCLONUS

Myoclonus is a nonspecific term used to define certain quick, involuntary muscle jerks (Fahn et al., 2002; Hallett and Shibasaki, 2008; Inoue et al., 2008). Myoclonus occurs with disorders involving all parts of the neuraxis and can usually be differentiated phenomenologically and electrophysiologically from other movement disorders, hyperreflexia, and fasciculations (Hallett et al., 1987). However, some forms of myoclonus and cerebellar dysmetria can be difficult to separate clinically but can be sorted out electrophysiologically. Relationships to normal and abnormal startle phenomena are discussed in Chapter 13. There is some disagreement regarding which forms of myoclonus are epileptic and which are nonepileptic, depending on the definition of epilepsy. For the purposes of this discussion, those myoclonic events that are regarded as fragments of epileptic seizures, as presented in the preceding sections on focal and generalized seizure types, will be called epileptic, and all other forms will be called nonepileptic, regardless of how they are classified by electrophysiological and etiological criteria (Hallett and Shibasaki, 2008; Inoue et al., 2008).

Myoclonus has been variously classified according to (1) the distribution of motor phenomena into focal, multifocal, unilateral, and generalized myoclonus, (2) the temporal features of the jerks, which may be random (*sporadic*) or rhythmic, (3) whether the jerks occur spontaneously or are provoked by voluntary movements (*action myoclonus*) or sensory stimulation (*reflex myoclonus*), and (4) the presumed anatomical substrates and pathophysiological mechanisms (Swanson et al., 1962; Halliday, 1967; Gastaut, 1968; Lance, 1968; Hallett, 1985; Fahn et al., 1986; Shibasaki and Hallett, 2005).

The phenomenological classification of myoclonus suggested by Gastaut (1968) over 40 years ago (Table 6–6) still provides useful concepts. The *massive and synchronous bilateral myoclonic jerk* of brief duration is the *massive myoclonic seizure* of the International Classification of Epileptic Seizures. The *long-duration* jerks of *infantile spasms* (Chapter 7) may be generated subcortically (Kellaway et al., 1983), and because of the long duration, most workers do not consider infantile spasms to be myoclonic phenomena. *Sporadic myoclonus* refers to multifocal jerks that occur randomly, affecting first one part of the body and then another. This is the cortical myoclonus seen in the progressive myoclonus epilepsies and in other myoclonic disorders unassociated with epilepsy (Chapter 7). Although cortical events appear to be involved in initiation, the pathological lesions are subcortical, and the mechanisms appear to be distinct from those of epilepsy. Therefore, persons with progressive myoclonus epilepsy might be viewed as having nonepileptic myoclonic disturbances reflecting subcortical mechanisms as well as epileptic disturbances reflecting cortical mechanisms. *Localized myoclonus* of cerebral origin is seen in two forms of epilepsia partialis continua, both of which may reflect epileptic mechanisms (Chapter 10). Localized myoclonus of spinal origin also occurs. *Rapid, rhythmic, bilateral myoclonus* usually repeats at two to eight jerks per second and is typified by *palatal myoclonus*. *Slow rhythmic* myoclonic jerks repeat at less than two per second and include the jerks of *Creutzfeldt-Jakob disease* and the acute postanoxic myoclonic symptoms associated with *pseudoperiodic* or *burst suppression* patterns on EEG (Chapters 10 and 13). Although the rhythmic movements of *subacute sclerosing panencephalitis* (SSPE) have also been placed in this category, most workers no longer consider this to be a form of myoclonus,

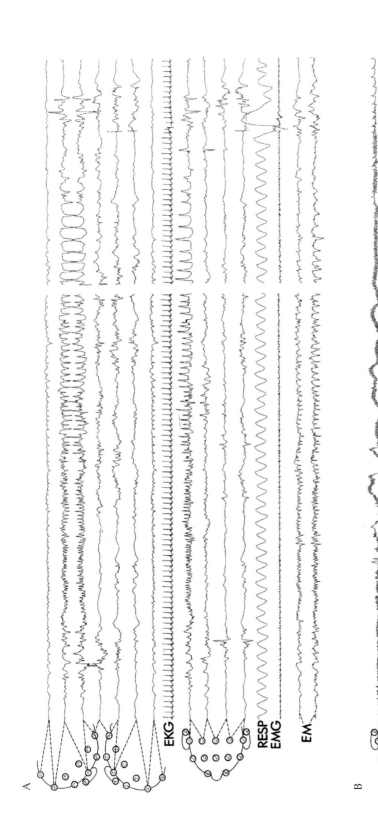

Figure 6–17. Segments from EEG recordings of newborn infants showing some unique features of neonatal seizures. None of these electrographic changes were associated with obvious clinical seizures, which illustrates the dissociations between EEG and behavioral ictal phenomena that occur in this age group. **A.** All the channels of an EEG recording of a full-term infant are shown to illustrate a typical montage, including electrocardiograph (*EKG*), respiration (*RESP*), electromyograph (*EMG*), and eye movement (*EM*) monitors. The first seven EEG channels consist of a "hatband" montage beginning and ending with O_1-O_2. For neonatal EEGs, FP_1 and FP_2 placement (channels 3, 4, and 5) is actually more posterior than shown here. Note the exquisite focality of this entire electrographic ictal event, even when it reaches high amplitude at the termination. The discharge is seen also in the channels used to record eye movement because eye monitor electrodes were referred to the right ear. Sixteen seconds have been removed at the gap in the tracing. **B.** Selected channels from an electrographic ictal event in a full-term infant demonstrate a prolonged period of highly regular 9-Hz sinusoidal activity, sometimes referred to as alphoid activity.

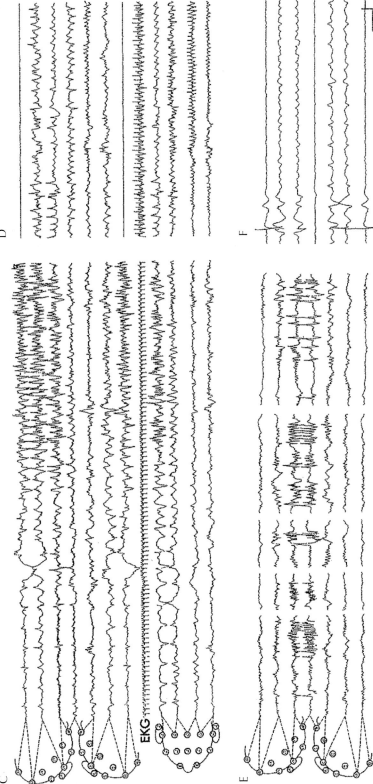

Figure 6–17. (Continued) C. An electrographic seizure begins in this full-term infant with a typical ictal pattern of slow, broad sharp waves, seen focally at C_4. After several seconds another typical ictal pattern, irregular mixed fast and sharp waves, appears posteriorly over the right hemisphere. **D.** Segment of an EEG showing another common feature of electrographic neonatal seizures, simultaneous independent focal discharges. In this full-term infant, continuous high-amplitude sharp waves are seen in the right temporal lobe, at the top of the tracing; then a lower-amplitude faster discharge begins independently in the left centrotemporal region, at the bottom of the tracing. Note that channels 1 and 7 are not recording. **E.** Five segments of a continuous tracing obtained from a full-term infant illustrate the variety of focal epileptiform discharges that can be seen from a single area of brain. The variability in duration as well as morphology of these events underlines the difficulty in distinguishing between interictal and ictal states in the neonate. **F.** Electrographic seizure recorded from a premature infant with a conceptual age of 30.5 weeks. The simple waveforms are typical of epileptiform EEG events in premature infants. Note the regular frequency and the independence of ictal patterns in the right and left temporal areas. All tracings were obtained at a paper speed of 15 mm/sec. Calibration: 2 seconds, 100 μV. (Courtesy of Dr. Alan Shewmon, University of California, Los Angeles.)

Table 6–6 Gastaut's Classification of Myoclonus

I. Spontaneous
  A. Intermittent
    1. Bilateral
      a. Massive and synchronous (*myoclonic jerk*)
        1) Brief duration (type A) (e.g., generalized familial, endogenous and exogenous toxins)
        2) Long duration (type B & C) (infantile spasms)
      b. Partial or segmental and asynchronous (*sporadic myoclonus*)
        1) With seizures (e.g., Lafora, some lipidoses, Unverricht-Lundborg)
        2) Without seizures (e.g., paramyoclonus multiplex of Friedreich)
    2. Unilateral (*localized myoclonus*)
      a. Cerebral origin (epilepsia partialis continua)
      b. Spinal origin
  B. Rhythmic
    1. Bilateral
      a. Rapid and partial (2–8 c/sec) (palatal, pharyngeal, laryngeal, diaphragmatic myoclonus)
      b. Massive and slow (<2 c/sec) (e.g., Creutzfeldt-Jakob, subacute sclerosing panencephalitis, acute postanoxic, some lipidoses)
    2. Unilateral
      a. Rapid and partial (asymmetrical form of bilateral)
      b. Massive and slow (asymmetrical form of bilateral, cerebral ischemia, and pseudoperiodic lateralized epileptiform discharges)

II. Provoked
  A. Massive bilateral provoked by light or sound (*reflex myoclonus*) (e.g., Tay-Sachs)
  B. Partial or segmental provoked by muscular activity (*action myoclonus*) (e.g., intoxication, posthypoxic, brain stem trauma, Wilson's, systems degeneration)

Neurological diseases in which myoclonus is an occasional feature:
  Encephalitis
  Cerebral atrophic and sclerosing diseases
  Miscellaneous degenerative diseases (e.g., Huntington's)
  Muscular diseases (e.g., McArdle's)

Adapted from Gastaut, 1968, with permission.

again because of the long duration. *Rhythmic unilateral myoclonus* occurs with acute focal brain damage and may be associated with *pseudoperiodic lateralized epileptiform discharges (PLEDs)* on the EEG (Chapter 13). *Reflex myoclonus* can be provoked by a variety of sensory modalities and overlaps with *hyperekplexia*, or *startle disease* (Chapter 13). The *action myoclonus of* acquired neurological disturbances such as *posthypoxic intention myoclonus (Lance-Adams syndrome)* (Chapter 7) may be due to lesions of subcortical structures such as cerebellum and thalamus.

Swanson et al. (1962) classified myoclonus as segmental or generalized. *Segmental myoclonus* is subcategorized as (1) brain stem myoclonus, involving the eyes, palate, jaw, face, neck, and tongue, and (2) spinal cord myoclonus, involving the limb, trunk, and diaphragm. Common causes of segmental myoclonus include vascular, infectious, demyelinating, neoplastic, and traumatic processes. *Generalized myoclonus* is subdivided into (1) acute and subacute, reflecting toxic, metabolic, and infectious disturbances of subcortical structures predominantly, and (2) chronic, including myoclonic symptoms of the progressive myoclonus epilepsies as well as *benign essential myoclonus*, which is likely a fragment of *dystonia*, and *periodic leg movements of sleep (PLMS)* (Chapter 7).

Electrophysiological features have also been used to differentiate myoclonic phenomena (Halliday, 1967; Hallett, 1985; Shibasaki, 1987; Shibasaki and Hallett, 2005). *Cortical myoclonus* can be focal or multifocal, SEPs are large, and the anatomical substrate is postulated to be hyperexcitability of motor cortex, sensory cortex, or both. Some forms of epilepsia partialis continua would be classified in this group.

Reticular reflex myoclonus involves the entire body (proximal muscles more than distal ones and flexor muscle groups more than extensors). Jerks are multifocal or generalized and can be provoked by somatosensory stimulation or action. The inconsistent temporal relationships between EEG discharges and electromyographic events, as well as the timing of activation of muscles innervated by cranial nerves, suggest a locus of hyperexcitability in the caudal brain stem. *Primary generalized epileptic myoclonus* can manifest as small, focal jerks resembling *minipolymyoclonus* similar to that seen with *motor neuron disease* or as massive bilaterally synchronous myoclonus. These are fragments of myoclonic seizures described above as a type of primarily generalized epileptic seizure and have a mechanism believed to be similar to that proposed for corticoreticular epilepsy (Gloor et al., 1982) (Chapter 4). As noted previously, the epilepsia partialis continua form of cortical reflex myoclonus and primary generalized epileptic myoclonus are considered to be epileptic phenomena here, but application of the term *epileptic* to reticular reflex myoclonus is based on evidence that the underlying neuronal mechanisms in the brain stem resemble those seen in the cortex with epilepsy.

There remains no clear basis for classifying all myoclonus mechanistically, for a variety of reasons, including (1) the phenomenological overlap between epileptic and myoclonic events, (2) the lack of definitive information concerning the anatomical substrates and pathophysiological mechanisms of most forms of myoclonus, and (3) the fact that myoclonic jerks, if they can be controlled at all by medication, generally respond to *clonazepam, valproic acid,* and occasionally *serotonin agonists* but not to other standard older antiseizure medications. Among the newer drugs, however, *levetiracetam, topiramate,* and *zonisamide* can be effective. A descriptive classification of myoclonic phenomena is useful, however, for categorizing and diagnosing specific myoclonic disorders that have known causes and outcomes (Chapter 7). Consequently, some familiarity with the variety of myoclonic phenomena and a common vocabulary to discuss them are necessary. Myoclonic phenomena that are clinically useful to recognize include (1) *massive and bilaterally synchronous myoclonic jerks,* which are often epileptic; (2) *sporadic*

myoclonus, which characterizes the nonepileptic myoclonic manifestations of benign essential myoclonus, posthypoxic myoclonus, and possibly the progressive myoclonus epilepsies, (3) *rapid rhythmic myoclonus,* which results from segmental myoclonic disturbances of the brain stem and spinal cord, and (4) myoclonic events that occur in association with bilateral or unilateral *periodic EEG discharges* in disorders such as Creutzfeldt-Jakob disease, some forms of epilepsia partialis continua, and acute cerebral hypoxia and ischemia.

SUMMARY AND CONCLUSIONS

The 1981 International Classification of Epileptic Seizures was based on descriptive phenomenology, necessitated by incomplete knowledge at the time concerning the pathophysiological basis and anatomical substrates of most human epileptic events. More recent efforts to revise this classification include attempts to define epileptic seizure types as unique diagnostic entities based on pathophysiological mechanisms and anatomical substrates. Diagnosis of a specific seizure type should inform etiology, therapy, and prognosis when a syndrome or disease diagnosis cannot be made. Whereas attempts to define seizure types as unique diagnostic entities have been relatively successful for most generalized ictal events, there remains no acceptable format for defining specific focal seizure types, although presumed pathophysiological mechanisms and underlying etiology will be more important than behavioral phenomenology for categorizing focal ictal events into unique diagnostic entities. An argument can be made for distinguishing neocortical from limbic seizures at a gross level; however, no other workable divisions have been accepted. It is clear that impairment of consciousness is not an appropriate criterion for classifying ictal events; however, it is an important descriptive factor for determining the disability associated with seizures in individual patients. Defining epileptic seizure types as unique diagnostic entities is important for several reasons:

1) Differential diagnosis between epileptic conditions and other disorders characterized by paroxysmal behavioral disturbances depends to a large extent on familiarity with the common

epileptic seizure patterns. A detailed understanding of seizure semiology helps physicians recognize epileptic phenomena, even if they have never seen them before.

2) Differential diagnosis between focal and generalized epileptic seizures in adolescents and adults is important because the former are more likely to result from discrete cerebral lesions that require specific treatment (e.g., brain tumors, vascular malformations, and localized infectious processes) and might indicate the need for a more detailed diagnostic evaluation. However, these pathological processes often cause generalized seizures in infants and children.

3) Current medical and surgical treatment of epilepsy is directed predominantly at the seizure type. Focal and generalized tonic-clonic seizures respond to one class of medications, absences to another, and myoclonic seizures to yet another. Certain forms of medically intractable focal and atonic seizures are likely to be amenable to surgical therapy, but surgery may also be an option for some causes of generalized seizures in infants and young children. The differential diagnosis between brief lapses of consciousness that might represent typical absences, atypical absences, or limbic seizures and the differential diagnosis between certain motor seizures and myoclonic phenomena are particularly important for determining prognosis as well as treatment. Consequently, a list of accepted epileptic seizure types as diagnostic entities can provide etiological, therapeutic, and prognostic information when a diagnosis of a specific epilepsy syndrome cannot be made.

4) Certain epilepsy syndromes are now recognized (Chapter 7). Their diagnosis, which carries etiological, prognostic, and therapeutic implications, depends heavily on accurate identification of specific ictal signs and symptoms of associated seizures.

The ultimate test of identifying specific epileptic seizure types as unique diagnostic entities is their clinical utility for determining etiology, prognosis, and management in individual patients. Efforts are aimed, therefore, at replacing phenomenological classifications with neurobiological ones. Research, however, is in turn determined to a large extent by the frames of reference imposed by existing approaches to classification and terminology. Consequently, premature acceptance of anatomical or pathophysiological schemes before

their accuracy is established could impede the conceptual development of both basic and clinical investigations of epilepsy.

REFERENCES

Ackermann, RF, Engel, J, Jr, and Baxter, L (1986). PET and autoradiographic studies of glucose utilization following electroconvulsive seizures in humans and rats. Ann N Y Acad Sci 462:263–269.

Ajmone-Marsan, C (1978). Clinical-electrographic correlations of partial seizures. In Modern Perspectives in Epilepsy: Proceedings of the Inaugural Symposium of the Canadian League Against Epilepsy. Edited by JA Wada. Montreal: Eden Press, pp. 76–98.

Ajmone-Marsan, C, and Ralston, BL (1957). The Epileptic Seizure: Its Functional Morphology and Diagnostic Significance: A Clinical-Electrographic Analysis of Metrazol-Induced Attacks. Springfield, IL: Charles C Thomas.

Bancaud, J, and Chauvel, P (1987). Commentary: Acute and chronic intracranial recording and stimulation with depth electrodes. In Surgical Treatment of the Epilepsies. Edited by J Engel, Jr. New York: Raven Press, pp. 289–296.

Bancaud, J, Talairach, J, Morel, P, Bresson, M, Bonis, A, Geier, S, Hemon, E, and Buser, P (1974). "Generalized" epileptic seizures elicited by electrical stimulation of the frontal lobe in man. Electroencephalogr Clin Neurophysiol 37:275–282.

Berg, AT, Berkovic, SF, Brodie, M, Buchhalter, J, Cross, JH, van Emde Boas, W, Engel, J, Jr, French, J, Glauser, TA, Mathern, GW, Moshé, SL, Nordli, D, Plouin, P, and Scheffer, IE (2010). Revidierte Terminologie und Konzepte zur Einteilung von epileptischen Anfällen und Epilepsien: Bericht der Klassifikations- und Terminologiekommission der Internationalen Liga gegen Epilepsie, 2005–2009. Akt Neurol 37:120–130.

Blume, WT, David, RB, and Gomez, MR (1973). Generalized sharp and slow wave complexes: Associated clinical features and long-term follow-up. Brain 96:289–306.

Blume, WT, Lüders, HO, Mizrahi, E, Tassinari, C, van Emde Boas, W, and Engel, J, Jr (2001). Glossary of descriptive terminology for ictal semiology: Report of the ILAE Task Force on Classification and Terminology. Epilepsia 42:1212–1218.

Blumenfeld, H (2011). Epilepsy and the consciousness system: Transient vegetative state? Neurol Clin 29:801–823.

Blumenfeld, H, and Coulter, DA (2008). Thalamocortical anatomy and physiology. In Epilepsy: A Comprehensive Textbook, 2nd ed. Edited by J Engel, Jr, and TA Pedley. Philadelphia: Lippincott Williams & Wilkins, pp. 353–366.

Browning, RA (1985). Role of the brain-stem reticular formation in tonic-clonic seizures: Lesion and pharmacological studies. Fed Proc 44:2425–2431.

Browning, RA (1994). Anatomy of generalized convulsive seizures. In Idiopathic Generalized Epilepsies: Clinical, Experimental and Genetic Aspects. Edited by A Malafosse, P Genton, E Hirsch, C Marescaux, et al. London: John Libbey, pp. 39–413.

Burnham, WM (1985). Core mechanisms in generalized convulsions. Fed Proc 44:2442–2445.

Caffi, J (1973). Zur Frage klinischer Anfallformen bei psychomotorischer Epilepsie. Schweiz Med Wochenschr 103:469–475.

Camfield, CS, and Camfield, PR (2010). Absence seizures. In Atlas of Epilepsies. Edited by CP Panayiotopoulos. London: Springer-Verlag, pp. 381–383.

Chadwick, D (1985). The discontinuation of antiepileptic therapy. In Recent Advances in Epilepsy 2. Edited by TA Pedley and BS Meldrum. New York: Churchill-Livingstone, pp. 111–124.

Commission on Classification and Terminology of the International League Against Epilepsy (1981). Proposal for revised clinical and electroencephalographic classification of epileptic seizures. Epilepsia 22:489–501.

Commission on Classification and Terminology of the International League Against Epilepsy (1985). Proposal for classification of epilepsies and epileptic syndromes. Epilepsia 26:268–278.

Dravet, C, and Seino, M (2008). Generalized clonic and hemiclonic seizures. In Epilepsy: A Comprehensive Textbook, 2nd ed. Edited by J Engel, Jr, and TA Pedley. Philadelphia: Lippincott Williams & Wilkins, pp. 563–571.

Duchowny, MD (1987). Complex partial seizures of infancy. Arch Neurol 44:911–914.

Duncan, JS, and Panayiotopoulos, CP (1996). Eyelid Myoclonia with Absences. London: John Libbey.

Eaton, RC (Ed) (1984). Neural Mechanisms of Startle Behavior. New York: Plenum Press.

Efron, R (1961). Post-epileptic paralysis: Theoretical critique and report of a case. Brain 84:381–394.

Engel, J, Jr (1987a). New concepts of the epileptic focus. In The Epileptic Focus. Edited by HG Wieser, E-G Speckmann, and J Engel, Jr. London: John Libbey, pp. 83–84.

Engel, J, Jr (Ed) (1987b). Surgical Treatment of the Epilepsies. New York: Raven Press.

Engel, J, Jr (2001). Classification of epileptic disorders. Epilepsia 42:316.

Engel, J, Jr (2006). Report of the ILAE Classification Core Group. Epilepsia 47:1558–1568.

Engel, J, Jr, and Crandall, PH (1983). Falsely localizing ictal onsets with depth EEG telemetry during anticonvulsant withdrawal. Epilepsia 24:344–355.

Engel, J, Jr, and Pedley, TA (Eds) (2008). Epilepsy: A Comprehensive Textbook, 2nd ed. Philadelphia: Lippincott Williams & Wilkins.

Engel, J, Jr, and Williamson, PD (2008). Limbic seizures. In Epilepsy: A Comprehensive Textbook, 2nd ed. Edited by J Engel, Jr, and TA Pedley. Philadelphia: Lippincott Williams & Wilkins, pp. 541–552.

Engel, J, Jr, and Wilson, CL (1986). Evidence for enhanced synaptic inhibition in epilepsy. In Neurotransmitters, Seizures and Epilepsy III. Edited by G Nistico, PL Morselli, KG Lloyd, RG Fariello, and J Engel, Jr. New York: Raven Press, pp. 1–13.

Engel, J, Jr, Ludwig, BI, and Fetell, M (1978). Prolonged partial complex status epilepticus: EEG and behavioral observations. Neurology 28:863–869.

Engel, J, Jr, Rausch, R, Lieb, JP, Kuhl, DE, and Crandall, PH (1981a). Correlation of criteria used for localizing epileptic foci in patients considered for surgical therapy of epilepsy. Ann Neurol 9:215–224.

Engel, J, Jr, Ackermann, RF, Caldecott-Hazard, S, and Kuhl, DE (1981b). Epileptic activation of antagonistic systems may explain paradoxical features of experimental and human epilepsy: A review and hypothesis. In Kindling 2. Edited by JA Wada. New York: Raven Press, 193–211.

Engel, J, Jr, Kuhl, DE, and Phelps, ME (1982). Patterns of human local cerebral glucose metabolism during epileptic seizures. Science 218:64–66.

Engel, J, Jr, Kuhl, DE, Phelps, ME, Rausch, R, and Nuwer, M (1983a). Local cerebral metabolism during partial seizures. Neurology 33:400–413.

Engel, J, Jr, Crandall, PH, and Rausch, R (1983b). The partial epilepsies. In The Clinical Neurosciences, Vol 2. Edited by RN Rosenberg. New York: Churchill Livingstone, pp. 1349–1380.

Engel, J, Jr, Lubens, P, Kuhl, DE, and Phelps, M (1985). Local cerebral metabolic rate for glucose during petit mal absences. Ann Neurol 17:121–128.

Fahn, S, Marsden, CD, and Van Woert, MH (1986). Definition and classification of myoclonus. Adv Neurol 43:1–5.

Fahn, S, Frucht, SJ, Hallett, M, and Truong, DD (Eds) (2002). Myoclonus and Paroxysmal Dyskinesias (Adv Neurol, Vol 89). Philadelphia: Lippincott Williams & Wilkins.

Falconer, MA, Driver, MV, and Serafetinides, EA (1962). Temporal lobe epilepsy due to distant lesions: Two cases relieved by operation. Brain 85:521–534.

Freeman, JL (2010). Gelastic seizures. In Atlas of Epilepsies. Edited by CP Panayiotopoulos. London: Springer-Verlag, pp. 479–481.

Freeman, JL, and Eeg-Olofsson, O (2008). Gelastic seizures. In Epilepsy: A Comprehensive Textbook, 2nd ed. Edited by J Engel, Jr, and TA Pedley. Philadelphia: Lippincott Williams & Wilkins, pp. 619–623.

Fromm, GH (1986). Role of inhibitory mechanisms in staring spells. J Clin Neurophysiol 3:297–311.

Fusco, L, Specchio, N, Yagi, K, Seino, M, and Vigevano, F (2008). Generalized tonic seizures. In Epilepsy: A Comprehensive Textbook, 2nd ed. Edited by J Engel, Jr, and TA Pedley. Philadelphia: Lippincott Williams & Wilkins, pp. 611–618.

Gastaut, H (1968). Semeiologie des myoclonies et nosologie analytique des syndromes myocloniques. Rev Neurol 119:1–30.

Gastaut, H, and Broughton, R (1972). Epileptic Seizures, Clinical and Electrographic Features, Diagnosis and Treatment. Springfield, IL: Charles C Thomas.

Gastaut, H, Gastaut, JL, Goncalves e Silva, GE, and Fernandez Sanchez, GR (1975). Relative frequency of different types of epilepsy: A study employing the classification of the International League Against Epilepsy. Epilepsia 16:457–461.

Gibbs, FA, and Gibbs, EL (1952). Epilepsy. Cambridge, MA: Addison-Wesley.

Gloor, P (1979). Generalized epilepsy with spike-and-wave discharge: A reinterpretation of its electrographic and clinical manifestations. Epilepsia 20:571–588.

Gloor, P, and Fariello, RG (1988). Generalized epilepsy: Some of its cellular mechanisms seem to differ from those of focal epilepsy. Trends Neurosci 11:63–68.

Gloor, P, Quesney, LF, and Zumstein, H (1977). Pathophysiology of generalized penicillin epilepsy in the cat: The role of cortical and subcortical structures. II. Topical applications of penicillin to the cerebral cortex and to subcortical structures. Electroencephalogr Clin Neurophysiol 43:79–94.

Gloor, P, Olivier, A, Quesney, LF, Andermann, F, and Horowitz, S (1982). The role of the limbic system in experimental phenomena of temporal lobe epilepsy. Ann Neurol 12:129–144.

Guerrini, R, Bonanni, P, Rothwell, L, et al. (2002). Myoclonus and epilepsy. In Epilepsy and Movement Disorders. Edited by R Guerrini, J Aicardi, F Andermann, et al. Cambridge, UK: Cambridge University Press, pp. 165–210.

Halgren, E, Walter, RD, Cherlow, DG, and Crandall, PH (1978). Mental phenomena evoked by electrical stimulation of the human hippocampal formation and amygdala. Brain 101:83–117.

Hallett, M (1985). Myoclonus: Relation to epilepsy. Epilepsia 26(suppl 1):S67–S77.

Hallett, M, and Shibasaki, H (2008). Myoclonus and myoclonic syndromes. In Epilepsy: A Comprehensive Textbook, 2nd ed. Edited by J Engel, Jr, and TA Pedley. Philadelphia: Lippincott Williams & Wilkins, pp. 2765–2770.

Hallett, M, Marsden, CD, and Fahn, S (1987). Myoclonus. In Handbook of Clinical Neurology, Vol 49 (Rev Ser, Vol 5). Edited by PJ Vinken, GW Bruyn, and HL Klawans. Amsterdam: Elsevier, pp. 609–625.

Halliday, AM (1967). The electrophysiological study of myoclonus in man. Brain 90:241–284.

Hausser-Hauw, C, and Bancaud, J (1987). Gustatory hallucinations in epileptic seizures: Electrophysiological, clinical, and anatomical correlates. Brain 110: 339–359.

Hirsch, E, Andermann, F, Chauvel, P, Engel, J, Jr, Lopes da Silva, F, and Lüders, H (Eds) (2006). Generalized Seizures: From Clinical Phenomenology to Underlying Systems and Networks. Montrouge, France: John Libbey Eurotext.

Holmes, GL (1987). Diagnosis and Management of Seizures in Children. Philadelphia: WB Saunders.

Holmes, GL, Dulac, O, and Vigevano, F (2008). Epileptic spasms. In Epilepsy: A Comprehensive Textbook, 2nd ed. Edited by J Engel, Jr, and TA Pedley. Philadelphia: Lippincott Williams & Wilkins, pp. 625–634.

Howe, JG, and Gibson, JD (1982). Uncinate seizures and tumors, a myth reexamined [letter]. Ann Neurol 12:227.

Hrachovy, RA, Frost, JD, and Kellaway, P (1984). Hypsarrhythmia: Variations on the theme. Epilepsia 25:317–325.

Inoue, Y, Terada, K, Dulac, O, Rubboli, G, and Tassinari, CA (2008). Generalized myoclonic seizures and negative myoclonus. In Epilepsy: A Comprehensive Textbook, 2nd ed. Edited by J Engel, Jr, and TA Pedley. Philadelphia: Lippincott Williams & Wilkins, pp. 585–599.

Jeavons, PM (1977). Nosological problems of myoclonic epilepsies in childhood and adolescence. Dev Med Child Neurol 19:3–8.

Jobst, BC (2010a). Focal tonic seizures. In Atlas of Epilepsies. Edited by CP Panayiotopoulos. London: Springer-Verlag, pp. 431–434.

Jobst, BC (2010b). Focal hyperkinetic seizures. In Atlas of Epilepsies. Edited by CP Panayiotopoulos. London: Springer-Verlag, pp. 437–440.

Jobst, BC (2010c). Focal seizures with auditory hallucinations. In Atlas of Epilepsies. Edited by CP Panayiotopoulos. London: Springer-Verlag, pp. 447–450.

Jobst, BC (2010d). Focal seizures with visual hallucinations. In Atlas of Epilepsies. Edited by CP Panayiotopoulos. London: Springer-Verlag, pp. 457–462.

Kellaway, P, and Mizrahi, EM (1987). Neonatal seizures. In Epilepsy: Electroclinical Syndromes. Edited by H Lüders and RP Lesser. London: Springer-Verlag, pp. 13–47.

Kellaway, P, Hrachovy, RA, Frost, JD, and Zion, T (1979). Precise characterization and quantification of infantile spasms. Ann Neurol 6:214–218.

Kellaway, P, Frost, JD, Jr, and Hrachovy, RA (1983). Infantile spasms. In Antiepileptic Drug Therapy in Pediatrics. Edited by PL Morselli, CE Pippenger, and JK Penry. New York: Raven Press, pp. 115–136.

Kotagal, P, and Lüders, HO (2008). Simple motor seizures. In Epilepsy: A Comprehensive Textbook, 2nd ed. Edited by J Engel, Jr, and TA Pedley. Philadelphia: Lippincott Williams & Wilkins, pp. 521–528.

Kotagal, P, Bleasel, A, Geller, E, Kankirawatana, P, Moorjani, BI, and Rybicki, L (2000). Lateralizing value of asymmetric tonic limb posturing observed in secondarily generalized tonic-clonic seizures. Epilepsia 41(4):457–462.

Lacy, JR, and Penry, JK (1976). Infantile Spasms. New York: Raven Press.

Lance, JW (1968). Myoclonic jerks and falls: Aetiology, classification and treatment. Med J Aust 1:113–120.

Lesser, RP, Lüders, H, Dinner, DS, and Morris, HH, III (1987). Simple partial seizures. In Epilepsy: Electroclinical Syndromes. Edited by H Lüders and RP Lesser. London: Springer-Verlag, pp. 223–278.

Lieb, JP, Joseph, JP, Engel, J, Jr, Walker, J, and Crandall, PH (1980). Sleep state and seizure foci related to depth spike activity in patients with temporal lobe epilepsy. Electroencephalogr Clin Neurophysiol 49:538–557.

Lieb, JP, Engel, J, Jr, and Babb, TL (1986). Interhemispheric propagation time of human hippocampal seizures: I. Relationship to surgical outcome. Epilepsia 27:286–293.

Liu, Y, Yang, T, Liao, W, et al. (2008). EEG-fMRI study of the ictal and interictal epileptic activity in patients with eyelid myoclonia with absences. Epilepsia 49:2078–2086.

Lombroso, CT (1983). A prospective study of infantile spasms: Clinical and therapeutic correlations. Epilepsia 24:135–158.

Lüders HO, Engel, J, Jr, and Munari, C (1993). General principles. In Surgical Treatment of the Epilepsies, 2nd ed. Edited by J Engel, Jr. New York: Raven Press, pp. 137–153.

Lüders, H, Acharya, J, Baumgartner, C, et al. (1998). Semiological seizure classification. Epilepsia 39:1006–1013.

McCormick, DA, and Contreras, D (2001). On the cellular and network bases of epileptic seizures. Annu Rev Physiol 63:815–846.

McLachlan, RS (1987). The significance of head and eye turning in seizures. Neurology 37:1617–1619.

Mellits, ED, Holden, KR, and Freeman, JM (1981). Neonatal seizures. II. Multivariate analysis of factors associated with outcome. Pediatrics 70:177–185.

Mizrahi, EM (2010). Neonatal seizures. In Atlas of Epilepsies. Edited by CP Panayiotopoulos. London: Springer-Verlag, pp. 493–502.

Mizrahi, EM, and Kellaway, P (1987). Characterization and classification of neonatal seizures. Neurology 37:1837–1844.

Mizrahi, EM, and Kellaway, P (1998). Diagnosis and Management of Neonatal Seizures. Philadelphia: Lippincott-Raven.

Mizrahi, EM, Plouin, P, and Clancy, RR (2008). Neonatal seizures. In Epilepsy: A Comprehensive Textbook, 2nd ed. Edited by J Engel, Jr, and TA Pedley. Philadelphia: Lippincott Williams & Wilkins, pp. 639–658.

Morales, MF, Chavali, M, Mishra, PK, et al. (2005). A comprehensive electrographic and behavioral analysis of generalized tonic-clonic seizures of GEPR-9s. Brain Res 1033:1–12.

Munari, C, Talairach, J, Bonis, A, Szikla, G, and Bancaud, J (1980). Differential diagnosis between temporal and "perisylvian" epilepsy in a surgical perspective. Acta Neurochir Suppl 30:97–101.

Munari C, Kahane P, Francione S, et al. (1995). Role of the hypothalamic hamartoma in the genesis of gelastic fits (a video-stereo-EEG study). Electroencephalogr Clin Neurophysiol 95:154–160.

Newmark, ME, and Penry, JK (1979). Photosensitivity and Epilepsy: A Review. New York: Raven Press.

Nordli, DR, Jr, Korff, CM, Goldstein, J, et al. (2007). Letter to the editor. Epilepsia 48:206–208.

Nordli, DR, Jr (2010a). Generalized myoclonic seizures. In Atlas of Epilepsies. Edited by CP Panayiotopoulos. London: Springer-Verlag, pp. 385–388.

Nordli, DR, Jr (2010b). Atonic seizures. In Atlas of Epilepsies. Edited by CP Panayiotopoulos. London: Springer-Verlag, pp. 395–398.

Nordli, DR, Jr (2010c). Generalized tonic seizures. In Atlas of Epilepsies. Edited by CP Panayiotopoulos. London: Springer-Verlag, pp. 399–402.

Nordli, DR, Jr (2010d). Generalized clonic seizures. In Atlas of Epilepsies. Edited by CP Panayiotopoulos. London: Springer-Verlag, pp. 403–405.

Nordli, DR, Jr (2010e). Epileptic spasms. In Atlas of Epilepsies. Edited by CP Panayiotopoulos. London: Springer-Verlag, pp. 417–422.

Ochs, R, Gloor, P, Quesney, F, Ives, J, and Olivier, A (1984). Does head-turning during a seizure have lateralizing or localizing significance? Neurology 34:884–890.

Ogren, JA, Bragin, A, Wilson, CL, et al. (2009). Three-dimensional hippocampal atrophy maps distinguish two common temporal lobe seizure-onset patterns. Epilepsia 50:1361–1370.

Oguni, H (2010). Epileptic drop attacks. In Atlas of Epilepsies. Edited by CP Panayiotopoulos. London: Springer-Verlag, pp. 407–415.

Panayiotopoulos, CP (Ed) (2010). Atlas of Epilepsies. London: Springer-Verlag.

Penfield, W, and Jasper, H (1954). Epilepsy and the Functional Anatomy of the Human Brain. Boston: Little, Brown & Co.

Penry, JK, Porter, RJ, and Dreifuss, FE (1975). Simultaneous recording of absence seizures with video tape and electroencephalography: A study of 374 seizures in 48 patients. Brain 98:427–440.

Porter, RJ, Penry, JK, and Dreifuss, FE (1973). Responsiveness at the onset of spike wave bursts. Electroencephalogr Clin Neurophysiol 34:239–245.

Quesney, LF, Gloor, P, Kratzenberg, E, and Zumstein, H (1977). Pathophysiology of generalized penicillin epilepsy in the cat: The role of cortical and subcortical structures. I. Systemic application of penicillin. Electroencephalogr Clin Neurophysiol 42:640–655.

Racine, RJ (1972). Modification of seizure activity by electrical stimulation. II. Motor seizure. Electroencephalogr Clin Neurophysiol 32:281–294.

Reeves, AG (1985). Epilepsy and the Corpus Callosum. New York: Plenum Press.

Risinger, MW, Engel, J, Jr, Van Ness, PC, Henry, TR, and Crandall, PH (1989). Ictal localization of temporal lobe seizures. Neurology 39:1288–1293.

Roger, J (chairman) (November 1987). Summary of discussion of Commission of Classification and Terminology of the International League Against Epilepsy, Esclimont, France.

Sato, S, Dreifuss, FE, and Penry, JK (1976). Prognostic factors in absence seizures. Neurology 26:788–796.

Schmidt, D, Tsai, JJ, and Janz, D (1983). Generalized tonic-clonic seizures in patients with complex partial seizures: Natural history and prognostic relevance. Epilepsia 24:43–48.

Schmidt, D, Einicke, I, and Haenel, F (1986). The influence of seizure type on the efficacy of plasma concentrations of phenytoin, phenobarbital and carbamazepine. Arch Neurol 43:263–265.

Semah, F, Picot, M-C, Adam, C, Broglin, D, Arzimanoglou, A, Bazin, B, Cavalcanti, D, and Baulac, M (1998). Is the underlying cause of epilepsy a major prognostic factor for recurrence? Neurology 51:1256–1262.

Shibasaki, H (1987). Progressive myoclonic epilepsy. In Epilepsy: Electroclinical Syndromes. Edited by H Lüders and RP Lesser. London: Springer-Verlag, pp. 187–206.

Shibasaki, H, and Hallett, M (2005). Electrophysiological studies of myoclonus. Muscle Nerve 31:157–174.

Skidmore, CT (2010a). Focal myoclonic seizures. In Atlas of Epilepsies. Edited by CP Panayiotopoulos. London: Springer-Verlag, pp. 435–436.

Skidmore, CT (2010b). Focal inhibitory seizures. In Atlas of Epilepsies. Edited by CP Panayiotopoulos. London: Springer-Verlag, pp. 441–442.

Spencer, DD, Spencer, SS, Williamson, PD, and Mattson, RH (1983). Sexual automatisms in complex partial seizures. Neurology 33:527–533.

Spencer, SS, Gates, JR, Reeves, AR, Spencer, DD, Maxwell, RE, and Roberts, D (1987). Corpus callosum section. In Surgical Treatment of the Epilepsies. Edited by J Engel, Jr. New York: Raven Press, pp. 425–444.

Spencer, SS, Guimaraes, P, Katz, A, Kim, J, and Spencer, D (1992). Morphological patterns of seizures recorded intracranially. Epilepsia 33:537–545.

Sperling, MR (2010a). Focal clonic seizures. In Atlas of Epilepsies. Edited by CP Panayiotopoulos. London: Springer-Verlag, pp. 425–430.

Sperling, MR (2010b). Autonomic seizures. In Atlas of Epilepsies. Edited by CP Panayiotopoulos. London: Springer-Verlag, pp. 467–470.

Sperling, MR, Mendius, JR, and Engel, J, Jr (1986). Mesial temporal spikes: A simultaneous comparison of sphenoidal, nasopharyngeal, and ear electrodes. Epilepsia 27:81–86.

Stefan, H, Snead, OC, III, and Eeg-Olofsson, O (2008). Typical and atypical absence seizures, myoclonic absences, and eyelid myoclonia. In Epilepsy: A

Comprehensive Textbook, 2nd ed. Edited by J Engel, Jr, and TA Pedley. Philadelphia: Lippincott Williams & Wilkins, pp. 573–584.

Stern, JM (2010a). Focal seizures with gustatory hallucinations. In Atlas of Epilepsies. Edited by CP Panayiotopoulos. London: Springer-Verlag, pp. 451–452.

Stern, JM (2010b). Focal seizures with olfactory hallucinations. In Atlas of Epilepsies. Edited by CP Panayiotopoulos. London: Springer-Verlag, pp. 453–454.

Stern, JM (2010c). Focal vertiginous seizures. In Atlas of Epilepsies. Edited by CP Panayiotopoulos. London: Springer-Verlag, pp. 463–465.

Stern, JM (2010d). Aphasic seizures. In Atlas of Epilepsies. Edited by CP Panayiotopoulos. London: Springer-Verlag, pp. 471–473.

Stern, JM (2010e). Dyscognitive seizures. In Atlas of Epilepsies. Edited by CP Panayiotopoulos. London: Springer-Verlag, pp. 475–477.

Swanson, PD, Luttrell, CN, and Magladery, JW (1962). Myoclonus—A report of 67 cases and review of the literature. Medicine 41:339–356.

Tassinari, CA, Michelucci, R, Shigematsu, H, and Seino, M (2008). Atonic and myoclonic-atonic seizures. In Epilepsy: A Comprehensive Textbook, 2nd ed. Edited by J Engel, Jr, and TA Pedley. Philadelphia: Lippincott Williams & Wilkins, pp. 601–609.

Tharp B (1980). Neonatal and pediatric electroencephalography. In Electrodiagnosis in Clinical Neurology. Edited by MJ Aminoff. New York: Churchill Livingstone, pp. 67–117.

Tharp, BR, Cukier, F, and Monod, N (1981). The prognostic value of the electroencephalogram in premature infants. Electroencephalogr Clin Neurophysiol 51:219–236.

Tinuper, P, D'Orsi, G, Bisulli, F, et al. (2003). Malformations of cortical development in adult patients. Epileptic Disorders 5:S85–S90.

Van Buren, JM (1963). The abdominal aura: A study of abdominal sensations occurring in epilepsy and produced by depth stimulation. Electroencephalogr Clin Neurophysiol 15:1–19.

Van Ness, PC, Lesser, RP, and Duchowny, MS (2008). Neocortical sensory seizures. In Epilepsy: A Comprehensive Textbook, 2nd ed. Edited by J Engel, Jr, and TA Pedley. Philadelphia: Lippincott Williams & Wilkins, pp. 529–539.

Velasco, AL, Wilson, CL, Babb, TL, and Engel, J, Jr (2000). Functional and anatomic correlates of two frequently observed temporal lobe seizure-onset patterns. Neural Plast 7:49–63.

Volpe, JJ (1987). Neurology of the Newborn, 2nd ed. Philadelphia: WB Saunders.

Wada, JA (1980). Unilateral blinking as a lateralizing sign of complex partial seizure of temporal lobe origin. In Advances in Epileptology. Edited by JA Wada and JK Penry. New York: Raven Press, p 533.

Wieser, HG (1983). Electroclinical Features of the Psychomotor Seizure: A Stereoelectroencephalographic Study of Ictal Symptoms and Chronotopographical Seizure Patterns Including Clinical Effects of Intracerebral Stimulation. London: Butterworths.

Wieser, HG, Hailemariam, S, Regard, M, and Landis, T (1985). Unilateral limbic epileptic status activity: Stereo EEG, behavioral and cognitive data. Epilepsia 26:19–29.

Wilkins, DE, Hallett, M, and Weiss, MM (1986). Audiogenic startle reflex of man and its relationship to startle syndromes: A review. Brain 109:561–573.

Williamson, PD, Spencer, DD, Spencer, SS, Novelly, RA, and Mattson, RH (1985). Complex partial status epilepticus: A depth electrode study. Ann Neurol 28:647–654.

Williamson, PD, Wieser, HG, and Delgado-Escueta, AV (1987). Clinical characteristics of partial seizures. In Surgical Treatment of the Epilepsies. Edited by J Engel, Jr. New York: Raven Press, pp. 101–123.

Wilson, CL, Isokawa-Akesson, M, Babb, TL, Engel, J, Jr, Cahan, LD, and Crandall, PH (1987). A comparative view of local and interhemispheric limbic pathways in humans: An evoked potential analysis. In Fundamental Mechanisms of Human Brain Function. Edited by J Engel, Jr, GA Ojemann, HO Lüders, and PD Williamson. New York: Raven Press, pp. 27–38.

Wyllie, E, Lüders, H, Morris, HH, Lesser, RP, and Dinner, DS (1986). The lateralizing significance of versive head and eye movements during epileptic seizures. Neurology 36:606–611.

Young, GB, and Blume, WT (1983). Painful epileptic seizures. Brain 106:537–554.

Zangaladze, A (2010). Focal somatosensory seizures. In Atlas of Epilepsies. Edited by CP Panayiotopoulos. London: Springer-Verlag, pp. 443–446.

Zifkin, BG (2010). Reflex seizures. In Atlas of Epilepsies. Edited by CP Panayiotopoulos. London: Springer-Verlag, pp. 485–489.

Zifkin, BG, and Andermann, F (2010). Generalized tonic-clonic seizures. In Atlas of Epilepsies. Edited by CP Panayiotopoulos. London: Springer-Verlag, pp. 389–394.

Zifkin, BG, and Dravet, C (2008). Generalized tonic-clonic seizures. In Epilepsy: A Comprehensive Textbook, 2nd ed. Edited by J Engel, Jr, and TA Pedley. Philadelphia: Lippincott Williams & Wilkins, pp. 553–562.

Chapter 7

Epilepsy Syndromes

NEONATAL PERIOD
Benign Familial Neonatal Epilepsy
Early Myoclonic Epilepsy
Ohtahara Syndrome

INFANCY
Epilepsy of Infancy with Migrating Focal
   Seizures
West Syndrome
Myoclonic Epilepsy in Infancy
Benign Infantile Epilepsy and Benign
   Familial Infantile Epilepsy
Dravet Syndrome
Myoclonic Encephalopathy in
   Nonprogressive Disorders

CHILDHOOD
Febrile Seizures Plus
Panayiotopoulos Syndrome
Epilepsy with Myoclonic-Atonic Seizures
Benign Epilepsy with Centrotemporal Spikes
Autosomal Dominant Nocturnal Frontal
   Lobe Epilepsy
Late Childhood Occipital Epilepsy (Gastaut
   Type)
Epilepsy with Myoclonic Absences
Lennox-Gastaut Syndrome

Epileptic Encephalopathy with Continuous
   Spike-and-Wave During Sleep
Landau-Kleffner Syndrome
Childhood Absence Epilepsy

ADOLESCENCE-ADULT
Juvenile Absence Epilepsy
Juvenile Myoclonic Epilepsy
Epilepsy with Generalized Tonic-Clonic
   Seizures Alone
Progressive Myoclonus Epilepsies
Autosomal Dominant Epilepsy with Auditory
   Features
Other Familial Temporal Lobe Epilepsies

**SYNDROMES WITH LESS SPECIFIC AGE
   RELATIONSHIPS**
Familial Focal Epilepsy with Variable Foci
Reflex Epilepsies

DISTINCTIVE CONSTELLATIONS
Mesial Temporal Lobe Epilepsy with
   Hippocampal Sclerosis
Rasmussen Syndrome
Gelastic Seizures with Hypothalamic
   Hamartoma
Hemiconvulsion-Hemiplegia-Epilepsy (HHE)
Head Nodding Syndrome

CONDITIONS WITH EPILEPTIC SEIZURES THAT ARE TRADITIONALLY NOT DIAGNOSED AS FORMS OF EPILEPSY PER SE
Benign Neonatal Seizures
Febrile Seizures

Reactive Seizures
Neonatal Seizures Due to Structural and
  Metabolic Disorders
MYOCLONIC SYNDROMES
SUMMARY AND CONCLUSIONS

An epilepsy syndrome is a *symptom complex* the primary feature of which is the occurrence of electroclinically characteristic epileptic seizures (Aicardi, 1986; Engel, 2001a) (Chapter 1). Epilepsy syndromes, therefore, have also been referred to as *electroclinical syndromes* (Lüders and Lesser, 1987; Berg et al., 2010). The International League against Epilepsy (ILAE) has recently suggested that electroclinical syndromes be limited to those conditions where there are strong developmental or genetic components to the symptom complex and refers to clinically distinctive disorders based on specific lesions or other causes as *constellations* (Berg et al., 2010) (Chapter 1). The occurrence of a particular seizure type or anatomical location alone is not a *symptom complex* and does not constitute a syndrome. Therefore, there is no such syndrome as *frontal lobe epilepsy* or *temporal lobe epilepsy*, although there are various temporal lobe syndromes and constellations, and frontal lobe as well as occipital and parietal lobe syndromes will undoubtedly be defined in the future based on additional clinical features. Electroclinical syndromes and constellations will both be considered here as epilepsy syndromes. Epilepsy syndromes are distinct from specific *disease states* or *pathologically defined disorders*, such as *tuberous sclerosis* or *Aicardi's syndrome*, which are usually but not always associated with epileptic seizures (Chapter 5). An epilepsy syndrome is empirically identified and does not imply a common etiology (Lüders and Lesser, 1987; Engel and Pedley, 2008; Panayiotopoulos, 2010; Bureau et al., 2012; see also the electronic textbook MedLink [www.medlink.com]).

The list of recognized epilepsy syndromes has changed considerably since the 1989 International Classification of the Epilepsies and Epileptic Syndromes (Commission on Classification and Terminology, 1989) (Chapter 1), and this chapter considers as epilepsy syndromes those conditions recognized most recently by the ILAE as electroclinical syndromes and constellations (Berg et al., 2010)

(see Table 1–9). Because there is as yet no accepted new approach to classifying or categorizing epilepsy syndromes, they are discussed here in order of age of onset. In addition, two common syndromes associated with epileptic seizures that are not considered to be epilepsy because seizures are not enduring, *benign neonatal seizures* and *febrile seizures*, as well as conditions associated with reactive seizures and other neonatal seizures are discussed separately. Myoclonic syndromes are also considered. Videos of epileptic phenomena associated with specific epilepsy syndromes can be seen at www.epilepticdisorders.com.

As more information becomes available concerning the multifactorial basis of various epilepsy syndromes (Chapter 5), it is likely that most of the currently recognized syndromes and new syndromes yet to be described will eventually be categorized into logical groupings based on their interrelationships as natural classes (Engel, 2001a, 2006; Berg et al., 2010). Our understanding of the epilepsies could eventually permit a comprehensive classification, as was attempted in the 1989 classification, that will include useful diagnostic categories for patients who do not have a recognized epilepsy syndrome. Until then, however, discussion of specific epilepsy conditions is limited to those that are currently accepted, acknowledging that many patients, including most of those with adult onset epilepsy, will not have a syndromic diagnosis as described here. For these patients, evaluation, treatment, and prognosis will be based on diagnosis of a specific seizure type (Chapter 6).

NEONATAL PERIOD

Benign Familial Neonatal Epilepsy

A rare autosomal dominant disorder with high penetrance, *benign familial neonatal epilepsy (BFNE)*, manifests as multifocal clonic seizures two or three days after birth (Rett and Teubel,

1964; Bjerre and Corelius, 1968; Tibbles, 1980; Plouin, 1985, 2008; Nordli, 2010b; Plouin and Neubauer, 2012). This condition has no characteristic clinical or EEG features and can be diagnosed on the basis of a family history, exclusion of other causes of neonatal seizures, and the disappearance of seizures within a day or two. Recurrence of seizures later in life occurs in approximately 14% of patients (Tibbles, 1980). Incidence is 14.4 per 100,000 live births, and there is no gender preference (Nordli, 2010b). BFNE was the first known "genetic epilepsy" (Leppert et al., 1989) and was later shown to be due to defects in either of two potassium channel genes, *KCNQ2* and *KCNQ3* (Charlier et al., 1998; Singh et al., 1998). Genetic testing for diagnosis is useful, particularly with *KCNQ2* defects (Ottman et al., 2010) (Chapter 12).

Early Myoclonic Encephalopathy

Early myoclonic encephalopathy (EME) is a very rare disorder characterized by onset of erratic and massive myoclonic jerks and focal seizures within the first three months of life (Aicardi, 1985; Djukic et al., 2008; Ohtahara and Yamatogi, 2010a; Mizrahi and Milh, 2012). There is arrest of psychomotor development, and death may occur within the first year. EEG demonstrates profound diffuse epileptiform disturbances consisting of suppression burst activity that evolves into hypsarrhythmia (see Fig. 6–15). One or more hereditary inborn errors of metabolism are suspected, because of the frequent familial nature of this disorder. Known causes are *nonketotic hyperglycinemia, D-glyceric acidemia, propionic acidemia, methylmalonic acidemia*, and *impaired mitochondrial glutamate transport*; however, the etiology is usually undetermined. Incidence could be as high as 2–3% of neonatal epilepsy (Watanabe et al., 1999), and there is a slight male preponderance (Djukic et al., 2008). *Benign neonatal sleep myoclonus* (Resnick et al., 1986), described in the section on myoclonic syndromes later in this chapter, should not be confused with the early malignant epilepsy disorders.

Ohtahara Syndrome

The *early infantile epileptic encephalopathy (EIEE)* described by Ohtahara (Ohtahara et al., 1976; Ohtahara, 1978) is now recognized by many workers as a syndrome discrete from EME, although others suggest that both conditions are on a spectrum of one disorder. Ohtahara syndrome (OS) is characterized by the onset of frequent tonic spasms, often in clusters, associated with a suppression burst EEG pattern, within the first few months of life (Ohtahara et al., 2008; Ohtahara and Yamatogi, 2010b; Mizrahi and Milh, 2012). OS can be clinically differentiated from EME by the fact that seizures are tonic spasms rather than myoclonias and focal seizures. Some workers have suggested that in OS, EEG burst suppression is not accentuated during sleep, as it is in EME, but this has not been universally accepted. When etiologies are identified in infants with OS, they are usually structural brain lesions rather than metabolic disturbances. More recently, genetic testing has been useful in patients with *STXBP1* and *ARX* defects (Ottman et al., 2010) (Chapter 12). Seizures of OS are intractable, there is a high mortality rate, and survivors experience severe psychomotor retardation with common evolution to *West syndrome* and *Lennox-Gastaut syndrome (LGS)*. Incidence is very low, perhaps 2.5% of West syndrome cases, and there is no gender preference (Ohtahara et al., 2008).

INFANCY

Epilepsy of Infancy with Migrating Focal Seizures

Epilepsy of infancy with migrating focal seizures, also known as *migrating partial seizures of infancy (MPSI)*. Originally described by Coppola et al. (1995), it is now recognized by the ILAE as a syndrome but is extremely rare, with scarcely 60 cases reported in the literature (Cilio et al., 2008; Plouin, 2010a; Mizrahi and Mihl, 2012). It has a unique presentation in otherwise normal children within the first six months of life, as early as the neonatal period, of focal clonic motor seizures that migrate from one part of the body to the other and that can involve one limb or half the body, with head and eye deviations, autonomic features, and oroalimentary automatisms. Seizures can cluster, become very frequent, or constitute status epilepticus. The interictal EEG is initially normal but develops slowing over time, with multifocal spikes in the temporal, parietal and occipital areas and fluctuating spatial distribution of ictal discharges, which correlate with ictal behavior. Burst suppression and hypsarrhythmia are never seen in these patients. It is important to distinguish this condition of multifocal, bilaterally migrating epileptiform abnormalities from focal seizures due to localized lesions that are surgically remediable. Magnetic resonance imaging (MRI) is initially normal, but patients develop atrophy and microcephaly. The cause is unknown, but de novo *SCN1A* mutations have been identified in a few patients (Rojo et al., 2011). Conventional antiseizure drugs are usually ineffective, and *vigabatrin* and *carbamazepine* may worsen seizures. Cognitive neurological deterioration and hypotonia develop during the first year, and long-term prognosis is poor with continuation of pharmacoresistant seizures. The progression is believed to be due to the seizures, and this condition is classified as an epileptic encephalopathy.

West Syndrome

CLINICAL DESCRIPTION

Technically, *West syndrome (WS)* (West, 1841) is defined as consisting of three features: (1) a specific seizure type, *infantile spasms* (Chapter 6), (2) arrest of psychomotor development, and (3) a characteristic EEG pattern, *hypsarrhythmia* (Gastaut, 1973) (Chapter 6). In common current usage, however, the terms *West syndrome* and *infantile spasms* are employed interchangeably to identify the syndrome, and two of the three features are sufficient to make the diagnosis (Dreifuss, 1983; Jeavons, 1985; Aicardi, 1986; Westmoreland and Gomez, 1987; Dulac et al., 2008; Korff and Nordli, 2010b; Fusco et al., 2012).

Using the old terminology, *symptomatic* and *cryptogenic* subgroups of WS are recognized (Lacy and Penry, 1976; Dulac et al., 2008). The symptomatic subgroup is the most common form, with characteristic infantile spasms (Chapter 6) that appear in infants who are known to have cerebral disease. Developmental delay precedes the onset of seizures. Spasms usually begin before the age of 6 months and always before 1 year. They may be associated with further psychomotor retardation. Almost all patients in this subgroup demonstrate hypsarrhythmia or other severe EEG abnormalities.

The cryptogenic subgroup accounts for approximately 15–32% of infants with infantile spasms (Dulac et al., 2008). Development is normal until the onset of spasms, and there is no identifiable underlying disease process. Spasms begin somewhat later than in the symptomatic group and may not always be associated with severe mental or neurological abnormalities or hypsarrhythmia. With increasing diagnostic sophistication, more patients with cryptogenic WS are being classified as symptomatic (Jeavons, 1985; Dulac et al., 2008), and it is possible that in all such cases the syndrome is due to as yet unidentified cerebral diseases that are less severe than those that cause the symptomatic form.

Perhaps as many as 50% of patients with WS also exhibit other seizure types (Westmoreland and Gomez, 1987). They occur most often with the symptomatic form and commonly consist of generalized tonic-clonic and focal seizures.

EPIDEMIOLOGY

The incidence of WS is 3–4.5% per 100,000 live births (Korff and Nordli, 2010b) with a male-to-female ratio of almost 1.5:1 (Jeavons, 1985; Brna et al., 2001).

ETIOLOGY

WS of the symptomatic type results from a variety of prenatal, perinatal, and postnatal cerebral disturbances, including toxic and infectious processes, perinatal hypoxia and other trauma, and a number of congenital and inherited conditions, such as *tuberous sclerosis, Down syndrome, Aicardi syndrome, neurofibromatosis, malformations of cortical development (MCDs), hemimegalencephaly,* and *phenylketonuria*. Workup, therefore, should include X-ray computed tomography (CT) for intracerebral calcifications, MRI for cerebral malformations, and metabolic screening, including biopsy if appropriate. Concerns that infantile spasms might be caused by diphtheria-pertussis-tetanus (DPT) immunization have not been substantiated (Bellman et al., 1983; Cendes and Sankar, 2011) (Chapter 5). A family history of WS can be elicited for some patients, which likely reflects inheritance of a particular underlying disease process rather than of WS per se. However, a few rare genetic mutations, including one that affects a sodium channel subunit, have been reported (Korff and Nordli, 2010b), which could be viewed as susceptibility genes. *STK9* and *CDKLS* defects are responsible in some early-onset cases, and an *ARX* defect causes a rare X-linked condition. Genetic testing is useful to diagnose these disorders (Ottman et al., 2010) (Chapter 12). In most patients, the etiology appears to be multifactorial and may reflect subcortical as well as cortical disturbances (Kellaway et al., 1979) (Chapter 6). Cholinergic and monoaminergic mechanisms have been implicated, and specific developmental as well as immunological defects have been suggested (Hrachovy and Frost, 1988). Positron emission tomography (PET) studies of WS usually show diffuse cortical hypometabolism with relatively preserved basal ganglia metabolism; however, localized areas of cortical hypometabolism, particularly involving posterior cerebrum, can be seen in some patients (Chugani and Conti, 1996).

DIFFERENTIAL DIAGNOSIS

In most cases, WS is distinguished from the benign and severe myoclonic epilepsies of infancy by the characteristic features of the ictal events and the presence of hypsarrhythmia on the EEG. However, hypsarrhythmia does not always occur with WS, particularly of the cryptogenic type, whereas hypsarrhythmia can occur with other disorders, for instance, *Dravet syndrome*. Phenomenological distinction between these disorders is of less practical clinical value than identification of the underlying disease process.

A nonfamilial syndrome of *benign myoclonus of early infancy*, also referred to as *benign infantile spasms*, beginning at three to nine months after birth, has been described (Lombroso and Fejerman, 1977; Fejerman, 2008a). The movements may superficially resemble infantile spasms in their clinical features and patterns of occurrence but are actually sporadic, multifocal, myoclonic jerks with no EEG correlates. Symptoms subside considerably within a few months and disappear by 2 years of age. Although some babies can have pre-, peri-, or postnatal risk factors, laboratory studies, including EEG, are normal, and there is no associated developmental arrest or regression. Treatment appears to be

unnecessary. This differential diagnosis may be difficult when infantile spasms present with a normal initial EEG. The EEG does not remain normal for long, however, in WS.

TREATMENT

Specific therapy for the underlying cause can be successful in controlling infantile spasms. Otherwise, *vigabatrin* and *adrenocorticotropic hormone (ACTH)* are the treatments of choice (Mackay et al., 2004; Dulac et al., 2008; Pellock et al., 2010; Go et al., 2012). Both are effective, but both have potential severe side effects. Continued treatment with vigabatrin for more than six months produces constriction of visual fields in 10–40% of patients, but it remains uncertain how often this represents a noticeable deficit (Krauss et al., 1997). Treatment with vigabatrin is usually discontinued at six months. Mortality rate from steroid therapy can be as high as 2–5%. Response can depend on etiology; for instance, vigabatrin may be more effective than steroids in tuberous sclerosis.

Although debate persisted in the past concerning the relative merits of ACTH and *corticosteroids* (Hrachovy et al., 1983; Snead et al., 1983), most workers today prefer ACTH (Dreifuss, 1983; Holmes, 1986; Westmoreland and Gomez, 1987; Mackay et al., 2004; Pellock et al., 2010). However, the dosage and duration of treatment are controversial. From 20 to over 100 units per day have been recommended, and treatment has been continued from one week to 10 months after seizures cease. High doses can cause hypertension, and there is no evidence that longer treatment reduces the risk of relapse (Holmes, 1986). A typical intermediate treatment protocol has been recommended (Holmes, 1986): Treatment is begun with 40 units a day of a nonsynthetic ACTH gel intramuscularly. If seizures persist after two weeks, the dose is increased by 10 units a week until seizures stop or until a maximum of 80 units a day is reached. If treatment is effective, it is continued for one month and then tapered by 10 units a week. If seizures relapse, ACTH is reinstituted at the maximum previous dose, and the protocol is repeated.

If seizures persist after vigabatrin and the 80 units per day dose of ACTH is reached, treatment with *prednisone, lamotrigine, topiramate, zonisamide, pyridoxine, sulthiame, nitrazepam,* or *valproic acid* can be tried

(Chapter 15). Valproic acid is used only as a last resort by many pediatric neurologists, because of the increased incidence of hepatotoxicity in this age group (Dreifuss et al., 1987).

In recent years, surgical resection has played an increasing role in the treatment of WS, as a result of PET and later MRI evidence of localized lesions, usually MCDs (Sankar et al., 1995; Chugani and Conti, 1996). These multilobar disturbances are usually posterior and are characterized on intraoperative *electrocorticography (ECoG)* by localized attenuation of epileptiform activity, which is referred to as the *zone of cortical abnormality*, because the lesion itself does not appear to be epileptogenic (Shields et al., 1993). Over 70% of carefully selected patients can expect to become seizure-free on five-year follow-up following large multilobar resections or hemispherectomies, and successful surgery is usually accompanied by reversal of developmental delay (Hemb et al., 2010). This observation is the best evidence that the developmental delay in at least some children with WS is a direct effect of the epileptic activity rather than a consequence of the underlying disease process, leading to the concept of *epileptic encephalopathy* (Engel, 2001a) (Chapter 11).

PROGNOSIS

The response to treatment may be dramatic, with complete cessation of spasms and normalization of EEG within two weeks (often within a few days). This occurs most often in the cryptogenic subgroup when treatment is begun early in the course of the disorder. Treatment is less likely to be effective in the symptomatic group or when instituted late. Over 50% of patients in the symptomatic group who respond to treatment experience relapse after medication withdrawal, and reinstitution usually has no effect.

WS is reputed to have a mortality rate of 6–22% (Lacy and Penry, 1976; Holmes, 1987; Westmoreland and Gomez, 1987). Even when medical treatment effectively stops spasms and normalizes the EEG, mental retardation usually ensues. Because mortality and disability are due at least in part to the underlying cause of WS, there is a great difference between the cryptogenic and symptomatic subgroups. In the cryptogenic group, symptoms spontaneously remit between 2 and 5 years of age. Early therapy provides the best chance for a good outcome, although less than half of children who receive such treatment will exhibit normal or near-normal intelligence (Jeavons, 1985). In the symptomatic group, spasms also disappear, but they are usually replaced by other seizure types, and the condition evolves into LGS in many patients. Whether or not a chronic epilepsy condition develops, almost all of the children in the symptomatic group are rendered moderately or severely retarded by the epileptic encephalopathy and the underlying disease process.

Risk factors for a poorer outcome with respect to mental development include onset of spasms before the age of 3 months, the presence of other seizure types, a severely abnormal EEG pattern other than hypsarrhythmia, a history of preceding seizures or abnormal development, neurological abnormalities, severe initial mental retardation, and a longer duration of illness (Lombroso, 1983a; Jeavons, 1985).

Myoclonic Epilepsy in Infancy

The very rare syndrome of *myoclonic epilepsy in infancy (MEI)* is characterized by brief, bilaterally synchronous myoclonic jerks occurring in the first three years of life (Dravet and Vigevano, 2008; Covanis, 2010a; Guerrini and Dravet, 2012). Jerks may be precipitated by sound or contact in some patients. There is often a family history of epilepsy, and there may also be febrile seizures. This condition belongs to a group of syndromes referred to as *idiopathic generalized epilepsy (IGE)*, but no specific genetic basis or other etiological factors have yet been determined. Jerks are associated with generalized spike-and-wave and polyspike-and-wave EEG discharges against a normal background, most commonly seen during the early stages of sleep and at times provoked by photic stimulation. This condition was initially termed *benign myoclonic epilepsy in infancy*, but the qualification of "benign" has now been removed. Children are generally normal at the onset of seizures, and seizures are usually easily controlled with proper medication and spontaneously remit within a few years. However, there may be mild developmental delay as well as other behavioral disturbances, and some children can develop other seizure types in adolescence. MEI represents approximately 2% of all seizures beginning in infancy, and there is a male-to-female prevalence of 2:1. *Valproic acid* is the drug of choice, but *ethosuximide, levetiracetam, topiramate,* and *benzodiazepines* can also be effective. Symptoms become worse with the use of *carbamazepine, oxcarbazepine, vigabatrin, gabapentin,* and *tiagabine*.

Benign Infantile Epilepsy and Benign Familial Infantile Epilepsy

Benign infantile epilepsy (BIE) and *benign familial infantile epilepsy (BFIE)* are a group of conditions characterized by seizure onset during the first two years of life in otherwise normal children (Vigevano et al., 2008; Vigevano and Specchio, 2010; Vigevano et al., 2012). This can be an autosomal dominant trait or sporadic, with the seizures in the familial form occurring earlier. Seizures are focal, with or without generalization, and tend to occur in clusters. The interictal EEG is normal, and seizures are associated with unilateral slow waves and epileptiform discharges in the parietooccipital region. A variety of chromosomal loci have been identified for the familial form, and a mutation in the *SCN2A* gene was identified in one family (Striano et al., 2006). Seizures resolve spontaneously with excellent outcome and often do not require treatment, although when treatment is indicated, virtually all antiseizure drugs are effective. These disorders may be the third most common type of epilepsy in the first two years of life.

Dravet Syndrome

Severe myoclonic epilepsy of infancy (SMEI) was originally described by Dravet (1978), but because myoclonic seizures are not a consistent feature of the disorder, the name has since been changed to *Dravet syndrome (DS)* (Dravet and Bureau, 2008; Bureau et al., 2010; Guerrini et al., 2011; Dravet et al., 2012). It is characterized by mixed generalized and focal seizures beginning during the first year of life in a child who is developmentally normal. It is classified as an epileptic encephalopathy with developmental delay, progressive cognitive deterioration, and behavioral disturbances. DS

is of particular interest because it has a course that would suggest what previously would have been classified as a severe symptomatic epilepsy, but there are no specific underlying structural or metabolic abnormalities. Seventy percent to 80% of children with DS carry mutations in the sodium channel gene *SCN1A* (Claes et al., 2001), a small percentage of females carry *PCDH19* mutations, and rare *GABARG2* and *SCN1B* mutations have also been identified (Marini et al., 2011). Consequently, DS would correctly be grouped as an IGE, making the point that such conditions are not necessarily benign. The first seizure often begins with fever, and the course typically consists of three phases: a *febrile phase* beginning in the first year, a *catastrophic phase* with frequent seizures and cognitive deterioration lasting through the fourth year, and a *sequelae phase*, when seizures decrease in frequency and there is a plateau of the behavioral disturbances. Generalized clonic, tonic, hemiclonic, and massive myoclonic seizures can occur, as well as atonic and adversive focal seizures with or without automatisms and altered consciousness. The EEG consists of generalized interictal spike-and-wave and polyspike discharges as well as focal and multifocal spikes that are often photosensitive, against a slow background. The incidence of DS is less than 1 per 40,000, and males are twice as afflicted as females. *Valproic acid, benzodiazepines,* and *topiramate* are commonly used, but other, newer drugs can be helpful; *carbamazepine* and *lamotrigine* can aggravate seizures. Prognosis is poor, with persistence of seizures and psychomotor retardation. Genetic testing can diagnose 70–80% of patients (Ottman et al., 2010) (Chapter 12). Although seizures are pharmacoresistant, early diagnosis and treatment is believed to reduce long-term disability.

Myoclonic Encephalopathy in Nonprogressive Disorders

First described by Dalla Bernardina et al. (1980), the very rare disorder of *myoclonic encephalopathy in nonprogressive disorders* is characterized by repeated myoclonic status in infants and young children who have a nonprogressive encephalopathy, most commonly *Angelman syndrome, Rett syndrome,* or *4p chromosomal aberration*, or who have suffered perinatal hypoxia (Dalla Bernardina, 2008; Zafeiriou, 2010; Guerrini and Dravet, 2012). Seizures can begin between the ages of 1 month and 7 years, and three forms have been identified (Caraballo et al., 2007): (1) with absences, sequences of rhythmic and arrhythmic myoclonic jerks, and myoclonic absences, (2) with absence status, continuous negative rhythmic myoclonus and dyskinetic movements, and (3) with bilateral rhythmic myoclonus associated with rolandic spikes. The first occurs mostly with *Angelman syndrome*, and the second has a female predominance. Prolonged myoclonias involve face, eyelids, and distal limb muscles, but brief hemiclonic and focal motor seizures as well as massive myoclonus also occur. Multifocal slow spike-and-wave discharges on EEG are predominantly posterior and correlate poorly with myoclonic jerks. MRI usually reveals cortical atrophy and various MCDs. Perhaps less than 1% of children with pharmacoresistant epilepsies have this condition. *ACTH, benzodiazepines, valproic acid, ethosuximide,* and *levetiracetam* can provide transient benefit, and seizures can improve or disappear with age, but most children are left with severe mental and neurological impairment.

CHILDHOOD

Febrile Seizures Plus

Febrile seizures plus (FS+) was originally described as *generalized epilepsy with febrile seizures plus (GEFS+)* by Scheffer and Berkovic (1997) as a cluster of poorly defined conditions characterized by a genetic etiology that causes febrile seizures and afebrile seizures in some family members, febrile seizures alone in others, and afebrile seizures alone in still others (Scheffer and Berkovic, 2008; Nordli, 2010a; Camfield et al., 2012). Because it is now known that some individuals in these families can have focal seizures, the qualifier *generalized* should be omitted and it is now better referred to as *genetic epilepsy with febrile seizures plus*. Indeed, GEFS+ could eventually be viewed as a category of epilepsy conditions including specific syndromes such as DS and even some forms of *mesial temporal lobe epilepsy with hippocampal sclerosis (MTLE with HS)*. The

genetic etiology is complex, and several mutations have been identified. The most common is a mutation of the gene encoding the alpha-1 subunit of SCN1A, but other mutations of sodium channels as well as γ-aminobutyric acid (GABA) receptors have now been documented in families with this condition (Chapter 5). Genetic testing is useful in 10–15% of patients (Ottman et al., 2010) (Chapter 12). Many types of generalized seizures, as well as focal seizures, appear following febrile ictal events in otherwise normal children; interictal EEG may be normal, while ictal EEGs correlate with the seizure type; and neuroimaging is normal. GEFS+ was originally recognized through studies of large family kindreds, and family history can be important for making a diagnosis in an individual patients. However, epidemiological data such as incidence, prevalence, and gender preponderance have not been determined. Febrile seizures occur during the usual period of childhood, but occasionally before the age of 3 months or after 6 years, and there may be a delay between febrile seizures and the onset of afebrile seizures. GEFS+ is generally viewed as a benign condition; seizures may not require treatment and usually remit by adolescence with no behavioral sequelae. There is, however, a spectrum to this disorder, and more severe phenotypes exist, especially if other recognized syndromes associated with early febrile seizures, such as DS and MTLE with HS, are included in the category of GEFS+.

Panayiotopoulos Syndrome

Panayiotopoulos syndrome (PS) is a relatively common, often misdiagnosed, condition that was previously referred to as *early-onset benign childhood occipital epilepsy (Panayiotopoulos type)*, to distinguish it from *late-onset childhood occipital epilepsy (Gastaut type)*. The condition was not recognized as a distinctive form of what was then considered *focal idiopathic epilepsy* until relatively recently (Panayiotopoulos, 1989a;b; Fejerman, 2008c; Covanis, 2010b; Panayiotopoulos et al., 2012). It is characterized by onset in otherwise normal children of primarily autonomic seizures with pallor, agitation, nausea, and vomiting, with peak incidence between 4 and 5 years of age. There is usually eye deviation, with or without head deviation, which may be followed by impairment of consciousness. Unilateral clonic or tonic seizures and secondarily generalized tonic-clonic seizures occur in some patients, and there may be visual symptoms, incontinence, and migraine-like headaches. Nocturnal events are more common than diurnal seizures, and in some patients seizures may occur only in sleep. They are usually prolonged, lasting longer than five minutes, and at times longer than 30 minutes, constituting a form of status epilepticus. Interictal EEG reveals bilateral, multifocal spike-and-wave activity more prevalent occipitally that is increased during sleep and, exceptionally, with eye closure. Ictal EEG consists of rhythmic theta and delta activity. Neuroimaging is normal. PS is now recognized as the second most common, after *benign childhood epilepsy with centrotemporal spikes (BECTS)*, of what were previously considered focal idiopathic epilepsies, representing 22% of children with those conditions and 13% of all afebrile seizures in children between the ages 3 and 6. PS is believed to be genetic, and an *SCN1A* mutation has been described in one family; it affects both genders equally. Seizures are infrequent and may occur only once, so treatment is often not necessary; however, autonomic seizures present a risk of cardiorespiratory arrest. *Carbamazepine* and *valproic acid* are the treatments of choice. If seizures do recur, they usually remit within a few years, but atypical, more severe courses can occur with transition to other forms of genetic focal epilepsy.

Epilepsy with Myoclonic-Atonic Seizures

In *epilepsy with myoclonic-atonic seizures (EMAS)*, also called *epilepsy with myoclonic-astatic seizures*, children develop normally until onset, between 6 months and 5 years of age, of myoclonic-atonic seizures (drop attacks associated with initial myoclonic jerks) as well as myoclonic and atonic seizures in isolation, brief absences with myoclonic jerks, tonic seizures, and tonic-clonic seizures (Doose, 1985; Dulac and Kaminska, 2008; Korff and Nordli, 2010a; Guerrini and Dravet, 2012). Status epilepticus of minor seizures is a characteristic. The EEG shows regular and irregular bilaterally synchronous 2- to 3-Hz spike-and-wave and polyspike patterns with a 4- to 7-Hz background. Neuroimaging is normal. A family

history is common, and the disorder is believed to have a polygenetic mode of inheritance, at times associated with acquired factors. This entity may represent 1–2% of all childhood epilepsies, with a 3:1 prevalence of boys. Where it fits between the so-called IGEs and LGS is unclear. Seizures are pharmacoresistant, but *valproic acid, lamotrigine, ethosuximide, topiramate, levetiracetam*, and *clobazam* are effective for myoclonic seizures and nonconvulsive status epilepticus. *Carbamazepine, phenytoin*, and *vigabatrin* can exacerbate seizures. Half of patients improve on the *ketogenic diet*, and *glucose-transporter-1 (GLUT1) deficiency* is suspected in some (Mullen et al., 2011). Prognosis is variable and is worse with frequent generalized tonic-clonic seizures, absence status, onset of generalized tonic-clonic seizures during the first year of life, and persistent epileptiform and nonepileptiform EEG abnormalities. Seizures decrease in frequency during the first year and eventually remit in most patients. Only a minority develop pharmacoresistant seizures and cognitive disturbances.

Benign Epilepsy with Centrotemporal Spikes

CLINICAL DESCRIPTION

Benign epilepsy with centrotemporal spikes (BECTS), also called *rolandic epilepsy*, is a common, well-described syndrome beginning at 3 to 13 years of age (Lombroso, 1967; Lerman and Kivity, 1975; Lüders et al., 1987; Fejerman, 2008b, 2010; Panayiotopoulos et al., 2012). In the majority of patients, generalized nocturnal tonic-clonic seizures are the only manifestation of this disorder, but some show occasional focal seizures during wakefulness. The focal seizures occur independently on either side and are usually characterized by lingual or perioral somatosensory symptoms on one side, followed by anarthria, excessive pooling of saliva, and tonic or clonic movements of facial muscles on the same side as the sensory symptoms. These focal seizures occasionally can spread to other limbs or become generalized. There may be speech arrest, but consciousness remains intact unless secondarily generalized seizures occur.

Diagnosis of BECTS is based on the unique EEG pattern. The interictal EEG shows normal baseline rhythms with characteristic centrotemporal discharges. They typically consist of high-amplitude broad spikes or sharp waves with a peculiar horizontal dipole, being negative in the temporal region and positive over the frontal region (Gregory and Wong, 1984), followed by a large slow wave of opposite polarity and a small slow wave of the same polarity (Lüders et al., 1987) (Fig. 7–1). These transients usually occur frequently, often in runs, are activated by sleep, and are attenuated by proprioceptive input. Neither their frequency nor their lateralization necessarily correlates with ictal events, and like the seizures, they can shift from side to side. The location and waveform of these EEG events makes them easily distinguishable from the more anterior temporal interictal spikes of temporal lobe epilepsy. Attempts at source localization using magnetoencephalography (MEG) and functional magnetic resonance imaging (fMRI) have yielded conflicting results concerning their origin. Neuroimaging is normal.

EPIDEMIOLOGY

BECTS has been reported to account for one-quarter of epilepsies in children of school age (Cavazzutti, 1980). Since nocturnal seizures are likely to be missed, prevalence might be much greater than recognized.

ETIOLOGY

The centrotemporal spike trait has an autosomal dominant pattern of inheritance with variable penetrance (Heijbel et al., 1975). Seizures develop in only 25%, or perhaps fewer, of persons with this EEG trait (Bray and Wiser, 1964; 1965; Lüders et al., 1987). There is a well-documented association with febrile seizures (Lu et al., 1987), and an association with the absence epilepsies may exist, because some patients also demonstrate 3-Hz spike-and-wave EEG discharges (Bray and Wiser, 1965; Blom et al., 1972) (Chapter 5). More recent studies suggest the mode of inheritance is more complex than previously believed (Vadlamudi et al., 2006).

DIFFERENTIAL DIAGNOSIS

BECTS must be distinguished from other, more serious conditions. The diagnosis is usually easily made from description of the characteristic seizures and the typical EEG pattern; however, the presence of a temporal lobe EEG spike focus may lead to an erroneous diagnosis of temporal lobe epilepsy if the specific features of the EEG spike and the history are not recognized. A diagnosis of a generalized epilepsy syndrome in patients with only nocturnal seizures can be ruled out by the focal EEG pattern. Patients with *cerebral palsy* and *Rett syndrome* can have similar centrotemporal spikes without seizures (Chapter 13), and patients with only the benign trait have identical spikes without any neurological symptoms (Chapter 5).

TREATMENT

Treatment is not considered to be necessary after a single or rare seizures; it is begun only when frequent seizures occur or seizures are disruptive. *Carbamazepine* has traditionally been considered the drug of choice for this condition, but virtually all antiseizure drugs have been used effectively, and *sulthiame* is preferred by some workers. Medication regimens should be instituted slowly and designed to have as little adverse effect on behavior as possible. Drugs may be discontinued after three seizure-free years if the EEG is normal or after age 15, although the prognostic value of a persistent centrotemporal spike after this age in a patient who no longer has seizures remains to be determined (Lu et al., 1987).

PROGNOSIS

The prognosis for BECTS is excellent. The seizures are easily controlled with antiseizure medication and almost invariably disappear before the age of 15. There are no other associated symptoms. An atypical evolution with severe neuropsychological impairment that can persist occurs in a minority of patients, associated with continuous spike-and-wave discharges on the EEG during slow sleep as well as development of atonic and myoclonic seizures or prolonged status. It has been suggested that such atypical evolution can be heralded by an exacerbation of EEG discharges with older antiseizure drugs and some new ones such as *lamotrigine, oxcarbazepine,* and *gabapentin,* and that if such EEG changes occur, alternative treatment with *benzodiazepines* or *sulthiame* should be considered.

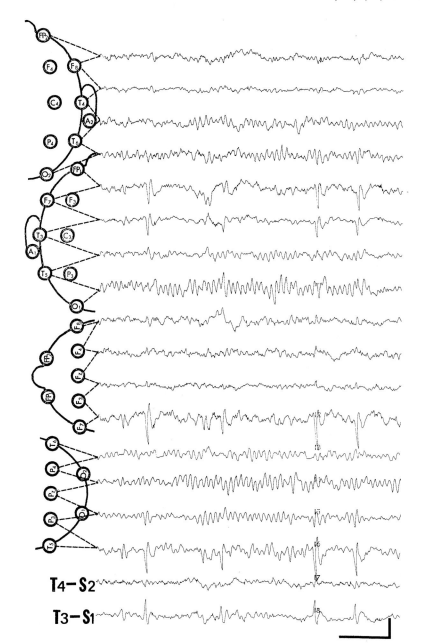

T4–S2

T3–S1

Figure 7–1. Typical EEG transients of benign childhood epilepsy with centrotemporal spikes. The left-sided spike is broad, with a horizontal dipole, negative in the midtemporal region and positive frontally. The sphenoidal channel at the bottom demonstrates that the negativity is lateral and not mesial. These spikes occur in children who have the characteristic seizure of this disorder and also in children with the genetic trait who do not have epileptic seizures. Calibration: 1 second, 100 μV. (From Engel, 1984, with permission.)

Autosomal Dominant Nocturnal Frontal Lobe Epilepsy

Autosomal dominant nocturnal frontal lobe epilepsy (ADNFLE) was originally described by

Lugaresi et al. (1986) as *nocturnal paroxysmal dystonia* and was only later recognized to be an epilepsy syndrome (Scheffer et al., 1994). It is extremely rare, with approximately 100 cases reported in the literature, but is important as the first epilepsy condition for which a specific genetic mutation was identified (Steinlein et al., 1995). Mutations have now been described in genes coding for three subunits, CHRNA4, CHRNB2, and CHRNA2, of the *nicotinic acetylcholine receptor* in a minority of ADNFLE families, and genetic heterogeneity is suspected. Animal studies suggest that activation of mutant nicotine receptors promote abnormal GABA-mediated hypersynchrony (Klaassen et al., 2006). ADNFLE is characterized by frequent nocturnal seizures beginning in childhood, although onset can range from infancy to adulthood. There are four seizure patterns: hyperkinetic seizures, asymmetric bilateral tonic seizures, paroxysmal arousal, and prolonged wandering episodes (Picard and Brodtkorb, 2008; 2010; Tinuper and Bisulli, 2010; Picard and Scheffer, 2012). Types of seizures and severity vary among patients, but seizures commonly occur at least once and sometimes several times each night, during non–rapid eye movement (non-REM) sleep. Interictal and sometimes ictal EEGs are normal, as is neuroimaging. Consequently, differential diagnosis from paroxysmal nonepileptic sleep disorders such as *parasomnias* and *REM behavior disorder* can be difficult (Chapter 13), particularly since approximately a third of patients have history of parasomnias, either in themselves or in a family member. Diagnosis is based on the characteristic ictal behaviors and may require video-EEG monitoring. Genetic testing is diagnostic in about 10% of patients (Ottman et al., 2010) (Chapter 12). *Carbamazepine* and *topiramate* can abolish seizures in a minority of patients and reduce the frequency in approximately half. Although surgical treatment can be beneficial in patients with some forms of nocturnal frontal lobe epilepsy (Nobile et al., 2007), there is no evidence to support its use in the genetic syndrome. Research is under way to determine whether approaches to administration of nicotine could be beneficial.

Late Childhood Occipital Epilepsy (Gastaut Type)

Late childhood occipital epilepsy (Gastaut type) is a rare familial disorder beginning in school-age children (Gastaut, 1982, 1985; Gobbi et al.,

2008; Kim and Nordli, 2010a; Panayiotopoulos et al., 2012). Ictal onset consists of stereotyped visual experiences, usually *positive elementary hallucinations* such as flashing colored lights or other unformed phenomena moving circularly in the periphery of one hemifield or *negative elementary hallucinations* such as unilateral blurring or hemianopsia. Either side can be involved. *Complex hallucinations* and *illusions* occur rarely, and temporooccipital connections appear to be involved in the pathophysiology. There may be associated eye findings such as blinking, eye deviation, or eye pain. These auras then evolve into hemiclonic motor seizures or automatisms with loss of consciousness. Postictally the patient often experiences headache, which has suggested a diagnosis of migraine rather than or in addition to epilepsy (Andermann and Lugaresi, 1987). Although the headaches are migrainous in nature, the auras are not typical of migraine (Chapter 13). High-amplitude EEG spike-and-wave discharges can be seen in the occipital region bilaterally or unilaterally with eye closure, and they spread to central and temporal regions during seizures. Neuroimaging is normal. This condition represents only about 2–3% of afebrile seizures in childhood. Treatment with most antiseizure drugs is effective. Sixty percent of patients experience complete control of seizures, which remit by late adolescence in over 95% (Gastaut and Zifkin, 1987). There is overlap between this syndrome, *childhood absence epilepsy (CAE)*, and BECTS (Gastaut and Zifkin, 1987). Some workers believe patients diagnosed with late childhood occipital epilepsy (Gastaut type) have either a variant form of BECTS or focal seizures due to an unrecognized occipital lesion (Lüders et al., 1987).

Epilepsy with Myoclonic Absences

In *epilepsy with myoclonic absences (EMA)*, absences associated with bilaterally synchronous rhythmic myoclonic jerks and tonic contractions begin between 11 months and 12 years of age (Tassinari and Bureau, 1985; Tassinari et al., 2008; Covanis, 2010f; Bureau and Tassinari, 2012). There may also be myoclonic jerks without absences. Seizures occur many times a day and can be precipitated by hyperventilation and occasionally by photic stimulation. Neuroimaging is normal. The

EEG shows bilaterally synchronous 3-Hz spike-and-wave discharges. This syndrome may account for 0.5–1% of all childhood epilepsies, with a preponderance in boys. The cause is unknown, but a family history is present in about 25% of patients. Combined treatment with *valproic acid* and either *ethosuximide* or *benzodiazepines* has been effective, but no clinical trials have been performed. Response to newer drugs, the *ketogenic diet*, and *vagus nerve stimulation (VNS)* (Chapter 16) is uncertain, but *phenytoin, carbamazepine, oxcarbazepine, gabapentin, tiagabine,* and *vigabatrin* can aggravate seizures. In contrast to CAE, seizures with EMA are not well controlled by medication and persist in about half of patients; mental deterioration occurs in about 70%; and symptoms may evolve into those of a more typical LGS.

Lennox-Gastaut Syndrome

CLINICAL DESCRIPTION

The symptom complex referred to as the *Lennox-Gastaut syndrome* (Lennox and Davis, 1950; Gastaut et al., 1966; Genton and Dravet, 2008; Kim and Nordli, 2010b; Crespel et al., 2012) has three features: (1) the occurrence of difficult-to-control multiple seizure types, almost always including drop attacks, atypical absences, and tonic seizures, but commonly also including myoclonic jerks and generalized tonic-clonic seizures, (2) some degree of psychomotor retardation, often with other evidence of neurological impairment, and (3) an interictal EEG pattern of generalized slow (less than 2.5 Hz) spike-and-wave discharges, usually with slowing of baseline rhythms and occasionally with focal features (Gastaut et al., 1966; Beaumanoir, 1985b; Aicardi, 1986; Blume, 1987). Although these signs and symptoms define a syndrome, this disorder represents a nonspecific response of the brain to a variety of diffuse and focal insults. Therefore, manifestations of LGS, responses to treatment, and prognosis vary considerably from one patient to another.

As with WS, cryptogenic and symptomatic forms are recognized. The former has a normal premorbid developmental history and no specific identified cause, whereas in the latter there is cerebral injury or maldevelopment preceding the onset of seizures. However, unlike in WS, the manifestations and prognosis for the cryptogenic form are not necessarily more benign, and the distinction between the cryptogenic and symptomatic groups is likely artificial. Undoubtedly, LGS comprises a number of subtypes that have different characteristics (Aicardi, 1986). For instance, EMAS and EMA are now considered to be separate syndromes that can be difficult to differentiate from LGS but appear to represent a transition between this disorder and IGE.

When onset is before the age of 2, the initial symptoms are absences with blinking and incomplete atonic seizures manifested by head drops (*epilepsia nutans*). Children can also have other peculiar seizures, such as laughter-like behaviors, and automatisms can be seen. After the age of 2, when children are more likely to be walking, the typical drop attacks appear (Chapter 6). These account for one of the major disabling features of this disorder, because the falls are sudden, occur without warning, and frequently cause lacerations, broken bones, and lost teeth if proper precautions are not taken.

Atypical absences usually do not begin until the age of 4; earlier onset heralds a more severe course. Prolonged absences (*spike-and-wave stupor, petit mal status, absence status*) are characteristic of this disorder, and patients can remain in a state of ictal dulled mentation for weeks or months (Chapter 10). Ictal impairment of consciousness may be minimal and apparent only with careful observation or specific testing by individuals who are familiar with the patient's usual interictal capabilities. One clue to the existence of absence status is the occurrence of repeated clonic movements—usually blinking of the eyes or facial twitching, but occasionally other muscles are involved. The diagnosis can sometimes be made by the EEG demonstration of continuous diffuse spike-and-wave discharges, although distinction between ictal and interictal EEG patterns is not always clear (Chapter 6).

Atypical absences and atonic seizures typically occur many times a day. Myoclonic jerks can also be frequent and can precede the drop attacks (*myoclonic-atonic seizures*). These seizures are not activated by hyperventilation and photic stimulation but may be activated by drowsiness and sleep and tend to occur when the individual goes to sleep at night or awakens in the morning.

The interictal EEG typically shows the *slow spike-and-wave* pattern, although this may be inconsistently present from one recording to another (Fig. 7–2). During sleep, the slow spike-and-wave is enhanced or may change into a polyspike pattern. An *independent multifocal spike discharge (IMSD)* pattern can also be seen and may fluctuate with the slow spike-and-wave (Noriega-Sanchez and Markand, 1976). Baseline EEG rhythms are usually diffusely slow, and both epileptiform and non-epileptiform abnormalities may have focal features. Many patients demonstrate brief runs (usually 2–5 seconds) of *generalized paroxysmal fast activity* (Fig. 7–3), which appear to be brief electrographic seizures resembling the EEG correlate of tonic convulsions (Brenner and Atkinson, 1982). These electrical phenomena are most common during sleep. Although they are not pathognomonic of LGS, they seem to be peculiar to patients with generalized seizures associated with diffuse encephalopathies and mental impairment.

Neuroimaging is important to help identify the underlying cause of LGS but is normal in the so-called cryptogenic cases.

EPIDEMIOLOGY

LGS accounts for 3–10% of all epilepsy in children, depending on the selectivity of the definition (Beaumanoir, 1985b). It affects boys three times more commonly than girls (Gastaut et al., 1975).

ETIOLOGY

The acquired and inherited causes of brain damage that give rise to the symptomatic form of LGS include trauma, intracranial hemorrhage, cerebral infections, MCDs, and inherited static and progressive encephalopathies, in particular tuberous sclerosis. By definition, etiology of the cryptogenic form is unknown, but a severe progressive encephalopathic process is inferred from the similarity of the course to that of the symptomatic form. Presumably, diffuse cortical and subcortical cerebral disturbances are necessary for the development of either form of the syndrome (Blume, 1987). A family history of epilepsy has been variably reported in 2.5–27% of cases (Erba and Browne, 1983); the higher figure appears to reflect an inherited predisposition for seizures rather than inheritance of the syndrome itself,

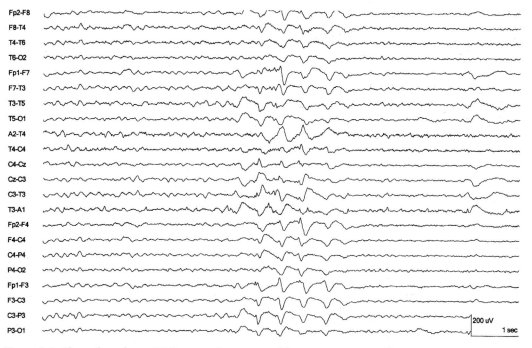

Figure 7–2. Slow spike-and-wave EEG pattern characteristic of the Lennox-Gastaut syndrome. (From Stern and Engel, 2005, with permission.)

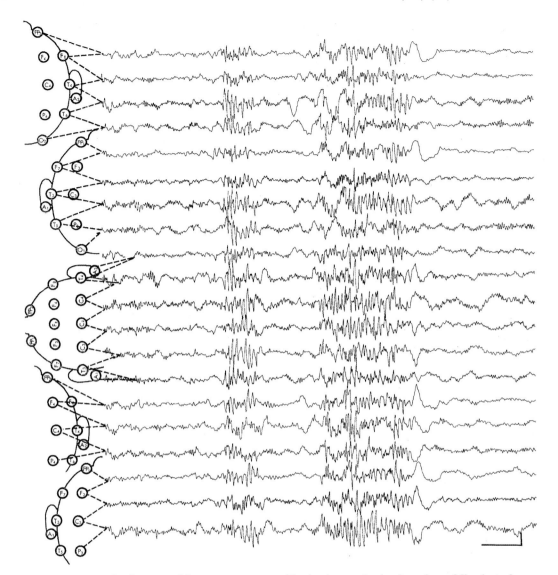

Figure 7–3. Generalized paroxysmal fast activity in a 3-year-old girl with generalized epilepsy due to diffuse brain damage. This particular electrographic event was not associated with any behavioral change. Calibration: 1 second, 100 μV.

because the cause of this condition is most likely multifactorial.

The evolution of WS to LGS is well known but is far from a necessary progression. Most patients with LGS do not have a history of WS, whereas many with WS either do not continue to have seizures or develop forms of epilepsy that would not be considered consistent with LGS. Consequently, this apparent progression likely reflects nonspecific age-dependent epileptic or epileptiform responses of the brain to insult (Chapter 8).

DIFFERENTIAL DIAGNOSIS

In the rare instance when patients present with absences only, LGS must be distinguished from CAE and MTLE characterized by limbic seizures with impaired consciousness only. This differential diagnosis is shown in Table 7–1. Atonic attacks must also be distinguished from other types of seizures that cause patients to fall but are not characteristic of LGS. These include the sudden collapse that can occur with focal seizures of frontal lobe origin, the gradual loss

Table 7–1 Differential Diagnosis of Disorders Manifesting as Lapses of Consciousness in Childhood

Seizure type	Typical absence	Atypical absence	Focal seizure with impairment of consciousness only
Duration	Usually < 10 seconds	Any duration	Usually > 10 seconds
Automatisms	Less elaborate	May be more elaborate	More elaborate
Aura	Never	Rare	Often
Other seizures	Rare grandma Synchronus myoclonic jerks or seizures can occur	Major motor Tonic and atonic Moclonic	Other complex partial Simple partial Secondarily generalized
Hyperventilation induced	Yes	No	Occasionally
Photic induced	Can be	No	No
Postictal	Normal	Either	Confused, automatisms
Baseline EEG	Normal	Focal or diffuse slowing	Maybe normal May have intermittent or continuous focal slowing
Paroxysmal EEG	Synchronous 3 c/sec spike-and -wave or faster Synchronous onset and ending Normal EEG immediately before and after paroxysm Some focal features occur	Atypical spike-and-wave 2.5 c/sec or slower May be asynchronous May begin and/or end asymmetrically May have slowing after paroxysm May have focal or multifocal spikes, fast activity, or suppression	May be normal May have unilateral, or bilaterally independent interictal mesial or anterior temporal spikes May have secondary bilateral synchrony Focal temporal theta at ictal onset common Postictal slowing common
Mental status	Normal	Low IQ	Memory deficit common
Neurological examination	Normal	Often abnormal	Usually normal
Family history	Usually positive	Usually negative	May be positive
Common syndromes	Childhood absence epilepsy Juvenile absence epilepsy Juvenile myoclonic epilepsy	Lennox-Gastaut syndrome	Temporal lobe epilepsy
Prognosis	Good	Poor	Variable
Treatment	Ethosuximide Valproate	Valproate All drugs Callosal section may benefit atonic sezures	Carbamazepine Phenytoin Primidone Phenobarbital Resective surgery

Adapted from Engel, 1984.

of postural control with automatic protective movements seen with some limbic seizures, and the retropulsive or propulsive tonic, and clonic movements that throw patients to the floor in association with generalized tonic-clonic seizures and massive myoclonus. *Juvenile myoclonic epilepsy (JME)* is sufficiently well defined that it should not be mistaken for LGS, even in those rare patients who have absences as well as myoclonic jerks and generalized tonic-clonic seizures. Differential diagnosis between LGS and the transitional syndromes of EMAS and EMA may be difficult, but accurate diagnosis in these cases is not essential, because treatment and prognosis in any event depend on a variety of additional factors.

TREATMENT

The traditional treatment of choice for LGS is *valproic acid*, because of its broad spectrum of action, but of the newer drugs, *levetiracetam*, *lamotrigine*, *topiramate*, *felbamate*, and *rufinamide* can also offer benefit. The latter two are specifically effective for atonic seizures. *Ethosuximide* is useful for atypical absences, and *benzodiazepines* for myoclonic seizures. The benzodiazepines, particularly *clonazepam*, have sedative side effects that further disable patients who are already mentally impaired. The development of tolerance to these drugs makes long-term use difficult. Rarely, intravenous benzodiazepines can cause tonic status epilepticus in LGS (Tassinari et al., 1972; Bittencourt and Richens, 1981). Treatment with two drugs, therefore, is often preferable to the use of benzodiazepines. Tonic and tonic-clonic seizures can be treated with antiseizure medications such as *carbamazepine* and *phenytoin*; however, carbamazepine may exacerbate atypical absences in some children (Snead and Hosey, 1985). Because seizures of LGS tend to cluster, evaluation of the efficacy of medical treatment can be difficult, and attempts to establish the appropriate regimen for individual patients can be extremely frustrating. The ketogenic diet and VNS (Chapter 16) are occasionally of some benefit for patients with this disorder.

Section of the corpus callosum became popular for LGS after this procedure was found to be particularly useful for controlling drop attacks (Chapter 16). The specific criteria for recommending corpus callosotomy have never been determined, but most investigators feel that medically refractory drop attacks and predominantly unilateral cerebral involvement are important indications (Reeves, 1985; Spencer et al., 1987). With the advent of VNS, which also is effective for drop attacks, there has been a marked decrease in the use of corpus callosotomies.

Treatment must take into account the need to prevent injury from frequent drop attacks. Preventing injury requires protective helmets and maintenance of a safe environment. It is also important to maximize the development of whatever intellectual and motor capabilities

the patient has in order to provide opportunities for the best psychosocial adjustment possible (Chapter 17).

PROGNOSIS

Prognosis for LGS is grim, because patients have many handicaps by definition, do not improve with time, and often become progressively more disabled for psychosocial as well as physical reasons. Less than one-third of patients have a good response to antiseizure medication, which may be effective against tonic and tonic-clonic seizures but not atonic and absence seizures or absence status. Even if seizures improve, children remain severely handicapped as a result of other neurological and mental impairment. Most of them eventually require institutional care (Douglass, 2011). Risk factors for poor outcome with respect to mental development include onset of seizures before the age of 2 years, tonic seizures, abnormal neuro-ophthalmological findings, and slow spike-and-wave at less than 1.5 Hz (Blume et al., 1973).

Epileptic Encephalopathy with Continuous Spike-and-Wave During Sleep

Epileptic encephalopathy with continuous spike-and-wave during sleep (CSWS), a rare epileptic encephalopathy of childhood, is actually a spectrum of disorders also known as *epilepsy with electrical status epilepticus during slow sleep (ESES)*. It is characterized by focal or generalized seizures occurring during sleep, atypical absences when awake, focal interictal EEG spikes, and continuous (>80%) generalized 1.5- to 3-Hz spike-and-wave discharges on the EEG during slow-wave sleep (Tassinari, 1982; Smith and Polkey, 2008; Striano and Capovilla, 2010; Tassinari et al., 2012). MRI is usually normal, but positron emission tomography with ^{18}F-fluorodeoxyglucose (FDG-PET) can show areas of increased and decreased metabolism in association cortex anatomically related to the location of focal EEG discharges and to the types of cognitive deterioration the child exhibits. Although epileptic seizures are pharmacosensitive and disappear within months or years, and some children never have seizures, neuropsychological disturbances develop that often persist. CSWS may account for some or most patients classified as having *Landau-Kleffner syndrome (LKS)* as well as atypical BECTS and other benign focal epilepsies of childhood. Some workers suggest that enduring behavioral deficits result from the electrical status and therefore might be avoided with prompt treatment (Tassinari, 1982). However, although many antiseizure medications are effective in controlling seizures, none are effective in abolishing the nocturnal EEG discharges, with the possible exception of ACTH (Tassinari, 1982). *Multiple subpial transection (MST)* has been helpful in some cases (Chapter 16). Diagnosis requires all-night sleep recordings. If an effective treatment is found that prevents the cognitive deficits, these studies would be appropriate in all children with progressive behavioral disturbances, aphasia, and evidence of epileptic seizures. Confusion with LGS is likely when polysomnography is not performed. There are insufficient data on the etiology of this syndrome; however, there is increasing evidence that it is an atypical evolution of BECTS.

Landau-Kleffner Syndrome

Focal neocortical seizures occurring in the dominant hemisphere can be associated with transient aphasia, and it is not uncommon for postictal language disturbances of varying durations to occur in patients with such focal seizures. A distinctly different association between epileptiform EEG discharges and aphasia was first described by Landau and Kleffner (1957), and *Landau-Kleffner syndrome (LKS)* is now recognized as a rare but definable syndrome (Beaumanoir, 1985a; Aicardi, 1986; Smith and Polkey, 2008; Covanis, 2010c; Tassinari et al., 2012). This epileptic encephalopathy is viewed as a subtype of CSWS. Symptoms begin in early childhood after the development of normal language and usually consist initially of an insidious deterioration of language function, taking the form of a verbal auditory agnosia. This is associated with interictal epileptiform EEG abnormalities, which may be bilaterally synchronous diffuse spike-and-wave discharges, often with a temporal preponderance, or focal spike-and-wave discharges in temporal or other areas. The language disturbance is progressive

for several years, during which time the epileptiform EEG abnormality is nearly continuous during slow-wave sleep. Epileptic seizures may not appear until several years after the aphasia is noted, and in 30% of patients, recognizable ictal events never occur. The seizures may be generalized or focal motor, are usually easily controlled by medication, and almost always remit spontaneously in adolescence. The aphasia, although often improved, persists to some extent in most patients.

As with CSWS, MRI is normal and FDG-PET can show focal hyper- and hypometabolism. The etiology of LKS is unknown. It is not clearly familial, and there are no intercurrent illnesses. A brain biopsy in one patient revealed chronic inflammatory changes similar to those seen in *Rasmussen syndrome* (Lou et al., 1977), but this is not a consistent finding (Cole et al., 1988). LKS comprises 0.2% of pediatric epilepsies, with predominance in girls. Acquired epileptic aphasia is not a benign disorder; although seizures are easily controlled with common antiseizure drugs and eventually disappear, nocturnal EEG discharges are pharmacoresistant, and most individuals continue to be disabled as a result of the persistent aphasia and other neuropsychological disturbances. MST has been effective in some children (Chapter 16). It is unclear whether LKS should be distinguished from CSWS, but like CSWS, it could represent atypical evolution of BECTS.

Childhood Absence Epilepsy

CLINICAL DESCRIPTION

Childhood absence epilepsy (CAE), also called *petit mal epilepsy*, is characterized by the occurrence of *typical absences* (Chapter 6) in otherwise normal children. It begins most often between the ages of 4 and 7, and rarely before the age of 3 (Loiseau, 1985; Hirsch et al., 2008, 2012; Covanis, 2010d).

It is now recognized that typical absences occur in childhood in association with a number of conditions, so that epilepsy with absence seizures of childhood onset is no longer considered synonymous with CAE. In addition to early onset of *juvenile absence epilepsy (JAE)* and JME, which can begin in childhood with infrequent absences, and EMA, there are other conditions that are not yet recognized as syndromes, such as *eyelid myoclonia with absences* (*Jeavons syndrome*) and *perioral myoclonia with absences*. Consequently, the definition of CAE has undergone an evolution in recent years, and many authors now adhere to specific inclusion and exclusion criteria for this syndrome (Table 7–2). Most important for this specific diagnosis is the presence of brief absences occurring many times a day (*pyknolepsy*), which may be associated with

Table 7–2 Inclusion and Exclusion Criteria for Childhood Absence Epilepsy

Inclusion Criteria for Childhood Absence Epilepsy
(1) Age at onset between 4 and 10 years and a peak at 5–7 years
(2) Normal neurologic state and development
(3) Brief (4–20 seconds, exceptionally longer) and frequent (tens per day) absence seizures with abrupt and severe impairment (loss) of consciousness. Automatisms are frequent but have no significance in the diagnosis.
(4) EEG ictal discharges of generalized high-amplitude single- and double (maximum occasional three spikes are allowed) spike-and-slow-wave complexes. They are rhythmic at around 3 Hz with a gradual and regular slowdown from the initial to the terminal phase of the discharge. Their duration varies from 4 to 20 seconds.

Exclusion Criteria for Childhood Absence Epilepsy
The following may be incompatible with childhood absence epilepsy:
(1) Other than typical absence seizures such as generalized tonic-clonic seizures or myoclonic jerks prior to or during the active stage of absences
(2) Eyelid myoclonia, perioral myoclonia, rhythmic massive limb jerking, and single arrhythmic myoclonic jerks of the head, trunk, or limbs. However, mild myoclonic elements of the eyes, eyebrows, and eyelids may be featured—particularly in the first 3 seconds of the absence seizure.
(3) Mild or no impairment of consciousness during the 3- to 4-Hz discharges
(4) Brief EEG 3- to 4-Hz spike-wave paroxysms of <4 seconds, multiple spikes (more than three), or ictal discharge fragmentations
(5) Visual (photic) and other sensory precipitation of clinical seizures

From Loiseau and Panayiotopoulos, 2000, with permission.

automatisms and mild periorbital myoclonia, but no other seizure types.

Brief absences can occur many times, sometimes hundreds of times, a day. They may interfere with school performance and be mistaken for *daydreaming* by teachers and parents. Absence seizures of CAE are classically induced by hyperventilation; are more common during relaxation, drowsiness, or, occasionally, stress; but are not induced by photic stimulation.

Approximately half of patients with CAE develop infrequent generalized tonic-clonic seizures in adolescence. These are seen less often in association with early onset of absence seizures and in patients treated with anticonvulsant medication (Loiseau, 1985). As many as one-quarter to one-half of persons with CAE ultimately have evidence of mild mental retardation (Sato et al., 1976), social maladjustment (Loiseau et al., 1983), or both, effects that indicate some degree of chronic cerebral dysfunction and contradict the supposedly benign nature of this disorder.

The interictal EEG in CAE is classically normal except for the paroxysmal features described for typical absences in Chapter 6. Bursts of generalized spike-and-wave discharges lasting longer than 4 seconds are usually associated with absences. Focal frontal spikes can occur, with equal frequency on either side. Abnormalities reported on MRI include thalamic atrophy and changes in cortical gray matter, including microdysgenesis, which has been confirmed on autopsy specimens; however, inconsistencies in numerous reports reflect the use of different diagnostic criteria for CAE. PET studies confirm the diffuse nature of this disorder by failing to show focal interictal abnormalities in cerebral metabolism (Engel et al., 1985) and by revealing generalized ictal hypermetabolism during absences (Engel et al., 1985), although fMRI suggests mesial frontal onset (Bai et al., 2010) (Chapter 6).

EPIDEMIOLOGY

Although reports of prevalence vary considerably from series to series because of differences in definition of the syndrome, CAE probably accounts for about 8–15% of childhood epilepsies. Two-thirds of those affected are female.

ETIOLOGY

Multiple factors appear to be responsible for the appearance of a 3-Hz spike-and-wave pattern, but a trait for this EEG disturbance is transmitted by an autosomal dominant gene with age-dependent penetrance (Metrakos and Metrakos, 1961) (Chapter 5). A mild degree of underlying brain damage may be necessary to trigger the manifestation of absence seizures in some persons predisposed to this disorder (Dalby, 1969; Loiseau, 1985). There is a high incidence of epileptic seizures as well as 3-Hz spike-and-wave discharges in relatives of persons with CAE (Newmark and Penry, 1980). A number of channelopathies and mutations in GABA receptors have been reported in families with CAE, but these most likely represent susceptibility genes. The relationship between CAE and the juvenile epilepsies that have previously been classified as IGE—JAE, JME, and *epilepsy with generalized tonic-clonic seizures only*, all of which can manifest with absences— is uncertain. Because families can have members with more than one type of syndrome, a neurobiological continuum has been suggested (Andermann and Berkovic, 2001) that could be called *idiopathic generalized epilepsy with variable phenotype* (Engel, 2001a). A relationship may exist between the CAE trait and BECTS (Bray and Wiser, 1965; Blom et al., 1972). Progress is being made in understanding the thalamocortical mechanisms of absence-like seizures in experimental animal models (Chapter 5), but this work has not been specifically related to the clinical disorder.

DIFFERENTIAL DIAGNOSIS

In addition to the need to distinguish the specific diagnostic entity of CAE from other absence epilepsies of childhood using the criteria in Table 7–2, it is important to distinguish typical absences from other seizure types that can mimic these events in childhood. Typical absence seizures in childhood must not be confused with focal dyscognitive seizures with impaired consciousness only and from atypical absences, which can be the sole initial presentation of LGS and other epilepsies associated with diffuse brain damage (see Table 7–1). In most cases, CAE can be easily recognized by history and EEG, including the observation of a hyperventilation-induced absence. However, diagnosis can be difficult when features of

more than one disorder are present as a result of multiple etiological factors and of overlap between syndromes (Chapter 5). Given that the presumed mechanisms, approaches to management, and prognoses are quite different for CAE, LGS, and focal dyscognitive seizures, inpatient EEG telemetry with video monitoring (Chapter 12) may be indicated for definitive diagnosis. A condition of *early absence epilepsy*, beginning before the age of 4, is recently recognized as a phenotype of GLUT1 deficiency (Roulet-Perez et al., 2008; Suls et al., 2009). Recognition of this condition is important. because it responds to the *ketogenic diet* (Chapter 16). Genetic testing is useful in 10% of patients with CAE (Ottman et al., 2010) (Chapter 12).

TREATMENT

The drug of choice for CAE is either *ethosuximide*, 20–40 mg/kg daily, to achieve a serum blood level of 40–100 µg/ml, or *valproic acid*, given at a dose of 20–60 mg/kg, to achieve a plasma level of 50–100 µg/ml. The latter is recommended for patients who also have generalized tonic-clonic seizures, because this single medication can control both seizure types. Some workers prefer valproic acid for patients who have only absences, to reduce the risk of subsequent tonic-clonic seizures (Loiseau, 1985). A recent randomized controlled trial demonstrated the superiority of valproate and ethosuximide over *lamotrigine* and found more cognitive deficits with valproic acid than with ethosuximide (Glauser et al., 2010). Medication can be withdrawn after a four-year seizure-free period, and very slow tapering of medication over six months to a year is recommended (Chapter 14).

PROGNOSIS

Remission rates reported for CAE vary considerably in the literature, undoubtedly because of difficulties in diagnosis. Although absence seizures tend to remit in adolescence, generalized tonic-clonic seizures often appear at this age. Risk factors for persistence of seizures include the occurrence of generalized tonic-clonic seizures, a positive family history, and mental or neurological deficits (Loiseau et al., 1983). An early onset of absence seizures and a rapid response to medication are good prognostic signs. There is disagreement about whether EEG features such as paroxysms that diverge from the classical 3-Hz spike-and-wave pattern, slow background rhythms, and focal interictal spikes should be considered unfavorable prognostic signs. Depending on the definition of the syndrome, complete remission may be expected in as few as half of patients with the diagnosis of CAE, but 90% of cases will remit if no risk factors are present (Sato et al., 1976). In addition to continuation of seizures, there is clearly an increased risk of mental subnormality and social maladjustment (Loiseau et al., 1983).

ADOLESCENCE-ADULT

Juvenile Absence Epilepsy

Juvenile absence epilepsy (JAE) accounts for 10% of all age-related epilepsies with absences and is, therefore, much less common than the childhood form (Wolf, 1985b; Hirsch et al., 2008; Thomas, 2010; Gélisse et al., 2012a). The sexes are affected equally, and the inheritance pattern has not been defined. The epileptic manifestations are the same as in CAE, with the exception that seizures begin at or after puberty, absences are less frequent (*spanioleptic*) or clustered (*cycloleptic*), and generalized tonic-clonic seizures are more likely to occur, particularly on awakening. Patients may also have myoclonic seizures, and there is a tendency for absence status. EEG spike-and-wave discharges during absence seizures may be faster than 3 Hz, and photic sensitivity is uncommon. Differential diagnosis between this disorder and epilepsy with generalized tonic-clonic seizures only can be arbitrary, because there is considerable overlap in the symptoms (Wolf, 1985b). Treatment is with *valproic acid* or *lamotrigine*, but *levetiracetam* is also effective and *ethosuximide* can be considered, although it is not effective against the generalized tonic-clonic seizures. Response to medication is good; however, complete remission by adulthood is not as likely as when absences begin earlier in life.

Juvenile Myoclonic Epilepsy

CLINICAL DESCRIPTION

Juvenile myoclonic epilepsy (JME) is characterized by the onset, usually between 12 and 19 years of age, of bilaterally synchronous single or repetitive massive myoclonic jerks (Janz

and Christian, 1957; Kobayashi et al., 2008b; Grünewald, 2010; Thomas et al., 2012). Jerks predominantly involve extensor muscles of the arms and may result in throwing objects held in the hand. At times the legs may also jerk, causing the person to fall if standing. Consciousness is preserved during brief myoclonic jerks, but confusion can occur during longer episodes. These *myoclonic seizures* occur most commonly in the morning shortly after awakening and occasionally evolve into generalized tonic-clonic seizures. Most persons with this disorder experience at least one generalized tonic-clonic seizure, usually after awakening, and 15–30% have absences. Sleep deprivation and alcohol are potent provocative influences. Thirty percent of patients are photosensitive (Goosses, 1984).

The most specific, but not necessarily most common, EEG abnormality is a frontally prominent, 4- to 6-Hz, bilaterally synchronous, irregular spike-and-wave or polyspike-and-wave discharge, which may appear at double or triple this frequency (Fig. 7–4). EEG spike discharges often occur without associated myoclonic jerks. Structural and functional neuroimaging have revealed frontal (predominantly mesial frontal) abnormalities.

Persons with JME may show cognitive features suggesting frontal lobe dysfunction (Wandschneider et al., 2010), and some authors have described a characteristic immature or feckless personality, but these patients are otherwise normal, with normal background EEG activity, neurological examination, intelligence, and behavioral adjustment.

EPIDEMIOLOGY

JME is the most common juvenile onset genetic epilepsy and represents perhaps 5% of persons with epilepsy (Wolf, 1985c). Boys and girls are affected equally.

ETIOLOGY

A number of channelopathies and GABA receptor mutations have been reported in JME, most likely representing susceptibility genes for a complex genetic disorder.

DIFFERENTIAL DIAGNOSIS

A diagnosis of JME, usually in an adolescent or young adult presenting with a generalized

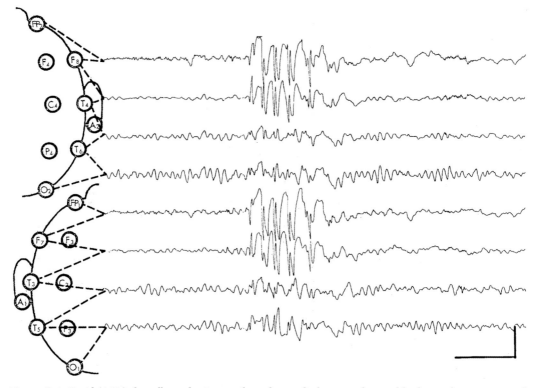

Figure 7–4. Rapid (4 Hz), frontally predominant spike-and-wave discharges and normal background in a patient with juvenile myoclonic epilepsy. Although this may be the most specific EEG paroxysm of this disorder, it is not necessarily the most common. Calibration: 1 second, 100 μV.

tonic-clonic seizure, is easily made when a history of typical early morning myoclonic jerks is elicited. This requires specific questions such as "Are you often clumsy in the morning?" and "Do your hands jerk so that you throw the soap in the shower or spill your coffee or orange juice at breakfast?" Most people with JME are not aware that these events are abnormal and assume that everyone does them, so these important symptoms are not likely to be spontaneously volunteered and will be missed if not pursued by the examiner. Distinction between these early morning myoclonic events, which occur minutes to hours after awakening, and normal myoclonic jerks that occur immediately on awakening (*hypnopompic*) or while going to sleep (*hypnogogic*) is also important.

When the predominant early morning phenomena are myoclonic jerks, one can rule out epilepsy with generalized tonic-clonic seizures only. Generalized tonic-clonic seizures that occur with JME usually evolve from myoclonic seizures. Although some patients with JAE have myoclonic seizures, these occur infrequently.

A spectrum may exist between these two syndromes and JME, with several unidentified factors determining which seizure types predominate. If these syndromes and CAE are considered variants of a single disorder, then prognosis is better when absences begin early and worse when generalized tonic-clonic seizures or myoclonic seizures are the most common or only seizure type.

JME begins at a later age than LGS, EMAS, and EMA. These childhood disorders are associated with more severe seizures and mental impairment. In the latter two, myoclonic jerks are likely to involve the face and are associated with absences rather than with preserved consciousness.

It is clinically most important to distinguish JME from many disorders characterized by nonepileptic myoclonus, which usually have a grave prognosis. In *progressive myoclonus epilepsies (PME)* and other degenerative disorders that give rise to myoclonus, as well as in *benign essential myoclonus*, the myoclonic jerks are more often sporadic, occurring multifocally and asynchronously, unlike the massive bilaterally synchronous jerks characteristic of epileptic myoclonus (Chapter 6). The myoclonic jerks of PME also are usually induced by movement (*action myoclonus*), occur spontaneously throughout the day rather than only after awakening, and are not as responsive to medication. Unlike JME, PME are often associated with dementia and cerebellar ataxia.

The typical EEG features of JME also help distinguish it from disorders associated with nonepileptic myoclonus. The latter show a variety of patterns, ranging from normal to multifocal or diffuse irregular spike-and-wave discharges. When other signs and symptoms of the progressive or degenerative diseases that give rise to myoclonus are present, they serve to rule out the diagnosis of JME. Familiarity with the typical features of JME makes it difficult to miss this diagnosis.

TREATMENT

Valproic acid is the drug of choice for treating the myoclonic jerks and generalized tonic-clonic seizures of JME, as well as absences when present. The teratogenic effects of valproic acid are problematic for women of childbearing age, so newer broad-spectrum antiseizure drugs such as *levetiracetam*, *lamotrigine*, and *topiramate* can be used; *primidone* is also effective for the first two seizure types. *Phenytoin*, *carbamazepine*, *oxcarbazepine*, *vigabatrin*, and *gabapentin* can exacerbate myoclonus and absences. Ensuring adequate sleep and reducing stress may improve control of the myoclonic jerks.

PROGNOSIS

Most patients can expect complete relief of all epileptic symptoms with appropriate treatment. Although relapse with medication withdrawal is extremely high (Janz, 1985), JME may remit spontaneously in a minority of patients (Camfield and Camfield, 2009).

Epilepsy with Generalized Tonic-Clonic Seizures Only

The original description of juvenile onset IGE included JAE, JME, and *epilepsy with generalized tonic-clonic seizures on awakening* (Wolf, 1985a; Janz, 1985). Many patients have

generalized tonic-clonic seizures only, usually in relationship to some structural brain abnormality; however, there are patients with genetic epilepsies in whom the predominant seizure type is a generalized tonic-clonic seizure, although absences and myoclonic phenomena can also occur. There is now debate as to whether patients with presumed genetic juvenile onset epilepsy whose generalized tonic-clonic seizures occur only on awakening constitute a specific syndrome, different from that of those with seizures that occur only in sleep or that have no relationship to the circadian cycle. Consequently, this rare genetic syndrome is recognized but poorly defined (Andermann and Berkovic, 2001; Iris et al., 2010; Gélisse et al., 2012b). Seizures begin in the second decade of life, and there is a familial predisposition. EEG shows typical 3-Hz spike-and-wave discharges, and neuroimaging is normal. Although in well over half of patients seizures can be controlled with standard antiseizure drugs, there is a high rate of relapse when attempts are made to discontinue treatment. There is some evidence that relapse is more likely in patients whose seizures occur on awakening than in those whose seizures occur during sleep.

Progressive Myoclonus Epilepsies

The *progressive myoclonus epilepsies (PME)* comprise a group of disorders characterized by the occurrence of both sporadic nonepileptic and epileptic myoclonic jerks and epileptic seizures that take the form of generalized tonic-clonic seizures, as well as by progressive dementia and neurological deficits that can include ataxia, neuropathy, and myopathy. In these disorders myoclonus and epilepsy coexist. Myoclonus is a disabling symptom, whereas the epileptic seizures are usually easily controlled by appropriate medication (Berkovic et al., 1986; Shibasaki, 1987; Berkovic, 2008; Serratosa, 2010; Genton et al., 2012).

The classic concept of PME includes two autosomal recessive progressive encephalopathies, one with and one without cerebral intracellular inclusions called *Lafora bodies* (Lafora, 1911). Both are characterized by sporadic myoclonus and generalized tonic-clonic convulsions associated with progressive intellectual deterioration and, later in the course, cerebellar signs. The EEG shows bilaterally synchronous irregular spikes and spike-and-wave discharges against a slow background and becomes increasingly abnormal as the disease progresses. Characteristically, the EEG spike-and-wave discharges are not time-locked to the myoclonic jerks and may reflect both epileptic and non-epileptic mechanisms. There are now a number of additional genetic disorders included in the syndrome of PME.

Lafora's disease, or *Lafora body encephalitis*, is the more rapidly progressive of the two forms. It usually begins in the second decade of life, with mental deterioration and myoclonic jerks, and severe disability and death ensue within several years (Lafora, 1911; Rapin, 1986; Giraldez and Serratosa, 2010a). The *periodic acid–Schiff-positive (PAS+) Lafora bodies* are intracytoplasmic concentric amyloid deposits seen throughout the nervous system, particularly in the dentate nucleus, red nucleus, substantia nigra, and hippocampus. Lafora bodies also occur in skeletal muscle, liver, and sweat glands, making definitive diagnosis possible without a brain biopsy. Most cases of this form of PME are caused by mutations of the *EPM2A* and *EPM2B* genes, which regulate glycogen synthesis.

The form of PME without Lafora bodies has been referred to as the *Unverricht-Lundborg syndrome* (Unverricht, 1895; Lundborg, 1903) or *Baltic myoclonus* (Koskiniemi et al., 1974a;b; Koskiniemi, 1986) and has been broken down into more discrete syndromes by some authors (Kälviäinen and Mervaala, 2010). The onset of symptoms in these disorders is later than in Lafora's disease, the mental deterioration less severe, and the course more prolonged, although patients may eventually become bed-ridden and the life span is shortened. This disorder is caused in most patients by mutations of the gene encoding *cystatin B*.

Neuronal storage disorders associated with myoclonus and epilepsy are commonly included under the heading of PME (Rapin, 1986; Shibasaki, 1987; Berkovic, 2008; Serratosa, 2010; Genton et al., 2012). These diseases are characterized by the same complex of symptoms, including sporadic myoclonus, generalized tonic-clonic seizures, intellectual deterioration, and a progressive course. In many patients, characteristic intracellular deposits are present outside the neuraxis, particularly in viscera, and a definitive diagnosis can sometimes be made without brain biopsy.

The *neuronal ceroid lipofuscinoses*, initially referred to as *familial amaurotic idiocy*, are genetic progressive neurodegenerative disorders characterized by the accumulation of intracellular material caused by a deficiency in certain lysosomal enzymes (Mole et al., 2010). There are congenital, infantile, juvenile, and adult forms, which have variable severity but are often associated with progressive severe visual impairment, movement disorders, and cognitive deterioration in addition to PME. Various eponyms have been attached to these disorders, such as *Jansky-* or *Batten-Bielschowsky*, *Hagberg-Santavuori*, and *Spielmeyer-Vogt* (Rapin, 1986).

Sialidosis with macular changes is also referred to as *cherry-red spot myoclonus* (Rapin, 1986; Franceschetti et al., 2010). Type 2 is diagnosed early in life, because of typical dysmorphic features and intellectual impairment, while Type 1 begins in adolescence or adulthood with seizures and myoclonus but no mental deterioration or dysmorphosis. Several mutations have been identified. It is important to recognize cherry-red spot myoclonus because patients usually exhibit little or no intellectual deterioration and have a relatively benign course with the exception of severe myoclonus, which can be seriously disabling (Engel et al., 1977; Rapin et al., 1978). A diagnosis of *late infantile ceroid lipofuscinosis* can be made from routine EEG when low-frequency (<3 Hz) photic stimulation gives rise to characteristic high-amplitude occipital sharp waves (Pampiglione and Harden, 1973) (Chapter 12). These disorders may be differentiated from each other and from Lafora's disease by their responses to stimulation (Table 7–3).

Myoclonus epilepsy with ragged red fibers (MERRF), also called *myoclonus epilepsy with mitochondrial myopathy*, is a mitochondrial disorder usually beginning in childhood and characterized by myoclonus, generalized seizures, ataxia, and ragged red fibers on muscle biopsy (Hirano, 2010). There is prominent neuronal cell loss in the cerebellum, brain stem, and spinal cord. Progression is variable but usually gradual, and blindness and cardiopathy are seen in addition to the PME. *Valproic acid* treatment is contraindicated in these patients (Chapters 5 and 15).

Other conditions causing PME include *GM gangliosidosis (Tay-Sachs disease)*, which usually affects infants and is rapidly progressive

Table 7–3 Differences in Precipitating Factors for Myoclonus Among Storage Disorders

Disease	Induced Myoclonus			Evoked Responses		
	Light	*Sound*	*Proprioception*	*All*	*VEP*	*SEP*
Tay-Sachs		+++		++	↓	
Juvenile Gaucher's	+++		++		↑	↑↑
sialidosis			+++		↓	↑↑
Ceroid lipofuscinosis						
Infantile				+++	↓	↓
Late infantile	++			++	↑↑	↑
Juvenile					↓	
Adult	+		+++		↑	↑↑
Lafora	++					

VEP = visual evoked potential; SEP = somatosensory evoked potential.

From Rapin, 1986, with permission.

(Kolodny and Sathe, 2011); *dentatorubral-pallidoluysian atrophy* (Bayreuther and Thomas, 2010); *Angelman syndrome* (Guerrini and Rosati, 2010); *noninfantile neuronopathic Gaucher's disease*; *action myoclonus–renal failure syndrome*; *autosomal recessive progressive myoclonus epilepsy–ataxia syndrome*; *juvenile Huntington's disease*; and *familial encephalopathy with neuroserpin inclusion bodies* (Giraldez and Serratosa, 2010b).

Autosomal Dominant Epilepsy with Auditory Features

Autosomal dominant epilepsy with auditory features (ADEAF), originally described by Ottman et al. (1995), is also referred to as *autosomal dominant lateral temporal lobe epilepsy* (Cendes et al., 2008; Nobile et al., 2010; Kahane et al., 2012). Onset can be at any age but most commonly occurs in late adolescence. Seizures typically begin with elementary or complex auditory auras, although other sensory, autonomic, and psychic auras can occur as well as aphasia. These may be followed by typical dyscognitive limbic seizures as well as secondarily generalized tonic-clonic seizures. Some patients may experience only the auditory auras. Seizure frequency ranges from several a month to a few a year, and approximately a quarter of patients have seizures that are triggered by auditory stimuli. EEG and neuroimaging studies, when abnormal, point to the left temporal lobe. Prevalence is uncertain. A mutation in the *leucine-rich, glioma-inactivated 1 (LGI1)* gene, which could result in malfunction of potassium channels or α-amino-3-hydroxy-5-methyl-4-isoxazole propionic acid (AMPA) receptors, is responsible for approximately half of the documented cases of this condition. Genetic testing is diagnostic in about half of patients with ADEAF (Ottman et al., 2010) (Chapter 12). Curiously, antibodies to this gene produce focal motor seizures (Irani et al., 2011) (Chapter 5). Seizures are usually easily controlled with standard antiseizure drugs, but there is a high rate of recurrence with drug withdrawal. Prognosis is good.

Other Familial Temporal Lobe Epilepsies

Familial mesial temporal lobe epilepsy is more common than ADEAF and has now been identified in families in North America, South America, Europe, and Australia (Cendes et al., 2008; Striano and Nobile, 2010; Kahane et al., 2012). The presentation is indistinguishable from that of sporadic MTLE, and it is diagnosed only by its familial pattern. It is, however, distinctly different from ADEAF. Most patients have seizures that are easily controlled by standard antiseizure medications, although some develop pharmacoresistant seizures and can be treated surgically. Many patients with this familial disorder have *hippocampal sclerosis*, suggesting that at least some cases of MTLE with HS may represent a sporadic form of the familial disorder. EEG demonstrates characteristic frontotemporal interictal spikes, while MRI shows hippocampal atrophy and other features of hippocampal sclerosis in many patients. Prevalence has not been determined, and no consistent genetic disturbance has been identified.

SYNDROMES WITH LESS SPECIFIC AGE RELATIONSHIPS

Familial Focal Epilepsy with Variable Foci

The recently described rare autosomal dominant condition of *familial focal epilepsy with variable foci* is recognized as a unique syndrome that, like GEFS+, is characterized by family history rather than by features of an individual patient (Kobayashi et al., 2008a; Wang and Xiao, 2010). Multiple members of families are affected with focal seizures, whose location varies from family member to family member but is consistent within individual members. Age of onset can vary from early infancy to midlife, with peaks at 5 and 25 years. Focal seizures, most commonly of frontal origin, with or without impaired consciousness and with or without secondarily generalized seizures, are less frequent than in ADNFLE and have no relationship to circadian cycles. Ictal semiology is dependent on the anatomical localization and is consistent with the interictal epileptiform abnormalities on the EEG. Interictal neuroimaging is normal, although ictal *single-photon emission computed tomography (SPECT)* reveals focal hyperperfusion. Prevalence has not been determined. Linkage analysis has defined at least two loci, but specific gene mutations have not been identified. Most patients respond to standard antiseizure medication with no sequelae, and seizures tend to remit spontaneously in midlife.

Reflex Epilepsies

Although a great variety of physical stimuli and even thought can induce seizures in many patients with epilepsy (Wilkins and Lindsay, 1985; Zifkin et al., 2008; Koutroumanidis, 2010) (Chapter 9), such provocation occurs for the most part in conditions in which epileptic seizures also occur spontaneously.

There are, however, rare reflex epilepsy syndromes, which the ILAE defines as conditions in which all epileptic seizures are precipitated by sensory stimuli (Engel, 2001a). The reflex epilepsies are a group of diverse conditions with a wide range of etiologies, anatomical localizations, and ictal manifestations, so there is very little pathophysiological basis for considering them together other than the fact that seizures are precipitated by specific stimuli.

Idiopathic photosensitive occipital lobe epilepsy (Parmeggiani and Guerrini, 2010) is characterized by visually induced focal and often secondarily generalized seizures in late childhood. Provocative stimuli are most commonly generated by television and video games, but other environmental visual patterns can be effective. Seizures consist of unformed visual phenomena such as multicolored patterns or flashing lights, which may move and can be lateralized. These can be followed by ictal blindness, although some seizures may begin with negative symptoms. Typically there is conscious head and eye deviation, usually to the side of visual hallucinations if they are unilateral, often with epigastric symptoms. This can evolve into a dyscognitive seizure with oroalimentary automatisms that can last for several minutes, and occasionally seizures will secondarily generalize. Postictal headache is common. Interictal EEG reveals bilateral spike-and-wave discharges, which are accentuated by eye closure and photic stimulation. Visual evoked potentials are enhanced, and low-frequency photic stimulation triggers occipital spikes. Ictal EEG can shift from one side to the other but appears to be restricted to calcarine cortex. Neuroimaging and visual fields are normal. The genetic basis of this disorder is unknown, but reports indicate possible phenotypic overlap with febrile seizures, JME, and BECTS. The abnormal photosensitivity manifests around puberty and usually remits spontaneously within a few years. Seizures usually respond to standard antiseizure medication, but many patients have only one or very infrequent seizures and require no treatment at all.

Other visual-sensitive epilepsies have been described, some of which at present are accepted as seizure types but not syndromes. They include *eyelid myoclonia and absences*, or *Jeavons syndrome*, which is induced by eye closure (Covanis, 2010e); *pattern-sensitive epilepsy* (Wilkins, 2010); and *fixation-off sensitivity* (Koutroumanidis and Tsiptsios, 2010) (Chapter 9).

Startle epilepsy is a rare condition of children, usually with diffuse brain damage and neurological deficits, who experience a variety of seizure types, including generalized myoclonus, tonic, and atonic seizures alone or in combination, that are induced by unexpected stimuli such as loud sounds or touch (Tibussek and Schmidt, 2010). Seizures may involve only half of the body, and focal seizures also occur. Interictal EEG is nonspecific with multifocal spikes and diffuse slowing, while ictal discharges consist of low-voltage fast activity as well as generalized spike-and-wave discharges. Neuroimaging reveals the underlying structural abnormalities. Seizures are often pharmacoresistant, and prognosis depends on the underlying etiology. When the abnormality is localized, some patients benefit from surgical therapy.

Primary reading epilepsy was originally believed to be a distinct syndrome but is now recognized as a heterogeneous group of conditions with seizures that can be precipitated not only by reading but, in different patients, by cognitive processes including other linguistic activities, calculation, and decision making (Bansal and Radhakrishnan, 2010). Seizures typically begin in adolescence, rather than earlier when patients begin learning to read, and consist of myoclonic movements of the jaw, tongue, lips, and other facial muscles without impaired consciousness, although patients may complain of ictal discomfort, anxiety, and confusion. Rarely, these events will lead to a secondarily generalized tonic-clonic seizure. The EEG can be normal or demonstrate spontaneous focal or generalized spike-and-wave discharges, but these are precipitated by reading or other specific cognitive activities, depending on the patient's sensitivity. Epileptiform discharges may be localized to the dominant hemisphere or bilateral. Neuroimaging is normal, and the etiology of this disorder is unknown, although approximately a third of patients have a family history of epilepsy. Boys are preferentially

affected. Antiseizure medication can control dyscognitive seizures, but the minor ictal symptomatology can be pharmacoresistant and controlled only by avoiding precipitating stimuli. Although seizures tend to persist, they may become less frequent with age.

Patients with musicogenic seizures usually have spontaneous seizures as well but occasionally have seizures induced only by specific musical stimuli, in which case they can be said to have the syndrome of *musicogenic epilepsy* (Zifkin et al., 2008). All types of music can be effective provocative stimuli, although the type of music tends to be consistently specific in each patient (Chapter 9). This disorder results from lesions of the temporal lobe, usually on the right side. When seizures do not respond to antiseizure medication and avoidance is difficult, surgical treatment can be effective.

Hot water epilepsy is a rare condition usually seen in infants and young children (Bebek, 2010). The syndrome was described in India, where bucket baths, in which warm water is poured over the head, are the most effective precipitating stimulus (Satishchandra, 2003). Seizures usually are dyscognitive, and when they occur in older children and adults, typical limbic auras and ictal pleasure are described. EEG findings are variable with focal or generalized discharges, although no abnormalities may be seen, and neuroimaging is usually normal. Etiology is undetermined, with some patients having a family history. Avoidance of provocative stimuli is the best treatment, but standard antiseizure drugs are effective, and seizures tend to remit spontaneously within a few years. There is also a rare, benign condition of infancy seen outside India where immersion in hot water precipitates seizures (Ioos et al., 2000) (Chapter 9).

DISTINCTIVE CONSTELLATIONS

Mesial Temporal Lobe Epilepsy with Hippocampal Sclerosis

CLINICAL DESCRIPTION

The term *mesial temporal lobe epilepsy (MTLE)* has been widely applied in the literature to describe a condition characterized by epileptic seizures that originate in or primarily involve mesial temporal limbic structures (Baldwin and Bailey, 1958; Lindsay et al., 1979a, 1979b, 1979c; Engel, 2001b). MTLE with HS is now recognized as a distinctive constellation (Engel et al., 2008; Alarcon and Valentin, 2010; Kahane et al., 2012); however, the term *mesial temporal lobe epilepsy* is also applied to conditions with mesial temporal lesions other than hippocampal sclerosis and even to conditions of neocortical epilepsy where seizures preferentially propagate to mesial temporal structures (Engel, 2001b; Williamson and Engel, 2008; Valentin and Alarcon, 2010). The concept of MTLE in the general sense implies that the characteristic ictal semiology (Chapter 6) depends primarily on activation of mesial temporal structures regardless of where the seizures actually originate. *Limbic epilepsy* is an acceptable alternative name, although there is no evidence that the characteristic seizure semiology can be generated by nontemporal limbic structures only. The term *psychomotor epilepsy* suggests the occurrence of psychic and motor symptoms although both are not necessarily present. The reason MTLE with HS is not considered a disease, or even a syndrome in the classic sense, is that there is clearly more than one type of hippocampal sclerosis that gives rise to this condition, and neither the etiologies of the various types of hippocampal sclerosis nor their specific relationship to epileptogenesis has been definitively demonstrated (Wieser et al., 2004).

MTLE with HS most often begins in late childhood, although it can appear at any age. Typical limbic seizures with and without altered consciousness are described in Chapter 6. Almost all patients experience dyscognitive seizures, but these are not essential for diagnosis. Limbic seizures in clear consciousness (auras) not only often precede dyscognitive seizures but also characteristically occur in isolation. This fact reflects the unique ability of the hippocampus to prevent propagation (Chapter 4). Approximately one-quarter of patients deny auras, but in some of these an aura may be missed because of retrograde amnesia and therefore not be recognized as an ictal event when it occurs alone.

The most common aura in this condition is a sensation of epigastric rising, sometimes associated with nausea. Psychic, autonomic, olfactory, and gustatory symptoms; emotional experiences (usually fear); and dysmnesic phenomena can occur alone or in combination. When the epileptogenic region is in neocortical areas that preferentially propagate to mesial structures, auditory and vertiginous experiences suggest lateral temporal lobe; mixed-formed illusions and hallucinations suggest the *temporal-parietal-occipital (TPO) junction*; and visual experiences suggest occipital cortex, usually below the calcarine fissure (see Fig. 8–2). Mesial temporal onsets, however, can sometimes be associated with nonspecific sensory sensations, usually bilateral or midline, such as tingling of the bridge of the nose or the fingers of both hands.

Typical limbic dyscognitive seizures of occipital lobe origin usually have initial visual symptoms or ocular signs and symptoms, such as nystagmus, periocular muscle twitching, or periocular sensations, before propagation to mesial temporal structures (Ludwig and Ajmone-Marsan, 1975). Typical limbic seizures of frontal lobe origin often begin with postural or other motor symptoms and can include falling, head and eye deviation, and incontinence. It is rare for typical limbic seizures to occur with perirolandic lesions and initial clonic motor or somatosensory symptoms.

Typical limbic dyscognitive seizures are usually followed by a period of postictal confusion. There is always amnesia for the ictal event and often some anterograde amnesia as well. Postictal reactive automatisms (Chapter 6) are occasionally associated with defensive combativeness that can be mistaken for violent or aggressive behavior. Prolonged postictal symptoms can be a particularly disabling aspect of MTLE.

Limbic auras in temporal lobe epilepsy can occur frequently, sometimes many times a day. Typical dyscognitive seizures are less frequent, ranging from one a year or less to one a day or more, but usually averaging a few a month. They can occur in clusters and are commonly exacerbated by stress, sleep deprivation, drowsiness, and menses.

Approximately half of patients experience infrequent secondarily generalized seizures. These do not always take the form of a classical grand mal tonic-clonic seizure (Chapter 6). Rather, they can involve asymmetrical or unilateral tonic or clonic movements and poorly coordinated thrashing movements of the limbs. Loss of tone with a drop to the ground (*temporal lobe syncope*) has been described as a rare event (Caffi, 1973), but a temporal origin of such seizures has never been proven. The infrequent occurrence of generalization is perhaps due to the effectiveness of antiseizure medication in preventing generalized motor symptoms.

The EEG features of MTLE with HS are those described for typical limbic seizures in Chapter 6. Unilateral or independently bilateral interictal anterior temporal spikes and a basal temporal ictal onset are the EEG hallmarks of this syndrome but are not present in all patients. Patients may also show focal temporal slow activity. Runs of *temporal intermittent rhythmic delta activity (TIRDA)* usually reflect electrographic ictal discharges in mesial temporal structures for which the spike activity is not projected to the surface (Chapter 12).

Other features that are commonly attributed to MTLE with HS include (1) normal neurological status, with the exception of memory deficit seen in most patients with poorly controlled dyscognitive seizures for many years, (2) unilateral or occasionally bilateral hippocampal atrophy, enhancement of T2 and fluid-attenuated

inversion recovery (FLAIR) signal (Fig. 7–5), or both (Jackson et al., 1990), (3) interictal unilateral temporal lobe hypometabolism on PET scans (Engel et al., 1982a, 1982b, 1982c; Henry and Chugani, 2008) (Fig. 7–6) and hyperperfusion on ictal SPECT (Bonte et al., 1983; Lee et al., 1986; Kazemi et al., 2008) (see Fig. 9–3), and (4) evidence of material-specific unilateral or bilateral temporal lobe dysfunction on neuropsychological testing, including the modified *intracarotid amobarbital procedure (IAP)* (Rausch, 1987; Wilson and Engel, 2010) (Chapter 12). Patients may also have a family history of epilepsy and prolonged febrile seizures in childhood (Falconer, 1971) as well as other initial precipitating insults within the first five years of life (Mathern et al., 1995) (Chapter 5). MTLE due to other causes can be identified when other structural lesions are apparent on MRI, and in the absence of such lesions, neocortical onset can be suspected by the presence of nonlimbic auras. Otherwise, differential diagnosis between MTLE with HS and other causes of epilepsy characterized by typical limbic seizures is difficult or impossible.

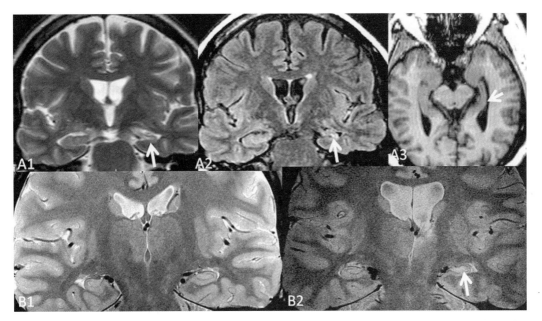

Figure 7–5. Left hippocampal sclerosis **A.** 1.5-T MRI. *A1:* Coronal T2-weighted image shows atrophy of the left hippocampal head (*arrow*), compared to the right side. *A2:* Coronal FLAIR image demonstrates high signal intensity within the atrophic left hippocampus (*arrow*). *A3:* T1 oblique axial image demonstrates atrophy of the left hippocampus (*arrow*) from head to tail. **B.** 3.0-T MRI. *B1:* Coronal proton density sequence demonstrates detailed anatomy of the hippocampus; Ammon's horn and dentate gyrus are well visualized. *B2:* Hyperintensity signal within the left dentate gyrus (*arrow*). (Courtesy of Dr. Noriko Salamon.)

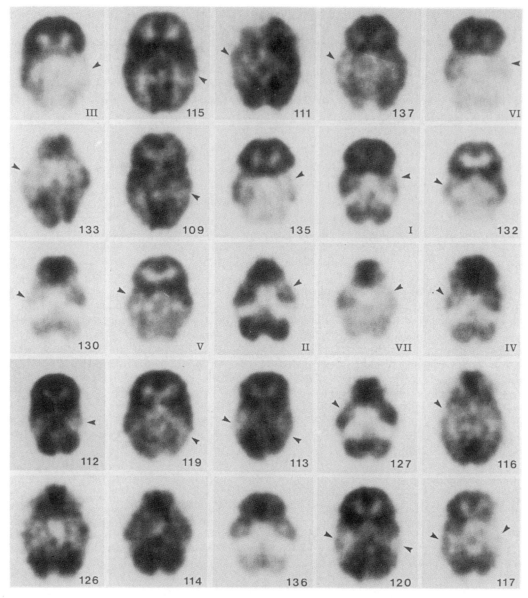

Figure 7–6. Representative planes of FDG-PET scans from 20 patients with temporal lobe seizures. Temporal lobe hypometabolic zones are indicated by *arrowheads*. In addition, left frontal hypometabolism is visible in patient 111, and the right occipital lobe appears to be abnormal in patient 133. In all cases indicated, hypometabolic zones were also seen on one or more adjacent sections. (From Engel et al., 1983b, with permission.)

Certain personality traits, with features that have been variously described as aggressive, emotional, overinclusive, sober, hypermoral, and hyposexual; affective disturbances, especially depression; and psychosis, particularly paranoid schizophrenia, have been considered by some workers to be more common in patients with limbic seizures than in patients with other types of epilepsy (Bear and Fedio, 1977; Blumer and Benson, 1982; Trimble, 1983). Because a relationship between these behavioral disorders and MTLE remains controversial (Chapter 11), however, they cannot be used to help characterize MTLE with HS specifically or MTLE in general.

EPIDEMIOLOGY

Forty percent of patients with epilepsy have dyscognitive seizures (Gastaut et al., 1975); however, the prevalence of MTLE with HS is unknown because only patients with pharmacoresistant seizures usually come to the attention of epilepsy centers where detailed diagnostic evaluations are performed. No data are available to determine the prevalence of this condition in patients whose seizures are well controlled, and for this reason, the natural history of MTLE with HS has not been determined. On the other hand, hippocampal sclerosis is the most common epileptogenic lesion identified on MRI scans of patients referred to epilepsy centers, and this is the most likely MRI finding to be associated with pharmacoresistance (Semah et al., 1998).

ETIOLOGY

Hippocampal sclerosis is readily identified on MRI in most patients, and the histopathology has been well studied (Armstrong and Bruton, 1987; Babb and Brown, 1987; Mathern et al., 2008; Blümcke et al., 2011) (Chapter 5). There are still arguments over whether this lesion is in fact the cause of epilepsy or merely a result of recurrent epileptic seizures (Chapter 10); however, both situations appear to apply, and undoubtedly multiple forms of hippocampal sclerosis exist (Armstrong and Bruton, 1987; Babb and Brown, 1987; Wieser et al., 2004; Ogren et al., 2009; Stefan et al., 2009) (Chapter 5). The relationship between sporadic MTLE with HS and familial MTLE, which can also be associated with hippocampal sclerosis and pharmacoresistant seizures (Cendes et al., 2008), is unclear. That patients with MTLE with HS often have a history of febrile seizures as well as a family history of epilepsy suggests a genetic predisposition, which could eventually place this disorder within the spectrum of epilepsies grouped as GEFS+. Other epileptogenic lesions commonly found in hippocampus, amygdala, or temporal neocortex of patients with MTLE, particularly those with seizures that begin in adolescence or later, include neoplasms; MCDs such as *focal cortical dysplasia*; *dysembryoplastic neuroepitheliomas (DNETs)*; *heterotopias*; cysts; *cavernous angiomas* and other vascular malformations; and occasionally

cicatrices induced by cerebral trauma, infection, or infarction (Chapter 5).

Hippocampal sclerosis is not necessarily unilateral and it rarely if ever occurs as an isolated lesion. Evidence of bilateral hippocampal sclerosis can be found in over 50% of patients and is equal on both sides in about 10% (Armstrong and Bruton, 1987; Babb and Brown, 1987). It is possible that some degree of enduring bilateral epileptiform dysfunction is necessary for limbic seizures to become manifest (Soper et al., 1978; Engel and Crandall, 1983; Babb and Brown, 1987) (Chapter 4). Hippocampal sclerosis can occur as part of more diffuse lesions such as MCDs as well as in association with discrete focal lesions adjacent to hippocampus, but even in classical MTLE with HS the pathological abnormality goes well beyond the hippocampus (Bonilha et al., 2012; Engel and Thompson, 2012). Pathological changes in the ipsilateral, and at times bilateral, thalamus and basal ganglia have long been observed (Margerison and Corsellis, 1966), and ipsilateral thalamic hypometabolism on PET is commonly seen (Henry and Chugani, 2008). Surgical outcome appears to depend more on the amount of parahippocampal tissue than on the amount of hippocampal and amygdala tissue removed (Siegel et al., 1990). MRI investigations using voxel-based morphometry have consistently demonstrated bilateral thinning in wide areas of neocortex (Lin et al., 2007) (Fig. 7–7). It appears, therefore, that MTLE with HS is in actuality a diffuse disease in which atrophy of one or both hippocampi is only the most obvious pathological finding (Wieser et al., 2004).

Prolonged febrile seizures in infancy and a family history of epileptic seizures both predict hippocampal sclerosis and a good outcome following anteromesial temporal lobe resection (Falconer, 1971; Engel et al., 1983a; 2008). This suggests a genetic lowered threshold to epileptic seizures as well as a predisposition to develop hippocampal sclerosis and subsequent epilepsy in response to an early insult (Chapter 5).

DIFFERENTIAL DIAGNOSIS

In addition to (1) distinction between MTLE with HS and MTLE due to other mesial temporal lobe lesions, which rarely alters prognosis and management, and (2) distinction between mesial temporal lesions that give rise to MTLE

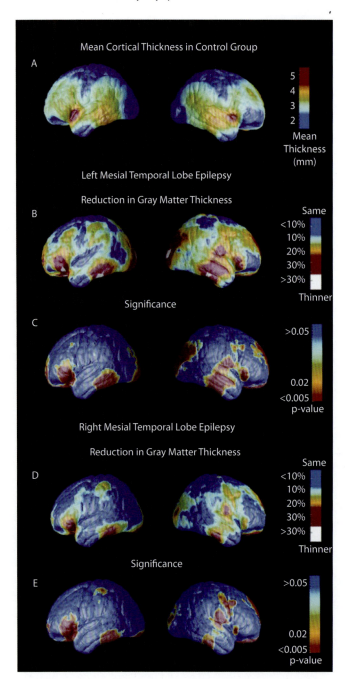

Figure 7–7. Cortical thickness maps show regional reduction, compared with controls (**a**), in groups with left MTLE (**b, c**) and right MTLE (**d, e**). Mean cortical thickness for controls (N = 19) is shown in millimeters on color bar (**a**); reds indicate a thicker cortex, and blues indicate a thinner cortex. Mean reductions in cortical thickness in MTLE groups as a percentage of the control average (**b, d**) show bilateral thickness decreases of up to 30% on average in the frontal poles, frontal operculum, orbital frontal, lateral temporal, and occipital regions, and the right angular gyrus and primary sensorimotor cortex surrounding the central sulcus. Maps of *p* values (**c, e**) show the statistical significance of these changes. (From Lin et al., 2007, with permission.)

and epiletogenic lesions in neocortex whose discharges preferentially propagate to mesial temporal structures, which does have practical importance when surgical treatment is considered, it is important to distinguish MTLE in general from other forms of epilepsy. MTLE in childhood should be distinguished from

BECTS because the latter has an invariably good prognosis. As noted previously, this differential diagnosis is usually made on the basis of the characteristic clinical presentation and EEG pattern of the benign syndrome. The differential diagnosis between MTLE initially manifested as impaired consciousness alone and epilepsy syndromes associated with absences has already been outlined (see Table 7–2).

MTLE must be distinguished from nonspecific epilepsy disorders with atypical dyscognitive seizures (Chapter 6) when resective surgical treatment is a consideration. Presurgical evaluation of suspected MTLE includes long-term video-EEG monitoring and in some cases intracranial recording (Chapters 12 and 16). Diffuse, multifocal, or bilaterally synchronous interictal EEG discharges and evidence of diffuse cerebral disturbance from neurological, neuropsychological, or imaging studies suggest a disorder other than MTLE. Normal MRI and absence of a focal ictal onset on scalp EEG, however, do not rule out a diagnosis of MTLE (Engel et al., 2008).

Migraine, particularly in children, may alter consciousness and be misdiagnosed as MTLE (Chapter 13). In some patients it is difficult to distinguish between MTLE and psychiatric disorders associated with intermittent symptoms such as psychotic delusions and hallucinations, fugue states, episodic dyscontrol, intermittent explosive disorder, and psychogenic seizures (Chapter 13). Prolonged limbic auras (*aura continua*) (Chapter 10) sometimes seen in MTLE can lead to erroneous diagnoses of neurotic and psychotic disorders. The diagnosis of MTLE in these situations, when suspected, is often made easily if routine EEG or long-term video-EEG monitoring reveals ictal epileptiform discharges or if *serum prolactin levels* are elevated (Chapter 12). However, definitive diagnosis of an ictal state may be impossible when consciousness is not impaired, the scalp EEG is normal (Wieser et al., 1985), and prolactin levels are not elevated (Sperling et al., 1986) (Chapter 13). In these situations, symptoms that resemble the patient's habitual auras are assumed to be seizures, whereas symptoms that have never been associated with obvious seizures, particularly those that are not stereotyped, are probably not epileptic.

TREATMENT

The most common treatment for MTLE is *carbamazepine* or *levetiracetam*, although many other antiseizure medications are also effective in most patients. Decisions about medication should be based on side effects, cost, ease of administration, and other considerations (Chapters 14 and 15). Medical control may require higher serum drug levels than are commonly used for other seizure types (Schmidt et al., 1986). Psychosocial intervention can also be necessary, because of the embarrassing nature of the seizures and associated interictal behavioral disturbances (Chapters 11 and 17). Patients with seizures that cannot be controlled medically are ideal candidates for resective surgical treatment. If the epileptogenic region can be localized accurately to one mesial temporal area, seizures can be abolished in 70–90% of patients and markedly reduced in most of the remainder (Engel, 1987; Engel et al., 2003; 2012; Wiebe et al., 2001; Spencer and Huh, 2008) (Chapter 16).

PROGNOSIS

Limbic seizures due to hippocampal sclerosis are often relatively refractory to available antiseizure medications (Semah et al., 1998). Older studies indicate that drugs control the epileptic seizures in less than half of patients with temporal lobe epilepsy, and disabling psychosocial disturbances may occur in at least a third (Rodin, 1968; Lindsay et al., 1979a, 1979b;sc), but some of the patients who did well in those early series probably had BECTS. One subsequent study, from a large epilepsy center in Paris, suggests that seizures associated with hippocampal sclerosis can be controlled in only a small minority of patients (Semah et al., 1998), while another, at a more community-based neurology clinic in Glasgow, found 42% to be seizure-free (Stephen et al., 2001). Both, however, found that hippocampal sclerosis was associated with the poorest seizure outcome of all MRI-identified lesions. The true natural history of MTLE with HS is unknown, as patients with a more benign course would not necessarily come to the attention of epilepsy centers (Labate et al., 2011). Remission of limbic seizures is less likely if secondarily generalized seizures are frequent (Schmidt et al., 1983). Progression of symptoms in this syndrome is suspected in some instances but difficult to prove definitively (Cascino, 2009) (Chapter 14). Outcome with surgery, on the other hand, is excellent (Chapter 16).

Rasmussen Syndrome

Rasmussen and colleagues first described chronic focal encephalitis associated with focal seizures, now known as *Rasmussen syndrome*, in 1958 (Rasmussen et al., 1958); this condition is also referred to as *Rasmussen's encephalitis*. Usually beginning in childhood, it is characterized by relentless progression of hemispheric atrophy, frequent contralateral focal seizures, and hemiparesis (Dubeau et al., 2008; Granata et al., 2012). The condition typically presents as unilateral seizures with variable semiology, although there are almost always motor components. These are pharmacoresistant and progress over several years before the development of hemiparesis and other neurological and cognitive deterioration associated with hemispheric atrophy. Symptoms eventually stabilize over a decade or more, and seizures may improve somewhat, but there can be secondary progression. There is evidence to suggest that early onset is associated with more rapidly progressive signs and symptoms than in the rare adolescent and early adult onset cases, where the course can be less severe. A number of variants have been described, including forms with bilateral hemispheric involvement, very early or very late onset, limited focal involvement that can remit, involvement of basal ganglia and brain stem, and dual pathology. The prevalence of this rare condition is unknown.

EEG reveals interictal spikes and slowing consistent with the location of atrophy and seizure semiology, and both structural and functional neuroimaging reveal the progressive hemispheric atrophy in typical cases (Fig. 7–8). Early on, MRI can be normal, but disturbances of perfusion and metabolism can be seen with SPECT and PET. Subsequently, hyperintense regions of cortex and caudate as well as areas of edema, that later become atrophic, can be seen on T2 and FLAIR MRI sequences. Most commonly, the initial disturbances involve temporal, frontal, and insular cortex, although disturbances can also begin posteriorly.

Detailed pathological evaluations on surgical specimens reveal perivascular cuffing, microglial proliferation, nodule formation, neuronal loss, and gliosis. The etiology of the inflammatory process is unknown, but both viral and autoimmune mechanisms are suspected, and autoimmunity could be provoked by a viral infection. Specifically, *anti-GluR3* antibodies were once implicated in some patients, and antibodies to other receptor subunits have now been reported (Chapter 5).

Antiseizure drugs are usually ineffective, and immune therapy, including interferon, steroids, other immunosuppressant agents, immunoglobulins, and plasmapheresis, have been tried with variable success. A few reports of benefit from antiviral therapy exist, but the definitive treatment is surgery, almost always involving hemispherectomy or hemispherotomy (Chapter 16). Because Rasmussen syndrome is a progressive disorder usually beginning in childhood, a surgical decision is difficult when hemiparesis has not progressed to the point where the hand is useless, particularly when the language-dominant hemisphere is involved. Removal or disconnection of the hemisphere in the absence of severe contralateral hemiparesis invariably introduces a new neurological deficit that can be profound; however, early intervention provides the best opportunity for transfer

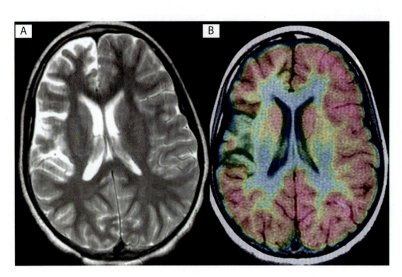

Figure 7–8. Rasmussen syndrome. **A.** Axial T2-weighted image of a patient with chronic Rasmussen's encephalitis. There is significant atrophy of the right perisylvian region. Left hemisphere is normal. **B.** PET-MRI coregistration demonstrates hypometabolism (*green*) in the right operculum, which is the most atrophic portion. The rest of the cortex shows normal metabolism (*red*). (Courtesy of Dr. Noriko Salamon.)

of language function, while the gradual contralateral deterioration that would invariably occur without surgery would delay later surgery so long that transfer of language function is no longer possible. Early surgery thus provides the best opportunity for a good outcome with respect to both elimination of seizures and maximal function.

Gelastic Seizures with Hypothalamic Hamartoma

Laughing, or *gelastic*, seizures are a rare seizure type (Chapter 6), and when associated with *hypothalamic hamartoma*, constitute a very rare epilepsy syndrome (Harvey et al., 2008). Precocious puberty and cognitive and developmental impairment can occur, particularly with larger tumors (Parvizi et al., 2011). Typically, the gelastic seizures begin in early childhood and may be associated with *dacrystic* (crying) seizures. Initially they are brief, frequent, and unassociated with impaired consciousness, but over time they may develop features of limbic seizures as well as secondarily generalized seizures. Cognitive deterioration, ranging from memory impairment to more severe attention and learning disorders, can occur, as well as behavioral disturbances and frank psychiatric comorbidity. The hamartomas originate from the mammillary bodies, in which case they are usually within the third ventricle, and from the tuber cinereum, in which case they usually lie below the third ventricle. Gelastic seizures commonly are associated with the intraventricular form, and electrophysiological studies have now definitively demonstrated that seizures originate within the hamartoma (Munari et al., 1995).

Early on and in mild cases, the interictal and even the ictal EEG may be normal, but variable abnormalities appear as the disease progresses, including focal, multifocal, and generalized spike-wave discharges, slowing, and paroxysmal fast activity. This change is believed to reflect propagation to mesial temporal structures, which likely become involved in the epileptogenic process as the seizure semiology progresses (Parvizi et al., 2011). Definitive diagnosis usually depends on identification of the hamartoma on MRI, and focal areas of hypoperfusion and hypometabolism can be seen with SPECT and PET (Fig. 7–9). Antiseizure medication is usually ineffective, as is surgical resection of cortex in most cases; however, surgical treatment that includes removal or ablation of the hamartoma is much more effective at eliminating seizures and improving behavior (Smith et al., 2009) (Chapter 16). Transcallosal resection is more effective than endoscopic and gamma knife procedures. Outcome is much better with surgery early in the course of the disorder, before neurological and cognitive sequelae develop.

Hemiconvulsion-Hemiplegia-Epilepsy

Occasionally, febrile seizures in infants, usually under the age of 2 years but as old as 4 years, can be unilateral and prolonged, at times alternating from one side of the body to the other. In this situation, the prolonged febrile seizure can be followed by hemiplegia, which can remain as a permanent neurological deficit. After one or several years, some of

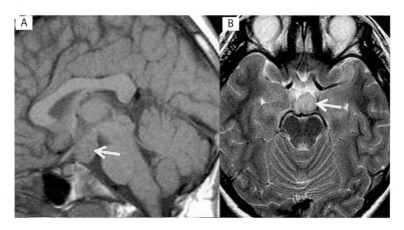

Figure 7–9. Hypothalamic hamartoma. **A.** Sagittal T1-weighted image demonstrates an inferiorly projecting round mass in the tuber cinereum (*arrow*), consistent with a hypothalamic hamartoma. **B.** Axial T2-weighted image shows high-intensity mass (*arrow*) in the interpeduncular cistern. (Courtesy of Dr. Noriko Salamon.)

these children can develop focal seizures in the damaged hemisphere, and this condition has been referred to as *hemiconvulsion-hemiplegia-epilepsy (HHE)* (Arzimanoglou et al., 2008; Arzimanoglou, 2010). The epilepsy syndrome exists only if spontaneous seizures occur. Whereas this was recognized as a rare but definite condition several decades ago, it has become almost nonexistent in the industrialized world, as a result of improved treatment for febrile status. HHE is more common, however, in developing countries and continues to be recognized by the ILAE as a specific syndrome. The etiology is unknown, but causes of the initial fever, such as viral infection, as well as preexisting cortical dysplasia, vascular mechanisms, and cytotoxic edema have been implicated. Most likely there are many reasons for this scenario to appear. The interictal EEG contains high-voltage delta activity and epileptiform discharges over the affected hemisphere, which appears atrophic on MRI. Prompt treatment of febrile status is an important preventive measure, but once the syndrome has developed, standard antiseizure drugs are often ineffective. Surgery, including hemispherectomy or hemispherotomy, can offer seizure relief (Chapter 16).

Head Nodding Syndrome

Although not recognized by ILAE, it is worth mention a condition peculiar to areas of Eastern sub-Saharan Africa, also called *nodding disease,* that has recently been considered by some workers to be an epilepsy syndrome (Winkler et al., 2008; Wadman, 2011). Originally described in Tanzania in the 1960's (Aall, 1962), the condition is most prevalent in South Sudan. It commonly affects children between the ages of 5 and 15 and is characterized by episodes of repetitive loss of neck tone causing head nodding, often brought on by eating. There is progressive impairment of growth and cognition, and premature death results from accidents and malnutrition. Whether these attacks are epileptic in nature remains disputed; hippocampal atrophy is seen on MRI and some patients have demonstrated interictal epileptiform abnormalities on EEG. A parasitic infection is suspected. Head nodding is responsive to antiseizure medication.

CONDITIONS WITH EPILEPTIC SEIZURES THAT ARE TRADITIONALLY NOT DIAGNOSED AS FORMS OF EPILEPSY PER SE

Benign Neonatal Seizures

The syndrome of *benign neonatal seizures (BNS)* begins, more or less, on the fifth day of life (*fifth-day fits*) in otherwise normal neonates without a family history. The diagnosis depends on exclusion of any specific underlying cause; consequently, this condition has also been referred to as *benign idiopathic neonatal seizures*, to distinguish it from benign neonatal seizures due to reversible metabolic disturbances such as hypocalcemia (Plouin, 2008, 2010b; Plouin and Neubauer, 2012). Seizures are focal clonic with or without apnea, but never tonic. They can alternate from side to side. Seizures are frequent and often lead to status epilepticus, which can persist from a few hours to a few days, after which there is rapid return to normalcy. EEG patterns are variable, with multifocal spikes as well as other abnormalities. BNS is rare and there is debate as to whether it still exists, given the increasing ability to identify specific causes of neonatal seizures. In any event, this condition is no longer considered, by ILAE, to meet the criteria for an epilepsy syndrome, because the seizures are not enduring.

Febrile Seizures

Febrile seizures (FS) is a well-defined reactive seizure condition that can be considered a syndrome. In keeping with the notion that reactive seizures are not epilepsy (Chapter 1), children with benign FS are not considered to have epilepsy, and this syndrome is not classified as an epilepsy syndrome. However, this disorder is the most common syndrome characterized by epileptic seizures.

CLINICAL DESCRIPTION

FS occurs in otherwise healthy children, usually between 3 months and 6 years of age. Peak incidence is 18–22 months (Nelson and

Ellenberg, 1983; Camfield et al., 2008; Nordli, 2010c). Generalized tonic-clonic seizures are induced during the rising phase of fever and, consequently, during the first day of a febrile illness. Seizures later in the course of a febrile illness should raise suspicion of another condition, unless a second infectious process is superimposed on the first. There is an increased risk for chronic epilepsy when febrile seizures last longer than 10–15 minutes or manifest focal features (Ellenberg and Nelson, 1978; Nelson and Ellenberg, 1981a;b). Febrile seizures that have these latter features are referred to as *complex*; isolated, brief tonic-clonic seizures are referred to as *simple*. Recent evidence supports a 10-minute duration as the upper limit of a simple febrile seizure (Hesdorffer et al., 2011).

Postictal EEG slowing is usually predominant in posterior head regions, may be asymmetrical, and can persist for several days. Interictal EEGs are most often normal, and the diagnostic value of an abnormal interictal EEG has not been established. Bilateral spike-and-wave discharges are common in the interictal EEG (Hauser, 1981), and centrotemporal spike foci can occur (Kajitani et al., 1981). These features are consistent with a diagnosis of benign FS and have no further diagnostic or prognostic value. Other laboratory tests are either normal or reflect the underlying febrile illness.

EPIDEMIOLOGY

Two percent to 5% of children in the United States experience one or more benign febrile seizures (Annegers et al., 1982), but the incidence is 7–8% in Japan and even higher in the Pacific Islands (Hauser, 1981), where children often sleep with their parents. Because febrile seizures occur before the febrile illness is recognized or late in the evening when the child is not being observed, the prevalence of this disorder may be much higher than reported.

ETIOLOGY

A predisposition to FS is an inherited trait, but the mode of inheritance is unknown. A family history of other types of epilepsy is common (Chapter 5). It is not known to what extent the polygenic trait is specific for epileptic seizures during fever and to what extent it involves nonspecific determinants of a lowered seizure threshold. Specific subunit mutations of the sodium channel and the $GABA_A$ receptor have been implicated in epilepsy syndromes, such as GEFS+ and Dravet syndrome, in which the habitual afebrile seizures are invariably preceded by febrile seizures; however, no clear relationship between the febrile seizures of these disorders and FS has been clearly demonstrated. The common febrile illnesses of childhood, such as *upper respiratory infections* and *otitis media*, are most often implicated in FS; however, fever of any cause can precipitate the typical ictal event in a susceptible infant or child.

DIFFERENTIAL DIAGNOSIS

The syndrome of FS must be distinguished from febrile illnesses that directly affect the brain and produce epileptic seizures, such as *meningitis* and *encephalitis*. Distinction from *cerebral malaria* presents a particular problem in some developing countries (Birbeck et al., 2010) (Chapter 5). When or whether to obtain a lumbar puncture after a first febrile seizure is a matter of clinical judgment (American Academy of Pediatrics, 1996). A lumbar puncture is obviously necessary if a central nervous system (CNS) infection is suspected for other reasons. Children under the age of 18 months, however, may not have signs of meningeal irritation. Meningitis or encephalitis should be considered when repeated seizures occur during a febrile illness or when seizures occur after the initial febrile peak. Although repeated generalized tonic-clonic seizures in adults may increase white cells in the cerebrospinal fluid (Schmidley and Simon, 1981), pleocytosis should not occur in FS. On the other hand, pleocytosis may not be present early in the course of an intracranial infectious process. Ictal events of FS can have focal clinical features; but both focal EEG changes apart from those mentioned above and focal neurological deficits suggest the presence of a localized brain disturbance. Seizures that occur in children during an immunization-induced fever represent FS and not an encephalopathic reaction to the immunization (Cendes and Sankar, 2011) (Chapter 5). The best evidence that a seizure during fever represents the first ictal event of a chronic seizure disorder is the subsequent occurrence of epileptic seizures without fever.

TREATMENT

Two aspects of therapy for FS are (1) the acute treatment of the seizure, which is usually accomplished with *benzodiazepines*, and (2) prophylaxis to prevent recurrence, which is no longer commonly recommended because these seizures are generally benign and the controversial effectiveness of seizure prevention with chronic antiseizure medication does not justify the risk of prolonged treatment.

PROGNOSIS

Based on retrospective studies indicating that patients with MTLE with HS have a relatively high incidence of prolonged febrile seizures in infancy, it was proposed that febrile seizures, particularly those that last longer than 30 minutes, lead to subsequent hippocampal sclerosis and chronic recurrent limbic seizures (Falconer, 1971). Subsequent prospective studies, however, have demonstrated that epileptic seizures without fever occur during later childhood in only 2–6% of patients with FS, and the incidence of other deleterious outcomes, such as mental retardation, neurological deficits, or death, is negligible (Ellenberg and Nelson, 1978; Nelson and Ellenberg, 1978; Hauser and Annegers, 1987). The incidence of later epilepsy appears to be only slightly higher when children are followed longer (Annegers et al., 1979), but this mildly increased risk persists into the fourth decade (Hauser and Annegers, 1987). There is now MRI evidence of hippocampal changes immediately following prolonged febrile seizures in infants and children, which could lead to hippocampal sclerosis; however, the relationship to later development of MTLE with HS in these situations has not been determined (Gomes and Shinnar, 2011).

Risk factors for subsequent epilepsy include a family history of nonfebrile epileptic seizures, preexisting neurological deficits and developmental delay, seizures lasting longer than 10–15 minutes, focal seizures, and multiple seizures occurring in one day (Ellenberg and Nelson, 1978; Nelson and Ellenberg, 1978). In a group of patients with FS followed to age 7, 60% had no major risk factors, and only 2% of that subgroup subsequently experienced nonfebrile epileptic seizures. The difference in nonfebrile seizure occurrence between this group and children who have not had FS is not statistically

significant. Thirty-four percent of patients had one risk factor, 3% of whom subsequently had nonfebrile epileptic seizures. Six percent of patients had two or more risk factors, and nonfebrile epileptic seizures occurred in 13% of this group. This nevertheless represents a relatively low incidence and probably reflects predisposing factors that would have given rise to epilepsy whether or not the child experienced febrile seizures (Fig. 7–10). Although the risk of nonfebrile epileptic seizures after two febrile seizures was twice the risk after one, there was no correlation between the further recurrence of febrile seizures and the ultimate appearance of nonfebrile epileptic seizures (Fig. 7–11). The conclusion of the Consensus Development Conference on Febrile Seizures (Nelson and Ellenberg, 1981a;b) was that a "rational approach to the management of febrile seizures should take into account that the long term prognosis is excellent, that prophylaxis reduces the risk of subsequent febrile seizures, and that there is no evidence that prophylaxis reduces the risk of subsequent nonfebrile seizures."

Reactive Seizures

Persons who have epileptic seizures resulting directly from transient stress or reversible

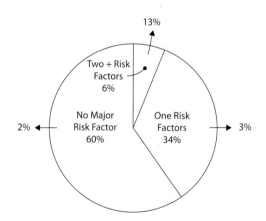

Figure 7–10. Incidence of risk factors among children with febrile seizures who also had nonfebrile seizures by age 7, based on results from the National Collaborative Perinatal Project on the outcome of 1,706 children. The risk factors evaluated were history of nonfebrile seizures in the immediate family, suspect or abnormal status in the child prior to first febrile seizure, and complex first febrile seizure. Numbers outside circle indicate percentages of all children with febrile seizures and indicated risk factors who had nonfebrile seizures. (From Ellenberg and Nelson, 1981, with permission.)

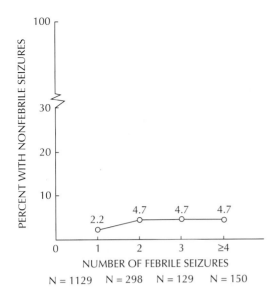

N = 1129   N = 298   N = 129   N = 150

Figure 7–11. Rate of later nonfebrile seizures among children with a first recurrence of febrile seizures was twice the rate in children with no recurrence. No additional increase in the rate of nonfebrile seizures was observed with further recurrence. (From Nelson and Ellenberg, 1981b, with permission.)

noxious insult to the brain are not considered to have epilepsy. Treatment consists of avoiding the precipitating factors when these are known (Wolf, 2008).

Seizures are the most common symptom of neurological disturbances in the newborn. Because these ictal events are unique to the neonate, they never constitute a chronic condition. Some neonatal seizures occur in response to transient and uncomplicated metabolic changes such as hypocalcemia, hypoglycemia, hyponatremia, and hypernatremia as well as to reversible toxic conditions such as drug withdrawal and intoxication (Chapter 5). Such seizures have a good prognosis and should be considered reactive. Neonatal seizures secondary to cerebral injury due to insults such as asphyxia, ischemia, congenital malformations, and hemorrhage have a much higher incidence of neurological sequelae, often including chronic seizures. Differential diagnosis of reactive neonatal seizure disorders is based largely on nonictal clinical data (Rose and Lombroso, 1970; Lombroso, 1983b; Aicardi, 1986; Holmes, 1986, 1987; Volpe, 1987).

Reactive ictal events induced in the more mature brain by physiological stress or systemic disturbances usually indicate a preexisting inherited or acquired low threshold for

seizures (Chapter 5). Reactive seizures are most often generalized tonic-clonic seizures, but absences and myoclonic jerks also occasionally occur. Focal reactive seizures can be seen when focal cerebral lesions are present that under ordinary circumstances do not give rise to spontaneous ictal events (Chapter 5). This can be a confusing point in differential diagnosis (Chapter 13). For instance, withdrawal seizures in alcoholics who have experienced serious head trauma in the past often manifest focal symptoms. Similarly, patients with severe unilateral brain damage can have reactive seizures that appear to be limited to the side of the body ipsilateral to the cerebral injury.

Neonatal Seizures Due to Structural and Metabolic Disorders

CLINICAL DESCRIPTION

Brain damage in the newborn can cause neonatal seizures that are indistinguishable from both (1) reactive seizures resulting from transient systemic disturbances and (2) benign neonatal seizures (BFNE, BNS) unrelated to an identifiable cerebral insult. Subtle, tonic, focal clonic, multifocal clonic, and myoclonic seizure types occur in all of these disorders, as do their various EEG correlates (Mizrahi et al., 2008) (Chapter 6). However, subtle and generalized tonic seizures, particularly those with poor EEG correlates, are more likely to reflect severe, irreversible cerebral dysfunction (Mizrahi and Kellaway, 1987; Mizrahi et al., 2008) (Chapter 6). Risk factors for subsequent neurological impairment include prematurity; evidence on examination of a focal or diffuse cerebral lesion; a history of asphyxia or trauma; and signs or symptoms of intracranial hemorrhage, cerebral malformations, or inborn errors of metabolism that cannot be corrected (Rose and Lombroso, 1970; Tharp et al., 1981; Lombroso, 1983b; Aicardi, 1986; Holmes, 1986, 1987; Volpe, 1987; Mizrahi et al., 2008). Onset of epileptic seizures before the third day of life and a severely abnormal background EEG rhythm are, in general, likely to indicate a condition associated with a poorer prognosis (Tharp et al., 1981; Holmes, 1987; Volpe, 1987). While a few specific syndromes have been proposed (Dulac et al., 1985), these disorders will be discussed here as a group.

EPIDEMIOLOGY

It is not possible to derive the incidence of sei-zures in the newborn from published reports. An overall incidence of neonatal seizures of 50 per 10,000 births was found in the National Collaborative Perinatal Project (Holden et al., 1982). Figures range from 15 per 10,000 for babies born at term (Eriksson and Zetterstrom, 1979) to over 2,000 per 10,000 for babies born prematurely (Seay and Bray, 1977). Perhaps 70–80% of all newborns with seizures have identifiable underlying causes (Lombroso, 1983b) (Chapter 5). These figures probably underestimate the incidence of seizures in the newborn; many seizures are undoubtedly missed because of subtle or absent clinical signs and the common use of muscle paralysis in treating respiratory distress.

ETIOLOGY

The most common causes of irreversible cere-bral injury associated with neonatal seizures are hypoxic-ischemic encephalopathy, intrac-ranial hemorrhage, intrauterine and postnatal infections, cerebral malformations, and inborn errors of metabolism (Chapter 5). Not all post-natal infections and inborn errors of metabo-lism, however, are irreversible.

DIFFERENTIAL DIAGNOSIS

Differential diagnosis and treatment of neo-natal seizures requires specialized skills and should be carried out by an expert in this field. The topic can be reviewed only briefly here and has been discussed in detail elsewhere (Lombroso, 1983b; Holmes, 1986, 1987; Volpe, 1987; Co et al., 2007; Mizrahi and Scher, 2008; Mizrahi et al., 2008). Management and progno-sis depend on the ability to distinguish epilepsy conditions due to irreversible structural and metabolic disorders from the reversible reac-tive seizures and BFNE or BNS. Commonly, more than one underlying cause of neonatal seizures can be identified; for instance, revers-ible metabolic disturbances often coexist with a chronic structural lesion. The diagnosis of BNS is made by exclusion and on the course. Seizures in the first three days of life are usu-ally due to hypoxic-ischemic encephalopathy, ischemia, intracranial bleeding, or congenital malformations; those beginning after the third

postnatal day are more likely due to postna-tally acquired infection and metabolic distur-bances. Early hypocalcemia, for instance, is almost always a complication of brain injury and not the primary cause of seizures, whereas late hypocalcemia (after three days) typically occurs in full-term infants fed cows' milk or formula with improper calcium-to-phosphorus and magnesium-to-phosphorus ratios (Volpe, 1987). This latter condition is completely reversible, without sequelae. Late hypocal-cemia has become rare where attention is paid to the preparation of infant formulas (Chapter 5).

Immediate recognition of reversible meta-bolic disturbances is paramount. This can be accomplished with available blood chemistry screening panels, including glucose, electro-lytes, blood urea nitrogen, calcium, magne-sium, and ammonia. It is also necessary to look for treatable chronic disorders, including the rare inborn errors of metabolism that respond to dietary manipulations, such as *pyridoxine dependency*, as well as infectious processes. *Herpes simplex encephalitis* has a particularly bad prognosis in the newborn and can be asso-ciated with a periodic EEG pattern (Mizrahi and Tharp, 1982), although this pattern may not be unique to herpes (E. M. Mizrahi, per-sonal communication, 1988).

Positive rolandic sharp waves in the new-born indicate *periventricular leukomalacia* and help to distinguish tonic events due to *intra-ventricular hemorrhage* from neonatal seizures (Novotny et al., 1987). *Jitteriness* is a nonspe-cific symptom of CNS dysfunction and also should not be mistaken for neonatal seizures (Chapter 13).

TREATMENT

Treatment of neonatal seizures consists first of acute management of epileptic symp-toms and specific therapy for the underlying cause or causes (Mizrahi and Scher, 2008). Ventilation should be ensured and blood glu-cose checked as soon as an IV line is opened. Hypoglycemia is treated immediately with 25% glucose (2–4 ml/kg IV) (Volpe, 1987). Controversy exists over whether or not the mild ictal symptoms of neonatal seizures lead to brain damage and need to be controlled by antiseizure drugs, which may also impair cerebral development (Chapters 8 and 10).

Most authors still recommend *phenobarbital* 20 mg/kg IV the first day, followed by daily maintenance of 5 mg/kg in two divided doses (Holmes, 1987; Volpe, 1987). Serum drug levels need to be monitored and should be in the range of 20–40 mg/ml. *Phenytoin* 20 mg/kg, *diazepam* 0.1–0.3 mg/kg, and *lorazepam* 0.05 mg/kg are also used. When present, hypocalcemia is treated with 5% *calcium gluconate* (4 ml/kg IV), and hypomagnesemia with 50% *magnesium sulfate* (0.2 ml/kg IM). *Pyridoxine* 50–100 mg IV should be given after administration of antiseizure medication if seizures continue and the cause remains unclear (Volpe, 1987).

PROGNOSIS

In the neonate, the prognostic issue is not whether seizures become chronic but rather whether seizures reflect a pathological process that is likely to give rise to chronic seizures at some point in the future. The outcome of neonatal seizure disorders, therefore, depends on the underlying cause (Watanabe et al., 1982) (Table 7–4). The National Collaborative Perinatal Project (Holden et al., 1982) carried out a seven-year follow-up study of 277 infants who experienced seizures, including those due to benign and reactive conditions as well as chronic brain disturbances, during the first 28 days of life. More than one-third died, but almost half appeared to be normal at age 7. Risk factors for a poor outcome included low Apgar scores, the need for resuscitation several minutes after birth, low birth weight, early

onset of seizures, and seizures lasting more than 30 minutes. Prognosis for neonatal seizures has improved greatly in the past 50 years. Mortality decreased from 40% to 15% between 1969 and 1987 (Volpe, 1987). For those infants who survive, the most common sequelae are mental retardation and motor deficits; in only 15–20% do chronic epileptic seizures develop. Recurrent epileptic conditions often take the form of WS, beginning during the first year of life, LGS, occurring later in childhood, or both.

MYOCLONIC SYNDROMES

The term *myoclonus* is used to describe several phenomena that occur in a variety of syndromes, many of which are not epileptic (Halliday, 1967; Gastaut, 1968; Hallett, 1985; Fahn et al., 1986, 2002; Hallett and Shibasaki, 2008) (Chapters 1 and 6). Nonepileptic myoclonus, as defined in Chapter 6, excludes myoclonic jerks that are believed to be due to cortical epileptic mechanisms (e.g., focal clonus of *epilepsia partialis continua* and *myoclonic seizures*). Nonepileptic myoclonus occurs in isolation and in association with a number of disease processes affecting the brain and spinal cord, but several conditions exist that are frequently referred to in the context of *myoclonic syndromes*. Startle disorders are considered separately in Chapter 13.

A myoclonic syndrome is a unique or readily recognizable symptom complex with the

Table 7–4 Incidence of Chronic Epilepsy After Neonatal Seizures

Main Etiological Factors	Number of Cases	Later Epilepsy (%)
Perinatal hypoxia and/or intracranial birth injury	140	41 (29.3)
Hypocalcemia		
Simple	20	0 (0.0)
Complicated	16	2 (12.5)
CNS infection	22	5 (22.7)
CNS dysgenesis	2	17 (81.0)
Hypoglycemia	8	1 (12.5)
Hyponatremia	2	0 (0.0)
Miscellaneous	7	0 (0.0)
Unknown	28	2 (7.1)
Total	264	68 (25.8)

From Watanabe et al., 1982, with permission.

occurrence of characteristic nonepileptic myoclonus as a principal feature. Some syndromes are inherited and have myoclonic symptoms as the only feature of the disorder, no identified pathological substrate, and a benign course. Others result from structural lesions of the CNS, although frequently these disorders are also inherited. A distinction is made here between nonepileptic myoclonic syndromes and those disorders characterized primarily by epileptic myoclonus (e.g., JME, discussed earlier), which are epilepsy syndromes.

The classic form of *benign essential myoclonus (paramyoclonus multiplex)* is inherited as an autosomal dominant trait. It is a rare disorder, characterized by sporadic myoclonic jerks (Chapter 6), that may be extremely mild or sufficiently severe to cause some degree of incapacitation (Halliday, 1967; Hallett et al., 1987). The EEG is usually unremarkable, and patients have normal intelligence and no other neurological deficits. Symptoms are not progressive, and prognosis is excellent. A nonfamilial form of benign essential myoclonus also exists. Disorders classified as benign essential myoclonus probably encompass more than one pathophysiological entity, including *essential tremor* and *myoclonus dystonia*. Some patients respond to *clonazepam*, others may experience relief from *5-hydroxytryptophan, propranolol, benztropine,* or *alcohol* (Hallett et al., 1987).

Several forms of *nocturnal myoclonus* are recognized. The *hypnic jerk* or *nocturnal start*, associated with arousal at sleep onset, and the small multifocal jerks, predominantly of hands and face, that occur during REM sleep are considered to be normal physiological phenomena (Hallett et al., 1987). At least four pathological syndromes are generally accepted (Hallett et al., 1987). *Periodic leg movements of sleep (PLMS)* consist of periodic (every 20 to 30 seconds), long-duration (500–2,000 msec), involuntary movements that predominantly involve leg flexors asynchronously or synchronously and occur during drowsiness and slow-wave sleep (Coleman et al., 1980). These events are usually more disturbing to the bed partner than the patient. *Restless legs syndrome (RLS)* is often familial and consists of a variety of nocturnal myoclonus symptoms, including PLMS. RLS is characterized by strange sensations of the lower extremities on attempting to go to sleep,

which cause a desire to move, and occasionally by a peripheral neuropathy (Lugaresi et al., 1986; Hallett et al., 1987). Movements are both voluntary and involuntary and can be due to a variety of disturbances, the most important of which is abnormal iron homeostasis (Catoire et al., 2011). *Excessive fragmentary myoclonus in non-REM sleep* is defined as multifocal sporadic myoclonic jerks occurring at a rate of five jerks or more per minute for at least 20 consecutive stages of non-REM sleep (Broughton et al., 1985). The clinical significance of this disorder is obscure (Hallett et al., 1987). *Benign neonatal sleep myoclonus* is characterized by multifocal and generalized myoclonic jerks during all stages of sleep. Jerks appear during the first month of life, do not occur during wakefulness, are not associated with EEG or developmental abnormalities, and disappear within a few months (Resnick et al., 1986).

A variety of other familial metabolic diseases can give rise to progressive symptoms and prominent myoclonus, including *juvenile neuroaxonal dystrophy, MERRF,* and *dentatorubral-pallidoluysianatrophy* (Berkovic et al., 1986; Shibasaki, 1987).

Posthypoxic myoclonus (Lance-Adams syndrome) is characterized by chronic, nonprogressive, sporadic, action myoclonus occurring some time after severe cerebral hypoxic insults such as those that may accompany cardiac arrest (Lance and Adams, 1963). Epileptic seizures can occur in this disorder, but it should not be considered in the category of PME. The specific anatomical sites of hypoxic damage responsible for this syndrome have not been identified, but several findings point to a disorder of serotonin metabolism (Fahn et al., 1986, 2002; Hallett and Shibasaki, 2008). Posthypoxic action myoclonus is a chronic syndrome, distinct from the condition of acute postanoxic myoclonus seen in comatose patients with *pseudoperiodic lateralized epileptiform discharges (PLEDs)* and burst suppression EEG patterns. *Valproic acid, clonazepam,* or *levetiracetam* are the treatments of choice for these forms of myoclonus. *Serotonergic* agents can also be effective in patients with posthypoxic action myoclonus but have more side effects than other agents.

Myoclonus is a prominent feature of the many conditions that constitute PME, as discussed in detail above.

SUMMARY AND CONCLUSIONS

An epilepsy syndrome is a symptom complex, the most important symptom being the occurrence of characteristic epileptic seizures of one or more types. When a condition is defined by a singular, specific pathological substrate, it is considered a disease associated with epileptic seizures and not an epilepsy syndrome. When the underlying disease process is unknown or could be due to several causes, diagnosis of a particular epilepsy syndrome informs the diagnostic evaluation and provides important insights into prognosis and management.

Any attempt to classify epilepsy syndromes must create artificial divisions, because all epilepsy disorders have multifactorial causes. Recognizing the necessary imprecision, however, it is arguably still clinically useful to distinguish three broad types of epileptic dysfunction: syndromes that are characterized by reactive seizures and should not be considered epilepsy; genetic, age-related epilepsy syndromes that are generally but not always benign and in which epileptic seizures are the only or principal disturbance; and epilepsy syndromes that result from acquired or genetically determined cerebral lesions or metabolic disorders, generally associated with other neurological and mental abnormalities and more refractory epileptic seizures. The old concepts of idiopathic and symptomatic, however, are no longer applied to define all epilepsies, because most recognized conditions have features of both. Susceptibility genes probably determine who is most likely to develop epilepsy given a specific acquired cerebral insult.

Not only is it not possible to logically categorize all epilepsy syndromes, but features of any individual patient often do not correspond to a precisely defined syndrome. Indeed, most adults with epileptic seizures cannot easily be diagnosed with one of the recognized syndromes discussed here. Rather than accept syndromes as discrete diagnostic entities, it is useful to see them as interrelated, with prognosis depending on where they lie within a spectrum of reactive, genetic, and specific structural or metabolic etiologies. Considering the disorder of an individual patient within this framework can provide a clinically useful perspective even if an exact diagnosis cannot be made.

Improved characterization and classification of specific epilepsy syndromes remains an important goal of clinical scientists. More sophisticated diagnostic tools and greater understanding of the genetic bases and pathophysiological mechanisms will allow syndromes to be more accurately described and relationships between syndromes to be more clearly defined. It is incorrect to state that a syndrome is either inherited or acquired. Rather, it must be determined to what extent genetic factors are involved and to what extent environmental factors are necessary for expression.

More precise characterization of epilepsy syndromes also stimulates relevant basic research. Improved definitions of clinical phenomena and their relationships to one another facilitate development of appropriate animal models and allow more homogeneous patient populations to be identified for clinical studies of fundamental mechanisms. Careful characterization, therefore, is a worthy pursuit that benefits the neuroscientist as well as the practicing physician.

REFERENCES

Aall, L (1962). Epilepsy in Tanganyika. Review and Newsletter—Transcultural Research in Mental Health Problems 13:54–57.

Aicardi, J (1985). Early myoclonic encephalopathy. In Epileptic Syndromes in Infancy, Childhood and Adolescence. Edited by J Roger, C Dravet, M Bureau, FE Dreifuss, and P Wolf. London: John Libbey, pp. 12–22.

Aicardi, J (1986). Epilepsy in Children. International Review of Child Neurology Series. New York: Raven Press.

Alarcon, G, and Valentin, A (2010). Mesial temporal lobe epilepsy with hippocampal sclerosis. In Atlas of Epilepsies. Edited by CP Panayiotopoulos. London: Springer-Verlag, pp. 1171–1176.

American Academy of Pediatrics (1996). Practice parameter: The neurodiagnostic evaluation of the child with a first simple febrile seizure. American Academy of Pediatrics, Provisional Committee on Quality Improvement, Subcommittee on Febrile Seizures. Pediatrics 97:769–772.

Andermann, F, and Berkovic, SF (2001). Idiopathic generalized epilepsy with generalized or other seizures in adolescence. Epilepsia 42:317–320.

Andermann, F, and Lugaresi, E (eds) (1987). Migraine and Epilepsy. Boston: Butterworths.

Annegers, JF, Hauser, WA, Elveback, LR, and Kurland, LT (1979). The risk of epilepsy following febrile convulsions. Neurology 29:297–303.

Annegers, JF, Hauser, WA, Anderson, VE, and Kurland, LT (1982). The risks of seizure disorders among relatives of patients with childhood onset epilepsy. Neurology 32:174–179.

Armstrong, DD, and Bruton, CJ (1987). Postscript: What terminology is appropriate for tissue pathology? How does it predict outcome? In Surgical Treatment of the Epilepsies. Edited by J Engel, Jr. New York: Raven Press, pp. 541–552.

Arzimanoglou, A (2010). Hemiconvulsion-hemiplegia-epilepsy syndrome. In Atlas of Epilepsies. Edited by CP Panayiotopoulos. London: Springer-Verlag, pp. 949–952.

Arzimanoglou, A, Dravet, C, and Chauvel, P (2008). Hemiconvulsion-hemiplegia-epilepsy syndrome. In Epilepsy: A Comprehensive Textbook, 2nd ed. Edited by J Engel, Jr, and TA Pedley. Philadelphia: Lippincott Williams & Wilkins, pp. 2355–2360.

Babb, TL, and Brown, WJ (1987). Pathological findings in epilepsy. In Surgical Treatment of the Epilepsies. Edited by J Engel, Jr. New York: Raven Press, pp. 511–540.

Bai, X, Vestal, M, Berman, R, Negishi, M, Spann, M, Vega, C, Desalvo, M, Novotny, EJ, Constable, RT, and Blumenfeld, H (2010). Dynamic time course of typical childhood absence seizures: EEG, behavior, and functional magnetic resonance imaging. J Neurosci 30:5884–5893.

Baldwin, M, and Bailey, P (eds) (1958). Temporal Lobe Epilepsy. Springfield, IL: Charles C Thomas.

Bansal, AR, and Radhakrishnan, K (2010). Primary reading epilepsy. In Atlas of Epilepsies. Edited by CP Panayiotopoulos. London: Springer-Verlag, pp. 1109–1114.

Bayreuther, C, and Thomas, P (2010). Dentatorubral-pallidoluysian atrophy. In Atlas of Epilepsies. Edited by CP Panayiotopoulos. London: Springer-Verlag, pp. 1251–1254.

Bear, DM, and Fedio P (1977). Quantitative analysis of interictal behavior in temporal lobe epilepsy. Arch Neurol 34:454–467.

Beaumanoir, A (1985a). The Landau-Kleffner syndrome. In Epileptic Syndromes in Infancy, Childhood and Adolescence. Edited by J Roger, C Dravet, M Bureau, FE Dreifuss, and P Wolf. London: John Libbey, pp. 181–191.

Beaumanoir, A (1985b). The Lennox-Gastaut syndrome. In Epileptic Syndromes in Infancy, Childhood and Adolescence. Edited by J Roger, C Dravet, M Bureau, FE Dreifuss, and P Wolf. London: John Libbey, pp. 89–99.

Bebek, N (2010). Hot water epilepsy. In Atlas of Epilepsies. Edited by CP Panayiotopoulos. London: Springer-Verlag, pp. 1119–1124.

Bellman, MH, Ross, EM, and Miller, DL (1983). Infantile spasms and pertussis immunization. Lancet 1:1031–1033.

Berg, AT, Berkovic, SF, Brodie, MJ, Buchhalter, J, Cross, JH, van Emde Boas, W, Engel, J, Jr, French, J, Glauser, TA, Mathern, GW, Moshé, SL, Nordli, D, Jr, Plouin, P, and Scheffer, IE (2010). Revised terminology and concepts for organization of seizures and epilepsies: Report of the ILAE Commission on Classification and Terminology, 2005–2009. Epilepsia 51:676–685.

Berkovic, SF, Andermann, F, Carpenter, S, and Wolfe, LS (1986). Progressive myoclonus epilepsies: Specific causes and diagnosis. N Engl J Med 315:296–305.

Berkovic, SF (2008). Progressive myoclonus epilepsies. In Epilepsy: A Comprehensive Textbook, 2nd ed. Edited by J Engel, Jr, and TA Pedley. Philadelphia: Lippincott Williams & Wilkins, pp. 2525–2535.

Birbeck, GL, Beare, N, Lewallen, S, Glover, SJ, Molyneux, ME, Kaplan, PW, and Taylor, TE (2010). Identification of malaria retinopathy improves the specificity of the clinical diagnosis of cerebral malaria: Findings from a prospective cohort study. Am J Trop Med Hyg 82:231–234.

Bittencourt, PRM, and Richens, A (1981). Anticonvulsant-induced status epilepticus in Lennox-Gastaut syndrome. Epilepsia 22:129–134.

Bjerre, I, and Corelius, E (1968). Benign familial neonatal convulsions. Acta Paediatr Scand 57:557–561.

Blom, S, Heijbel, J, and Bergfors, PG (1972). Benign epilepsy of children with centro-temporal EEG foci: Prevalence and follow-up study of 40 patients. Epilepsia 13:609–619.

Blümcke, I, Thom, M, Aronica, E, et al. (2011). The clinicopathologic spectrum of focal cortical dysplasias: A consensus classification proposed by an ad hoc task force of the ILAE Diagnostic Methods Commission. Epilepsia 52:158–174.

Blume, WT (1987). Lennox-Gastaut syndrome. In Epilepsy: Electroclinical Syndromes. Edited by H Lüders and RP Lesser. London: Springer-Verlag, pp. 73–92.

Blume, WT, David, RB, and Gomez, MR (1973). Generalized sharp and slow wave complexes: Associated clinical features and long-term follow-up. Brain 96:289–306.

Blumer, D, and Benson, DF (1982). Psychiatric manifestations of epilepsy. In Psychiatric Aspects of Neurologic Disease, Vol II. Edited by DF Benson and DF Blumer. New York: Grune & Stratton, pp. 25–48.

Bonilha, L, Matz, GU, Glazier, SS, and Edwards, JC (2012). Subtypes of medial temporal lobe epilepsy: Influence on temporal lobectomy outcomes? Epilepsia 53:1–5.

Bonte, FJ, Stokely, EM, Devous, MD, Sr, and Homan, RW (1983). Single-photon tomographic study of regional cerebral blood flow in epilepsy: A preliminary report. Arch Neurol 40:267–270.

Bray, PF, and Wiser, WC (1964). Evidence for a genetic etiology of temporalcentral abnormalities in focal epilepsy. N Engl J Med 271:926–933.

Bray, PF, and Wiser, WC (1965). The relation of focal to diffuse epileptiform EEG discharges in genetic epilepsy. Arch Neurol 13:223–237.

Brenner, RP, and Atkinson, R (1982). Generalized paroxysmal fast activity: Electroencephalographic and clinical features. Ann Neurol 11:386–390.

Brna, PM, Gordon, KE, Dooley, JM, and Wood, EP (2001). The epidemiology of infantile spasms. Can J Neurol Sci 28:309–312.

Broughton, R, Tolentino, MA, and Krelina, M (1985). Excessive fragmentary myoclonus in NREM sleep. A report of 38 cases. Electroencephalogr Clin Neurophysiol 61:123–133.

Bureau, M, and Tassinari, CA (2012). Myoclonic absences and absences with myoclonias. In Epileptic Syndromes in Infancy, Childhood and Adolescence. Edited by M Bureau, P Genton, C Dravet, A Delgado-Escueta, CA Tassinari, P Thomas, and P Wolf. London: John Libbey.

Bureau, M, Genton, P, and Dravet, C (2010). Dravet syndrome. In Atlas of Epilepsies. Edited by CP Panayiotopoulos. London: Springer-Verlag, pp. 891–898.

Bureau, M, Genton, P, Dravet, C, Delgado-Escueta, A, Tassinari, CA, Thomas, P, and Wolf, P (eds) (2012). Epileptic Syndromes in Infancy, Childhood and Adolescence. London: John Libbey.

Caffi, J (1973). Zur Frage klinischer Anfallformen bei psychomotorischer Epilepsie. Schweiz Med Wochenschr 103:469–475.

Camfield, CS, and Camfield, PR (2009). Juvenile myoclonic epilepsy 25 years after seizure onset. Neurology 73:1041–1045.

Camfield, CS, Camfield, PR, and Neville, BG (2008). Febrile seizures. In Epilepsy: A Comprehensive Textbook, 2nd ed. Edited by J Engel, Jr, and TA Pedley. Philadelphia: Lippincott Williams & Wilkins, pp. 659–664.

Camfield, P, Scheffer, I, and Marini, C (2012). Febrile seizures and GEFS+. In Epileptic Syndromes in Infancy, Childhood and Adolescence. Edited by M Bureau, P Genton, C Dravet, CA Tassinari, A Delgado-Escueta, P Thomas, and P Wolf. London: John Libbey.

Carabello, RH, Cersosimo, RO, Espeche, A, Arroyo, HA, and Fejerman, N (2007). Myoclonic status in nonprogressive encephalopathies: Study of 29 cases. Epilepsia 48:107–113.

Cascino, GD (2009). Temporal lobe epilepsy is a progressive neurologic disorder. Neurology 72:1718–1719.

Catoire, H, Dion, PA, Xiong, L, Amari, M, Gaudet, R, Girard, SL, Noreau, A, Gaspar, C, Turecki, G, Montplaisir, JY, Parker, JA, and Rouleau, GA (2011). Restless legs syndrome-associated MEIS1 risk variant influences iron homeostasis. Ann Neurol 70:170–175.

Cavazzutti, GB (1980). Epidemiology of different types of epilepsy in school-age children of Modena, Italy. Epilepsia 21:57–62.

Cendes, F, and Sankar, R (2011). Vaccinations and febrile seizures. Epilepsia 52(suppl 3):23–25.

Cendes, F, Kobayashi, E, Lopes-Cendes, I, Andermann, F, and Andermann, E (2008). Familial temporal lobe epilepsies. In Epilepsy: A Comprehensive Textbook, 2nd ed. Edited by J Engel, Jr, and TA Pedley. Philadelphia: Lippincott Williams & Wilkins, pp. 2487–2493.

Charlier, C, Singh, NA, Ryan, SG, et al. (1998). A pore mutation in a novel KQT-like potassium channel gene in an idiopathic epilepsy family. Nat Genet 18:53–55.

Chugani, HT, and Conti, JR (1996). Etiologic classification of infantile spasms in 140 cases: Role of positron emission tomography. J Child Neurol 11:44–48.

Cilio, MR, Dulac, O, Guerrini, R, and Vigevano, F (2008). Migrating partial seizures in infancy. In Epilepsy: A Comprehensive Textbook, 2nd ed. Edited by J Engel, Jr, and TA Pedley. Philadelphia: Lippincott Williams & Wilkins, pp. 2323–2328.

Claes, L, Del-Favero, J, Ceulemand, B, Lagae, L, Van Broeckhoven, C, and De Jonghe, P (2001). De novo mutations in the sodium-channel gene SCN1A cause severe myoclonic epilepsy of infancy. Am J Hum Genet 68:1327–1332.

Co, JPT, Elia, M, Engel, J, Jr, Guerrini, R, Mizrahi, EM, Moshé, SL, and Plouin, P (2007). Proposal of an algorithm for diagnosis and treatment of neonatal seizures in developing countries. Epilepsia 48:1158–1164.

Cole, AJ, Andermann, F, Taylor, L, Olivier, A, Rasmussen, T, Robitaille, Y, and Spire, J-P (1988). The Landau-Kleffner syndrome of acquired epileptic aphasia: Unusual clinical outcome, surgical experience and absence of encephalitis. Neurology 38:31–38.

Coleman, RM, Pollak, CP, and Weitzman, ED (1980). Periodic movements in sleep (nocturnal myoclonus): Relation to sleep disorders. Ann Neurol 8:416–421.

Commission on Classification and Terminology of the International League Against Epilepsy (1989). Proposal for revised classification of epilepsies and epileptic syndromes. Epilepsia 30:389–399.

Coppola, G, Plouin, P, Chiron, C, Robain, O, and Dulac, O (1995). Migrating partial seizures in infancy: A malignant disorder with developmental arrest. Epilepsia 36:1017–1024.

Covanis, A (2010a). Myoclonic epilepsy in infancy. In Atlas of Epilepsies. Edited by CP Panayiotopoulos. London: Springer-Verlag, pp. 871–878.

Covanis, A (2010b). Panayiotopoulos syndrome. In Atlas of Epilepsies. Edited by CP Panayiotopoulos. London: Springer-Verlag, pp. 965–972.

Covanis, A (2010c). Landau-Kleffner syndrome. In Atlas of Epilepsies. Edited by CP Panayiotopoulos. London: Springer-Verlag, pp. 905–912.

Covanis, A (2010d). Childhood absence epilepsy. In Atlas of Epilepsies. Edited by CP Panayiotopoulos. London: Springer-Verlag, pp. 1013–1024.

Covanis, A (2010e). Jeavons syndrome. In Atlas of Epilepsies. Edited by CP Panayiotopoulos. London: Springer-Verlag, pp. 1081–1092.

Covanis, A (2010f). Epilepsy with myoclonic absences. In Atlas of Epilepsies. Edited by CP Panayiotopoulos. London: Springer-Verlag, pp. 1025–1028.

Crespel, A, Ferlazzo, E, Nikanorova, M, Ferlazzo, E, and Genton, P (2012). The Lennox-Gastaut syndrome. In Epileptic Syndromes in Infancy, Childhood and Adolescence. Edited by M Bureau, P Genton, C Dravet, A Delgado-Escueta, CA Tassinari, P Thomas, and P Wolf. London: John Libbey.

Dalby, MA (1969). Epilepsy and 3 per second spike and wave rhythms: A clinical, electroencephalographic and prognostic analysis of 346 patients. Acta Neurol Scand 45(suppl 40):183.

Dalla Bernardina, B (2008). Myoclonic status in nonprogressive encephalopathy. In Epilepsy: A Comprehensive Textbook, 2nd ed. Edited by J Engel, Jr, and TA Pedley. Philadelphia: Lippincott Williams & Wilkins, pp. 2361–2364.

Dalla Bernardina, B, Trevisan, C, Bondavalli, S, et al. (1980). Une forme particulière d'epilepsies myoclonique chez des enfants porteurs d'encéphalopathie fixée. Boll Lega Ital Epil 29–30:183–187.

Djukic, A, Vigevano, F, Plouin, P, and Moshé, SL (2008). Early myoclonic encephalopathy (neonatal myoclonic encephalopathy). In Epilepsy: A Comprehensive Textbook, 2nd ed. Edited by J Engel, Jr, and TA Pedley. Philadelphia: Lippincott Williams & Wilkins, pp. 2297–2301.

Doose, H (1985). Myoclonic astatic epilepsy of early childhood. In Epileptic Syndromes in Infancy, Childhood and Adolescence. Edited by J Roger, C Dravet, M Bureau, FE Dreifuss, and P Wolf. London: John Libbey, pp. 78–88.

Douglass, L (ed) (2011). Long-term outlook of Lennox-Gastaut syndrome and related epilepsies: Care for a lifetime. Epilepsia 52(suppl 5).

Dravet, C (1978). Les epilepsies grave des de l'enfant. Vie Med 8:543–548.

Dravet, C, and Bureau, M (2008). Severe myoclonic epilepsy in infancy (Dravet syndrome). In Epilepsy: A

Comprehensive Textbook, 2nd ed. Edited by J Engel, Jr, and TA Pedley. Philadelphia: Lippincott Williams & Wilkins, pp. 2337–2342.

Dravet, C, and Vigevano, F (2008). Idiopathic myoclonic epilepsy in infancy. In Epilepsy: A Comprehensive Textbook, 2nd ed. Edited by J Engel, Jr, and TA Pedley. Philadelphia: Lippincott Williams & Wilkins, pp. 2343–2348.

Dravet, C, Bureau, M, Oguni, H, Cokar, O, and Guerrini, R (2012). Dravet syndrome. In Epileptic Syndromes in Infancy, Childhood and Adolescence. Edited by M Bureau, P Genton, C Dravet, CA Tassinari, A Delgado-Escueta, P Thomas, and P Wolf. London: John Libbey.

Dreifuss, FE (1983). Infantile spasms. In Pediatric Epileptology. Edited by FE Dreifuss. Boston: John Wright, pp. 97–108.

Dreifuss, FE, Santilli, N, Langer, DH, Sweeney, KP, Moline, KA, and Menander, KB (1987). Valproic acid hepatic fatalities: A retrospective review. Neurology 37:379–385.

Dubeau, F, Andermann, F, Wiendl, H, and Bar-Or, A (2008). Rasmussen's encephalitis (chronic focal encephalitis). In Epilepsy: A Comprehensive Textbook, 2nd ed. Edited by J Engel, Jr, and TA Pedley. Philadelphia: Lippincott Williams & Wilkins, pp. 2439–2453.

Dulac, O, and Kaminska, A (2008). Epilepsy with myoclonic astatic seizures. In Epilepsy: A Comprehensive Textbook, 2nd ed. Edited by J Engel, Jr, and TA Pedley. Philadelphia: Lippincott Williams & Wilkins, pp. 2349–2354.

Dulac, O, Aubourg, P, and Plouin, P (1985). Other epileptic syndromes in neonates. In Epileptic Syndromes in Infancy, Childhood and Adolescence. Edited by J Roger, C Dravet, M Bureau, FE Dreifuss, and P Wolf. London: John Libbey, pp. 23–29.

Dulac, O, Dalla Bernardina, B, and Chiron, C (2008). West syndrome. In Epilepsy: A Comprehensive Textbook, 2nd ed. Edited by J Engel, Jr, and TA Pedley. Philadelphia: Lippincott Williams & Wilkins, pp. 2329–2335.

Ellenberg, JH, and Nelson, KB (1978). Febrile seizures and later intellectual performance. Arch Neurol 35:17–21.

Ellenberg, JH, and Nelson, KB (1981). Long-term clinical trials on the use of prophylaxis for prevention of recurrences of febrile seizures and epilepsy. In Febrile Seizures. Edited by KB Nelson and JH Ellenberg. New York: Raven Press, pp. 267–278.

Engel, J, Jr (1984). A practical guide for routine EEG studies in epilepsy. J Clin Neurophysiol 1:109–142.

Engel, J, Jr (1987). Outcome with respect to epileptic seizures. In Surgical Treatment of the Epilepsies. Edited by J Engel, Jr. New York: Raven Press, pp. 553–572.

Engel, J, Jr (2001a). A proposed diagnostic scheme for people with epileptic seizures and with epilepsy: Report of the ILAE Task Force on Classification and Terminology. Epilepsia 42:796–803.

Engel, J, Jr (2001b). Mesial temporal lobe epilepsy: What have we learned? The Neuroscientist 7:340–352.

Engel, J, Jr (2006). Report of the ILAE Classification Core Group. Epilepsia 47:1558–1568.

Engel, J, Jr, and Pedley, TA (eds) (2008). Epilepsy: A Comprehensive Textbook, 2nd ed. Philadelphia: Lippincott Williams & Wilkins.

Engel, J, Jr, and Thompson, PM (2012). Going beyond hippocampocentricity in the concept of mesial temporal lobe epilepsy. Epilepsia 53:220–223.

Engel, J, Jr, Rapin, I, and Giblin, DR (1977). Electrophysiological studies in two patients with the cherry red spot–myoclonus syndrome. Epilepsia 18:73–87.

Engel, J, Jr, Brown, WJ, Kuhl, DE, Phelps, ME, Mazziotta, JC, and Crandall, PH (1982a). Pathological findings underlying focal temporal lobe hypometabolism in partial epilepsy. Ann Neurol 12:518–528.

Engel, J, Jr, Kuhl, DE, Phelps, ME, and Crandall, PH (1982b). Comparative localization of epileptic foci in partial epilepsy by PCT and EEG. Ann Neurol 12:529–537.

Engel, J, Jr, Kuhl, DE, Phelps, ME, and Mazziotta, JC (1982c). Interictal cerebral glucose metabolism in partial epilepsy and its relation to EEG changes. Ann Neurol 12:510–517.

Engel, J, Jr, Crandall, PH, and Rausch, R (1983a). The partial epilepsies. In The Clinical Neurosciences, Vol 2. Edited by RN Rosenberg. New York: Churchill Livingstone, pp. 1349–1380.

Engel, J, Jr, Kuhl, DE, Phelps, ME, Rausch, R, and Nuwer, MR (1983b). Local cerebral metabolism during partial seizures. Neurology 33:400–413.

Engel, J, Jr, Lubens, P, Kuhl, DE, and Phelps, M (1985). Local cerebral metabolic rate for glucose during petit mal absences. Ann Neurol 17:121–128.

Engel, J, Jr, Wiebe, S, French, J, Gumnit, R, Spencer, D, Sperling, M, Williamson, P, Zahn, C, Westbrook, E, and Enos, B (2003). Practice parameter: Temporal lobe and localized neocortical resections for epilepsy. Neurology 60:538–547.

Engel, J, Jr, Williamson, PD, and Wieser, HG (2008). Mesial temporal lobe epilepsy with hippocampal sclerosis. In Epilepsy: A Comprehensive Textbook, 2nd ed. Edited by J Engel, Jr, and TA Pedley. Philadelphia: Lippincott Williams & Wilkins, pp. 2479–2486.

Engel, J, Jr, McDermott, MP, Wiebe, S, Langfitt, JT, Stern, JM, Dewar, S, Sperling, MR, Gardiner, I, Erba, G, Fried, I, Jacobs, M, Vinters, HV, Mintzer, S, and Kieburtz, K (2012). Early surgical therapy for drug-resistant temporal lobe epilepsy: a randomized trial. JAMA 307:922–930.

Erba, G, and Browne, TR (1983). Atypical absence, myoclonic, atonic, and tonic seizures, and the "Lennox-Gastaut Syndrome." In Epilepsy, Diagnosis and Management. Edited by TR Browne and RG Feldman. Boston: Little, Brown & Co, pp. 75–94.

Eriksson, M, and Zetterstrom, R (1979). Neonatal convulsions: Incidence and causes in the Stockholm area. Acta Paediatr Scand 68:807–811.

Fahn, S, Marsden, CD, and Van Woert, MH (eds) (1986). Myoclonus. Adv Neurol 43.

Fahn, S, Frucht, SJ, Hallett, M, and Truong, DD (eds) (2002). Myoclonus and paroxysmal dyskinesias. Adv Neurol 89.

Falconer, MA (1971). Genetic and related aetiological factors in temporal lobe epilepsy: A review. Epilepsia 12:13–31.

Fejerman, N (2008a). Nonepileptic neurologic paroxysmal disorders and episodic symptoms in infants. In Epilepsy: A Comprehensive Textbook, 2nd ed. Edited by J Engel, Jr, and TA Pedley. Philadelphia: Lippincott Williams & Wilkins, pp. 2783–2791.

Fejerman, N (2008b). Benign childhood epilepsy with centrotemporal spikes. In Epilepsy: A Comprehensive Textbook, 2nd ed. Edited by J Engel, Jr, and TA Pedley. Philadelphia: Lippincott Williams & Wilkins, pp. 2369–2377.

Fejerman, N (2008c). Early-onset benign childhood occipital epilepsy (Panayiotopoulos type). In Epilepsy: A Comprehensive Textbook, 2nd ed. Edited by J Engel, Jr, and TA Pedley. Philadelphia: Lippincott Williams & Wilkins, pp. 2379–2386.

Fejerman, N (2010). Benign childhood epilepsy with centrotemporal spikes. In Atlas of Epilepsies. Edited by CP Panayiotopoulos. London: Springer-Verlag, pp. 957–964.

Franceschetti, S, Canafoglia, L, and Panzica, F (2010). Sialidoses (Types I and II). In Atlas of Epilepsies. Edited by CP Panayiotopoulos. London: Springer-Verlag, pp. 1243–1246.

Fusco, L, Chiron, C, Trivisano, M, Chugani, H, and Vigevano, F (2012). Infantile spasms. In Epileptic Syndromes in Infancy, Childhood and Adolescence. Edited by M Bureau, P Genton, C Dravet, A Delgado-Escueta, CA Tassinari, P Thomas, and P Wolf. London: John Libbey.

Gastaut, H (1968). Séméiologie des myoclonies et nosologie analytique des syndromes myocloniques. Rev Neurol 119:1–30.

Gastaut, H (1973). Dictionary of Epilepsy. Part I. Definitions. Geneva: World Health Organization.

Gastaut, H (1982). A new type of epilepsy: Benign partial epilepsy of childhood with occipital spike waves. In Advances in Epileptology: XIIIth Epilepsy International Symposium. Edited by H Akimoto, H Kazamatsuri, M, Seino, and AA Ward, Jr. New York: Raven Press, pp. 19–24.

Gastaut, H (1985). Benign epilepsy of childhood with occipital paroxysms. In Epileptic Syndromes in Infancy, Childhood and Adolescence. Edited by J Roger, C Dravet, M Bureau, FE Dreifuss, and P Wolf. London: John Libbey, pp. 159–170.

Gastaut, H, and Zifkin, BG (1987). Benign epilepsy of childhood with occipital spike and wave complexes. In Migraine and Epilepsy. Edited by F Andermann and E Lugaresi. Boston: Butterworths, pp. 47–81.

Gastaut, H, Roger, J, Soulayrol, R, Tassinari, CA, Regis, H, Dravet, C, Bernard, R, Pinsard, N, and Saint-Jean, M (1966). Childhood epileptic encephalopathy with diffuse slow spike-waves (otherwise known as petit mal variant) or Lennox syndrome. Epilepsia 7:139–179.

Gastaut, H, Gastaut, JL, Goncalves e Silva, GE, and Fernandez Sanchez, GR (1975). Relative frequency of different types of epilepsy: A study employing the classification of the International League Against Epilepsy. Epilepsia 16:457–461.

Gélisse, P, Wolf, P, and Inoue, Y (2012a). Juvenile absence epilepsy. In Epileptic Syndromes in Infancy, Childhood and Adolescence. Edited by M Bureau, P Genton, C Dravet, A Delgado-Escueta, CA Tassinari, P Thomas, and P Wolf. London: John Libbey.

Gélisse, P, Crespel, A, Del Socorro Gonzalez, M, Thomas, P, and Genton, P (2012b). IGE with grand mal seizures only. In Epileptic Syndromes in Infancy, Childhood and Adolescence. Edited by M Bureau, P Genton, C Dravet, A Delgado-Escueta, CA Tassinari, P Thomas, and P Wolf. London: John Libbey.

Genton, P, and Dravet, C (2008). Lennox-Gastaut syndrome. In Epilepsy: A Comprehensive Textbook, 2nd ed. Edited by J Engel, Jr, and TA Pedley. Philadelphia: Lippincott Williams & Wilkins, pp. 2417–2427.

Genton, P, Michelucci, R, Serratosa, JM, and Delgado-Escueta, A (2012). Progressive myoclonus epilepsies. In Epileptic Syndromes in Infancy, Childhood and Adolescence. Edited by M Bureau, P Genton, C Dravet, A Delgado-Escueta, CA Tassinari, P Thomas, and P Wolf. London: John Libbey.

Giraldez, BG, and Serratosa, JM (2010a). Lafora disease. In Atlas of Epilepsies. Edited by CP Panayiotopoulos. London: Springer-Verlag, pp. 1231–1234.

Giraldez, BG, and Serratosa, JM (2010b). Other progressive myoclonic epilepsies. In Atlas of Epilepsies. Edited by CP Panayiotopoulos. London: Springer-Verlag, pp. 1265–1270.

Glauser, TA, Cnaan, A, Shinnar, S, et al. (2010). Ethosuximide, valproic acid, and lamotrigine in childhood absence epilepsy. N Engl J Med 362:790–799.

Go, CY, Mackay, MT, Weiss, SK, Stephens, D, Adams-Webber, T, Ashwal, S, and Snead, OC, III (2012). Evidence-based guideline update: Medical treatment of infantile spasms. Neurology 78:1974–1980.

Gobbi, G, Guerrini, R, and Grosso, S (2008). Late-onset childhood occipital epilepsy (Gastaut type). In Epilepsy: A Comprehensive Textbook, 2nd ed. Edited by J Engel, Jr, and TA Pedley. Philadelphia: Lippincott Williams & Wilkins, pp. 2387–2395.

Gomes, WA, and Shinnar, S (2011). Prospects for imaging-related biomarkers of human epileptogenesis: A critical review. Biomarkers Med 5:599–606.

Goosses, R (1984). Die Beziehung der Fotosensibilität zu den verschiedenen epileptischen Syndromen. Thesis, West Berlin.

Granata, T, Hart, Y, and Andermann, F (2012). Rasmussen's syndrome. In Epileptic Syndromes in Infancy, Childhood and Adolescence. Edited by M Bureau, P Genton, C Dravet, A Delgado-Escueta, CA Tassinari, P Thomas, and P Wolf. London: John Libbey.

Gregory, DL, and Wong, PK (1984). Topographical analysis of the centrotemporal discharges in benign rolandic epilepsy of childhood. Epilepsia 25:705–711.

Grünewald, RA (2010). Juvenile myoclonic epilepsy. In Atlas of Epilepsies. Edited by CP Panayiotopoulos. London: Springer-Verlag, pp. 1033–1040.

Guerrini, R, and Dravet, C (2012). Idiopathic myoclonic epilepsies in infancy and early childhood. In Epileptic Syndromes in Infancy, Childhood and Adolescence. Edited by M Bureau, P Genton, C Dravet, A Delgado-Escueta, CA Tassinari, P Thomas, and P Wolf. London: John Libbey.

Guerrini, R, and Rosati, A (2010). Angelman syndrome. In Atlas of Epilepsies. Edited by CP Panayiotopoulos. London: Springer-Verlag, pp. 1255–1264.

Guerrini, R, Bureau, M, Dalla Bernardina, B, and Dravet, C (eds) (2011). Severe myoclonic epilepsy—Dravet syndrome, thirty years later. Epilepsia 52(suppl 2).

Hallett, M (1985). Myoclonus: Relation to epilepsy. Epilepsia 26(suppl 1):S67–S77.

Hallett, M, and Shibasaki, H (2008). Myoclonus and myoclonic syndromes. In Epilepsy: A Comprehensive Textbook, 2nd ed. Edited by J Engel, Jr, and TA Pedley. Philadelphia: Lippincott Williams & Wilkins, pp. 2765–2770.

Hallett, M, Marsden, CD, and Fahn, S (1987). Myoclonus. In Handbook of Clinical Neurology, Vol 49 (Rev Ser, Vol 5). Edited by PJ Vinken, GW Bruyn, and HL Klawans. Amsterdam: Elsevier, pp. 609–625.

Halliday, AM (1967a). The clinical incidence of myoclonus. In Modern Trends in Neurology, Vol 4. Edited by D Williams. London: Butterworths, pp. 69–103.

Halliday, AM (1967b). The electrophysiological study of myoclonus in man. Brain 90:241–284.

Harvey, AS, Eeg-Olofsson, O, and Freeman; JL (2008). Hypothalamic hamartoma with gelastic seizures. In Epilepsy: A Comprehensive Textbook, 2nd ed. Edited by J Engel, Jr, and TA Pedley. Philadelphia: Lippincott Williams & Wilkins, pp. 2503–2509.

Hauser, WA (1981). The natural history of febrile seizures. In Febrile Seizures. Edited by KB Nelson and JH Ellenberg. New York: Raven Press, pp. 5–17.

Hauser, WA, and Annegers, JF (1987). Prognosis of children with febrile seizures. In Advances in Epileptology, Vol 16. Edited by P Wolf, M Dam, D Janz, and FE Dreifuss. New York: Raven Press, pp. 155–161.

Heijbel, J, Blom, S, and Rasmuson, M (1975). Benign epilepsy of childhood with centrotemporal EEG foci: A genetic study. Epilepsia 16:285–293.

Hemb, M, Velasco, TR, Parnes, MS, et al. (2010). Improved outcomes in pediatric epilepsy surgery. The UCLA experience, 1986–2008. Neurology 74:1768–1775.

Henry, TR, and Chugani, HT (2008). Positron emission tomography. In Epilepsy: A Comprehensive Textbook, 2nd ed. Edited by J Engel, Jr, and TA Pedley. Philadelphia: Lippincott Williams & Wilkins, pp. 945–964.

Hesdorffer, DC, Benn, EKT, Bagiella, E, Nordli, D, Pellock, J, Hinton, V, and Shinnar, S, for the FEBSTAT Study Team (2011). Distribution of febrile seizure duration and associations with development. Ann Neurol 70:93–100.

Hirano, M (2010). Myoclonus epilepsy with ragged-red fibers. In Atlas of Epilepsies. Edited by CP Panayiotopoulos. London: Springer-Verlag, pp. 1247–1250.

Hirsch, E, Thomas, P, and Panayiotopoulos, CP (2008). Childhood and juvenile absence epilepsies. In Epilepsy: A Comprehensive Textbook, 2nd ed. Edited by J Engel, Jr, and TA Pedley. Philadelphia: Lippincott Williams & Wilkins, pp. 2397–2411.

Hirsch, E, Delgado-Escueta, A, and Medina, M (2012). Childhood absence epilepsy. In Epileptic Syndromes in Infancy, Childhood and Adolescence. Edited by M Bureau, P Genton, C Dravet, A Delgado-Escueta, CA Tassinari, P Thomas, and P Wolf. London: John Libbey.

Holden, KR, Mellits, ED, and Freeman, JM (1982). Neonatal seizures I. Correlation of prenatal and perinatal events with outcomes. Pediatrics 70:165–176.

Holmes, GL (1986). Morphological and physiological maturation of the brain in the neonate and young child. J Clin Neurophysiol 3:209–238.

Holmes, GL (1987). Diagnosis and Management of Seizures in Children. Philadelphia: WB Saunders.

Hrachovy, RA, and Frost, JD (1988). Infantile spasms. Cleve Clin J Med 56(suppl 1):S10–S16.

Hrachovy, RA, Frost, JD, Jr, Kellaway, P, and Zion, TE (1983). Double blind study of ACTH vs prednisone therapy in infantile spasms. J Pediatr 103:641–645.

Ioos, C, Fohlen, M, Villeneuve, N, et al. (2000). Hot water epilepsy: A benign and unrecognized form. J Child Neurol 15:125–128.

Irani, SR, Michell, AW, Lang, B, Pettingill, P, Waters, P, Johnson, MR, Schott, JM, Armstrong, RJE, Zagami, AS, Bleasel, A, Somerville, ER, Smith, SMJ, and Vincent, A (2011). Faciobrachial dystonic seizures precede Lgi1 antibody limbic encephalitis. Ann Neurol 69:892–900.

Iris, U, Gerhard, B, and Eugen, T (2010). Epilepsy with generalized tonic-clonic seizures only. In Atlas of Epilepsies. Edited by CP Panayiotopoulos. London: Springer-Verlag, pp. 2041–2050.

Jackson, GD, Berkovic, SF, Tress BM, Kalnins, RM, Fabinyi, G, and Bladin, PF (1990). Hippocampal sclerosis can be reliably detected by magnetic resonance imaging. Neurology 40:1869–1875.

Janz, D (1985). Epilepsy with impulsive petit mal (juvenile myoclonic epilepsy). Acta Neurol Scand 72:449–459.

Janz, D, and Christian, W (1957). Impulsiv-Petit Mal. Dtsch Z Nervenheilkd 176:346–386.

Jeavons, PM (1985). West syndrome: Infantile spasms. In Epileptic Syndromes in Infancy, Childhood and Adolescence. Edited by J Roger, C Dravet, M Bureau, FE Dreifuss, and P Wolf. London: John Libbey, pp. 42–50.

Kahane, P, Bartolomei, F, and Trottier, S (2012). Temporal lobe epilepsy syndromes. In Epileptic Syndromes in Infancy, Childhood and Adolescence. Edited by M Bureau, P Genton, C Dravet, A Delgado-Escueta, CA Tassinari, P Thomas, and P Wolf. London: John Libbey (in press).

Kajitani, T, Ueoka, K, Nakamura, M, and Kumanomidou, Y (1981). Febrile convulsions and rolandic discharges. Brain Dev 3:351–359.

Kälviäinen, R, and Mervaala, E (2010). Unverricht-Lundborg disease (EPM1). In Atlas of Epilepsies. Edited by CP Panayiotopoulos. London: Springer-Verlag, pp. 1225–1230.

Kazemi, NJ, O'Brien, TJ, Cascino, GD, and So, EL (2008). Single photon emission computed tomography. In Epilepsy: A Comprehensive Textbook, 2nd ed. Edited by J Engel, Jr, and TA Pedley. Philadelphia: Lippincott Williams & Wilkins, pp. 965–973.

Kellaway, P, Hrachovy, RA, Frost, JD, and Zion, T (1979). Precise characterization and quantification of infantile spasms. Ann Neurol 6:214–218.

Kim, AJ, and Nordli, DR, Jr (2010a). Idiopathic childhood occipital epilepsy of Gastaut. In Atlas of Epilepsies. Edited by CP Panayiotopoulos. London: Springer-Verlag, pp. 973–976.

Kim, A, and Nordli, DR, Jr (2010b). Lennox-Gastaut syndrome. In Atlas of Epilepsies. Edited by CP Panayiotopoulos. London: Springer-Verlag, pp. 899–904.

Klaassen, A, Glykys, J, Maguire, J, Labarca, C, Mody, I, and Boulter, J (2006). Seizures and enhanced cortical GABAergic inhibition in two mouse models of human autosomal dominant nocturnal frontal lobe epilepsy. Proc Natl Acad Sci U S A 103:19152–19157.

Kobayashi, E, Andermann, F, and Andermann, E (2008a). Familial partial (focal) epilepsy with variable foci. In Epilepsy: A Comprehensive Textbook, 2nd ed. Edited by J Engel, Jr, and TA Pedley. Philadelphia: Lippincott Williams & Wilkins, pp 2549–2552.

Kobayashi, E, Zifkin, BG, Andermann, F, and Andermann, É (2008b). Juvenile myoclonic epilepsy. In Epilepsy: A Comprehensive Textbook, 2nd ed. Edited by J Engel, Jr, and TA Pedley. Philadelphia: Lippincott Williams & Wilkins, pp 2455–2460.

Kolodny, EH, and Sathe, S (2011). Lysosomal disorders and Menkes syndrome. In The Causes of Epilepsy: Common and Uncommon Causes in Adults and Children. Edited by SD Shorvon, F Andermann, and R Guerrini. Cambridge, UK: Cambridge University Press, pp 206–211.

Korff, CM, and Nordli, DR, Jr (2010a). Epilepsy with myoclonic-astatic seizures. In Atlas of Epilepsies. Edited by CP Panayiotopoulos. London: Springer-Verlag, pp 1007–1012.

Korff, CM, and Nordli, DR, Jr (2010b). West syndrome. In Atlas of Epilepsies. Edited by CP Panayiotopoulos. London: Springer-Verlag, pp 885–890.

Koskiniemi, M, Donner, M, Majuri, H, Haltia, M, and Nario, R (1974a). Progressive myoclonus epilepsy: A clinical histopathological study: Acta Neurol Scand 50:307–332.

Koskiniemi, M, Toivakka, E, and Donner, M (1974b). Progressive myoclonus epilepsy: Electroencephalographical findings. Acta Neurol Scand 50:333–359.

Koskiniemi, ML (1986). Baltic myoclonus. Adv Neurol 43:57–64.

Koutroumanidis, M (2010). Reflex seizures and reflex epilepsies. In Atlas of Epilepsies. Edited by CP Panayiotopoulos. London: Springer-Verlag, pp 1067–1068.

Koutroumanidis, M, and Tsiptsios, D (2010). Fixation-off sensitivity. In Atlas of Epilepsies. Edited by CP Panayiotopoulos. London: Springer-Verlag, pp. 1099–1104.

Krauss, GL, Johnson, MA, and Miller, NR (1997). Vigabatrin-associated retinal cone dysfunction. Electroretinogram and ophthalmologic findings. Neurology 50:614–618.

Labate, A, Gambardella, A, Andermann, E, Aguglia, U, Cendes, F, Berkovic, SF, and Andermann, F (2011). Benign mesial temporal lobe epilepsy. Nat Rev Neurol 7:237–240.

Lacy, JR, and Penry, JK (1976). Infantile Spasms. New York: Raven Press.

Lafora, GR (1911). Uber das Vorkommen amyloider Körperchen im Innern der Ganglienzellen: Zugleich ein Beitrag zum Studium der amyloiden Substanz im Nerven System. Virchows Arch Pathol Anat 205:295–303.

Lance, JW, and Adams, RD (1963). The syndrome of intention or action myoclonus as a sequel to hypoxic encephalopathy. Brain 86:111–136.

Landau, WM, and Kleffner, FR (1957). Syndrome of acquired aphasia with convulsive disorder in children. Neurology 7:523–530.

Lee, BI, Markand, ON, Siddiqui, AR, Park, HM, Mock, B, Wellman, HH, Worth, RM, and Edwards, MK (1986). Single photon emission computed tomography (SPECT) brain imaging using N,N,N-trimethyl-N'-(2-hydroxy-3-methyl-5-(123)I-iodobenzyl)-1,3-propanediamine 2 HCL (HIPDM): Intractable complex partial seizures. Neurology 36:1471–1477.

Lennox, WG, and Davis, JP (1950). Clinical correlates of the fast and the slow spike-wave electroencephalogram. Pediatrics 5:626–644.

Leppert, M, Anderson, VE, Quattlebaum, T, et al. (1989). Benign familial neonatal convulsions linked to genetic markers on chromosome 20. Nature 337:647–648.

Lerman, P, and Kivity, S (1975). Benign focal epilepsy of childhood: A follow up study of 100 recovered patients. Arch Neurol 32:261–264.

Lin, JJ, Salamon, N, Lee, AD, Dutton, RA, Geaga, JA, Hayashi, KM, Lüders, E, Toga, AW, Engel, J, Jr, and Thompson, PM (2007). Reduced neocortical thickness and complexity mapped in mesial temporal lobe epilepsy with hippocampal sclerosis. Cereb Cortex 17:2007–2018.

Lindsay, J, Ounsted, C, and Richards, P (1979a). Long-term outcome in children with temporal lobe seizures. I. Social outcome and childhood factors. Dev Med Child Neurol 21:285–298.

Lindsay, J, Ounsted, C, and Richards, P (1979b). Long-term outcome in children with temporal lobe seizures. II. Marriage, parenthood and sexual indifference. Dev Med Child Neurol 21:433–440.

Lindsay, J, Ounsted, C, and Richards, P (1979c). Long-term outcome in children with temporal lobe seizures. III. Psychiatric aspects in childhood and adult life. Dev Med Child Neurol 21:630–636.

Loiseau, P (1985). Childhood absence epilepsy. In Epileptic Syndromes in Infancy, Childhood and Adolescence. Edited by J Roger, C Dravet, M Bureau, FE Dreifuss, and P Wolf. London: John Libbey, pp. 106–120.

Loiseau, P, and Panayiotopoulos, CP (2000). Childhood absence epilepsy. In Neurobase. Edited by S Gilman. San Diego: Arbor.

Loiseau, P, Pestre, M, Dartigues, JF, Commenges, D, Barberger-Gateau, C, and Cohadon, S (1983). Long-term prognosis in two forms of childhood epilepsy: Typical absence seizures and epilepsy with rolandic (centrotemporal) EEG foci. Ann Neurol 13:642–648.

Lombroso, CT (1967). Sylvian seizures and midtemporal spike foci in children. Arch Neurol 17:52–59.

Lombroso, CT (1983). A prospective study of infantile spasms: Clinical and therapeutic correlations. Epilepsia 24:135–158a.

Lombroso, CT (1983). Neonatal seizures. In Epilepsy Diagnosis and Management. Edited by TR Browne and RG Feldman. Boston: Little, Brown & Cob, pp. 297–313.

Lombroso, CT, and Fejerman, N (1977). Benign myoclonus of early infancy. Ann Neurol 1:138–143.

Lou, HC, Brandt, S, and Bruhn, P (1977). Progressive aphasia and epilepsy with a self-limited course. In Epilepsy: The Eighth International Symposium. Edited by JK Penry. New York: Raven Press, pp 295–303.

Lüders, H, and Lesser, RP (eds) (1987). Epilepsy: Electroclinical Syndromes. London: Springer-Verlag.

Lüders, H, Lesser, RP, Dinner, DS, and Morris, HH, III (1987). Benign focal epilepsy of childhood. In Epilepsy: Electroclinical Syndromes. Edited by H Lüders and RP Lesser. London: Springer-Verlag, pp. 303–346.

Ludwig, BI, and Ajmone-Marsan, C (1975). Clinical ictal patterns in epileptic patients with occipital electroencephalographic foci. Neurology 25:463–471.

Lugaresi, E, Cirignotta, F, Coccagna, G, and Montagna, P (1986). Nocturnal myoclonus and restless leg syndrome. Adv Neurol 43:295–307.

Lundborg, H (1903). Die progressive Myoklonus-Epilepsie (Unverrichts Myoclonie). Uppsala: Almqvist and Wiksell.

Mackay, MT, Weiss, SK, Adams-Webber, T, Ashwal, S, Stephens, D, Ballaban-Gill, K, Baram, TZ, Duchowny, M, Hirtz, D, Pellock, JM, Shields, WD, Shinnar, S, Wyllie, E, and Snead, OC, III (2004). Practice parameter: Medical treatment of infantile spasms. Neurology 62:1668–1681.

Margerison, JH, and Corsellis, JA (1966). Epilepsy and the temporal lobes: A clinical, electroencephalographic and neuropathological study of the brain in epilepsy, with particular reference to the temporal lobes. Brain 89:499–530.

Marini, C, Scheffer, IE, Nabbout, R, Suls, A, De Jonghe, P, Zara, F, and Guerrini, R (2011). The genetics of Dravet syndrome. Epilepsia 52:24–29.

Mathern, GW, Pretorius, JK, and Babb, TL (1995). Influence of the type of initial precipitating injury and at what age it occurs on course and outcome in patients with temporal lobe seizures. J Neurosurg 82:220–227.

Mathern, GW, Wilson, CL, and Beck, H (2008). Hippocampal sclerosis. In Epilepsy: A Comprehensive Textbook, 2nd ed. Edited by J Engel, Jr, and TA Pedley. Philadelphia: Lippincott Williams & Wilkins, pp. 121–136.

Metrakos, K, and Metrakos, JD (1961). Genetics of convulsive disorders. II. Genetic and electroencephalographic studies in centrencephalic epilepsy. Neurology 11:474–483.

Mizrahi, EM, and Kellaway, P (1987). Characterization and classification of neonatal seizures. Neurology 37:1837–1844.

Mizrahi, E, and Milh, M (2012). Early severe neonatal and infantile epilepsies. In Epileptic Syndromes in Infancy, Childhood and Adolescence. Edited by M Bureau, P Genton, C Dravet, A Delgado-Escueta, CA Tassinari, P Thomas, and P Wolf. London: John Libbey.

Mizrahi, EM, and Scher, MS (2008). Treatment of neonatal seizures. In Epilepsy: A Comprehensive Textbook, 2nd ed. Edited by J Engel, Jr, and TA Pedley. Philadelphia: Lippincott Williams & Wilkins, pp. 1335–1343.

Mizrahi, EM, and Tharp, BR (1982). A characteristic EEG pattern in neonatal herpes simplex encephalitis. Neurology 32:1215–1220.

Mizrahi, EM, Plouin, P, and Clancy, RR (2008). Neonatal seizures. In Epilepsy: A Comprehensive Textbook, 2nd ed. Edited by J Engel, Jr, and TA Pedley. Philadelphia: Lippincott Williams & Wilkins, pp. 639–658.

Mole, SE, Goyal, S, and Williams, RE (2010). The neuronal ceroid lipofuscinoses. In Atlas of Epilepsies. Edited by CP Panayiotopoulos. London: Springer-Verlag, pp. 1235–1242.

Mullen, SA, Marini, C, Suls, A, Mei, D, Della Giustina, E, Buti, D, Arsov, T, Damiano, J, Lawrence, K, De Jonghe, P, Berkovic, SF, Scheffer, IE, and Guerrini, R (2011). Glucose transporter 1 deficiency as a treatable cause of myoclonic astatic epilepsy. Arch Neurol 68:1152–1155.

Munari, C, Kahane, P, Francione, S, et al. (1995). Role of the hypothalamic hamartoma in the genesis of gelastic fits (a video-stereo EEG study). Electroencephalogr Clin Neurophysiol 95:154–160.

Nelson, KB, and Ellenberg, JH (1978). Prognosis in children with febrile seizures. Pediatrics 61:720–727.

Nelson, KB, and Ellenberg, JH (eds) (1981a). Febrile Seizures. New York: Raven Press.

Nelson, KB, and Ellenberg, JH (1981b). The role of recurrences in determining outcome in children with febrile seizures. In Febrile Seizures. Edited by KB Nelson and JH Ellenberg. New York: Raven Press, pp. 19–25.

Nelson, KB, and Ellenberg, JH (1983). Febrile seizures. In Pediatric Epileptology. Edited by FE Dreifuss. Boston: John Wright, pp. 173–198.

Newmark, ME, and Penry, JK (1980). Genetics of Epilepsy: A Review. New York: Raven Press.

Nobile, C, Francioni, S, Mai, R, Cardinale, F, Castana, L, Tassi, L, Sartori, I, Didato, G, Citterio, A, Colombo, N, Galli, C, Lo Russo, G, and Cossu, M (2007). Surgical treatment of drug resistant nocturnal frontal lobe epilepsy. Brain 130:561–573.

Nobile, C, Pasini, E, and Michelucci, R (2010). Familial lateral temporal lobe epilepsy. In Atlas of Epilepsies. Edited by CP Panayiotopoulos. London: Springer-Verlag, pp. 1139–1146.

Nordli, DR, Jr (2010a). Generalized epilepsy with febrile seizures plus (GEFS+). In Atlas of Epilepsies. Edited by CP Panayiotopoulos. London: Springer-Verlag, pp. 861–864.

Nordli, DR, Jr (2010b). Neonatal epileptic syndromes: Overview. In Atlas of Epilepsies. Edited by CP Panayiotopoulos. London: Springer-Verlag, p 833.

Nordli, DR, Jr (2010c). Febrile seizures. In Atlas of Epilepsies. Edited by CP Panayiotopoulos. London: Springer-Verlag, pp. 855–860.

Noriega-Sanchez, A, and Markand, ON (1976). Clinical and electroencephalographic correlation of independent multifocal spike discharges. Neurology 26:667–672.

Novotny, EJ, Jr, Tharp, BR, Coen, RW, Bejar, R, Enzmann, D, and Vaucher, YE (1987). Positive rolandic sharp waves in the EEG of the premature infant. Neurology 37:1481–1486.

Ogren, JA, Bragin, A, Wilson CL, et al. (2009). Three-dimensional hippocampal atrophy maps distinguish two common temporal lobe seizure-onset patterns. Epilepsia 50:1361–1370.

Ohtahara, S (1978). Clinico-electrical delineation of epileptic encephalopathies in childhood. Asian Med J 21:7–17.

Ohtahara, S, and Yamatogi, Y (2010a). Early myoclonic encephalopathy. In Atlas of Epilepsies. Edited by CP Panayiotopoulos. London: Springer-Verlag, pp. 843–846.

Ohtahara, S, and Yamatogi, Y (2010b). Ohtahara syndrome. In Atlas of Epilepsies. Edited by CP Panayiotopoulos. London: Springer-Verlag, pp. 847–850.

Ohtahara, S, Ishida, T, Oka, E, Yamatogi, Y, Inique, H, Ohtsuka, Y, and Kanda, S (1976). On the age-dependent epileptic syndromes: The early infantile encephalopathy with suppression-burst. Brain Dev 8:270–288.

Ohtahara, S, Yamatogi, Y, and Ohtsuka, Y (2008). Early myoclonic encephalopathy (neonatal myoclonic encephalopathy). In Epilepsy: A Comprehensive Textbook, 2nd ed. Edited by J Engel, Jr, and TA Pedley. Philadelphia: Lippincott Williams & Wilkins, pp. 2303–2307.

Ottman, R, Risch, N, Hauser, WA, Pedley, TA, Lee, JH, Barker-Cummings, C, Lustenberger, A, Nagle, KJ, Lee, KS, Scheuer, ML, et al. (1995). Localization of a gene for partial epilepsy to chromosome 10q. Nat Genet 10:56–60.

Ottman, R, Hirose, S, Jain, S, Lerche, H, Lopes-Cendes, I, Noebels, JL, Serratosa, J, Zara, F, and Scheffer, IE (2010). Genetic testing in the epilepsies—Report of the ILAE Genetics Commission. Epilepsia 51:655–670.

Pampiglione, G, and Harden, A (1973). Neurophysiological identification of a late infantile form of neuronal lipidosis. J Neurol Neurosurg Psychiatry 36:68–74.

Panayiotopoulos, CP (1989a). Benign childhood epilepsy with occipital paroxysms: A 15-year prospective study. Ann Neurol 26:51–56.

Panayiotopoulos, CP (1989b). Benign nocturnal childhood occipital epilepsy: A new syndrome with nocturnal seizures, tonic deviation of the eyes, and vomiting. J Child Neurol 4:43–49.

Panayiotopoulos, CP (ed.) (2010). Atlas of Epilepsies. London: Springer-Verlag.

Panayiotopoulos, CP, Bureau, M, Dalla Bernardina, B, Caraballo, RH, and Valeta, T (2012). Idiopathic focal epilepsies in childhood. In Epileptic Syndromes in Infancy, Childhood and Adolescence. Edited by M Bureau, P Genton, C Dravet, A Delgado-Escueta, CA Tassinari, P Thomas, and P Wolf. London: John Libbey.

Parmeggiani, L, and Guerrini, R (2010). Idiopathic photosensitive occipital lobe epilepsy. In Atlas of Epilepsies. Edited by CP Panayiotopoulos. London: Springer-Verlag, pp. 1077–1080.

Parvizi, J, Scheherazade, L, Foster, BL, Bourgeois, B, Riviello, JJ, Prenger, E, Saper, C, and Kerrigan, JF (2011). Gelastic epilepsy and hypothalamic hamartomas: Neuroanatomical analysis of brain lesions in 100 patients. Brain 134:2960–2968.

Pellock, JM, Hrachovy, R, Shinnar, S, Baram, TZ, Bettis, D, Dlugos, DJ, Gaillard, WD, Gibson, PA, Holmes, GL, Nordli, DR, O'Dell, C, Shields, WD, Trevathan, E, and Wheless, JW (2010). Infantile spasms: A U.S. consensus report. Epilepsia. 51:2175–2189.

Picard, F, and Brodtkorb, E (2008). Familial frontal lobe epilepsies. In Epilepsy: A Comprehensive Textbook, 2nd ed. Edited by J Engel, Jr, and TA Pedley. Philadelphia: Lippincott Williams & Wilkins, pp. 2495–2502.

Picard, F, and Brodtkorb, E (2010). Familial frontal lobe epilepsies. In Atlas of Epilepsies. Edited by CP Panayiotopoulos. London: Springer-Verlag, pp. 2495–2502.

Picard, F, and Scheffer, I (2012). Genetically determined focal epilepsies. In Epileptic Syndromes in Infancy, Childhood and Adolescence. Edited by M Bureau, P Genton, C Dravet, A Delgado-Escueta, CA Tassinari, P Thomas, and P Wolf. London: John Libbey.

Plouin, P (1985). Benign neonatal convulsions (familial and non-familial). In Epileptic Syndromes in Infancy, Childhood and Adolescence. Edited by J Roger, C Dravet, M Bureau, FE Dreifuss, and P Wolf. London: John Libbey, pp. 2–11.

Plouin, P (2008). Benign familial neonatal seizures and benign idiopathic neonatal seizures. In Epilepsy: A Comprehensive Textbook, 2nd ed. Edited by J Engel, Jr, and TA Pedley. Philadelphia: Lippincott Williams & Wilkins, pp. 2287–2295.

Plouin, P (2010a). Malignant migrating partial seizures in infancy. In Atlas of Epilepsies. Edited by CP Panayiotopoulos. London: Springer-Verlag, pp. 943–948.

Plouin, P (2010b). Benign idiopathic neonatal seizures. In Atlas of Epilepsies. Edited by CP Panayiotopoulos. London: Springer-Verlag, pp. 839–842.

Plouin, P, and Neubauer, B (2012). Benign neonatal seizures and epilepsies. In Epileptic Syndromes in Infancy, Childhood and Adolescence. Edited by M Bureau, P Genton, C Dravet, A Delgado-Escueta, CA Tassinari, P Thomas, and P Wolf. London: John Libbey.

Rapin, I (1986). Myoclonus in neuronal storage and Lafora diseases. Adv Neurol 43:65–85.

Rapin, I, Goldfischer, S, Katzman, R, Engel, J, Jr, and O'Brien, JS (1978). The cherry-red spot-myoclonus syndrome. Ann Neurol 3:234–242.

Rasmussen, T, Olszewski, J, and Lloyd-Smith, D (1958). Focal seizures due to chronic localized encephalitis. Neurology 8:435–445.

Rausch, R (1987). Neurophysiological evaluation. In Surgical Treatment of the Epilepsies. Edited by J Engel, Jr. New York: Raven Press, pp. 181–196.

Reeves, AG (1985). Epilepsy and the Corpus Callosum. New York: Plenum Press.

Resnick, TJ, Moshé, SL, Perotta, L, and Chambers, HJ (1986). Benign neonatal sleep myoclonus: Relationship to sleep states. Arch Neurol 43:266–268.

Rett, AR, and Teubel, R (1964). Neugeborenenkrämpfe im Rahmen einer epileptisch belasten Familie. Wien Klin Wochenschr 76:609–613.

Rodin, EA (1968). The Prognosis of Patients with Epilepsy. Springfield, IL: Charles C Thomas.

Rojo, DC, Hamiwka, L, McMahon, JM, Dibbens, LM, Arsov, T, Suls, A, Stödberg, T, Kelley, K, Wirrell, E, Appleton, B, Mackay, M, Freeman, JL, Yendle, SC, Berkovic, SF, Bienvenu, T, De Jonghe, P, Thorburn, DR, Mulley, JC, Mefford, HC, and Scheffer, IE (2011). De novo SCN1A mutations in migrating partial seizures of infancy. Neurology 77:380–383.

Rose, AL, and Lombroso, CT (1970). Neonatal seizure states: A study of clinical, pathological and electroencephalographic features in 137 full-term babies with a long-term follow-up. Pediatrics 45:404–425.

Roulet-Perez, E, Ballhausen, D, Bonafé,, L, Cronel-Ohayon, S, and Maeder-Ingvar, M (2008). Glut-1 deficiency syndrome masquerading as idiopathic generalized epilepsy. Epilepsia 49:1955–1958.

Sankar, R, Curran, JG, Kevill, JW, Rintahaka, PJ, Shewmon, DA, and Vinters, HV: Microscopic cortical dysplasia in infantile spasms (1995). Evolution of white matter abnormalities. AJNR Am J Neuroradiol 16:1265–1272.

Satishchandra, P (2003). Hot-water epilepsy. Epilepsia 44(suppl 1): 29–32.

Sato, S, Dreifuss, FE, and Penry, JK (1976). Prognostic factors in absence seizures. Neurology 26:788–796.

Scheffer, IE, and Berkovic, SF (1997). Generalized epilepsy with febrile seizures plus. A genetic disorder with heterogeneous clinical phenotypes. Brain 120:479–490.

Scheffer, IE, and Berkovic, SF (2008). Generalized (genetic) epilepsy with febrile seizures plus. In Epilepsy: A Comprehensive Textbook, 2nd ed. Edited by J Engel, Jr, and TA Pedley. Philadelphia: Lippincott Williams & Wilkins, pp. 2553–2558.

Scheffer, IE, Bhatia, KP, Lopes-Cendes, I, Fish, DR, Marsden, CD, Andermann, F, Andermann, E, Desbiennes, R, Cendes, F, Manson, JI, et al. (1994). Autosomal dominant frontal lobe epilepsy misdiagnosed as a sleep disorder. Lancet 343:515–517.

Schmidley, JW, and Simon, RP (1981). Postictal pleocytosis. Ann Neurol 9:81–84.

Schmidt, D, Tsai, JJ, and Janz, D (1983). Generalized tonic-clonic seizures in patients with complex partial seizures: Natural history and prognostic relevance. Epilepsia 24:43–48.

Schmidt, D, Einicke, I, and Haenel, F (1986). The influence of seizure type on the efficacy of plasma concentrations of phenytoin, phenobarbital and carbamazepine. Arch Neurol 43:263–265.

Seay, AR, and Bray, PF (1977). Significance of seizures in infants weighing less than 2500 grams. Arch Neurol 34:381–382.

Semah, F, Picot, M-C, Adam, C, Broglin, D, Arzimanoglou, A, Bazin, B, Cavalcanti, D, and Baulac, M (1998). Is the underlying cause of epilepsy a major prognostic factor for recurrence? Neurology 51:1256–1262.

Serratosa, JM (2010). Progressive myoclonic epilepsies: Overview. In Atlas of Epilepsies. Edited by CP Panayiotopoulos. London: Springer-Verlag, pp. 1221–1224.

Shibasaki, H (1987). Progressive myoclonic epilepsy. In Epilepsy: Electroclinical Syndromes. Edited by H Lüders and RP Lesser. London: Springer-Verlag, pp. 187–206.

Shields, WD, Duchowny, MS, and Holmes, GL (1993). Surgically remediable syndromes of infancy and early childhood. In Surgical Treatment of the Epilepsies, 2nd ed. Edited by J Engel, Jr. New York, Raven Press, pp. 35–48.

Siegel, AM, Wieser, HG, Wichmann, W, and Yasargil, GM (1990). Relationships between MR-imaged total amount of tissue removed, resection scores of specific mesiobasal limbic subcompartments and clinical outcome following selective amygdalohippocampectomy. Epilepsy Res 6:56–65.

Singh, NA, Charlier, C, Stauffer, D, et al. (1998). A novel potassium channel gene, KCNQ2, is mutated in an inherited epilepsy of newborns. Nat Genet 18:23–29.

Smith, MC, and Polkey, CE (2008). Landau-Kleffner syndrome and CSWS. In Epilepsy: A Comprehensive Textbook, 2nd ed. Edited by J Engel, Jr, and TA Pedley. Philadelphia: Lippincott Williams & Wilkins, pp. 2429–2437.

Smith, MC, Byrne, R, and Kanner, AM (2009). Hypothalamic hamartoma and multiple subpial transection. In The Treatment of Epilepsy, 3rd ed. Edited by S Shorvon, E Perucca, and J Engel, Jr. West Sussex, UK: Wiley-Blackwell, pp. 951–957.

Snead, OC, and Hosey, LC (1985). Exacerbation of seizures in children by carbamazepine. N Engl J Med 313:916–921.

Snead, OC, Benton, JW, and Myers, GJ (1983). ACTH and prednisone in childhood seizure disorders. Neurology 33:966–970.

Soper, HV, Strain, GM, Babb, TL, Lieb, JP, and Crandall, PH (1978). Chronic alumina temporal lobe seizures in monkeys. Exp Neurol 62:99–121.

Spencer, S, and Huh, L (2008). Outcomes of epilepsy surgery in adults and children. Lancet Neurol 7:525–537.

Spencer, SS, Gates, JR, Reeves, AR, Spencer, DD, Maxwell, RE, and Roberts, D (1987). Corpus callosum section. In Surgical Treatment of the Epilepsies. Edited by J Engel, Jr. New York: Raven Press, pp. 425–444.

Sperling, MR, Pritchard, PB, III, Engel, J, Jr, Daniel, C, and Sagel, J (1986). Prolactin in partial epilepsy: An indicator of limbic seizures. Ann Neurol, 20:716–722.

Stefan, H, Hildebrandt, M, Kerling, F, Kasper, BS, Hammen, T, Dörfler, A, Weigel, D, Buchfelder, M, Blümcke, I, and Pauli, E (2009). Clinical prediction of postoperative seizure control: Structural, functional findings and disease histories. J Neurol Neurosurg Psychiatry 80:196–200.

Steinlein, OK, Magnusson, A, Stoodt, J, Bertrand, S, Weiland, S, Berkovic, SF, Nakken, KO, Propping, P, and Bertrand, D (1997). An insertion mutation of the CHRNA4 gene in a family with autosomal dominant nocturnal frontal lobe epilepsy. Hum Mol Genet 6:943–947.

Stephen, LJ, Kwan, P, and Brodie, MJ (2001). Does the cause of localisation-related epilepsy influence the response to antiepileptic drug treatment? Epilepsia 42:357–362.

Stern, J, and Engel, J, Jr (2005). Atlas of EEG Patterns. Philadelphia: Lippincott, Williams & Wilkins.

Striano, P, and Capovilla, G (2010). Epileptic encephalopathy with continuous spike-and-wave during sleep. In Atlas of Epilepsies. Edited by CP Panayiotopoulos. London: Springer-Verlag, pp. 913–918.

Striano, P, and Nobile, C (2010). Familial mesial temporal lobe epilepsy. In Atlas of Epilepsies. Edited by CP Panayiotopoulos. London: Springer-Verlag, pp. 1135–1138.

Striano, P, Bordo, L, Lispi, ML, Specchio, N, Minetti, C, Vigevano, F, and Zara, F (2006). A novel SCN2A mutation in family with benign familial infantile seizures. Epilepsia 47:218–220.

Suls, A, Mullen, SA, Weber, YG, et al. (2009). Early-onset absence epilepsy caused by mutations in the glucose transporter GLUT1. Ann Neurol 66:415–419.

Tassinari, CA (1982). Electrical status epilepticus during sleep in children (ESES). In Sleep and Epilepsy. Edited by MB Sterman, MN Shouse, and P Passouant. New York: Academic Press, pp. 465–479.

Tassinari, CA, and Bureau, M (1985). Epilepsy with myoclonic absences. In Epileptic Syndromes in Infancy, Childhood and Adolescence. Edited by J Roger, C Dravet, M Bureau, FE Dreifuss, and P Wolf. London: John Libbey, pp. 121–129.

Tassinari, CA, Dravet, C, Roger, J, Cano, JP, and Gastaut, H (1972). Tonic status epilepticus precipitated by intravenous benzodiazepine in five patients with Lennox-Gastaut syndrome. Epilepsia 13:421–435.

Tassinari, CA, Michelucci, R, Gardella, E, and Rubboli, G (2008). Epilepsy with myoclonic absences. In Epilepsy: A Comprehensive Textbook, 2nd ed. Edited by J Engel, Jr, and TA Pedley. Philadelphia: Lippincott Williams & Wilkins, pp. 2413–2416.

Tassinari, CA, Canatlupo, G, Bureau, M, Cirelli, C, and Tononi, G (2012). CSWS and related syndromes. In Epileptic Syndromes in Infancy, Childhood and Adolescence. Edited by M Bureau, P Genton, C Dravet, A Delgado-Escueta, CA Tassinari, P Thomas, and P Wolf. London: John Libbey.

Tharp, BR, Cukier, F, and Monod, N (1981). The prognostic value of the electroencephalogram in premature infants. Electroencephalogr Clin Neurophysiol 51:219–236.

Thomas, P (2010). Juvenile absence epilepsy. In Atlas of Epilepsies. Edited by CP Panayiotopoulos. London: Springer-Verlag, pp. 1029–1032.

Thomas, P, Genton, P, Medina, M, Steinhoff, B, and Benbadis, S (2012). JME and IGE in adolescence and adulthood. In Epileptic Syndromes in Infancy, Childhood and Adolescence. Edited by M Bureau, P Genton, C Dravet, A Delgado-Escueta, CA Tassinari, P Thomas, and P Wolf. London: John Libbey.

Tibbles, JAR (1980). Dominant benign neonatal seizures. Dev Med Child Neurol 22:664–667.

Tibussek, D, and Schmitt, B (2010). Startle epilepsy. In Atlas of Epilepsies. Edited by CP Panayiotopoulos. London: Springer-Verlag, pp. 1115–1118.

Tinuper, P, and Bisulli, F (2010). Autosomal dominant nocturnal frontal lobe epilepsy. In Atlas of Epilepsies. Edited by CP Panayiotopoulos. London: Springer-Verlag, pp. 1127–1134.

Trimble, MR (1983). Personality disturbances in epilepsy. Neurology 33:1332–1334.

Unverricht, H (1895). Über familiäre Myoclonie. Dtsch Z Nervenheilkd 7:32–67.

Vadlamudi, L, Kjeldsen, MJ, Corey, LA, Solaas, MH, Friis, ML, Pellock, JM, Nakken, KO, Milne, RL, Scheffer, IE, Harvey, AS, Hopper, JL, and Berkovic, SF (2006). Analyzing the etiology of benign rolandic epilepsy: A multicenter twin collaboration. Epilepsia 47:550–555.

Valentin, A, and Alarcon, G (2010). Mesial temporal lobe epilepsy due to etiologies other than hippocampal sclerosis. In Atlas of Epilepsies. Edited by CP Panayiotopoulos. London: Springer-Verlag, pp. 1177–1182.

Vigevano, F, and Specchio, N (2010). Benign infantile seizures or Watanabe-Vigevano syndrome. In Atlas of Epilepsies. Edited by CP Panayiotopoulos. London: Springer-Verlag, pp. 865–870.

Vigevano, F, Bureau, M, and Watanabe, K (2012). Idiopathic focal epilepsies in infants. In Epileptic Syndromes in Infancy, Childhood and Adolescence. Edited by M Bureau, P Genton, C Dravet, A Delgado-Escueta, CA Tassinari, P Thomas, and P Wolf. London: John Libbey.

Vigevano, F, Specchio, N, Caraballo, R, and Watanabe, K (2008). Benign familial and nonfamilial seizures. In Epilepsy: A Comprehensive Textbook, 2nd ed. Edited by J Engel, Jr, and TA Pedley. Philadelphia: Lippincott Williams & Wilkins, pp. 2313–2321.

Volpe, JJ (1987). Neurology of the Newborn, 2nd ed. Philadelphia: WB Saunders.

Wadman, M (2011). African outbreak stumps experts. Nature 475:148–149.

Wandschneider, B, Kopp, UA, Kliegel, M, Stephani, U, Kurlemann, G, Janz, D, and Schmitz, B (2010). Prospective memory in patients with juvenile myoclonic epilepsy and their healthy siblings. Neurology 75:2161–2167.

Wang, X, and Xiao, F (2010). Familial focal epilepsy with variable foci. In Atlas of Epilepsies. Edited by CP Panayiotopoulos. London: Springer-Verlag, pp. 1147–1152.

Watanabe, K, Kuroyanagi, M, Hara, K, and Miyazaki, S (1982). Neonatal seizures and subsequent epilepsy. Brain Dev 4:341–346.

Watanabe, K, Miura, K, Natsume, J, et al. (1999). Epilepsies of neonatal onset: Seizure type and evolution. Dev Med Child Neurol 41:318–322.

West, WJ (1841). On a peculiar form of infantile convulsions. Lancet I:724–725.

Westmoreland, BF, and Gomez, M (1987). Infantile spasms (West syndrome). In Epilepsy: Electroclinical Syndromes. Edited by H Lüders and RP Lesser. London: Springer-Verlag, pp. 49–71.

Wiebe, S, Blume, WT, Girvin, JP, and Eliasziw, M (2001). A randomized, controlled trial of surgery for temporal lobe epilepsy. N Engl J Med 345:311–318.

Wieser, HG, Hailemariam, S, Regard, M, and Landis, T (1985). Unilateral limbic epileptic status activity: Stereo EEG, behavioral and cognitive data. Epilepsia 26:19–29.

Wieser, H-G, Özkara, Ç, Engel, J, Jr, Hauser, AW, Moshé, SL, Avanzini, G, Helmstaedter, C, Henry, TR, and Sperling, MR (2004). Mesial temporal lobe epilepsy with hippocampal sclerosis: Report of the ILAE Commission on Neurosurgery of Epilepsy. Epilepsia 45:695–714.

Wilkins, A (2010). Pattern-sensitive epilepsy. In Atlas of Epilepsies. Edited by CP Panayiotopoulos. London: Springer-Verlag, pp. 1093–1098.

Wilkins, A, and Lindsay, J (1985). Common forms of reflex epilepsy: Physiological mechanisms and the techniques for treatment. In Recent Advances in Epilepsy 2. Edited by TA Pedley and BS Meldrum. New York: Churchill Livingstone, pp. 239–271.

Williamson, PD, and Engel, J, Jr (2008). Anatomic classification of focal epilepsies. In Epilepsy: A Comprehensive Textbook, 2nd ed. Edited by J Engel, Jr, and TA Pedley. Philadelphia: Lippincott Williams & Wilkins, pp. 2465–2477.

Wilson, SJ, and Engel, J, Jr (2010). Diverse perspectives on developments in epilepsy surgery. Seizure 19:659–668.

Winkler, AS, Friedrich, K, Konig, R, Meindl, M, Helbok, R, Unterberger, I, Gotwald, T, Dharsee, J, Velicheti, S, Kidunda, A, Jilek-Aall, L, Matuja, M, and Schmutzhard, E (2008). The head nodding syndrome—Clinical classification and possible causes. Epilepsia 49:2008–2015.

Wolf, P (1985a). Epilepsy with grand mal on awakening. In Epileptic Syndromes in Infancy, Childhood and Adolescence. Edited by J Roger, C Dravet, M Bureau, FE Dreifuss, and P Wolf. London: John Libbey, pp. 259–270.

Wolf, P (1985b). Juvenile absence epilepsy. In Epileptic Syndromes in Infancy, Childhood and Adolescence. Edited by J Roger, C Dravet, M Bureau, FE Dreifuss, and P Wolf. London: John Libbey, pp. 242–246.

Wolf, P (1985c). Juvenile myoclonic epilepsy. In Epileptic Syndromes in Infancy, Childhood and Adolescence. Edited by J Roger, C Dravet, M Bureau, FE Dreifuss, and P Wolf. London: John Libbey, pp. 247–258.

Wolf, P (2008). Isolated seizures. In Epilepsy: A Comprehensive Textbook, 2nd ed. Edited by J Engel, Jr, and TA Pedley. Philadelphia: Lippincott Williams & Wilkins, pp. 2543–2548.

Zafeiriou, DI (2010). Myoclonic status epilepticus in nonprogressive encephalopathy. In Atlas of Epilepsies. Edited by CP Panayiotopoulos. London: Springer-Verlag, pp. 919–922.

Zifkin, BG, Guerrini, R, and Plouin, P (2008). Reflex seizures. In Epilepsy: A Comprehensive Textbook, 2nd ed. Edited by J Engel, Jr, and TA Pedley. Philadelphia: Lippincott Williams & Wilkins, pp. 2559–2572.

Chapter 8

Epileptogenesis

THE DEVELOPMENT OF EPILEPSY
Phenomenology
Character of the Lesion
Location of the Lesion
Genetic Factors
Practical Considerations
   Prophylaxis for Early Seizures
   Prophylaxis for Chronic Epilepsy

THE PROGRESSIVE NATURE OF EPILEPSY
Secondary Epileptogenesis

Clinical Evidence for Progression
Practical Considerations
EPILEPTIC SEIZURES AND BRAIN DEVELOPMENT
Epileptic Susceptibility of the Immature Brain
Evolution of Epilepsy Syndromes
Migration of the Interictal EEG Spike
Practical Considerations

SUMMARY AND CONCLUSIONS

Epileptogenesis is defined as "the development and extension of tissue capable of generating spontaneous seizures, including development of an epilepsy condition, and progression after the condition is established" (Chapter 1). Considerable interest in recent years has focused on developing interventions that prevent or retard epileptogenesis. *Antiepileptogenesis*, therefore, can be *complete*, preventing the development of an epilepsy condition, or *partial*, resulting in a delay in the development of epilepsy, or a reduction in its severity. Antiepileptogenesis can also

prevent or reduce the progression of epilepsy after it has been established. The complete reversal of an epilepsy condition after it has been established is referred to as a *cure*. Partial prevention, or alteration of the progression that is less than a cure, is referred to as *seizure modification* (Chapter 1). Antiepileptogenesis is one aspect of *disease or syndrome modification*, which refers to processes that also alter the development or progression of the neurobiological, cognitive, psychological, and social consequences of epilepsy or the pathological substrates of an epilepsy condition. Both basic

296

and clinical research in this area have been hampered by imprecise and conflicting use of descriptive terms; therefore, a standardized terminology for these processes has been proposed (Table 8–1).

As discussed in Chapter 4, the *National Institute of Neurological Disorders and Stroke (NINDS) benchmarks* have identified epileptogenesis and antiepileptogenesis as high priorities for basic research on epilepsy (Kelly et al., 2009; Jacobs et al., 2001). This chapter is

Table 8–1 Proposed Terminology

Epileptogenesis: The development and extension of tissue capable of generating spontaneous seizures, including
- development of an epilepsy condition
- progression after the condition is established

Disease or syndrome modification: A process that alters the development or progression of a "disease," in this case epilepsy (either epilepsy disease or epilepsy syndrome). Disease- or syndrome-modifying interventions can be antiepileptogenic. They can also modify comorbidity by reducing or preventing deleterious nonepileptic functional changes in the brain. They can also modify the pathological changes underlying epileptogenesis or comorbidities. That is, such interventions can act by
- antiepileptogenesis
- comorbidity modification
- reversal of pathology (related to either one)

Antiepileptogenesis: A process that counteracts the effects of epileptogenesis, including
- prevention
- seizure modification
- cure

Prevention (treatment given prior to epilepsy occurrence): The process of completely preventing the development of epilepsy. *Partial prevention* can delay the development of epilepsy.

Seizure modification (treatment given prior to or after epilepsy occurrence): A process after which seizures occur but may be lower in frequency, shorter, or of milder seizure type. Antiepileptogenesis can also prevent or reduce the progression of epilepsy after it has already been established or change epilepsy from drug-resistant to drug-sensitive.

Cure: The complete and permanent reversal of epilepsy such that no seizures occur after treatment withdrawal.

Modified from Pitkänen, 2010, with permission.

concerned with the clinical relevance of epileptogenesis and antiepileptogenesis as it relates to (1) development of an epilepsy condition, (2) progression of an epilepsy condition once it is established, and (3) the interaction between epileptic phenomena and cerebral maturation. Disease modification as it is concerned with the behavioral consequences of epilepsy is discussed in Chapter 11.

THE DEVELOPMENT OF EPILEPSY

Phenomenology

Mechanisms that are responsible for or influence the development of a chronic epilepsy condition differ from those that actually precipitate acute or chronic epileptic seizures (Chapter 4). It is well known from studies with patients as well as with experimental animal models that there is a latent period between induction of a localized epileptogenic cerebral insult and the appearance of a chronic epilepsy condition. Penfield and Jasper (Penfield and Jasper, 1954) referred to this period as "ripening of the scar." Presumably, the acute structural changes produced in a region of cortical tissue are not in themselves adequate to cause chronic seizures, even if a reactive epileptic seizure ensues. Reorganization of neuronal integration predisposing to enhanced excitation and synchronization must occur before recurrent spontaneous ictal discharges appear.

Animal models of focal epilepsy (Chapter 4) reveal a characteristic course in the development of chronic epileptogenic lesions. First, localized interictal EEG spikes occur in cortical areas immediately adjacent to the experimental intervention; later, in some but not all cases, spontaneous epileptic seizures are seen. The process does not necessarily stop at that point: epileptic seizures may become progressively more elaborate, with larger areas of brain involvement or the appearance of secondary epileptogenic regions. The time between the initial insult and the development of spontaneous seizures depends on many factors, including the type of epileptogenic intervention, the cortical location manipulated, the degree of phylogenetic and ontogenetic development of the experimental animal, and the genetic predisposition of the animal for specific types of epilepsy.

The *kindling model* of epilepsy (Goddard et al., 1969) (Chapter 4) demonstrates a relatively consistent evolution of epileptic phenomena and has been used to study the alterations in function, structure, or both that are responsible for the development of chronic seizures in human focal epilepsy following specific cortical insults (Goddard, 1983; Wada, 1986; Wada, 1981; Wada, 1976; Corcoran and Moshé, 2005; McIntyre, 2006; Morimoto et al., 2004). However, the kindling stimulus mimics an epileptic seizure rather than an epileptogenic lesion and more correctly can be considered to simulate the progression of an epilepsy condition once seizures have occurred, rather than primary epileptogenesis. Furthermore, kindling, as used by most investigators, terminates with the development of epileptic seizures induced by electrical stimulation. When the tedious process of *overkindling* (kindling until spontaneous seizures appear) is carried out, the site of origin of the spontaneous epileptic seizures is not where intermittent electrical stimulation was applied; rather, it is a cortical area one or more synapses removed from that location (Pinel and Rovner, 1978). Consequently, the mechanisms responsible for kindled *spontaneous* epileptic seizures may not be relevant to the development of a chronic epileptogenic zone *in the immediate vicinity* of structural cortical damage (Engel and Cahan, 1986). Rather, kindling models the development of secondary epileptogenesis responsible for progression of an epilepsy condition.

There are a number of animal models of chronic epilepsy, induced by a variety of epileptogenic interventions, including excitotoxic and stimulation-induced status epilepticus, which cause hippocampal damage; *traumatic brain injury (TBI)*; specific irritants, usually applied to neocortex, such as certain metals, tetanus toxin, and freezing; and neonatal manipulations such as hypoxia and hyperthermia (Chapter 4). Experimental animal models of TBI and *posttraumatic epilepsy (PTE)* (Pitkänen et al., 2006) are of particular recent interest, because of the increasing prevalence of these conditions in veterans of the Iraq and Afghan wars (Chapter 4). Changes that occur in the brain during the latent period between the application of epileptogenic insults in these models and the appearance of spontaneous seizures are more directly related to the initial epileptogenic process in human epilepsy than is kindling. Studies of these changes are complicated, however, by the fact that the duration of the latent period is variable, not only from one model to another, but from animal to animal within the same model, and for most of these conditions not all animals develop spontaneous seizures. Consequently, when investigations during the latent period require sacrifice of the animal, it is not possible to know which animals would eventually have developed chronic epilepsy. Factors such as age and genetic predisposition greatly influence the epileptogenic process. Research with these animals has revealed a large number of neuronal disturbances that can be considered potential targets for development of antiepileptogenic agents (Chapter 4).

Studies of animal models of epilepsies that result from genetic disturbances are problematic, because there is no clear time of initial insult that marks the beginning of the epileptogenic process. Nevertheless, recognition of the importance of the *mammalian target of rapamycin (mTOR) signaling pathway* in the development of seizures with *tuberous sclerosis* has led to an antiepileptogenic intervention in a mouse model of this condition (Zeng et al., 2008), and similar mechanisms may be relevant to other types of acquired epilepsy. Also, the demonstration that early treatment with *ethosuximide* in a genetic rat model of spike-wave epilepsy can prevent the later age-specific onset of spontaneous seizures (Blumenfeld et al., 2008) holds promise for the elucidation of specific epileptogenic mechanisms in human genetic epilepsies.

It is difficult to study the evolutionary processes leading to the appearance of chronic seizures in humans. Although many distinct pathological disturbances give rise to focal epilepsy (Chapter 5), for the most part they reflect lesions such as congenital malformations and brain tumors, where the epileptogenic process has no specific time of onset. PTE provides the best opportunity to examine the course of epileptogenesis, because the time of the initial focal insult can be most easily documented (Temkin, 2003; 2009; Pitkänen, 2010). Jennett's (Jennett, 1975) classic studies of epilepsy after nonmissile head injuries provide evidence for a pathophysiological distinction between *early seizures* occurring in the first or second

Table 8–2 Risk Factors for Epileptic Seizures and Epilepsy After Nonmissile Head Trauma

Early seizures
  Intracranial hematoma
  Focal neurological signs
  Posttraumatic amnesia > 24 hours
  Any neurological signs
  Depressed skull fracture
  Subarachnoid hemorrhage
  Injury before 5 years of age
  Linear skull fracture
Late seizures
  Intracranial hematoma
  Early seizures, especially when delayed
  Depressed skull fracture
  Posttraumatic amnesia > 24 hours
  Injury after 16 years of age
  Glasgow Coma Scale score of 3 to 8
  Dural penetration
  At least one nonreactive pupil
  Time to following commands of a week or more
  Parietal lesion on CT

Adapted from Jennett, 1975 and Temkin, 2003.

posttraumatic week and those occurring subsequently. The risk factors for, and therefore the mechanisms of, early reactive seizures are different from those that determine the appearance of chronic epilepsy at a later date (Table 8–2). This work, and others, confirmed that the latent period between the initial injury and the first late spontaneous epileptic seizure can range from months to more than 10 years (Raymont et al., 2010) (Table 8–3). Similar data have been obtained from studies of patients with thromboembolic cerebrovascular disease (Lesser et al., 1985) and penetrating head injuries (Salazar et al., 1985).

Character of the Lesion

It is well known that certain cortical insults are more likely to result in chronic epileptic seizures than others (Temkin, 2003). Blood, in particular, has an extremely irritating effect on cortical neurons; it not only induces acute seizures but also causes chronic epilepsy, perhaps due to hemosiderin deposits (Willmore et al., 1978). An acute hematoma presents the most potent risk for the development of chronic epilepsy following closed head trauma (Jennett, 1975). Other highly epileptogenic lesions are those that produce chronic irritation of the cortex with minimal cortical destruction, such as depressed skull fractures, meningiomas, meningioparenchymal cicatrices resulting from cerebral contusions or infections, cortical granulomas, and other noninfiltrating masses such as hamartomas, abscesses, and vascular malformations (Chapter 5). Chronic irritation could give rise to structural changes in adjacent neurons and their surrounding glia that predispose

Table 8–3 Time of First Late Seizure in 481 Patients with Late Posttraumatic Epilepsy

Interval after Injury	Cases with Onset In Each Period		Cumulative % That Have Begun by End of Year	
First 3 months	130	27%	1	56%
4–12 months	138	29%		
1–2 years	62	13%	2	69%
2–3 years	40	8%	3	77%
3–4 years	20	4%	4	81%
4–5 years	18	4%	5	85%
5–6 years	14	3%	6	88%
6–7 years	18	4%	7	92%
7–8 years	8	2%	8	93%
8–9 years	7	2%	9	95%
9–10 years	11	2%	10	97%
>10 years	15	3%		

From Jennett, 1975, with permission.

to epileptiform discharges (Chapter 4). In some situations, however, such as hypothalamic hamartoma, seizures appear to originate within an alien tissue lesion (Munari et al., 1995).

Depth electrode recording from human sclerotic hippocampus has revealed that seizures originate in cell-sparse areas, not in the adjacent, more normal-appearing tissue (Babb et al., 1984). Pathological processes that destroy some neurons while leaving others untouched in the same region would necessarily give rise to synaptic reorganization within the disrupted neuronal aggregate; this could induce changes that predispose to hypersynchronization and hyperexcitability (Chapter 4). Consequently, irritating lesions and pathological processes that result in patchy cell loss appear to be more epileptogenic than those that completely destroy discrete areas of tissue or infiltrate the brain without disrupting connections.

The severity and extent of the lesion can also be a factor. The incidence of PTE is directly correlated with the severity of TBI (Frey, 2003) and the volume of brain tissue lost (Salazar et al., 1985). However, when a chronic seizure disorder develops, the severity of seizures decreases with increasing volume of tissue lost (Salazar et al., 1985). This finding agrees with other evidence, discussed previously, that mechanisms for development of a chronic seizure disorder are not exactly the same as mechanisms for the occurrence of an ictal event. Perhaps the greater the extent of the lesion, the more opportunity exists for synaptic integration to become epileptogenically reorganized in some area of damaged cortex; however, extensive loss of brain tissue reduces the available anatomical substrates for clinical manifestations of ictal electrographic discharges.

Location of the Lesion

Analysis of regional differences in epileptic potential must distinguish between propensity for epileptic excitability and predisposition for the development of a chronic epileptogenic lesion. Results of studies on variations of acute epileptic responses to noxious insults from one brain region to another, therefore, may not be relevant to the risk of developing chronic epilepsy from injury to these regions.

Regional differences in chronic epileptogenic potential might be partially revealed by

Table 8–4 Incidence of Epileptic Seizures in Children Aged 1–16 According to Location of Epileptic Spike Foci

Central foci	38%
Occipital foci	54%
Frontal foci	75%
Temporal foci	91%
Multiple foci	76%

From Kellaway. 1980 with permission.

the incidence of epileptic seizures associated with interictal EEG spikes in various cortical areas. For instance, the fact that children with occipital spikes are much less likely to have spontaneous seizures than those with anterior temporal spikes (Kellaway, 1980) (Table 8–4) could reflect a greater tendency for epileptogenic insults of the temporal lobe to cause spontaneous recurrent ictal events. The lowered incidence of seizures in children with central spikes, however, does not necessarily indicate a resistance of this region to the behavioral manifestations of epilepsy. Rather, the data are skewed by inclusion of a large percentage of patients with the EEG trait of *benign epilepsy of childhood with centrotemporal spikes* (Chapter 7) or *centroparietal (CP) spikes* (Stillerman et al., 1952) (Chapter 13). In both of those conditions, the dipole peculiarities of the centrotemporal spike appear to indicate a more diffuse or poorly localized functional cortical generator rather than a specific lesion in the neocortex adjacent to the rolandic fissure. In fact, experimental findings in primates indicate that application of alumina to sensorimotor cortex easily induces chronic focal motor seizures (Ward, 1972), whereas this does not appear to be true with hippocampus unless bilateral lesions are induced (Soper et al., 1978). However, focal motor seizures in animals with experimental precentral cortical lesions often consist of localized clonic movements associated with isolated EEG spikes and could represent mechanisms that would be considered interictal in other brain regions that do not mediate obvious behaviors. Manifestations of ictal discharges in the hippocampus are much more difficult for an observer to identify until widespread propagation occurs.

Kindling data do not help resolve this issue. Ictal behavioral symptoms often appear earlier with hippocampal than with neocortical kindling, but neocortical kindling is inconsistent and may produce no behavioral changes before the generalized seizure stage (Goddard et al., 1969; Seki and Wada, 1986; Wada, 1980). The amygdala is among the easiest brain structures to kindle in animals (Goddard et al., 1969), but only rarely is it the site of ictal onset in human temporal lobe epilepsy (Wieser, 1983). These observations indicate that regional differences in epileptogenicity reflect complicated mechanisms that vary depending on the epileptogenic agent, the epileptiform response measured, and probably the species studied.

A more clinically relevant approach to this question again comes from studies of PTE. Although Jennett (1975) noted that the incidence of late epilepsy was relatively high for patients with skull fractures over frontal and temporal lobes and relatively low for those with fractures over occipital areas, the relevance of these data can be questioned, because of the uncommon occurrence of fractures of the temporal bone in his series and the difficulty in determining the importance of contrecoup injuries. However, these findings are consistent with clinical impressions derived from the incidence of epileptic seizures after penetrating wounds of the brain (Caveness and Liss, 1961; Russell and Whitty, 1952) (Fig. 8–1) and with brain tumors (Penfield and Jasper, 1954). PTE may be more common when there are parietal lesions on computed tomography (CT) (Temkin, 2003). In all of these studies, lesions near the central fissure are associated with a high incidence of epileptic seizures. In one large series of Vietnam veterans, all patients with anterior temporal or central spike foci had PTE (Jabbari et al., 1986). As with monkey alumina foci, the latter observation could reflect the increased likelihood that brief epileptiform discharges near the motor strip will produce symptoms attracting clinical attention. Interictal spikes in less epileptogenic areas, such as occipital lobe, can also be shown to induce functional disturbances when measuring techniques are sufficiently sensitive to detect them (Shewmon and Erwin, 1988).

Specific cortical connections and preferential propagation pathways could be determining factors in the development of chronic seizures. Intracerebral electrode recordings

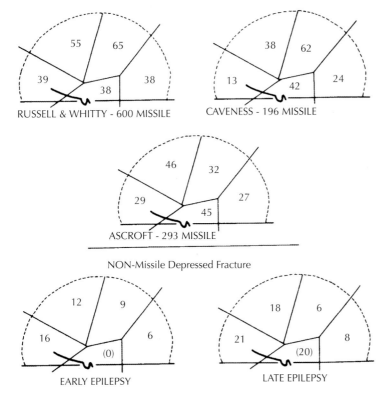

RUSSELL & WHITTY - 600 MISSILE

CAVENESS - 196 MISSILE

ASCROFT - 293 MISSILE

NON-Missile Depressed Fracture

EARLY EPILEPSY

LATE EPILEPSY

Figure 8–1. Incidence of epilepsy by lobe involved in head trauma (frontal to left, occipital to right). The term "early epilepsy" used for the nonmissile series refers to early transient seizures. Parentheses in lower figures indicate that fractures over the temporal lobe usually involved parietal, not temporal, bone. (From Jennett, 1975, with permission.)

from patients with medically intractable focal epilepsy demonstrate widespread areas capable of generating interictal epileptiform discharges and occasionally more than one site of ictal generation (Bancaud and Chauvel, 1987; Engel et al., 1981; Morrell, 1985; Wieser, 1983). In some patients with multiple regions of epileptogenicity, resection of the primary epileptogenic region abolishes habitual ictal events, even if contralateral seizures occurred preoperatively (Engel and Crandall, 1983; Morrell, 1985). In other such patients, auras and sometimes habitual seizures persist, even when the apparent site of ictal origin is completely resected and a discrete pathological lesion has been demonstrated in resected tissue (Engel, 1987a; Morrell, 1985). Although distant, presumably *secondary*, epileptogenic zones undoubtedly exist in patients with medically intractable focal epilepsy, it is not clear whether or to what degree distant kindling-like transsynaptic changes must occur before the *secondary* epileptogenic zone can give rise to spontaneous seizures.

The hippocampus may play a prominent role in establishing distant excitability changes necessary for epileptogenesis. It appears to participate in generalized tonic-clonic as well as focal seizures (Wieser, 1983), and it receives epileptiform propagation from many neocortical regions (Fig. 8–2). Contralateral spread of ictal discharges from one hippocampus to the other is quite slow (Lieb et al., 1986) and may not occur at all. Although that observation was believed to reflect a sparse or absent hippocampal commissure in the human (Wilson et al., 1987), contralateral propagation is also impaired in rodents, which have massive hippocampal commissures. Consequently, the hippocampus appears to have inherent homeostatic mechanisms that oppose propagation, perhaps involving the *dentate gate* (Engel et al., 2003; 2008a) (Chapter 4). In humans, bilaterally synchronous EEG spikes are common

with frontal lobe epileptogenic regions but not hippocampal epileptogenic regions; however, important communications between limbic structures must exist, because bilaterally *independent* spike foci occur commonly in the anterior temporal regions (Hughes, 1985) and are almost invariably encountered on depth electrode evaluations of patients with severe *mesial temporal lobe epilepsy (MTLE)* (Engel et al., 1981; Wieser, 1983).

Genetic Factors

Genetic factors in epileptogenesis are discussed in detail in Chapter 5. The importance of genetic factors was first clearly demonstrated in primate kindling experiments. Amygdaloid kindling in the rhesus monkey requires hundreds of trials, and generalized seizures never occur (Wada et al., 1978). Amygdaloid kindling of the genetically photosensitive baboon *Papio papio*, however, results in generalized seizures in less than 100 trials (Wada and Osawa, 1976). Presumably, the genetic trait responsible for photosensitive seizures in this baboon also predisposes to kindled limbic seizures. Subsequently, lines of rapid-kindling and slow-kindling rats have been developed (Racine et al., 1999), and more recently, variable sensitivities to kainate-induced epileptogenesis have been described for different mouse strains (Schauwecker, 2002). Advances in genetic screening have now revealed numerous susceptibility genes, predominantly involving ion channels and GABA receptors, that appear to play an important role in the manifestation of acquired epilepsy in humans (Chapter 5).

According to Jennett (Jennett, 1975), the incidence of a family history of epilepsy in patients with closed head trauma who develop late seizures is 6–17%, compared with only 3–4% in those who do not. Furthermore, the risk for late epilepsy is greater and the latency

---

Figure 8–2. Ictal EEG activity recorded from depth and surface (including sphenoidal) electrodes. In this patient, the epileptogenic zone was in the right occipital cortex (*ROC*), as indicated by the ictal onset seen at the beginning of the upper segment. Ictal EEG discharge remained confined to this area during the period that the patient stated she was seeing "butterflies," which were actually unformed colored visions. The bottom tracing is continuous with the top and shows that the focal ictal discharge disappears several seconds before the regional onset of rapid spiking in right mesial temporal structures. Several seconds after this, the ictal discharge propagates to left mesial temporal structures, and the patient loses consciousness. *R*, right; *L*, left; *AMYG*, amygdala; *AP*, anterior hippocampal pes; *MG*, *PG*, mid- and posterior hippocampal gyrus; *PTC*, posterior temporal cortex; *OC*, occipital cortex. Calibration: 1 second.

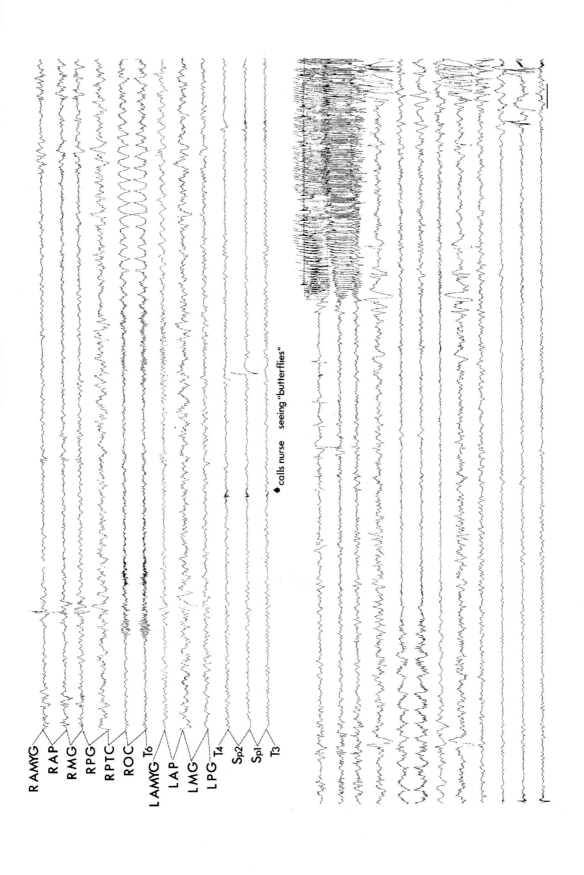

R AMYG
RAP
R MG
RPG
RPTC
ROC
L AMYG
T6
LAP
LMG
LPG
T4
Sp2
Sp1
T3

calls nurse   seeing "butterflies"

between head injury and the first late spontaneous seizure is shorter for patients who experience early reactive seizures (Jennett, 1975). These findings strongly suggest that innate, presumably genetically determined, predisposing factors (Chapter 5) contribute to the development of PTE. That a family history of epilepsy may not be a significant risk factor for late epilepsy following penetrating head injuries (Salazar et al., 1985) could indicate that this influence is relatively weak compared with the effects of extensive intracranial trauma in this particular patient population.

Genetic traits may also influence the types of seizures that result from an acquired epileptogenic lesion. A patient whose temporal lobe epilepsy is heralded by a generalized tonic-clonic seizure is much more likely to have a family history of epilepsy than one whose disorder begins with focal seizures (Schmidt et al., 1983). A genetic predisposition could explain the inconsistent occurrence of secondarily generalized seizures among patients with focal epilepsies, the prognostic value of this finding with respect to outcome after surgical treatment, and the occasional continuation of generalized seizures following resective surgery that abolishes habitual focal ictal events (Engel, 1987b).

Over half the patients who develop late epilepsy following closed head injury (Jennett, 1975) and 30% of those with penetrating wounds (Salazar et al., 1985) have generalized rather than focal seizures. However, this could reflect a high incidence of frontal lobe involvement and generalized tonic-clonic seizures of frontal lobe origin (Bancaud et al., 1974) (Chapter 6) rather than inheritance of a specific predisposition for generalized epilepsy.

Bilaterally synchronous spike-and-wave discharges in the EEGs of patients with temporal lobe epilepsy predict a poor outcome following anterior temporal lobectomy (Engel et al., 1975; Lieb et al., 1981) and presumably indicate frontal or other neocortical, rather than mesial temporal, epileptogenic lesions. However, some patients with these EEG patterns do have a specific epileptogenic lesion in one temporal lobe and do benefit from temporal lobe resection. In these patients, a genetic trait for a generalized epileptic disorder could account for the EEG findings and also help predispose to the development of limbic seizures (Andermann, 1982).

Practical Considerations

Posttraumatic seizures provide an excellent model for discussing the clinical implications of epileptogenesis. Prophylactic drug treatment following head injury has been instituted to protect patients from both early epileptic seizures occurring one to two weeks post insult and the development of subsequent chronic epilepsy. Those two issues need to be clearly distinguished, because clinical studies so far show that prophylactic treatments prevent the occurrence of early seizures but have no effect on epileptogenesis (Temkin et al., 1990; Temkin, 2009). Antiepileptogenic interventions would have tremendous clinical value and are an area of intensive investigation.

PROPHYLAXIS FOR EARLY SEIZURES

Early seizures are reactive (acute symptomatic) seizures that occur within a week or so of an injury (Beghi et al., 2010). Certain risk factors following closed head injury predispose to early seizures: (1) an intracranial hematoma, intradural bleeding being more important than extradural bleeding, (2) the presence of neurological signs or symptoms, focal findings being more important than nonfocal ones, (3) posttraumatic amnesia lasting more than 24 hours, (4) depressed skull fracture, (5) injury before the age of 5 years, and (6) linear skull fracture (Jennett, 1975) (see Table 8–2). Early seizures rarely follow trivial head injury except in patients under 5 years of age, but early status epilepticus is more common with severe head injury in this age group (22%) than in older patients (8%). More than half of the early seizures occur within 24 hours of the injury, but early seizures induced by intracerebral hematomas are usually delayed and repeated. Early epileptic seizures are rarely the only or first sign of a developing hematoma, and an uncomplicated seizure should not be considered evidence of an acute change in the neurological condition (Jennett, 1975). More than half of early posttraumatic epileptic seizures have focal features, most being focal motor. Focal seizures in children do not increase the risk of later PTE.

Posttraumatic early seizures complicate management, particularly when postictal depression obscures alterations in consciousness that might indicate an acute change in neurological status that could be life-threatening. It is important, therefore, to anticipate the occurrence of these early seizures and, if possible, prevent them. A large controlled study with *phenytoin* (Young et al., 1983) indicated that plasma concentrations above the usual therapeutic range (which is 25–30 µg/ml) may be necessary to prevent early posttraumatic seizures. Because such high levels are needed, the study's authors recommend prophylactic treatment with phenytoin only after an initial seizure has occurred. Prophylactic treatment at these levels might also be reasonable, however, when there is a great risk for early repeated seizures or status, as in children under the age of 5 and patients with posttraumatic amnesia of more than 24 hours, a depressed skull fracture, or an intracranial hematoma (Jennett, 1975).

Further information is available from studies of prophylactic treatment following craniotomy. In another large controlled series, phenytoin prevented postoperative early seizures at usual plasma concentrations (North et al., 1983). The reason for this apparent discrepancy between phenytoin's effectiveness against early seizures after trauma and after brain surgery may relate to a difference in potential epileptogenicity between those insults. Trauma is more likely to produce residual intracortical blood and therefore might require higher levels of medication. For patients undergoing craniotomy, prophylactic treatment is recommended when there is a high risk of early postoperative seizures, as occurs with surgery for meningiomas, trauma, aneurysms, and abscesses. If surgery is elective, prophylaxis should begin one week preoperatively.

PROPHYLAXIS FOR CHRONIC EPILEPSY

Phenytoin, the prophylactic medication still most commonly used for head trauma, was reported to prevent the development of chronic seizures following experimental focal neocortical lesions induced by alumina in the cat (Rapport and Ojemann, 1975) but does not appear to prevent amygdaloid kindling in this animal (Wada et al., 1976). *Phenobarbital* and *carbamazepine* do exert a prophylactic effect on amygdaloid kindling in the cat (Wada et al., 1976), and a differential action between the neocortex and the limbic system may exist for some drugs (Burnham et al., 1980). Animal

studies on the whole, however, have yielded negative results for commonly used antiseizure drugs, a not surprising observation given that these compounds were developed to suppress ictogenesis, not epileptogenesis.

Clinically, antiseizure medication can be continued indefinitely, but in this situation the symptomatic antiseizure effects would mask any antiepileptogenic effects. Although this would be the most effective treatment, it is not justified by the relatively low yearly incidence of seizures after 1 year (see Table 8–3). Current debate, therefore, concerns when to continue treatment for a year. Any clinical assumption that epileptogenic processes can be adequately dampened by antiseizure medications within a year appears to be unfounded; however, basic research continues to investigate potential antiepileptogenic effects of some new antiseizure drugs, immunosuppressants, rapamycin, anti-inflammatory agents, and drugs that interfere with proliferation and plasticity (Galanopoulou et al., 2012; Löscher and Brandt, 2010; Pitkänen, 2010). On the other hand, stroke studies indicate that phenytoin and some other antiseizure drugs impair neural repair and may do more harm than good for patients with TBI (Goldstein, 1998).

Whether and how long antiseizure medication should be continued after initial prophylactic administration for head trauma is determined by the risk of subsequent recurrent epileptic seizures, but evidence concerning the effectiveness of longer treatment to prevent the later development of chronic epilepsy remains lacking. Treatment can be instituted for a few weeks to protect against early seizures, but continuous treatment with *phenytoin, phenobarbital, valproic acid, carbamazepine, zonisamide, diazepam*, and *magnesium* has not prevented epileptogenesis; that is, the recurrence of late seizures after medication is discontinued in clinical studies of TBI, intracranial surgery, neonatal hypoxia, or febrile status epilepticus (Chang and Lowenstein, 2003; Temkin, 2009).

The failure of clinical trials to identify an antiepileptogenic intervention might be attributed to several factors: (1) antiseizure drugs used may not be antiepileptogenic, (2) patient populations tested may be inappropriate for demonstrating an antiepileptogenic effect, (3) dosing regimens, timing, and duration of studies may be suboptimal, (4) effective serum levels may not have been achieved because of noncompliance (people are unlikely take drugs faithfully for disorders they do not have), and (5) study designs may have been inadequate.

Clinical trials of antiepileptogenesis are difficult and expensive to perform, for a variety of reasons, which is why so few have been conducted. To overcome interindividual variability, it is necessary to choose as homogeneous a patient population as possible. Even with conditions such as severe TBI, this variability would undoubtedly require large, multicenter studies of 1,000 to 2,000 patients to obtain statistically significant results. Demonstration of an antiepileptogenic effect, as opposed to an antiseizure effect, requires withdrawal of the potential antiepileptogenic intervention after a period of time for comparison with an untreated control group, and this could raise ethical issues. End-point measures are also difficult to define, particularly given that some patients may develop seizures 10 years or more after an epileptogenic insult.

Only 5% of patients in Jennett's series (Jennett, 1975) developed chronic late epilepsy following nonmissile head injury, but it occurred in 31% of patients with hematomas, 25% with early seizures, and 15% with depressed skull fractures. The incidence of late epilepsy after missile wounds of the head is 28–53% (Caveness and Liss, 1961; Jennett, 1975; Russell and Whitty, 1952; Salazar et al., 1985) and appears to correlate with the extent of cortical disruption and retained metal fragments (Salazar et al., 1985). Consequently, the population of high-risk patients with such injuries is well suited for clinical trials of novel antiepileptogenic interventions .

PTE is a consequence of brain surgery, especially supratentorial interventions (Foy et al., 1992). In one large retrospective study with prolonged follow-up, the incidence of epilepsy after supratentorial craniotomy was 17% (Shaw and Foy, 1991). The incidence was greater than 20% for vascular lesions, hemorrhage, meningioma, and abscess. Because the latent period for PTE after surgery is shorter than for TBI (Foy et al., 1981), this patient population is also appropriate for trials of antiseizure treatments.

Identification of reliable biomarkers of epileptogenesis and epileptogenicity would greatly facilitate such clinical trials, by (1) identifying those patients who will develop epilepsy following a specific insult without antiepileptogenic intervention, (2) staging the epileptogenic

Table 8–5 Potential Biomarkers

- Hippocampal changes on MRI
- Interictal spike features, including on functional MRI
- Pathological high-frequency oscillations (pHFOs)
- Excitability—transcranial magnetic stimulation (TMS)
- AMT-PET imaging
- Gene expression profiles

process in a standardized fashion so progress can be measured, and (3) establishing a reliable end-point by permitting definitive evidence at some time after the intervention that epileptogenesis is not occurring or that epileptogenicity does not exist to a degree that might cause chronic epileptic seizures in the future (Engel, 2011a;b). Biomarkers of epileptogenesis could also lead to development of more cost-effective, rapid-throughput experimental screening models that would greatly facilitate identification of potential antiepileptogenic treatments. Candidate biomarkers that might serve as outcome measures for clinical trials assessing antiepileptogenesis and disease modification in epilepsy are shown in Table 8–5. Research into the fundamental mechanisms of epileptogenesis has revealed early changes that might be targets for the development of biomarkers (Table 8–6) (Chapter 4). Several biomarkers are under investigation, including *pathological high-frequency oscillations (pHFOs)* (Worrell and Gotman, 2011), *positron emission tomography with α-methyl-tryptophan (AMT-PET)* (Kumar et al., 2011), and *hippocampal changes with magnetic resonance imaging (MRI)* (Gomes and Shinnar, 2011) (Chapter 12).

Of potential practical interest is the fact that one animal study has demonstrated a

Table 8–6 Potential Target Mechanisms for Biomarkers of Epileptogenesis

Altered excitability and synchrony
Altered neuronal function (e.g., gene expression profiles, protein products)
Cell loss (e.g., hippocampal atrophy)
Axonal sprouting
Synaptic reorganization
Neurogenesis
Altered glial function and gliosis
Angiogenesis
Inflammatory changes

Modified from Engel, 2011b, with permission.

potentially important phenomenon referred to as *conditioned inefficacy* (Weiss and Post, 1991). When chronic carbamazepine is administered to rats at doses too low to prevent the development of kindled seizures, the subsequent seizures are refractory to adequate levels of carbamazepine. Research on conditioned inefficacy could contribute valuable clinically relevant information, because the data suggest that inadequate prophylaxis may be worse than no prophylaxis.

THE PROGRESSIVE NATURE OF EPILEPSY

Secondary Epileptogenesis

The progressive nature of epilepsy and the adverse effect of seizures on the brain have been best demonstrated in the animal laboratory, but supporting clinical evidence, at least for some forms of epilepsy, also exists (Engel, 2002; Heinemann et al., 1996; Sutula and Pitkänen, 2002). Secondary epileptogenesis is readily demonstrated in animals by kindling (Corcoran and Moshé, 2005; Goddard et al., 1969; Wada, 1986; Wada, 1981; Wada, 1976) and the *mirror focus phenomenon* (Morrell 1959/60) (Chapter 4). At least two accidental occurrences of electrical kindling in patients have been reported (Monroe, 1970; Sramka et al., 1977), but focal brain stimulation is certainly not a major cause of human epilepsy. Some studies of spontaneous epileptic seizures following repeated *electroconvulsive shock treatment (ECT)* have indicated a small increased incidence, consistent with a kindling effect (Devinsky and Duchowny, 1983). This relationship is disputed (Small et al., 1981), however, and of more theoretical than practical importance, because 50 to 70 repeated ECT trials appear to be necessary before there is an increased risk of inducing spontaneous epileptic seizures (Blumenthal, 1955; Naoi, 1959).

Arguments for the clinical relevance of secondary epileptogenesis must account for discrepancies between the kindling animal model and human focal epilepsy (Engel and Cahan, 1986) (Table 8–7). As noted previously, the amygdala is one of the most easily kindled structures in the animal brain but is rarely the site of ictal onset in patients. Furthermore, afterdischarge thresholds decrease and duration progressively increases during kindling (Racine, 1972a), but duration of the electrographic seizure is variable from one seizure to another in the human. Afterdischarge threshold decreases in kindling but may actually be elevated at the site of ictal onset in human hippocampus (Cherlow et al., 1977). There is a stereotyped progression of limbic symptoms over time in the kindling model (Racine, 1972b) that does not occur in patients, and *2-deoxyglucose (2DG)* autoradiography in the kindled animal demonstrates a consistent ictal propagation pattern, without interictal abnormalities (Engel et al., 1978); whereas studies using PET with *fluorodeoxyglucose (FDG)* in patients with temporal lobe epilepsy usually show a zone of hypometabolism interictally (Engel et al., 1982a;b;c) and variable patterns of ictal propagation (Engel et al., 1982d; Engel et al., 1983). These differences, however, could reflect the greater complexity of cerebral organization in the human, variable genetic factors, and the influence of antiseizure drugs (Engel and Cahan, 1986).

On the other hand, certain features of limbic seizures in patients with temporal lobe epilepsy resemble aspects of amygdaloid kindling in animals (Racine, 1972b). Behavioral similarities include an initial arrest reaction and oroalimentary automatisms (Chapter 6). Both also demonstrate transsynaptic alterations in excitability such as spontaneous interictal spikes and enhanced evoked potentials in distant structures (Buser and Bancaud, 1983; Racine et al., 1975) and paired pulse suppression with perforant path stimulation (Engel and Wilson, 1986; Tuff et al., 1983).

There has been considerable controversy concerning the nature of secondary epileptogenic phenomena in humans and their relevance to the practice of clinical epileptology (Engel and Cahan, 1986; Goldensohn, 1984; Morrell et al., 1987; Engel and Shewmon, 1991; Engel, 1998; Engel et al., 2001; Engel, 2005). Those who reject the importance of secondary epileptogenesis argue that distant epileptogenic areas encountered in patients are only rarely capable of independently and spontaneously giving rise to epileptic seizures (Goldensohn, 1984). However, these distant pathophysiological disturbances frequently occur (Engel and Cahan, 1986; Morrell et al., 1987) and may have other profound effects on cerebral function even when they fail to generate seizures. For instance, a focal irritative lesion that is already a generator of epileptiform discharges

Table 8–7 **Comparisons between Kindling and Human Epilepsy**

Amygdaloid-Kindled Animal	Human Limbic Epilepsy	Similar
Behavioral		
Stereotyped progression of limbic symptoms over time	Symptoms do not progress with time in a stereotyped fashion	No
Arrest reaction and chewing occur initially	Arrest reaction and chewing are common early symptoms of complex partial seizures	Yes
Anatomical		
Microanatomy of neurons normal	Hippocampal cell loss, dendritic changes, and spine loss	No
Mossy fiber sprouting	Mossy fiber sprouting	Yes
Amygdala most susceptible to kindling	Amygdala rarely the site of onset of seizures	No
Distant interictal hypometabolism not seen with 2DG autoradiography	Distant interictal hypometabolism common on PET scans with FDG	No
Consistent pattern of ictal propagation seen with 2DG autoradiography	Pattern of ictal propagation seen on PET scans with FDG variable from patient to patient but consistent from seizure to seizure in the same patient	No
Electrophysiological		
Afterdischarge duration progressively increases	Afterdischarge duration variable from one seizure to another	No
Afterdischarge threshold progressively decreases	Afterdischarge threshold elevated	No
Spontaneous interictal spikes appear in distant structures	Spontaneous interictal spikes occur commonly in distant structures	Yes
Excitability is enhanced in distant structures	Excitability may be enhanced in contralateral hippocampus	Yes
Potentials evoked in distant structures by stimulation of the focus can be enhanced	Potentials evoked in distant structures by stimulation of the focus can be enhanced	Yes
Paired pulse suppression occurs ipsilateral to the primary focus	Paired pulse suppression occurs ipsilateral to the primary focus	Yes
Neurochemical		
No consistent enduring change identified	No consistent enduring change identified	—

Adapted from Engel and Cahan, 1986.

might kindle adjacent or distant brain structures to (1) convert subclinical into clinical epileptic events (Engel, 1987b), (2) change the character of epileptic seizures, rendering them more disabling and more refractory to treatment (Engel, 1987b), and (3) disrupt normal neuronal integration in other ways, giving rise to interictal behavioral disturbances (Chapter 11) (Adamec, 1975; Engel et al., 1986; Griffith et al., 1987). This view, then, holds that at least some forms of human epilepsy are progressive; the occurrence of epileptic seizures, and perhaps even subclinical epileptiform events, might adversely influence the subsequent course of the disorder. This possibility was proposed as long ago as 1881 by Gowers (Gowers, 1881), who stated, "The effect of a convulsion...is such as to render the occurrence of another more easy, to intensify

the predisposition that already exists." Indeed, the International League Against Epilepsy has now recognized a number of epilepsy syndromes as *epileptic encephalopathies*, indicating that the seizures themselves appear to be responsible for progression of epileptic activity as well as cerebral dysfunction (Engel, 2001) (Chapter 7), although a relationship between these progressive disorders and kindling has not been demonstrated.

Clinical Evidence for Progression

Information on the natural history of the epilepsies is confounded almost inevitably by therapeutic intervention that alters the clinical course. However, in some situations the timing of this therapeutic intervention itself provides important information. A major study on prognosis in epilepsy listed the following among the risk factors for an adverse outcome: a young age at onset, more seizures prior to first visit to a physician, and a longer duration of illness (Rodin, 1968). Most subsequent studies have confirmed these findings. In a very large series from Japan (Okuma and Kumashiro, 1981) outcome was best when therapy was begun less than one year after the onset of seizures. In several studies, seizure-free children experienced relapse more often after drug withdrawal when the duration of illness before control was longer, more seizures occurred before control, and seizures were more severe (Holowach et al., 1972; Holowach-Thurston et al., 1982; Todt, 1984). A common view, therefore, was that "seizures may predispose to further seizures, and...effective treatment may be important to prevent evolution into chronic and more intractable epilepsy" (Shorvon and Reynolds, 1982).

It can be argued, however, that the poor prognosis for patients whose seizures take longer to control or who have more frequent seizures is due to more severe epilepsy initially rather than the occurrence of seizures per se. Prognosis in these studies also depended on other features, such as neurological deficits and an organic etiology, that clearly reflect the severity of the epileptogenic process from the start. Consequently, the data from these studies do not directly address the possible progressive nature of epilepsy.

The concept of symptom progression was supported by examination of two older extensive studies of the natural history of temporal lobe epilepsy, involving 666 patients from London (Currie et al., 1971) and 100 from Oxford (Lindsay et al., 1979a;b;c; Ounsted et al., 1966). In both series, a large percentage of patients who continued to have seizures demonstrated a grim prognosis, worsening of their epilepsy, and a deterioration in function. Both series, however, also included a subset of patients with medically refractory seizures who underwent anterior temporal lobectomy. When seizures were reduced or abolished by surgery, their conditions did not deteriorate. It is interesting to speculate that many of the patients in these series whose seizures resolved spontaneously actually had *rolandic epilepsy*, a condition that was not yet well recognized.

Additional evidence for secondary epileptogenesis in human epilepsy has been derived from EEG data and surgical series. It is well known that in children the appearance of EEG spikes in the temporal region increases with age and with duration of an epileptic disorder (Trojaborg, 1966). This finding is consistent with the concept of increased epileptic excitability in mesial temporal structures as a result of preferential involvement of the hippocampi in focal limbic and generalized seizures, even when the primary epileptogenic lesion is elsewhere. Thus the classical behavioral and electrographic presentation of temporal lobe epilepsy can occur as a result of structural lesions in other parts of the brain (Chapters 6 and 7). Although habitual seizures may be relieved by resection of these neocortical lesions (Falconer et al., 1962), more commonly seizures persist to some degree when the hippocampus is not removed (Crandall, 1987).

In one large series of patients with EEG follow-up of from 15 to 40 years, (Hughes, 1985), an increase in bilateral, as opposed to unilateral, spike foci occurred at a rate of almost 1% per year; the pattern of developing bilateral temporal foci was seen in 34% of patients. Bilateral independent interictal temporal lobe spike foci are present in almost all patients with medically intractable temporal lobe epilepsy who are studied with depth electrodes for surgical resection, but most have habitual attacks originating from only one temporal lobe, even though the other may be hyperexcitable (Engel et al., 1981; Gloor, 1975; Morrell, 1985). When spontaneous seizures occasionally arise in this contralateral region, it is not necessarily an indication that these will continue after the removal of the epileptogenic lesion (Engel and Crandall, 1983; Morrell, 1985).

It has been argued that bilaterally independent epileptogenic mesial temporal abnormalities may be due to bilateral mesial temporal insults and not a mirror focus phenomenon. This issue was investigated by Morrell (Morrell, 1985; Morrell et al., 1987) in a series of patients with focal epilepsy resulting from neoplastic lesions that would be unlikely to occur bilaterally. Of 123 patients with temporal lobe epilepsy, 36% demonstrated unequivocal evidence of independent interictal or ictal epileptiform discharges contralateral to and homotopic with the tumor. Fifteen percent had epileptic seizures that were documented to occur from the contralateral site. Twenty-one percent of 57 patients with frontal lobe tumors had similar evidence of secondary epileptogenesis, and in a third group of 47 patients with isolated brain tumors, 34% had evidence of secondary epileptogenesis (Morrell et al., 1987). All patients underwent surgical resection of the primary epileptogenic region, and only in approximately one-third of the patients with evidence of secondary epileptogenesis did seizures continue to arise from the secondary area. Morrell and colleagues postulated that both reversible and irreversible forms of secondary epileptogenesis exist. Irreversibility was positively correlated with a longer duration of seizures and a higher frequency of seizure occurrence before surgical intervention. This finding suggests progressive development of first the reversible and then the irreversible form of secondary epileptogenesis.

In another study attempting to elucidate the clinical relevance of kindling (Engel and Cahan, 1986), the influence of preoperative duration of illness and seizure frequency on postoperative outcome was assessed for 106 patients who underwent anterior temporal lobectomy for medically intractable seizures. In patients who improved after surgery, there was a direct correlation between the degree of improvement and the duration of illness. Patients who were completely seizure-free had the shortest preoperative course, those who experienced only auras had a somewhat longer course, those with rare seizures had an even longer course, and those with more than rare seizures had the longest course. In contrast, patients who did not improve after surgery had an intermediate duration of illness prior to surgery. The researchers concluded that the epileptogenic lesion was not completely removed in the last group of patients, while in the others a kindling effect, which increased the epileptogenic potential of cortex outside the resected temporal lobe, determined the degree of residual symptoms following complete removal of the epileptogenic lesion. Frequency of seizures in this study did not appear to influence outcome, perhaps because some auras and subclinical electrographic discharges, which could not be counted, also contributed to the kindling effect. More recent surgical series, now that neuroimaging greatly reduces the likelihood that an epileptogenic lesion is missed and not resected, appear to confirm duration of epilepsy as a risk factor for poorer prognosis

(McLachlan et al., 1997; Engel, 1999; Janszky et al., 2005).

The advent of high-resolution structural as well as functional neuroimaging has contributed importantly to arguments that certain forms of epilepsy are progressive. Increases in hippocampal atrophy, for instance, can be demonstrated to occur over time in patients with MTLE (Cendes, 2005). Identification of focal structural lesions, usually cortical dysplasia, in infants and young children with severe generalized epilepsies such as *West syndrome* has led to successful surgical treatment in such patients (Chugani et al., 1990) (Chapter 14). When such surgery results in elimination of epileptic seizures, there is usually a reduction or reversal in developmental delay, and children who were otherwise destined for an institutional existence can recoup much of their normal function (Hemb et al., 2010; Mathern, 2010). This strongly suggests that the functional deterioration almost invariably encountered in these children without surgery results from recurrent seizures and not from some progressive underlying neurological disease process, leading directly to the concept of epileptic encephalopathy. *Landau-Kleffner syndrome* and *epileptic encephalopathy with continuous spike-and-wave during sleep* (CSWS) are the classic examples of epileptic encephalopathies (Chapter 7); however, because there are no structural abnormalities associated with these conditions and the underlying cause is unknown, and also because it is extremely difficult to eliminate the epileptiform EEG activity during sleep, it remains unproven that the progressive behavioral disturbances are in fact due to epileptic activity and not to some other etiological process. Nevertheless, the concept that repeated epileptic seizures, at least in some conditions, can lead to worsening of the epileptic condition as well as nonepileptic cerebral dysfunction is now universally accepted. Progression in the recognized epileptic encephalopathies is not disputed.

Although there are no adequate longitudinal studies of the natural history of MTLE or other acquired focal epilepsies, individuals with pharmacoresistant seizures who are referred to epilepsy centers often have a characteristic pattern of seizures that are easily treated initially, with prolonged periods of remission, followed by recurrence of seizures, but now more severe ones that do not respond to medication

(Berg et al., 2003). This pattern strongly suggests a progressive disorder. Furthermore, with continued seizures these patients develop worsening behavioral disturbances, typically involving memory and learning dysfunction (Hermann et al., 2006), and depression (Kanner and Blumer, 2008), changes that could, at least in part, reflect functional and perhaps structural disruption due to recurrent seizures (Engel et al., 2008b). Evidence also exists that some single seizures could cause actual structural brain damage (Sutula and Pitkänen, 2002) (Chapter 9) and that the cerebellar atrophy commonly seen in patients with epilepsy may be due to seizures and not phenytoin therapy, as previously believed (Oyegbile et al., 2011).

Practical Considerations

From the foregoing discussion, there appears to be little doubt that at least some patients with epilepsy demonstrate progressive symptoms resembling secondary epileptogenesis in animals and that epileptic encephalopathies exist. Given that epileptogenesis develops over time following a specific epileptogenic insult, it is unreasonable to assume that this process stops as soon as spontaneous seizures occur. Consequently, it is more likely than not that most epilepsy disorders that arise as a result of progressive epileptogenic mechanisms continue to progress to some degree once seizures occur, but it is equally likely that, at least in some patients, this process does eventually stop and may actually be reversed, resulting in spontaneous remissions. In the genetic, age-related epilepsy syndromes, the epileptogenic process differs from that after an acquired insult, so progression was not thought to occur. However, some genetic syndromes, such as *Dravet syndrome*, are epileptic encephalopathies where progressive deterioration, presumably due to recurrent seizures, is a characteristic feature. Even if progression of the epileptogenic mechanisms does not result in a worsening of epileptic seizures, these effects or the homeostatic protective mechanisms that develop to maintain the interictal state could negatively influence normal brain functions and worsen the course of an epilepsy condition. More research is necessary before we can determine what clinical phenomena can be attributed

to epileptogenic progression, the risk factors for developing these disturbances, and their relevance to long-term prognosis and management for individual patients with epilepsy. Furthermore, the possibility that some forms of apparent intractable epilepsy "burn out," or remit spontaneously, has not been adequately investigated.

In the past, proponents of secondary epileptogenesis suggested that focal seizures should be treated with *barbiturates* rather than phenytoin. Barbiturates, which prevent formation of mirror foci in animals (Morrell and Baker, 1961), are no longer a drug of choice for epilepsy, for a variety of reasons (Chapter 14). Today, acceptance that some forms of epilepsy can be progressive has underlined the need for early aggressive treatment, as exemplified by the mantra "No seizures, no side effects, as soon as possible." This means not only institution of appropriate antiseizure medication at maximal effective doses but referral to specialized epilepsy centers after trials of two antiseizure medications have failed, to identify patients who might be surgical candidates (Engel, 2008) (Chapter 14).

At this point in our understanding of the epileptogenic mechanisms underlying progression, it would be inappropriate to try to abolish all auras or subclinical EEG discharges with antiseizure medication, and for some patients, continuation of occasional seizures may be preferable to the side effects induced by further increasing serum drug levels (Chapter 14). In particular, there is no indication at present for an aggressive approach to the treatment of certain benign epilepsy conditions associated with absences and epileptic myoclonus, as well as rolandic epilepsy, *Panayiotopoulos syndrome*, or other nondebilitating focal seizures. Common practice is also not to treat most first seizures (Chapter 14) or benign febrile seizures (Chapter 7).

No studies have been performed to demonstrate the effects of any potential antiepileptogenic intervention other than surgery to reverse the progression of an epilepsy condition once the diagnosis is established. Two studies, the Multicenter Study of Early Epilepsy and Single Seizures (MESS) (Marson et al., 2005) and the First Seizure Trial Group (FIRST) (Musicco et al., 1997), evaluated the benefit of instituting standard antiseizure medications after a single epileptic seizure when the diagnosis of epilepsy remains in doubt. Early treatment with these medications did not affect long-term remission in those patients who ultimately were diagnosed with epilepsy, and therefore the conclusion of these studies was that standard antiseizure medication appeared to have no antiepileptogenic effect at this early stage of the condition. Future studies to identify and validate potential antiepileptogenic interventions to arrest or reverse progression would benefit greatly from the development of appropriate biomarkers, as already discussed (Engel, 2011a;b).

EPILEPTIC SEIZURES AND BRAIN DEVELOPMENT

Epileptic Susceptibility of the Immature Brain

Discussion of the susceptibility of the immature brain to epilepsy must distinguish between reactive seizures and the development of chronic epilepsy. The immature brain is generally considered to be more epileptogenic than the mature brain. The incidence of seizures is high during the first year of life (Hauser and Kurland, 1975). This phenomenon reflects the high risk of exposure to cerebral insult in the neonatal period as well as the higher susceptibility of the immature brain to generate acute epileptic seizures in reaction to injury (Rakhade and Jensen, 2009; Galanopoulou and Moshé, 2009) (Chapter 5). Animal studies in general confirm the clinical impression of greater epileptic excitability of the immature brain (Chapter 3), but the few that have addressed chronic epileptogenesis have found immature animals to be less likely than adults to develop recurrent spontaneous seizures (Holmes et al., 1984; Moshé and Albala, 1982; Okada et al., 1984) (Chapter 3). A similar pattern emerges from the clinical literature.

Vulnerability of the neonatal brain to epileptic brain damage is not well defined (Haut et al., 2004; Scantlebury et al., 2007). Reactive seizures, such as those induced in the neonate by hypocalcemia and febrile seizures in infancy, commonly leave no sequelae (Freeman, 1983; Holmes, 1987; Holmes, 1985; Nelson and Ellenberg, 1981; Rose and Lombroso, 1970;

Volpe, 1987) (Chapter 6). Chronic epilepsy that begins within the first year of life often carries a poor prognosis, because it is usually due to severe cerebral injury. Perhaps severe injury is necessary for chronic epileptogenesis at this stage because the immature brain is less susceptible to developing epilepsy than the more mature brain. Furthermore, although children under the age of 5 are the most likely to develop early seizures and status epilepticus following head trauma, there is no increased incidence of late PTE in this age group (Jennett, 1975). On the contrary, children under the age of 16 are less likely to develop late seizures following head trauma than older patients (Jennett, 1975) (see Table 8–2).

Epidemiological studies indicate that seizure onset below the age of 10 is a good prognostic sign (Okuma and Kumashiro, 1981), and later-onset epilepsy is a risk factor for relapse with drug withdrawal following a seizure-free period (Holowach-Thurston et al., 1982). These findings probably reflect inclusion in these series of age-related benign genetic epilepsies of childhood, however, and cannot be legitimately used to support the argument that epileptogenesis is decreased for the immature brain.

Evolution of Epilepsy Syndromes

There is controversy concerning whether some unique ictal behaviors typical of *neonatal seizures* as well as *infantile spasms* are due to epileptic mechanisms in neocortex similar to those in the more mature brain or to subcortical mechanisms related to myoclonus or movement disorders (Kellaway and Mizrahi, 1987). The latter concept is supported by the poor relationship in the newborn between epileptiform EEG discharges recorded from the scalp, which presumably reflect primarily cortical activity, and clinical seizures (Mizrahi and Kellaway, 1987; Tharp, 1980; Mizrahi et al., 2008). Although some patients demonstrate evolution from severe neonatal seizures to infantile spasms and then to the *Lennox-Gastaut syndrome* (Chapter 7), there is no known mechanistic relationship among these phenomena. These syndromes reflect nonspecific age-dependent responses of the developing brain to severe insult, rather than some progressive pathophysiological process.

The percentage of neonates with seizures who develop chronic epilepsy varies from 7% to 26% across series, depending on the incidence of benign reactive seizures such as those that occur with late hypocalcemia (Volpe, 1987; Watanabe et al., 1982). In one study of neonates with seizures, 80% with central nervous system dysgenesis, 30% with perinatal hypoxia, and 23% with meningitis subsequently developed chronic epileptic conditions (Watanabe et al., 1982). Neonates with the most severe brain damage were more likely to exhibit myoclonic jerks and ultimately to progress to infantile spasms; those with less severe neonatal seizures who developed chronic epilepsy most often had generalized or focal motor seizures later (Watanabe et al., 1982). Neonatal seizures do not become chronic; they are transient, age-dependent symptoms of cerebral dysfunction, at times due to irreversible injury that later gives rise to chronic seizures.

Only about one-third of *slow spike-and-wave* EEG patterns evolve from a pattern of *hypsarrhythmia*, whereas almost three-fourths of hypsarrhythmic patterns ultimately become slow spike-and-wave (Hughes, 1985). Similarly, infants with infantile spasms are highly likely to develop a Lennox-Gastaut syndrome in childhood, whereas most patients with the Lennox-Gastaut syndrome have no history of infantile spasms. Therefore, the transition from infantile spasms to the Lennox-Gastaut syndrome is certainly not an obligatory one. As children with the slow spike-and-wave pattern become older, the EEG has a tendency to change to nonspecific irregular spike-and-wave discharges as well as multifocal spiking (Hughes, 1985). These EEG and behavioral stages all presumably depend on cerebral maturational factors, rather than a specific evolutionary disease process.

Migration of the Interictal EEG Spike

A common maturational change in epileptiform EEG activity is the anterior migration of interictal spike activity from occipital to frontotemporal regions (Hughes, 1985; Trojaborg, 1966). This also does not reflect evolution of a specific pathophysiological process, but rather results from properties of the maturing brain that influence the manifestation of epileptiform discharges. In early childhood, interictal spikes tend to show spatial fluctuation and are

not necessarily localized to the site of the epileptogenic lesion. With sequential EEGs, spike foci may appear to switch from side to side or from one part of the brain to another almost at random. With increasing age there is greater localizing specificity of the interictal EEG spike focus to the region of the epileptogenic lesion. Serial EEGs spaced widely in time often show posterior spiking initially and more anterior spiking later in life, giving the illusion of anterior migration. This pattern is due to a relatively greater capacity of the posterior portions of the immature brain to generate epileptiform EEG potentials, coupled with the relatively high tendency for chronic epileptogenic lesions to be located in frontotemporal regions. As the child matures, posteriorly predominant epileptiform EEG potentials are more likely to become restricted to the area over the actual lesion.

Practical Considerations

Certain diagnostic decisions must take maturational factors into account. Shifting spike foci with serial EEGs in children under the age of 12 do not necessarily indicate a multifocal pathological process. Similarly, an interictal spike focus on a single EEG unreliably identifies the site of the epileptogenic region in this age group. If localizing information is clinically important in children, consistent findings on multiple serial EEGs and confirmation from independent structural and functional tests (Chapters 12 and 16) are needed. When lateralization is important, asymmetrical nonepileptiform EEG activity such as *sleep spindles* and *vertex sharp waves* can be useful.

Although acute reactive seizures are more common in the immature than in the mature brain, experimental and clinical evidence suggests a comparatively decreased risk for epileptogenesis, that is, a lowered propensity for the development of chronic seizures, in the immature brain. Prognosis depends on the underlying pathological process and not the recurrence of ictal events per se.

Debate about the treatment of epileptic seizures in neonates and infants is less concerned with epileptogenesis than with whether epileptic seizures or antiseizure drugs are more likely to damage the maturing brain. Animal studies have demonstrated epilepsy-induced disruption of brain growth in newborn rats

(Wasterlain et al., 1980), but these animals are significantly more immature at birth than humans. Developmental disturbances have not been clearly attributed to epileptic seizures in the human infant and neonate. Based on the fact that barbiturates retard brain growth in the immature rat (Diaz and Schain, 1978), other chronic antiseizure medications may be more disruptive to brain development than are some types of epileptic seizures. Consequently, controversy exists over when febrile seizures (Nelson and Ellenberg, 1981) and neonatal seizures (Freeman, 1983) need to be treated, if at all (Chapter 7).

Current consensus is against treatment of febrile seizures unless specific risk factors are present (Chapter 7). On the other hand, risk factors have not been well developed for neonatal seizures, apart from the underlying pathological process. The subtle character of some neonatal seizures combined with the absence of EEG correlates, as well as the presence of EEG discharges without behavioral seizures, makes it difficult even to know when epileptic seizures are occurring. Consequently, until epileptic phenomena can be better defined in the neonatal period and the risk factors for a poor prognosis resulting from recurrent seizures can be better identified, the consensus is to treat in most cases (Chapter 7). When treatment is instituted, however, it remains unclear whether the goal should be to abolish only behavioral manifestations or all ictal EEG events. The latter is often much more difficult to achieve.

SUMMARY AND CONCLUSIONS

The latent period between the occurrence of a cerebral insult and the appearance of chronic recurring epileptic seizures reflects the development of specific epileptogenic disturbances. Undoubtedly, several types of epileptogenesis exist. Mechanisms underlying these processes are under investigation, but the risk factors for acute early epileptic seizures are different from those for the development of later chronic epilepsy. Although prophylactic treatment with high levels of antiseizure drugs can prevent early seizures, clinical research has so far failed to demonstrate that prophylactic treatment retards epileptogenesis in patients.

Secondary epileptogenesis has been well documented in experimental animals, and there is evidence that similar phenomena occur in some forms of human epilepsy. Such secondary processes could increase the severity of ictal symptoms and perhaps contribute to the development of interictal behavioral disturbances. Progression of epilepsy, as well as ensuing nonepileptic cerebral dysfunction, in those epilepsy syndromes referred to as *epileptic encephalopathies*, is now believed to be due to recurrent seizures. Clinical observations suggest that early and aggressive medical or surgical treatment positively influences the outcome for patients with disabling focal and generalized tonic-clonic seizures. There is, as yet, little to no definitive evidence that recurrent absences, myoclonic seizures, or nondebilitating focal seizures associated with genetic epilepsy syndromes result in progressive dysfunction.

The immature brain is more susceptible than the mature brain to acute reactive seizures; however, it appears to have a decreased potential for the development of chronic epilepsy. The increased incidence of chronic epilepsy beginning in early childhood more likely reflects greater exposure to severe cerebral insult at this age than it does enhanced propensity for epileptogenesis. This supports the prevailing attitude against prophylactic treatment of benign febrile seizures and suggests that indications for aggressive or prolonged treatment of reactive neonatal seizures should be reevaluated, particularly because antiseizure medications may have adverse effects on cerebral development.

Research on epileptogenesis is receiving higher priority today than it has received in the past. Both experimental animal and clinical studies are necessary to determine (1) the mechanisms by which a structural cerebral lesion becomes epileptogenic, (2) the specific effects of repeated epileptic seizures on subsequent ictal manifestations, interictal cerebral function, and development, and (3) the risk factors for these adverse consequences. Results should provide better guidelines for determining prognosis for epilepsy following acute injury and for identifying potentially progressive epileptic phenomena that require prompt and aggressive treatment. Reliable biomarkers of epileptogenesis will greatly facilitate the search for antiepileptogenic interventions. Such biomarkers would permit better identification of populations at risk, establishment of valid end points for clinical trials, and development of cost-effective, high-throughput animal models for screening potential antiepileptogenic interventions.

REFERENCES

Adamec, R (1975). Behavioral and epileptic determinants of predatory attack behavior in the cat. Can J Neurol Sci 2:457–466.

Andermann, E (1982). Multifactorial inheritance of generalized and focal epilepsy. In Genetic Basis of the Epilepsies. Edited by VE Anderson, WA Hauser, JK Penry, and CF Sing. Raven Press: New York, pp. 355–374.

Babb, TL, Lieb, JP, Brown, WJ, Pretorius, J, and Crandall, PH (1984). Distribution of pyramidal cell density and hyperexcitability in the epileptic human hippocampal formation. Epilepsia 25:721–728.

Bancaud, J, and Chauvel, P (1987). Commentary: Acute and chronic intracranial recording and stimulation with depth electrodes. In Surgical Treatment of the Epilepsies. Edited by J Engel, Jr. New York: Raven Press, pp. 289–296.

Bancaud, J, Talairach, J, Morel, P, Bresson, M, Bonis, A, Geier, S, Hemon, E, and Buser, P. "Generalized" epileptic seizures elicited by electrical stimulation of the frontal lobe in man. Electroencephalogr Clin Neurophysiol 37 (1974).275–282.

Beghi, E, Carpio, A, Forsgren, L, Hesdorffer, DC, Malmgren, C, Sander, JW, Tomson, T, and Hauser, WA (2010). Recommendation for a definition of acute symptomatic seizure. Epilepsia 51:671–675.

Berg, AT, Langfitt, J, Shinnar, S, Vickrey, BG, Sperling, MR, Walczak, T, Bazil, C, Pacia, SV, and Spencer, SS (2003). How long does it take for partial epilepsy to become intractable? Neurology 60:186–190.

Blumenfeld, H, Klein, JP, Schridde, U, Vestal, M, Rice, T, Khera, DS, Bashyal, C, Giblin, K, Paul-Laughinghouse, C, Wang, F, Phadke, A, Mission, J, Agarwal, RK, Englot, DJ, Motelow, J, Nersesyan, H, Waxman, SG, and Levin, AR (2008). Early treatment suppresses the development of spike-wave epilepsy in a rat model. Epilepsia 49:400–409.

Blumenthal, IJ (1955). Spontaneous seizures and related electroencephalographic findings following shock therapy. J Nerv Ment Dis 122:581–588.

Burnham, WM, Lynchacz, B, Avila, J, Livingston, KE, and Racine, RJ (1980). Differential anticonvulsant response of cortex- and amygdala-kindled seizures. In Limbic Epilepsy and the Dyscontrol Syndrome. Edited by M Girgis and L Kiloh. New York: Elsevier, pp. 161–170.

Buser, P, and Bancaud, J (1983). Unilateral connections between amygdala and hippocampus in man: A study of epileptic patients with depth electrodes. Electroencephalogr Clin Neurophysiol 55:1–12.

Caveness, WF, and Liss, HR (1961). Incidence of post-traumatic epilepsy. Epilepsia 2:123–129.

Cendes, F (2005). Progressive hippocampal and extra-hippocampal atrophy in drug resistant epilepsy. Curr Opin Neurol 18:173–177.

Chang, BS, and Lowenstein, DH (2003). Practice parameter: Antiepileptic drug prophylaxis in severe traumatic brain injury. Neurology 60:10–16.

Cherlow, DG, Dymond, AM, Crandall, PH, Walter, RD, and Serafetinides, EA (1977). Evoked response and after-discharge thresholds to electrical stimulation in temporal lobe epileptics. Arch Neurol 34:527–531.

Chugani, HT, Shields, WD, Shewmon, DA, Olson, DM, Phelps, ME, and Peacock, WJ (1990). Infantile spasms: I. PET identifies focal cortical dysgenesis in cryptic cases for surgical treatment. Ann Neurol 27:406–413.

Corcoran, ME, and Moshé, SL (eds) (2005). Kindling 6. New York: Springer Science.

Crandall, PH (1987). Cortical resection. In Surgical Treatment of the Epilepsies. Edited by J Engel, Jr. New York: Raven Press, pp. 377–404.

Currie, S, Heathfield, WG, Henson, RA, and Scott, DF (1971). Clinical course and prognosis of temporal lobe epilepsy—A survey of 666 patients. Brain 94:173–190.

Devinsky, O, and Duchowny, MS (1983). Seizures after convulsive therapy: A retrospective case survey. Neurology 33:921–925.

Diaz, J, and Schain, RJ (1978). Phenobarbital: Effects of long-term administration on behavior and brain of artificially reared rats. Science 199:90–91.

Engel, J, Jr (1987a). Outcome with respect to epileptic seizures. In Surgical Treatment of the Epilepsies. Edited by J Engel, Jr. New York: Raven Pressa, pp. 553–572.

Engel, J, Jr (1987b). New concepts of the epileptic focus. In The Epileptic Focus. Edited by HG Weiser, E-J Speckmann, and J Engel, Jr. London: John Libbey, pp. 83–94.

Engel, J, Jr (1998). The syndrome of mesial temporal lobe epilepsy: A role for kindling. In Kindling 5. Edited by M Corcoran and S Moshé. New York: Plenum Press, pp. 469–480.

Engel, J, Jr (1999). The timing of surgical intervention for mesial temporal lobe epilepsy: A plan for a randomized clinical trial. Arch Neurol 56:1338–1341.

Engel, J, Jr (2001). A proposed diagnostic scheme for people with epileptic seizures and with epilepsy: Report of the ILAE Task Force on Classification and Terminology. Epilepsia 42:796–803.

Engel, J, Jr (2002). So what can we conclude—Do seizures damage the brain? Prog Brain Res 135:509–512.

Engel, J, Jr (2005). Natural history of mesial temporal lobe epilepsy with hippocampal sclerosis: How does kindling compare with other commonly used animal models? In Kindling 6. Edited by ME Corcoran and SL Moshé. New York: Springer Science, pp. 371–384.

Engel, J, Jr (2008). Surgical treatment for epilepsy: Too little too late? JAMA 300:2548–2550.

Engel, J, Jr (ed) (2011a). Biomarkers in epilepsy. Biomarkers Med 5:529–664.

Engel, J, Jr (2011b). Biomarkers in epilepsy—Introduction. Biomarkers Med 5:537–544.

Engel, J, Jr, and Cahan, L (1986). Potential relevance of kindling to human partial epilepsy. In Kindling 3. Edited by J Wada. New York: Raven Press, pp. 37–51.

Engel, J, Jr, and Crandall, PH (1983). Falsely localizing ictal onsets with depth EEG telemetry during anticonvulsant withdrawal. Epilepsia 24:344–355.

Engel, J, Jr, and Shewmon, DA (1991). Impact of the kindling phenomenon on clinical epileptology. In Kindling and Synaptic Plasticity: The Legacy of

Graham Goddard. Edited by F. Morrell. Cambridge, MA: Birkhäuser Boston, pp. 195–210.

Engel, J, Jr, and Wilson, CL: Evidence for enhanced synaptic inhibition in epilepsy. In Neurotransmitters, Seizures and Epilepsy III. Edited by G Nistico, PL Morselli, KG Lloyd, RG Fariello, and J Engel, Jr. New York (1986). Raven Press, pp. 1–13.

Engel, J, Jr, Driver, MV, and Falconer, MA (1975). Electrophysiological correlates of pathology and surgical results in temporal lobe epilepsy. Brain 98:129–156.

Engel, J, Jr, Wolfson, L, and Brown L (1978). Anatomical correlates of electrical and behavioral events related to amygdaloid kindling. Ann Neurol 3:538–544.

Engel, J, Jr, Rausch, R, Lieb, JP, Kuhl, DE, and Crandall, PH (1981). Correlation of criteria used for localizing epileptic foci in patients considered for surgical therapy of epilepsy. Ann Neurol 9:215–224.

Engel, J, Jr, Brown, WJ, Kuhl, DE, Phelps, ME, Mazziotta, JC, and Crandall, PH (1982a). Pathological findings underlying focal temporal lobe hypometabolism in partial epilepsy. Ann Neurol 12:518–528.

Engel, J, Jr, Kuhl, DE, Phelps, ME, and Crandall, PH (1982b). Comparative localization of epileptic foci in partial epilepsy by PCT and EEG. Ann Neurol 12:529–537.

Engel, J, Jr, Kuhl, DE, Phelps, ME, and Mazziotta, JC (1982c). Interictal cerebral glucose metabolism in partial epilepsy and its relation to EEG changes. Ann Neurol 12:510–517.

Engel, J, Jr, Kuhl, DE, and Phelps, ME (1982d). Patterns of human local cerebral glucose metabolism during epileptic seizures. Science 218:64–66.

Engel, J, Jr, Kuhl, DE, Phelps, ME, Rausch, R, and Nuwer, M (1983). Local cerebral metabolism during partial seizures. Neurology 33:400–413.

Engel, J, Jr, Caldecott-Hazard, S, and Bandler, R (1986). Neurobiology of behavior: Anatomic and physiologic implications related to epilepsy. Epilepsia 27(suppl 2): S3–S11.

Engel, J, Jr, Schwartzkroin, PA, Moshé, SL, and Lowenstein, DH (eds) (2001). Brain Plasticity and Epilepsy: A Tribute to Frank Morrell. San Diego: Academic Press.

Engel, J, Jr, Wilson, C, and Bragin, A. Advances in understanding the process of epileptogenesis based on patient material (2003). What can the patient tell us? Epilepsia 44(suppl 12):60–71.

Engel, J, Jr, Dichter, MA, and Schwartzkroin, PA (2008a). Basic mechanisms of human epilepsy. In Epilepsy: A Comprehensive Textbook, 2nd ed. Edited by J Engel, Jr, and TA Pedley. Philadelphia: Lippincott Williams & Wilkins, pp. 495–507.

Engel, J, Jr, Taylor, DC, and Trimble, MR (2008b). Neurobiology of behavioral disorders. In Epilepsy: A Comprehensive Textbook, 2nd ed. Edited by J Engel, Jr, and TA Pedley. Philadelphia: Lippincott Williams & Wilkins, pp. 2077–2083.

Falconer, MA, Driver, MV, and Serafetinides, EA (1962). Temporal lobe epilepsy due to distant lesions: Two cases relieved by operation. Brain 85:521–534.

Foy, PM, Copeland, GP, and Shaw, MD (1981). The natural history of postoperative seizures. Acta Neurochir (Wien) 57:15–22.

Foy, PM, Chadwick, DW, Rajgopalan, N, Johnson, AL, and Shaw, MD (1992). Do prophylactic anticonvulsant drugs alter the pattern of seizures after craniotomy? J Neurol Neurosurg Psychiatry 55:753–757.

Freeman, JM (1983). Neonatal seizures. In Pediatric Epileptology. Edited by FE Dreifuss. Boston: John Wright, pp. 159–172.

Frey, LC (2003). Epidemiology of posttraumatic epilepsy: A critical review. Epilepsia 44(suppl 10):11–17.

Galanopoulou, AS, and Moshé, SL (2009). Age-specific responses to antiepileptic drugs. In Encyclopedia of Basic Epilepsy Research. Edited by PA Schwartzkroin. Amsterdam: Elsevier, pp. 1025–1033.

Galanopoulou, AS, Buckmaster, P, Staley, K, Moshé, SL, Perucca, E, Engel, J, Jr, Löscher, W, Noebels, JL, Pitkänen, A, Stables, J, White, SH, O'Brien, TJ, and Simonato, M (2012). Identification of new epilepsy treatments: Issues in preclinical methodology. Epilepsia 53:571–582.

Gloor, P (1975). Contributions of electroencephalography and electro-corticography to the neurosurgical treatment of the epilepsies. Adv Neurol 8:59–105.

Goddard, GV (1983). The kindling model of epilepsy. Trends Neurosci 6:275–279.

Goddard, GV, McIntyre, DC, and Leech, CK (1969). A permanent change in brain function resulting from daily electrical stimulation. Exp Neurol 25:295–330.

Goldensohn, ES (1984). The relevance of secondary epileptogenesis to the treatment of epilepsy: Kindling and the mirror focus. Epilepsia 25 (suppl 2):S156–S173.

Goldstein, LB (1998). Potential effects of common drugs on stroke recovery. Arch Neurol 55:454–456.

Gomes, WA, and Shinnar, S (2011). Prospects for imaging-related biomarkers of human epileptogenesis: A critical review. Biomarkers Med 5, 599–606.

Gowers, WR (1881). Epilepsy and Other Chronic Convulsive Diseases. London: Churchill.

Griffith, N, Engel, J, Jr, and Bandler, R (1987). Ictal and enduring interictal disturbances in emotional behavior in an animal model of temporal lobe epilepsy. Brain Res 400:360–364.

Hauser, WA, and Kurland, LT (1975). The epidemiology of epilepsy in Rochester, Minnesota, 1935 through 1967. Epilepsia 16:1–66.

Haut, SR, Velisková, J, and Moshé, SL (2004). Relative vulnerability of immature and adult brain to seizures. Lancet Neurol 3:608–617.

Heinemann, U, Engel, J, Jr, Meldrum, BS, Wasterlain, C, Avanzini, G, Mouritzen-Dam, A (eds) (1996). The Progressive Nature of Epilepsy. Epilepsy Res(suppl 12). Amsterdam: Elsevier.

Hemb, M, Velasco, TR, Parnes, MS, Wu, JY, Lerner, JT, Matsumoto, JH, Yudovin, S, Shields, WD, Sankar, R, Salamon, N, Vinters, HV, and Mathern, GW (2010). Improved outcomes in pediatric epilepsy surgery: The UCLA experience, 1986–2008. Neurology 74:1768–1775,.

Hermann BP, Seidenberg M, Dow C, et al. (2006). Cognitive prognosis in chronic temporal lobe epilepsy. Ann Neurol 60(1):80–87.

Holmes, GL (1985). Neonatal seizures. In Recent Advances in Epilepsy 2. Edited by TA Pedley and BS Meldrum. New York: Churchill Livingstone, pp. 207–235.

Holmes, GL (1987). Diagnosis and Management of Seizures in Children. Philadelphia: WB Saunders.

Holmes, GL, Albala, BJ, and Moshé, SL (1984). Effect of a single brief seizure on subsequent seizure susceptibility in the immature rat. Arch Neurol 41:853–855.

Holowach, J, Thurston, DL, and O'Leary, J (1972). Prognosis in childhood epilepsy. N Engl J Med 286:169–174.

Holowach-Thurston, J, Thurston, DL, Hixon, BB, and Keller, A (1982). Prognosis in childhood epilepsy: Additional followup of 148 children 15 to 23 years after withdrawal of anticonvulsant therapy. N Engl J Med 306:831–836.

Hughes, JR (1985). Long-term clinical and EEG changes in patients with epilepsy. Arch Neurol 42:213–223.

Jabbari, B, Vengrow, MI, Salazar, AM, Harper, MG, Smutok, MA, and Amin, D (1986). Clinical and radiological correlates of EEG in the late phase of head injury: A study of 515 Vietnam veterans. Electroencephalogr Clin Neurophysiol 64:285–293.

Jacobs, MP, Fischbach, GD, Davis, MR, Dichter, MA, Dingledine, R, and Lowenstein, DH (2001). Future directions for epilepsy research. Neurology 57:1536–1542.

Janszky, J, Janszky, I, Schulz, R, et al. (2005). Temporal lobe epilepsy with hippocampal sclerosis: Predictors for long-term surgical outcome. Brain 128:395–404.

Jennett, B (1975). Epilepsy after Non-missile Head Injuries, 2nd ed. Chicago: William Heinemann.

Kanner, AM, and Blumer, D (2008). Affective disorders. In Epilepsy: A Comprehensive Textbook, 2nd ed. Edited by J Engel, Jr, and TA Pedley. Philadelphia: Lippincott Williams & Wilkins, pp. 2123–2138.

Kellaway, P (1980). The incidence, significance and natural history of spike foci in children. In Current Clinical Neurophysiology: Update on EEG and Evoked Potentials. Edited by C Henry. Amsterdam: Elsevier/North Holland, pp. 151–175.

Kellaway, P, and Mizrahi, EM (1987). Neonatal seizures. In Epilepsy: Electroclinical Syndromes. Edited by H Lüders and RP Lesser. London: Springer-Verlag, pp. 13–47.

Kelly, MS, Jacobs, MP, and Lowenstein, DH (2009). The NINDS epilepsy research benchmarks. Epilepsia 50:579–582.

Kumar, A, Asano, E, and Chugani, HT (2011). α-[^{11}C]-methyl-l-tryptophan PET for tracer localization of epileptogenic brain regions: Clinical studies. Biomarkers Med 5, 577–584.

Lesser, RP, Lüders, H, Dinner, DS, and Morris, HH (1985). Epileptic seizures due to thrombotic and embolic cerebrovascular disease in older patients. Epilepsia 26:622–630.

Lieb, JP, Engel, J, Jr, Gevins, AS, and Crandall, PH (1981). Surface and deep EEG correlates of surgical outcome in temporal lobe epilepsy. Epilepsia 22:51–538.

Lieb, JP, Engel, J, Jr, and Babb, TL (1986). Interhemispheric propagation time of human hippocampal seizures. I. Relationship to surgical outcome. Epilepsia 27:286–293.

Lindsay, J, Ounsted, C, and Richards, PL (1979a). Long-term outcome in children with temporal lobe seizures. I. Social outcome and childhood factors. Dev Med Child Neurol 21:285–298.

Lindsay, J, Ounsted, C, and Richards, P (1979b). Long-term outcome in children with temporal lobe seizures. II. Marriage, parenthood and sexual indifference. Dev Med Child Neurol 21:433–440.

Lindsay, J, Ounsted, C, and Richards, P (1979c). Long-term outcome in children with temporal lobe seizures. III. Psychiatric aspects in childhood and adult life. Dev Med Child Neurol 21:630–636.

Löscher, W, and Brandt, C (2010). Prevention or modification of epileptogenesis after brain insults: Experimental approaches and translational research. Pharmacol Rev 62:668–700.

Marson, A, Jacoby, A, Johnson, A, et al. (2005). Immediate versus deferred antiepileptic drug treatment for early epilepsy and single seizures: A randomized controlled trial. Lancet 365:2007–2013.

Mathern, GW (2010). Cerebral hemispherectomy: When half a brain is good enough. Neurology 75:1578–1580.

McIntyre DC (2006). The kindling phenomenon. In Models of Seizures and Epilepsy. Edited by A Pitkänen, PA Schwartzkroin, and SL Moshé. Burlington, MA: Elsevier Academic Press, pp. 351–353.

McLachlan, RS, Rose, KJ, Derry, PA, Bonnar, C, Blume, WT, and Girvin, JP (1997). Health-related quality of life and seizure control in temporal lobe epilepsy. Ann Neurol 41:482–489.

Mizrahi, EM, and Kellaway, P (1987). Characterization and classification of neonatal seizures. Neurology 37:1837–1844.

Mizrahi, EM, Plouin, P, and Clancy, RR (2008). Neonatal seizures. In Epilepsy: A Comprehensive Textbook, 2nd ed. Edited by J Engel, Jr, and TA Pedley. Philadelphia: Lippincott Williams & Wilkins, pp. 639–658.

Monroe, RR (1970). Episodic Behavioral Disorders: A Psychodynamic and Neurophysiologic Analysis. Cambridge, MA: Harvard University Press.

Morimoto, K, Fahnestock, M, and Racine, RJ (2004). Kindling and status epilepticus models of epilepsy: Rewiring the brain. Prog Neurol 73:1–60.

Morrell, F (1959/1960). Secondary epileptogenic lesions. Epilepsia 1:538–560.

Morrell, F (1985). Secondary epileptogenesis in man. Arch Neurol 42:318–335.

Morrell, F, and Baker, L (1961). Effects of drugs on secondary epileptogenic lesions. Neurology 11:651–664.

Morrell, F, Wada, JA, and Engel, J, Jr (1987). Potential relevance of kindling and secondary epileptogenesis to the consideration of surgical treatment for epilepsy. In Surgical Treatment of the Epilepsies. Edited by J Engel, Jr. New York: Raven Press, pp. 699–705.

Moshé, SL, and Albala, BJ (1982). Kindling in developing rats: Persistence of seizures into adulthood. Brain Res 256:67–71.

Munari, C, Kahane, P, Francione, S, Hoffman, D, Tassi, L, Cusmai, R, Vigevano, F, Pasquier, B, and Betti, OO (1995). Role of the hypothalamic hamartoma in the genesis of gelastic fits (a video-stereo-EEG study). Electroencephalogr Clin Neurophysiol 95:154–160.

Musicco, M, Beghi, E, Solari, A, and Viani, F (1997). Treatment of first tonic-clonic seizure does not improve the prognosis of epilepsy. First Seizure Trial Group (FIRST Group). Neurology 49:991–998.

Naoi, T (1959). EEG assessment of electroconvulsive treatment. Psychiat Neurol Jpn (Seishin Shinkeigaku) 61:871–881. (In Japanese)

Nelson, KB, and Ellenberg, JH (eds) (1981). Febrile Seizures. New York: Raven Press.

North, JB, Penhall, RK, Hanieh, A, Frewin, DB, and Taylor, WB (1983). Phenytoin and postoperative epilepsy. J Neurosurg 58:672–677.

Okada, R, Moshé, SL, and Albala, BJ (1984). Infantile status epilepticus and future seizure susceptibility in the rat. Dev Brain Res 15:177–183.

Okuma, T, and Kumashiro, H (1981). Natural history and prognosis of epilepsy: Report of a multi-institutional study in Japan. Epilepsia 22:35–53.

Ounsted, C, Lindsay, L, and Norman, R (1966). Biological Factors in Temporal lobe Epilepsy (Clinics in Developmental Medicine, No 22). London: Spastics Society of Medical Education and Information Unit in association with William Heinemann Medical Books.

Oyegbile, TO, Bayless, K, Dabbs, K, Jones, J, Rutecki, P, Pierson, R, Seidenberg, M, and Hermann, B (2011). The nature and extent of cerebellar atrophy in chronic temporal lobe epilepsy. Epilepsia 52:698–706.

Penfield, W, and Jasper, H (1954). Epilepsy and the Functional Anatomy of the Human Brain. Boston: Little, Brown & Co.

Pinel, JPJ, and Rovner, LI (1978). Experimental epileptogenesis: Kindling-induced epilepsy in rats. Exp Neurol 58:190–202.

Pitkänen, A (2010). Therapeutic approaches to epileptogenesis—Hope on the horizon. Epilepsia 51(suppl 3): 2–17.

Pitkänen, A, Kharatishvili, I, Nissinen, J, and McIntosh, TK (2006). Posttraumatic epilepsy induced by lateral fluid-percussion brain injury in rats. In Models of Seizures and Epilepsy. Edited by A Pitkänen, PA Schwartzkroin, and SL Moshé. Burlington, MA: Elsevier Academic Press, pp. 465–476.

Racine, RJ (1972a). Modification of seizure activity by electrical stimulation: I. Afterdischarge threshold. Electroencephalogr Clin Neurophysiol 32:269–279.

Racine, RJ (1972b). Modification of seizure activity by electrical stimulation. II. Motor seizure. Electroencephalogr Clin Neurophysiol 32:281–294.

Racine, R, Newberry, F, and Burnham, WM (1975). Post-activation potentiation and the kindling phenomenon. Electroencephalogr Clin Neurophysiol 39:261–271.

Racine, RJ, Steingart, M, and McIntyre, DC (1999). Development of kindling-prone and kindling-resistant rat: Selective breeding and electrophysiological studies. Epilepsy Res 35:183–195.

Rakhade, SN, and Jensen, FE (2009). Epileptogenesis in the immature brain: Emerging mechanisms. Nat Rev Neurol 5:380–391.

Rapport, RL, II, and Ojemann, GA (1975). Prophylactically administered phenytoin: Effects on the development of chronic cobalt induced epilepsy in the cat. Arch Neurol 32:539–548.

Raymont, V, Salazar, AM, Lipsky, R, Goldman, D, Tasick, G, and Grafman, J (2010). Correlates of posttraumatic epilepsy 35 years following combat brain surgery. Neurology 75:224–229.

Rodin, EA (1968). The Prognosis of Patients with Epilepsy. Springfield, IL: Charles C Thomas.

Rose, AL, and Lombroso, CT (1970). Neonatal seizure states: A study of clinical, pathological and electroencephalographic features in 137 full-term babies with a long-term follow-up. Pediatrics 45:404–425.

Russell, WR, and Whitty, CWM (1952). Studies in traumatic epilepsy. I. Factors influencing the incidence of epilepsy after brain wounds. J Neurol Neurosurg Psychiatry 15:93–98.

Salazar, AM, Jabbari, B, Vance, SC, Grafman, J, Amin, D, and Dillon, JD (1985). Epilepsy after penetrating head injury. I. Clinical correlates: A report of the Vietnam head injury study. Neurology 35:1406–1414.

Scantlebury, MH, Heida, JG, Hasson, HJ, Velisková, J, Velísek, L, Galanopoulou, AS, and Moshé, SL (2007). Age dependent consequences of status epilepticus: Animal models. Epilepsia 48:75–82.

Schauwecker, PE (2002). Complications associated with genetic background effects in models of experimental epilepsy. Prog Brain Res 135:139–148.

Schmidt, D, Tsai, JJ, and Janz, D (1983). Generalized tonic-clonic seizures in patients with complex partial seizures: Natural history and prognostic relevance. Epilepsia 24:43–48.

Seki, K, and Wada, JA (1986). Kindling of cortical association area 5 in the cat. In Kindling 3. Edited by JA Wada. New York: Raven Press, pp. 429–446.

Shaw, MD, and Foy, PM (1991). Epilepsy after craniotomy and the place of prophylactic anticonvulsant drugs: Discussant paper. J R Soc Med 84:221–223.

Shewmon, DA, and Erwin, RJ (1988). Focal spike-induced cerebral dysfunction is related to the after-coming slow wave. Ann Neurol 23:131–137.

Shorvon, SD, and Reynolds, EH (1982). Early prognosis of epilepsy. Br Med J 285:1699–1701.

Small, J, Milstein, V, Small, IF, and Sharpley, PH (1981). Does ECT produce kindling? Biol Psychiatry 16:773–778.

Soper, HV, Strain, GM, Babb, TL, Lieb, JP, and Crandall, PH (1978). Chronic alumina temporal lobe seizures in monkeys. Exp Neurol 62:99–121.

Sramka, M, Sedlack, P, and Nadvornik, P (1977). Observation of the kindling phenomenon in treatment of pain by stimulation in the thalamus. In Neurosurgical Treatment in Psychiatry, Pain and Epilepsy. Edited by WH Sweet, S Obrador, and JG Martin-Rodriguez. Baltimore: University Park Press, pp. 651–654.

Stillerman, ML, Gibbs, EL, and Perlstein, MA (1952). Electroencephalographic changes in strabismus. Am J Ophthalmol 35:54–63.

Sutula, T, and Pitkänen, A (eds). Do seizures damage the brain? Prog Brain Res 135. Amsterdam (2002). Elsevier.

Temkin, NR (2003). Risk factors for posttraumatic seizures in adults. Epilepsia 44(suppl 10):18–20.

Temkin NR (2009). Preventing and treating posttraumatic seizures: The human experience. Epilepsia 50 (suppl 2): 10–13.

Temkin, NR, Dikmen, SS, Wilensky, AJ, Keihm, J, Chabal, S, and Winn, HR (1990). A randomized double-blind study of phenytoin for the prevention of post-traumatic seizures. N Engl J Med 323:497–502.

Tharp B (1980). Neonatal and pediatric electroencephalography. In Electrodiagnosis in Clinical Neurology. Edited by MJ Aminoff. New York: Churchill Livingstone, pp. 67–117.

Todt, H (1984). The late prognosis of epilepsy in childhood: Results of a prospective follow-up study. Epilepsia 25:137–144.

Trojaborg, W (1966). Focal spike discharges in children, a longitudinal study. Acta Paediatr Scand Suppl 168:1–113.

Tuff, LP, Racine, RJ, and Adamec, R (1983). The effects of kindling on GABA-mediated inhibition in the dentate gyrus of the rat. I. Paired-pulse depression. Brain Res 277:79–90.

Volpe, JJ (1987). Neurology of the Newborn, 2nd ed. Philadelphia: WB Saunders.

Wada, JA (ed) (1976). Kindling. New York: Raven Press.

Wada, JA (1980). Amygdaloid and frontal cortical kindling in subhuman primates. In Limbic Epilepsy and the Dyscontrol Syndrome. Edited by M Girgis and LG Kiloh. Amsterdam: Elsevier, pp. 133–147.

Wada, JA (ed) (1981). Kindling 2. New York: Raven Press.

Wada, JA (ed) (1986). Kindling 3. New York: Raven Press.

Wada, JA, and Osawa, T (1976). Spontaneous recurrent seizure state induced by daily electrical amygdaloid stimulation in Senegalese baboons, Papio papio. Neurology 26:273–286.

Wada, JA, Sato, M, Wake, A, Green, JR, and Troupin, AS (1976). Prophylactic effects of phenytoin, phenobarbital, and carbamazepine examined in kindling cat preparations. Arch Neurol 33:426–434.

Wada, JA, Mizoguchi, T, and Osawa, T (1978). Secondarily generalized convulsive seizures induced by daily amygdaloid stimulation in rhesus monkeys. Neurology 28:1026–1036.

Ward, AA, Jr (1972). Topical convulsant metals. In Experimental Models of Epilepsy—A Manual for the Laboratory Worker. Edited by DP Purpura, JK Penry, DB Tower, and RD Walter. New York: Raven Press, pp. 13–35.

Wasterlain, CG, Fando, JM, and Subhas, BS (1980). Epilepsy and brain development. In Neurochemistry and Clinical Neurology. Edited by L Battistin, G Hakim, and A Lajtha. New York: Alan R Liss, pp. 101–122.

Watanabe, K, Kuroyanagi, M, Hara, K, and Miyazaki, S (1982). Neonatal seizures and subsequent epilepsy. Brain Dev 4:341–346.

Weiss, SRB, and Post, RM (1991). Development and reversal of contingent inefficacy and tolerance to the anticonvulsant effects of carbamazepine. Epilepsia 32:140–145.

Wieser, HG (1983). Electroclinical Features of the Psychomotor Seizure: A Stereoelectroencephalographic Study of Ictal Symptoms and Chronotopographical Seizure Patterns Including Clinical Effects of Intracerebral Stimulation. London: Butterworths.

Willmore, LS, Sypert, GW, and Munson, JB (1978). Recurrent seizures induced by cortical iron injection: A model of post-traumatic epilepsy. Ann Neurol 4:329–336.

Wilson, CL, Isokawa-Akesson, M, Babb, TL, Engel, J, Jr, Cahan, LD, and Crandall, PH (1987). A comparative view of local and interhemispheric limbic pathways in humans: An evoked potential analysis. In Fundamental Mechanisms of Human Brain Function. Edited by J Engel, Jr, GA Ojemann, HO Lüders, and PD Williamson. New York: Raven Press, pp. 27–38.

Worrell, G, and Gotman, J (2011). High-frequency oscillations and other electrophysiological biomarkers of epilepsy: Clinical studies. Biomarkers Med 5:557–566.

Young, B, Rapp, RP, Norton, JA, Haack, D, Tibbs, PA, and Bean, JR (1983). Failure of prophylactically administered phenytoin to prevent early post-traumatic seizures. J Neurosurg 58:236–241.

Zeng, LH, Xu, L, Gutmann, DH, and Wong, M (2008). Rapamycin prevents epilepsy in a mouse model of tuberous sclerosis complex. Ann Neurol 63:444–453.

Chapter 9

Periictal Phenomena

ICTAL INITIATION
Mechanisms
Clinical Considerations
POSTICTAL SYMPTOMS
Mechanisms
Clinical Considerations

MORTALITY
Comorbidity
Sudden Unexpected Death
Drowning
SUMMARY AND CONCLUSIONS

Traditionally, the epileptic seizure has been the major focus of interest for diagnosis, treatment, and research in the field of epilepsy. Much useful information can be gained, however, from studying events that precede and follow the ictus as well as physiological consequences of epileptic seizures that may not always be readily apparent to patients or their physicians. This chapter is concerned with factors that precipitate epileptic seizures and might be manipulated or avoided, aspects of postictal symptoms that contribute greatly to disability in many patients, and consequences of ictal events, some of which are potentially life-threatening.

ICTAL INITIATION

The characteristic feature of epilepsy is the spontaneous occurrence of epileptic seizures, often without warning and for no apparent reason. Although the events that determine when a seizure will begin may not be readily appreciated, fluctuations in internal milieu and external environment continually influence epileptic excitability. Knowledge of the mechanisms that generate seizures makes it possible to understand how some specific and nonspecific factors affect patterns of their occurrence. This information may then be useful for patient management. Failure to understand

320

precipitating factors in individual patients is perhaps the single greatest cause of disability associated with epilepsy.

Mechanisms

Two physiological factors primarily influence the transition from the interictal to ictal state: neuronal *synchronization* and neuronal *excitability* (Chapters 3 and 4).

Conditions that enhance *synchronization* increase the opportunity for an ictal event to occur (Chapters 3 and 4). In some situations the effective synchronizing input may be extremely specific. For example, flickering light within a certain frequency range can precipitate photosensitive seizures (Newmark and Penry, 1979; Zifkin et al., 1998; 2008). Visual evoked potentials at these frequencies may be altered in photosensitive patients (Broughton et al., 1969; Faught and Lee, 1984), which suggests that the seizure results from increased sensitivity of occipital cortex to appropriately spaced visual stimuli. Mechanisms may be more complicated, however. In some disorders the proprioceptive feedback that results from photic-induced myoclonic responses may provoke the epileptic seizure. This mechanism has been demonstrated in the photosensitive baboon *Papio papio*, where photic-induced eye blinking appears to trigger epileptiform discharges in motor cortex that can be abolished by muscle paralysis (Naquet and Meldrum, 1972). Intermittent light at the red end of the spectrum has been reported to be more potent than other colors (Takahashi, 1987). This effect appears to be due to enhanced sensitivity to monochromatic light (Binnie et al., 1984), because red, green, and blue cones mutually inhibit each other when stimulated simultaneously. White and other mixed-spectra light are, therefore, less effective than monochromatic light at inducing photosensitive responses. Red light in the environment is more likely to be monochromatic than green or blue.

Other highly synchronizing influences that induce epileptic seizures in susceptible individuals may be less specific. For instance, in patients with *startle epilepsy* (Alajouanine and Gastaut, 1955; Zifkin et al., 1998; 2008), seizures can be precipitated by any sudden, unexpected stimulus, such as a loud noise or pinprick. The neuronal mechanisms of normal startle behavior have been studied in detail (Eaton, 1984), but how these events precipitate an epileptogenic process remains unknown. Proprioceptive input from the startle movement may be the actual epileptogenic stimulus (Bancaud et al., 1975). Synchronization may also be enhanced by intrinsic influences, as occur, for instance, during slow-wave sleep and drowsiness. Not only do these states precipitate certain epileptic phenomena, but epileptic seizures can induce sleep disturbances that in turn can exacerbate the epileptic condition (Sterman et al., 1982; Shouse and Quigg, 2008; Shouse et al., 2008). These potentially important, complicated interactions are poorly understood.

Chaos theory, the physical-mathematical theory of nonlinear dynamics, has recently been applied to computerized analysis of EEGs preceding epileptic seizures in patients (Lehnertz et al., 2008). This technology is intended to identify EEG changes that predict seizure occurrence, which would have important implications for developing feedback methods for seizure prevention. The results of these studies, however, seem contradictory to current theories of hypersynchronous hippocampal ictogenesis (Chapter 4): there is an increase in chaos, indicating desynchronization, prior to seizure onset. One way to reconcile this observation would be to assume that the technology is identifying widespread natural homeostatic protective mechanisms engaged to counteract the onset of a focal hypersynchronous discharge (Bragin and Engel, 2008). Recent basic research, however, indicates a reduction in neuronal firing rate at the onset of some animal and human seizures (Gnatkovsky et al., 2008; DeCurtis and Gnatkovsky, 2009; Truccolo et al., 2010), suggesting synchronization through inhibition as a mechanism of ictogenesis (Chapter 4).

Endogenous and exogenous factors that modulate neuronal *excitability* also influence the timing of seizure occurrence (Chapter 3). Normal and pathological biorhythms as well as other endogenous processes, such as metabolic imbalance or fever, affect the probability of seizure generation. Environmental factors that enhance epileptic excitability include emotional excitation, sleep deprivation, psychological stress, the use of stimulant or proconvulsant drugs, and withdrawal from sedative and hypnotic substances such as alcohol (Chapter 5).

Clinical Considerations

REFLEX SEIZURES

Precipitating factors determine when epileptic seizures occur (Chapter 5), but it is often impossible to determine why a seizure occurs at a particular time. In some patients, however, the precipitating factors may be not only apparent but strikingly consistent, in which case avoidance, when possible, becomes the most effective treatment. Ictal events, when precipitated by specific environmental stimuli or behaviors, are referred to as *reflex seizures*. Reflex seizures can occur in the context of established epilepsy conditions, in which case spontaneous seizures also occur, but when only reflex seizures occur, the condition is known as a *reflex epilepsy* (Zifkin et al., 1998; 2008; Wolf et al., 2004). Reflex epilepsies that are recognized as syndromes (Chapter 7) are listed in Table 9–1, and common reflex stimuli are listed in Table 9–2.

Reflex seizures and epilepsies can occur in the context of a genetic epilepsy syndrome, most commonly *juvenile myoclonic epilepsy (JME)*, or as a result of a focal or diffuse cerebral lesion. In genetic syndromes, there appear to be regional differences in epileptogenicity, resulting in the susceptibility of specific brain areas to certain environmental stimuli. Although the resultant ictal events are usually generalized tonic-clonic seizures, there may be initial focal signs or symptoms related to the susceptible area. The various photic-induced epilepsies, reading epilepsy, seizures induced by thinking and praxis, and head tapping are examples of these genetic conditions. Musicogenic and startle epilepsy, as well as seizures induced by eating, proprioception, somatosensory stimuli, and hot water, are examples of conditions associated with localized lesions of the brain, and the resultant focal ictal events

Table 9–1 Reflex Epilepsy Syndromes

Genetic cause
Idiopathic photosensitive occipital lobe epilepsy
Other visual-sensitive epilepsies
Reading epilepsy
Structural lesions
Startle epilepsy
Musicogenic epilepsy
Hot water epilepsy

Table 9–2 Reflex Seizure Stimuli

Visual stimuli
  Flickering light
  Patterns
Reading
Thinking
Praxis
Startle
Music
Eating
Proprioceptive
Somatosensory
Hot water

reflect the functions of those areas (Zifkin et al., 2008).

GENETIC REFLEX EPILEPSIES

The most potent epileptogenic sensory stimulus is *photic stimulation* (Newmark and Penry, 1979; Zifkin et al., 2008). It is estimated that 3% of all persons with epilepsy are susceptible to visually induced seizures (Jeavons and Harding, 1975). *Intermittent-light photosensitivity* is the characteristic feature of *idiopathic photosensitive occipital lobe epilepsy*, and is particularly common in JME and *Dravet syndrome*, but it can also be seen in the myoclonic syndromes of *progressive myoclonus epilepsy* and, rarely, with occipital lesions (Chapter 7). A number of environmental stimuli commonly cause these photosensitive epileptic seizures. These include (1) sunlight passing through trees or other regularly spaced objects as seen from a moving vehicle, (2) stroboscopic illumination, (3) flickering of the television set, which has its greatest effect when the patient is close to the screen and the image is out of focus (*television epilepsy*), and (4) video games (Daneshmend and Campbell, 1982; Rushton, 1981).

Forty percent of patients with photosensitive seizures have seizures only with photic stimulation (Zifkin et al., 2008). This condition is likely much more common than previously suspected, as evidenced by the *Pocket Monsters (Pokémon)* incident in Japan in 1997, when 685 Japanese children and a few adults were hospitalized for seizures induced by prolonged flashing red and blue lights shown in an episode of a popular animated television program for children (Ishida et al., 1998).

Intermittent-light photosensitivity is highest in school-age children who spend a considerable amount of time watching television and playing computer games. Consequently, communications and trade commissions that regulate television programming and video games have established guidelines for avoiding frequencies and colors of images that would provoke photosensitive epileptic seizures.

This type of photosensitivity can be easily demonstrated in the EEG laboratory with intermittent-light stimulation. The most effective frequency is 15–20 Hz, although the frequency can vary considerably from patient to patient. Flickering light through a pattern can be more effective than diffuse light for some patients (Jeavons and Harding, 1975), but not for all (Engel, 1974). Red light is the most epileptogenic, and a better response with eyes closed than open has been attributed to red light passing through the eyelids (Takahashi, 1987). Photic stimulation is not epileptogenic when presented monocularly.

Photosensitive seizures that are environmentally induced are most often generalized tonic-clonic seizures, whereas in the EEG laboratory they are absences or myoclonic jerks. Because exposure to effective visual stimulation in the environment is relatively rare, it may be that only patients who experience generalized tonic-clonic seizures are likely to come to the attention of physicians, whereas in the EEG laboratory photic stimulation is routinely discontinued before a generalized tonic-clonic seizure occurs. Although the epileptic manifestation of intermittent-light photosensitivity is almost always generalized, occasionally focal visual symptoms such as blurring, elementary hallucinations, and even blindness, as well as limbic and versive features, headache, nausea, and vomiting, can occur as the initial or only ictal symptom.

The EEG pattern associated with intermittent-light photosensitivity is referred to as a *photoparoxysmal (photoconvulsive)* response. It consists of a diffuse spike-and-wave discharge that is not time-locked to the frequency of the photic stimulation and that usually persists after the stimulus is discontinued (Takahashi, 1987). Some investigators maintain that photoparoxysmal responses that are self-limited and do not outlast the stimulus are much less likely to indicate an epileptic condition than are those of longer duration (Reilly and Peters, 1973). A brief photoparoxysmal EEG event usually has no clinical correlate. This pathological response must be distinguished from the *photomyogenic (photomyoclonic) response* (Bickford et al., 1952) and other nonepileptic time-locked photic-induced EEG patterns (see Figs. 3–17 to 3–19).

An EEG photoparoxysmal response occurs in 20–50% of close relatives of patients with photosensitive epilepsy (Newmark and Penry, 1979), many of whom have no history of epileptic seizures. The expression of this hereditary trait (Chapter 5) depends on age and sex; it is found more frequently in females and manifests most often in childhood (Pedley, 2008) (Fig. 9–1). Although photosensitivity is common in certain genetic epilepsies, such as JME, the gene for the photosensitive trait is different from those responsible for the epilepsy (Zifkin et al., 2008).

Variations of photosensitive epilepsy include seizures on eye closure, seizures on viewing

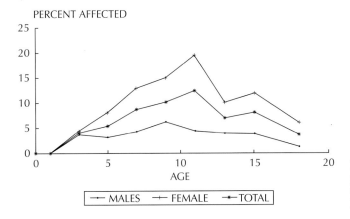

Figure 9–1. Prevalence of photoparoxysmal responses in normal children. (From Pedley, 2008, with permission.)

specific visual patterns, and *self-induced seizures*. Seizures on eye closure may represent a response to eye movement, because the effect can also occur in the dark (Gastaut and Tassinari, 1966) and is often seen in *eyelid myoclonia*, where the resultant ictus is an absence. There is considerable overlap between intermittent-light photosensitivity and *visual pattern sensitivity* (Newmark and Penry, 1979; Zifkin et al., 2008). Effective stimuli for the latter have spatial frequencies that appear to impose synchronizing influences and typically include striped patterns (as seen on picket fences or imprinted on clothing) and checkered patterns (as occur on screen doors or tablecloths). Self-induced seizures are most commonly caused by waving a hand with open fingers in front of a light source, blinking, or staring at a television set. The view that self-induction is an involuntary part of the seizure itself and not intentional (Ames, 1974) has been disproven (Zifkin et al., 2008). Seizures on eye closure, visual pattern sensitivity, and self-induced seizures are characterized most commonly by generalized tonic-clonic behaviors that occur spontaneously as well as with appropriate stimulation. All three conditions demonstrate age, sex, and inheritance patterns similar to those of intermittent-light photosensitivity.

These photosensitive seizures can be prevented by avoiding precipitating stimuli or, if this is not possible, patching one eye. In patients who appear to be particularly sensitive to monochromatic (red) intermittent light, blue-colored glasses may be of benefit. Self-induction can sometimes be treated by avoidance conditioning (Forster, 1977).

Reading epilepsy is a recognized genetic syndrome and also is seen with JME. In this condition, reading elicits jerking movements or clicking of the jaw, which can then lead to a generalized tonic-clonic seizure (Zifkin et al., 2008; Wolf et al., 2004) (Chapter 7). The initial symptoms can be mistaken for simple tics or stuttering when the generalized tonic-clonic seizures do not occur. Approximately one-third of the patients show bilaterally synchronous EEG spike-and-wave discharges, one-third show asymmetrical discharges, and one-third show unilateral discharges; however, there are no associated lesions on MRI. In related conditions, seizures are precipitated by thinking and praxis, which also can sometimes occur

with JME (Zifkin et al., 2008). Doing arithmetic, solving puzzles, making decisions, drawing, and other cognitive functions cause bilateral myoclonic jerks, which can evolve to generalized tonic-clonic seizures. Praxis is defined as physical activity involving spatial and sequential decisions, such as writing, and causes the same bilateral myoclonic jerks and generalized tonic-clonic seizures seen with reading and thinking sensitivity.

Tapping the head in infants and small children ages 6 months to 3 years can produce blinking, bilateral myoclonic jerks, and falling (Zifkin et al., 2008). These are unassociated with structural lesions, should not be confused with startle epilepsy (see below), and are believed to be related to the genetic epilepsies.

REFLEX EPILEPSIES DUE TO STRUCTURAL LESIONS

Epileptic seizures *in startle epilepsy* (Alajouanine and Gastaut, 1955) can be provoked by any sudden unexpected somatosensory, visual, or auditory stimulus that gives rise to a startle response (Andermann and Andermann, 1986). The epileptic seizure follows the initial startle, which may be unusually marked. This type of epilepsy usually occurs in patients with severe unilateral or diffuse brain damage, usually involving frontal and perisylvian regions (Zifkin et al., 2008). In patients with unilateral lesions, the epileptic startle seizure consists of tonic posturing of the contralateral limbs, similar to *supplementary motor area seizures* (Chapter 6), whereas generalized tonic-clonic seizures occur with bilateral cerebral involvement. Usually paroxysmal EEG discharges distinguish this syndrome from *startle disease (hyperekplexia)* (Kirstein and Silfveskiold, 1958), which is an inherited nonepileptic disorder in otherwise normal individuals (Chapter 13). When hyperekplexia and startle epilepsy are present in the same patient, *clonazepam, valproic acid*, and sometimes *carbamazepine* may be effective in controlling the epileptic seizure, but not necessarily the exaggerated startle (Saenz-Lope et al., 1984).

Musicogenic epilepsy is recognized as an epilepsy syndrome in which specific forms of music initiate focal and secondarily generalized seizures (Zifkin et al., 2008) (Chapter 7). This condition is caused by lesions of the temporal lobe, more often in the right hemisphere, and patients may also experience spontaneous seizures (see Fig. 12–22). The ictal events have limbic semiology appropriate to the location of the structural lesion. Patients with pharmacoresistant seizures can often be treated surgically.

Seizures with lesional epilepsies can also rarely be provoked by eating, proprioception, and somatosensory stimuli (Zifkin et al., 2008). Eating-induced seizures are easily provoked by chewing and swallowing food, but in some patients even the sight or smell of food can be effective. The ictal events consist of clonus or paralysis of the muscles of swallowing. These are most often associated with relatively large lesions involving limbic and suprasylvian areas, but there have been reports of eating-induced seizures in nonlesional genetic epilepsies. Eating-induced seizures rarely occur in infants, but when they do they can be life threatening. Proprioceptive seizures induced by movement are most common in *nonketogenic hyperglycemia* and are associated with lesions in the sensorimotor cortex. Proprioceptive seizures induced by gait typically cause drop attacks. Writing causes chronic jerking of the writing hand. Seizures induced by sensorimotor stimulation usually begin with a sensory aura, which can have Jacksonian features, followed by tonic supplementary motor area ictal events, occasionally associated with pain and autonomic features. Sensorimotor seizures may be self-induced in children with developmental delay. Seizures provoked by emotional thoughts or emotional stimuli have been referred to as *psychogenic epileptic seizures*, not to be confused with *psychogenic nonepileptic seizures* (Chapter 13).

Hot water epilepsy is now recognized as a syndrome (Chapter 7). It was originally described in southern India, where bathing involves the repeated pouring of hot water over the head (Satishchandra, 2003). Seizures are typically seen in infants and small children and have a limbic semiology. The reflex seizures usually remit spontaneously; however, children may later develop temporal lobe epilepsy. Although the etiology is unknown, it is not believed to be a genetic condition. A different form of hot water epilepsy has been reported in non-Indian children, usually beginning in infancy and triggered by immersion in hot bathwater (Ioos et al., 2000); that is, the hot water is on the bottom, not the top. This is a benign condition treated by lowering the temperature of the bathwater and does not indicate a structural or metabolic abnormality.

SIMPLE VERSUS COMPLEX REFLEX EPILEPSIES

Forster (1977) has classified the reflex epilepsies and seizures into *simple* and *complex* types (Table 9–3). This classification does not correspond directly with the division of reflex epilepsies and seizures into those associated with

Table 9–3 Simple and Complex Reflex Epilepsies

	Simple Type	Complex Type
Visually induced	Photosensitivity Pattern-evoked Eye closure–induced	Color-induced
Auditory evoked	Evoked by nonspecific startling sounds	Specific but nonverbal sounds without startle Specific voices
Movement-induced	Evoked by startling passive movement	Evoked by active movement or concept of movement
Communications/reading Decision making	Due to eye movement or patterns	Due to acquisition of knowledge Sequential decision-making under stress
Somatosensory evoked	Evoked by startling tap stimulation	Evoked by prolonged nonstartle stimulation
Eating	Myoclonic attacks with swallowing	With eating, but obscure evoking stimulus

From Forster, 1977, with permission.

lesions and those associated with nonlesional genetic epilepsies, but rather identifies components of the different types of stimuli that provoke either simple or complex ictal semiology.

The *simple reflex epilepsies* are typified by *photosensitive epilepsy*, when seizures occur only with effective stimulation. They include, predominantly, the hereditary generalized disorders. Simple stimuli evoke generalized seizures and generalized EEG discharges within seconds of presentation. Patients usually demonstrate sensitivity limited to specific stimulus features. Synchronizing ability and intensity are of paramount importance. Effective stimuli may be repetitive, as with a flickering light or pattern, or may involve sudden presentation of any modality, including movement. Unilateral stimulation and stimulation during sleep are not effective.

The *complex reflex epilepsies* appear to reflect an entirely different mechanism of action. They often require a certain degree of cognitive or emotional appreciation of the stimulus but, curiously, can sometimes be induced during sleep. Complex reflex seizures are usually focal, with focal epileptiform EEG discharges localized over cerebral areas appropriate to the provoking stimulation. The intensity of the stimulus is not important, but other features may be specifically effective: for example, only one particular piece of music may induce a seizure. The effective stimulation must be presented for a certain period before a seizure develops. Once a complex reflex seizure occurs, there is a prolonged refractory period, during which a second presentation of the same stimulus is ineffective.

Simple reflex seizures can often be controlled by *clobazam*, valproic acid, and the new broad-spectrum drugs, whereas the complex reflex seizures are more effectively treated by carbamazepine and *phenytoin*. Behavioral therapy can also be effective in some patients (Forster, 1977) (Chapter 16).

REFLEX MYOCLONUS

Reflex myoclonus is most often precipitated by proprioceptive input caused by movement (*action* or *intention myoclonus*). Action myoclonus is classically seen with the *progressive myoclonus epilepsies* and *posthypoxic myoclonus* (Chapter 7). The multifocal jerks of action myoclonus can usually be distinguished

from action-induced epileptic seizures by the more pronounced motor signs and paroxysmal EEG discharges of the latter. Other movement-induced conditions, such as *paroxysmal kinesigenic choreoathetosis* and *paroxysmal dystonia*, have distinguishing clinical characteristics (Chapter 13) and no EEG correlates. Nonspecific or specific startling stimuli may also precipitate myoclonus, as in the *acoustic startle* jerks seen with *Tay-Sachs disease* and other lipidoses (Chapter 7). Startle-induced myoclonus lacks the ictal EEG changes seen with startle epilepsy.

ABORTIVE STIMULI

Sensory stimuli can be used to abort seizures in certain circumstances. In ancient times, progression of a focal motor or sensory seizure beginning in one hand was prevented by plunging the arm into cold water or tying a ligature around the arm to disrupt the flow of evil spirits (Chapter 2) (Temkin, 1945). Strong or painful stimuli interfere with early ictal hypersynchrony, particularly when applied to an anatomical area projecting to the site of ictal generation. For instance, rubbing or pinching the body part involved in focal clonic motor or sensory seizures can occasionally avert a Jacksonian march, and presenting a strong smell has been reported to abort *uncinate fits*. In one published case study, operant conditioning was used to pair the effective smell with the sight of a bracelet, and eventually even the thought of the bracelet could abort the seizure (Efron, 1957). It is rare, however, for an aura to be sufficiently prolonged and so consistently disrupted by easily applied specific stimulation to allow abortive input to be practically useful for controlling evolution to disabling seizures (Chapter 16). More commonly, some patients report that concentration at the earliest recognition of an ictal symptom at times can disrupt progression of an epileptic seizure.

SLEEP-WAKE CYCLES AND CHRONOBIOLOGY

Changes occurring during the *sleep-wake cycle* commonly modulate epileptic activity. Twenty-four-hour *circadian rhythms* controlled by the *suprachiasmatic nuclei* of the *anterior hypothalamus* and other hypothalamic influences result in hormonal alterations as well as brain activity, but the circadian rhythm and the sleep-wake cycle are not necessarily identical (Shouse and Quigg, 2008). The occurrence of epileptic seizures in some patients only during certain phases of the sleep-wake cycle has been well documented (Janz, 1974). The degree to which 24-hour fluctuations in interictal EEG spike activation and epileptic seizure occurrence are dependent on the sleep-wake cycle, as opposed to the endogenous circadian rhythm, is unclear. In addition, there are *ultradian cycles* (cycles of less than 24 hours), such as the *basic rest activity cycle (BRAC)*, which lasts 90–120 minutes. The BRAC is responsible for alterations between *rapid eye movement (REM)* and *non-REM (NREM)* sleep, but it also occurs throughout waking. The briefer *cyclic alternating pattern (CAP)*, which results in periodic *microarousals*, is another ultradian rhythm (Shouse and Quigg, 2008). *Infradian rhythms* (with periods greater than 24 hours) also exist, such as the *menstrual cycle*, which is associated with alterations in seizure susceptibility and *catamenial epilepsy*.

REM and NREM sleep behavior are mediated through basal forebrain, diencephalic, and brain stem mechanisms (Chapter 3). NREM sleep is divided into three stages. *Stage 1* is initial drowsiness with slow eye movements and EEG changes consisting of *theta activity* and *vertex sharp waves*. *Stage 2* is deeper sleep associated with EEG *sleep spindles* and *K-complexes*. *Stage 3*, which is a condensation of Stages 3 and 4 in the 1968 classification (Rechtschaffen and Kales, 1968), is deep sleep, or slow-wave sleep, associated with 1- to 2-Hz delta activity on the EEG (Iber et al., 2007). The basic mechanisms underlying the delta activity of slow-wave sleep are not clearly understood, but it correlates with fluctuations in neuronal activity referred to as the *up-down state (UDS)* (Steriade et al., 1993) (Chapter 3). The up phase is characterized by an increase in neuronal activity, and the down phase by a decrease or cessation in neuronal activity. The UDS has been observed with invasive EEG recordings at the onset of epileptic seizures in some patients (Bragin et al., 2007). It is abnormal in an experimental animal model of mesial temporal lobe epilepsy, showing increased neuronal activity and *up spikes* during the up phase; these changes could provide insights into interactions between sleep and epileptic mechanisms and perhaps ultimately serve as a biomarker for epilepsy (He et al., 2010).

Seizures on awakening usually occur within 10 minutes to two hours after awakening during a period of postawakening drowsiness. These are most commonly seen in the age-related genetic generalized epilepsies. Nocturnal seizures are more likely to occur during the first two stages of NREM sleep and are characteristic of certain genetic syndromes, such as *autosomal dominant nocturnal frontal lobe epilepsy*, *childhood epilepsy with centrotemporal spikes*, and *Panayiotopoulos syndrome*. Interictal spikes are predominant during slow-wave sleep in *epileptic encephalopathy with continuous spike-and-wave during sleep* and the related *Landau-Kleffner syndrome*. Focal seizures due to neocortical lesions, particularly in the frontal lobe, also are more likely to occur during NREM sleep than during wakefulness, but limbic seizures of mesial temporal lobe origin are more likely to occur during wakefulness (Shouse et al., 2008). Secondarily generalized seizures, however, are more likely to occur during NREM sleep in both neocortical and mesial temporal conditions, indicating that mechanisms responsible for initiation of limbic seizures are not the same as mechanisms responsible for propagation. Similarly, in these focal epilepsies, interictal spikes may be more frequent during Stage 3 NREM sleep, while seizures are more likely to occur during Stage 1 and 2 NREM sleep, indicating that mechanisms underlying interictal spike generation are not the same as those responsible for ictogenesis (Shouse et al., 2008).

Natural and sedated sleep are used to activate focal interictal epileptiform discharges in the EEG laboratory (Chapter 12), but spikes during wakefulness are more likely to be localized to the site of the epileptogenic region than those that occur during NREM sleep, and spikes during REM are the most localizing (Lieb et al., 1980; Montplaisir et al., 1985). This phenomenon, where the most localizing interictal EEG spikes are those that are least affected by changes in state, is referred to as *spike autonomy*. The frequency of interictal spikes is increased during slow-wave sleep and reduced during REM sleep in the genetic epilepsies; in some patients with absences, the 3-Hz spike-and-wave does not occur during REM sleep (Billiard, 1982). For purposes of EEG diagnosis, night sleep is a more potent activator of interictal spike activity in patients with all forms of epilepsy than is daytime nap sleep, but the yield from the latter can be enhanced by sleep deprivation (Arne-Bes et al., 1982; Ellingson et al., 1984). Sleep deprivation is a powerful activator of epileptic seizures in the genetic generalized epilepsies such as JME, and sleep deprivation can also be used to activate focal seizures during presurgical evaluation with video-EEG telemetry (Shouse et al., 2008). Sleep deprivation increases interictal spike frequency more in children than in adults and more in genetic epilepsies than in lesional epilepsies.

The BRAC, which is responsible for the highly stable rhythmic oscillations between REM and the three stages of NREM sleep (Shouse et al., 2008) and also continues during wakefulness, is accompanied by rhythmic variations in interictal EEG spike frequency (Billiard, 1982; Kellaway, 1985). Interaction between the circadian 24-hour sleep-wake cycle and this ultradian cycle produces characteristic patterns of interictal spike discharge (Kellaway, 1985; Kellaway et al., 1980) (Fig. 9–2). It is unclear, however, what relationship exists between this ultradian fluctuation and interictal spike occurrence or the potential for ictogenesis. Similarly, spontaneous arousals in sleep mediated by CAP oscillations provoke interictal spikes and also seizures in JME (Shouse et al., 2008).

Circadian fluctuations in hormones such as *cortisol* (Weitzman, 1976; Weitzman et al., 1979; 1983) influence the temporal patterns of seizure occurrence but less so than neuronal mechanisms underlying the particular level of consciousness (Chapter 3). The latter include activation of *GABAergic* and *galaninergic* cells of the anterior *hypothalamus/preoptic basal forebrain* responsible for inducing sleep and of *histamine-*, *acetylcholine-*, and *hypocretin-secreting* cells of the *posterior, anterior*, and *lateral hypothalamus* responsible for inducing wakefulness (Shouse and Quigg, 2008; Shouse et al., 2008). These arousal mechanisms promote synchronized thalamocortical discharges, effects that might be exacerbated by BRAC and CAP rhythms deriving from *norepinephrine, serotonin*, and *cholinergic* influences in the *pontine tegmentum* and *ascending reticular activating system*. Seizures, therefore, appear to be more often *state-dependent* than truly *circadian*. For instance, epileptic myoclonic seizures that occur after awakening in JME

are even more likely to occur with nighttime awakening than with morning awakening. The critical period for these events is not limited to the moment of awakening but sometimes persists for several hours afterward. Therefore, this phenomenon cannot be attributed to the synchronizing influences of arousal and must involve other, more slowly adapting endogenous factors related to the transition from sleep to wakefulness.

Recognition of these state-dependent predisposing or precipitating factors is of clinical importance for three reasons: (1) sleep, drowsiness, or sleep deprivation can be used to provoke electrographic or clinical epileptiform events in the EEG laboratory for diagnostic purposes, (2) a history of epileptic seizures that occur only or predominantly during sleep and after awakening suggests a genetic epilepsy with a good prognosis, and (3) knowledge of specific patterns of seizure occurrence can dictate schedules for antiseizure medication and daily activities to reduce the chance of injury or embarrassment at times of particular risk.

Not only does the sleep-wake cycle influence epileptic seizures, but epileptic seizures can influence the sleep-wake cycle. Patients with certain types of focal epilepsy can have disturbed sleep architecture (specifically, reduced REM sleep time), and nocturnal seizures disrupt sleep, which not only causes increased daytime sleepiness but can exacerbate epilepsy conditions (Shouse et al., 2008). Antiseizure drugs can improve sleep if they eliminate nocturnal seizures, but essentially all antiseizure medications have some direct effect on sleep, increasing sleepiness or even causing insomnia (Shouse et al., 2008). Finally, patients with epilepsy may have other sleep disturbances, such as *sleep apnea* or *periodic limb movements*, that adversely affect control of their epileptic seizures. *Hypersomnia* due to sleep disturbances is diagnosed by the *Multiple Sleep Latency Test (MSLT)*, but results from simple instruments such as the *Epworth Sleepiness Scale* can identify the existence of sleep disturbances and correlate well with the results of the MSLT (Foldvary-Schaefer, 2002).

A number of nonepileptic events that occur during sleep (*parasomnias*), such as *night terrors, somnambulism, enuresis, jactatio capitis nocturnus (head banging)*, and *REM sleep behavior disorder*, can occasionally be mistaken for nocturnal seizures (Chapter 13).

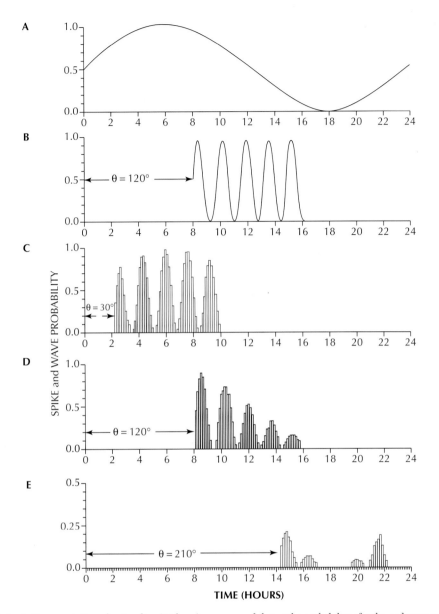

Figure 9–2. A. Representation of a circadian (24-hour) process modulating the probability of spike-and-wave production. **B.** Representation of an 8-hour sleep period showing the 100-minute sleep cycle as a modulator of spike-and-wave production. **C–E.** Joint probabilities of spike-and-wave production obtained by interaction of the processes represented in **A** and **B** at different sleep onset times (θ). (From Kellaway et al., 1980, with permission.)

Some authors believe that particular forms of nocturnal wandering may be epileptic (Pedley and Guilleminault, 1977).

METABOLIC AND TOXIC INFLUENCES

Although it is rare for epileptic seizures in women to occur only around the time of *menses*

(*catamenial epilepsy*), all types of epileptic seizures are commonly exacerbated immediately preceding and during the menstrual period and occasionally at the time of ovulation (Backström, 2008). This phenomenon usually reflects alterations in the balance between the anticonvulsant effects of *progesterone* and the convulsant effects of *estrogen*, and perhaps water retention during menses (Chapter 3), but in some patients it is due to changes in antiseizure drug levels (Rosciszewska et al., 1986). Drug levels, therefore, should be checked and adjusted as required. *Acetazolamide*, 250 or 500 mg a day beginning 10 days prior to the expected onset of menses and continued until bleeding stops, can be effective adjunctive therapy (Chapter 14). Alternatively, antiseizure medication can be increased to provide higher serum drug levels during this period. Some patients may also benefit from regulation of the menstrual cycle with oral contraceptives or parenteral *depomedroxyprogesterone* (Herzog, 2008; Herzog et al., 2012) (Chapter 16).

During pregnancy, epileptic seizures can increase (*gravidic epilepsy*) or decrease (Backström, 2008; Dalessio, 1985; Schmidt, 1982). Poor seizure control at this time can be due to increased clearance of antiseizure medication rather than to hormonal changes. This increased clearance is a result of *hypoalbuminemia* associated with pregnancy, which results in reduced protein binding and increased free levels of antiseizure drugs. Consequently, although increased free drug results in increased clearance, it also results in an increased amount passing into the brain, so serum drug free levels, and not total levels, are necessary to determine whether an increase in seizures is due to decreased drug availability (Chapter 14).

Ultradian seizure patterns during wakefulness most often result from extrinsic environmental influences imposed by work or school. *Hypoglycemia* related to meal schedules can increase susceptibility to seizures at specific times in some patients. Intrinsic 90- to 120-minute epileptic excitability cycles have been described in some patients (Stevens et al., 1971), corresponding to the BRAC fluctuations described in the preceding section.

Endocrinological influences seem to play an important role in the age-related onset and disappearance of many types of epileptic seizures (Chapter 7). After puberty, absence seizures commonly disappear, whereas generalized tonic-clonic seizures become more prominent or occur for the first time, often as a result of a disorder that has been present since birth (Backström, 2008). The effect of *menopause* and *hormone replacement* on seizure frequency is inconsistent (Backström, 2008).

Many *toxic states* influence normal excitability and predispose to epileptic seizure occurrence (Chapter 5). Of particular clinical concern is the withdrawal of sedative and hypnotic drugs, particularly alcohol, minor tranquilizers, sleeping pills, and perhaps cannabis. Some patients are exquisitely sensitive to withdrawal effects of alcohol and experience seizure exacerbation consistently after only small doses (Mattson, 1983; Brust, 2008). These individuals should avoid the use of alcohol altogether. Most patients, however, can tolerate social alcohol intake and an occasional minor tranquilizer or sleeping pill without difficulty, as long as they are not used consistently for some time and then stopped abruptly. Certain drugs (see Table 5–10) and excessive amounts of commonly used stimulants such as coffee, tea, and cola drinks can lower the threshold for epileptic seizures. Again, some patients are extremely sensitive and must avoid these stimulants and drugs, but most can tolerate them in moderation. There is no contraindication to the use of neuroleptics in adequately treated patients with epilepsy, because provocation of an ictal event with these agents is rare (Logothetis, 1967). Cocaine is used experimentally to produce epileptic seizures, and single or repeated use can provoke seizures in patients (Baxter et al., 1988; Pritchard et al., 1985).

PSYCHOLOGICAL STRESS

Psychological stress is often noted by patients to be a potent precipitating factor for seizures, second perhaps only to drowsiness. When this observation is made, the actual time of seizure occurrence is more likely to be the period of relaxation following stress than the stressful situation itself. In some patients, the combination of stress and exercise or exercise alone will provoke seizures. A term applied to seizures that are induced by psychological factors is *psychogenic epileptic seizures*, which should not be confused with *psychogenic nonepileptic seizures* (Chapter 13). Hyperventilation during stress could play a part in seizure initiation, although increased respiration in this case corrects a metabolic imbalance and should not induce alkalosis (Chapter 3). An important but rare condition is *convulsive syncope* (Gastaut, 1974), in which vasovagal or other forms of syncope are accompanied by generalized tonic-clonic symptoms (Chapter 13). This reactive phenomenon is not considered to be epileptic.

POSTICTAL SYMPTOMS

Epileptic seizures are terminated by the ictal engagement of active inhibitory mechanisms rather than by neuronal exhaustion (Caspers and Speckmann, 1972) (Chapter 4). Several types of seizure arrest exist; for instance, the neuronal processes that terminate generalized tonic-clonic seizures do not appear to be active at the end of absences (Engel et al., 1981; 1985; 2008). Forms of active inhibition that arrest generalized tonic-clonic and some focal seizures induce a period of postictal depression with characteristic behavioral and electroencephalographic features. Focal seizures can also cause localized postictal dysfunction (Efron, 1961). Different types of epileptic seizures induce a variety of cerebral and systemic dysfunctions. Although status epilepticus can cause brain damage, it remains unclear if, and under what circumstances, structural disturbances can result from single ictal events (Sutula and Pitkänen, 2002).

Mechanisms

After most focal and generalized tonic-clonic seizures, there is a postictal refractory period, when the threshold for provoking a second seizure is extremely high. This postictal threshold elevation can be experimentally demonstrated in the kindled rat by *recycling*, where an electrical stimulus produces the habitual seizure, and stimuli are then repeated at regular intervals until a second seizure occurs (Engel and Ackermann, 1980). Inherent differences in the duration of the postictal refractory period exist from one rat to another, and this duration is markedly shorter in rat pups (Moshé et al., 1983). This observation suggests that stable intrinsic factors influence postictal inhibitory mechanisms, which are poorly developed in the immature brain. The effectiveness of these mechanisms can also be experimentally manipulated; for instance, repeated seizures can increase the epileptic seizure threshold for several days (Mucha and Pinel, 1977).

After kindled epileptic seizures in animals, as with generalized tonic-clonic and some focal seizures in patients, there is a period of behavioral depression that is associated with EEG slow waves and an increase in EEG spike activity (Frenk et al., 1979; Gotman and Marciani, 1985). Postictal depression in rats can be measured by noting suppression of specific behaviors such as grasping reflexes, food consumption, memory, and affective pain responses (Caldecott-Hazard et al., 1983). Explosive motor behavior can also occur postictally in these animals (Caldecott-Hazard et al., 1983). Such postictal behaviors in rats may be analogous to postictal motor, cognitive, and affective symptoms seen following some limbic and generalized tonic-clonic seizures in patients (Caldecott-Hazard and Engel, 1987).

Although the mechanisms of seizure termination, the postictal refractory period, and other postictal behaviors are incompletely understood, it appears that some share a common pathophysiological basis (Chapter 4). Disturbances in *endogenous opiate* function have been implicated, because pretreatment of rats with *morphine* or *naloxone* can increase or decrease, respectively, the duration of some postictal behaviors. Seizure suppression, frequency of EEG spikes (Caldecott-Hazard et al., 1982; Frenk et al., 1979; Holaday and Belenky, 1980), and intensity of the trilevel pain response (which is believed to involve higher cognitive function) (Caldecott-Hazard et al., 1983) appear to be opiate-sensitive. Conversely, postictal explosive motor behavior in rats is enhanced by naloxone-precipitated morphine withdrawal (Caldecott-Hazard et al., 1983). Postictal changes in the trilevel pain response and explosive motor behavior could represent rat equivalents of clinical postictal confusion and combative behavior, respectively. It is postulated, therefore, that the disabling postictal symptoms that occur in patients are necessary consequences of the protective mechanisms that stop seizures and prevent repeated seizures from occurring. Some of these mechanisms could be mediated by endogenous opioids. An ultimate goal is to dissociate these various effects in order to reduce postictal symptoms without increasing the risk of producing status epilepticus.

Clinical Considerations

SPECIFIC POSTICTAL CEREBRAL DYSFUNCTION

Specific negative symptoms frequently occur after focal seizures and are referable to the particular function involved in the ictal event (Efron, 1961). Thus a focal seizure with classic motor symptoms of one arm can be followed by paralysis of that arm (*Todd's paralysis*) (Todd, 1855). Although this symptom can last for varying periods of time, it typically is gone within 48 hours. Less commonly, similar Todd's phenomena consisting of localized sensory deficits such as numbness, blindness, or deafness follow focal seizures with somatosensory, visual, or auditory symptoms. Todd's phenomena can be associated with focal EEG slowing over the appropriate cortical region. The anterograde amnesia following some dyscognitive limbic seizures can be considered a Todd's phenomenon involving the hippocampi bilaterally. Postictal aphasias can occur after seizures beginning almost anywhere in the language-dominant hemisphere. Focal postictal dysfunction indicates a focal seizure disorder and provides information about the brain areas involved in the ictal discharge. However, the area of dysfunction is not necessarily the site of ictal onset.

Focal neurological deficits appearing immediately after focal seizures do not reflect permanent structural damage but rather represent transient postictal disruption of function that will resolve within minutes or hours. These focal functional postictal changes account for the local cerebral hypoperfusion seen on postictal *single-photon emission computed tomography (SPECT)* (Berkovic et al., 1993) (Fig. 9–3) and could contribute to some extent to the appearance of interictal hypometabolism on *positron emission tomography with fluorodeoxyglucose (FDG-PET)* (Engel, 1984; 1983). This concept is reinforced by PET studies in patients with limbic seizures that reveal an interictal increase in μ-*opiate receptor* binding in the hypometabolic temporal lobe (Frost et al., 1988). If borne out, such data support the suggestion that endogenous opioids not only contribute to postictal dysfunction but also might play a role in the development of interictal behavioral disturbances (Engel et al., 1984) (Chapter 11).

Occasionally, postictal deficits last weeks or months after focal status epilepticus. In particular, prolonged short-term memory deficits are common after limbic status epilepticus (Engel et al., 1978). A new homonymous hemianopia was reported to persist for almost a year in one patient after an episode of limbic status epilepticus originating from an epileptogenic lesion in the contralateral occipital cortex; this deficit eventually resolved completely (Engel et al., 1983) (Fig. 9–4). Such enduring postictal neurological deficits are unlikely to involve the same transient functional mechanisms that give rise to Todd's paralysis and might reflect actual seizure-induced structural damage that ultimately is compensated for by neuronal reorganization (Engel et al., 1978; Engel et al., 1983).

NONSPECIFIC POSTICTAL CEREBRAL DYSFUNCTION

Ictal events associated with impaired consciousness give rise to less specific postictal symptoms that reflect transient dysfunction over wider areas of the brain bilaterally. These changes can be seen as diffuse hypometabolism on FDG-PET scans obtained during and after such seizures (Engel et al., 1982; Engel et al., 1983) (see Figs. 6–4, 6–7, and 6–11). Postictal disorientation and confusion, whether or not associated with fatigue or lethargy, represent dysfunction of memory and higher cortical cognitive processes. Reactive automatisms that commonly occur during the postictal period (Chapter 6) appear to be purposeless or semipurposeful motor behaviors released as a result of suppression of cortical control. These postictal behaviors are much more likely to appear after limbic dyscognitive seizures than after generalized convulsions, presumably because higher cortical functions are depressed but motor functions are relatively spared after the former. At times reactive automatisms can be violent, usually in response to stimuli that appear threatening or to attempts at restraint, but these behaviors are not voluntary. Similarly, associated verbal or other affective display is reflex, not premeditated, behavior. Rarely, postictal aggressive behavior, as well as postictal hypersexuality, can have tragic consequences (Chapter 11).

Patients who are aware of increased depression or tension prior to generalized tonic-clonic or limbic seizures occasionally report a feeling of euphoria or release during the postictal period. This may reflect the same physiological or biochemical changes induced in the brain that are responsible for the well-known therapeutic effect of *electroconvulsive shock therapy (ECT)* on clinical depression. Patients can also report depression as a consistent consequence of these epileptic seizures or can

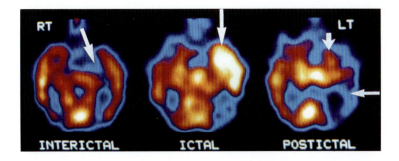

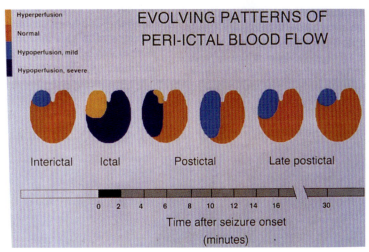

Figure 9–3. *Top:* Interictal, ictal, and postictal [99]Tc – hexamethylpropyleneamine oxime (HM-PAO) single photon emission tomography (SPECT) images of the temporal lobes in a patient with left temporal lobe epilepsy. The interictal study shows relatively symmetrical temporal lobe perfusion with a minor decrease in the left anteromesial temporal region (*arrow*). The ictal study shows marked left temporal *hyperperfusion* involving the mesial and especially the lateral temporal regions (*arrow*). The postictal study shows *hyper*perfusion of the left mesial temporal region (*short arrow*) with relative *hypo*perfusion of the lateral temporal cortex (*long arrow*). This change from the ictal to the postictal state is the "postictal switch." (From Newton et al., 1992). *Bottom:* Evolution of blood flow changes in temporal lobe epilepsy. In the interictal state there may be mild *hypo*perfusion of the epileptogenic temporal lobe. During the seizure there is marked *hyper*perfusion of the temporal lobe. In the early postictal period there is mesial temporal *hyper*perfusion and extensive lateral *hypo*perfusion. The mesial hyperperfusion disappears within a few minutes, whereas lateral hypoperfusion may persist for 10–20 minutes postictally before returning to the interictal state. (From Berkovic et al., 1993, with permission; modified from Rowe et al.,1991).

exhibit postictal psychotic behavior, usually with a latent period of several days after single or recurrent generalized tonic-clonic or limbic seizures (Chapter 11). In rare instances, this behavior can last days or weeks (Penfield and Jasper, 1954; Alper et al., 2008) and require antipsychotic medication. Postictal delirium associated with clouded consciousness and a normal EEG also occurs after repeated seizures. The typical 3-Hz spike-and-wave EEG pattern identifies *absence status*, which rarely can follow a generalized tonic-clonic seizure and responds to antiabsence medication (Bauer et al., 1982) (Chapter 10). Some investigators believe that prolonged *fugue states* or

twilight states (*poriomania*) (Mayeux et al., 1979) and other bizarre behaviors occurring in patients with known epilepsy may be postictal phenomena (Chapter 13). More enduring postictal behavioral disturbances are discussed in detail in Chapter 11.

SYSTEMIC POSTICTAL DYSFUNCTION

Patients frequently complain of a headache after generalized tonic-clonic and, less commonly, after limbic seizures (D'Alessandro et al., 1987). Headache after generalized tonic-clonic seizures could be accounted for by systemic hypertension; however, diffuse

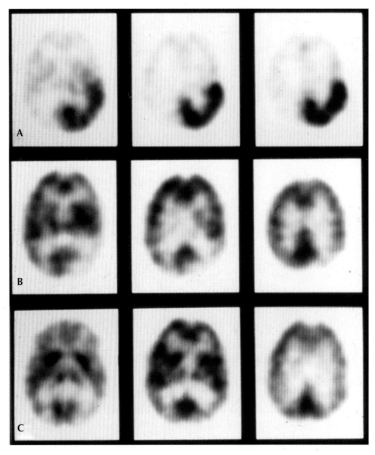

Figure 9–4. Representative sections of three FDG-PET scans from a patient with occipital-onset focal dyscognitive seizures. **A.** Ictal scan shows increased metabolic activity in right occipital and temporal lobes, and decreased activity in the rest of the brain. **B.** One month later, the patient still demonstrated a postictal left homonymous hemianopia and hypometabolism involving the right occipital and temporal lobes, including the calcarine cortex. **C.** One year later, after the visual field deficit had resolved, a small zone of hypometabolism was still present at the right occipitotemporal junction, but the right calcarine cortex was metabolically normal. (Note that older PET scans in this book are not reversed, right is on the right side and left is on the left side.) (From Engel et al., 1983, with permission.)

metabolic disturbances involving subcortical structures may be necessary for headache after limbic seizures (D'Alessandro et al., 1987; Engel et al., 1983). Some postictal headaches after focal seizures may represent ictal cephalgia (Young and Blume, 1983), and activation of trigeminal fibers has been postulated to explain occasional pain ipsilateral to the epileptogenic zone (Lesser et al., 1987).

Elevated blood pressure during a generalized tonic-clonic seizure can cause intracerebral bleeding (Tabaddor and Balagura, 1981). Postictal pulmonary edema (Simon et al., 1982) may be neurogenic and rarely can occur unilaterally (Koppel et al., 1987). The intense muscular contractions of generalized tonic-clonic seizures give rise to muscle soreness and exhaustion in the postictal period and may be sufficiently severe to cause joint dislocation and fractures, particularly of the spine.

Laboratory tests following a generalized tonic-clonic seizure usually show elevated blood glucose levels of up to 200 mg/dL (Simon, 1985). Cerebrospinal fluid pleocytosis is rare, but as many as 80 cells per mm³ have been reported after major motor status epilepticus (Schmidley and Simon, 1981). However, a cell count above 10/cmm³ (Andermann and Andermann, 1986) should initiate a search for an intracranial inflammatory process. Strenuous muscular activity during generalized tonic-clonic seizures elevates muscle enzymes measured in the blood and induces *lactic acidosis*. The arterial pH may go below 7.0 after a single generalized tonic-clonic seizure but normalizes within an hour, largely by metabolism of lactate (Orringer et al., 1977). Epileptic seizures also elevate many of the neurohumoral substances of the brain, which could influence interictal behavior (Engel et al., 1984) (Chapter 11). *Prolactin* has gained the greatest clinical attention. The finding that prolactin elevation may be specific for epileptic seizures involving mesial temporal structures has been useful for differentiating limbic from nonepileptic psychogenic seizures (Collins et al., 1983; Pritchard et al., 1985) (Chapter 14). Prolactin determinations also may help to distinguish typical limbic seizures involving mesial temporal limbic structures from atypical events that predominantly involve extratemporal areas (Sperling et al., 1986).

MORTALITY

Comorbidity

People with epilepsy have an increased risk of premature death, which begins soon after the onset of seizures and persists for many decades (Sperling, 2004; Sillanpää and Shinnar, 2010; Nelligan et al., 2011). The mortality rate has been estimated to be at least three times as high as that expected in the general population after adjusting for age and sex and is increased in patients with pharmacoresistant seizures due to structural causes. This elevated mortality can be explained to some extent by the significantly higher prevalence of chronic comorbid conditions, including disorders such as stroke, cancer, heart disease, and diabetes, in people with epilepsy (Téllez-Zenteno et al., 2005; Gaitatzis et al., 2004), which undoubtedly accounts for many premature deaths in the epilepsy population. Mortality for single seizures depends on the underlying cause (Hesdorffer et al., 2009) (Chapter 2); mortality from status epilepticus is discussed in Chapter 9. Accidents, particularly drowning, and suicides are also relatively common causes of seizure-related mortality; however, deaths attributable directly to seizures are rare. Approximately 30% of deaths are unexplained and fall into the category of *sudden unexpected (or unexplained) death (SUD)*.

Sudden Unexpected Death

SUD is not unique to epilepsy, but people with epilepsy have an increased susceptibility to this condition, which has now been referred to as *SUD in epilepsy (SUDEP)* (Jay and Leestma, 1981; Leestma et al., 1984; Nashef and Tomson, 2008; Hirsch et al., 2011; Devinsky, 2011). Although SUDEP accounts for approximately 30 percent of deaths among people with epilepsy, the true incidence remains uncertain; rates of 1 per 200–300 person-years have been estimated, and this increases to 1 per 100 person-years in patients with pharmacoresistant seizures (Nashef and Tomson, 2008). Typically, patients are between 20 and 40 years old and have had epileptic seizures for at least one year. They are likely to have subtherapeutic or no levels of antiseizure medications in the blood and a structural cerebral lesion, often frontal or temporal, underlying their condition. Risk factors include a nongenetic epilepsy, polydrug therapy, frequent generalized tonic-clonic seizures, and a childhood onset (Sillanpää and Shinnar, 2010; Hesdorffer et al., 2011). A recent meta-analysis of antiseizure drug trials found SUDEP to be seven times more common among patients in the add-on placebo group than in the efficacious antiseizure drug group (Ryvlin et al., 2011), strongly suggesting that poor seizure control is a significant contributing factor. Prolonged postictal EEG depression might also be a risk factor for SUDEP (Lhatoo et al., 2010). Patients are usually found dead in bed with no evidence that an epileptic seizure occurred or on the floor in the bedroom, bathroom, or elsewhere, suggesting a sudden catastrophic event. Autopsy provides no clues to the cause of death (Hirsch and Martin, 1971; Leestma et al., 1984; Terrence et al., 1975).

In addition to the well-known effects of generalized tonic-clonic seizures on heart rate, blood pressure, respiration, and a variety of other functions (Chapter 6), some ictal and even interictal epileptiform events have more subtle autonomic influences (Delgado et al., 1960; Van Buren, 1958; Goodman et al., 2008). The higher centers for control of cardiorespiratory function include the amygdala and orbital frontal regions (Galosy et al., 1981), structures that are commonly involved in limbic seizures. These limbic areas also have direct projections to the hypothalamus. Experimentally induced interictal as well as ictal epileptiform events in animals can alter cardiac responses to changes in blood pressure, increase the variability of cardiac sympathetic and parasympathetic discharges, and induce arrhythmias (Lathers and Schraeder, 1982). The most common cardiac abnormality in patients with epilepsy is reduced heart rate variability (Nashef and Tomson, 2008), reflecting an inability to adjust to alterations in cardiac demand, though some studies suggest that SUDEP is more likely to be a failure in respiratory control (Nashef and Tomson, 2008).

It is reasonable to assume that more than one mechanism for SUDEP exists. Chronic epileptic activity might produce a state of cardiorespiratory instability that the patient does not perceive and that is not necessarily associated with behavioral manifestations of an epileptic seizure. Although isolated ictal arrhythmias (Pritchett et al., 1980) and seizure-related neurogenic pulmonary edema (Koppel et al., 1987) have been reported, of more concern is the influence this instability might have on responses of the cardiovascular system to normal compromise that might occur, for instance, during sleep transitions (Guilleminault et al., 1984) or after a seizure (Nashef and Tomson, 2008). Recently, a mutation in the SCN5A gene, which codes for sodium channels in the heart, has been linked to SUDEP; this gene is also present in the brain, suggesting a common cerebrocardiac disturbance (Hartmann et al., 1999; Crompton and Berkovic, 2009; Goldman et al., 2009). Undoubtedly, further research will reveal multiple causes of SUDEP.

The prevailing view is that most patients die of sudden, irreversible cardiac or respiratory arrest. In a few cases such arrest has actually occurred in an emergency room or intensive care setting (in the absence of an apparent epileptic seizure), and attempts at cardiopulmonary resuscitation were ineffective (Dasheiff and Dickinson, 1986; Leestma et al., 1984). There is reason to believe that certain types of epileptic seizures that influence control of cardiorespiratory function increase the risk of sudden cardiac or respiratory arrest, particularly during sleep or after a seizure. Repeated epileptiform discharges into orbital frontal, amygdala, and hypothalamic structures responsible for cardiorespiratory control could create instability (Frysinger et al., 1987; 1993) similar to that demonstrated for some forms of *sudden infant death syndrome (SIDS)* (Tilden et al.,

1983). Brief ictal or interictal discharges propagating to cardiorespiratory control centers during a critical period of sleep might then be able to precipitate irreversible cardiac or respiratory arrest. It is conceivable that such events might even occur spontaneously.

Data are relatively consistent indicating that SUDEP is more common among patients with pharmacoresistant focal and secondarily generalized tonic-clonic seizures, raising the question of whether surgical treatment might be protective. A number of studies have shown a reduction in mortality rate, and specifically SUDEP, among patients who become seizure-free following surgical treatment as compared with those who continue to experience seizures postoperatively (Sperling, 2004; Nashef and Tomson, 2008). Whether this difference reflects the beneficial effects of surgery per se or a difference in the pathophysiology of patients who respond to surgical treatment remains to be determined.

Research to improve identification of patients at risk for SUDEP and to develop preventive interventions is a high priority (Hirsch et al., 2011). Reliable biomarkers for SUDEP have not yet been clearly identified, and all-night polysomnography to screen for sleep-related cardiorespiratory abnormalities is obviously not practical for every patient. There is currently no recommended approach to reduce the incidence of these events other than to maximize seizure control. If spontaneous or ictal high-risk cardiac arrhythmias are noted in patients with epilepsy, it may be possible to use monitoring devices similar to those used for SIDS to alert family members when an arrest occurs. However, evidence from patients who experienced SUDEP in a hospital setting suggests that even with the best available cardiopulmonary resuscitation, the damage is irreversible.

An important issue is whether the risk of SUDEP should be discussed with patients and their families when a diagnosis of epilepsy is made. On the one hand, there is fear that such a discussion can cause anxiety, precipitate stress reactions, and be misinterpreted with respect to the relative risk. On the other hand, a frank discussion of the actual risk and risk factors improves the doctor-patient relationship and helps patients and their relatives contribute to setting treatment goals, including the reduction of risk factors, which would include a concerted effort to control habitual seizures

(Ryvlin et al., 2011). One case-controlled study has found that the risk of SUDEP is reduced when patients are monitored or when another person 10 years old or older sleeps in the same room (Langan et al., 2005). Education about SUDEP is now recommended, not only for patients, their families, and care providers but also the public in general, to communicate the seriousness of epilepsy and the need for further research (Hirsch et al., 2011).

Drowning

Drowning is an unusually common cause of death in persons with epilepsy and has generally been ascribed to the occurrence of an epileptic seizure while swimming or in the bath. An alternative explanation should be considered, however. On submersion, diving mammals exhibit a *dive reflex* consisting of bradycardia, diminished peripheral blood flow, and other autonomic changes, which conserve oxygen and protect cerebral metabolism. A remnant of this reflex occurs in humans when the face is immersed in water (Hurwitz and Furedy, 1986). Although it is an entirely speculative notion, epilepsy-related autonomic disturbances might exaggerate this primitive reflex and increase the risk of drowning.

SUMMARY AND CONCLUSIONS

The major cause of disability associated with epilepsy is the unpredictability of seizure occurrence. Management of epileptic seizures should be influenced, when possible, by identification of normal and abnormal preictal events that act as precipitating factors. These include specific exogenous or endogenous stimuli that can directly provoke an epileptic seizure; nonspecific functional states, such as drowsiness, emotional excitation, or menses, that lower seizure thresholds; and intermittent physiological disturbances caused by perturbations such as sedative and hypnotic drug withdrawal and sleep deprivation. With uncomplicated reactive epileptic seizures, effective control can be achieved simply by removal or avoidance of the precipitating factors. In the chronic reflex epilepsies, identification of precipitating factors can aid in making management plans. If precipitating factors are unavoidable—as

is clearly the case, for instance, with seizures induced during sleep—medication schedules can be devised to provide peak serum levels of the drug at times of greatest risk.

Postictal symptoms following generalized tonic-clonic seizures and some focal seizures, particularly of the limbic type, can greatly increase the overall disability suffered by some patients. The degree to which disability is due to postictal dysfunction may not always be apparent to observers or even to the patient. Identification of such disturbances can suggest useful supportive measures during this time.

Mortality in people with epilepsy is triple that in the general population. This can be accounted for in large part by increased comorbidity of serious chronic conditions. Thirty percent of deaths in epilepsy, however, are due to SUDEP, which can occur at any time following onset of epilepsy. Risk factors include early onset of a nongenetic epilepsy condition, pharmacoresistance, polytherapy, and frequent generalized tonic-clonic seizures. Research suggests that certain types of epilepsy disrupt the central mechanisms of cardiorespiratory control in a manner similar to that seen in SIDS. Because there are no effective approaches for prognosis or treatment of SUDEP, this is currently a high-priority area for research. Education of patients, their families, care providers, and the general public about SUDEP gives them a realistic understanding of the seriousness of epilepsy and could help to generate more resources for research.

Priority research issues should also include the following: (1) the role of specific circulating hormones and other factors related to normal and abnormal biorhythms in establishing patterns of seizure occurrence, (2) the interrelationships between sleep- and sleep-deprivation-induced epileptic phenomena and the adverse effects of epileptic seizures on sleep, (3) the characteristics of specific simple and complex stimuli that allow them to precipitate seizures in the reflex epilepsies, (4) the potential for therapeutic exploitation of natural seizure-suppressing neuronal processes that act to maintain the interictal state, limit ictal spread once seizures have begun, and terminate the ictal event, and (5) the neuronal mechanisms of the various forms of postictal dysfunction and the relationship of those mechanisms to those that terminate ictal discharges, induce interictal behavioral disturbances, or both.

REFERENCES

Alajouanine, T, and Gastaut, H (1955). La syncinésie-sursaut et l'épilepsie-sursaut a déclanchement sensoriel ou sensitif inopiné. I. Les faits anatomo-cliniques; 15 observations. Rev Neurol 93:29–41.

Alper, K, Kuzniecky, R, Carlson, C, Barr, WB, Vorkas, CK, Patel, JG, Carrelli, AL, Starner, K, Flom, PL, and Devinsky, O (2008). Postictal psychosis in partial epilepsy: A case-control study. Ann Neurol 63:602–610.

Ames, FR (1974). Cinefilm and EEG recording during "hand-waving" attacks of an epileptic, photosensitive child. Electroencephalogr Clin Neurophysiol 37:301–304.

Andermann, F, and Andermann, E (1986). Excessive startle syndromes: Startle disease, jumping and startle epilepsy. Adv Neurol 43:321–338.

Arne-Bes, MC, Calvet, U, Thiberge, M, and Arbus, L (1982). Effects of sleep deprivation in an EEG study of epileptics. In Sleep and Epilepsy. Edited by MB Sterman, MN Shouse, and P Passouant. New York: Academic Press, pp. 441–452.

Backström, T. Effects of hormones on seizure expression. In Epilepsy (2008). A Comprehensive Textbook, 2nd ed. Edited by J Engel, Jr, and TA Pedley. Philadelphia: Lippincott Williams & Wilkins, pp. 2043–2052.

Bancaud, J, Talairach, J, Lamarche, M, Bonis, A, and Trottier, S (1975). Hypothéses neurophysiopathologiques sur l'épilepsie-sursaut chez l'homme. Rev Neurol 131:559–571.

Bauer, G, Aichner, F, and Mayr, U (1982). Nonconvulsive status epilepticus following generalized tonic-clonic seizures. Eur Neurol 21:411–419.

Baxter, LR, Jr, Schwartz, JM, Phelps, ME, Mazziotta, JC, Barrio, J, Rawson, RA, Engel, J, Jr, Ackerman, R, Guze, BH, Selin, C, and Sumida, R (1988). Localization of the neurochemical effects of cocaine and other stimulants in the human brain. J Clin Psychiatry 49(suppl 2): 23–26.

Berkovic, SF, Newton, MR, Chiron, C, and Dulac, O (1993). Single photon emission tomography. In Surgical Treatment of the Epilepsies, 2nd ed. Edited by J Engel, Jr. New York: Raven Press, pp. 233–243.

Bickford, RG, Sem-Jacobsen, CW, White, PT, and Daly, D (1952). Some observations on the mechanism of photic and photo-Metrazol activation. Electroencephalogr Clin Neurophysiol 4:275–282.

Billiard, M (1982). Epilepsies and the sleep-wake cycle. In Sleep and Epilepsy. Edited by MB Sterman, MN Shouse, and P Passouant. New York: Academic Press, pp. 269–286.

Binnie, CD, Estevez, O, Kasteleijn-Nolst Trenite, DGA, and Peters, A (1984). Colour and photosensitive epilepsy. Electroencephalogr Clin Neurophysiol 58:387–391.

Bragin, A, and Engel, J,Jr (2008). Is prediction of the time of a seizure onset the only value of seizure-prediction studies? In Seizure Prediction in Epilepsy: From Basic Mechanisms to Clinical Applications. Edited by B Schelter, J Timmer, and A Schulze-Bonhage. Berlin: Wiley-VCH, pp. 163–168.

Bragin, A, Claeys, P, Vonck, K, Van Roost, D, Wilson, C, Boon, P, and Engel, J, Jr (2007). Analysis of initial slow waves (ISWs) at the seizure onset in patients with drug resistant temporal lobe epilepsy. Epilepsia 48:1883–1894.

Broughton, R, Meier-Ewert, KH, and Ebe, M (1969). Evoked visual, somatosensory and retinal potentials in photosensitive epilepsy. Électroencephalogr Clin Neurophysiol 27:373–386.

Brust, JCM (2008). Alcohol and drug abuse. In Epilepsy: A Comprehensive Textbook, 2nd ed. Edited by J Engel, Jr, and TA Pedley. Philadelphia: Lippincott Williams & Wilkins, pp. 2683–2687.

Caldecott-Hazard, S, and Engel, J, Jr (1987). Limbic postictal events: Anatomical substrates and opioid receptor involvement. Prog Neuropsychopharmacol Biol Psychiatry 11:389–418.

Caldecott-Hazard, S, Shavit, Y, Ackermann, RF, Engel, J, Jr, Frederickson, RCA, and Liebeskind, JC (1982). Behavioral and electrographic effects of opioids on kindled seizures in rats. Brain Res 251:327–333.

Caldecott-Hazard, S, Yamagata, N, Hedlund, J, Camacho, H, and Liebeskind, JC (1983). Changes in simple and complex behaviors following kindled seizures in rats: Opioid and nonopioid mediation. Epilepsia 24:539–547.

Caspers, H, and Speckmann, E-J (1972). Cerebral pO2, pCO2 and pH: Changes during convulsive activity and their significance for spontaneous arrest of seizures. Epilepsia 13:699–725.

Collins, WC, Lanigan, O, and Callaghan, N (1983). Plasma prolactin concentrates following epileptic and pseudo seizures. J Neurol Neurosurg Psychiatry 46:505–508.

Crompton, DE, and Berkovic, SF (2009). The borderland of epilepsy: Clinical and molecular features of phenomena that mimic epileptic seizures. Lancet Neurol 8:370–381.

D'Alessandro, R, Sacquegna, T, Pazzaglia, P, and Lugaresi, E (1987). Headache after partial complex seizures. In Migraine and Epilepsy. Edited by F Andermann and E Lugaresi. Boston: Butterworths, pp. 273–278.

Dalessio, DJ (1985). Current concepts: Seizure disorders and pregnancy. N Engl J Med 312:559–563.

Daneshmend, TK, and Campbell, MJ (1982). Dark warrior epilepsy. Br Med J 284:1751–1752.

Dasheiff, RM, and Dickinson, LJ (1986). Sudden unexpected death of epileptic patient due to cardiac arrhythmia after seizure. Arch Neurol 43:194–196.

deCurtis, M, and Gnatkovsky, V (2009). Reevaluating the mechanisms of focal ictogenesis: The role of low-voltage fast activity. Epilepsia 50:2514–2525.

Delgado, JM, Mihailovic, L, and Sevillano, M (1960). Cardiovascular phenomena during seizure activity. J Nerv Ment Dis 130:477–487.

Devinsky, O (2011). Sudden, unexplained death in epilepsy. N Engl J Med 365:1801–1811.

Eaton, RC (ed) (1984). Neural Mechanisms of Startle Behavior. New York: Plenum Press.

Efron, R (1957). The conditioned inhibition of uncinate fits. Brain 80:251–262.

Efron, R (1961). Post-epileptic paralysis: Theoretical critique and report of a case. Brain 84:381–394.

Ellingson, RJ, Wilken, K, and Bennett, DR (1984). Efficacy of sleep deprivation as an activation procedure in epileptic patients. J Clin Neurophysiol 1:83–101.

Engel, J, Jr (1974). Selective photoconvulsive responses to intermittent diffuse and patterned photic stimulation. Electroencephalogr Clin Neurophysiol 37: 283–292.

Engel, J, Jr (1984). The use of positron emission tomographic scanning in epilepsy. Ann Neurol 15(suppl 1): S180–S191.

Engel, J, Jr, and Ackermann, RF (1980). Interictal EEG spikes correlate with decreased, rather than increased epileptogenicity in amygdaloid kindled rats. Brain Res 190:543–548.

Engel, J, Jr, Ludwig, BI, and Fetell, M (1978). Prolonged partial complex status epilepticus: EEG and behavioral observations. Neurology 28:863–869.

Engel, J, Jr, Ackermann, RF, Caldecott-Hazard, S, and Kuhl, DE (1981). Epileptic activation of antagonistic systems may explain paradoxical features of experimental and human epilepsy. A review and hypothesis. In Kindling 2. Edited by JA Wada. New York: Raven Press, pp. 193–211.

Engel, J, Jr, Kuhl, DE, and Phelps, ME (1982). Patterns of human local cerebral glucose metabolism during epileptic seizures. Science 218:64–66.

Engel, J, Jr, Kuhl, DE, Phelps, ME, Rausch, R, and Nuwer, M (1983). Local cerebral metabolism during partial seizures. Neurology 33:400–413.

Engel, J, Jr, Caldecott-Hazard, S, Chugani, HT, and Ackermann, RF (1984). Neuropeptides, seizures and epilepsy. In Advances in Epileptology: XVth Epilepsy International Symposium. Edited by RJ Porter, RH Mattson, AA Ward, and M Dam. New York: Raven Press, pp. 25–30.

Engel, J, Jr, Lubens, P, Kuhl, DE, and Phelps, M (1985). Local cerebral metabolic rate for glucose during petit mal absences. Ann Neurol 17:121–128.

Engel, J, Jr, Dichter, MA, and Schwartzkroin, PA (2008). Basic mechanisms of human epilepsy. In Epilepsy: A Comprehensive Textbook, 2nd ed. Edited by J Engel, Jr, and TA Pedley. Philadelphia: Lippincott Williams & Wilkins, pp. 495–507.

Faught, E, and Lee, SI (1984). Pattern-reversal visual evoked potentials in photosensitive epilepsy. Electroencephalogr Clin Neurophysiol 59:125–133.

Foldvary-Schaefer, N (2002). Sleep complaints and epilepsy: The role of seizures, antiepileptic drugs and sleep disorders. J Clin Neurophysiol 19:514–541.

Forster, FM (1977). Reflex Epilepsy, Behavioral Therapy and Conditional Reflexes. Springfield, IL: Charles C Thomas.

Frenk, H, Engel, J, Jr, Ackermann, RF, Shavit, Y, and Liebeskind, JC (1979). Endogenous opioids may mediate post-ictal behavioral depression in amygdaloid-kindled rats. Brain Res 167:435–440.

Frost, JJ, Mayberg, HS, Fisher, RS, Douglass, KH, Dannals, RF, Links, JM, Wilson, AA, Ravert, HT, Rosenbaum, AE, Snyder, SH, and Wagner, HN (1988). Mu-opiate receptors measured by positron emission tomography are increased in temporal lobe epilepsy. Ann Neurol 23:231–237.

Frysinger, RC, Harper, RM, and Hackel, RJ (1987). State-dependent cardiac and respiratory changes associated with complex partial epilepsy. In Fundamental Mechanisms of Human Brain Function. Edited by J Engel, Jr, GA Ojemann, HO Lüders, and PD Williamson. New York: Raven Press, pp. 219–226.

Frysinger, RC, Engel, J, Jr, and Harper, RM (1993). Interictal heart rate patterns in partial seizure disorders. Ann Neurol 43:2136–2139.

Gaitatzis, A, Carroll, K, Majeed, A, and Sander, JW (2004). The epidemiology of the comorbidity of epilepsy in the general population. Epilepsia 45:1613–1622.

Galosy, RA, Clarke, LK, Vasko, MR, and Crawford, IL (1981). Neurophysiology and neuropharmacology of cardiovascular regulation and stress. Neurosci Biobehav Rev 5:137–175.

Gastaut, H (1974). Syncopes: Generalized anoxic cerebral seizures. In The Epilepsies (Handbook of Clinical Neurology, Vol 15). Edited by O Magnus and AM Lorentz de Haas. Amsterdam: North Holland, pp. 815–835.

Gastaut, H, and Tassinari, CA (1966). Triggering mechanisms in epilepsy: The electroclinical point of view. Epilepsia 7:85–138.

Gnatkovsky, V, Librizzi, L, Trombin, F, and deCurtis, M (2008). Fast activity at seizure onset is mediated by inhibitory circuits in the entorhinal cortex in vitro. Ann Neurol 64:674–686.

Goldman, AM, Glasscock, E, Yoo, J, Chen, TT, Klassen, TL, and Noebels, JL (2009). Arrhythmia in heart and brain: KCNQ1 mutations link epilepsy and sudden unexplained death. Sci Transl Med 14:1–11.

Goodman, JH, Stewart, M, and Drislane, FW (2008). Autonomic disturbances. In Epilepsy: A Comprehensive Textbook, 2nd ed. Edited by J Engel, Jr, and TA Pedley. Philadelphia: Lippincott Williams & Wilkins, pp. 1999–2005.

Gotman, J, and Marciani, MG (1985). Electroencephalographic spiking activity, drug levels, and seizure occurrence in epileptic patients. Ann Neurol 17:597–603.

Guilleminault, C, Pool, P, Malta, J, and Gillis, AM (1984). Sinus arrest during REM sleep in young adults. N Engl J Med 311:1006–1010.

Hartmann, HA, Colom, LV, Sutherland, ML, and Noebels, JL (1999). Selective localization of cardiac SCN5A sodium channels in limbic regions of rat brain. Nat Neurosci 2:593–595.

He, DF, Ma, DL, Tang, YC, Engel, J, Jr, Bragin, A, and Tang, FR (2010). Morpho-physiologic characteristics of dorsal subicular network in mice after pilocarpine induced status epilepticus. Brain Pathol 20:80–95.

Herzog, AG (2008). Sex-hormone treatment. In Epilepsy: A Comprehensive Textbook, 2nd ed. Edited by J Engel, Jr, and TA Pedley. Philadelphia: Lippincott Williams & Wilkins, pp. 1387–1394.

Herzog, AG, Fowler, KM, Smithson, SD, Kalayjian, LA, Heck, CN, Sperling, MR, Liporace, JD, Harden, CL, Dworetzky, BA, Pennel, PB, and Massaro, JM, for the Progesterone Trial Study Group (2012). Progesterone vs. placebo for women with epilepsy: A randomized clinical trial. Neurology 78:1959–1966.

Hesdorffer, DC, Benn, EKT, Cascino, GD, and Hauser, WA (2009). Is a first acute symptomatic seizure epilepsy? Mortality and risk for recurrent seizure. Epilepsia 50:1102–1108.

Hesdorffer, DC, Tomson, T, Benn, E, Sander, JW, Nilsson, L, Langan, Y, Walczak, TS, Beghi, E, Brodie, MJ, and Hauser, A, for the ILAE Commission on Epidemiology, Subcommission on Mortality. Combined analysis of risk factors for SUDEP. Epilepsia 52 (2011). 1150–1159.

Hirsch, CS, and Martin, DL (1971). Unexpected death in young epileptics. Neurology 21:682–690.

Hirsch, LJ, Donner, EJ, So, EL, Jacobs, M, Nashef, L, Noebels, JL, and Buchhalter, JR (2011). Abbreviated report of the NIH/NINDS workshop on sudden unexpected death in epilepsy. Neurology 76:1932–1938.

Holaday, JW, and Belenky, GL (1980). Opiate-like effects of ECS in rats: A differential effect of naloxone on nociceptive measures. Life Sci 27:1929–1938.

Hurwitz, BE, and Furedy, JJ (1986). The human drive reflex: An experimental topographical and physiological analysis. Physiol Behav 36: 287–294.

Iber, C, Ancoli-Israel, S, Chesson, A, and Quan, S, for the American Academy of Sleep Medicine (2007). BAAS Manual for Scoring of Sleep and Associated Events: Rules, Terminology and Technical Specifications, 1st ed. Westchester, IL: American Academy of Sleep Medicine.

Ioos, C, Fohlen, M, Villeneuve, N, et al. (2000). Hot water epilepsy: A benign and unrecognized form. J Child Neurol 15:125–128.

Ishida, S, Yamashita, Y, Matsuishi, T, Ohshima, M, Ohshima, H, Kato, H, and Maeda, H (1998). Photosensitive seizures provoked while viewing "Pocket Monsters," a made-for-television animation program in Japan. Epilepsia 39:1340–1344.

Janz, D (1974). Epilepsy and the sleeping-waking cycle. In The Epilepsies (Handbook of Clinical Neurology, Vol 15). Edited by O Magnus and AM Lorentz de Haas. Amsterdam: North Holland, pp. 457–490.

Jay, GW, and Leestma, JE (1981). Sudden death in epilepsy: A comprehensive review of the literature and proposed mechanisms. Acta Neurol Scand Suppl 82:1–66.

Jeavons, PM, and Harding, GFA (1975). Photosensitive Epilepsy: A Review of the Literature and a Study of 460 Patients (Clinics in Developmental Medicine, No 56). Philadelphia: JB Lippincott, p 121.

Kellaway, P (1985). Sleep and epilepsy. Epilepsia 26(suppl 1): S15–S30.

Kellaway, P, Frost, JD, and Crawley, JW (1980). Time modulation of spike-and-wave activity in generalized epilepsy. Ann Neurol 8:491–500.

Kirstein, L, and Silfveskiold, BP (1958). A family with emotionally precipitated "drop seizures." Acta Psychiatr Neurol Scand 33:471–476.

Koppel, BS, Pearl, M, and Perla, E (1987). Epileptic seizures as a cause of pulmonary edema. Epilepsia 28:41–44.

Langan, Y, Nashef, L, and Sander, JW (2005). Case-control study of SUDEP. Neurology 64:1131–1133.

Lathers, CM, and Schraeder, PL (1982). Autonomic dysfunction in epilepsy: Characterization of autonomic cardiac neural discharge associated with pentylenetetrazol-induced epileptogenic activity. Epilepsia 23:633–647.

Leestma, JE, Kalelkar, MB, Teas, SS, Jay, GW, and Hughes, JR (1984). Sudden unexpected death associated with seizures: Analysis of 66 cases. Epilepsia 25:84–88.

Lehnertz, K, Le Van Quyen, M, and Litt, B (2008). Seizure prediction. In Epilepsy: A Comprehensive Textbook, 2nd ed. Edited by J Engel, Jr, and TA Pedley. Philadelphia: Lippincott Williams & Wilkins, pp. 1011–1024.

Lesser, RP, Lüders, H, Dinner, DS, and Morris, HH, III (1987). Simple partial seizures. In Epilepsy: Electroclinical Syndromes. Edited by H Lüders and RP Lesser. London: Springer-Verlag, pp. 223–278.

Lhatoo, SD, Faulkner, HJ, Dembny, K, Trippick, K, Johnson, C, and Bird, JM (2010). An electroclinical case-control study of sudden unexpected death in epilepsy. Ann Neurol 68:787–796.

Lieb, JP, Joseph, JP, Engel, J, Jr, Walker, J, and Crandall, PH (1980). Sleep state and seizure foci related to depth spike activity in patients with temporal lobe epilepsy. Electroencephalogr Clin Neurophysiol 49:538–557.

Logothetis, J (1967). Spontaneous epileptic seizures and electroencephalographic changes in the course of phenothiazine therapy. Neurology 17:869–877.

Mattson, RH (1983). Seizures associated with alcohol use and alcohol withdrawal. In Epilepsy, Diagnosis and Management. Edited by TR Browne and RG Feldman. Boston: Little, Brown & Co, pp. 325–332.

Mayeux, R, Alexander, MD, Benson, DF, Brandt, J, and Rosen, J (1979). Poriomania. Neurology 29:1616–1619.

Montplaisir, J, Laverdiere, M, and Saint-Hilaire, JM (1985). A study of epileptic patients investigated with depth electrodes during sleep. Union Med Can 114:1019–1020.

Moshé, SL, Albala, BJ, Ackermann, RF, and Engel, J, Jr (1983). Increased seizure susceptibility of the immature brain. Dev Brain Res 7:81–85.

Mucha, RF, and Pinel, JPJ (1977). Postseizure inhibition of kindled seizures. Exp Neurol 54: 266–282.

Naquet, R, and Meldrum, BS (1972). Photogenic seizures in baboon. In Experimental Models of Epilepsy. Edited by DP Purpura, JK Penry, DB Tower, DM Woodbury, and RD Walter. New York: Raven Press, pp. 373–406.

Nashef, L, and Tomson, T (2008). Sudden death in epilepsy. In Epilepsy: A Comprehensive Textbook, 2nd ed. Edited by J Engel, Jr, and TA Pedley. Philadelphia: Lippincott Williams & Wilkins, pp. 1991–1998.

Nelligan, A, Bell, GS, Johnson, AL, Goodridge, DM, Shorvon, SD, and Sander, JW (2011). The long-term risk of premature mortality in people with epilepsy. Brain 134:388–395.

Newmark, ME, and Penry, JK (1979). Photosensitivity and Epilepsy: A Review. New York: Raven Press.

Newton, MR, Berkovic, SF, Austin, MC, Rowe, CC, McKay, WJ, and Bladin, PF (1992). Postictal switch in blood flow distribution and temporal lobe seizures. J Neurol Neurosurg Psychiatry 55:891–894.

Orringer, CE, Eustace, JC, Wunsch, CD, and Gardner, LB (1977). Natural history of lactic acidosis after grand mal seizures: A model for the study of an anion-gap acidosis not associated with hyperkalemia. N Engl J Med 297:796–799.

Pedley, TA (2008). EEG traits. In Epilepsy: A Comprehensive Textbook, 2nd ed. Edited by J Engel, Jr, and TA Pedley. Philadelphia: Lippincott Williams & Wilkins, pp. 171–181.

Pedley, TA, and Guilleminault, C (1977). Episodic nocturnal wanderings responsive to anticonvulsant drug therapy. Ann Neurol 2:30–35.

Penfield, W, and Jasper, H (1954). Epilepsy and the Functional Anatomy of the Human Brain. Boston: Little, Brown &Co.

Pritchard, PB, III, Wannamaker, BB, Sagel, J, and Daniel CM (1985). Serum prolactin and cortisol levels in evaluation of pseudoepileptic seizures. Ann Neurol 18:87–89.

Pritchett, EL, McNamara, JO, and Gallagher, JJ (1980). Arrhythmogenic epilepsy: An hypothesis. Am Heart J 100:683–688.

Rechtschaffen, A, and Kales, A (1968). A Manual of Standardized Technology, Techniques and Scoring System for Sleep Stages of Human Subjects. US Department of Health, Education, and Welfare, National Institutes of Health.

Reilly, EL, and Peters, JF (1973). Relationship of some varieties of electroencephalographic photosensitivity to clinical convulsive disorders. Neurology 23:1050–1057.

Rosciszewska, D, Buntner, B, Guz, I, and Zawisza, L (1986). Ovarian hormones, anticonvulsant drugs, and seizures during the menstrual cycle in women with epilepsy. J Neurol Neurosurg Psychiatry 49:47–51.

Rowe, CC, Berkovic, SF, Austin, MC, McKay, WJ, and Bladin, PF (1991). Patterns of postictal cerebral blood flow in temporal lobe epilepsy: Qualitative and quantitative analysis. Neurology 41:1096–1103.

Rushton, DN (1981). "Space Invader" epilepsy [letter]. Lancet 1(8218):501.

Ryvlin, P, Cucherat, M, and Rheims, S (2011). Risk of sudden unexplained death in epilepsy in patients given adjunctive antiepileptic treatment for refractory seizures: Ameta-analysis of placebo-controlled randomised trials. Lancet Neurol 10:961–968.

Saenz-Lope, E, Herranz, FJ, and Masdeu, JC (1984). Startle epilepsy: A clinical study. Ann Neurol 16:78–81.

Satishchandra, P (2003). Hot-water epilepsy. Epilepsia 44(suppl 1):29–32.

Schmidley, JW, and Simon, RP (1981). Postictal pleocytosis. Ann Neurol 9:81–84.

Schmidt, D (1982). The effect of pregnancy on the natural history of epilepsy: Review of the literature. In Epilepsy, Pregnancy and the Child. Edited by D Janz, M Dam, A Richen, L Bossi, H Helge, and D Schmidt. New York: Raven Press, pp. 3–14.

Shouse, MN, and Quigg, MS (2008). Chronobiology. In Epilepsy: A Comprehensive Textbook, 2nd ed. Edited by J Engel, Jr, and TA Pedley. Philadelphia: Lippincott Williams & Wilkins, pp. 1961–1974.

Shouse, MN, Bazil, CW, and Malow, BA (2008). Sleep. In Epilepsy: A Comprehensive Textbook, 2nd ed. Edited by J Engel, Jr, and TA Pedley. Philadelphia: Lippincott Williams & Wilkins, pp. 1975–1990.

Sillanpää, M, and Shinnar, S (2010). Long-term mortality in childhood-onset epilepsy. New Engl JMed 363:2522–2529.

Simon, RP, Bayne, LL, Tranbaugh, RF, and Lewis, FR (1982). Elevated pulmonary lymph flow and protein content during status epilepticus in sheep. J Appl Physiol Respir Environ Exerc Physiol 52:91–95.

Simon, RP (1985). Management of status epilepticus. In Recent Advances in Epilepsy 2. Edited by TA Pedley and BS Meldrum. New York: Churchill Livingstone, pp. 137–160.

Sperling, MR (2004). The consequences of uncontrolled epilepsy. CNS Spectr 9:98–109.

Sperling, MR, Pritchard, PB, III, Engel, J, Jr, Daniel, C, and Sagel, J (1986). Prolactin in partial epilepsy: An indicator of limbic seizures. Ann Neurol 20:716–722.

Steriade, M, McCormick, DA, and Sejnowski, TJ (1993). Thalamocortical oscillations in the sleeping and aroused brain. Science 262:679–685.

Sterman, MB, Shouse, MN, and Passouant, P (eds) (1982). Sleep and Epilepsy. New York: Academic Press.

Stevens, JR, Kodama, H, Lonsbury, B, and Mills, L (1971). Ultradian characteristics of spontaneous seizure discharges recorded by radio telemetry in man. Electroencephalogr Clin Neurophysiol 31:313–325.

Sutula, T, and Pitkänen, A (eds) (2002). Do Seizures Damage the Brain? (Progress in Brain Research, Vol 135). Amsterdam: Elsevier.

Tabaddor, K, and Balagura, S (1981). Acute epidural hematoma following epileptic seizures. Arch Neurol 38:198–199.

Takahashi, T (1987). Activation methods. In Electroencephalography: Basic Principles, Clinical Applications and Related Fields, 2nd ed. Edited by E Niedermeyer and F Lopes da Silva. Baltimore: Urban & Schwarzenberg, pp. 209–227.

Téllez-Zenteno, JF, Matijevic, S, and Wiebe, S (2005). Somatic comorbidity of epilepsy in the general population in Canada. Epilepsia 46:1955–1962.

Temkin, O (1945). The Falling Sickness: A History of Epilepsy from the Greeks to the Beginnings of Modern Neurology. Baltimore: Johns Hopkins University Press.

Terrence, CF, Jr, Wisotzkey, HM, and Perper, JA (1975). Unexpected, unexplained death in epileptic patients. Neurology 25:594–598.

Tilden, JT, Roeder, LM, and Steinschneider, A (eds) (1983). Sudden Infant Death Syndrome. New York: Academic Press.

Todd, RB (1855). Clinical Lectures on Paralysis, Disease of the Brain and Other Affections of the Nervous System. Philadelphia: Lindsay & Blakiston.

Truccolo, W, Donoghue, JA, Hochberg, LR, Eskandar, EN, Madsen, JR, Anderson, WS, Brown, EN, Halgren, E, and Cash, SS (2010). Single-neuron dynamics in human focal epilepsy. Nat Neurosci 14:635–641.

Van Buren, JM (1958). Some autonomic concomitants of ictal automatism: A study of temporal lobe attacks. Brain 81:505–528.

Weitzman, ED (1976). Circadian rhythms and episodic hormone secretion in man. Annu Rev Med 27:225–243.

Weitzman, ED, Czeisler, CA, and Moore-Ede, MC (1979). Sleep-wake neuroendocrine and body temperature circadian rhythms under entrained and nonentrained (free-running) conditions in man. In Biological Rhythms and Their Central Mechanisms. Edited by M Suda, O Hayaishi, and H Nakagawa. Amsterdam: Elsevier, pp. 199–227.

Weitzman, ED, Czeisler, CA, Zimmermann, JC, Moore-Ede, MC, and Ronda, JM (1983). Biological rhythms in man: Internal physiological organization during non-entrained (free-running) conditions and application to delayed sleep phase syndrome. In Sleep Disorders: Basic and Clinical Research. Edited by MH Chase and ED Weitzman. New York: SP Medical and Scientific Books, pp. 153–171.

Wolf, P, Inoue, Y, and Zifkin, BG (eds) (2004). Reflex Epilepsies (Current Problems in Epilepsy, Vol 19). Paris: John Libbey Eurotext.

Young, B, and Blume, WT (1983). Painful epileptic seizures. Brain 106:537–554.

Zifkin, BG, Andermann, F, Beaumanoir, A, et al. (eds) (1998). Reflex Epilepsies and Reflex Seizures (Advances in Neurology, Vol 75). Philadelphia: Lippincott-Raven Publishers.

Zifkin, BG, Guerrini, R, and Plouin, P (2008). Reflex seizures. In Epilepsy: A Comprehensive Textbook, 2nd ed. Edited by J Engel, Jr, and TA Pedley. Philadelphia: Lippincott Williams & Wilkins, pp. 2559–2573.

Chapter 10

Status Epilepticus

GENERALIZED CONVULSIVE STATUS EPILEPTICUS
Clinical Description
Epidemiology
Etiology
Treatment
Prognosis

ABSENCE STATUS EPILEPTICUS
Clinical Description
Epidemiology
Etiology
Differential Diagnosis
Treatment
Prognosis

EPILEPSIA PARTIALIS CONTINUA
Clinical Description
Epidemiology
Etiology
Differential Diagnosis

Treatment
Prognosis

FOCAL DYSCOGNITIVE (COMPLEX PARTIAL) STATUS EPILEPTICUS
Clinical Description
Epidemiology
Etiology
Differential Diagnosis
Treatment
Prognosis

SUBTLE STATUS EPILEPTICUS

FEBRILE STATUS EPILEPTICUS

NEONATAL STATUS EPILEPTICUS

EPILEPTIC BRAIN DAMAGE

SUMMARY AND CONCLUSIONS

There is no consensus on a definition for status epilepticus, but the traditional conceptual definition is: an epileptic seizure that is so frequently repeated or so prolonged as to create a fixed and lasting epileptic condition. Practically speaking, status epilepticus is a pathophysiological state where the natural homeostatic mechanisms that limit the duration or frequent repetition, of seizures fail. Determining when this is the case is the diagnostic challenge.

342

Status is not necessarily fixed and lasting and the terms "frequently repeated" and "prolonged" need to be quantified. Operationally, most investigators agree that repeated seizures associated with impaired consciousness should be considered status epilepticus when the recurrence rate does not permit full return of consciousness between events.

Although it is often stated in the literature that a fixed and lasting epileptic condition should continue for 30 minutes before it is called status epilepticus, this is not a functionally useful concept except for certain epidemiological studies. Clinically, it is not appropriate to wait 30 minutes before treating a condition as status epilepticus. Depending on the type of seizure, *impending status* can be diagnosed much more quickly. It is unusual, for instance, for a generalized tonic-clonic seizure in adults to last more than one minute, so if such a seizure persists for two or three minutes it can be considered impending status, and preparation for aggressive treatment might begin at this point. Focal dyscognitive seizures, however, can go on for two or three minutes, so the important diagnostic feature here is recurrence of a seizure before consciousness returns. Focal dyscognitive and generalized tonic-clonic seizures occurring in rapid succession with return of consciousness during the interictal state are called *serial seizures*. Consequently, a few generalized tonic-clonic seizures with prolonged postictal depression might meet these criteria for status epilepticus, whereas serial seizures can occur much more frequently and not be considered status. From a practical clinical point of view, however, serial seizures should be considered in the same category as status epilepticus and should be treated aggressively, because they can evolve into status and might cause serious complications in themselves.

Most types of epileptic seizures (Chapter 6) can manifest as status epilepticus. These different forms often require different approaches to management and have different prognoses. There is no official classification of status epilepticus, but a practical scheme for categorizing these disorders was suggested by Gastaut (1983), and an adaptation is the basis for the discussion here (Table 10–1). Although Gastaut classified *absence status* as *generalized nonconvulsive status*, some authors classify all status as either *convulsive*—generalized tonic-clonic, tonic, or clonic—or *nonconvulsive*,

including absence status and focal status with or without impaired consciousness. Others, however, consider focal motor status to be convulsive. In addition, the term *nonconvulsive status* is occasionally used to define a state of generalized epileptiform EEG discharges without gross motor manifestations in comatose patients, sometimes called *subtle status*. Because of this ambiguity, the term *nonconvulsive status epilepticus* will not be used here. Status can evolve to a point where generalized EEG discharges persist but there are no ictal motor movements at all, in which case it is referred to as *electrographic status epilepticus*. Electrographic status epilepticus can also occur without preceding clinical status epilepticus, as with the characteristic sleep EEG patterns of *continuous spike-and-wave during sleep (CSWS)*, and the associated *Landau-Kleffner syndrome* (Chapter 7). Furthermore, some patients with atypical absence and focal dyscognitive status can have continuous generalized spike-and-wave EEG patterns with only minimal behavioral impairment (*spike-wave stupor*).

Status epilepticus occurs because of the failure of those protective homeostatic mechanisms that normally act to terminate ictal events (Chapter 4). There are many reasons why this may occur for individual seizure types and given clinical circumstances; however, the important aspect of status epilepticus is that further changes can occur over a period of 30 minutes or so that cause the ictogenic process to become self-sustained and progressively pharmacoresistant (Wasterlain and Chen, 2008). Recent research in animal models of status epilepticus, confirmed to some extent in patients, indicates maladaptive receptor trafficking involving the internalization of γ-*aminobutyric acid A (GABA$_A$) receptors* and externalization of N-*methyl-D-aspartate (NMDA) receptors*. This explains why status becomes resistant to benzodiazepines and other GABA agonist drugs. Other alterations include structural rearrangement in the subunit composition of the GABA receptor; alterations in calcium and *calmodulin-dependent kinase II*; reduced chloride gradient across the neuronal membrane; depletion of inhibitory neuropeptides such as *dynorphin, galanin, somatostatin*, and *neuropeptide Y*; and increased expression of proconvulsant neuropeptides such as *tachykinins, substance P*, and *neurokinin B* (Wasterlain and Chen, 2008).

Table 10–1 **Classification of Status Epilepticus**

1. Generalized status epilepticus
    A. Convulsive status
        1. Tonic-clonic (grand mal)
        2. Tonic
        3. Clonic
        4. Myoclonic
2. Focal status epilepticus
    A. Epilepsia partialis continua
        1. Somatomotor
        2. Dysphasic or aphasic
        3. Adversive
        4. Somatosensory
        5. Elementary visual
        6. Autonomic
    B. Focal dyscognitive status
3. Neonatal status epilepticus

Based on the classification of Gastaut, 1983.

Some or most of these effects may be important in developing the self-sustained nature of several different types of status epilepticus.

GENERALIZED CONVULSIVE STATUS EPILEPTICUS

Clinical Description

TONIC-CLONIC STATUS EPILEPTICUS

The *tonic-clonic* form of *generalized convulsive status epilepticus*, also called *grand mal* or *major motor status epilepticus*, is the most common and serious of all status conditions (Treiman, 2008; Towne, 2010). Recurrent generalized tonic-clonic seizures (Chapter 6) occur with no return of consciousness during the interictal state. Most persons with generalized tonic-clonic status epilepticus have localized cerebral disturbances and, therefore, have secondarily generalized focal seizures (Hauser, 1983). Some have discrete, identifiable initial focal ictal symptoms, but others may experience generalization so quickly that the focal onset is missed.

Tonic-clonic status epilepticus is a medical emergency, because brain damage and death can result from systemic consequences of repeated tonic-clonic seizures. Epileptic cerebral activity itself can also disrupt brain structure

or otherwise cause enduring neurological and intellectual deficits (discussed in the final section of this chapter). Therapeutic intervention, therefore, must be directed at stopping the epileptic process, as recorded on EEG, and not just the behavioral manifestations.

The initial recurrent ictal events of tonic-clonic status epilepticus resemble the isolated tonic-clonic seizures described in Chapter 6. Over time, however, as status continues, a natural progression is reported to occur that can be characterized by a sequence of EEG patterns: (1) discrete seizures, (2) merging seizures with a waxing and waning amplitude and frequency of EEG rhythms, (3) continuous ictal activity, (4) continuous ictal activity punctuated by isoelectric "flat periods," and (5) pseudoperiodic epileptiform discharges on a flat background (Treiman et al., 1990; Treiman, 2008) (Fig. 10–1). This last stage is characteristic of *subtle status*, an acute epileptic encephalopathy associated with coma and intermittent subtle ictal motor movements such as nystagmus and clonic twitches, which can be unilateral or multifocal (Treiman, 1987; Hirsch and Friedman, 2011). Differential diagnosis between this end stage of tonic-clonic status epilepticus and acute anoxic, toxic, and metabolic nonepileptic encephalopathies associated with coma, myoclonic jerks, and pseudoperiodic (Fig. 10–2) or burst suppression (Fig. 10–3) EEG patterns, is often necessary in comatose patients in the intensive care unit and can be difficult when the more obvious preceding generalized tonic-clonic seizures have not been documented (Chapter 13). Because the term *subtle status* has been used inconsistently, including for other conditions that do not necessarily have an epileptic etiology, an alternative term, *status epilepticus terminans*, has been proposed (Hirsch and Friedman, 2011).

The frequent recurrence and subsequent progression of tonic-clonic seizures creates unique and life-threatening systemic disturbances (Table 10–2). *Hyperpyrexia* commonly occurs as a result of excessive muscular activity and is a preventable cause of permanent brain damage. Rectal temperature must be monitored, and paralyzing drugs instituted if necessary.

Cerebrovascular autoregulation fails during tonic-clonic status epilepticus, and cerebral blood flow becomes dependent on systemic

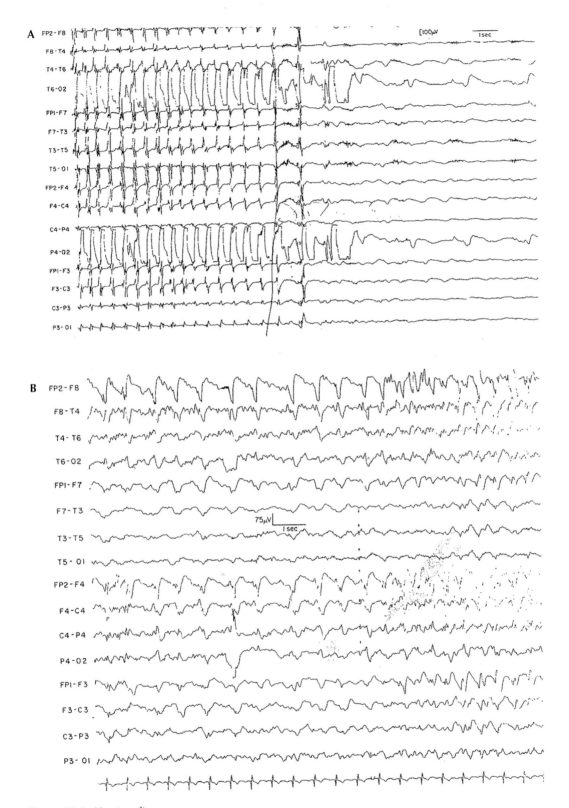

Figure 10–1. (Continued)

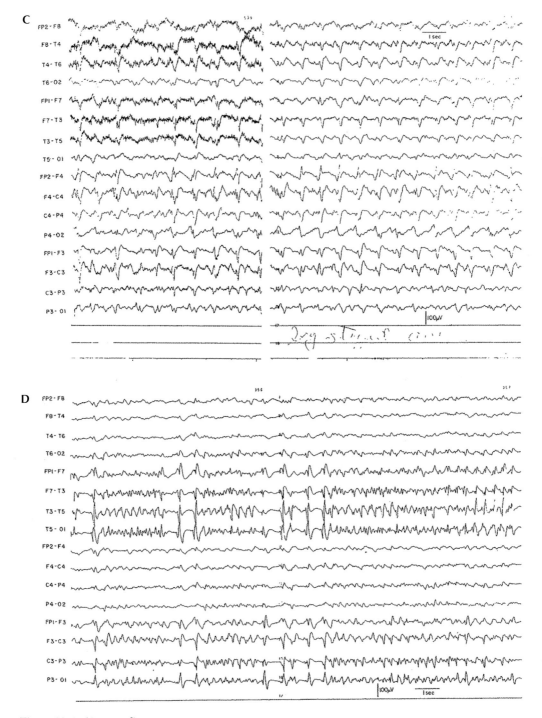

Figure 10–1. (Continued)

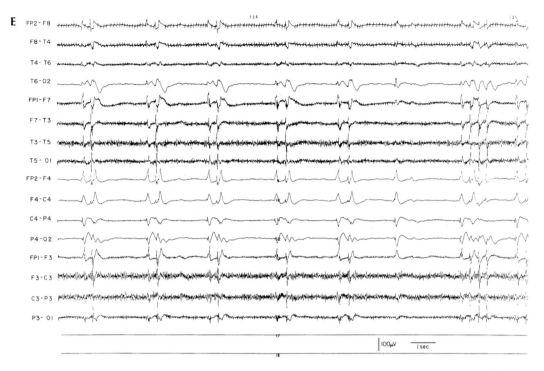

Figure 10–1. Characteristic EEG patterns for five stages of tonic-clonic status epilepticus. **A.** Discrete generalized tonic-clonic seizures with interictal slowing, recorded prior to treatment in a 39-year-old man. Example shows end of clonic phase of the seizure and the appearance of postictal slowing. **B.** Merging of discrete seizures, recorded prior to treatment in a 64-year-old man. Ictal discharges are continuous, but with waxing and waning of frequency and amplitude. An increase in frequency and amplitude can be seen beginning on the right side of the recording. **C.** Continuous ictal discharges recorded prior to treatment in a 68-year-old man. Examples are 16 minutes apart. Continuous ictal activity persisted for 101 minutes, stopping only after phenytoin infusion was completed and 4 minutes after the end of lorazepam infusion. **D.** Continuous ictal discharges with flat periods recorded prior to treatment in 68-year-old man. The seizure focus is clearly in the left hemisphere, but spread of ictal activity to the right hemisphere can be seen as well. **E.** Periodic epileptiform discharges on a flat background recorded prior to treatment in a 64-year-old man. (From Treiman et al., 1990, with permission.)

blood pressure (Plum et al., 1968), which initially rises and then falls. The early increase in cerebral perfusion compensates for increased metabolic demand, but the later hypoperfusion results in cerebral hypoxia (Ingvar and Siesjo, 1983; Meldrum and Nilsson, 1976). Hypoxia contributes to neuronal cell death, particularly in structures also subject to epileptic brain damage, such as the hippocampus, cerebellum, and neocortex (Meldrum, 1983). Consequently, maintenance of systemic blood pressure during major motor status epilepticus is important.

Although mild cerebral *edema* is a consequence of prolonged tonic-clonic status, initial increased intracranial pressure is related to arterial pressure and appears to reflect increased intravascular blood volume (Wasterlain, 1974). If markedly increased

intracranial pressure is present in the face of normal or low blood pressure, a mass lesion such as an abscess, a tumor, or a hematoma is likely.

Blood glucose can initially rise to 200 mg/dl, but after 15–30 minutes *hypoglycemia* can ensue. Controversy exists over whether hypoglycemia has a deleterious effect on the brain in status epilepticus. Raising the blood sugar level can prevent brain damage in newborn rats in status (Wasterlain and Duffy, 1976), but this effect is unique to the immature brain and occurs only when circulation is maintained. Hyperglycemia, on the other hand, appears to worsen ischemic brain damage in more mature animals, including rats (Blennow et al., 1978), monkeys (Myers and Yamaguchi, 1976), and humans (Pulsinelli et al., 1982). Nevertheless, the common practice of giving glucose initially

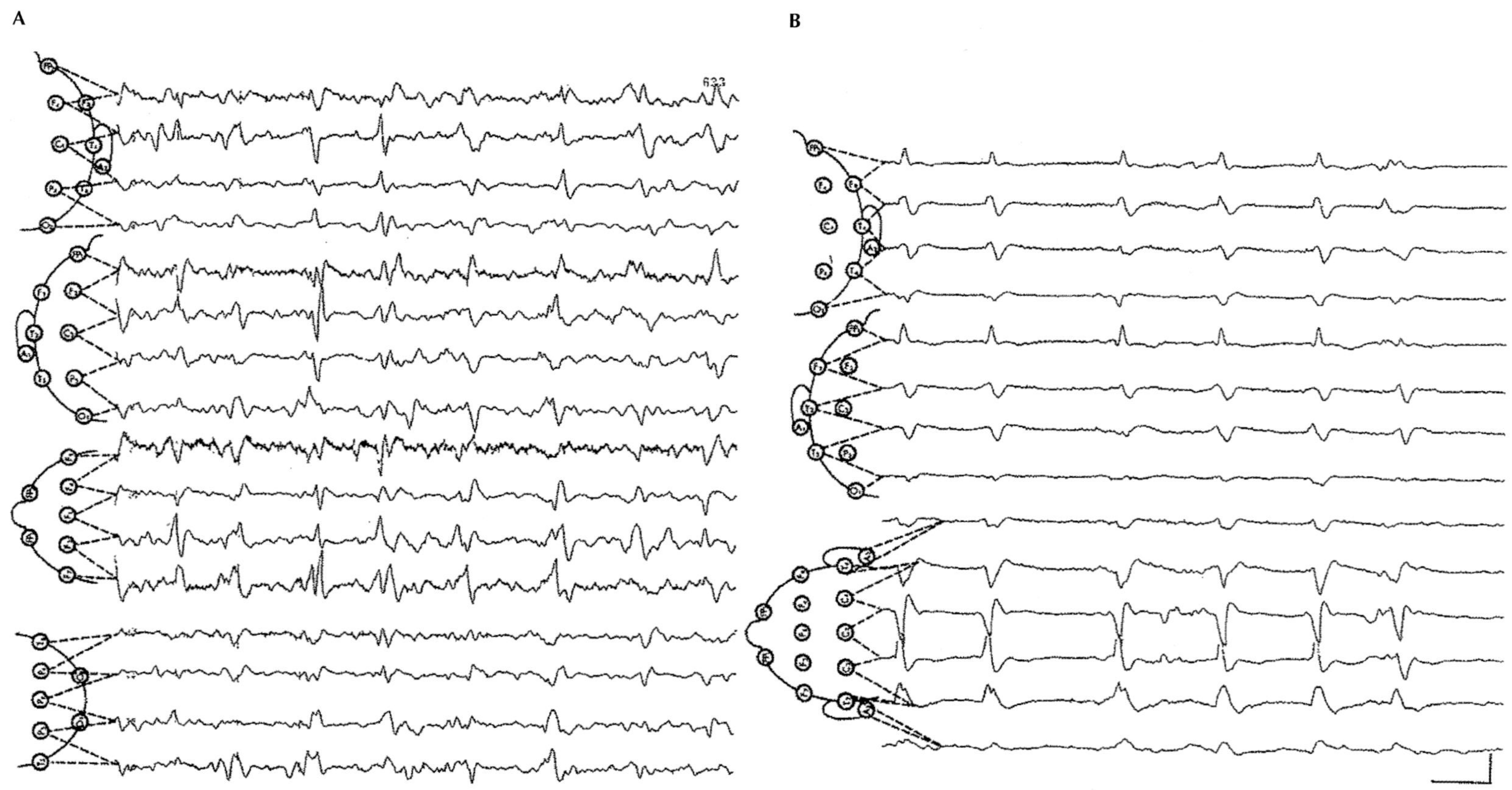

Figure 10–2. Segments of EEG tracings illustrating nonepileptic pseudoperiodic patterns. **A.** Pseudoperiodic discharges recorded from a 68-year-old man following a severe hypoglycemic insult. **B.** Recording from the same patient 6 days later shows progressive deterioration with loss of all background EEG activity and reduction in the frequency of pseudoperiodic transients. Intravenous pancuronium bromide was given to abolish muscle artifact. Note the similarities between these pseudoperiodic patterns and some of the electrographic correlates of generalized convulsive status epilepticus shown in Figure 10–1. Calibration: 1 second, 100 μV.

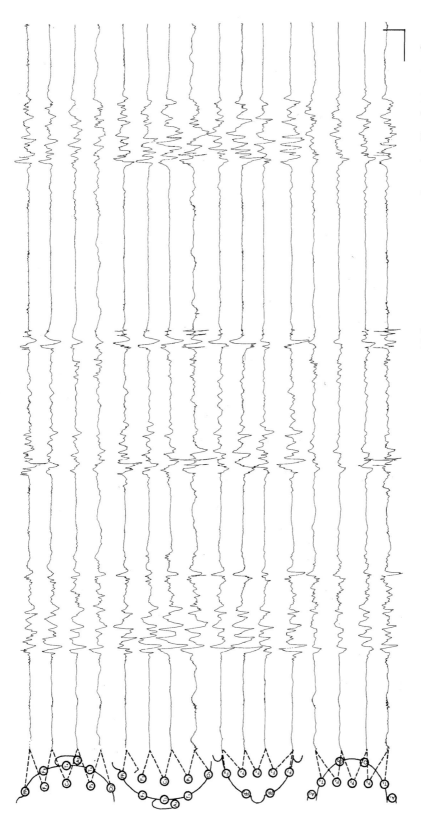

Figure 10–3. Segment of an EEG from a 30-year-old man showing a burst suppression pattern. Reversible burst suppression patterns may be produced by administration of anesthetic agents. This pattern should not be confused with patterns of generalized convulsive status epilepticus, seen in Figure 10–1. Calibration: 1 second, 100 μV.

Table 10–2 Medical Complications of Major Motor Status Epilepticus

Metabolic	Lactic acidosis
	CO_2 narcosis
	Hyperkalemia
	Hypoglycemia, hypertension, shock
Cardiopulmonary	Arrhythmias
	High output failure
	Pulmonary edema
	Pneumonia, aspiration
Renal	Acute tubular necrosis and myoglobinuria secondary to rhabdomyolysis
Autonomic	Hyperpyrexia
	Vomiting, loss of electrolytes and fluids
	Hypersecretions: sweat, salivation, tracheobronchial

in the treatment of generalized tonic-clonic status, in case the status was precipitated by hypoglycemia, is currently considered safe and appropriate.

Acidosis results from increases in lactic acid production and Pco_2. The latter can be due to apneic episodes during the seizures but is intensified if there is respiratory obstruction from soft tissue or secretions. There is also controversy concerning the importance of treating acidosis during status. Mild acidosis does not contribute to brain damage, and it exerts an antiseizure effect. Current practice, therefore, is not to give bicarbonate routinely. More severe acidosis, however, causes circulatory collapse and requires correction (Wasterlain, 1974).

Early reports that *hypoxia*, like hypoglycemia, may exert a protective effect (Blennow et al., 1978) have been retracted (Blennow et al., 1985; Soderfeldt et al., 1983). Status epilepticus–induced brain damage takes longer to develop when baboons are paralyzed and ventilated (Meldrum, 1983). Mild hypoxia may not be dangerous if cerebral perfusion is maintained, but severe hypoxia causes *hypotension* and cerebral hypoperfusion. Consequently, it is important that the airway be protected during generalized tonic-clonic status epilepticus, and nasal oxygen is routinely administered.

Morbidity associated with generalized tonic-clonic status epilepticus is also due to postictal complications, including cardiac and

circulatory collapse, pulmonary edema, electrolyte disturbances, aspiration pneumonia, and complications of medication (Simon, 1985). Myoglobinuria can result from massive muscular contractions and lead to renal dysfunction.

Consequences of the underlying disease processes constitute another source of potentially preventable morbidity and mortality. Intracerebral hemorrhage, contusion with edema, abscess, or other rapidly expanding space-occupying lesions can present as status epilepticus, and patients can die from cerebral herniation if these conditions are missed due to preoccupation with treatment of seizures. Toxic and metabolic causes of status epilepticus, such as severe hypoglycemia, can also be life threatening if not recognized early and treated specifically. In some instances, specific treatment of the underlying cause is sufficient to stop seizures.

OTHER FORMS OF GENERALIZED CONVULSIVE STATUS EPILEPTICUS

Tonic status epilepticus (Gastaut, 1983; Hartman, 2010) occurs most frequently in children and adolescents with epilepsy due to diffuse structural abnormalities, characteristically the *Lennox-Gastaut syndrome*. The seizures are less severe but repeated more frequently than in generalized tonic-clonic status and occasionally can be so mild as to be missed. Tonic status epilepticus is not usually associated with the life-threatening systemic changes of generalized tonic-clonic status epilepticus and may continue for days or weeks. The EEG typically shows *electrodecremental* events (Chapter 6) or generalized fast activity during tonic spasms. Intravenous benzodiazepines have been reported to cause tonic status, rarely, in patients with the Lennox-Gastaut syndrome (Bittencourt and Richens, 1981; Tassinari et al., 1972).

Clonic status epilepticus occurs mostly in infants and very young children; one-quarter of cases are due to an acute brain lesion, one-quarter due to a chronic encephalopathy, and one-half due to unknown causes but often associated with fever (Gastaut, 1983). The regularly recurring clonic movements are usually weak, bilateral but asymmetrical and asynchronous, and associated with generalized high-amplitude spike-and-wave discharges or low-voltage fast activity on the EEG. A unilateral form of clonic status epilepticus, usually with preserved consciousness, has been described following acute hemispheric insults in infants and young children with the *hemiconvulsions, hemiplesia, and epilepsy HHE syndrome* (Gastaut et al., 1960; Arzimanoglou, 2010; Arzimanoglou et al., 2008) (Chapter 7). Subsequently, there is transient or permanent hemiplegia on the affected side of the body, and later a chronic partial seizure disorder develops on that side.

Two types of *myoclonic status epilepticus* are recognized (Gastaut, 1983). First, prolonged episodes of bilaterally synchronous myoclonic jerks associated with preserved consciousness and multiple spike-and-wave discharges on the EEG occur rarely with *juvenile myoclonic epilepsy* (Chapter 7). There is no specified duration for which repeated myoclonic seizures must occur to be considered status epilepticus, but they must happen frequently and long enough to significantly impair function. It has been suggested that the criterion should at least be once every 10 seconds for longer than 10 minutes or once a minute for longer than 30 minutes (Gerard and Hirsch, 2010).

Second, and more commonly, bilateral asymmetrical and asynchronous myoclonic jerks associated with clouding of consciousness and irregular spike-and-wave and slow activity on the EEG occur in the generalized epilepsies associated with diffuse brain damage and are believed to be a variant of atypical absence status. Myoclonic status is a feature of the rare infantile epilepsy condition *myoclonic encephalopathy in nonprogressive disorders* (Dalla Bernardina et al., 1980; Dalla Bernardina, 2008) (Chapter 7). Continuous multifocal myoclonic jerks, which are not necessarily epileptic, can occur with a variety of myoclonic conditions (Chapter 7). Acute postanoxic myoclonus is the most common (Chapter 7), but others include *Creutzfeldt-Jakob disease* and acute toxic, metabolic, and infectious processes. Prolonged bursts of nonepileptic myoclonic jerks in these conditions should not be referred to as status epilepticus and have been called *myoclonic status* or *myoclonic storms*. As mentioned previously, however, these conditions in comatose patients may be difficult to distinguish from the end stages of generalized convulsive status epilepticus if the immediately preceding events are unknown (Chapter 13). When doubt exists,

it is best to treat these patients for generalized convulsive status.

Epidemiology

The annual incidence of generalized tonic-clonic status epilepticus is reported to be 0.18–0.28 per 1,000 in the United States and much higher in developing countries. Peaks in incidence occur in children and in the elderly (Treiman, 2008). Some form of status has been reported in 1.3–16% of patients with epilepsy (Hauser, 1983). More than half of these patients have generalized convulsive status, with most having had focal seizures that secondarily generalized. In children, generalized convulsive status epilepticus, including tonic and clonic status, is most common (Aicardi and Chevrie, 1970). Hauser and Kurland (Hauser and Kurland, 1975) have reported that 12% of initial epileptic seizures last longer than 30 minutes and that 5% of children with febrile seizures experience an ictal event lasting longer than 30 minutes.

Etiology

Most patients with generalized convulsive status epilepticus have cerebral lesions (Hunter, 1959/60; Janz, 1961; Oxbury and Whitty, 1971; Treiman, 2008; Towne, 2010). Etiologies differ for adults and children. Children tend to have static or progressive encephalopathies; adults have localized lesions, most often in the frontal lobe (Janz, 1961). The common lesions in adults are those that cause focal epileptic disorders, particularly CNS infections, vascular insults, trauma, and brain tumors (Chapters 5 and 7). Numerous uncommon causes of status epilepticus have been documented, including immune-mediated conditions such as *NMDA receptor encephalitis* and *Hashimoto's disease*; mitochondrial diseases; opportunistic infections; and toxins such as *domoic acid* and certain GABAergic drugs, specifically *tiagabine* and *vigabatrin* (Tan et al., 2010; Shorvon et al., 2011). Diagnosis of cause can be particularly difficult and important in children, and there are no accepted assessment standards for performing diagnostic tests such as lumbar puncture, neuroimaging, blood cultures, toxicology, or metabolic studies (Riviello et al., 2006; Tan et al., 2010; Shorvon et al., 2011).

In patients with epilepsy, generalized convulsive status epilepticus is commonly triggered by the same precipitating factors that induce reactive epileptic seizures in nonepileptic individuals (Chapter 5). Therefore, frequently repeated seizures can develop in persons with epilepsy as a result of acute nonspecific and transient cerebral insults. The most common precipitating factor is a fall in the plasma level of an antiseizure drug for a variety of reasons, including noncompliance and drug-drug interactions. Other factors include fever; metabolic disturbances such as hypoglycemia, hypocalcemia, and hyponatremia, particularly when the fall in sodium is rapid; hyperosmolality due to hyperglycemia, hypernatremia, and uremia, although these can often cause focal motor status (Berkovic et al., 1982; Singh and Strobos, 1980); exposure to convulsant drugs; toxins; infections; and withdrawal from sedative and hypnotic drugs, including alcohol. Status epilepticus also commonly presents in people without a prior diagnosis of epilepsy, as a result of an acute cerebral insult or as the first presentation of an epilepsy condition.

Treatment

Because generalized tonic-clonic status epilepticus becomes increasingly pharmacoresistant with time, response to treatment is dependent on the timing of the therapeutic intervention. In one large study, treatment was effective in 56% of patients overall but in only 15% of patients with late-stage pseudoperiodic epileptiform discharges (Treiman et al., 1998). With failure to respond to the first treatment, only generalized anesthesia offered substantial improvement. The best prognosis is obtained with effective prehospital intervention by paramedics. Recent data suggest that *intramuscular (IM) midazolam* is at least as effective as *intravenous (IV) lorazepam*, because of the greater ease of IM administration (Silbergleit et al., 2012). The efficacy of *buccal midazolam,* commonly used in some countries, is under investigation (McIntyre et al., 2005).

A number of approaches to in-hospital treatment of generalized tonic-clonic status epilepticus all follow the same general principles: (1) restoration of homeostasis, (2) specific medical treatment of the epileptic seizures, and (3) institution of maintenance therapy. It is more important to be prepared with a particular therapeutic schedule in mind before this medical emergency arises than to try to determine what might be the best therapeutic schedule every time an admission occurs (Alldredge et al., 2008; Walker and Shorvon, 2009). One standard protocol is shown in Table 10–3, but others may be preferred. Management guidelines for treatment of status epilepticus in adults have been published by the European Federation of Neurological Societies (Meierkord et al., 2010) and the Neurocritical Care Society (Brophy et al., 2012).

The first step in treating tonic-clonic status is to secure an airway. The nasopharynx should be cleared and suctioned if necessary. It is usually inappropriate to attempt to intubate the patient at this point, because intubation is difficult and time-consuming during active seizures. However, preparation must be made to rapidly carry out the procedure later if indicated. A quick neurological examination is then required for evaluating critical forebrain and brain stem functions and ruling out acute intracerebral lesions causing herniation or other life-threatening conditions. Blood pressure should also be checked initially, and nasal oxygen given. Before the intravenous drip is begun, blood should be drawn for a complete blood count and measurement of glucose, urea nitrogen, electrolytes, and serum levels of antiseizure drugs as well as other drugs if there is a possibility that neuroactive agents are contributing to the condition. The intravenous line should be kept open with a slow drip of isotonic saline solution for subsequent administration of drugs. Hypoglycemia is a rare precipitating factor in status epilepticus; therefore, administration of 50 ml of a 50% glucose solution intravenously is recommended. In this case, 100 mg of *thiamine* intramuscularly or intravenously must be given before the glucose infusion to avoid precipitating *Wernicke's encephalopathy.* Stopping the seizure is the most effective means of correcting acidosis; however, if blood pressure falls, blood gases should be measured and pH imbalance corrected as appropriate (Engel et al., 1982).

In general, drugs should be injected directly into the vein by the physician, but many drugs can now also be administered as an IV drip. It is useful to have one favored drug regimen

Table 10–3 **Treatment Protocol for Generalized Convulsive Status Epilepticus**

Time (min)

0 Establish the diagnosis by observing one additional seizure in a patient with recent seizures or impaired consciousness or by observing continuous behavioral and/or electrical seizure activity for >10 minutes.

Start the EEG as soon as possible, but do not delay treatment unless EEG verification of the diagnosis is necessary.

5 Establish intravenous (IV) catheter with normal saline (dextrose solutions may precipitate phenytoin)— with fosphenytoin either dextrose or saline is acceptable.

Draw blood for serum chemistry, hematologic values, and antiseizure drug concentrations. Check for hypoglycemia by finger stick. If hypoglycemia is present, administer 100 mg of thiamine (if indicated) followed by 50 ml of 50% glucose by direct push into the IV line.

10 Administer lorazepam (0.1 mg/kg) by IV push (<2 mg/min).

25 If status continues, start fosphenytoin (20 mg/kg PE) by fast IV push (up to 150 mg PE/min) directly into the IV port nearest to patient; if only phenytoin is available, give by slow IV push (<50 mg/min); with either preparation monitor blood pressure and electrocardiogram during infusion. If status continues after 20 mg PE/kg fosphenytoin (or 20 mg/kg phenytoin), administer an additional 5 mg/kg and, if necessary, another 5 mg/kg, to a maximum dose of 30 mg/kg.

Alternatively give valproic acid (30 mg/kg) IV, at a rate up to 500 mg/min. If status epilepticus continues, administer an additional 15 mg/kg and, if necessary, another 15 mg/kg.

60 If status persists, support respiration by endotracheal intubation; give phenobarbital (20 mg/kg) by IV push (<100 mg/min) or, preferably, start barbiturate coma: give pentobarbital (5–15 mg/kg) slowly as an initial IV dose to suppress all epileptiform activity and continue 0.5–5 mg/kg/hour to maintain suppression; slow infusion rate periodically to determine cessation of seizure activity; monitor blood pressure, electrocardiogram and respiratory function. If unable to suppress all epileptiform activity, change to continuous infusions of propofol (1 mg/kg given over 5 min, then 2–4 mg/kg/hour; adjust to 1–15 mg/kg/hour) or midazolam (0.2 mg/kg bolus injection, followed by infusion of 0.05–0.5 mg/kg/h).

Maintain full suppression of epileptiform activity (not a burst-suppression pattern) for 48–72 hours before beginning to slow the infusion rate. Before beginning withdrawal of intravenous anesthesia, adjust phenytoin serum concentration to 30 μg/ml; load phenobarbital to achieve 100–150 μg/ml serum concentration. If VPA (valproic acid) has been used in the initial treatment, adjust VPA serum concentration to 150 μg/ml. Maintain these levels as the anesthetic agent is slowed. Intravenous levetiracetam (LEV) and/or lacosamide (LCM) are alternatives if PHT (phenytoin), VPA and/or PB (phenobarbitol) are contraindicated. Load LEV with 4 grams IV, maintain with up to 1000 mg q 6 hrs; load LCM with 400 mg IV, maintain with 100 mg q 6 hrs. Target 150 μg/ml of VPA; target serum concentrations for LEV and LCM are not known.

If epileptiform activity returns during lightening of the induced coma, increase the infusion rate of the anesthetic agent (pentobarbital, propofol, or midazolam) to suppress all epileptiform activity for another 48–72 hours before attempting anesthesia withdrawal again.

Repeat as many times as necessary. Do not give up. Patients have recovered consciousness after >2 months of coma.

From Seif-Eddeine and Treiman, 2011, with permission.

rather than switching from one drug to another on the basis of the most recent journal article or anecdotal report. Differences in efficacy of the various accepted practices (Treiman et al., 1998; Chen and Wasterlain, 2006) are often small, and the opportunities for serious errors when using unfamiliar drugs are great. There are, however, reasons for preferring particular drug strategies in individual situations (Table 10–4).

Ideally, antiseizure medications should act rapidly to terminate seizures as quickly as possible and have a long duration of action to prevent recurrence. The important pharmacokinetic values for drugs commonly used to treat status epilepticus are shown in Table 10–5. As can be seen, there is no single drug with both these ideal characteristics. Only one randomized controlled trial comparing the four most common initial treatment

Table 10–4 Drug Treatments for Generalized Convulsive Status Epilepticus

Drug	Dose/Route	Comments
Lorazepam	0.1 mg/kg IV, <2 mg/min	Fast acting, but can wait 12 hours before giving maintenance drug orally or IV fosphenytoin if necessary. May cause respiratory depression, apnea, or hypotension.
Diazepam	0.15 mg/kg IV, <5 mg/min	Fast acting, but must be followed immediately by fosphenytoin. May cause respiratory depression, apnea, or hypotension.
Fosphenytoin (Phenytoin)	20 mg/kg PE IV, <150 mg/min with ECG monitoring (<50 mg/min for phenytoin)	Takes 6–10 minutes to infuse (20–30 minutes for phenytoin). Slower to take effect than lorazepam or diazepam. Used to follow diazepam or lorazepam. Can be used alone if needed to preserve consciousness. May cause cardiac arrhythmia or hypotension.
Phenobarbital	20 mg/kg IV, <100 mg/min	Slower to take effect than lorazepam or diazepam, but also acts as a maintenance drug. Consciousness is impaired for a much longer period of time than with the benzodiazepines. May cause respiratory depression and hypotension.

PE = phenytoin equivalent (fosphenytoin PE dose = phenytoin dose multiplied by 1.5).

regimens for generalized tonic-clonic status epilepticus has been performed (Treiman et al., 1998). In that trial, *lorazepam* alone was successful in 65% of patients, *phenobarbital* was effective in 58%, *diazepam followed by phenytoin* was effective in 56%, and *phenytoin* was effective in 44%, leading to a recommendation against the use of phenytoin alone. There were no differences among these treatments with respect to adverse effects or outcome at 30 days after status. Lorazepam is currently the preferred choice because of its long duration of action, but diazepam and phenytoin have the advantage that consciousness can return more quickly when this might be of diagnostic importance. Phenobarbital is still preferred by some doctors, despite the fact that the therapeutic effect takes longer

Table 10–5 Pharmacokinetic Properties of Drugs Used to Treat Generalized Convulsive Status Epilepticus

	Diazepam	Lorazepam	Fosphenytoin Phenytoin	Phenobarbital
Route of administration	IV	IV	IV	IV
Time to enter brain	10 sec	2–3 min	1 min	20 min
Time to peak brain concentration		30 min	15–30 min	30 min
Effective serum concentration (μg/ml)	0.2–0.8	0.2	25	35–40
Time to stop status	1 min	<5 min	15–30 min	20 min
Effective half-life	15 min	14 hr	22+ hr	50–120 hr

Adapted from Treiman, 1983, with permission.

than with benzodiazepines and consciousness returns more slowly. Phenytoin is preferred by some doctors for serial seizures, but not for status, when there is a diagnostic reason to preserve consciousness. *Paraldehyde* was not tested in the randomized controlled trial and is no longer readily available in the United States for parenteral administration, but it can be an effective second-line drug under certain circumstances where it is available. Today, *fosphenytoin*, a water-soluble prodrug of phenytoin, is preferred for intravenous injection when a central line is not available, because it does not require formulation with *propylene glycol*, which causes severe tissue damage if extravasated (Chapter 15). Because fosphenytoin is not always available, the following discussion refers to either fosphenytoin or phenytoin, and fosphenytoin doses are given as *phenytoin-equivalent (PE)* dose (phenytoin dose multiplied by 1.5).

LORAZEPAM

Lorazepam is a benzodiazepine that has a smaller volume of distribution and therefore a longer duration of action than diazepam (Chapter 15). Lorazepam is given intravenously at a rate of 2 mg/min or less to a total dose of 0.1 mg/kg (Treiman, 2008). In a small percentage of patients, the administration of lorazepam leads to respiratory depression or arrest, hypotension, or both. The risk is greatest in the elderly or when barbiturates or other sedatives have already been given. Maintenance fosphenytoin need not begin as soon as the lorazepam infusion is completed because lorazepam will remain effective for at least 12 hours. If the patient regains consciousness within a few hours, additional intravenous medications may not be necessary. The advantage of lorazepam over diazepam, therefore, is its longer duration of action. Intravenous benzodiazepines should be given with caution in patients who are elderly or severely ill or who have already received sedative drugs.

DIAZEPAM

When beginning with an intravenous bolus of diazepam (Chapter 15), the recommended dose is 0.15 mg/kg at a rate of 5 mg/min or less (Treiman et al., 1998). In adults the usual practice is to give 10 mg over 2 minutes, repeating

the dose once if necessary. If an intravenous line is not obtained within 5 minutes in a small child, the appropriate dose of diazepam can be administered rectally. Diazepam is absorbed from the blood within seconds and from the rectum within minutes; failure of adequate response is rare unless a large structural lesion, such as hemorrhage or brain tumor, is present (Browne and Penry, 1973).

Because the effect of diazepam is often short, administration should be followed immediately with 20 mg/kg of fosphenytoin PE given intravenously. When two intravenous lines are in place, fosphenytoin can be given simultaneously with diazepam. An additional 7 mg/kg of fosphenytoin PE can be given if necessary to stop seizures. The recommended safe rate of administration of phenytoin is 50 mg/min or less, but fosphenytoin can be given at as much as 150 mg/min. Although fosphenytoin can be infused much faster than phenytoin, it is a prodrug of phenytoin and there is a delay for conversion to the active metabolite. Consequently, the time to antiseizure action is approximately the same for both drugs. Both require *electrocardiography (ECG)* and blood pressure monitoring. In small children, the infusion rate should be adjusted to allow complete administration over 10–20 minutes. At a maximum infusion rate it takes approximately 15–30 minutes after administration is complete for the serum level of phenytoin in the brain to peak at 25–30 µg/ml, the same time that the diazepam effect is dissipating. Maintenance therapy with fosphenytoin PE is usually begun the following day with a dose of 4–6 mg/kg/day divided into two or three portions.

Risks of respiratory depression and hypotension are the same as for lorazepam. Hypotension and cardiac arrhythmias may result from intravenous fosphenytoin administration. Infusion of fosphenytoin should be slowed or stopped if blood pressure drops below 90/60, the Q-T interval widens, or arrhythmias appear. *Dopamine* or other pressor agents may be necessary to support blood pressure in elderly or severely ill patients.

The advantages of this approach are the rapid institution of adequate levels of an effective anticonvulsant and maintenance of control with an equally effective longer-acting anticonvulsant that reaches peak levels as the first disappears from the brain. Intravenous fosphenytoin is contraindicated in patients with heart block, sinus bradycardia, hypotension, severe cardiac insufficiency, or fosphenytoin allergy and in patients with *progressive myoclonus epilepsy* or *juvenile myoclonic epilepsy*. These patients should be treated with phenobarbital as described below.

FOSPHENYTOIN

Fosphenytoin (Chapter 15) can be given as indicated above as the only treatment for serial seizures when it is important to preserve consciousness, but it is an inferior treatment for status epilepticus. Fosphenytoin alone, therefore, may be recommended for serial seizures resulting from severe head trauma or intracerebral hemorrhage when continuous neurological assessment is necessary and rapid termination of seizures is not the primary concern.

PHENOBARBITAL

Phenobarbital (Chapter 15) is an older method of treating tonic-clonic status epilepticus. It is given intravenously no faster than 100 mg/min to a dose of 20 mg/kg or until seizures stop. This is sufficient to achieve a serum level of 30–40 μg/ml. The main disadvantage of phenobarbital is its relatively slow time to reach peak brain concentrations, approximately 30 minutes, although seizure control can be achieved within 10–15 minutes. Sudden respiratory depression and hypotension during the initial phases of administration may be less likely with phenobarbital than with the benzodiazepines, but delayed respiratory and circulatory depression are common. These complications inevitably develop with higher doses, and intubation is necessary if seizures are not easily controlled early. After control with an intravenous bolus, serum drug levels will remain high for 24 hours; thereafter maintenance therapy can be instituted. With this approach, consciousness remains impaired for some time after the initial treatment, which makes adequate neurological examination impossible. Phenobarbital is generally recommended as a second-line drug if lorazepam or the combination of diazepam and phenytoin fails. It is still used as a first-line drug by a few doctors (Shaner et al., 1988) and is preferred when the precipitating factor is phenobarbital withdrawal, in patients in whom benzodiazepines

and phenytoin are contraindicated, and in the treatment of neonatal status (Chapter 7).

PARALDEHYDE

Parenteral paraldehyde (Chapter 15) (which is unavailable in the United States) rapidly peaks in the brain when administered intravenously as a 4% solution diluted in normal saline. The intravenous dose can be titrated, beginning with 50–100 ml/hr and increased by 50–100 ml/hr if needed. It reaches a peak level in 20 minutes after intramuscular injection, 5–10 ml (5 cc per site), and can also be given rectally, 5–10 ml as a 2:1 dilution in mineral oil or in 200 ml of 0.9% NaCl. It is dangerous to give paraldehyde by nasogastric tube, because aspiration can cause pulmonary hemorrhage, but 5–10 cc can be safely administered by this route if the patient is intubated and the cuff is inflated. The effective half-life is approximately 6 hours. Laryngospasm can be a problem with rapid intravenous injections. Plastic syringes cannot be used, because they are dissolved by the drug, but modern plastic intravenous infusion sets are safe with a 4% solution. The drug decomposes with prolonged storage, especially when exposed to light, and can then induce profound acidosis. It has a shelf life of 36 months but should not be kept more than 24 hours after opening. Paraldehyde was particularly useful in severe renal or hepatic failure, because it is predominantly excreted through the lungs; when intramuscular administration was necessary or preferable; and for status due to alcohol withdrawal (Mattson, 1983). Unfortunately, the production of sterile injectable paraldehyde has been discontinued in the United States, and its future in this country is unknown.

OTHER DRUGS

Valproic acid (Chapter 15) is available in an intravenous formulation and has efficacy against status epilepticus (Wasterlain and Chen, 2008; Walker and Shorvon, 2009). Potential advantages are a low incidence of respiratory and cardiac depression, but there is a risk of prolonged bleeding time, hepatic dysfunction, pancreatitis, and hyperammonemia. The usual dose is 20 mg/kg over 2–5 minutes followed by 10 mg/kg 10 minutes later, then by infusion at 5 mg/kg/hr. Valproic acid is contraindicated in patients with mitochondrial myopathies. *Levetiracetam* (Chapter 15) is also available in intravenous formulation and has been used to treat status epilepticus in doses ranging from 500 to 7,500 mg (Wasterlain and Chen, 2008); however, the usual dose is 4,000 mg. The major advantage of levetiracetam is the lack of hepatic metabolism and drug interactions. Valproic acid or levetiracetam are preferred to fosphenytoin by some doctors for use with diazepam. Several case studies have found *topiramate* (Chapter 15) to be effective in treating status epilepticus when administered via nasogastric tube at 300–1,600 mg/day in adults or 3–10 mg/kg/day in children (Wasterlain and Chen, 2008). Because of the enhanced availability of NMDA receptors in late pharmacoresistant status epilepticus, NMDA antagonists have been used to treat this condition (Wasterlain and Chen, 2008). Most of these drugs have prohibitive toxic effects, particularly psychosis, and are not recommended for clinical use; however, *ketamine* at 1.5 mg/kg/day intravenously has been considered for short-term use. *Lacosamide* may also be a treatment option for status (Chen et al., 2010).

GENERAL ANESTHESIA

At some point after failure of two drugs (including benzodiazepines, fosphenytoin, phenobarbital, and more recently also valproic acid and levetiracetam), a condition called *refractory status*, it becomes necessary to consider *general anesthesia*. The common agents used for drug-induced coma as a treatment for generalized tonic-clonic status epilepticus are *pentobarbital*, *midazolam*, and *propofol*. There are no comparison trials, and the literature is inconsistent concerning relative efficacy (Claassen et al., 1992; Shorvon and Ferlisi, 2011). Inhalant anesthetics are not considered first-line drugs for treatment of refractory status epilepticus. Coma is carried out under EEG control to achieve EEG silence or *burst suppression* (see Fig. 10–3). There are no data to support preferring EEG silence over burst suppression; however, because it can be difficult to discriminate burst suppression from ongoing epileptic activity, complete EEG silence is a safer option. The patient can be maintained in this state with ventilatory support for hours or days, if necessary. The usual practice is to begin to reduce the drug infusion

after 24 hours to determine whether or not epileptiform discharges and epileptic seizures recur (Simon, 1985; Alldredge et al., 2008; Walker and Shorvon, 2009; Meierkord et al., 2010). It is generally a good idea to administer a loading dose of fosphenytoin, phenobarbital, or other maintenance antiseizure medication before attempting to reduce the rate of infusion of the coma-inducing drug. Decerebrate posturing and burst suppression EEG patterns occur as patients are coming out of barbiturate coma and should not be mistaken for recurrence of epileptic seizures.

ALTERNATIVE TREATMENTS

When all else fails and a surgically resectable lesion can be identified, surgical treatment may be effective (Chapter 16) (Gorman et al., 1992). Anecdotal reports of novel therapies exist in the literature. These include the successful use of serial *electroconvulsive therapy (ECT)* (Kamel et al., 2010) and hypothermia (Corry et al., 2008). Other than surgery when appropriate, however, the place of alternative therapies for refractory status epilepticus has not been established.

EEG MONITORING, VENTILATION, AND FOLLOW-UP

As the initial treatment plan proceeds, respiration should be closely monitored; depression indicates the immediate need for intubation and ventilatory support. If intubation is required while seizures continue or if laryngospasm occurs, it is occasionally necessary to paralyze the patient. Rectal temperature should be monitored, because hyperpyrexia can lead to brain damage. Body temperature can be controlled by cooling and paralysis. Although EEG monitoring during the initiation of treatment for generalized tonic-clonic status epilepticus would be ideal, this is not always possible, and treatment should never be delayed until EEG is available. An EEG should be obtained, however, if patients do not begin to regain consciousness after effective therapy has been instituted, especially if sedative drugs are used. EEG monitoring is essential if general anesthesia or muscular paralysis is required, because electroclinical dissociations occur. Results of blood studies drawn before treatment was begun, careful history, and other evaluations, including structural imaging studies, might indicate a cause of status that requires specific treatment. Serum *neuron-specific enolase (NSE)* has been proposed as a prognostic marker of brain injury in status epilepticus (DeGiorgio et al., 1995).

The objective of treatment for generalized tonic-clonic status epilepticus is to intervene as rapidly as possible with the appropriate medication at adequate doses. Inadequate response to treatment most commonly results from giving too little medication, giving a drug too slowly or by the wrong route, failing to repeat the dose if the initial dose is not effective, failing to identify a treatable underlying cause, and failing to institute maintenance treatment once the status is initially broken. Mortality and morbidity in status epilepticus are directly related to the duration of time before seizures stop. Once the status has been effectively controlled, maintenance therapy should be instituted. If control has been achieved with a drug that can also be given as chronic therapy, this drug can be continued as indicated earlier. If the patient has been taking long-term antiseizure medication, however, it is usually best to reinstitute the previous regimen. Every effort must be made to identify the precipitating factors responsible for status and to take steps to prevent their recurrence.

Tonic, clonic, and myoclonic status epilepticus in an unconscious patient should be treated according to the same protocol as generalized tonic-clonic status. Nonepileptic myoclonic status in a conscious patient, however, is not an emergency. This is not generalized convulsive status epilepticus; although jerks may respond to benzodiazepines, more aggressive treatment with anesthetics is inappropriate.

Prognosis

Morbidity and mortality in generalized tonic-clonic status epilepticus is largely determined by the underlying etiology and appropriate treatment. Mortality rates have been reported to range from 1% to 50%, reflecting variability in the populations under study, and depend to a large extent on the underlying cause (Treiman, 2008). One study comparing mortality rates in the community to those at a university center found them to be 31% and 27%, respectively, and not significantly different (DeLorenzo et al., 2009). The risk of death with status epilepticus

of unknown cause is also high, particularly in the elderly (Logroscino et al., 1997; 2008). Morbidity and mortality are lower in children than in adults (Maytal et al., 1989). The severity of brain damage following status epilepticus depends on the duration of status, with neurological sequelae more common if status lasts longer than 2 hours (Aminoff and Simon, 1980; Rowan and Scott, 1970). Approximately two-thirds to three-quarters of patients who survive generalized tonic-clonic status epilepticus have no permanent sequelae. In one study, subsequent neurological or mental impairment was attributed to the underlying lesion in two-thirds of patients and to the seizures in one-third (Aminoff and Simon, 1980). *Acute hemiplegia, mental deficiency,* and *chronic recurrent seizures* are most often cited as sequelae of prolonged status in infants and children (Aicardi and Chevrie, 1983; Dalla Bernardina, 2008), but it is difficult to determine when these problems are a direct result of epileptic activity.

ABSENCE STATUS EPILEPTICUS

Clinical Description

Absence status (*spike-wave stupor*) refers to a condition of continuous clouding of consciousness associated with bilaterally synchronous spike-and-wave discharges on the EEG (Pulsinelli et al., 1982; Thomas and Snead, 2008; Koutroumanidis et al., 2010). The term *twilight state* has been applied to absence status but is also used to refer to *focal dyscognitive (complex partial) status epilepticus* and prolonged confusional states that might be postictal (Chapter 9). The term *petit mal status* (Lennox, 1945) is also used, but absence status occurs with lesional generalized epilepsies, such as the Lennox-Gastaut syndrome, and not only with *petit mal epilepsy*. When absence status occurs in patients with a diagnosis of a genetic absence epilepsy, usually of the juvenile type (Chapter 7), the EEG usually demonstrates irregular, slower spike-and-wave discharges that cannot be distinguished phenomenologically from atypical absence status of the lesional generalized epilepsies. Absence status can also occur sporadically as an acute confusional state in older adults with no prior history of epilepsy and no apparent cause (Ellis and Lee, 1978), and a similar pattern is seen as a manifestation of focal lesions, usually of the frontal lobe (Williamson et al., 1985).

The predominant behavioral manifestation of absence status in all cases is invariably depression in mental state, which may be so minimal as to go unnoticed by most observers who do not know the patient well. Other features of absences can occur, such as blinking and clonic movements of facial muscles or automatisms. Absence status can persist for days or even months.

Epidemiology

Eighty to 90% of patients with absence status have a genetic generalized epilepsy, usually an absence epilepsy (Thomas and Snead, 2008). Three percent of all patients with a genetic generalized epilepsy and 10% who continue to have absences into adulthood will experience absence status (Hauser, 1983). Fifteen to 40% of patients with generalized epilepsies due to diffuse encephalopathic disturbances will experience absence status (Thomas and Snead, 2008). Absence status is rare before the age of 10.

Etiology

There is undoubtedly more than one cause of absence status epilepticus, and the mechanistic relationship between the typical absence status epilepticus seen in the genetic generalized epilepsies, particularly juvenile absence epilepsy, and the atypical absence status epilepticus that is a manifestation of the lesional generalized epilepsies is unknown. Some forms of absence status can have a focal onset (Niedermeyer et al., 1979; Rothner and Morris III, 1987; Williamson et al., 1985). Some studies suggest that the distinction between absence status and focal dyscognitive status, particularly of frontal lobe origin, may not be well defined (Williamson et al., 1985). The etiology of the sporadic form of absence status occurring in adulthood is unknown (Ellis and Lee, 1978). In most cases, no clear precipitating factors have been identified; however, hormonal factors associated with the menstrual cycle, childbirth, and menopause in women, as well as drug-related factors, appear to be important (Thomas and Snead, 2008). Several psychotropic drugs; some antiseizure drugs, including *carbamazepine*, phenytoin, and GABA agonists such as *tiagabine* and *vigabatrin*; and *metrizamide* used for myelography have been reported to precipitate absence status epilepticus in some patients (Pritchard and O'Neal, 1984; Rumpl and Hinterhuber, 1981; Thomas and Snead, 2008). Generalized tonic-clonic seizures, either generalized from the start or secondarily generalized from a focal seizure, can occasionally be followed by an electroclinical state that resembles absence status (Bauer et al., 1982). This condition may be similar to the end stage of tonic-clonic status epilepticus described earlier or to the adult sporadic and pharmacologically induced forms of absence status.

Differential Diagnosis

Absence status epilepticus can usually be diagnosed easily by the characteristic EEG pattern, but ordering an EEG requires a high degree of suspicion. This condition is readily recognized when it occurs in a patient who has a history of generalized epilepsy. However, when it occurs as an initial symptom, particularly in later life or as a result of therapeutic intervention with a drug, it can easily be mistaken for psychiatric or toxic metabolic disturbances (Chapter 13). When an absence-like status occurs after a generalized tonic-clonic seizure, distinction from postictal confusion is important so that specific treatment can be instituted. An EEG should be obtained in any case of unexplained prolonged confusion, and absence status should be particularly suspected if blinking, automatisms, or other behaviors characteristic of absences (Chapter 6) are part of the clinical picture. Differential diagnosis between some forms of absence status and some prolonged atypical dyscognitive focal seizures may not be possible, because these might be variations of the same phenomenon (Chapter 6).

Treatment

Absence status epilepticus can be aborted early by antiabsence drugs such as *ethosuximide* and *valproic acid*. Once the condition is well under way, however, it is effectively treated with intravenous benzodiazepines or valproic acid (Browne and Penry, 1973; Dreifuss, 1983;

Walker and Shorvon, 2009). The adult form of absence status without a previous history and the postictal absence-like status respond to the protocol outlined for convulsive status epilepticus, indicating that the pathophysiological mechanisms underlying these disorders are different from those that produce childhood absences. Usually, the sporadic adult onset and postictal forms of absence status can be treated easily, but the forms in children with lesional generalized epilepsies can be extremely refractory to medication. Because the seizures are not life-threatening and permanent damage is unproven, treatment of these children with general anesthesia is usually not recommended. However, persistent absence-like status of adults with clouded consciousness may be difficult to differentiate from end-stage tonic-clonic status epilepticus. In this situation, seizures should be treated aggressively.

Prognosis

The prognosis for patients with absence status is variable and depends more on the underlying disease process than the epileptic manifestation. Although some forms of absence status in children may contribute to mental impairment (Doose, 1984), the prognosis is excellent for patients who have no identifiable cause for their absence status, regardless of how similar it may appear behaviorally and electroencephalographically to that associated with the lesional generalized epilepsies.

EPILEPSIA PARTIALIS CONTINUA

Clinical Description

The term *epilepsia partialis continua* (*simple partial status* in the 1981 terminology) can be used for all forms of focal status in clear consciousness, but it is most often applied to the continuous clonic focal motor seizures of *Kojewnikow syndrome* (Kojewnikow, 1895; Wieser and Chauvel, 2008; Sinha, 2010a;b), which is now considered a seizure type rather than a syndrome (Engel, 2006). Less common forms of epilepsia partialis continua include (1) *dysphasic* or *aphasic status epilepticus*, which consists of repeated or continuous language disturbances, sometimes associated with alexia and agraphia, (2) *adversive status epilepticus*, which may involve head and eye turning or oculoclonic seizures alone, (3) *somatosensory status epilepticus* with persistent dysesthesias, (4) *elementary visual status epilepticus* with continuous scintillating phosphenes, (5) *autonomic status epilepticus* with continuous or recurrent episodes of abdominal pain or vomiting, headache, or other autonomic symptoms (Gastaut, 1983), and (6) continuous phenomena such as vertiginous, auditory, and psychic symptoms typically associated with limbic seizures. Another term for epilepsia partialis continua unassociated with motor signs is *aura continua*. Aura continua typically is unassociated with EEG alterations, leading to misdiagnosis, and in the case of continuous psychic ictal symptoms can be confused with psychiatric disorders (Wieser et al., 1985).

The focal motor seizures of Kojewnikow syndrome (Kojewnikow, 1895) can be caused by focal, multifocal, or diffuse brain lesions and undoubtedly include a number of subtypes. Two specific syndromes are recognized: one involves a diffuse unilateral chronic encephalitic process, and the other has a more focal origin (Wieser and Chauvel, 2008).

The *focal form* can begin at any age. The unifying feature is the presence of continuous, clonic, well-localized focal motor symptoms or *myoclonias*, without other disturbances or progression. The EEG shows a normal background with focal spike-and-wave discharges in the contralateral rolandic region, where a well-localized structural lesion usually exists.

The *encephalitic form* begins almost exclusively in childhood and is the principal feature of *Rasmussen syndrome* (Aguilar and Rasmussen, 1960) (Chapter 7). It is characterized by unilateral continuous or frequent intermittent focal motor seizures, usually with clonic components that can be exquisitely focal myoclonias or can evolve into dyscognitive focal or sometimes secondarily generalized seizures. The EEG can show focal spike discharges in the appropriate contralateral brain area. More often, however, there are multifocal abnormalities or only unilateral or diffuse slow-wave activity, with poorly defined or no focal or epileptiform features (Fig. 10–4). Brain tissue from the affected hemisphere reveals nonspecific inflammatory changes, and an autoimmune process is suspected (Chapter 7). In over half the patients,

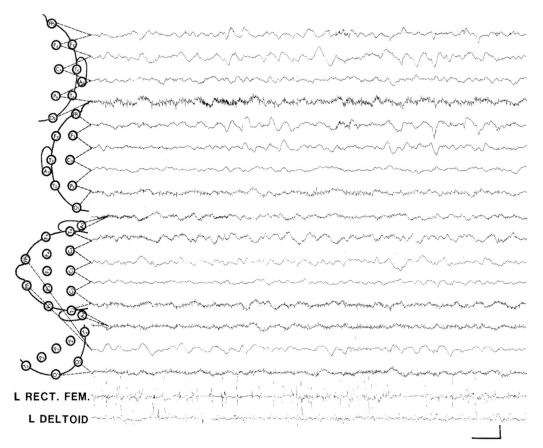

Figure 10–4. Representative segment of an EEG recorded from a patient with epilepsia partialis continua involving the left arm and leg. Bilateral high-voltage irregular slow activity is seen, somewhat more pronounced on the right. There is poor temporal correlation between these slow waves and the EMG activity (last two channels) recorded from muscles involved in the seizure. Calibration for EEG channels: 1 second, 100 μV. (From Engel et al., 1983, with permission.)

the *cerebrospinal fluid (CSF)* examination is normal (Rasmussen, 1978). Progressive focal motor deficits and mental deterioration usually occur.

Epidemiology

There are no well-documented statistics on the incidence of epilepsia partialis continua, but it is considered to be very rare (Wieser and Chauvel, 2008).

Etiology

The focal form of epilepsia partialis continua is likely to be associated with a discrete epileptogenic lesion such as a scar, brain tumor, or vascular compromise in or adjacent to the precentral gyrus. Pathological studies suggest that some degree of more diffuse or subcortical disturbance may also be necessary for manifestation of this syndrome (Juul-Jensen and Denny-Brown, 1966; Wieser and Chauvel, 2008). The common appearance of continuous focal motor seizures in elderly patients with postanoxic coma supports this possibility.

The encephalitic form is associated with a diffuse unilateral chronic inflammatory process (*Rasmussen syndrome*) (Chapter 7) and, historically, with the rare tick-borne virus of *Russian spring-summer encephalitis*. Inflammatory changes can be found throughout the affected hemisphere, and diffuse dysfunction may be necessary for symptoms to appear. Ictal metabolic patterns

A

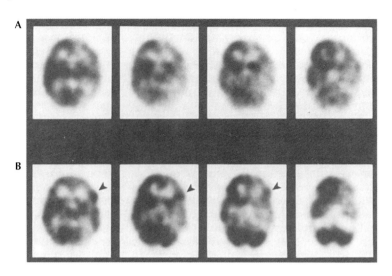

B

Figure 10–5. Interictal (**A**) and ictal (**B**) FDG-PET scans from the patient whose EEG is shown in Figure 10–4. The right hemisphere is relatively hypometabolic. In **B**, there appears to be a small area of increased uptake in the right frontal lobe (*arrowheads*). Quantitative analysis, however, revealed that there was increased metabolism of many areas in both hemispheres ictally, indicating diffuse participation in the seizure. (Note that older PET scans in this book are not reversed, right is on the right side and left is on the left side.) (From Engel et al., 1983, with permission.)

demonstrated by *positron emission tomography with* ^{18}F-*fluorodeoxyglucose (FDG-PET)* during continuous focal clonic discharges in one child with suspected Rasmussen syndrome substantiated diffuse cerebral involvement (Fig. 10–5), although more focal changes appeared in other such children (Engel et al., 1983). Why the inflammatory process should affect only one hemisphere of the brain is unknown.

Focal motor status can also be a manifestation of metabolic disturbances, most often *nonketotic hyperglycemia* (Singh and Strobos, 1980) and other hyperosmolar states. Presumably any structural lesion that can cause focal seizures in clear consciousness can cause epilepsia partialis continua. No particular precipitating factors exist in most cases.

Differential Diagnosis

Continuous sensory, autonomic, or psychic ictal phenomena may be extremely difficult to recognize as epileptic, and the scalp EEG may fail to identify an ictal discharge (Wieser et al., 1985). When these symptoms occur in a patient with a history of epileptic seizures and their features are consistent with previous, self-limited behavioral seizures, epilepsia partialis continua can be assumed. The diagnosis may be missed, however, in the rare situation when these symptoms are the only manifestation of an epilepsy disorder and the EEG fails to demonstrate a clear epileptiform abnormality (Chapter 13).

In some cases the distinction between epilepsia partialis continua of cortical origin and a subcortical myoclonic process is not clear. In fact, this condition has been called a form of cortical myoclonus by some authors (Gastaut, 1968; Hallett, 1985) (Chapter 6). It is conceivable that epilepsia partialis continua requires the presence of both a region of localized cortical irritability and diencephalic or brain stem disturbances similar to those seen with myoclonic disorders. The postulated necessity for both cortical and subcortical dysfunction is consistent with observations that cortical resections are not uniformly beneficial and EEGs frequently show diffuse or nonfocal abnormalities, at least in the encephalitic form.

It is particularly important to distinguish Rasmussen syndrome from other forms of focal epilepsy and from the focal form of epilepsia partialis continua, because of the relatively poor prognosis of the former and its general failure to respond to localized resective surgery. Evidence of symptom progression, such as development of focal paresis, other neurological and mental deficits, or cerebral hemiatrophy, suggests Rasmussen syndrome. A normal CSF examination does not rule out this diagnosis (Chapter 7). Recognition of the focal form is at least of theoretical clinical value because some patients with this condition might be candidates for neocortical surgical resection. Epilepsia partialis continua can usually be easily distinguished from movement disorders, tremors, asterixis, hemifacial spasm, and fasciculations by its abnormal EEG and by characteristic clinical features of the latter, nonepileptic phenomena (Chapter 13). When continuous focal clonic motor activity occurs during coma in acute encephalopathy, particularly when the pattern of muscle involvement is not proportional to representation in the motor homunculus, the condition is more likely to be a form of nonepileptic myoclonus or the end stage of generalized tonic-clonic status than epilepsia partialis continua. By definition, these latter events cannot be epilepsia partialis continua, because they involve impaired consciousness.

Treatment

Institution of treatment with intravenous *diazepam* or *lorazepam* followed by *fosphenytoin* is more effective in breaking epilepsia partialis continua than is slowly building an adequate therapeutic level with oral medication. The former should be tried if symptoms are particularly disturbing. When medication is ineffective, patients with focal lesions may be candidates for resective surgical therapy (Chapter 16). Focal status due to nonketotic hyperglycemia will respond to *insulin*, but may not to antiseizure drugs. Because epilepsia partialis continua is not a life-threatening condition, it usually does not require aggressive treatment. In some patients the symptoms are so mild that treatment or alteration in treatment may not be necessary at all.

Both forms of epilepsia partialis continua are notoriously refractory to medical treatment. Some patients experience meaningful improvement with the antiseizure drugs used for treating focal seizures, but complete control is rare. Hemispherectomy is the treatment of choice for Rasmussen syndrome (Chapters 7 and 16).

Prognosis

Response to treatment for epilepsia partialis continua is usually dependent on the cause, and not the epileptic manifestations. Some conditions, particularly the focal motor status associated with Rasmussen syndrome, can be extremely refractory to all reasonable attempts at therapy except surgery. There is no definitive

evidence that epilepsia partialis continua itself leads to focal brain damage.

FOCAL DYSCOGNITIVE (COMPLEX PARTIAL) STATUS EPILEPTICUS

Clinical Description

Focal dyscognitive status epilepticus usually consists of frequently repeated episodes of typical or atypical limbic seizures (Chapter 6) without full clearing of consciousness during the interictal state (Williamson, 2008). This causes a fluctuating mental state with least responsiveness during the ictal episodes and varying degrees of confusion in between. Occasionally, recurrent epileptic seizures cycle independently in both temporal lobes, producing an even greater variety of fluctuating symptoms (Engel et al., 1978). Rarely, dyscognitive focal status exists as a continuous clouding of consciousness, and this condition is difficult to differentiate clinically from absence status (Lugaresi et al., 1971; Williamson et al., 1985; Williamson, 2008).

Dyscognitive focal status epilepticus can continue for hours, days, or even weeks; is often followed by anterograde memory impairment; and occasionally gives rise to other postictal deficits if neocortical structures are involved. When status is prolonged, neurological sequelae can persist for months but can ultimately resolve (Engel et al., 1978; Engel et al., 1983) (Chapter 9).

A variety of focal features can be seen at the onset of focal dyscognitive status if seizures begin outside the temporal lobe. For instance, an occipital lobe origin can be associated with initial visual symptoms, such as hallucinations (Engel et al., 1983) or blindness (Engel et al., 1978). There are no reports of features that distinguish patients with dyscognitive focal seizures who are at risk for status from those who are not. The only clear risk factor appears to be previous occurrence of status. In some patients, dyscognitive focal status has been the presenting symptom of the epileptic disorder.

The EEG during the ictal phase may show unilateral or bilateral temporal low-voltage rhythmic activity, usually in the 5- to 7-Hz range, as described for typical limbic seizures, or more diffuse slow and sharp activity with focal features, as described for atypical limbic seizures (Chapter 6). If seizures begin extratemporally, the initial ictal EEG pattern may reflect onset at the appropriate cortical area. Typically, the ictal EEG discharge evolves, becoming higher in amplitude and slower, and ends with transitions to more diffuse, irregular slow activity during the interictal phase. The ictal EEG discharge may alternate from one side to the other, occur synchronously on both sides, or cycle independently on either side, but bilateral involvement to some extent is presumably necessary to produce impaired consciousness (Fig. 10–6). In the continuous form of dyscognitive focal status epilepticus, there are no clearly differentiated ictal and postictal EEG patterns.

Epidemiology

There are no data on the incidence of focal dyscognitive status epilepticus, and this condition was at one time believed to be exceedingly rare. However, with the proliferation of epilepsy centers, it has now been frequently documented (Williamson, 2008), although it is likely to go unrecognized in the community (Tomson et al., 1986; Williamson et al., 1985).

Etiology

The epileptogenic lesions that give rise to focal dyscognitive status epilepticus appear to be the same as those that cause dyscognitive focal seizures. Although these lesions are generally assumed to involve mesial temporal structures, a depth electrode study of eight patients suggested that focal dyscognitive status epilepticus often results from epileptic activity in the frontal lobes, at times with no mesial temporal involvement at all (Williamson et al., 1985). These patients had scalp EEG patterns indicating atypical, rather than typical, focal dyscognitive seizures (Chapter 6); without depth electrode recordings, some might even have been classified as having absence status. Consequently, some forms of absence status might actually be focal status of frontal lobe origin. In some cases of focal dyscognitive status epilepticus, there are identifiable precipitating factors, such as a fall in antiseizure drug level.

Differential Diagnosis

Differential diagnosis is essentially the differential diagnosis of confusional states (Table 10–6). The form of dyscognitive focal status epilepticus that consists of repeated epileptic seizures usually can be distinguished clinically from absence status, encephalopathies, and psychotic states (Chapter 13) by the fluctuating level of consciousness. The less common, continuous form can usually be recognized on an EEG examination, which requires a high degree of suspicion. Rare patients, however, cannot be reliably classified as having clear absence status or clear atypical dyscognitive focal status. When temporal low-voltage rhythmic activity is difficult to identify, prominent slowing can cause the condition to be confused with toxic, metabolic, and other nonictal organic disturbances. In this situation, the diagnosis may be aided by the use of sphenoidal or true temporal electrodes and paradoxical clearing of consciousness following intravenous *diazepam* or *lorazepam* injection (Chapter 13).

Treatment

Dyscognitive focal status epilepticus is treated initially as generalized tonic-clonic status; however, there has been controversy in the past concerning whether treatment should include general anesthesia if initial approaches fail. When standard therapies fail, the European Federation of Neurological Sciences guidelines (Meierkord et al., 2010) recommend treating with *phenobarbital, valproic acid, levetiracetam*, or some combination before considering general anesthesia. Although focal dyscognitive status epilepticus is not life-threatening, the prolonged postictal cognitive deficits cannot be explained on the basis of simple Todd's phenomena and may reflect actual structural changes that require reorganization before symptoms resolve (Chapter 9). Evidence is insufficient to indicate the risk of these deficits becoming permanent; however, many epileptologists believe that dyscognitive focal status epilepticus can produce enduring memory disturbances and lead to other types of cognitive impairment. Consequently, an argument can be made for terminating this condition as quickly as possible. Surgical therapy can be an

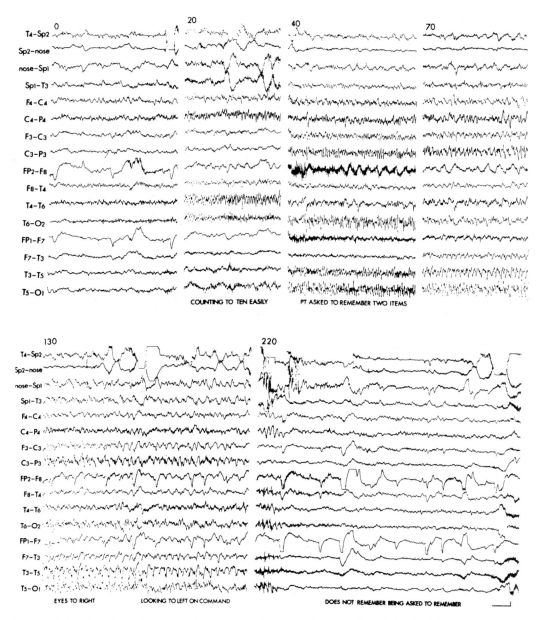

Figure 10–6. Selected samples from a sphenoidal-scalp EEG recording carried out during focal dyscognitive status epilepticus in a patient who demonstrated temporally independent ictal and postictal cycles of the left and right hemispheres. Numbers in the upper left corner of each EEG segment indicate the number of seconds elapsed from the beginning of the first segment. *0:* Fast activity begins to build up in the right temporooccipital area, while slow waves are seen on the left. *20:* Well-developed fast activity is seen on the right, and low-voltage fast activity is beginning to build up on the left; however, the patient is able to perform simple tasks. *40:* Fast activity is now well developed bilaterally, and the patient is asked to remember two items. *70:* Bilateral fast activity gives way to 4- to 6-Hz sharp waves, and the patient no longer responds to questions. *130:* Slowing appears on the right, while sharp waves are still present in the left temporooccipital area and the patient's eyes turn to the right; however, she is able to look to the left on command. *220:* Sharp activity is replaced by low-voltage slowing bilaterally, and the patient is responsive but has been amnesic for the past 3 minutes. Calibration: 1 second, 50 µV. (From Engel et al., 1978, with permission.)

Table 10–6 **Differential Diagnosis of Focal Dyscognitive Status Epilepticus**

1. Absence status epilepticus or spike-wave stupor
2. Other "epileptiform" causes of confusion
   Prolonged postictal confusion
   Delirium in cerebral infarction
   Confusion associated with PLEDs
   Poriomania
3. Organic encephalopathies
   Toxic-metabolic encephalopathies, especially hypoglycemia
   Alcohol and other drug intoxication or withdrawal
   Transient ischemic attacks
   Transient global amnesia
   Posttraumatic amnesia
4. Psychiatric syndromes
   Dissociative reactions
   Hysterical conversion reactions
   Acute psychotic reactions

PLEDs = pseudoperiodic lateralized epileptiform discharges.
Adapted from Treiman and Delgado-Escueta, 1983, with permission.

effective last resort if status is not broken by general anesthesia (Chapter 16).

Prognosis

There are insufficient case reports to make general statements concerning the prognosis of focal dyscognitive status epilepticus, although most patients do extremely well. Patients who experience one episode appear to have an increased susceptibility to recurrent episodes and are at risk for enduring postictal cognitive deficits.

SUBTLE STATUS EPILEPTICUS

As noted earlier, the term *subtle status epilepticus* has been used to define a variety of events characterized by continuous or frequent epileptiform EEG abnormalities in a comatose patient who may or may not manifest myoclonic jerks (Treiman, 1987; Hirsch and Friedman, 2011; Bauer and Trinka, 2010). This phenomenon can occur as a nonepileptic consequence of severe encephalopathy, as commonly occurs with post–cardiac arrest,

cerebral hypoxia, or other diffuse brain injuries; does not respond to antiseizure medications; and has an extremely poor prognosis. The nonepileptic nature of the myoclonic jerks can usually be identified by their anatomical distribution, corresponding to areas of the body, such as the *rectus abdominis* or *sternocleidomastoid*, with small representation in the motor homunculus of the precentral cortex. Focal epileptic myoclonus, by contrast, usually involves areas with large representation in the precentral cortex, such as the face and hands. Also, the motor activity in nonepileptic myoclonus is typically not temporally correlated with the epileptiform EEG transients, which are usually *pseudoperiodic lateralized epileptiform discharges (PLEDs)*. Although benzodiazepines may obliterate the movements and the EEG abnormalities, patients do not wake up from this condition, because their coma is due to the underlying brain insult. This situation is also seen as a very late stage of generalized tonic-clonic status epilepticus, as noted previously, and the term *status epilepticus terminans* has been recommended (Hirsch and Friedman, 2011).

Treatment is indicated for status epilepticus terminans; however, there is mounting evidence that this condition reflects profound brain damage caused by the prolonged status, rather than an epileptic process, because it has the same features seen in the severe posthypoxic states, it does not respond to antiseizure medications, and prognosis is extremely poor. Whether and when to treat, however, remains a controversial issue. When patients present with this scenario and it is undetermined whether they may have been in prolonged generalized tonic-clonic status epilepticus, treatment is also indicated until additional evidence becomes available to support the view that the condition is not epileptic. Frequent epileptic seizures and various forms of status epilepticus are encountered, however, in patients in coma. This has only become appreciated with routine use of EEG monitoring in intensive care units (Friedman et al., 2009; Vespa et al., 2010; Bleck et al., 2008). These seizures should be treated, and prognosis depends on the underlying cause; however, in this case, the altered consciousness could be due to status epilepticus and may be reversed by administration of benzodiazepines or other antiseizure medications.

FEBRILE STATUS EPILEPTICUS

Febrile status epilepticus in infancy is of increasing interest, because of the accumulating evidence that it could be a cause of *hippocampal sclerosis* and *mesial temporal lobe epilepsy* (MTLE). Febrile seizures occur in 2–5% of children, and in 5% of these they are prolonged beyond 30 minutes, meeting criteria for status epilepticus (Lewis and Shinnar, 2008). In a study of first febrile seizures, 14% lasted longer than 10 minutes, 9% longer than 15 minutes, and 5% longer than 30 minutes, and in another study, of those with febrile status epilepticus, 58% of seizures lasted 30–59 minutes, 24% from 60–119 minutes, 15% from 120–239 minutes, and 3% over 240 minutes (Lewis and Shinnar, 2008; Yoong and Scott, 2010). The bimodal distribution of febrile seizure duration supports defining 10 minutes as the upper limit of a simple febrile seizure and considering seizures longer than 10 minutes to represent febrile status epilepticus (Hesdorffer et al., 2011). Postictal *magnetic resonance imaging (MRI)* has now demonstrated that many patients with febrile status epilepticus will have hippocampal edema, and in some this goes on to become hippocampal sclerosis (Gomes and Shinnar, 2011). It remains to be seen how often these patients develop MTLE and how the development of this disorder relates to the presence of postictal hippocampal MRI changes. It is unclear whether febrile status epilepticus is itself a cause of hippocampal sclerosis as opposed to a symptom of an underlying disturbance that gives rise to both; perhaps status epilepticus in addition to an underlying disturbance is necessary for the manifestation of hippocampal sclerosis and subsequent chronic epilepsy. Seizure semiology is similar to the semiology of febrile seizures. Although retrospective studies suggest that febrile status epilepticus has a low morbidity and mortality, it is considered to be a serious medical emergency in infancy, and aggressive medical management is indicated (Lewis and Shinnar, 2008).

A new, rare condition referred to as *febrile infection-related epilepsy syndrome (FIRES)* is associated with therapy-refractory status epilepticus in previously healthy children 3–15 years old (Van Baalen et al., 2010). This is a nonencephalitic encephalopathy that is presumed to have an infection-related etiology, and there may be a genetic predisposition. Epileptiform EEG discharges are focal and multifocal, MRI can show atrophy or hyperintensity, mortality rate is over 10%, and prognosis is poor for survivors with a high incidence of mental retardation and other neurological disturbances.

NEONATAL STATUS EPILEPTICUS

Neonatal status epilepticus manifests with the subtle, multifocal, clonic, tonic, and myoclonic features typical of *neonatal seizures* (Mizrahi, 2010; Mizrahi et al., 2008) (Chapter 6). As with neonatal seizures in general, there is often dissociation between electrographic and clinical phenomena, and EEG monitoring is necessary for full evaluation of the condition (Kellaway and Mizrahi, 1987; Mizrahi and Kellaway, 1987). Treatment of neonatal status epilepticus is essentially the same as that for neonatal seizures discussed in Chapter 7. Attention is paid first to correcting the underlying cause. Controversy exists, however, regarding the indications for, and end points of, therapy for the seizures. Animal studies indicate that the immature brain is less susceptible than the adult brain to epileptic damage (Okada et al., 1984) (Chapters 4 and 8). Although mortality is reported to be higher with neonatal status than with status in children or adults, and the incidence of sequelae is equivalent (Dreyfus-Brisac and Monod, 1964), both mortality and sequelae in neonatal status are often thought to be due to the underlying causes rather than to the seizures themselves (Chapter 7). Nevertheless, increased cerebral blood flow during status in preterm and posthypoxic term infants may present a risk of intracerebral hemorrhage (Perlman and Volpe, 1983; Volpe, 1987), and evidence for brain damage from neonatal seizures themselves is more convincing if seizures last longer than 30 minutes (Vert and Wasterlain, 1990). Consequently, the current recommendation is to treat neonatal status, and *phenobarbital* 20 mg/kg IV is generally preferred (Chapter 7). If this fails, *lorazepam*, 0.1 mg/kg IV; *diazepam*, 0.3–0.5 mg/kg IV; *fosphenytoin*, 20 mg/kg IV; and even pentobarbital coma can be used. Diazepam and lorazepam are contraindicated in jaundiced neonates. It is now accepted that treatment should not stop once behavioral seizures are controlled, but should be continued until all ictal EEG discharges are suppressed (McBride et al., 2000).

EPILEPTIC BRAIN DAMAGE

The morbidity and mortality of status epilepticus are determined to a large extent by the underlying disease process. In the absence of an acute insult, morbidity and mortality are relatively low and have progressively declined over the past several decades (Shinnar et al., 2008). While definitive data are not available, children are less likely to suffer persistent deficits than adults, and motor and cognitive sequelae are rare. The occurrence of status epilepticus in isolation does not necessarily indicate the presence of an epilepsy condition, but one-third of patients will experience recurrence of status (Hesdorffer et al., 2007).

In addition to such systemic factors as hyperpyrexia and cerebral hypoperfusion, which contribute to the destruction of cerebral neurons during status epilepticus, there is incontrovertible evidence that epilepsy itself can cause structural damage in the brain (epileptic brain damage). Bouchet and Cazauvieilh (Bouchet and Cazauvieilh, 1825) postulated almost 200 years ago that the sclerotic mesial temporal lesions found in postmortem brain tissue of epileptic patients represented changes induced by epileptic seizures. Subsequently, it was demonstrated that prolonged generalized motor seizures in baboons (Meldrum et al., 1974) produce hippocampal lesions that resemble *mesial temporal sclerosis*, the most common pathological finding in patients with MTLE (Chapters 5 and 7).

Although availability of surgically resected temporal lobe tissue has focused attention on sclerosis of the hippocampus, postmortem studies show that this may be only part of a more diffuse pathological picture with cell loss also in other limbic structures, cortex, thalamus, and cerebellum (Norman, 1964). More recently, MRI studies have confirmed the presence of diffuse neocortical thinning in patients with typical MTLE (Lin et al., 2007). Questions have not been resolved concerning the role of repeated epileptic seizures in producing these lesions and the possibility that these lesions

subsequently become epileptogenic or lead to interictal behavioral disturbances. Many patients with epilepsy who exhibit typical sclerotic lesions have no history of generalized tonic-clonic seizures; consequently, if these pathological changes are considered to represent epileptic brain damage, then repeated focal seizures must be sufficient to cause structural disturbances.

Animal studies have demonstrated that excessive excitatory synaptic activity can produce brain damage similar to that seen in human epilepsy. Hippocampal sclerosis can result from seizures induced by cytotoxic agents such as *kainic acid*, noncytotoxic agents such as *pilocarpine* in combination with *lithium* (Olney et al., 1983), and repeated electrical stimulation (Handforth and Ackerman, 1989; McIntyre et al., 1982; Sloviter and Damiano, 1981) (Chapter 4). The mechanism of action does not appear to require cytotoxic agents, generalized motor seizures, or occurrence of systemic factors leading to hypoxia, ischemia, or hypothermia. Synaptic activation appears to be a necessary but not sufficient factor (Engel, 1983; Meldrum, 1986). It is interesting that hippocampal damage is not extensive in immature animals with kainic acid–induced status (Okada et al., 1984).

Evidence indicates that the endogenous excitatory amino acids, particularly *glutamate*, mediate damage to hippocampal neurons via the NMDA receptor (Chapter 4). Resultant Ca^{2+} influx activates *proteases* (Lopez-Meraz et al. 2010) and *lipases* and leads to mitochondrial dysfunction (Meldrum, 1986; Meldrum, 1983; Rothman and Olney, 1987). Although Cl^- influx causes neuronal swelling and could also contribute to cell damage, seizure-induced cell death can be prevented experimentally by competitive NMDA antagonists (Rothman and Olney, 1987; Thompson and Wasterlain, 1997). Similar drugs may ultimately prove to be of clinical value.

Because the majority of patients with epilepsy do not have obvious progressive cerebral degeneration, it is unwise to suggest that repetitive focal ictal events must lead to permanent brain damage in humans. However, there is evidence that hippocampal sclerosis, at least, can be progressive (Cendes, 2005) (Chapter 8). The animal studies mentioned in the previous paragraph strongly suggest that brain damage can result from some types of intermittent focal epileptic seizures and perhaps even sub-clinical events. Exactly what types of seizures might destroy cerebral neurons remains to be determined, as does how many of these ictal events must take place and how severe they must be before damage becomes clinically apparent. Treatment with general anesthesia is certainly not indicated for every patient with status epilepticus, nor is it appropriate to recommend pharmacological therapy at toxic levels to stop all recurrent seizures. Until these important questions have been answered, however, it is reasonable to argue for prompt intervention with all forms of status, effective control of epileptic seizures at drug doses that do not produce unacceptable side effects, and early consideration of surgical therapy where indicated.

SUMMARY AND CONCLUSIONS

Generalized tonic-clonic status epilepticus can result in permanent brain damage or death. It is important to recognize when this dangerous situation exists or is imminent and to know how to institute appropriate treatment. Management begins with restoration of homeostasis, followed by intravenous administration of rapidly active anticonvulsant drugs, institution of maintenance pharmacological therapy, and specific treatment for the cause of the condition when known. Because this is an emergency situation, it is best for the physician to find one particular approach that can be executed comfortably and expediently on a routine basis except in those rare situations where it might be contraindicated. Common errors that account for an inadequate response to treatment include initial administration of the anticonvulsant medication at too slow a rate, at too low a dose, or by some route other than intravenous; failure to repeat the dose when the first is ineffective; failure to identify a treatable underlying cause; and failure to institute appropriate maintenance therapy. Because outcome depends on early intervention, prehospital treatment by paramedics can be critical.

Typical absence status that does not respond to oral medication is treated with intravenous benzodiazepines and valproic acid, but the atypical and the adult forms can be managed as generalized tonic-clonic status. The typical childhood forms can be extremely difficult to control, but there appear to be no long-term deleterious consequences. There is also no definitive evidence that permanent structural damage to the brain results from epilepsia partialis continua. Dyscognitive focal status epilepticus, however, can cause enduring disruption of memory and other cognitive functions. Consequently, general anesthesia is not appropriate for absence status and epilepsia partialis continua but may be for dyscognitive focal status if control is not obtained by standard approaches; surgery can be considered in particularly refractory cases of focal dyscognitive status.

The electroclinical distinctions among the types of status epilepticus described here are not always clear, and pathophysiological overlap exists. The end-stage of generalized tonic-clonic status epilepticus is characterized by coma with pseudoperiodic EEG discharges and myoclonic jerks. This end-stage condition most likely reflects the resultant encephalopathy rather than epileptic seizures per se, although the issue remains controversial. The EEG discharges and clonic symptoms may also have focal features that resemble nonepileptic myoclonus in a comatose patient. Persons with dyscognitive focal status epilepticus often have recurrent or continuous ictal events that reflect atypical rather than typical limbic seizures. In some cases, these events resemble absence status, which suggests that some forms of dyscognitive focal status, particularly of frontal lobe origin, and atypical absence status might share common mechanisms. Better data are needed on the differential diagnosis and long-term consequences of these various forms of status before they can be accurately classified for purposes of treatment and prognosis.

Febrile status epilepticus affects approximately 5% of infants with febrile seizures and is of increasing concern because of accumulating evidence that it could be a cause of hippocampal sclerosis and MTLE. In any event, febrile status epilepticus is considered to be a medical emergency of infancy and should be treated aggressively.

Neonatal seizures that last longer than 30 minutes are more likely to cause cerebral damage than briefer events. The endpoint for treatment is cessation of ictal EEG rather than clinical activity.

The circumstances under which epileptiform discharges induce structural changes in the brain have not been entirely determined, and the mechanisms of epileptic brain damage are incompletely understood. NMDA receptors have been implicated, and NMDA antagonists may exert a protective action. Except for generalized tonic-clonic and particularly refractory dyscognitive focal status epilepticus, current approaches to treatment of status involve balancing control of disabling ictal events against unacceptable side effects of drugs, and treatment should not be influenced by fear that seizures might induce epileptic brain damage.

Elucidation of the neuronal mechanisms of natural seizure-suppressing influences is necessary for understanding how these mechanisms fail in status epilepticus and how they might be exploited for therapy. Identification of the conditions that lead to epileptic brain damage is essential for preventing deleterious consequences of status and perhaps of some forms of chronic recurrent seizures. These should be priority goals for future research.

REFERENCES

Aguilar, MJ, and Rasmussen, T (1960). Role of encephalitis in pathogenesis of epilepsy. Arch Neurol 2:663–676.

Aicardi, J, and Chevrie, JJ (1970). Convulsive status epilepticus in infants and children: A study of 239 cases. Epilepsia 11:187–197.

Aicardi, J, and Chevrie, JJ (1983). Consequences of status epilepticus in infants and children. Adv Neurol 34:115–125.

Alldredge, BK, Treiman, DM, Bleck, TP, and Shorvon, SD (2008). Treatment of status epilepticus. In Epilepsy: A Comprehensive Textbook, 2nd ed. Edited by J Engel, Jr, and TA Pedley. Philadelphia: Lippincott Williams & Wilkins, pp. 1357–1363.

Aminoff, MJ, and Simon, RP (1980). Status epilepticus: Causes, clinical features and consequences in 98 patients. Am J Med 69:657–666.

Arzimanoglou, A (2010). Hemiconvulsion-hemiplegia-epilesy syndrome. In Atlas of Epilepsies. Edited by CP Panayiotopoulos. London: Springer-Verlag, pp. 949–952.

Arzimanoglou, A, Dravet, C, and Chauvel, P (2008). Hemiconvulsion-hemiplegia-epilepsy syndrome. In Epilepsy: A Comprehensive Textbook, 2nd ed. Edited by J Engel, Jr, and TA Pedley. Philadelphia: Lippincott Williams & Wilkins, pp. 2355–2360.

Bauer, G, and Trinka, E (2010). Nonconvulsive status epilepticus and coma. Epilepsia 51:177–190.

Bauer, G, Aichner, F, and Mayr, U (1982). Nonconvulsive status epilepticus following generalized tonic-clonic seizures. Eur Neurol 21:411–419.

Berkovic, SF, Johns, JA, and Bladin, PF (1982). Focal seizures and systemic metabolic disorders. Aust NZ J Med 12:620–623.

Bittencourt, PRM, and Richens, A (1981). Anticonvulsant-induced status epilepticus in Lennox-Gastaut syndrome. Epilepsia 22:129–134.

Bleck, TP, Hirsch, LJ, and Vespa, PM (2008). Electroencephalography in the intensive care unit. In Epilepsy: A Comprehensive Textbook, 2nd ed. Edited by J Engel, Jr, and TA Pedley. Philadelphia: Lippincott Williams & Wilkins, pp. 855–862.

Blennow, G, Brierly, JB, Meldrum, BS, and Siesjo, BK (1978). Epileptic brain damage: The role of systemic factors that modify cerebral energy metabolism. Brain 101:687–700.

Blennow, G, Nilsson, B, and Siesjo, BK (1985). Influence of reduced oxygen availability on cerebral metabolic changes during bicuculline-induced seizures in rats. J Cereb Blood Flow Metab 5:439–445.

Bouchet, C, and Cazauvieilh, JB (1825). De l'épilepsie considerée dans ses rapports avec l'alienation mentale. Arch Gen Med 9:510–542.

Brophy, GM, Bell, R, Claassen, J, Alldredge, B, Bleck, TP, Glauser, T, LaRoche, SM, Riviello, JJ, Jr, Shutter, L, Sperling, MR, Treiman, DM, and Vespa, P (2012). Guidelines for the evaluation and management of status epilepticus. Neurocrit Care, online.

Browne, TR, and Penry, JK (1973). Benzodiazepines in the treatment of epilepsy: A review. Epilepsia 14:277–310.

Cendes, F (2005). Progressive hippocampal and extra-hippocampal atrophy in drug resistant epilepsy. Curr Opin Neurol 18:173–177.

Chen, JWY, and Wasterlain, CG (2006). Status epilepticus: Pathophysiology and management in adults. Lancet 5:246–256.

Chen, LL, Haneef, Z, Dorsch, A, Keselman, I, and Stern JM (2010). Successful treatment of refractory simple motor status epilepticus with lacosamide and levetiracetam. Seizure 20:263–265.

Claassen, J, Hirsch, LJ, Emerson, RG, et al. (2002). Treatment of refractory status epilepticus with pentobarbital, propofol, or midazolam: A systematic review. Epilepsia 43:146–153.

Corry, JJ, Dhar, R, Murphy, T, and Diringer, MN (2008). Hypothermia for refractory status epilepticus. Neurocrit Care 9:189–197.

Dalla Bernardina, B (2008). Myoclonic status in nonprogressive encephalopathy. In Epilepsy: A Comprehensive Textbook, 2nd ed. Edited by J Engel, Jr, and TA Pedley. Philadelphia: Lippincott Williams & Wilkins, pp. 2361–2364.

Dalla Bernardina, B, Trevisan, C, Bondavalli, S, et al. (1980). Une forme particulière d'epilepsies myoclonique chez des enfants porteurs d'encéphalopathie fixée. Boll Lega Ital Epil 29–30:183–187.

DeGiorgio, CM, Correale, JD, Gott, PS, Ginsburg, DL, Bracht, KA, Smith, T, Boutros, R, Loskota, WJ, and Rabinowicz, AL (1995). Serum neuron-specific enolase in human status epilepticus. Neurology 45:1134–1137.

DeLorenzo, RJ, Kirmani, B, Deshpande, LS, Jakkampudi, V, Waterhouse, E, Garnett, L, and Ramakrishnan, V (2009). Comparisons of the mortality and clinical presentations of status epilepticus in private practice community and university hospital settings in Richmond, Virginia. Seizures 18:405–411.

Doose, H (1984). Nonconvulsive status epilepticus in childhood: Clinical aspects and classification. Adv Neurol 34:115–125.

Dreifuss, FE (1983). Status epilepticus. In Pediatric Epileptology. Edited by FE Dreifuss. Boston: John Wright, pp. 221–230.

Dreyfus-Brisac, C, and Monod, N (1964). Electroclinical studies of status epilepticus and convulsions in the newborn. In Neurological and Electroencephalographic Correlative Studies in Infancy. Edited by P Kellaway and I Peterson. New York: Grune & Stratton, pp. 250–271.

Ellis, JM, and Lee, SI (1978). Acute prolonged confusion in later life as an ictal state. Epilepsia 19:119–128.

Engel, J, Jr (1983). Epileptic brain damage: How much excitement can a limbic neuron take? Trends Neurosci 6:356–357.

Engel, J, Jr (2006). Report of the ILAE Classification Core Group. Epilepsia 47:1558–1568.

Engel, J, Jr, Ludwig, BI, and Fetell, M (1978). Prolonged partial complex status epilepticus: EEG and behavioral observations. Neurology 28:863–869.

Engel, J, Jr, Troupin, AS, Crandall, PH, Sterman, MB, and Wasterlain, CG (1982). Recent developments in the diagnosis and therapy of epilepsy. Ann Intern Med 97:584–598.

Engel, J, Jr, Kuhl, DE, Phelps, ME, Rausch, R, and Nuwer, M (1983). Local cerebral metabolism during partial seizures. Neurology 33:400–413.

Friedman, D, Claassen, J, and Hirsch, LJ (2009). Continuous electroencephalogram monitoring in the intensive care unit. Anesth Analg 109:506–523.

Gastaut, H (1968). Séméiologie des myoclonies et nosologie analytique des syndromes myocloniques. Rev Neurol 119:1–30.

Gastaut, H (1983). Classification of status epilepticus. Adv Neurol 34:15–35.

Gastaut, H, Poirer, F, Payan, H, Salamon, G, Toga, M, and Vigouroux, M (1960). H.H.E. syndrome: Hemiconvulsion, hemiplegia, epilepsy. Epilepsia 1:418–447.

Gerard, EE, and Hirsch, LJ (2010). Generalized myoclonic status epilepticus. In In Atlas of Epilepsies. Edited by CP Panayiotopoulos. London: Springer-Verlag, pp. 523–531.

Gomes, WA, and Shinnar, S (2011). Prospects for imaging-related biomarkers of human epileptogenesis: Acritical review. Biomarkers Med 5, 599–606.

Gorman, DG, Shields, WD, Shewmon, DA, Chugani, HT, Finkel, R, Comair, YG, and Peacock, WJ (1992). Neurosurgical treatment of refractory status epilepticus. Epilepsia 33:546–549.

Hallett, M (1985). Myoclonus: Relation to epilepsy. Epilepsia 26(suppl 1):S67–S77.

Handforth, A, and Ackerman, RF (1989). Limbic status and kindled seizures. In Anatomy of Epileptogenesis. Edited by BS Meldrum, JA Ferendelli, and HG Wieser. London: John Libbey, pp. 71–87.

Hartman, AL (2010). Generalized tonic status epilepticus. In Atlas of Epilepsies. Edited by CP Panayiotopoulos. London: Springer-Verlag, pp. 519–522.

Hauser, WA (1983). Status epilepticus: Etiology and neurological sequelae. Adv Neurol 34:3–14.

Hauser, WA, and Kurland, LT (1975). The epidemiology of epilepsy in Rochester, Minnesota, 1935 through 1967. Epilepsia 16:1–66.

Hesdorffer, DC, Logroscino, G, Cascino, GD, and Hauser, WA (2007). Recurrence of afebrile status epilepticus in a population-based study in Rochester, Minnesota. Neurology 69:73–78.

Hesdorffer, DC, Benn, EKT, Bagiella, E, Nordli, D, Pellock, J, Hinton, V, and Shinnar, S, for the FEBSTAT Study Team (2011). Distribution of febrile seizure duration and associations with development. Ann Neurol 70:93–100,.

Hirsch, LJ, and Friedman, D (2011). Subtle Status Epilepticus. San Diego: MedLink.

Hunter, RA (1959/1960): Status epilepticus: History, incidence and problems. Epilepsia 1:162–188.

Ingvar, MH, and Siesjo, BK (1983). Local blood flow and oxygen consumption in the rat brain during sustained bicuculline-induced seizures. Acta Neurol Scand 68:128–144.

Janz, D (1961). Conditions and causes of status epilepticus. Epilepsia 2:170–177.

Juul-Jensen, P, and Denny-Brown, D (1966). Epilepsia partialis continua. Arch Neurol 6:23–39.

Kamel, H, Comes, SB, Hegde, M, Hall, SE, and Josephson, A (2010). Electroconvulsive therapy for refractory status epilepticus. Neurocrit Care 12:204–210.

Kellaway, P, and Mizrahi, EM (1987). Neonatal seizures. In Epilepsy: Electroclinical Syndromes. Edited by H Lüders and RP Lesser. London: Springer-Verlag, pp. 13–47.

Kojewnikow, L (1895). Eine besondere Form von corticaler Epilepsie. Neurologisches Centralblatt 14:47–48.

Koutroumanidis, M, Tsatsou, K, and Tsiptsios, D (2010). Absence status epilepticus. In Atlas of Epilepsies. Edited by CP Panayiotopoulos. London: Springer-Verlag, pp. 537–544.

Lennox, WG (1945). The petit mal epilepsies: Their treatment with Tridione. JAMA 129:1069–1074.

Lewis, DV, and Shinnar, S (2008). Febrile status epilepticus. In Epilepsy: A Comprehensive Textbook, 2nd ed. Edited by J Engel, Jr, and TA Pedley. Philadelphia: Lippincott Williams & Wilkins, pp. 731–736.

Lin, JJ, Salamon, N, Lee, AD, Dutton, RA, Geaga, JA, Hayashi, KM, Luders, E, Toga, AW, Engel, J, Jr, and Thompson, PM (2007). Reduced neocortical thickness and complexity mapped in mesial temporal lobe epilepsy with hippocampal sclerosis. Cereb Cortex 17:2007–2018.

Logroscino, G, Hesdorffer, DC, Cascino, G, Annegers, JF, and Hauser, WA (1997). Short-term mortality after a first episode of status epilepticus. Epilepsia 38:1344–1349.

Logroscino, G, Hesdorffer, DC, Cascino, G, and Hauser, WA (2008). Status epilepticus without an underlying cause and risk of death. Arch Neurol 65:221–224.

Lopez-Meraz, ML, Niquet, J, and Wasterlain, CG (2010). Distinct caspase pathways mediate necrosis and apoptosis in subpopulations of hippocampal neurons after status epilepticus. Epilepsia 51(suppl 3):56–60.

Lugaresi, E, Pazzaglia, P, and Tassinari, CA (1971). Differentiation of "absence status" and "temporal lobe status." Epilepsia 12:77–87.

Mattson, RH (1983). Seizures associated with alcohol use and alcohol withdrawal. In Epilepsy: Diagnosis and Management. Edited by TR Browne and RG Feldman. Boston: Little, Brown & Co, pp. 325–332.

Maytal, J, Shinnar, S, Moshé, SL, and Alvarez, LA (1989). Low morbidity and mortality of status epilepticus in children. Pediatrics 83:323–331.

McBride, MC, Laroia, N, and Guillet, R (2000). Electrographic seizures in neonates correlate with poor neurodevelopmental outcome. Neurology 55:506–513.

McIntyre, DC, Nathanson, D, and Edson, N (1982). A new model of partial status epilepticus based on kindling. Brain Res 250:53–63.

McIntyre, J, Robertson, S, Norris, E, Appleton, R, Whitehouse, WP, Phillips, B, Martland, T, Berry, K, Collier, J, Smith, S, and Choonara, I (2005). Safety and efficacy of buccal midazolam versus rectal diazepam for emergency treatment of seizures in children: A randomised controlled trial. Lancet 66:205–210.

Meierkord, H, Boon, P, Engelsen, B, Göcke, K, Shorvon, S, Tinuper, P, and Holtkamp, M (2010). EFNS guideline on the management of status epilepticus in adults. Eur J Neurol 17:348–355.

Meldrum, BS (1983). Metabolic factors during prolonged seizures and their relation to nerve cell death. Adv Neurol 34:261–275.

Meldrum, BS (1986). Cell damage in epilepsy and the role of calcium in cytotoxicity. Adv Neurol 44:275–299.

Meldrum, BS, and Nilsson, B (1976). Cerebral blood flow and metabolic rate early and late in prolonged epileptic seizures induced in rats by bicuculline. Brain 99:523–542.

Meldrum, BS, Horton, RW, and Brierley, JB (1974). Epileptic brain damage in adolescent baboons following seizures induced by allylglycine. Brain 97:407–418.

Mizrahi, EM (2010). Neonatal seizures. In Atlas of Epilepsies. Edited by CP Panayiotopoulos. London: Springer-Verlag, pp. 493–502.

Mizrahi, EM, and Kellaway, P (1987). Characterization and classification of neonatal seizures. Neurology 37:1837–1844.

Mizrahi, EM, Plouin, P, and Clancy, RR: Neonatal seizures. In Epilepsy (2008). A Comprehensive Textbook, 2nd ed. Edited by J Engel, Jr, and TA Pedley. Philadelphia: Lippincott Williams & Wilkins, pp. 639–658.

Myers, RE, and Yamaguchi, S (1976). Nervous system effects of cardiac arrest in monkeys: Preservation of vision. Arch Neurol 34:65–74.

Niedermeyer, E, Fineyre, R, Riley, T, and Vematsu, T (1979). Absence status (petit mal status) with focal characteristics. Arch Neurol 36:417–421.

Norman, RM (1964). The neuropathology of status epilepticus. Med Sci Law 4:46–51.

Okada, R, Moshé, SL, and Albala, BJ (1984). Infantile status epilepticus and future seizure susceptibility in the rat. Dev Brain Res 15:177–183.

Olney, JW, de Gubareff, T, and Labruyere, J (1983). Seizure-related brain damage induced by cholinergic agents. Nature 301:520–522.

Oxbury, JM, and Whitty, CWM (1971). Causes and consequences of status epilepticus in adults: A study of 86 cases. Brain 94:733–744.

Perlman, JM, and Volpe, JJ (1983). Seizures in the preterm infant: Effects on cerebral blood flow velocity, intracranial pressure, and arterial blood pressure. J Pediatr 102:288–293.

Plum, F, Posner, JB, and Troy, B (1968). Cerebral metabolic and circulatory responses to induced convulsions in animals. Arch Neurol 18:1–13.

Pritchard, PB, III, and O'Neal, DB (1984). Nonconvulsive status epilepticus following metrizamide myelography. Ann Neurol 16:252–254.

Pulsinelli, WA, Brierley, JB, and Plum, F (1982). Temporal profile of neuronal damage in model of transient forebrain ischemia. Ann Neurol 11:491–498.

Rasmussen, T (1978). Further observations on the syndrome of chronic encephalitis and epilepsy. Appl Neurophysiol 41:1–12.

Riviello, JJ, Ashwal, S, Hirtz, D, Glauser, T, Balaban-Gil, K, Kelley, K, Morton, LD, Phillips, S, Sloan, E, and Shinnar, S (2006). Practice parameter: Diagnostic assessment of the child with status epilepticus (an evidence-based review). Neurology 67:1542–1550.

Rothman, SM, and Olney, JW (1987). Excitotoxicity and the NMDA receptor. Trends Neurosci 10:299–302.

Rothner, AD, and Morris, HH, III (1987). Generalized status epilepticus. In Epilepsy: Electroclinical Syndromes. Edited by H Lüders and R Lesser. London: Springer-Verlag, pp. 207–222.

Rowan, AJ, and Scott, DF (1970). Major status epilepticus: A series of 42 patients. Acta Neurol Scand 146:573–584.

Rumpl, E, and Hinterhuber, H (1981). Unusual "spike-wave stupor" in a patient with manic-depressive psychosis treated with amitriptyline. J Neurol 226:131–135.

Seif-Eddeine, H, and Treiman, DM (2011). Problems and controversies in status epilepticus: A review and recommendations. Expert Rev Neurother 11:1747–1758.

Shaner, DM, McCurdy, SA, Herring, MO, and Gabor, AJ (1988). Treatment of status epilepticus: A prospective comparison of diazepam and phenytoin versus phenobarbital and optional phenytoin. Neurology 38:202–207.

Shinnar, S, Babb, TL, Moshé, SL, and Wasterlain, CG (2008). Long term sequelae of status epilepticus. In Epilepsy: A Comprehensive Textbook, 2nd ed. Edited by J Engel, Jr, and TA Pedley. Philadelphia: Lippincott Williams & Wilkins, pp. 751–759.

Shorvon, S, and Ferlisi, M (2011). The treatment of super-refractory status epilepticus: A critical review of available therapies and a clinical treatment protocol. Brain 134:2802–2818.

Shorvon, SD, Tan, RYL, and Neligan, A (2011). Uncommon causes of status epilepticus. In The Causes of Epilepsy: Common and Uncommon Causes in Adults and Children. Edited by SD Shorvon, F Andermann, and R Guerrini. Cambridge, UK: Cambridge University Press, pp. 745–751.

Silbergleit, R, Durkalski, V, Lowenstein, D, Conwit, R, Pancioli, A, Palesch, Y, and Barsan, W (2012). Intramuscular versus intravenous therapy for prehospital status epilepticus. N Engl J Med 366:591–600.

Simon, RP (1985). Management of status epilepticus. In Recent Advances in Epilepsy 2. Edited by TA Pedley and BS Meldrum. New York: Churchill Livingstone, pp. 137–160.

Singh, BM, and Strobos, RJ (1980). Epilepsia partialis continua associated with non-ketotic hyperglycemia: Clinical and biochemical profile of 21 patients. Ann Neurol 8:155–160.

Sinha, SR (2010a) Focal status epilepticus. In Atlas of Epilepsies. Edited by CP Panayiotopoulos. London: Springer-Verlag, pp. 545–552.

Sinha, SR (2010b). Epilepsia partialis continua of Kozhevnikov. In Atlas of Epilepsies. Edited by CP Panayiotopoulos. London: Springer-Verlag, pp. 553–558.

Sloviter, RS, and Damiano, BP (1981). Sustained electrical stimulation of the perforant path duplicates kainate-induced electrophysiological effect and hip-pocampal damage in rats. Neurosci Lett 24:279–284.

Soderfeldt, B, Blennow, G, Kalimo, H, Olsson, Y, and Siesjo, BK (1983). Influence of systemic factors on experimental epileptic brain injury: Structural changes accompanying bicuculline-induced seizures in rats following manipulations of tissue oxygenation or γ-tocopherol levels. Acta Neuropathol 60:81–91.

Tan, RYL, Neligan, A, and Shorvon, SD (2010). The uncommon causes of status epilepticus: A systematic review. Epilepsy Res 91:111–122.

Tassinari, CA, Dravet, C, Roger, J, Cano, JP, and Gastaut, H (1972). Tonic status epilepticus precipitated by intravenous benzodiazepine in five patients with Lennox-Gastaut syndrome. Epilepsia 13:421–435.

Thomas, P, and Snead, OC, III (2008). Absence status epilepticus. In Epilepsy: A Comprehensive Textbook, 2nd ed. Edited by J Engel, Jr, and TA Pedley. Philadelphia: Lippincott Williams & Wilkins, pp. 693–703.

Thompson, KW, and Wasterlain, CG (1997). Partial protection of hippocampal neurons by MK-801 during perforant path stimulation in the immature brain. Brain Res 751:96–101.

Tomson, T, Svanborg, E, and Wedlund, J-E (1986). Nonconvulsive status epilepticus: High incidence of complex partial status. Epilepsia 27:276–285.

Towne, A (2010). Generalized tonic-clonic status epilepticus. In Atlas of Epilepsies. Edited by CP Panayiotopoulos. London: Springer-Verlag, pp. 507–518.

Treiman, DM (1983). General principles of treatment: Responsive and intractable status epilepticus in adults. Adv Neurol 34:377–384.

Treiman, DM (1987). Status epilepticus. In Current Therapy in Neurologic Disease 2. Edited by RT Johnson. Philadelphia: CB Decker, pp. 38–42.

Treiman, DM (2008). Generalized convulsive status epilepticus. In Epilepsy: A Comprehensive Textbook, 2nd ed. Edited by J Engel, Jr, and TA Pedley. Philadelphia: Lippincott Williams & Wilkins, pp. 665–676.

Treiman, DM, and Delgado-Escueta, AV (1983). Complex partial status epilepticus. Adv Neurol 34:69–81.

Treiman, DM, Walton, NY, and Kendrick, C (1990). A progressive sequence of electroencephalographic changes during generalized convulsant status epilepticus. Epilepsy Res 5:49–60.

Treiman, DM, Meyers, PD, Walton, NY, et al. (1998). A comparison of four treatments for generalized convulsive status epilepticus. N Engl J Med 339:792–798.

Van Baalen, A, Hausler, M, Boor, R, Rohr, A, Sperner, J, Kurlemann, G, Panzer, A, Stephani, U, and Kluger, G (2010). Febrile infection-related epilepsy syndrome (FIRES): Anonencephalic encephalopathy in childhood. Epilepsia 51:1323–1328.

Vert, P, and Wasterlain, CG (eds) (1990). Neonatal Seizures: Pathophysiology and Pharmacologic Management. New York: Raven Press.

Vespa, PM, McArthur, DL, Xu, Y, Eliseo, M, Etchepare, M, Dinov, I, Alger, J, Glenn, TP, and Hovda, D (2010). Nonconvulsive seizures after traumatic brain injury are associated with hippocampal atrophy. Neurology 75:792–798.

Volpe, JJ (1987). Neurology of the Newborn, 2nd ed. Philadelphia: WB Saunders.

Walker, MC, and Shorvon, SD (2009). Emergency treatment of seizures and status epilepticus. In The Treatment of Epilepsy, 3rd ed. Edited by S Shorvon, E Perucca, and J Engel, Jr. Oxford: Wiley-Blackwell, pp. 231–247.

Wasterlain, CG (1974). Mortality and morbidity from serial seizures: An experimental study. Epilepsia 15:155–174.

Wasterlain, CG, and Chen, JWY (2008). Mechanistic and pharmacologic aspects of status epilepticus and its treatment with new antiepileptic drugs. Epilepsia 49:63–73.

Wasterlain, CG, and Duffy, TE (1976). Status epilepticus in immature rats: Protective effects of glucose on survival and brain development. Arch Neurol 33:831–837.

Wieser, HG, and Chauvel, P (2008). Simple partial status epilepticus and epilepsia partialis continua of Kozhevnikov. In Epilepsy: A Comprehensive Textbook, 2nd ed. Edited by J Engel, Jr, and TA Pedley. Philadelphia: Lippincott Williams & Wilkins, pp. 705–723.

Wieser, HG, Hailemariam, S, Regard, M, and Landis, T (1985). Unilateral limbic epileptic status activity: Stereo EEG, behavioral and cognitive data. Epilepsia 26:19–29.

Williamson, PD (2008). Complex partial status epilepticus. In Epilepsy: A Comprehensive Textbook, 2nd ed. Edited by J Engel, Jr, and TA Pedley. Philadelphia: Lippincott Williams & Wilkins, pp. 677–692.

Williamson, PD, Spencer, DD, Spencer, SS, Novelly, RA, and Mattson, RH (1985). Complex partial status epilepticus: A depth electrode study. Ann Neurol 28:647–654.

Yoong, M, and Scott, RC (2010). Febrile status epilepticus. In Atlas of Epilepsies. Edited by CP Panayiotopoulos. London: Springer-Verlag, pp. 533–536.

Chapter 11

Chronic Behavioral Disturbances

EPIDEMIOLOGY OF PSYCHIATRIC COMORBIDITY IN EPILEPSY

PHENOMENOLOGY OF BEHAVIORAL DISTURBANCES IN EPILEPSY
Ictal and Periictal Behavior
Psychosocial Adaptation
Neurological, Intellectual, and Cognitive Function
Personality
Mood and Affect
Anxiety
Attention Deficit Hyperactivity Disorder

Psychosis
Classification of Neuropsychiatric Disorders in Epilepsy
Autism Spectrum Disorders

MECHANISMS OF INTERICTAL BEHAVIORAL DISTURBANCES IN EPILEPSY
Psychosocial Factors: The Predicament
Neuropathological Factors
Effects of Treatment
Epilepsy-Induced Neurobiological Factors

SUMMARY AND CONCLUSIONS

Throughout history epilepsy has been associated with negative images (Berrios, 1984; Jilek, 1979; Temkin, 1945), which continue to create misconceptions and compromise the lives of those who suffer from epileptic seizures. In almost all cultures, these people are stigmatized not only in the eyes of the public but also in their own minds (Chapter 17). Because of fear that genuine scientific interests in examining possible relationships between epilepsy and socially unacceptable behavior could exacerbate this problem, up until a few decades ago such

studies were a source of heated controversy (Bear and Fedio, 1977; Dodrill and Batzel, 1986; Engel et al., 1991; Engel et al., 2008; Gastaut et al., 1955; Gibbs, 1951; Hermann et al., 1982a; Hermann et al., 1982b; Hill et al., 1957; Mungas, 1982; Perez and Trimble, 1980; Perini and Mendius, 1984; Rodin and Schmaltz, 1984; Schiffer and Babigian, 1984; Slater et al., 1963; Stevens, 1966; Stevens and Hermann, 1981; Taylor, 1972; Trimble, 1983).

Today, not only is psychiatric comorbidity of epilepsy accepted as a major cause of potentially treatable disability, but it also has become one of the more important areas of epilepsy research (Ettinger and Kanner, 2007). Indeed, epilepsy is now defined by the *International League Against Epilepsy (ILAE)* not only on the basis of the occurrence of epileptic seizures but also by "the neurobiological, cognitive, psychological, and social consequences of this disorder" (Fisher et al., 2005), and the ILAE has recently published clinical practice guidelines for the treatment of neuropsychiatric conditions associated with epilepsy (Kerr et al., 2011). Furthermore, behavioral disturbance are now considered a high priority for research on epilepsy by the *National Institute of Neurological Disorders and Stroke (NINDS)* (Kelly et al., 2009).

Certain epilepsy syndromes are recognized as *epileptic encephalopathies*, defined as conditions in which progression of nonepileptic, as well as epileptic, dysfunction is directly related to the recurrence of epileptic seizures. These conditions are discussed individually in Chapter 7. The psychiatric condition of *psychogenic nonepileptic seizures (PNES)* encountered in people without epilepsy presents problems of differential diagnosis and is discussed in Chapter 13, but it is important to recognize that PNES is also a psychiatric comorbidity of epilepsy. This chapter is concerned with the more common ictal and postictal behavioral disturbances as well as interictal behavioral disturbances that occur to a greater extent in people with epilepsy than in the general population (Tellez-Zenteno et al., 2007; Gaitatzis et al., 2004; Hesdorffer and Hauser, 2007). There is great interest today in the potential shared mechanisms that might underlie certain types of behavioral disorders and epilepsy, particularly those involving the *limbic system* (Engel et al., 2002) and the *hypothalamic-pituitary-adrenal axis* (Kanner, 2011). Common genetic variants have been identified between epilepsy and autism, schizophrenia, and intellectual disability (Mefford et al., 2010). Questions that remain include: (1) when are these disturbances caused by epilepsy per se rather than by the underlying neuropathological process, environmental pressures, or treatment, (2) when are certain specific behavioral symptoms related to particular forms of epilepsy, in some cases constituting a syndrome, (3) how often might these disturbances be expected to occur or to be progressive, and (4) to what extent does the pathophysiology of psychiatric disorders contribute to epileptogenicity?

EPIDEMIOLOGY OF PSYCHIATRIC COMORBIDITY IN EPILEPSY

Studies of the point prevalence of behavioral disturbances among people with epilepsy have yielded results ranging from a low of less than 6% (Forsgren, 1992) to a high of over 54% (Gudmundsson, 1966). These vast discrepancies have been ascribed to differences in ascertainment as well as in the measures and definitions used (Tellez-Zenteno et al. 2007). Large population-based studies indicate that one-quarter to one-third of people with epilepsy have a lifetime risk for coexistent mental health disorders, approximately twice the prevalence in the general population (Gaitatzis et al., 2004; Tellez-Zenteno et al., 2007). These figures vary with the type of epilepsy, being highest in most studies with temporal lobe epilepsy, and with the psychiatric diagnosis (Fig. 11–1). Most studies have found *mood disorders*, in particular *depression* and its most serious complication, *suicidality*, to be the most common psychiatric comorbidity, and *anxiety disorder* and *panic disorder* to be the the be the next most common (Hesdorffer and Hauser, 2007). The epidemiology of *personality disorders, bipolar disorder, schizophrenia*, and other psychoses has not been well established for people with epilepsy.

Psychiatric comorbidities are not limited to patients with structural or metabolic epileptogenic disturbances; they can also occur in patients with no demonstrable lesions, in some cases presumably with genetic conditions (Austin and Dunn, 2002; Hermann and Jones, 2006; McAfee et al., 2007). These comorbidities are often associated with a reduced quality of life (Gilliam, 2002; Baca et al., 2011), increased economic burdens to the family and society (Cramer et al., 2004), and an increased risk of suicide (Christensen et al., 2007).

Psychiatric comorbidity can precede or follow the development of epilepsy, and there is increasing evidence that this bidirectionality, well described for depression (Kanner, 2011), also exists for other conditions, such as *anxiety disorder* (Petrovski et al., 2010). Not only are people with epilepsy more likely to develop depression and certain other psychiatric

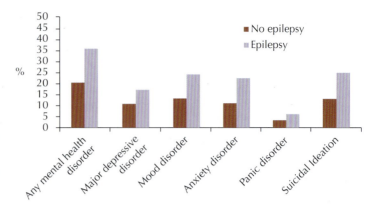

Figure 11–1. Psychiatric comorbidity from a population-based study comparing the prevalences of specific psychiatric disorders in matched populations with and without epilepsy. (Graph prepared by Anne Berg from data in Tellez-Zenteno et al., 2007, with permission.)

conditions, but these mental health disorders predispose to the development of epilepsy and predict a poor prognosis for seizure control with both medical and surgical therapy (Kanner, 2011). Evidence exists to support the view that such bidirectionality reflects the existence of common mechanisms underlying both epilepsy and psychopathology involving *frontotemporal limbic structures* and increased *cortisol* production due to a *hyperactive hypothalamic-pituitary-adrenal axis* (Kanner, 2011).

Ictal and periictal behavioral disturbances that are direct consequences of epileptogenic mechanisms are transient events, traditionally considered as different from enduring interictal behavioral disorders.

Postictal psychosis accounts for approximately 25% of psychosis associated with epilepsy, and the annual incidence of such episodes in patients with focal epilepsy who are undergoing video-EEG monitoring was reported to be over 6% (Kanner et al., 1996). Because they typically occur one to five days after a seizure or a flurry of seizures, postictal psychotic episodes are often missed or misdiagnosed in the community. Although transient, these events, like some other behavioral disturbances, are predictive of a poorer seizure outcome (Alper et al., 2008).

PHENOMENOLOGY OF BEHAVIORAL DISTURBANCES IN EPILEPSY

Ictal and Periictal Behavior

Transient prodromal, ictal, and postictal behavioral changes are directly related to epileptic seizures, as opposed to chronic, persistent interictal disturbances (Table 11–1). It may occasionally be difficult, however, to distinguish periictal from ictal phenomena.

Prodromal behavioral changes can be brief or last hours or days (Chapter 9). Complaints commonly include anxiety, withdrawal, irritability, and other emotional aberrations. These behavioral disturbances probably reflect fluctuations in predisposing factors that lower the epileptic threshold or the appearance of endogenous precipitating factors responsible for ictal initiation (Chapters 5 and 9). By definition, prodromal symptoms are not the same as auras, which are focal ictal events (Chapters 1 and 6).

Ictal events can resemble or precisely mimic psychiatric symptoms (Chapter 6). Such behavior is readily recognized as epileptic when it is brief and intermittent, or when, on occasion, it evolves into a more obvious epileptic seizure. The correct diagnosis may easily be missed, however, in those rare circumstances when the disturbed behavior is long-lasting or repetitive and more familiar epileptic symptoms never occur. Although features of *absence status* and *focal dyscognitive status epilepticus* may be mistaken for psychotic behavior, the existence of impaired consciousness, EEG abnormalities, amnesia, and postictal confusion usually makes the diagnosis obvious (Chapter 10). On the other hand, forms of *focal limbic status epilepticus* can consist of prolonged emotional symptoms (Henriksen, 1973) or more profound personality and psychotic disturbances in clear consciousness, and scalp EEG changes are usually not present in this situation (Wieser et al., 1985). In these cases, diagnosis may be impossible unless intravenous administration of diazepam consistently abolishes symptoms

Table 11–1 **Behavioral Disturbance in Epilepsy**

Prodromal (Chapter 9)	Systemic or cerebral state that predisposes to epileptic seizures
Ictal (Chapters 6 and 10)	Bilateral involvement: impaired consciousness; abnormal EEG
	Unilateral involvement: clear consciousness; EEG can be normal
Postictal (Chapter 9)	Todd's phenomenon (focal deficit); consciousness may be clear; focally abnormal
	Confused state with or without reactive automatisms: impaired consciousness; EEG
	Psychosis: latent phase, clear consciousness; normal EEG
Interictal	Inadequate psychological adaptation
	Neurological, intellectual, and cognitive deficits
	Aberrant personality traits
	Affective disorders
	Psychoses

on repeated occasions (Chapter 13); however, even this is not absolutely diagnostic, because diazepam can also disrupt psychotic behaviors. Some behavioral experts believe that bizarre dissociative behaviors such as *multiple personality disorders* (Benson et al., 1986; Mesulam, 1981), *possession states* (Mesulam, 1981), and *fugue states* (*poriomania*) (Mayeux et al., 1979) may at times reflect continuous or serial epileptic seizures. When there is clouded consciousness, an abnormal EEG, and postictal amnesia for the entire event, these might be ictal. In most cases, however, an ictal state has not been substantiated, and when these events occur in people with known epilepsy, they have been referred to as *seizure related*. Fear is a common ictal symptom in limbic epilepsy, and patients with fearful auras appear to be predisposed to interictal panic disorder, suggesting a common pathological substrate (Mintzer and Lopez, 2002).

The unfortunate use of epilepsy as an inappropriate legal defense (Chapter 17) has derived from misconceptions about aggression during seizures. Ictal violence (Saint-Hilaire et al., 1981) is extremely rare, and when it occurs it takes the form of nondirected automatisms followed by complete amnesia (Delgado-Escueta et al., 1981). Explosive and violent reactive automatisms can also occur during *postictal confusion* following limbic dyscognitive and, rarely, generalized convulsive seizures (Chapter 9). These reactive postictal behaviors are nondirected and are usually responses to stimulation perceived as threatening or attempts at restraint. Intermittent violent behavior characterizes the so-called

episodic dyscontrol syndrome (Monroe, 1970; Rickler, 1982) (Chapter 13), now referred to as *intermittent explosive disorder* (American Psychiatric Association, 2000), which is not considered to be an epileptic disorder. This condition occasionally occurs in patients with epilepsy, however, and intermittent outbursts in some may be controlled by anticonvulsant drugs (Monroe, 1975; Rickler, 1982).

Postictal dysfunction can cause neurological deficits such as aphasia and anterograde amnesia, as well as less specific confusion, with or without impaired consciousness, automatisms, emotional changes, and psychosis (Chapter 9). Most of these disturbances are associated with EEG slowing. Although the postictal state usually resolves over minutes or hours, some symptoms can last for days or weeks. That persistent memory deficits frequently improve after successful surgical treatment of *mesial temporal lobe epilepsy (MTLE)* (Rausch and Crandall, 1982; Bell et al., 2011) suggests that these apparent interictal disturbances might reflect enduring, but reversible, postictal disruption. Motor function is impaired during the postictal phase of generalized tonic-clonic seizures, but it is not unusual for patients to react defensively to perceived threat during the postictal confusion that follows a focal dyscognitive seizure when motor function remains intact. Postictal psychiatric symptoms in patients with pharmacoresistant seizures, including depression, anxiety, and hypomania, are much more frequent than generally appreciated; the occurrence of postictal anxiety may be as high as 50% (Kanner et al., 2004). Very rarely, aggressive postictal sexual behavior can occur (Blumer, 1970). Although at odds with the concept that epilepsy should not be used as a legal defense, postictal, rather than ictal, violent outbursts can be directed and destructive.

Postictal psychosis is a well-described prolonged psychotic episode that is often underdiagnosed or mistaken for interictal psychosis. It occurs most often after a flurry of generalized tonic-clonic or focal dyscognitive seizures, and there is usually a latent period of 24–120 hours before symptoms occur (Blumer and Benson, 1982; Kanner et al., 1996; Alper et al., 2008). The existence of this *lucid interval*, in addition to the fact that the EEG is normal, accounts for the frequent failure to recognize postictal psychosis as a direct consequence of an epileptic seizure. This condition cannot be attributed to a Todd's phenomenon or an ictal status and is treated as a delirious state. Postictal psychosis must be distinguished from postictal absence-like status, which begins immediately after the seizure and responds to anticonvulsant drugs (Chapter 10).

Postictal psychosis lasts hours to days or, rarely, weeks. It consists of affect-laden delusions, hallucinations, delusions, and thought disorders that respond to low-dose antipsychotic medication and, for rapid therapy, benzodiazepines. Insomnia and agitation can precede these events by a day or two. Prophylactic treatment with low-dose atypical antipsychotic drugs such as *risperidone* or *quetiapine* can reduce the subsequent occurrence of postictal psychosis. Risk factors for postictal psychosis include focal epilepsy with diffuse or bilateral pathology, secondarily generalized tonic-clonic seizures, a family history of psychiatric disorders, and a history of encephalitis (Alper et al., 2008). The diffuse or bilateral pathophysiology could explain why postictal psychosis is predictive of more severe epilepsy and a relatively poor postoperative prognosis for seizures. Although it should not be considered a contraindication to surgery per se, patients exhibiting postictal psychosis might be warned that they are more likely to experience mania or depression during the first few postoperative months (Kanemoto et al., 2001).

These periictal behavioral disturbances should be recognized and distinguished from interictal disorders, although patients who experience postictal psychosis are at an increased risk for developing interictal psychosis (Kanner

and Ostrovskaya, 2008). The remainder of this chapter deals with truly interictal disturbances of behavior, which can be divided into difficulties with psychosocial adaptation, neurological and cognitive deficits, aberrant personality traits, affective disorders, anxiety disorders, psychosis, and autism.

Psychosocial Adaptation

The literature reports that many people with epilepsy experience problems with psychosocial adaptation. These are, above all else, a measure of the disability associated with epilepsy. The effectiveness of therapeutic intervention in individual patients must ultimately depend on the degree of psychosocial adjustment rather than absolute reduction in seizure frequency, because the two are not necessarily related (Taylor, 1987; Engel et al., 2008). Indeed, in epilepsy, prognosis for psychosocial adjustment is known to relate more to intellectual limitations, organic and psychological disturbances, and motivation than to epileptic seizure type or frequency (Rodin, 1968).

A major difficulty in evaluating psychosocial adaptation in the past was the absence of accepted quantitative criteria and the dangers inherent in relying on subjective data from patients, relatives, or associates. Taylor (1972) overcame this latter problem with an exhaustive study of 100 patients treated surgically for temporal lobe epilepsy. He visited each patient in his or her home and verified records relating to schooling and employment. This objective study was carried out on a highly selected group of patients, and the approach has not been replicated with a broader population. Help from sociologists is clearly required if such studies are ever to be adequately accomplished on a larger scale.

A second quantitative approach, more applicable to surveys of large populations, was taken by Dodrill and colleagues (Dodrill, 1983; Dodrill et al., 1980;1984a;1984b). They devised the *Washington Psychosocial Seizure Inventory (WPSI)* to sample patients' concerns about family background, emotional adjustment, interpersonal adjustment, vocational adjustment, financial status, adjustment to seizures, and medicine and medical management. Five groups of patients in different regions of the

United States (Dodrill et al., 1984a) and similar groups in Canada, Finland, and the German Democratic Republic were studied (Dodrill et al., 1984b). For all groups tested, concerns were highest about emotional adjustment. In the United States, concerns about family background, vocational adjustment, and financial status were less apparent for patients who had routine appointments than for those with special needs. Comparing data from different countries, lack of governmental responsibility for financial and vocational support negatively influenced concerns about emotional and vocational adjustment in the United States especially. Concerns about family background and medical management were least common in all groups. This approach offers an objective means of studying factors that influence various aspects of psychosocial adjustment and, for the most part, can be used to follow patient response to intervention. The family background scale, however, is based largely on historical information and so should not change as a result of intervention. Two serious family-related problems encountered by patients with epilepsy, a reduced rate of successful marriage and increased dependency on family (Batzel and Dodrill, 1984), are reflected in the emotional adjustment and financial status scale of the WPSI.

The Epilepsy Surgery Inventory-55 (ESI-55) (Vickrey et al., 1992) is a *health-related quality of life (HRQOL)* instrument adapted for an epilepsy population specifically to assess outcome after epilepsy surgery. This scale was subsequently expanded to create a more broad-based instrument that could be used in a wide range of epilepsy studies. A group of instruments referred to as the *Quality of Life in Epilepsy (QOLIE)* instruments consists of the *QOLIE-89* (with 89 items sampling 17 scales), the *QOLIE-31* (31 items from 7 scales), and *QOLIE-10* (10 items from 7 scales) (Devinsky et al., 1995). Table 11–2 shows the scales sampled in the QOLIE instruments. A 48-item questionnaire has also been developed for use in adolescents (*QOLIE-AD-48*) (Cramer et al., 1999). With the advent of these instruments, HRQOL has become an essential measure for all epilepsy outcome studies as well as a variety of other investigations that depend on analysis of the burden of disease borne by people with epilepsy (Baker et al., 2008). More recently, quantitative measurements of HRQOL in

Table 11–2 The Quality of Life in Epilepsy Scales

Scale	Number of items
Health Perceptions	6
Seizure Worry°	5
Physical Function	10
Role Limitation, Physical	5
Role Limitation, Emotional	5
Pain	2
Overall Quality of Life°	2
Emotional Well-being°	5
Energy/Fatigue°	4
Attention/Concentration°	9
Memory	6
Language	5
Medication Effects°	3
Social Function, Work, Driving°	11
Social Support	4
Social Isolation	2
Health Discouragement	2
Sexual Function	1
Change in Health	1
Overall Health	1

The QOLIE-89 contains 87 questions from these 17 scales. The QOLIE-31 and QOLIE-10 respectively contain 31 and 10 questions from the seven scales marked with an asterisk.
From Baker et al., 2008, with permission.

outcome studies of epilepsy have been supplemented by additional instruments that measure social adjustment to identify reasons for either improvement or worsening of quality of life (Austin et al., 2008; Rubin and Wiebe, 2008) (Chapter 17).

Although, as a group, patients with epilepsy have poorer prospects for leading a fulfilling life than the population at large, many have no problems with psychosocial adjustment, even when their seizures are not well controlled. Some factors that influence adaptation can be derived from follow-up studies of patients who have undergone surgical treatment. A good psychosocial outcome following successful resective surgery can be predicted by (1) a supportive family, (2) early therapeutic intervention (i.e., surgery), and (3) absence of an addictive personality type (Crandall et al., 1987). Adjusting to the *burden of normality* presents its own set of challenges to patients and their families who have lived for many years with chronic disease (Wilson et al., 2004).

Much more research is needed, however, to identify risk factors for psychosocial dysfunction, as well as to characterize specific problems in psychosocial adaptation that might afflict persons with epilepsy more than those with other chronic disabilities.

Neurological, Intellectual, and Cognitive Function

In persons with epilepsy, neurological deficits are important in determining prognosis (Rodin, 1968). They are presumed to reflect underlying *structural* lesions, but focal *functional* disturbances, as demonstrated by interictal *positron emission tomography (PET)* (Chugani et al., 1987; Engel et al., 1982; Henry and Chugani, 2008), may also account for neurological impairment and could be reversible. Neurological deficits are common in patients with structural or metabolic generalized epilepsy disorders (Chapter 7), particularly those with Lennox-Gastaut syndrome. Focal neurological deficits in patients with focal seizures, due to destructive effects of a lesion, to a postictal Todd's phenomenon, or perhaps to other reversible interictal dysfunction, can also be disabling.

Of particular concern in assessing disability in association with epilepsy, however, have been aspects of *intellectual* and *cognitive* impairment (Loring et al., 2008; Rankin and Vargha-Khadem, 2008; Bell et al., 2011). The appreciation of this problem depends largely on the types of studies carried out and the population evaluated. Specific dysfunctions such as memory deficits are commonly encountered in patients with medically intractable MTLE (Delaney et al., 1980). Learning disabilities have been identified in children with epilepsy (Stores, 1981). In a large study on the Isle of Wight, children between the ages of 9 and 11 with epilepsy were much more likely to show reading retardation than those without epilepsy (Rutter and Yule, 1973). On subtests of the *Wechsler Intelligence Scales* that measure abilities such as attention, visuospatial problem solving, and sequencing, persons who have focal seizures perform better than those who have generalized seizures (Giordani et al., 1985). Reliable conclusions cannot be drawn from such studies, however, without controlling

for other factors that influence performance, such as antiseizure drug regimen, severity of the underlying pathophysiological process, and aspects of the seizure disorder including age of onset, types of seizures, and frequency of attacks (Lesser et al., 1986). It is, therefore, of little value to attempt to enumerate data on IQ performance in various forms of epilepsy or epilepsy as a whole. As will be discussed later, it is sufficient to conclude that IQ is most often depressed in patients with generalized epilepsy syndromes associated with diffuse or multifocal structural lesions of the brain and who have high levels of antiseizure medications, particularly those that produce sedative effects, such as the barbiturates and benzodiazepines. With focal seizures, cognitive deficits reflect the location of the epileptogenic region. Of particular concern are verbal memory deficits in patients with MTLE due to seizures arising in the language-dominant hemisphere (Loring et al., 2008). Such cognitive disturbances are likely to be less severe if seizures begin early in life, when brain function is sufficiently plastic to permit compromised functions to transfer to the contralateral hemisphere.

Personality

The association between specific personality traits or disorders and epilepsy has been a subject of controversy since Gibbs (Gibbs, 1951) first suggested that patients with psychomotor seizures have an increased incidence of psychiatric disturbances. A relationship between amygdala irritability and temporal lobe seizures was postulated, creating what some workers considered to be a *reverse Klüver-Bucy syndrome* (Gastaut et al., 1955). Although other investigators failed to identify behavioral disturbances peculiar to temporal lobe epilepsy (Stevens, 1966) personality disturbances are common, and often unrecognized, among people with epilepsy and are the result of biological as well as social and emotional factors (Devinsky et al., 2008).

Many investigators have attempted to assess various aspects of psychopathology in the context of epilepsy using the *Minnesota Multiphasic Personality Index (MMPI)*, but such attempts have been criticized on the basis of the state-dependent nature of this test and its lack of specificity for the particular behavioral disturbances in question (Dodrill and Batzel, 1986). The MMPI failed to identify differences in the incidence of psychopathology between patients with epilepsy and those with other chronic medical and neurological disorders or in patients with limbic versus other seizure types; however, abnormal profiles in the epilepsy population were of greater severity (Whitman et al., 1984; Dikmen et al., 1983) and more common with limbic seizures that secondarily generalized (Hermann et al., 1982b). A use for personality inventories has been to assist in the evaluation of patients with epilepsy and nonepileptic seizures, where the Personality Assessment Inventory has some discrimination (Locke et al., 2011).

An interictal *aggressive personality trait* has been variably associated in the literature with epilepsy, particularly MTLE. It is reported to be characterized by irritability, explosiveness, and at times intense anger due to a combination of impulsive tendencies and what has been referred to as *deepened emotions* (Blumer and Benson, 1982). Such aggressive behavior was noted to be most prominent in male patients with an early onset of epileptic seizures and a low IQ (Taylor, 1969). Although an increased incidence of epileptic seizures was found among prisoners (Gunn, 1969), this can be explained by a high risk of head trauma in this population, and a prospective study of patients with epilepsy revealed no increase in crime rate (Alstrom, 1950). Despite claims of increased aggressiveness, there is no evidence that persons with epilepsy have an unusually high incidence of premeditated violent or antisocial acts (Treiman, 1986). On the other hand, after adjustment for psychiatric comorbidity, people with epilepsy were reported to be 1.5 times more likely than the general population to be victims of aggression (Kwon et al., 2011). Whether this victimization reflects some aspect of a personality trait or the stigma of epilepsy was not determined.

A subject that was controversial in the past that is worth mentioning for historical purposes is the concept of an *epileptic personality*, usually considered in the context of temporal lobe epilepsy. *Hypergraphia, hyposexuality,* and *hyperreligiosity* were proposed as an interictal syndrome characteristic of temporal lobe epilepsy (Waxman and Geschwind, 1974) while numerous other features have also been associated with temporal lobe epilepsy in the

literature (Bear and Fedio, 1977). The *Bear-Fedio Personality Inventory* (Bear and Fedio, 1977) was developed to assess the 18 personality traits most often ascribed to a temporal lobe epilepsy personality in published reports (Table 11–3). These traits were conveniently condensed to include hyposexuality, hypometamorphosis, and deepened emotionality (Blumer and Benson, 1982). *Hyposexuality* refers to failure to develop an interest in sexual activity when seizure onset is before puberty and loss of sexual interest or sexual habits such as *homosexuality, fetishism,* or *transvestism* when the onset of epileptic seizures is later. *Hypometamorphosis* refers to a quality of *viscosity, adhesiveness,* or *stickiness* and is defined as an overinclusiveness or excessive attention to detail, with the verbal manifestation being circumstantiality in speech and writing. A particular feature of this language trait is that the patient does not lose track of thought and eventually returns to the point. *Deepened emotionality* refers to a certain degree of sobriety and interest in issues of a moral, religious, or philosophical nature. Traits subsumed under this heading also include *anger, moodiness,* and

Table 11–3 Characteristics Claimed to Be Due to Interictal Behavior in Temporal Lobe Epilepsy*

Emotionality
Elation, euphoria
Sadness
Anger
Aggression
Altered sexual interest
Guilt
Hypermoralism
Obsessionalism
Circumstantiality
Viscosity
Sense of personal destiny
Hypergraphia
Religiosity
Philosophical interest
Dependence, passivity
Humorlessness, sobriety
Paranoia

*This table lists the 18 personality traits most often associated with temporal lobe epilepsy in the literature; however, no such association has been definitively proven for any of these traits.

From Bear and Fedio, 1977, with permission.

explosiveness, which may fluctuate in individual patients.

The Bear-Fedio test has been used with varying results (Bear and Fedio, 1977; Hermann and Riel, 1981; Nielson and Kristensen, 1981). Considerable evidence suggests that the test measures nonspecific psychopathology related to factors such as intelligence, gender, and antiseizure drug levels (Mungas, 1982; Rodin and Schmaltz, 1984). Differences between patients presumed to have left and right temporal lobe disturbances were also reported on the initial studies with the Bear-Fedio inventory, with left temporal lobe patients tending to exaggerate their problems ("tarnishers") and right temporal lobe patients tending to deemphasize them ("polishers") (Bear and Fedio, 1977). These results are not subject to the criticisms concerning patient selection, but studies of hemispheric specialization in patients with focal seizures during this period must take into account the potential for considerable error in lateralization of the epileptogenic region (Mendius and Engel, 1985). This finding has not been replicated; however, if true, it has interesting implications for brain function and for treatment; tarnishers may be more amenable to psychiatric intervention than polishers.

The Bear-Fedio test has essentially been replaced over the last two decades with a variety of more focused personality instruments (Devinsky et al., 2008; Broicher et al., 2012). Studies of social cognition and *theory of mind*, which refers to the ability to recognize the emotions, attitudes, intentions, desires, and beliefs of others, define an individual's ability to develop complex interpersonal relationships. This is an active new area of research, particularly in identifying disturbances responsible for behavioral disorders associated with autism, but similar disturbances may exist in MTLE (Broicher et al., 2012). Just as recurrent epileptic seizures in mesial temporal structures of the language-dominant hemisphere can lead to disabling verbal memory deficits, it is probable that similar epileptic activity, perhaps in the non-language-dominant hemisphere, can lead to progressive disturbances in social cognition leading to the development of problematic personality traits like those described in earlier studies. Questions remain unresolved concerning whether specific personality traits (1) are unusually prevalent among people with epilepsy, (2) occur individually or together in some form to create a syndrome, and (3) constitute characteristic features of temporal lobe epilepsy. The bulk of evidence indicates that certain personality disturbances may well be associated with some forms of epilepsy, particularly those that involve mesial temporal limbic structures. Reliable identification of the patient population at risk for these behaviors, however, is difficult, because mesial temporal structures are also commonly involved in generalized tonic-clonic seizures. Furthermore, comorbid mood, anxiety, and attention deficit disorders, which are common in epilepsy, can easily be mistaken for personality disorders.

Mood and Affect

Mood disturbances may be limited to disorders of feeling tone or may constitute a *major depressive syndrome* with somatic symptoms such as disturbances of sleep, appetite, libido, and neuroendocrine rhythms (American Psychiatric Association, 2000). Alterations in mood can occur interictally or as ictal or postictal symptoms of epilepsy (Betts, 1981; Henriksen, 1973), but *depression* is now recognized as perhaps the most important interictal comorbidity of epilepsy (Mendez et al., 1986; Robertson and Trimble, 1983; Kanner and Blumer, 2008). The suicide rate among patients with epilepsy has been reported to be five times higher than that in the general population and 25 times higher in those with a diagnosis of temporal lobe epilepsy (Barraclough, 1981). Suicide occurs for reasons other than depression, however, and implications of a direct relationship are not justified. Some workers have argued that depression is no greater among patients with epilepsy than among patients with other severe diseases (Dodrill and Batzel, 1986; Schiffer and Babigian, 1984), consistent with the notion that this affective disturbance reflects a reaction to illness. This view, however, was clearly refuted by a controlled study in which depression was almost twice as common, and suicide attempts more than four times as common, for people with as for people without epilepsy matched for vocational disability (Mendez et al., 1986).

Table 11–4 shows a classification of the relationship of depressive symptoms to seizures. *Ictal depressed mood* is usually associated with an aura of fear, can persist for long periods of time (Henriksen, 1973), and, rarely,

Table 11–4 **Depressive Symptoms in Epilepsy**

Ictal (Chapters 6 and 10)	Simple partial symptoms, usually associated with fear; EEG may be normal
Postictal (Chapter 9)	More common than believed
Interictal	Reactive to life situation
	Drug-induced; related to specific changes in medication
	Chronic dysphoria with apathy, hopelessness, and worthlessness
	Chronic dystonia with poor self-image and depersonalization

Adapted from material in Benson et al., 1986

may result in suicide attempts (Betts, 1981). *Postictal depressed mood* is more often than not unrecognized but in fact can be relatively frequent in patients with treatment-resistant focal epilepsy. Indeed, in one study of 100 consecutive patients, 43 endorsed postictal depressive symptoms, with a median duration of 24 hours (Kanner et al., 2004). Among these 43 patients, 15 endorsed more than five symptoms that, except for the duration, could mimic a major depressive episode. Thirteen endorsed habitual postictal suicidal ideation. Likewise, patients with interictal or preictal depression can report relief or euphoria postictally, which is consistent with the well-known beneficial effect of *electroconvulsive shock therapy (ECT)*. Postictal *hypomania* can occur, particularly after repeated limbic seizures. *Interictal depression* may be reactive, clearly related to despondency over restrictions in lifestyle, or coincide with the institution of a particular medication. Chronic mood disorders can take the form of minor or major depression or bipolar affective disorder, all of which do not differ in character from these conditions in people without epilepsy (Krishnamoorthy et al., 2007). Two other chronic forms of interictal depression have been noted (Benson et al., 1986). One is a long-standing *dysphoria* characterized by apathy, hopelessness, and a state of psychomotor retardation. The other, referred to as *depersonalized dystonia*, is described by patients as a "spaced-out," "unreal," or "out of control" sensation (Benson et al., 1986; Blumer et al., 2004). This latter condition can also be seen, however, in patents with diffuse cerebral dysfunction from any cause.

The recognition of a bidirectional relationship between epilepsy and depression provides insights into possible shared mechanisms (Kanner, 2011). Not only have population-based and experimental animal studies supported an increased incidence of depression associated with epilepsy, but people with depression have a three to seven times higher risk of developing epilepsy than the general population (Forsgren and Nystrom, 1990; Hesdorffer et al., 2006). Furthermore, people with epilepsy who are depressed are less likely to become seizure-free following pharmacological and surgical treatment (Kanner, 2011). Having etiologies in common could explain these observations. Neuroimaging studies have revealed bilateral temporal lobe atrophy in depression, and patients with unilateral temporal lobe epilepsy are more likely to have contralateral hippocampal atrophy if they are depressed (Finegersh et al., 2011). Hippocampal atrophy in patients with depression has been attributed to the cytotoxic effects of high serum cortisol (Sapolsky et al., 2000), and corticosteroids facilitate amygdaloid kindling in rats (Kumar et al., 2007). This work has implicated hypothalamic-pituitary-adrenal hyperactivity as a mechanism of treatment-resistant epileptic seizures in patients with comorbid depression and perhaps with other psychiatric disorders (Kanner, 2011). Studies of time order in suicidality, which is not the same as depression, have also revealed bidirectionality (Hecimovic et al., 2011).

Anxiety

Anxiety disorders are the second most common psychiatric comorbidity in epilepsy (Tellez-Zenteno et al., 2007; Brandt et al. 2010). Like mood disorders, they are associated with a poorer therapeutic response to both antiseizure drugs and surgery (Petrovski et al., 2010; Kanner et al., 2009). In addition, patients with epilepsy who also have anxiety disorders have a reduced quality of life (Gilliam, 2002) and are at increased risk for suicide (Christensen et al., 2007). Anxiety disorders manifest in many forms, including panic disorder, social phobia, specific phobia, generalized anxiety disorder, obsessive-compulsive disorder, and posttraumatic stress disorder. Social phobia, agoraphobia, and generalized anxiety are most common among people with epilepsy, who often have more than one form and can have a simultaneous mood disorder (Kanner et al., 2009). In one population-based study a lifetime prevalence of comorbid anxiety and mood disorder was found in 34% of people with epilepsy (Tellez-Zenteno et al., 2007). Evidence suggests that the coexistence of anxiety and mood disorders is the strongest predictor of a poor quality of life (Johnson et al., 2004), and anxiety disorders increase the risk of suicide attempts in patients with mood disorders (Christensen et al., 2007).

The implication of these findings is that diagnosis and treatment of anxiety disorders, especially when they exist in association with mood disorders, could improve seizure control and quality of life and reduce the risk of suicide in people with epilepsy. An easy-to-use screening instrument widely employed by general practitioners is the *Patient's Health Questionnaire–Generalized Anxiety Disorder-7 (GAD-7)* (Spitzer et al. 2006). Standard treatment for anxiety disorder includes the use of *selective serotonin reuptake inhibitors (SSRIs)* and *selective norepinephrine reuptake inhibitors (SNRIs)* along with initial benzodiazepines for four to eight weeks, because of the delay in SSRI and SNRI action. *Cognitive behavioral therapy (CBT)* is also beneficial. Although no studies have evaluated therapies of this kind specifically in patients with epilepsy, it is generally agreed that these approaches are effective and safe in this population (Kerr et al., 2011).

Attention Deficit Hyperactivity Disorder

Attention deficit hyperactivity disorder (ADHD) occurs in approximately 5% of children and is characterized by a greater degree of inattention, hyperactivity-impulsivity, or both

than is normal for the child's age (Hesdorffer and Hauser, 2007). There is a familial susceptibility to ADHD, and symptoms can persist into adulthood in up to 50% of patients with primary ADHD. Nonetheless, the prevalence of ADHD in adults with epilepsy has not been determined. Symptoms of ADHD exist in a third of children with epilepsy and are sufficient for a diagnosis of ADHD in almost half of these children—three times the prevalence in children without epilepsy (Hesdorffer and Hauser, 2007; Dunn et al., 2009). The common belief that ADHD in this population was merely a side effect of antiseizure drugs was refuted by a study that found ADHD to be 2.5 times more common in children with newly diagnosed epilepsy than in matched controls (Hesdorffer et al., 2004). Not only does this observation establish ADHD as an epilepsy-related comorbidity, but evidence exists that ADHD, like depression and anxiety disorders, is a risk factor for the development of epilepsy.

Psychosis

Table 11–5 shows a classification of the relationship of psychotic disturbances to seizures. *Ictal* phenomena, particularly focal dyscognitive and absence status epilepticus (Chapter 10), can masquerade as psychotic states. As discussed earlier, *postictal psychosis* (Chapter 9), which can go on for days or even weeks in rare instances, can be distinguished from focal dyscognitive and absence status epilepticus by the clear consciousness and normal EEG and from interictal psychosis by the temporal relationship to repeated epileptic seizures and lack of a chronic course.

Interictal psychosis associated with epilepsy can be episodic or continuous. In some patients it is a toxic effect of antiseizure drugs, as discussed later in this chapter, whereas in others it reflects an endogenous process. Furthermore, prolonged focal seizures with psychic symptoms can occur in clear consciousness without scalp-recorded EEG changes (Wieser et al., 1985) (Chapter 6) and be mistaken for interictal intermittent psychosis.

Questions concerning continuous interictal psychosis associated with epilepsy have received much attention and are as controversial as those about personality traits and epilepsy. Psychosis is generally believed to

Table 11–5 **Psychosis in Epilepsy**

Ictal (Chapter 10)	
Temporal lobe status	Usually fluctuating level of consciousness with focal temporal ictal and/fusely slow EEG
Absence status	Usually continuous clouded consciousness with diffuse spike-and-wave discharges on EEG
Postictal (Chapter 9)	May have lucid interval of 12–24 hrs; usually clear consciousness, normal EEG
Interictal	
Toxic (Chapters 14 and 15)	Confused, organic, due to drugs; slow EEG
Episodic (Chapter 13)	May be unrelated to epileptic condition or may be ictal with normal scalp EEG
Continuous	May alternate with epileptic seizures or be unrelated; clear consciousness; schizophreniform paranoia reported; normal EEG

Derived from Blumer and Benson, 1982.

be more common among patients with epilepsy than in the population at large, although sampling bias has not been definitely ruled out (Stevens, 1966; Trimble and Schmitz, 2008; Hesdorffer and Hauser, 2007). Some researchers have calculated the prevalence of psychosis to be as high as 10–15% in severe uncontrolled temporal lobe epilepsy (Sherwin et al., 1982), compared with 5–9% for epilepsy in general. (Gudmundsson, 1966; Ounsted and Lindsay, 1981).

Reports that schizophrenia is more common with left temporal epilepsies and mood disorder with right temporal epilepsies (Flor-Henry, 1976; Flor-Henry, 1969) have been replicated inconsistently. Most of the older studies suffer from failure to identify the side of the epileptogenic lesion with certainty (Mendius and Engel, 1985).

Psychosis alternating with epileptic seizures has been noted on occasion. Some patients were observed to develop psychotic behaviors only when their seizures stopped and their EEG became normal (*forced normalization*) (Landolt, 1958). This finding suggested that epilepsy and psychosis are mutually exclusive and provided a rationale for ECT. (Sackheim et al., 1986). Although such an alternating relationship may occur in some patients, it has not been a common finding (Ramani and Gumnit, 1982). An alternative explanation for forced normalization is that these psychotic behaviors are actually ictal events associated with epileptiform discharges in deeper structures that are not reflected in surface EEG, during which time interictal activity would cease (Wolf, 1991).

A *schizophreniform paranoid psychosis* has been described as peculiar to epileptic conditions of long duration (Slater et al., 1963). Patients with this condition are said to lack the flattened affect that commonly occurs with schizophrenia, to be warm, and to relate personally. There is considerable disagreement, however, whether such a psychotic profile is unique to patients with epilepsy. A study comparing psychotic patients with and without epilepsy found that half the patients with epilepsy had schizophrenic symptoms indistinguishable from those without epilepsy. The other half, all of whom had temporal lobe epilepsy, were mostly manic, while paranoia was rare (Perez and Trimble, 1980).

Although there appears to be a higher risk for psychosis in patients with epilepsy than in the nonepileptic population, major areas of debate concern the assertions discussed above that (1) patients with temporal lobe epilepsy are even more susceptible to psychosis than those with other forms of epilepsy, (2) laterality of the epilepsy influences the manifestation of psychosis, (3) an antagonistic relationship exists between occurrence of epileptic seizures and the manifestations of psychotic illness, and (4) a characteristic schizophreniform psychosis is present in people with epilepsy that differs from other types of schizophrenia.

Classification of Neuropsychiatric Disorders in Epilepsy

The classification and terminology of psychiatric conditions encountered in people with epilepsy remains uncertain because of the lack of data, the atypical manifestations of many disorders, and the failure to consistently meet criteria established by the fourth edition of the *Diagnostic and Statistical Manual of Mental Disorders* (DSM-IV) (American Psychiatric Association, 2000). The *Commission on Neuropsychiatric Aspects of Epilepsy* of the ILAE has attempted to define the forms of neuropsychiatric disturbances encountered in people with epilepsy, preparing a classification (Table 11–6), based in part on the DSM-IV, that distinguishes comorbidity that should be diagnosed in the same fashion as for patients without epilepsy, implying no *organic* etiology, and conditions that appear to be epilepsy-related (Krishnamoorthy et al., 2007).

Autism Spectrum Disorders

Autism spectrum disorders are increasingly recognized as an important neurodevelopmental cause of disability (Amaral et al., 2011). Autism, like epilepsy, is a complex disorder with many manifestations and etiologies; however, the common coexistence of autism and epilepsy suggests not only involvement of similar pathophysiological processes and anatomical disturbances but also shared genetic and molecular mechanisms (Mefford et al., 2010). The prevalence of epilepsy among individuals with autism spectrum disorders and intellectual disabilities is 20% (Tuchman, 2011), while autism develops in 14% of infants with onset of epilepsy in the first year of life, 46% of patients

Table 11–6 ILAE Classification of Neuropsychiatric Disorders: Key Categories, Clinical Features, and Conclusions

Category	Special Features	Key Conclusions in Draft Classification Proposal
The problem of comorbidity	• Anxiety and phobic disorders • Minor and major depression • Obsessive-compulsive disorder • Other somatoform, dissociative, and neurotic disorders	No different from the range of common mental disorders prevalent in the community and in clinic/hospital populations. Classification should be as per ICD-10 and DSM-IV
Psychopathology as presenting symptom of epileptic seizures	Altered awareness, confusion, disorientation, memory disturbances, anxiety, dysphoria, hallucinations, and paranoid syndromes	Complex partial, simple partial, and absence status and other epilepsy syndromes can be diagnosed; clinically supported by EEG
Interictal psychiatric disorders that are specific to epilepsy	• Cognitive dysfunction including memory complaints • Psychoses of epilepsy • Affective somatoform disorders • Personality disorders • Anxiety and phobias specific to epilepsy	• May be general or specific; diagnosed with standard neuropsychological tests • To be classified based on the relationship to seizure—prodromal, interictal, postictal, and alternating • Hyperethical, viscous, labile, mixed, and other • Both trait accentuation and disorder to be coded • Fear of seizures recognized as a distinct and disabling entity
Other information of relevance	• Relationship to antiseizure drug therapy • Relationship to EEG change	Coded as not documented; associated with institution and/or withdrawal with specified time periods for both Presence or absence of associated EEG change documented

DSM-IV = *Diagnostic and Statistical Manual of Mental Disorders*, 4th ed. (American Psychiatric Association, 2000).
From Krishnamoorthy et al., 2007, with permission.

with infantile spasms, and 69% of infants with seizures caused by acquired or congenital brain insults (Tuchman and Cuccaro, 2011). Epilepsy is more than twice as common in girls with autism than boys (Tuchman et al., 1991). Although there is no direct evidence that epilepsy causes autism or that autism causes epilepsy, the bidirectional relationship, as with the psychiatric disorders noted previously, has stimulated research into shared mechanisms that could lead to improved treatment or prevention and also elucidate potential mechanisms underlying disturbances in social cognition experienced by people with epilepsy, particularly MTLE, who do not have autism (Broicher et al., 2012).

MECHANISMS OF INTERICTAL BEHAVIORAL DISTURBANCES IN EPILEPSY

Interictal behavioral disturbances can have psychosocial, neuropathological, and therapeutic causes and may result from effects of epilepsy itself (Table 11–7).

Table 11–7 **Causes of Behavior Disturbances in Epilepsy**

Psychosocial factors
  Stigmata associated with epilepsy
  Learned helplessness
Neuropathological factors
  Extent of the lesion
  Location of lesion
    Specific anatomical site
    Hemispheric specialization
  Pathological substrates
  Hereditary components
Effects of treatment
  Cerebral toxicity of drugs
    Dose related
    Hypersensitive
    Idiopathic
  Indirect drug effects on other systems
  Surgically induced disturbances
  Abrupt cessation of epileptic seizures
Epilepsy-induced disturbances
  Disruption of normal activity
  Potentiation of abnormal activity (e.g., kindling-altered receptor sensitivity, physiological dependency)
  Indirect effects (neuroendocrine, sleep)

Psychosocial Factors: The Predicament

Taylor (1982) has written eloquently about the *predicament* of the patient with epilepsy. Parental overprotection and guilt, underachievement due to restricted school and work opportunities, and resultant dependence and feelings of inadequacy can be consequences of many serious medical conditions. The stigmata associated with epilepsy and the inability to predict the occurrence of a seizure, however, create psychosocial problems that are peculiar to this disorder (Jacoby et al., 2008).

A feeling of lack of control undoubtedly affects patients' abilities to deal with their medical conditions and with life in general. This disturbing mental attitude may resemble *learned helplessness* (Seligman and Maier, 1967), in which psychological disturbances are produced experimentally when animals or humans are placed in a situation of temporarily unavoidable electric shock. Similar psychological problems might develop when people with epilepsy are unable to avoid or even predict their epileptic seizures (McIntyre, 1982). Indeed, identification of precipitating factors (Chapter 9) might greatly reduce the disabling mental disturbances associated with epilepsy.

In the past, epileptic seizures have been singularly identified with numerous socially unacceptable conditions (Temkin, 1945) (Chapter 2). To some degree in all cultures, people with epilepsy have been considered outcasts because of misconceptions relating symptoms to demonic possession, punishment for sins, contagious diseases (Jilek, 1979), and insanity (Berrios, 1984). It is difficult to appreciate the extent to which such superstition continues to influence attitudes about epilepsy. Self-image as well as ability to cope in society is necessarily determined by the degree to which these beliefs are prevalent in a patient's own mind and in the minds of those with whom daily contact is necessary or important. It is a sad commentary on the medical sophistication of modern society when almost all persons with epilepsy would rather keep their disorder a secret whenever possible (Chapter 17).

Reports that behavioral disturbances are more prevalent among people with epilepsy than among patients with other, equally disabling medical conditions do not necessarily indicate that neurobiological factors play a prominent role. Such comparative studies cannot rule out psychosocial influences until it is possible to control for the unique predicament created by epilepsy.

Neuropathological Factors

Disability and prognosis in epilepsy correlate strongly with the degree of neurological and mental impairment caused by underlying structural lesions of the brain (Rodin, 1968); however, these handicaps may also be associated with more severe epilepsy. For instance, the risks of seizures persisting in children who are clumsy, have severe hypotonia, or have cerebral palsy are two, five, and ten times greater, respectively, than in those without a motor handicap (Sillanpaa, 1975). Furthermore, there is an inverse relationship between the incidence and severity of epileptic seizures and IQ; the incidence of epilepsy is 50% in patients with an IQ below 20 (Corbett, 1981). Because behavioral disturbances that appear to correlate with the extent of structural pathology often correlate equally well with the severity of associated epileptic seizures, independent contributions of these two factors cannot be easily assessed.

Of more interest has been the possible correlation between specific behavioral disturbances and the location or pathological characteristics of a small well-localized epileptogenic lesion. Controversial observations that aberrant personality traits and psychoses are more commonly associated with mesial temporal limbic lesions than with other lesion sites have already been mentioned. This relationship is reported to be most likely when areas of the limbic system responsible for generating fear responses are involved (Hermann et al., 1982a). Given the importance of the limbic system in the development of human behavior, it is reasonable to postulate that the location of a structural lesion in one mesial temporal lobe could be a causal factor in the later development of personality disturbances and psychosis. At present, the contribution of functional disruption induced by epileptiform activity in these areas cannot be dissected from purely ablative effects of a lesion. The incidence of similar behavioral disturbances in individuals with small, nonepileptogenic lesions in mesial

temporal structures cannot be determined easily, because such minor defects generally do not come to the attention of physicians unless they cause epileptic seizures. The relative contribution of ablative versus epileptiform irritative disturbances to the development of interictal behavioral disorders could be resolved by careful follow-up studies after early surgical intervention. If further ablation that eliminates epileptogenic influences prevents or reverses specific behavioral disturbances, this would clearly implicate a direct effect of recurrent seizures. Although studies of surgical outcome in infants and young children with diffuse lesions limited to one hemisphere have confirmed an important role of recurrent seizures in the developmental delay associated with epileptic encephalopathies (Chapter 7), it has been much more difficult to carry out similar studies following more localized surgical procedures such as anteromesial temporal resections.

Controversy over the role of hemispheric specialization in the manifestation of interictal behavioral disorders has also been mentioned. The most reliable studies involve patients with definitely identified epileptogenic regions; those who undergo surgical resection for temporal lobe epilepsy have a well-defined structural abnormality in the resected temporal lobe and unequivocally benefit from this procedure (Mendius and Engel, 1985). One such study has revealed a weak relationship between an epileptogenic region in the left temporal lobe and psychosis (Sherwin et al., 1982), but an additional confounding factor exists. The relatively high incidence of right hemispheric dominance for language in patients with long-standing epilepsy of left temporal lobe origin (Rausch and Walsh, 1984) suggests that inconsistent pathological shifting of a variety of functions could be common.

An interesting example of imaginative speculation resulted from the observation that there is a statistically significant increased risk for schizophrenia among people with epilepsy who have *hamartomas*, particularly if these lesions occur in the left mesial temporal lobes of left-handed women (Taylor, 1975). This intriguing finding was explained by postulating a language-dependent thought disorder due to functional disruption, but not destruction, of language-specific cortex during a gender-dependent critical period in development. This peculiar pathological association is supported by more recent evidence of an unusual risk for depression after resections of a *dysembryoplastic neuroepithelial tumor (DNET)*, a lesion that in the past was diagnosed as a *hamartoma*, or of a *ganglioglioma* (Andermann et al., 1999; Shaw et al., 2004).

Another interesting hypothesis derives from controversial work relating specific karyotype abnormalities, such as an extra Y chromosome, with psychopathology, because individuals with these defects also demonstrate *ectodermal dysplasias* (Razavi, 1975). Hamartomas and other malformations of cortical development are ectodermal dysplasias, and the mesial temporal structures are highly epileptogenic; therefore, there could be a related genetic determinant for psychosis and dysplastic brain tissue, whereas the epileptic seizures would be merely an unrelated consequence when cortical dysplasia develops fortuitously in one mesial temporal lobe. The first hypothesis would account for the location of the lesion and the second for its specific pathological features.

Effects of Treatment

Antiseizure medications often cause dose-related or idiosyncratic behavioral side effects (Hirtz and Nelson, 1985; Parnas et al., 1980;

Reynolds, 1983; Rivinus, 1982; Schmidt and Schachter, 2008; Pirmohamed and Arroyo, 2008) (Table 11–8; Chapter 14). Sedation, cognitive impairment, and a depressed mood are dose-related side effects of all antiseizure drugs (Chapter 15). These effects are most often seen with the *barbiturates* and *benzodiazepines* and are usually minimal with *carbamazepine*, *valproic acid*, and the newer antiseizure drugs (Mattson et al., 1985; Trimble and Thompson, 1983; Schmidt and Schachter, 2008). Rarely, aphasia, deficits in recent memory, and other specific disturbances in cognitive function occur as reversible dose-related drug effects, in direct relation to the antiseizure medications' ability to cause nonspecific sedation and mental impairment. These effects presumably reflect unmasking of preexisting subclinical localized disturbances. Therefore, the appearance of focal features in patients with known cerebral compromise does not necessarily indicate a progressive neurological disorder. Differential diagnosis is helped by the coexistence of other common dose-related toxic signs and symptoms, such as nystagmus, slurred speech, ataxia, and diplopia (Chapters 12 and 14).

In children, the barbiturates are known to produce reversible *hyperkinetic* behavior characterized by irritability, tantrums, disobedience, lethargy, or insomnia and have

Table 11–8 Adverse Behavioral Effects of Some Antiseizure Drugs

Adrenocorticotropic hormone and steroids	Depression, irritability, labile mood (personality change and psychosis rare under the age of 12)
Benzodiazepines	Aggression, anorexia, confusion, depression, drowsiness, dysarthria, excitation, hallucinations, irritability
Bromides	Drowsiness, hyposexuality, personality change, psychosis
Carbamazepine	Anorexia, depression, dizziness, drowsiness, psychosis
Ethosuximide	Anorexia, dizziness, drowsiness, insomnia, irritability, personality change, psychosis
Lamotrigine	Insomnia
Levetiracetam	Irritability, aggressive behavior
Phenobarbital	Drowsiness, dysarthria, excitation, and, especially in children, hyperactivity
Phenytoin	Anorexia, dementia, dizziness, drowsiness, dysarthria, hyperactivity, organic brain syndrome, personality change, progressive encephalopathy
Primidone	Anorexia, dizziness, drowsiness, hyperactivity and excitement, personality change, psychosis, sexual dysfunction and impotence
Topiramate	Affective symptoms, cognitive disturbances
Valproic acid	Aggression, depression, hyperactivity, psychosis
Vigabatrin	Psychosis, depression

been found to cause or exacerbate preexisting depression (Ferrari et al., 1983). Barbiturates can also produce confusion in older individuals. Similar behavioral side effects are encountered with the benzodiazepines, although less commonly. Aggressive behavior has been a particular problem in children, as has depression in adults. *Primidone* is less likely to cause hyperactivity than *phenobarbital* but can induce an idiosyncratic personality change and psychosis.

Phenytoin occasionally gives rise to a reversible encephalopathy without associated nystagmus or ataxia (Trimble and Reynolds, 1976). The resulting picture of progressive deterioration may be mistakenly diagnosed as a degenerative disorder. In most of these cases the serum blood level of phenytoin is in the toxic range. *Valproic acid* can lead to a similar progressive encephalopathy (Reynolds, 1983), but dose-related behavioral disturbances are less frequent than with most other antiseizure drugs. Valproic acid–induced hyperammonemia causes lethargy, sedation, and coma. Behavioral disturbances associated with *carbamazepine* are relatively rare and minimal; improvement of cognitive function can often be seen when carbamazepine is substituted for other antiseizure drugs (Mattson et al., 1985; Trimble and Thompson, 1983).

Psychosis occurs rarely with *ethosuximide*, usually in young adults with a history of a psychiatric disorder (Chapter 15). The psychosis may alternate with epileptic seizures (Wolf, 1980). Depression and psychosis are common side effects of *phenacemide* and a major drawback in the clinical use of this drug.

Psychiatric side effects do occur with the new antiseizure drugs (Schmitz, 2008). *Vigabatrin* has the highest incidence of psychosis (2.5%) and depression (12%); *topiramate* can cause affective symptoms as well as cognitive disturbances with higher doses; *levetiracetam* provokes aggressive behavior and irritability, particularly in patients with preexisting dysphoria; and *lamotrigine* can induce insomnia, which in turn can result in psychiatric disturbances. Behavioral side effects of the other newer antiseizure drugs are rare except in patients with preexisting cognitive and psychiatric disorders.

Positive psychotropic effects were claimed for certain older antiseizure medications (Table 11–9) (Parnas et al., 1980), but very few have been substantiated in controlled

Table 11–9 Positive Psychotropic Effects Claimed for Antiseizure Drugs

Benzodiazepines	Reduce anxiety
Carbamazepine	Antidepressant; antimanic; reduces hyperactivity and irritability
Phenytoin	Antiaggressive; reduces anxiety, hyperactivity, irritability, and compulsive eating; improves concentration, nervousness, auditory perception (all unsubstantiated)

trials (Table 11–10) (Schmitz, 2008; Ettinger, 2006). Of interest are the potential *antimanic* and *antidepressant* effects of *carbamazepine*, *oxcarbazepine*, *lamotrigine*, and *valproic acid* (Post et al., 1984; Schmitz, 2008), making them, at least theoretically, drugs of choice for patients with focal or generalized tonic-clonic seizures who have or are at risk for affective disturbances.

Antiseizure drugs can influence behavior by a number of mechanisms other than their direct pharmacological action on the brain (Rivinus, 1982; Schmidt and Schachter, 2008; Pirmohamed and Arroyo, 2008). Mental symptoms can result from drug-induced *hypocalcemia*, autoimmune disturbances, *hyper-* and *hypoparathyroid disease*, and *systemic lupus erythematosus*. Long-term therapy influences neuroendocrine function (Franceschi et al., 1984; Toone, 1987), perhaps via GABAergic and biogenic amine mechanisms. Lowering of *folic acid* and *vitamin B$_{12}$* levels due to antiseizure medication received considerable attention in the past (Reynolds, 1967); the importance of this effect in the development of behavioral disturbances remains controversial. Claims that replacement of folic acid may reduce the efficacy of antiseizure drugs (Carl and Smith, 1983) have not been substantiated. Rare side effects of phenytoin, such as *hyperglycemia*, *pseudolymphoma*, and *hepatic necrosis* all might alter mental performance. Antiseizure drugs, particularly the barbiturates, exacerbate symptoms of *porphyria*, which is associated with psychiatric symptoms. Behavioral disturbances in some patients might be attributed to benzodiazepine- or barbiturate-induced sleep disorders such as deprivation of *rapid eye movement (REM) sleep*, particularly because these sedative drugs are commonly given at

Table 11–10 **Psychotropic Effects of Antiseizure Drugs Demonstrated in Controlled Trials**

	Depression	Mania	Bipolar Disorder	Anxiety
Carbamazepine	0	+	+	0
Oxcarbazepine	0	+	0	0
Valproic acid	0	+	+	0
Lamotrigine	0	0	+	0
Gabapentin	0	−	−	+/−
Topiramate	0	−	0	0
Tiagabine	0	−	0	0
Levetiracetam	0	0	0	−
Pregabalin	0	0	0	+
Zonisamide	0	0	0	0

+, positive results; −, negative results; 0, no published data.
From Schmitz, 2008, with permission.

bedtime. This possibility has not been adequately studied (Engel et al., 1986). Finally, the well-known cosmetic side effects of phenytoin (Falconer and Davison, 1973) can contribute powerfully to a patient's poor self-image and lack of confidence.

Risk factors for the development of behavioral side effects of antiseizure drugs include a history of psychiatric problems; the presence of diffuse brain damage; early age of onset of epileptic seizures; long duration of antiseizure drug treatment, particularly with prolonged toxicity; polypharmacy; malnutrition; pregnancy; and intercurrent illness (Rivinus, 1982; Schmitz, 2008). Administration of multiple drugs can cause unexpected problems, most often resulting from inhibition of liver enzymes (Chapter 14). A common example is valproic acid–induced reduction in barbiturate metabolism. The sudden appearance of lethargy or coma when valproic acid is added to the regimen of a patient on barbiturates can create considerable diagnostic confusion until the grossly elevated barbiturate plasma level is discovered.

Recognizing that behavioral disturbances are due to antiseizure drug administration is relatively easy when the onset of symptoms is temporally related to addition of or increase in a particular drug or when there are other signs of toxicity, such as nystagmus, slurred speech, and ataxia. It is much more difficult, however, when the onset is insidious and other signs of toxicity are absent, as with phenytoin encephalopathy, or when the effect is not dose-related, as in the psychoses that occur with primidone and ethosuximide. In these cases diagnosis requires a high degree of suspicion. Symptoms almost always resolve when the offending medication is decreased or removed.

Behavioral disturbances associated with *surgical treatment* of epilepsy are also well recognized (Chapter 16). When resective surgery, particularly anteromesial temporal lobe resection, is successful in relieving habitual seizures, there is often an improvement in intellectual and memory function (Rausch and Crandall, 1982). Anteromesial temporal lobe resection in the language-dominant and nondominant hemispheres can, however, give rise to deficits in verbal and nonverbal memory, respectively, that may only be elicited by special testing (Milner, 1975). Nonverbal memory deficits following mesial temporal resections of the non-language-dominant hemisphere are usually not noticeable or disabling; however, verbal memory deficits following mesial temporal resections of the language-dominant hemisphere can be more severe and disabling. These are much more likely to occur when there is no verbal memory deficit prior to surgery, suggesting that a normally functioning hippocampus was removed; however, when onset of epilepsy was early in life and memory function was transferred to the contralateral hemisphere, patients may be spared postoperative verbal memory deficits (Loring et al., 2008) (Chapter 16). Evaluation of patients undergoing surgery for refractory MTLE has yielded important insights into the anatomical substrates of memory (Bell et al., 2011).

The appearance of transient postoperative depression, or occasionally hypomania or psychosis, in approximately one-quarter to one-third of patients who undergo anterior temporal lobectomy (Hill et al., 1957; Horowitz and Cohen, 1968; Koch-Stoecker and Kanemoto, 2008) is of theoretical as well as practical interest. This phenomenon is most common in patients whose seizures were abolished by surgery but cannot be easily explained on the basis of difficulty adapting to a life without epilepsy. Symptoms usually disappear over the first postoperative year. Suicide is a risk, however, even after many years, in patients who have been surgically cured of epilepsy (Taylor and March, 1979). ECT was even prescribed in some cases in the past (Hill et al., 1957). Behavioral disturbances in these patients might result from cessation of seizures per se, as discussed in a later section of this chapter. This raises the intriguing possibility that some apparent side effects of antiseizure drugs are due to seizure control rather than direct pharmacological action. Conversely, the appearance of hypomanic behavior following successful surgery can occasionally be attributed to discontinuation of carbamazepine.

Corpus callosum section gives rise to an *acute hemispheric disconnection syndrome* characterized by mutism, apraxia, apathy, confusion, infantile behavior, and alternating focal motor seizures (Roberts, 2008) (Chapter 16). These symptoms resolve over days to months.

Vagus nerve stimulation is reported to have a beneficial effect on mood and may improve daytime alertness and vigilance (Schachter and Boon, 2008) (Chapter 16). Deep-brain stimulation and transcranial magnetic stimulation are other neuromodulatory interventions that may have an impact on mood, but further research is needed (Fregni et al., 2005; Miatton et al., 2011) (Chapter 16).

Epilepsy-Induced Neurobiological Factors

Perhaps the most interesting and potentially important factor to be considered as a cause of behavioral disturbances in epilepsy is the epileptic process itself. This suggestion has been controversial, because of concern that it could cause additional anxiety for people with epilepsy and their families; however, those arguments are similar to the ones that were levied against the view that epileptic disorders are progressive, a concept that is now clearly recognized for the epileptic encephalopathies and increasingly acknowledged for other forms of epilepsy as well (Chapter 7). Exploring this suggestion might reveal preventable or treatable causes of behavioral disturbances in epilepsy that should not be overlooked.

Evidence that epilepsy itself gives rise to reversible interictal, as well as ictal and postictal, alterations in behavior can be inferred from results of surgery. When anteromesial temporal lobe resection is effective in abolishing epileptic seizures, intellectual function, including memory, and in some cases aggression, hyposexuality, and problems with interpersonal relationships, can improve (Hill et al., 1957; Rausch and Crandall, 1982; Taylor, 1972; Walker and Blumer, 1977). On the other hand, personality traits such as hyperreligiosity, viscosity (Walker and Blumer, 1977), and psychosis (Taylor, 1972) may not resolve even when seizures no longer occur.

Postoperative improvement in intellectual function, particularly memory, is striking in some patients, especially in view of the fact that the surgical procedure involves removal of one hippocampus, which supposedly subserves memory. The interpretation is inescapable that the diseased hippocampus was not only malfunctioning but adversely influencing the contralateral hippocampus and other cerebral structures to produce the observed behavioral deficit. For the personality traits, however, it can be argued that improvement, when it occurs, is the result of decreased psychosocial stress consequent upon becoming seizure-free. Conversely, it could also be argued that persistence of abnormal behavior reflects an epilepsy-induced enduring alteration in cerebral function or structure.

Support for the concept of epilepsy-induced behavioral changes is also provided by observations that personality disturbances usually do not appear until sometime after the onset of an epileptic condition, and psychosis develops even later (Slater et al., 1963). More studies are needed to determine whether behavioral disturbances can be avoided if successful surgical treatment is performed early in the course of the disorder (Davidson and Falconer, 1975; Dreifuss, 1987; Rausch and Crandall, 1982).

Results from a number of epilepsy surgery centers indicate that the most rewarding outcomes with respect to ultimate psychosocial adaptation occur when patients undergo surgery in early adolescence or within a few years after the onset of the epilepsy disorder (Engel, 1987).

Epilepsy may be uniquely capable of producing enduring functional disruption of cerebral activity. Structural lesions cause deficits, and plasticity of the central nervous system can often compensate for effects of ablation. Particularly when static lesions occur early in childhood, transfer of function can allow development to progress normally. The intermittent nature of epileptic activity, however, could make epileptogenic disturbances much more potent factors in abnormal development than are purely structural defects. Intermittent epileptiform discharges might disrupt function locally and at a distance without inducing compensatory plastic changes. Normal development of responses of lateral geniculate neurons to visual stimulation can be prevented by corticofugal projections from epileptic lesions in immature rabbit visual cortex (Baumbach and Chow, 1981; Chow et al., 1978). Such a mechanism might explain why early onset of an epileptic disturbance in the left temporal lobe can produce a persistent disorder of language-dependent thought rather than causing initial aphasia and subsequent shift of language functions to the right side (Taylor, 1975).

In addition to interfering with normal function, epileptic mechanisms might actually potentiate the development of abnormal function. Animal experiments suggest that kindling-like changes along the pathways that propagate epileptic activity in temporal lobe epilepsy might mediate commonly encountered behavioral disorders (Engel and Cahan, 1986; Engel et al., 1986). The amygdala and its projection fields have been shown to modulate aggressive behavior in the cat (Flynn et al., 1970), and kindling of the amygdala and hippocampus has been reported to produce enduring suppression or facilitation of predatory behavior in this species (Adamec, 1975). Explosive motor behavior and reactive biting are seen postictally in amygdala- and hippocampus-kindled rats (Pinel et al., 1977), effects that may be mediated in part by opioid mechanisms (Caldecott-Hazard et al., 1983). Defensive rage behavior can be produced in normal cats by stimulation of the midbrain central gray (Bandler, 1982), which receives afferent input from the amygdala and is rich in opioid-containing cell bodies. Amygdaloid kindling in cats can alter the threshold for this stimulation-induced defensive rage (Siegel, 1985/86). Chronic temporal lobe seizures induced in cats by kainic acid injected into hippocampus produce an enduring interictal state of irritability, inappropriate defensive reactions to mild threat, and lowered thresholds to stimulation-induced defensive rage that can occur only when the animal is approached contralateral to the epileptic hippocampus (Engel et al., 1985/86; 1986; 1991; 2008; Griffith et al., 1987) (Fig. 11–2). Collectively these studies demonstrate that enduring alterations in the excitability of neuronal circuits mediating affective display in animals can be induced by experimental limbic epilepsy and reinforce the belief that similar mechanisms exist in the human condition. In the more evolved human brain, however, these effects are unlikely to manifest as defensive rage and perhaps give rise to more sophisticated behaviors such as depression, insecurity, and paranoia. Future studies using functional neuroimaging and magnetoencephalography (Chapter 12) may elucidate abnormal neuronal connectivity responsible for epilepsy-related behavioral disturbances in patients.

Acquired dependency on endogenous opioids might also account for some behavioral disturbances (Caldecott-Hazard and Engel, 1987; Engel et al., 1986). In rats, these substances are released during epileptic seizures (Hong et al., 1979) and appear to mediate certain postictal behaviors (Caldecott-Hazard and Engel, 1987). Endogenous opioids are believed to function as natural mood elevators (Kline et al., 1977) and may partially account for the beneficial effect of ECT on clinical depression. It has been suggested that patients with recurrent epileptic seizures become physiologically dependent on intermittent high levels of endogenous opioids and experience depression as a response to reduction of these abnormal levels when seizures do not occur at regular intervals (Engel et al., 1984a;b; 1986; 1991; 2008). This concept might be directly tested now that PET has demonstrated altered opioid binding in the epileptic temporal lobes of patients with MTLE (Frost et al., 1988; Mayberg et al., 1994).

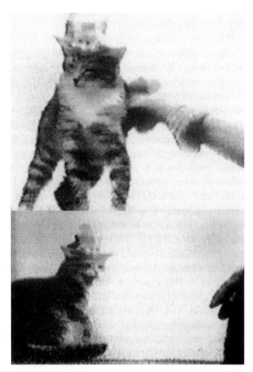

Figure 11–2. Demonstration of lateralized hyperreactivity. Photographs were taken from a videotape recording of a cat with a chronic, kainic acid–induced epileptogenic lesion in the left hippocampus. *Top:* When the cat was approached on the left (ipsilateral) side, it responded by rubbing up against the offered hand and purring. *Bottom:* When an attempt was made to touch the cat on the right (contralateral) side, it assumed a defensive posture (ears back, piloerection, and pupillary dilatation), hissed, and struck at the offered hand with the right paw. (From Engel et al., 1991, with permission.)

Another possible mechanistic explanation for the common occurrence of depression among people with epilepsy is suggested by the bidirectional relationship between these two conditions (Kanner, 2011). As discussed earlier, high cortisol levels are believed to play a role in the manifestation of depression and in hippocampal atrophy, suggesting a role in epileptogenesis. Corticosteroids facilitate amygdaloid kindling in rats (Kumar et al., 2007). This mechanism is being studied in a rat model of temporal lobe epilepsy. High steroid levels during the interictal period promote symptoms equivalent to depression in these animals and also facilitate epileptogenicity (Mazarati et al., 2009). The associated seizures could cause hyperactivity of the hypothalamic-pituitary-adrenal axis, which

would also decrease the metabolism of serotonin, a neurotransmitter implicated in protection against both depression and epilepsy (Kanner, 2011). Interrelationships between this process and noradrenergic, GABAergic, and glutamatergic neurotransmitter systems have also been implicated in the bidirectional relationship between depression and epilepsy (Kanner, 2011).

Altered receptor sensitivity has been invoked to explain psychiatric behaviors (Engel et al., 1986; 1991; 2008). Current hypotheses of schizophrenia postulate enhanced catecholamine-mediated effects in the same limbic structures involved in temporal lobe epilepsy (Stevens, 1973). Catecholamines are known to inhibit most experimental epileptic conditions (Ehlers et al., 1980; Engel and Katzman, 1977; Engel and Sharpless, 1977; Maynert et al., 1975) (Chapters 3 and 4). This relationship would be expected if an antagonistic relationship exists between epilepsy and psychosis, as discussed previously (Lesser et al., 1986). However, a schizophrenia-like state has been reported in cats as a result of kindling catecholaminergic afferent input into limbic structures (Stevens and Livermore, 1978). Furthermore, amygdaloid kindling causes a long-lasting enhancement of *methamphetamine* stereotypy (Sato, 1983; Sato and Ogawa, 1984), implying an epilepsy-induced upregulation of dopamine receptors. Such an enduring alteration in receptor sensitivity could conceivably develop as a protective mechanism in response to epileptic seizures (Engel and Wilson, 1986; Frost et al., 1988) and account for the development of chronic psychosis in epileptic patients.

Epileptic seizures might indirectly give rise to other chronic behavioral disturbances by their effects on the neuroendocrine systems and on sleep (Engel et al., 1986; 1991; 2008). Epileptic seizures induce changes in prolactin release, which appear to be specifically related to ictal discharges in limbic structures that project to hypothalamus (Sperling et al., 1986). Chronic abnormalities in sex hormones have been demonstrated in patients with temporal lobe epilepsy, and these have been postulated to play a role in the occurrence of sexual disturbances (Herzog et al., 1982; Toone, 1987; Herzog, 2008; Harden and Frye, 2008). Epileptic seizures are also known to have adverse effects on sleep patterns (Sterman et al., 1982; Shouse et al., 2008) (Chapter 9). Chronic epilepsy in experimental animals as well as in humans alters night sleep, particularly causing a reduction in the percentage of REM time. Chronic REM deficits cause progressive behavioral changes (Dement et al., 1967). These potential areas of investigation have received too little attention and could conceivably provide insights into reversible causes of progressive changes in behavior associated with certain epileptic disorders.

Epileptic mechanisms undoubtedly give rise to interictal psychiatric comorbidity in patients with epilepsy, particularly those with epileptogenic lesions in the limbic system. An important question that needs to be addressed is the extent to which these effects of epileptogenesis are actually side effects of powerful homeostatic mechanisms that develop in response to epileptogenesis and epileptogenicity to maintain the interictal state and therefore should not be antagonized. Equally important for future research is to elucidate mechanisms by which psychiatric disorders promote epileptogenicity and common substrates that underlie the bidirectional relationship between epilepsy and behavioral disturbances. Further studies are needed not only to identify targets for therapies intended to reverse or prevent these disturbing and disabling conditions but also to elucidate when and why such therapeutic interventions might actually suppress or prevent epileptogenic processes.

SUMMARY AND CONCLUSIONS

Behavioral disturbances in people with epilepsy present considerable diagnostic and treatment issues for patients, families, and clinicians. Although fear of exacerbating the damaging and erroneous negative stereotypes associated for centuries with epilepsy once caused a reluctance to study the incidence, characteristics, and causes of interictal behavioral disturbances in patients, these concerns no longer constitute a valid argument to ignore the often treatable causes of such disabilities. Psychiatric comorbidity among people with epilepsy is now generally acknowledged to be common and is becoming increasingly well defined. Furthermore, these psychiatric conditions have a major negative impact on seizure control, quality of life, and cost of health care. Continued research on this subject will not only help to identify targets for prevention and treatment of these comorbid disorders but also provide knowledge of common underlying mechanisms of psychiatric disturbances and epilepsy that could lead to improved approaches to preventing and treating epilepsy.

Behavioral disturbances can reflect the psychosocial predicament of the patient with epilepsy who is subjected to overprotection, restriction on activities, discrimination, and unpredictable ictal events. The cerebral lesions underlying an epilepsy condition can produce neurological and mental dysfunctions that are related only indirectly to the epilepsy condition but are responsible in a major way for the degree of disabilities suffered by some patients. Behavior can also be adversely affected by antiseizure medications that cause sedation, depression, cognitive impairment, and psychiatric symptoms, and by surgical therapy. Some of the newer antiseizure medications, surgery, and vagus nerve stimulation, however, can also ameliorate certain behavioral disturbances.

Prodromal, ictal, and postictal behavioral disturbances can masquerade as interictal symptoms. Postictal psychiatric symptoms, including postictal psychosis, are more common and disabling than is generally appreciated, and morbidity can be reduced by timely diagnosis and treatment.

Claims of a characteristic epileptic personality are no longer generally accepted, although some personality traits may occur more often than expected in people with epilepsy, particularly those with mesial temporal involvement. An increased incidence of depressed mood and suicidality in people with epilepsy is well documented, and cannot be accounted for entirely by reaction to illness.

Depression is the most important comorbidity of epilepsy, and the relationship is bidirectional, in that depression is associated with a poor response of seizures to both drug and surgical therapy. Common underlying mechanisms appear to exacerbate both depression and epileptogenicity. Anxiety disorders are the second most common comorbidity of epilepsy and also appear to have a bidirectional relationship with it, again implying common mechanisms. ADHD is common in children with epilepsy and is not merely a side effect of antiseizure medications. While ictal and postictal psychosis have been well documented in epilepsy and carry considerable morbidity, a relationship between specific interictal psychotic disturbances and epilepsy has not been definitively demonstrated. In particular, the existence of a schizophreniform psychosis peculiar to people with epilepsy has yet to be proven. There is also a special relationship between epilepsy and autism spectrum disorder.

Epileptogenic mechanisms are clearly responsible for cognitive disturbances and developmental delay in the epileptic encephalopathies and for memory disturbances in temporal lobe epilepsy. Evidence from animal as well as clinical research has led to neurobiological hypotheses linking epilepsy-induced disturbances in limbic excitability, endogenous opioid mechanisms, hyperactivity of the hypothalamic-pituitary-adrenal axis, glutamatergic and GABAergic mechanisms, and catecholamine receptor supersensitivity to enduring alterations in behavior as well as to more severe epilepsy. Some of these behavioral disturbances, however, could reflect the effects of homeostatic protective mechanisms that exist to maintain the interictal state. Epileptic seizures might also influence interictal behavior by disrupting sleep and endocrine functions.

Assessment of behavioral comorbidities is an essential component of caring for the patient with epilepsy. Relative ignorance of many forms of interictal behavioral disturbances suffered by people with epilepsy and of their causes, coupled with the potential that improved understanding in this area has for relieving considerable discomfort and disability, makes this a high-priority area for future research.

REFERENCES

Adamec, R (1975). Behavioral and epileptic determinants of predatory attack behavior in the cat. Can J Neurol Sci 2:457–466.

Alper, K, Kuzniecky, R, Carlson, C, Barr, WB, Vorkas, CK, Patel, JG, Carrelli, AL, Starner, K, Flom, PL, and Devinsky, O (2008). Postictal psychosis in partial epilepsy: A case-control study. Ann Neurol 63:602–610.

Alstrom, CH (1950). A study of epilepsy in its clinical, social and genetic aspects. Acta Psychiatr Neurol Suppl 63:1–284.

Amaral, DG, Dawson, G, and Geschwind, DH (eds) (2011). Autism Spectrum Disorder. Oxford: Oxford University Press.

American Psychiatric Association (2000). Diagnostic and Statistical Manual of Mental Disorders, 4th ed, with text revision (DSM–IV-TR). Washington, DC: American Psychiatric Association.

Andermann, LF, Savard, G, Meencke, HJ, McLachlan, R, Moshé, S, and Andermann, F (1999). Psychosis after resection of ganglioglioma or DNET: Evidence for an association. Epilepsia 40:83–87.

Austin, JK, and Dunn, DW (2002). Progressive behavioral changes in children with epilepsy. Prog Brain Res 135:419–427.

Austin, JK, de Boer, HM, and Shafer, PO (2008). Disruptions in social functioning and services facilitating adjustment for the child and the adult. In Epilepsy: A Comprehensive Textbook, 2nd ed. Edited by J Engel, Jr, and TA Pedley. Philadelphia: Lippincott Williams & Wilkins, pp. 2237–2245.

Baca, CB, Vickrey, BG, Caplan, R, Vassar, SD, and Berg, AT (2011). Psychiatric and medical comorbidity and quality of life outcomes in childhood-onset epilepsy. Pediatrics 128:e1532–1543.

Baker, GA, Devinsky, O, Taylor, J, and Cramer, JA (2008). Quantitative measures of assessment. In Epilepsy: A Comprehensive Textbook, 2nd ed. Edited by J Engel, Jr, and TA Pedley. Philadelphia: Lippincott Williams & Wilkins, pp. 1133–1140.

Bandler, R (1982). Induction of rage following microinjections of glutamate into midbrain but not hypothalamus of cats. Neurosci Lett 30:183–188.

Barraclough, B (1981). Suicide and epilepsy. In Epilepsy and Psychiatry. Edited by EH Reynolds and MR Trimble. London: Churchill Livingstone, pp. 72–76.

Batzel, LW, and Dodrill, CB (1984). Neuropsychological and emotional correlates of marital status and ability to live independently in individuals with epilepsy. Epilepsia 25:594–598.

Baumbach, HD, and Chow, KL (1981). Visuocortical epileptiform discharges in rabbits: Differential effects on neuronal development in the lateral geniculate nucleus and superior colliculus. Brain Res 209:61–76.

Bear, DM, and Fedio, P (1977). Quantitative analysis of interictal behavior in temporal lobe epilepsy. Arch Neurol 34:454–467.

Bell, B, Lin, JJ, Seidenberg, M, and Hermann, B (2011). The neurobiology of cognitive disorders in temporal lobe epilepsy. Nat Rev Neurol 7:154–164.

Benson, DF, Miller, BL, and Signer, SF (1986). Dual personality associated with epilepsy. Arch Neurol 43:471–474.

Berrios, GE (1984). Epilepsy and insanity during the early 19th century: A conceptual history. Arch Neurol 41:978–981.

Betts, TA (1981). Depression, anxiety and epilepsy. In Epilepsy and Psychiatry. Edited by EH Reynolds and MR Trimble. London: Churchill Livingstone, pp. 60–71.

Blumer, D (1970). Hypersexual episodes in temporal lobe epilepsy. Am J Psychiatry 126:1099–1106.

Blumer, D, Benson, DF (1982). Psychiatric manifestations of epilepsy. In Psychiatric Aspects of Neurologic Disease, Vol II. Edited by D Benson and DF Blumer. New York: Grune &Stratton, pp. 25–48.

Blumer, D, Montouris, G, and Davies, K (2004). The interictal dysphoric disorder: Recognition, pathogenesis, and treatment of the major psychiatric disorders of epilepsy. Epilepsy Behav 5:826–840.

Brandt, C, Schoendienst, M, Trentowska, M, May, TW, Pohlmann-Eden, B, Tuschen-Caffier, B, Schrecke, M, Fueratsch, N, and Witte-Boelt, K (2010). Prevalence of anxiety disorders in patients with refractory focal epilepsy—A prospective clinic based survey. Epilepsy Behav 17:259–263.

Broicher, SD, Kuchukhidze, G, Grunwald, T, Günter, K, Kurthen, M, and Jokeit, H (2012). "Tell me how do I feel"—Emotion recognition and theory of mind in symptomatic mesial temporal lobe epilepsy. Neuropsychologia 50:118–128.

Caldecott-Hazard, S, and Engel, J, Jr (1987). Limbic postictal events: Anatomical substrates and opioid receptor involvement. Prog Neuropsychopharmacol Biol Psychiatry 11:389–418.

Caldecott-Hazard, S, Yamagata, N, Hedlund, J, Camacho, H, and Liebeskind, JC (1983). Changes in simple and complex behaviors following kindled seizures in rats: Opioid and nonopioid mediation. Epilepsia 24:539–547.

Carl, GF, and Smith, DB (1983). Interaction of phenytoin and folate in the rat. Epilepsia 24:494–501.

Chow, KL, Baumbach, HD, and Glanzman, DL (1978). Abnormal development of lateral geniculate neurons in rabbit subjected to either eyelid closure or corticofugal paroxysmal discharges. Brain Res 146:151–158.

Christensen, J, Vestergaard, M, Mortensen, P, Sidenius, P, and Agerbo, E (2007). Epilepsy and risk of suicide: A population-based case-control study. Lancet Neurol 6:693–698.

Chugani, HT, Mazziotta, JC, Engel, J, Jr, and Phelps, ME (1987). The Lennox-Gastaut syndrome: Metabolic subtypes determined by 2-deoxy-2[(18)F]fluoro-D-glucose positron emission tomography. Ann Neurol 21:4–13.

Corbett, J (1981). Epilepsy and mental retardation. In Epilepsy and Psychiatry. Edited by EH Reynolds and MR Trimble. London: Churchill Livingstone, pp. 138–146.

Cramer, JA, Westbrook, LE, Devinsky, O, et al. (1999). Development of the Quality of Life in Epilepsy Inventory for Adolescents: The QOLIE-AD-48. Epilepsia 40:1114–1121.

Cramer, JA, Blum, D, Fanning, K, and Reed, M (2004). The impact of comorbid depression on health resource utilization in a community sample of people with epilepsy. Epilepsy Behav 5:337–342.

Crandall, PH, Rausch, R, and Engel, J, Jr (1987). Preoperative indicators for optimal surgical outcome for temporal lobe epilepsy. In Presurgical Evaluation of Epileptics: Basics, Techniques, and Implications. Edited by HG Weiser and CE Elger. Berlin: Springer-Verlag, pp. 325–334.

Davidson, S, and Falconer, MA (1975). Outcome of surgery in 40 children with temporal lobe epilepsy. Lancet 1:1260–1263.

Delaney, RC, Rosen, AJ, Mattson, RH, and Novelly, RA (1980). Memory function in focal epilepsy: A comparison of non-surgical unilateral temporal lobe and frontal lobe samples. Cortex 16:103–117.

Delgado-Escueta, AV, Mattson, RH, King, L, Goldensohn, ES, Spiegel, H, Madsen, J, Crandall, P, Dreifuss, F, and Porter, RJ (1981). Special report: The nature of aggression during epileptic seizures. N Engl J Med 305:711–716.

Dement, W, Henry, P, Cohen, H, and Ferguson, J (1967). Studies on the effect of REM deprivation in humans and in animals. In Sleep and Altered States of Consciousness (Research Publications, Association for Research in Nervous and Mental Diseases, Vol XLV). Edited by S Kety, E Evarts, and H Williams. Baltimore: Williams and Wilkins, pp. 456–468.

Devinsky, O, Vickrey, BG, Perrine, K, et al. (1995). Development of the Quality of Life in Epilepsy Inventory. Epilepsia 36:1089–1104.

Devinsky, O, Vorkas, C, Barr, WB, and Hermann, BP (2008). Personality disorders in epilepsy. In Epilepsy: A Comprehensive Textbook, 2nd ed. Edited by J Engel, Jr, and TA Pedley. Philadelphia: Lippincott Williams & Wilkins, pp. 2105–2112.

Dikmen, S, Hermann, BP, Wilensky, AJ, and Rainwater, G (1983). Validity of the Minnesota Multiphasic Personality Inventory (MMPI) to psychopathology in patients with epilepsy. J Nerv Ment Dis 171:114–122.

Dodrill, CB (1983). Development of intelligence and neuropsychological impairment scales for the Washington Psychosocial Seizure Inventory. Epilepsia 24:1–10.

Dodrill, CB, Batzel, LW, Queisser, HR, and Temkin, NR (1980). An objective method for the assessment of psychological and social problems among epileptics. Epilepsia 21:123–135.

Dodrill, CB, Breyer, DN, Diamond, MB, Dubinsky, BL, and Geary, BB (1984a). Psychosocial problems among adults with epilepsy. Epilepsia 25:168–175.

Dodrill, CB, Beier, R, Kasparick, M, Tacke, I, Tacke, U, and Tan, S-Y (1984b). Psychosocial problems in adults with epilepsy: Comparison of findings from four countries. Epilepsia 25:176–183.

Dodrill, CB, and Batzel, LW (1986). Interictal behavioral features of patients with epilepsy. Epilepsia 27(suppl 2): S64–S76.

Dreifuss, FE (1987). Goals of surgery for epilepsy. In Surgical Treatment of the Epilepsies. Edited by J Engel, Jr. New York: Raven Press, pp. 31–50.

Dunn, DW, Austin, JK, and Perkins, SM (2009). Prevalence of psychopathology in childhood epilepsy: Categorical and dimensional measures. Dev Med Child Neurol 55:364–372.

Ehlers, CL, Clifton, DK, and Sawyer, CH (1980). Facilitation of amygdala kindling in the rat by transecting ascending noradrenergic pathways. Brain Res 189:274–278.

Engel, J, Jr (1987). Outcome with respect to epileptic seizures. In Surgical Treatment of the Epilepsies. Edited by J Engel, Jr. New York: Raven Press, pp. 553–572.

Engel, J, Jr, and Cahan, L (1986). Potential relevance of kindling to human partial epilepsy. In Kindling 3. Edited by J Wada. New York: Raven Press, pp. 37–51.

Engel, J, Jr, and Katzman, R (1977). Facilitation of amygdaloid kindling by lesions of the stria terminalis. Brain Res 122:137–142.

Engel, J, Jr, and Sharpless, NS (1977). Long-lasting depletion of dopamine in the rat amygdala induced by kindling stimulation. Brain Res 136:381–386.

Engel, J, Jr, and Wilson, CL (1986). Evidence for enhanced synaptic inhibition in epilepsy. In Neurotransmitters, Seizures and Epilepsy III. Edited by G Nistico, PL Morselli, KG Lloyd, RG Fariello, and J Engel, Jr. New York: Raven Press, pp 1–13.

Engel, J, Jr, Kuhl, DE, Phelps, ME, and Mazziotta, JC (1982). Interictal cerebral glucose metabolism in partial epilepsy and its relation to EEG changes. Ann Neurol 12:510–517.

Engel, J, Jr, Ackermann, RF, Caldecott-Hazard, S, and Chugani, HT (1984a). Do altered opioid mechanisms play a role in human epilepsy? In Neurotransmitters, Seizures, and Epilepsy II. Edited by RG Fariello, PL

Morselli, K Lloyd, LF Quesney, and J Engel, Jr. New York: Raven Press, pp. 263–274.

Engel, J, Jr, Caldecott-Hazard, S, Chugani, HT, and Ackermann, RF (1984b). Neuropeptides, seizures and epilepsy. In Advances in Epileptology: XVth Epilepsy International Symposium. Edited by RJ Porter, RH Mattson, AA Ward, and M Dam. New York: Raven Press, pp. 25–30.

Engel, J, Jr, Bandler, R, and Caldecott-Hazard, S (1985/1986). Modification of emotional expression induced by clinical and experimental epileptic disturbances. Int J Neurol 19/20:21–29.

Engel, J, Jr, Caldecott-Hazard, S, and Bandler, R (1986). Neurobiology of behavior: Anatomic and physiologic implications related to epilepsy. Epilepsia 27(suppl 2): S3–S11.

Engel, J, Jr, Bandler, R, Griffith, NC, et al. (1991). Neurobiological evidence for epilepsy-induced interictal disturbances. In Advances in Neurology, Vol 55. Edited by D Smith, D Treiman, and M Trimble. New York: Raven Press, pp. 97–111.

Engel, J, Jr, Wilson, C, and Lopez-Rodriguez, F (2002). Limbic connectivity: Anatomical substrates of behavioral disturbances in epilepsy. In The Neuropsychiatry of Epilepsy. Edited by M Trimble and B Schmitz. Cambridge, UK: Cambridge University Press, pp. 18–37.

Engel, J, Jr, Taylor, DC, and Trimble, MR (2008). Neurobiology of behavioral disorders. In Epilepsy: A Comprehensive Textbook, 2nd ed. Edited by J Engel, Jr, and TA Pedley. Philadelphia: Lippincott Williams & Wilkins, pp. 2077–2083.

Ettinger, AB (2006). Psychotropic effects of antiepileptic drugs. Neurology 67:1916–1925.

Ettinger, AB, and Kanner, AM (eds) (2007). Psychiatric Issues in Epilepsy: A Practical Guide to Diagnosis and Treatment. Philadelphia: Lippincott, Williams & Wilkins.

Falconer, MA, and Davison, S (1973). Coarse features in epilepsy as a consequence of anticonvulsant therapy. Lancet 2:1112–1114.

Ferrari, M, Barabas, G, and Matthews, WS (1983). Psychologic and behavioral disturbance among epileptic children treated with barbiturate anticonvulsants. Am J Psychiatry 140:112–113.

Finegersh, A, Avedissian, C, Shamim, S, Dustin, I, Thompson, PM, and Theodore, WH (2011). Bilateral hippocampal atrophy in temporal lobe epilepsy: Effect of depressive symptoms and febrile seizures. Epilepsia 52:689–697.

Fisher, RS, van Emde Boas, W, Blume, W, Elger, C, Engel, J, Jr, Genton, P, and Lee, P (2005). Epileptic seizures and epilepsy: Definitions proposed by the International League Against Epilepsy (ILAE) and the International Bureau for Epilepsy (IBE). Epilepsia 46:470–472.

Flor-Henry, P (1969). Psychosis and temporal lobe epilepsy. A controlled investigation. Epilepsia 10:363–395.

Flor-Henry, P (1976). Epilepsy and psychopathology. In Recent Advances in Clinical Psychiatry, No 2. Edited by K Granville-Grossman. London: Churchill Livingstone, pp. 262–295.

Flynn, JP, Vanegas, H, Foote, W, and Edwards, S (1970). Neural mechanisms involved in a cat's attack on a rat. In The Neural Control of Behavior. Edited by RE Whalen. New York: Academic Press, pp. 135–173.

Forsgren, L (1992). Prevalence of epilepsy in adults in northern Sweden. Epilepsia 33:450–458.

Forsgren, L, and Nystrom, L (1990). An incident case-referent study of epileptic seizures in adults. Epilepsy Res 6:66–81.

Franceschi, M, Perego, L, Cavagnini, F, Cattaneo, AG, Invitti, C, Caviezel, F, Strambi, LF, and Smirne, S (1984). Effects of long-term antiepileptic therapy on the hypothalamic-pituitary axis in man. Epilepsia 25:46–52.

Fregni, F, Schachter, SC, and Pascual-Leone, A (2005). Transcranial magnetic stimulation treatment for epilepsy: Can it also improve depression and vice versa? Epilepsy Behav 7:182–189.

Frost, JJ, Mayberg, HS, Fisher, RS, Douglass, KH, Dannals, RF, Links, JM, Wilson, AA, Ravert, HT, Rosenbaum, AE, Snyder, SH, and Wagner, HN (1988). Mu-opiate receptors measured by positron emission tomography are increased in temporal lobe epilepsy. Ann Neurol 23:231–237.

Gaitatzis, A, Carroll, K, Majeed, A, and Sander, JW (2004). The epidemiology of the comorbidity of epilepsy in the general population. Epilepsia 45:1613–1622.

Gastaut, H, Morin, G, and Lesevre, N (1955). Étude du comportement des épileptiques psycho-moteurs dans l'intervalle de leurs crises. Les troubles de l'activité globale et de la sociabilité. Ann Med Psychol (Paris)113:1–27.

Gibbs, FA (1951). Ictal and nonictal psychiatric disorders in temporal lobe epilepsy. J Nerv Ment Dis 113:522–528.

Gilliam, FG (2002). Optimizing health outcomes in active epilepsy. Neurology 58(suppl 5):S9–S19.

Giordani, B, Berent, S, Sackellares, JC, Rourke, D, Seidenberg, M, O'Leary, DS, Dreifuss, FE, and Brell, TJ (1985). Intelligence test performance of patients with partial and generalized seizures. Epilepsia 26:37–42.

Griffith, N, Engel, J, Jr, and Bandler, R (1987). Ictal and enduring interictal disturbances in emotional behaviour in an animal model of temporal lobe epilepsy. Brain Res 400:360–364.

Gudmundsson, G (1966). Epilepsy in Iceland. Acta Neurol Scand 43(suppl 25):1–24.

Gunn, JC (1969). The prevalence of epilepsy among prisoners. Proc R Soc Med 62:60–63.

Harden, CL, and Frye, CA (2008). Hormone changes in epilepsy. In Epilepsy: A Comprehensive Textbook, 2nd ed. Edited by J Engel, Jr, and TA Pedley. Philadelphia: Lippincott Williams & Wilkins, pp. 2037–2041.

Hecimovic, H, Salpekar, J, Kanner, AM, and Barry, JJ (2011). Suicidality and epilepsy: A neuropsychobiological perspective. Epilepsy Behav 22:77–84.

Henriksen, GF (1973). Status epilepticus partialis with fear as clinical expression: Report of a case and ictal EEG findings. Epilepsia 14:39–46.

Henry, TR, and Chugani, HT (2008). Positron emission tomography. In Epilepsy: A Comprehensive Textbook, 2nd ed. Edited by J Engel, Jr, and TA Pedley. Philadelphia: Lippincott Williams & Wilkins, pp. 945–964.

Hermann, BP, and Jones, JE (2006). Intractable epilepsy and patterns of psychiatric comorbidity. Adv Neurol 97:367–374.

Hermann, BP, and Riel, P (1981). Interictal personality and behavioral traits in temporal lobe and generalized epilepsy. Cortex 17:125–128.

Hermann, BP, Dikmen, S, Schwartz, MS, and Karnes, WE (1982a). Interictal psychopathology in patients with ictal fear: A quantitative investigation. Neurology 32:7–11.

Hermann, BP, Dikmen, S, and Wilensky, AJ (1982b). Increased psychopathology associated with multiple seizure types: Fact or artifact? Epilepsia 23:587–596.

Herzog, AG (2008). Disorders of reproduction and fertility. In Epilepsy: A Comprehensive Textbook, 2nd ed. Edited by J Engel, Jr, and TA Pedley. Philadelphia: Lippincott Williams & Wilkins, pp. 2053–2059.

Herzog, AG, Russell, V, Vaitukaitis, JL, and Geschwind, N (1982). Neuroendocrine dysfunction in temporal lobe epilepsy. Arch Neurol 39:133–135.

Hesdorffer, DC, and Hauser, AW (2007). Epidemiologic considerations. In Psychiatric Issues in Epilepsy: A Practical Guide to Diagnosis and Treatment. Edited by AB Ettinger and AM Kanner. Philadelphia: Lippincott, Williams & Wilkins, pp. 1–16.

Hesdorffer, DC, Ludvigsson, P, Olafsson, E, Gudmundsson, G, Kjartansson, O, and Hauser, WA (2004). ADHD as a risk factor for incident unprovoked seizures and epilepsy in children. Arch Gen Psychiatry 61:731–736.

Hesdorffer, D, Hauser, WA, Olafsson, E, Ludvigsson, P, and Kjartansson, O (2006). Depression and suicide attempt as risk factors for incident unprovoked seizures. Ann Neurol 59:35–41.

Hill, D, Pond, DA, Mitchell, W, and Falconer, MA (1957). Personality changes following temporal lobectomy for epilepsy. J Ment Sci 103:18–27.

Hirtz, DG, and Nelson, KB (1985). Cognitive effects of antiepileptic drugs. In Recent Advances in Epilepsy 2. Edited by TA Pedley and BS Meldrum. New York: Churchill Livingstone, pp. 161–181.

Hong, JS, Gillin, JC, Yang, HY, and Costa, E (1979). Repeated electroconvulsive shocks and the brain content of endorphins. Brain Res 177:273–278.

Horowitz, MJ, and Cohen, FM (1968). Temporal lobe epilepsy: Effect of lobectomy on psychosocial functioning. Epilepsia 9:23–41.

Jacoby, A, Snape, D, and Baker, GA (2008). Social aspects: Epilepsy stigma and quality of life. In Epilepsy: A Comprehensive Textbook, 2nd ed. Edited by J Engel, Jr, and TA Pedley. Philadelphia: Lippincott Williams & Wilkins, pp. 2229–2236.

Jilek, WG (1979). The epileptic's outcast role and its background: A contribution to the social psychiatry of seizure disorder. J Oper Psychiatry 10:127–133.

Johnson, EK, Jones, JE, Seidenberg, M, and Hermann, BP (2004). The relative impact of anxiety, depression, and clinical seizure features on health-related quality of life in epilepsy. Epilepsia 45:544–550.

Kanemoto, K, Kim, Y, Miyamoto, T, and Kawasaki, J (2001). Presurgical postictal and acute interictal psychoses are differentially associated with postoperative mood and psychotic disorders. J Neuropsychiatry Clin Neurosci 13:243–247.

Kanner, AM (2011). Depression and epilepsy: A bidirectional relation? Epilepsia 52(suppl 1):21–27.

Kanner, AM, and Blumer, D (2008). Affective disorders. In Epilepsy: A Comprehensive Textbook, 2nd ed. Edited by J Engel, Jr, and TA Pedley. Philadelphia: Lippincott Williams & Wilkins, pp. 2123–2138.

Kanner, AM, and Ostrovskaya, A (2008). Long-term significance of postictal psychotic episodes II. Are they predictive of interictal psychotic episodes? Epilepsy Behav 12:154–156.

Kanner, AM, Stagno, S, Kotagal, P, and Morris, HH (1996). Postictal psychiatric events during prolonged video-electroencephalographic monitoring studies. Arch Neurol 53:258–263.

Kanner, AM, Soto, A, and Gross-Kanner, H (2004). Prevalence and clinical characteristics of postictal psychiatric symptoms in partial epilepsy. Neurology 62:708–713.

Kanner, AM, Byrne, RW, Chicharro, AV, Wuu, J, and Frey, M (2009). Is a lifetime psychiatric history predictive of a worse postsurgical seizure outcome following a temporal lobectomy? Neurology 72:793–799.

Kelly, MS, Jacobs, MP, and Lowenstein, DH (2009). The NINDS epilepsy research benchmarks. Epilepsia 50:579–582.

Kerr, MP, Menash, S, Besag, F, de Toffol, B, Ettinger, A, Kanemoto, K, Kanner, A, Kemp, S, Krishnamoorthy, E, LaFrance, WC, Jr, Mula, M, Schmitz, B, van Elst, LT, Trollor, J, and Wilson, SJ (2011). International consensus clinical practice statements for the treatment of neuropsychiatric conditions associated with epilepsy. Epilepsia 52:2133–2138.

Kline, NS, Li, CH, Lehmann, HE, Lajtha, A, Laski, E, and Cooper, T (1977). Beta-endorphin-induced changes in schizophrenic and depressed patients. Arch Gen Psychiatry 34:1111–1113.

Koch-Stoecker, SC, and Kanemoto, K (2008). Psychiatry and surgical treatment. In Epilepsy: A Comprehensive Textbook, 2nd ed. Edited by J Engel, Jr, and TA Pedley. Philadelphia: Lippincott Williams & Wilkins, pp. 2169–2178.

Krishnamoorthy, ES, Trimble, MR, and Blumer, D (2007). The classification of neuropsychiatric disorders in epilepsy: A proposal by the ILAE Commission on Psychobiology of Epilepsy. Epilepsy Behav 10:349–353.

Kumar, G, Couper, A, O'Brien, TJ, Salzberg, MR, Jones, NC, Rees, SM, and Morris, MJ (2007). The acceleration of amygdala kindling epileptogenesis by chronic low-dose corticosterone involves both mineralocorticoid and glucocorticoid receptors. Psychoneuroendocrinology 32:834–842.

Kwon, C, Liu, M, Quan, H, Thoo, V, Wiebe, S, and Jetté, N (2011). Motor vehicle accidents, suicides, and assaults in epilepsy. Neurology 76:801–806.

Landolt, H (1958). Serial encephalographic investigations during psychotic episodes in epileptic patients and during schizophrenic attacks. In Lectures on Epilepsy. Edited by AM Lorentz de Haas. Amsterdam: Elsevier, pp. 91–133.

Lesser, RP, Lüders, H, Wyllie, E, Dinner, DS, and Morris, HH (1986). Mental deterioration in epilepsy. Epilepsia 27(suppl 2):S105–S123.

Locke, DE, Kirlin, KA, Wershba, R, Osborne, Drazkowski, JF, Sirven, JI, and Noe, KH (2011). Randomized comparison of the Personality Assessment Inventory and the Minnesota Multiphasic Personality Inventory-2 in the epilepsy monitoring unit. Epilepsy Behav 21:397–401.

Loring, DW, Barr, WB, Hamberger, M, and Helmstaedter, C (2008). Neuropsychology evaluation—Adults. In Epilepsy: A Comprehensive Textbook, 2nd ed. Edited by J Engel, Jr, and TA Pedley. Philadelphia: Lippincott Williams & Wilkins, pp. 1057–1065.

Mattson, RH, Cramer, JA, Collins, JF, Smith, DB, Delgado-Escueta, A, Brown, TR, Williamson, PD, Treiman, DM, McNamara, JO, McCutchen, DB, Homan, RW, Crill, WE, Lubozynski, MF, Rosenthal, NP, and Mayerdorf, A (1985). Comparison of carbamazepine, phenobarbital, phenytoin and primidone in partial and secondarily generalized tonic-clonic seizures. N Engl J Med 313:145–151.

Mayberg, HS, Lewis, PJ, Regenold, W, and Wagner, HNJ (1994). Paralimbic hypoperfusion in unipolar depression. Journal of Nuclear Medicine 35:929–934.

Mayeux, R, Alexander, MD, Benson, DF, Brandt, J, and Rosen, J (1979). Poriomania. Neurology 29:1616–1619.

Maynert, EW, Marczynski, TJ, and Browning, RA (1975). The role of the neurotransmitters in the epilepsies. Adv Neurol 13:79–147.

Mazarati, AM, Shin, D, Kwon, YS, Bragin, A, Pineda, E, Tio, D, Taylor, AN, and Sankar, R (2009). Elevated plasma corticosterone level and depressive behavior in experimental temporal lobe epilepsy. Neurobiol Dis 34:457–461.

McAfee, AT, Chilicott, KE, Johannes, CB, Hornbuckle, K, Hauser, WA, and Walker, AM (2007). The incidence of first unprovoked seizure in pediatric patients with and without psychiatric diagnosis. Epilepsia 48:1075–1082.

McIntyre, HB (1982). The Primary Care of Seizure Disorders. Boston: Butterworths.

Mefford, HC, Muhle, H, Ostertag, P, von Spiczak, S, Buysse, K, Baker, C, Franke, A, Malafosse, A, Genton, P, Thomas, P, Gurnett, CA, Schreiber, S, Bassuk, AG, Guipponi, M, Stephani, U, Helbig, I, and Eichler, EE (2010). Genome-wide copy number variation in epilepsy: Novel susceptibility loci in idiopathic generalized and focal epilepsies. PLoS Genet6:e1000962.

Mendez, MF, Cummings, JL, and Benson, DF (1986). Depression in epilepsy: Significance and phenomenology. Arch Neurol 43:766–770.

Mendius, JR, and Engel, J, Jr (1985). Studies of hemispheric lateralization in patients with partial epilepsy. In The Dual Brain. Edited by DF Benson and E Zaidel. New York: Guilford Press, pp. 263–276.

Mesulam, MM (1981). Dissociative states with abnormal temporal lobe EEG: Multiple personality and the illusion of possession. Arch Neurol 38:176–181.

Miatton, M, Van Roost, D, Thiery, E, Carrette, E, Van Dycke, A, Vonck, K, Meurs, A, Vingerhoets, G, and Boon, P (2011). The cognitive effects of amygdalohippocampal deep brain stimulation in patients with temporal lobe epilepsy. Epilepsy Behav 22:759–764.

Milner, B (1975). Psychological aspects of focal epilepsy and its neurosurgical management. Adv Neurol 8:299–321.

Mintzer, S, and Lopez, F (2002). Comorbidity of ictal fear and panic disorder. Epilepsy Behav 3:330–337.

Monroe, RR (1970). Episodic Behavioral Disorders: A Psychodynamic and Neurophysiologic Analysis. Cambridge, MA: Harvard University Press.

Monroe, RR (1975). Anticonvulsants in the treatment of aggression. J Nerv Ment Dis 160:119–126.

Mungas, D (1982). Interictal behavioral abnormality in temporal lobe epilepsy: A specific syndrome or nonspecific psychopathology? Arch Gen Psychiatry 39:108–111.

Nielson, H, and Kristensen, O (1981). Personality correlates of sphenoidal EEG-foci in temporal lobe epilepsy. Acta Neurol Scand 64:289–300.

Ounsted, C, and Lindsay, J (1981). The long-term outcome of temporal lobe epilepsy in childhood. In Epilepsy and Psychiatry. Edited by EH Reynolds and MR Trimble. London: Churchill Livingstone, pp. 185–215.

Parnas, J, Gram, L, and Flachs, H (1980). Psychopharmacological aspects of antiepileptic treatment. Prog Neurobiol 15:119–138.

Perez, MM, and Trimble, MR (1980). Epileptic psychosis—Diagnostic comparison with process schizophrenia. Br J Psychiatry 137:245–249.

Perini, GI, and Mendius, R (1984). Depression and anxiety in complex partial seizures. J Nerv Ment Dis 172:287–290.

Petrovski, CEI, Szoecke, NC, Jones, NC, Salzberg, LJ, Sheffield, RM, Huggins, RM, and O'Brien, TJ (2010). Neuropsychiatric symptomatology predicts seizure recurrence in newly treated patients. Neurology 75:1015–1021.

Pinel, JPJ, Treit, D, and Rovner, LI (1977). Temporal lobe aggression in rats. Science 197:1088–1089.

Pirmohamed, M, and Arroyo, S (2008). Idiosyncratic adverse reactions. In Epilepsy: A Comprehensive Textbook, 2nd ed. Edited by J Engel, Jr, and TA Pedley. Philadelphia: Lippincott Williams & Wilkins, pp. 1201–1208.

Post, RM, Ballenger, JC, Uhde, TW, and Bunney, WE, Jr (1984). Efficacy of carbamazepine in manic-depressive illness: Implication for underlying mechanisms. In Neurobiology of Mood Disorders. Edited by RM Post and J Ballenger. Baltimore: Williams & Wilkins, pp. 777–816.

Ramani, V, and Gumnit, RJ (1982). Intensive monitoring of interictal psychosis in epilepsy. Ann Neurol 11:613–622.

Rankin, PM, and Vargha-Khadem, F (2008). Neuropsychological evaluation—Children. In Epilepsy: A Comprehensive Textbook, 2nd ed. Edited by J Engel, Jr, and TA Pedley. Philadelphia: Lippincott Williams & Wilkins, pp. 1067–1076.

Rausch, R, and Crandall, PH (1982). Psychological status related to surgical control of temporal lobe seizures. Epilepsia 23:191–202.

Rausch, R, and Walsh, GO (1984). Right-hemisphere language dominance in right-handed epileptic patients. Arch Neurol 41:1077–1080.

Razavi, L (1975). Cytogenetic and somatic variations in the neurobiology of violence: Epidemiological, clinical and morphogenetic considerations. In Neurological Bases of Violence and Aggression. Edited by WS Fields and WH Sweet. St Louis: Warren H Green, pp. 205–270.

Reynolds, EH (1967). Effects of folic acid on the mental state and fit-frequency of drug-treated epileptic patients. Lancet 1:1086–1088.

Reynolds, EH (1983). Mental effects of antiepileptic medication: A review. Epilepsia 24(suppl 2):S85–S95.

Rickler, KC (1982). Episodic dyscontrol. In Psychiatric Aspects of Neurological Disease, Vol II. Edited by DF Benson and D Blumer. New York: Grune & Stratton, pp. 49–73.

Rivinus, TM (1982). Psychiatric effects of the anticonvulsant regimens. J Clin Psychopharmacol 2:165–192.

Roberts, DW (2008). Corpus callosotomy. In Epilepsy: A Comprehensive Textbook, 2nd ed. Edited by J Engel,

Jr, and TA Pedley. Philadelphia: Lippincott Williams & Wilkins, pp. 1907–1913.

Robertson, MM, and Trimble, MR (1983). Depressive illness in patients with epilepsy: A review. Epilepsia 24(suppl 2): S109–S116.

Rodin, EA (1968). The Prognosis of Patients with Epilepsy. Springfield, IL: Charles C Thomas.

Rodin, EA, and Schmaltz, S (1984). The Bear-Fedio personality inventory and temporal lobe epilepsy. Neurology 34:591–596.

Rubin, ZA, and Wiebe, S (2008). Issues in health outcome assessment. In Epilepsy: A Comprehensive Textbook, 2nd ed. Edited by J Engel, Jr, and TA Pedley. Philadelphia: Lippincott Williams & Wilkins, pp. 2267–2275.

Rutter, M, and Yule, W (1973). Specific reading retardation. In The First Review of Special Education, Vol 2. Edited by L Mann and D Sabatino. Philadelphia: JSE Press, pp. 1–50.

Sackheim, HA, Decina, P, Prohovnik, S, Kanzler, M, and Malitz, S,1986: Dosage, seizure threshold, and the antidepressant efficacy of electroconvulsive therapy. Ann N Y Acad Sci 462:398–410.

Saint-Hilaire, JM, Gilbert, M, Bouvier, G, and Barbeau, A (1981). Épilepsie avec manifestations agressives: Deux cas etudiés avec électrodes en profondeur. Rev Neurol 3:161–179.

Sapolsky, RM (2000). Glucocorticoids and hippocampal atrophy in neuropsychiatric disorders. Arch Gen Psychiatry 57:925–935.

Sato, M (1983). Long-lasting hypersensitivity to methamphetamine following amygdaloid kindling in cats: The relationship between limbic epilepsy and the psychotic state. Biol Psychiatry 18:525–536.

Sato, M, and Ogawa, T (1984). Abnormal behavior in epilepsy and catecholamines. In Neurotransmitters, Seizures and Epilepsy II. Edited by RG Fariello, PL Morselli, KG Lloyd, LF Quesney, and J Engel, Jr. New York: Raven Press, pp. 1–9.

Schachter, SC, and Boon, P (2008). Vagus nerve stimulation. In Epilepsy: A Comprehensive Textbook, 2nd ed. Edited by J Engel, Jr, and TA Pedley. Philadelphia: Lippincott Williams & Wilkins, pp. 1395–1399.

Schiffer, RB, and Babigian, HM (1984). Behavioral disorders in multiple sclerosis, temporal lobe epilepsy, and amyotrophic lateral sclerosis. Arch Neurol 41:1067–1069.

Schmidt, D, and Schachter, SC (2008). Dose-related side effects. In Epilepsy: A Comprehensive Textbook, 2nd ed. Edited by J Engel, Jr, and TA Pedley. Philadelphia: Lippincott Williams & Wilkins, pp. 1193–1200.

Schmitz, B (2008). Psychiatric side effects of antiepileptic drugs. In Epilepsy: A Comprehensive Textbook, 2nd ed. Edited by J Engel, Jr, and TA Pedley. Philadelphia: Lippincott Williams & Wilkins, pp. 2163–2167.

Seligman, ME, and Maier, SF (1967). Failure to escape traumatic shock. J Exp Psychol 74:1–9.

Shaw, P, Mellers, J, Henderson, M, Polkey, C, David, AS, and Toone, BK (2004). Schizophrenia-like psychosis arising de novo following a temporal lobectomy: Timing and risk factors. J Neurol Neurosurg Psychiatry 75:1003–1008.

Sherwin, I, Peron-Magnan, P, and Bancaud, J (1982). Prevalence of psychosis in epilepsy as a function of the laterality of the epileptogenic lesion. Arch Neurol 39:621–625.

Shouse, MN, Bazil, CW, and Malow, BA (2008). Sleep. In Epilepsy: A Comprehensive Textbook, 2nd ed. Edited by J Engel, Jr, and TA Pedley. Philadelphia: Lippincott Williams & Wilkins, pp. 1975–1990.

Siegel, A, 1985/1986: Experimental induced seizure disturbances of the temporal lobe and aggressive behavior. Int J Neurol 19/20:59–72.

Sillanpää, M (1975). The significance of motor handicap in the progression of childhood epilepsy. Dev Med Child Neurol 17:52–57.

Slater, E, Beard, AW, and Glithero, E (1963). The schizophrenia-like psychoses of epilepsy. Br J Psychiatry 109:95–150.

Sperling, MR, Pritchard, PB, III, Engel, J, Jr, Daniel, C, and Sagel, J (1986). Prolactin in partial epilepsy: An indicator of limbic seizures. Ann Neurol 20:716–722.

Spitzer, RL, Kroenke, K, Williams, JB, and Lowe, B (2006). A brief measure for assessing generalized anxiety disorder: The GAD-7. Arch InternMed 166:1092–1097.

Sterman, MB, Shouse, MN, and Passouant, P (eds) (1982). Sleep and Epilepsy. New York: Academic Press.

Stevens, JR (1966). Psychiatric implications of psychomotor epilepsy. Arch Gen Psychiatry 14:461–471.

Stevens, JR (1973). An anatomy of schizophrenia? Arch Gen Psychiatry 29:117–189.

Stevens, JR, and Hermann, BP (1981). Temporal lobe epilepsy, psychopathology and violence: The state of the evidence. Neurology 31:1127–1132.

Stevens, JR, and Livermore, A, Jr (1978). Kindling of the mesolimbic dopamine system: Animal model of psychosis. Neurology 28:36–46.

Stores, G (1981). Problems of learning and behaviour in children with epilepsy. In Epilepsy and Psychiatry. Edited by EH Reynolds and MR Trimble. New York: Churchill Livingstone, pp. 33–48.

Taylor, DC (1969). Aggression and epilepsy. J Psychosom Res 13:229–236.

Taylor, DC (1972). Mental state and temporal lobe epilepsy. A correlative account of 100 patients treated surgically. Epilepsia 13:727–765.

Taylor, DC (1975). Factors influencing the occurrence of schizophrenia-like psychosis in patients with temporal lobe epilepsy. Psychol Med 5:249–254.

Taylor, DC (1982). The components of sickness: Disease, illness and predicaments. In One Child. Edited by J Apley and C Ounsted. London: William Heinemann Medical Books, pp. 1–13.

Taylor, DC (1987). Psychiatric and social issues in measuring the input and output of epilepsy surgery. In Surgical Treatment of the Epilepsies. Edited by J Engel, Jr. New York: Raven Press, pp. 485–504.

Taylor, DC, and March, SM (1979). Implications of long-term follow-up studies in epilepsy: With a note on the cause of death. In Epilepsy: The Eighth International Symposium. Edited by JK Penry. New York: Raven Press, pp. 27–34.

Tellez-Zenteno, JF, Patten, SB, Jetté, N, Williams, J, and Wiebe, S (2007). Psychiatric comorbidity in epilepsy: A population-based analysis. Epilepsia 48:2336–2344.

Temkin, O (1945). The Falling Sickness: A History of Epilepsy from the Greeks to the Beginnings of Modern Neurology. Baltimore: Johns Hopkins University Press.

Toone, B (1987). Sexual disorders in epilepsy. In Recent Advances in Epilepsy 3. Edited by TA Pedley and

BS Meldrum. New York, Churchill Livingstone, pp. 233–259.

Treiman, DM (1986). Epilepsy and violence: Medical and legal issues. Epilepsia 27(suppl 2):S77–S104.

Trimble, MR (1983). Personality disturbances in epilepsy. Neurology 33:1332–1334.

Trimble, MR, and Reynolds, EH (1976). Anticonvulsant drugs and mental symptoms: A review. Psychol Med 6:169–178.

Trimble, MR, and Schmitz, B (2008). Schizophrenia and other psychoses. In Epilepsy: A Comprehensive Textbook, 2nd ed. Edited by J Engel, Jr, and TA Pedley. Philadelphia: Lippincott Williams & Wilkins, pp. 2113–2121.

Trimble, MR, and Thompson, PJ (1983). Anticonvulsant drugs, cognitive function, and behavior. Epilepsia 24(suppl 1): S55–S63.

Tuchman, R (2011). Epilepsy and electroencephalography in autism spectrum disorders. In Autism Spectrum Disorders. Edited by DG Amaral, G Dawson, and DH Geschwind. Oxford: Oxford University Press, pp. 381–394.

Tuchman, R, and Cuccaro, M (2011). Epilepsy and autism: Neurodevelopmental perspective. Curr Neurol Neurosci Rep 11:428–434.

Tuchman, R, Rapin, I, and Shinnar, S (1991). Autistic and dysphasic children. II: Epilepsy. Pediatrics 88:1219–1225.

Vickrey, BG, Hays, RD, Graber, J, et al. (1992). A health-related quality of life instrument for patients evaluated for epilepsy surgery. Med Care 30:299–319.

Walker, AE, and Blumer, D (1977). Long-term behavioral effects of temporal lobectomy for temporal lobe epilepsy. McLean Hosp J(special issue):85–103.

PART 4

Management

Chapter 12

Diagnostic Evaluation

HISTORY
Seizure History
Antiseizure Drug History
Past Medical History
Family History
Psychosocial History

PHYSICAL EXAMINATION
General Physical Examination
Neurological Examination
Epileptic Seizure Observation

LABORATORY EXAMINATION
Clinical Laboratory Tests
Electroencephalography
Magnetoencephalography
Transcranial Magnetic Stimulation
Structural Neuroimaging
Functional Neuroimaging

PSYCHOLOGICAL EVALUATION

BIOMARKERS

SUMMARY AND CONCLUSIONS

The evaluation of the patient with suspected epilepsy addresses five separate diagnostic issues: (1) Does an *epilepsy condition* exist? (2) Is there a *treatable underlying cause*? (3) What types of *epileptic seizures* occur, and do they have specific precipitating and predisposing factors? (4) Do the clinical features constitute an *epilepsy syndrome*? (5) What aspects of the epileptic seizures, interictal neurological and psychosocial impairments, and environmental factors are responsible for the patient's *predicament* (Chapter 11)? Table 12–1

indicates the general diagnostic approach used to answer these questions and provides an outline for the following discussion.

HISTORY

The diagnosis of epilepsy usually depends on historical information, particularly an accurate description of seizures (Aicardi and Taylor, 2008). Consequently, the initial interview with

Table 12–1 General Diagnostic Approach to the Patient with Epileptic Seizures

A. History (from patient and reliable observer)
  1. Epileptic seizure history (for each seizure type)
    a. Aura or prodromal symptoms
    b. Clinical seizure
    c. Postictal symptoms
    d. Patterns of occurrence and precipitating factors
    e. Frequency
    f. Age of onset
    g. Progression of symptoms
    h. Response to antiseizure drugs
  2. Past medical history
    a. Possible causative factors
    b. Other predisposing factors
  3. Family history
  4. Psychosocial history
B. Physical examination
  1. General examination for underlying disease processes, stigmata, and asymmetries
  2. Neurological examination for specific neurological disorders, focal deficits, and evidence of diffuse cerebral dysfunction
C. Observation of an epileptic seizure, if possible
D. Laboratory examination
  1. Routine laboratory tests for diagnosis and baseline (lumbar puncture only if necessary to provide adequate prognosis or determine effective management)
  2. Electroencephlography (EEG)
    a. Routine for diagnosis and baseline
    b. Special electrodes, activation, long-term monitoring, or computer enhancement only if necessary to provide adequate prognosis or determine effective management.
  3. Tests of cerebral structure
    a. X-ray computed tomography (CT), magnetic resonance imaging (MRI), or both for diagnosis and baseline
    b. Special radiographic studies only if necessary for effective management
  4. Other tests of cerebral function
    a. Psychological evaluations
    b. Positron emission tomography (PET), single-photon emission computed tomography (SPECT), radionuclide brain scan, visual fields, or routine evoked-potential mapping when available, only if necessary for effective management
    c. Magnetoencephalography (MEG)
    d. Magnetic resonance spectroscopy (MRS)
    e. Functional magnetic resonance imaging (fMRI)

the patient should include a close relative or friend who has observed ictal and periictal phenomena and who is familiar with other medical and personal details of the patient's life. For patients with childhood onset epilepsy or an early childhood insult, historical information is best obtained from a parent.

The history can help reveal a treatable underlying cause, but most patients require specific therapy for their seizures. In this instance, knowledge of the seizure type or syndrome determines the appropriate treatment and prognosis, whereas understanding the predicament caused by the epilepsy condition is necessary for achievement of satisfactory psychosocial adjustment.

Seizure History

The seizure history should include a careful description of (1) an aura or prodromal symptoms if present, (2) the clinical seizure, and (3) postictal symptoms. It is also useful to elicit a detailed description of the first seizure and the circumstances under which it occurred and to then clearly define any age- or treatment-related changes in seizure character, frequency, or pattern. When several seizure types exist, this information should be obtained for each type. Given the prevalence of cell phones with video cameras, it is not uncommon today for patients to bring a video of their or their child's ictal events to the consultation.

AURA OR PRODROME

Many patients fail to recognize an aura as such. Consequently, it is best to ask first if the patient knows when a seizure will occur and then to request a precise description of the perceptions that constitute the warning. An aura usually consists of stereotyped sensory, autonomic, or psychic phenomena that can herald the onset of more dramatic ictal manifestations. Auras represent the beginning of focal seizures and must be distinguished from prodromal symptoms, such as vague uneasiness or irritability beginning many minutes or hours before the onset of an epileptic seizure. Prodromal warnings probably reflect physiological state changes that alter seizure threshold and predispose to ictal onset rather than focal ictal symptoms (Chapter 9). Therefore, they do not provide localizing information, nor do they distinguish between focal and generalized epileptic seizures. Once recognized as reliable warnings, auras and prodromal symptoms often provide an opportunity for the patient to avoid injury or embarrassment during an epileptic attack.

A well-defined aura immediately preceding the behavioral epileptic seizure is pathognomonic of a diagnosis of a focal seizure. The characteristics of this aura can provide important clues to the cerebral localization of the epileptogenic lesion, although this structure-function correlation is not absolute (Chapters 6 and 16). Persons with typical *mesial temporal lobe epilepsy (MTLE)* and *focal dyscognitive seizures* that begin with auras almost invariably also have auras that are not followed by these ictal events (*auras in isolation*). Auras that never occur in isolation should raise concern that the condition is not MTLE (Chapter 7). The duration of the aura or warning provides information about the rapidity of progression of the ictal process, which is typically slow for seizures of mesial temporal lobe origin (Lieb et al., 1986a; 1987) and more rapid for seizures of frontal lobe origin (Williamson et al., 1987). Often, the degree of disability is inversely related to the duration of the aura, because the aura provides an opportunity to take precaution against injury during the behavioral seizure.

CLINICAL SEIZURES

As noted above, the onset of observable ictal behavior should be described in detail by a reliable witness. This description should include the temporal sequence of any arrest of movement, autonomic changes, alteration in consciousness, the part of the body and side involved in initial clonic or tonic movements, any spread or progression of these movements, and the degree of consistency from one seizure to another (*stereotypy*). Ictal onset patterns can provide lateralizing and localizing information (see Table 6–3) when this is needed, as might be the case for surgical candidates (Chapter 16).

Features of specific seizure types described in Chapter 6 can usually be distinguished. For instance, the tonic or clonic movements more characteristic of neocortical seizures can be distinguished from the semipurposeful or automatic movements that occur with limbic seizures, often in association with oroalimentary automatisms. The oroalimentary automatisms of limbic seizures typically occur while consciousness is impaired, although some responsiveness to the environment is usually retained. An ictal fall can cause injury when it is due to a sudden loss of tone's causing collapse (*atonic seizure*) or to sudden forceful movements (*tonic-clonic, tonic, clonic,* and *myoclonic seizures*). More coordinated loss of upright posture with appropriate protective reactions that prevent injury usually indicates a *focal seizure*. Some ictal automatic behaviors, such as running or combativeness, may present a risk to the patient or others. Description of the ictal event should include duration of the entire epileptic seizure and of individual sequential manifestations. The frequency of occurrence of urinary and fecal incontinence, oral lacerations, and injuries from falling provide an index of the degree of handicap the seizures produce.

Stereotyped seizures suggest a single epileptogenic process, but variable ictal manifestations do not always indicate a multifocal disturbance. Often when a person with epilepsy and observers report what appear to be several seizure types, on closer questioning these are attributable to a unitary process. For instance, an aura that does not progress can be identified as one type of seizure. When the aura progresses to include altered consciousness, motor manifestations, or both, it can be perceived as a second ictal episode, particularly when the aura is not recalled. Rapid progression on occasion to a secondarily generalized tonic-clonic seizure can easily be perceived as a third type of ictal event. Careful description by a competent observer of the initial manifestations of these seizures would help to establish that all three actually originated from the same epileptogenic region.

POSTICTAL PERIOD

Nonspecific postictal symptoms, such as confusion and headache, as well as *reactive automatisms*, contribute greatly to the disability caused by seizures. Postictal nondirected combative behavior is not unusual after some types of seizures (Chapters 9 and 10) and can have serious adverse consequences when mistaken for purposeful antisocial behavior, particularly when law enforcement is involved. Often, patients and observers are unable to distinguish the ictal from the postictal period and report the entire process as a single event. Indeed, whether problematic automatisms, for instance, are ictal or postictal makes little difference with respect to their impact on the patient's predicament. Specific features of the postictal period may have diagnostic value. Focal neurological deficits indicate a focal seizure disorder and may help lateralize or localize the epileptogenic region, while amnesia for the ictal event may be the only evidence of ictal impaired consciousness (Chapters 6 and 9). Knowledge of stereotypical postictal signs and symptoms helps patients determine that a seizure has occurred when the ictal event itself was not observed and informs approaches to management during the postictal period. For instance, patients known to have combative reactive automatisms should not be constrained or approached in a manner that could be perceived as threatening, and the expense of time and money for unnecessary trips to the emergency room for prolonged postictal obtundation only adds to the disability of patients for whom this is a typical aftereffect of their habitual seizures.

PRECIPITATING FACTORS AND PATTERN

It is important to elucidate precipitating factors and nonspecific influences that modulate ictal occurrence or establish characteristic frequency patterns (Chapters 5 and 9). Examples of the former are sensory or emotional stimuli; examples of the latter are sleep-wake cycles, toxic and metabolic disturbances, and physiological states such as menses and pregnancy. Knowledge of precipitating factors or patterns of seizure occurrence can suggest beneficial modifications in daily routine.

FREQUENCY

The frequency of each type of epileptic seizure should be noted. The number of seizures that occur during a convenient period, such as a week, month, or year, may not be a realistic measure of disability for patients who experience seizures in clusters. In that case, especially when disturbing postictal symptoms last for several hours or days, tabulation of the number of *seizure* or *symptomatic days* is a more reasonable means of assessing disability and monitoring the effectiveness of therapy.

Often persons with focal dyscognitive or absence seizures are unaware that seizures have occurred. Thus an accurate measure of seizure frequency may be impossible unless the patient is under constant observation. Patients who sleep alone may also have undetected nocturnal seizures. They should be aware that a wet bed, blood on the pillow, and symptoms such as headache, muscle soreness, or a sore mouth on awakening often indicate that a nocturnal generalized tonic-clonic seizure has occurred.

For some patients, it is helpful to keep a seizure log, usually with the aid of a pocket calendar. This allows the frequency of each type of seizure or consequent disability to be quantified or correlated with changes in antiseizure drug regimens and serum drug levels. On the other hand, seizure logs can be a poor idea if they are unnecessary for monitoring results of therapeutic intervention and serve only to increase patient or parental preoccupation with ictal signs and symptoms.

AGE OF ONSET

Information about age of onset is diagnostically useful because many causes of epilepsy (Chapter 5) (Table 12–2) and most specific epilepsy syndromes (Chapter 7) are age-related. A history of prior specific cerebral insults should also be elucidated. A report of head trauma, however, must be interpreted with caution.

Table 12–2 **Diagnostic Considerations by Age of Onset of Epileptic Seizures**

Common Etiological Factors (Chapter 5)

Neonatal Period

Early (0–3 days)	Intracranial infection
	Perinatal asphyxia
	Intracranial hemorrhage
	Drug withdrawal
Late (after 3 days)	Primary metabolic
	Developmental defects
Infancy and childhood	Trauma
	Intracranial infection
	Developmental defects (e.g., cerebral dysgenesis, vascular malformation)
	Inherited CNS disorders (e.g., degenerative, metabolic, phakomatoses)
	Hippocampal sclerosis
Adolescence	Trauma
	Intracranial infection
Adulthood	Trauma
	Intracranial infection
	Neoplasm
	Vascular occlusion

Occasionally an apparently accidental traumatic event preceding the onset of chronic epilepsy is actually the first seizure. Also, the initial ictal episode is commonly attributed to a previous minor head injury when this is not actually warranted. Head trauma unassociated with loss of consciousness is a potential cause of acute epileptic seizures only in children below the age of 5 (Jennett, 1975), and it is rarely if ever the cause of a chronic epileptic disorder.

PROGRESSION OF SYMPTOMS

Symptoms of epileptic seizures can change with time. The evolution of symptoms may suggest progression of the underlying pathophysiological process (Chapter 8) but more often can be related to age, particularly puberty (Chapters 5 and 9); to alterations in environmental conditions, including living habits; and to specific therapeutic interventions. Documentation of the influences of environmental factors and therapeutic intervention provides important clues for effective management.

Antiseizure drugs that retard the spread of epileptic discharge can alter *ictal* manifestations. An aura might become recognized because the patient is no longer amnestic for initial symptoms, or secondarily generalized tonic-clonic seizures might be aborted. Consequently, current epileptic seizures can appear to be entirely different from the initial ictal episodes experienced by the patient. On the other hand, new ictal manifestations could also indicate an enlarging epileptogenic lesion, such as a neoplasm, or the development of secondary epileptogenesis (Chapter 8). Loss of a limbic aura could reflect the development of a contralateral mesial temporal epileptogenic region and more rapid transhemispheric propagation.

Apparent worsening of *interictal* symptoms might reflect postictal changes, unrecognized seizures, medication effects, psychogenic disturbances, or progression of the underlying cerebral disease process (Table 12–3) (Chapter 11). Repeated or prolonged focal seizures in clear consciousness and unrecognized nocturnal seizures are occasionally the cause of new interictal behavioral disturbances.

Antiseizure Drug History

When patients have been treated previously for epileptic seizures, an appropriate drug history includes as much of the following as possible: (1) a complete list of all the antiseizure drugs used, along with their highest doses, serum levels, dose schedules, combinations, and the length of time they were tried, and (2) any beneficial effects of specific drugs on seizure severity or frequency, the duration of these effects, and toxic side effects. If an antiseizure drug was discontinued, the reason should be noted.

Improper use or unnecessary termination of effective drugs is a frequent cause of apparent medical intractability (Porter et al., 1977). Commonly, the drug of choice has not been given at correct dosage intervals, sufficiently high serum levels have not been obtained, or it has been used only in combination with other medications (Chapter 14). Antiseizure drugs are also unnecessarily discontinued because of fear of toxic effects. Unpleasant dose-related side effects, such as nausea, sedation, or ataxia, often can be avoided by alterations in dosage schedules or resolve spontaneously. Mild *leukopenia* or elevated *alkaline phosphatase* should not be considered evidence of impending *blood dyscrasia* or *hepatotoxicity* (Chapter 14).

Table 12–3 Differential Diagnosis of Progressive Interictal Symptoms

	Progression of a Pathological Lesion	Drug Effect	Postictal	Unrecognized Ictal	Psychogenic
Common symptoms and signs	New neurological deficit, focal or diffuse dysfunction.	Focal or diffuse dysfunction, often associated with specific toxic side effects such as sedation, fatigue, nystagmus, disequilibrium. Ataxia and nystagmus may be absent with phenytoin and valproate encephalopathy.	Focal or diffuse dysfunction.	Focal or diffuse dysfunction; may have myoclonic jerks or blinking if mentation is altered.	Mental status disturbances, only rarely specific neurological deficit.
Temporal pattern	Static or progressive, related to features of underlying disease process.	Can be static, progressive, or fluctuating, related to high serum drug levels or institution of a specific drug.	Fluctuation in relation to seizure frequency or time since last seizure.	Fluctuating; may be related to low serum drug levels.	Can be static, progressive, or fluctuating; may be related to drugs or seizures.
EEG findings	May have focal or diffuse slowing or no change.	Focal or diffuse slowing; may have increased fast activity with barbiturates or benzodiazepines.	May have focal or diffuse slowing or no change.	May have characteristic ictal EEG pattern or, if focal, without impairment of consciousness, no change.	No change.
CT or MRI	May see new structural lesions or progression of previously noted lesion.	No change.	No change.	No change.	No change.

Past Medical History

Past medical history provides clues to etiology. Seizure onset at any age can represent sequelae of brain injury that occurred many years earlier or malformations present since before birth. Complications during gestation, birth trauma, postnatal intracranial infections, and serious head injury are common causes of epileptogenic lesions. Patients who have mesial temporal sclerosis may have a history of a febrile seizure lasting over 30 minutes, although the possible causal relationship remains uncertain (Chapters 5, 7, and 8). Brief febrile seizures in infancy, however, indicate a lowered threshold to the development of chronic epilepsy, given other cerebral insults (Chapter 5), and should be listed as a risk factor. In many cases, the risk factor is a mutation of the gene encoding the SCN1A subunit of voltage-gated sodium channels or some other genetic mutation (Chapter 5). In children, the developmental history helps to distinguish between a progressive degenerative neurological disorder and a static lesion. In the elderly, it is particularly necessary to look for specific disorders common in this age group, such as cerebrovascular disease and metastatic carcinoma (Chapter 5).

Family History

Documentation of similar epileptic seizures or neurological symptoms in other family members may aid in the identification of a specific genetic epilepsy syndrome (Chapter 7) or one of the many inherited diseases associated with epileptic seizures (Chapter 5). Some patients report family members with a variety of dissimilar epilepsy disorders, ranging from febrile seizures in infancy to late-onset epileptic seizures in association with brain tumors or strokes. Such a history suggests a familial lowered threshold to the development of epilepsy, as occurs with *genetic epilepsy with febrile seizures plus (GEFS+)* due to gene mutations that encode for sodium channel and GABA receptor subunits (Chapter 7). Left-handedness, in the absence of a family history of sinistrals, raises the suspicion of early injury to the left cerebral hemisphere (Satz et al., 1985).

Psychosocial History

A careful psychosocial history is essential for planning management, because psychosocial disturbances created by the seizure disorder contribute considerably to the degree of disability (Chapters 11 and 17), and coexistent life adjustment problems or psychiatric disorders can further influence outcome.

Questions about schooling, employment, and social life are necessary in determining whether a patient could benefit from additional counseling or available social services (Chapter 17). Management is facilitated if family and friends constitute a reliable support group for the patient and if the physician has regular contact with members of this group. Patients may be more concerned about interpersonal relationships, financial status, personal esteem, and health than about their seizures. Interictal neuroses, affective disorders, or psychoses complicate management and require special attention. All of the elements that make up the patient's predicament must be understood and taken into account before an effective treatment plan can be instituted.

Psychological information can be of diagnostic value. A history of a specific, persistent, interictal cognitive deficit, such as aphasia, suggests a focal lesion, whereas more generalized mental impairment can indicate a diffuse process. When evidence of progressive psychological dysfunction exists, this may be due to recurrent seizures, toxic symptoms of overmedication, or an underlying degenerative disease process (see Table 12–3). Historical features, as well as other studies discussed in later sections of this chapter, can help to elucidate the cause of such progression.

PHYSICAL EXAMINATION

Although modern diagnostic testing, particularly neuroimaging, is highly effective in identifying structural and metabolic causes of epileptic seizures, a careful physical examination can occasionally reveal unsuspected findings that call for additional, or reevaluation of, existing diagnostic testing. It is still useful, therefore, to discuss the physical examination in patients with epilepsy (Aicardi and Taylor, 2008).

General Physical Examination

The general physical examination of patients with epilepsy should be directed toward finding the physical signs of specific disease processes or malformations that cause epileptic seizures (Chapter 5). Infants and young children with multifocal or generalized seizures and diffuse disruption of cerebral function may have *hepatosplenomegaly* and *fundoscopic abnormalities* (Fig. 12–1) suggestive of a storage disorder or stigmata of a specific congenital syndrome. Children and young adults should be examined for the characteristic dermatological abnormalities of the *phakomatoses*, such as the *axillary freckling, nevus anemicus*, and *café au lait spots* associated with *neurofibromatoses* (Fig. 12–2), the *port wine stain of Sturge-Weber syndrome*, and the facial *sebaceous adenoma* (Fig. 12–3), *ash leaf spots* and *shagreen patch* (Fig. 12–4) of *tuberous sclerosis*. Diagnosis of tuberous sclerosis can be facilitated by the use of a *Wood's lamp* to identify areas of hypopigmentation. Patients with late-onset epileptic seizures may have signs of cardiovascular disease or neoplasm. Many of the specific acquired metabolic, toxic, and infectious processes that can present with chronic epilepsy in all age groups

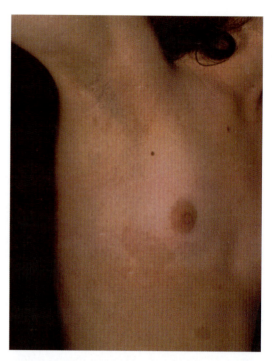

Figure 12–2. Café au lait spots and axillary freckling in a patient with neurofibromatosis. (Courtesy of Dr. V. Newcomer, UCLA.)

(Chapter 5) are associated with characteristic physical findings.

The general physical examination can also provide evidence for fixed lesions of the brain, although these are better diagnosed today by the structural imaging studies described later

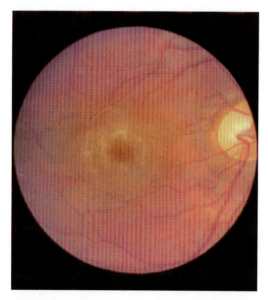

Figure 12–1. Fundoscopic view demonstrates a cherry-red spot. (Used with permission from J.D. Kivlin, Wisconsin Eye Institute.)

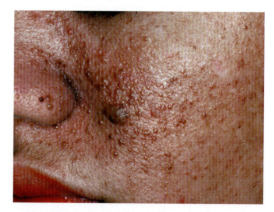

Figure 12–3. Adenoma sebaceum in a patient with tuberous sclerosis. (Courtesy of the Victor D. Newcomer, MD collection at UCLA and Logical Images, Inc.)

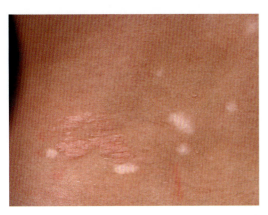

Figure 12–4. Hypomelanotic spots, including some with a characteristic ash leaf pattern, and a shagreen patch (*arrow*) on the lower back of a patient with tuberous sclerosis. (Used with permission from VisualDx. (c) Logical Images, Inc.)

in this chapter. Asymmetries of the hands, feet, and face suggest early lateralized cerebral injury (Satz et al., 1985). Careful examination of the head can reveal other asymmetries that reflect underlying abnormalities of cerebral development or evidence of old or recent trauma, including past surgery, that may not have been reported during the historical interview. Transillumination is a helpful way of identifying gross cerebral malformations in babies. Examination of the head in children should include measurement of head size for correlation with body weight and height. Auscultation of the head for bruits is appropriate in patients of all ages.

Evidence of systemic antiseizure drug effects (Chapter 15) should be noted, particularly the cosmetic side effects of *phenytoin*, such as *gingival hyperplasia*, coarsening of facial features, and *hirsutism*. The physical examination can also reveal evidence of jaundice, anemia, bleeding, adenopathy, or chronic infection due to drug-induced hematological, renal, or hepatic toxicity. Signs of rickets in children can indicate a phenytoin-induced disturbance in calcium metabolism (Chapters 14 and 15).

Neurological Examination

The neurological examination is often normal in patients with epilepsy, but diagnosis is aided when focal or generalized neurological impairment can be demonstrated. The presence of abnormal findings suggests a diffuse structural or metabolic epilepsy disorder. Focal or lateralized features suggest a structural lesion and might provide localizing information when this is important. Specific motor and sensory deficits are seen with disturbances in primary cortical regions, but a mild central facial paresis, manifest as flattening of the nasolabial fold, occasionally occurs with lesions in the contralateral mesial temporal lobe (Remillard et al., 1977). Superior quadrantic visual field defects are encountered rarely and can indicate a lesion in the posterior temporal lobe. Careful examination during the immediate postictal period may reveal diagnostically useful focal or lateralized dysfunction that otherwise is not apparent. Evidence of focal impairment involving the posterior fossa or spinal cord as well as the cerebral hemispheres suggests a multifocal neurological disease process such as neurofibromatosis. Mild peripheral neuropathies encountered in patients with epilepsy are most often due to the effects of antiseizure drugs (Chapters 14 and 15).

Diagnosis of a structural or metabolic, rather than genetic, generalized epilepsy disorder is supported by findings of minimal brain dysfunction such as clumsiness, synkinesis, abnormal posturing of the hands, hyperreflexia, and mild mental retardation or dementia. When such nonspecific generalized neurological and mental disturbances are encountered, static or progressive signs and symptoms of an underlying disease process must be distinguished from toxic side effects of antiseizure drugs. Slurred speech, ataxia, nystagmus, and poor attention span due to sedation are more characteristic of the latter (see Table 12–3) (Chapters 11, 14, and 15). However, focal deficits such as aphasia can also result from toxic drug levels in patients with otherwise asymptomatic localized lesions. Fluctuations in these findings on repeated examination suggest medication effects, particularly if the fluctuations can be correlated with alterations in serum levels of specific antiseizure drugs.

Impairment of memory function is common in patients with generalized tonic-clonic and focal dyscognitive seizures. Memory disturbances can result from the underlying lesion and are exacerbated by antiseizure drug effects.

Most often, however, memory disturbances reflect reversible dysfunction induced by the epileptic seizures (Rausch and Crandall, 1982) (Chapter 11). Deterioration of memory function in patients with generalized tonic-clonic or focal dyscognitive seizures who report no change in frequency or severity of ictal events may indicate the occurrence of subclinical or unrecognized nocturnal ictal events.

Focal or generalized neurological and mental impairment may reflect ictal or postictal, rather than interictal, disturbances (see Table 12–3) (Chapter 9). Repeating the neurological examination at intervals of hours or days may be necessary to distinguish postictal effects from static interictal deficits. In general, a postictal Todd's phenomenon does not last more than 48 hours, but some neurological or mental disabilities may slowly resolve over weeks or months after status epilepticus (Chapter 9). Consequently, it is not always possible to distinguish transient from fixed disturbances except by following their course.

In some epileptic disorders, notably atypical absence status (Chapter 10), the continuous ictal state may be considered interictal until a neurological and mental status examination reveals slightly dulled mentation with or without minor clonic movements such as eye blinking. In other conditions, such as focal dyscognitive status epilepticus (Chapter 10), bizarre behavior should not be mistaken for psychosis or delirium when examination reveals characteristic fluctuating alterations in mental status with associated automatisms.

Epileptic Seizure Observation

Direct observation of a seizure is the best way to document behavioral features. This is certainly possible during the evaluation of status epilepticus, but the opportunity is also available when patients have spontaneous epileptic seizures in the presence of a physician and when relatively benign seizures can be provoked (e.g., absences by hyperventilation). Provocation of epileptic seizures, however, should not be routinely attempted if a generalized tonic-clonic seizure might occur. When trained personnel are present during a spontaneous or provoked epileptic seizure, this opportunity to characterize the ictal and postictal events should be

exploited. It is necessary, therefore, to know in advance how to examine a patient during a seizure (Table 12–4). Attention should be paid to (1) the form and anatomical distribution of movements at the beginning of the epileptic seizure, (2) initial alterations in consciousness, (3) responsiveness and memory during the ictal event, and (4) postictal neurological and mental deficits (Chapters 6 and 7). When a patient is given a specific phrase to remember during the ictus and cannot recall it afterward, amnesia is documented (unless a focal seizure in clear consciousness with receptive aphasia occurred). Failure to respond to command during an ictal event is not always evidence of impaired consciousness; patients with ictal receptive aphasia may not understand a command, patients with a negative motor seizure may be able to understand the command but unable to execute it, and patients may be

Table 12–4 Clinical Examination During Epileptic Seizures

A. Ictal phase
  1. Mental status
     a. Determine responsiveness to commands, orientation, language function.
     b. Present a phrase for later recall, to determine amnesia.
  2. Motor
     a. Note site of initiation and pattern of motor symptoms, clonic and/or postural.
     b. Note focal or lateralizing motor deficits during spontaneous movements, and if possible, provoke movements to confirm deficits.
  3. Sensory
     In special situations it may be useful to demonstrate a general analgesia to pin prick, or to document a specific sensory deficit, such as ictal blindness.
B. Postictal phase
  1. Observe spontaneous abnormal behavior, e.g., automatisms, combativeness, and unresponsiveness; determine time course of resolution.
  2. Examine for specific focal or lateralizing neurological deficits, including cognitive deficits.
  3. Test for recall of phrase given in 1b, to determine amnesia for ictal event.
  4. Elicit description, if possible, of aura, behavioral seizure, and postictal symptoms.

inattentive for various reasons. Conversely, patients may respond to single commands during focal dyscognitive seizures and still have impaired consciousness. Demonstration of ictal amnesia is the critical piece of information needed for the diagnosis of focal dyscognitive seizures. The reliability of the historical description of seizures can be assessed by asking the patient and any friends or relatives in the office to describe what occurred and to indicate whether this was a habitual ictal event. More sophisticated video and *electroencephalogram (EEG)* monitoring of epileptic seizures may be necessary for diagnosis, as discussed later in this chapter.

LABORATORY EXAMINATION

Clinical Laboratory Tests

Specific *hematological* and *chemical* laboratory studies might be indicated to confirm underlying disease processes suggested by historical information or physical examination. Otherwise, a complete blood count, including differential white cell and platelet count; standard clinical chemistry evaluation, including electrolytes, calcium, and tests of liver and renal function; and a routine urinalysis should be obtained initially. These tests provide baseline values for assessing possible side effects of antiseizure drug treatment or other subsequent changes in medical status (Leppik, 2008). A *lumbar puncture* is not routinely performed unless the history and physical examination suggest the presence of a specific disorder associated with characteristic findings in the *cerebrospinal fluid (CSF)*. A lumbar puncture performed after a generalized tonic-clonic seizure may show mild pleocytosis caused by the epileptic seizure rather than by an intracranial inflammatory process (Chapter 9). Elevated CSF *glutamine* levels can be useful for diagnosing *valproate*-related hyperammonemic encephalopathy when serum ammonia levels are normal (Vossler et al., 2002).

Serum *prolactin* is elevated after focal dyscognitive and generalized tonic-clonic seizures and may aid in the differential diagnosis between epileptic and nonepileptic events (Pritchard et al., 1985; Sperling et al., 1986a).

When indicated, prolactin levels should be drawn within 20 minutes of the ictal episode and compared with levels drawn at the same time on another day, not with laboratory standards.

A few genetic epilepsy syndromes and a number of genetic diseases that cause epilepsy can be diagnosed by genetic testing (Ottman et al., 2010) (Table 12–5). This is particularly important for the epileptic encephalopathies (Chapter 7), where mutations in the *SCN1A* gene can be diagnostic of *Dravet syndrome*, *PCDH19* mutations cause a condition known as *epilepsy limited to females with mental retardation*, and spasms in infancy can be related to *ARX* mutations in boys and *CDKL5* mutations in girls (Scheffer, 2011) (Chapter 7). *Early-onset absence*s (i.e., absences first occurring under the age of 4 years) can be caused by a mutation of the *SLC2A1* gene that causes GLUT1 deficiency and can be treated with the *ketogenic diet* (Scheffer, 2011) (Chapter 7). Genetic testing is now standard for diagnosing specific genetic diseases, but because mendelian epilepsies all have incomplete penetrance, a positive or negative result is not an absolute indication of risk, and using genetic testing for counseling of individuals who do not have a disease but may be at risk raises serious ethical concerns when the disease cannot be prevented or modified (Elmslie, 2008). This issue is particularly important when parents want to know the risk in a sibling of an affected child, in which case the child's right not to know must be taken into account. In the future, however, genetic screening might provide not only disease diagnosis but also information about a patient's susceptibility to drug efficacy and toxicity (Glauser, 2011), while gene expression profiles could serve as biomarkers of epileptogenesis and epileptogenicity (Engel, 2011a;b).

Electroencephalography

WHEN TO USE EEG

Routine EEG remains the single most informative laboratory test for the diagnosis of epilepsy, (Cooper et al., 1980; Ebersole and Pedley, 2003; Fisch and Spehlmann, 1999; Goldensohn et al., 1999; Kiloh et al., 1981; Krauss and Fisher, 2006; Schomer and Lopes da Silva, 2011; Stern

Table 12–5 **Clinical Utility of Genetic Testing in Affected Individuals**

Syndrome or Condition	Genes	Proportion with Mutations	Clinical Utility
Benign familial neonatal seizures	KCNQ2 KCNQ3	60% ~7%	Somewhat useful
Benign familial neonatal-infantile seizures	SCN2A	?	Somewhat useful
Ohtahara syndrome	STXBP1 ARX	~35% ?	Very useful
Early-onset spasms	STK9/CDKLS	10–17%	Very useful
X-linked infantile spasms	ARX	<5% of males	Very useful
Dravet syndrome*	SCN1A	70–80%	Very useful
Epilepsy and mental retardation limited to females*	PCDH19	?	Very useful
Early-onset absence epilepsy	SLC2A1	~10%	Very useful
Autosomal dominant nocturnal frontal lobe epilepsy	CHRNA4	<10%	Very useful
	CHRNB2 CHRNA2	<5% ?	
Autosomal dominant focal epilepsy with auditory features	LGI1	~50%	Not very useful
Epilepsy with paroxysmal exercise-induced dyskinesia	SLC2A1	?	Very useful

*Also very useful in unaffected relatives of affected individuals.
Adapted from Ottman et al., 2010, with permission.

and Engel, 2005; Walczak et al., 2008) but it is easily misused. Most importantly, overinterpretation of the EEG recording is the most common cause of an unwarranted diagnosis of epilepsy (Chapter 13), and unnecessary EEG procedures result in avoidable expense and inconvenience. Much is now known about the neuronal mechanisms that generate EEG signals (Chapter 3), but the clinical interpretation of EEG recordings and application of EEG findings to the diagnosis and treatment of epilepsy remain more an art than a science (Engel, 1984a).

EEG procedures should be performed to answer specific questions of therapeutic or prognostic value. Because routine EEGs are noninvasive, benign, and relatively inexpensive, at least one EEG should be obtained for all patients with epilepsy or suspected epilepsy to provide baseline data that can be used if the clinical picture changes. Because the diagnosis of epilepsy is usually made clinically, however, repeat EEGs, especially those using more sophisticated techniques that are time-consuming, expensive, and occasionally invasive, should be carried out only if expected results would alter patient management or provide new prognostic information. There is no justification for routinely repeated EEGs at yearly or any intervals. The four most important questions that the EEG can help to answer are as follows:

1. *Does the patient have epilepsy?* Interictal and ictal EEG abnormalities help to distinguish epilepsy conditions from other disorders with intermittent symptoms. However, a number of normal spike-like EEG events may be overinterpreted, leading to a mistaken diagnosis of epilepsy (Chapter 13). In addition, approximately 2% of the population (Zivin and Ajmone-Marsan, 1968) and 3% of children (Cavazzuti et al., 1980) have abnormal epileptiform spike-and-wave complexes in their EEGs but never experience seizures. On the other hand, approximately 50% of patients with epilepsy do not demonstrate epileptic abnormalities on one routine EEG, (Ajmone-Marsan and Zivin, 1970; Salinsky et al., 1987) and 10–20% remain negative even after serial routine studies (Salinsky et al., 1987). In those rare circumstances when repeat EEGs are clinically required, the diminishing yield does not justify

more than four (Salinsky et al., 1987). The likelihood of obtaining epileptiform abnormalities on an interictal EEG depends in part on the epilepsy condition (Chapter 7). There is no reason to routinely decrease antiseizure medication before obtaining an EEG (Ajmone-Marsan and Zivin, 1970).

2. *What kind of epilepsy does the patient have?* Characteristic interictal and ictal EEG patterns can help identify types of epileptic seizures and specific epilepsy syndromes (Chapters 6 and 7). The EEG findings of use in the differential diagnosis of epilepsy are discussed in Chapter 13.

3. *How good is therapy?* The EEG can be useful for distinguishing dose-related side effects of antiseizure drugs (which are often associated with EEG slowing) from exacerbation of epileptic symptoms. The frequency of interictal spikes can also provide an indication of the efficacy of antiseizure drug therapy for patients with typical absences (Kellaway et al., 1979), but interictal spike frequency does not correlate with epileptic seizure control for other seizure types. The EEG is essential for monitoring the progress of therapy during status epilepticus when clinical behavior is not a reliable guide (Chapter 10).

4. *Where is the lesion?* Accurate localization of an interictal EEG spike focus is an interesting challenge for the electroencephalographer but of little practical importance for most patients. Interictal spikes in some areas are more likely to be associated with epileptic seizures than interictal spikes in other areas, particularly in children (Kellaway, 1980) (Chapter 8), but this is usually due to their association with specific syndromes that are easily recognized on the basis of other clinical data. For instance, anterior temporal spikes are highly correlated with *mesial temporal lobe epilepsy*, whereas centrotemporal spikes are characteristic of *benign focal epilepsy of childhood* (Chapter 7) and are also seen in children with *cerebral palsy*, who do not have seizures (Chapter 13). Precise localization of the epileptogenic region is essential in patients with focal seizures who are candidates for resective surgical therapy, because the results of this treatment depend on accurate identification of the brain tissue to be removed (Chapter 16). Although neuroimaging, particularly *magnetic resonance imaging (MRI)*, is now the most important test for localizing structural lesions in the brain, EEG is still

important for demonstrating that these lesions are epileptogenic.

SPECIAL EEG APPROACHES

Additional Electrodes

It is impossible to determine whether a focal epileptiform transient is of cerebral origin when no topographical field distribution is demonstrated. Consequently, if EEG spikes appear at only one electrode, additional scalp electrodes between the standard 10–20 placements (Fig. 12–5) are used to prove that a field exists.

The standard 10–20 placements do not adequately cover the temporal lobes. Therefore, *basal electrodes* are often used to clarify inferior and mesial temporal epileptiform EEG activity. In the past, *nasopharyngeal electrodes* (Mavor and Hellen, 1964) (see Fig. 12–5) were inserted through the nose to record from the roof of the nasopharynx, but these are no longer recommended. *Sphenoidal electrodes* (King et al., 1986; Rovit et al., 1961a; Sperling and Engel, 1986) (Fig. 12–6) are inserted through the skin and usually record from the region of the *foramen ovale*. These electrodes must be placed by a physician. Electrodes on the *ear lobes* (A_1 and A_2), on the *mastoid* (M_1 and M_2), over the *zygoma*, or at T_1 and T_2 (*true*

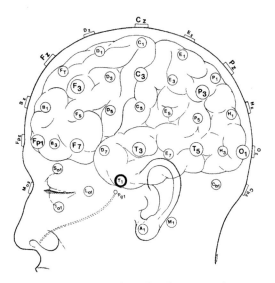

Figure 12–5. EEG electrode placement relative to underlying regions of the brain. (Modified courtesy of Dr. G. E. Chatrian, University of Washington. From Sperling and Engel, 1985, with permission.)

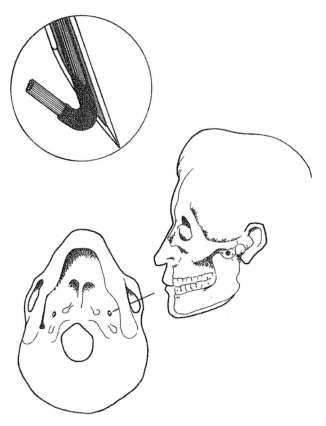

Figure 12–6. Illustration to show the placement of sphenoidal electrodes. The needle is inserted approximately 1 inch anterior to the tragus immediately under the zygomatic arch (*black dot on lateral view*). The tip of the electrode should lie close to the foramen ovale (*basilar view*). *Inset* shows how multistranded Teflon-coated wire protrudes from the tip of the insertion needle and is bent backward on the Teflon coating for prevention of breakage of wire strands. Inner lip of the needle can also be beveled to further ensure that breakage of the sphenoidal wire does not occur. See text for details.

temporals) (Silverman, 1960) (see Fig. 12–5) also record basal epileptiform events.

The most effective and efficient approach for basal electrode recording during routine EEG is to use the standard ear electrode placements or true temporals with an appropriate basal montage (Table 12–6) on all patients with epilepsy or suspected epilepsy. Because modern digital recording techniques allow post hoc adjustment of filter settings and recording parameters, the accuracy of true temporal electrodes for localizing interictal spikes and ictal onsets in mesial temporal lobe epilepsy is not appreciably different from that of sphenoidal electrodes (Mintzer et al., 2002); the former are generally used for routine long-term monitoring, and sphenoidal electrodes are employed only when they might resolve equivocal findings. There is no indication for the use of nasopharyngeal electrodes. Pharyngeal muscle contraction and movement produce artifacts that confound interpretation, and the closely spaced electrode tips, joined by wet mucous membrane, make lateralization

difficult (Sperling and Engel, 1985; Sperling et al., 1986b) (Fig. 12–7). In addition, these electrodes are uncomfortable, reduce the likelihood that a natural sleep recording can be obtained, and cannot be left in for long periods of time.

Sphenoidal electrodes for long-term monitoring are usually constructed from Teflon-coated, braided, multistranded stainless steel wire. These electrodes are tough and flexible and provide stable recordings for up to six weeks (Sperling and Engel, 1986). Sphenoidal electrodes are commercially available but can be easily "homemade": wires are bared for 3–4 mm at the tip, threaded through a standard 22-gauge 1.5-inch hypodermic needle, and bent backward just proximal to the bared portion (see Fig. 12–6). The skin is disinfected with alcohol, and no anesthetic is necessary. The sterilized needle assembly is inserted perpendicular to the surface of the skin through the mandibular notch with the mouth closed. The notch can be located by palpation just under the zygomatic arch, approximately 1 inch

Table 12–6 Montage Strategy for Basal Electrode Recordings

First Nine Channels Always*	Basal Short Chain†		Options for Longer Basal Chains‡	
$FP_1–F_7$	$T_3–B_1$	$C_3–B_1$	$C_z–C_3$	$C_z–C_3$
$F_7–T_3$	$B_1–B_2$ or $B_1–B_2$		$C_3–T_3$	$C_3–T_3$
$T_3–T_5$	$B_2–T_4$	$B_2–C_4$	$T_3–B_1$	$T_3–B_1$
$T_5–O_1$			$B_1–N_z$	$B_1–B_2$
$FP_2–F_8$	Additional coverage‡		$N_z–B_2$ or	$B_2–T_4$
$F_8–T_4$	$F_3–P_3$ $F_7–F_3$ $F_7–F_3$		$B_2–T_4$	$T_4–C_4$
$T_4–T_6$	$P_3–C_3$ $F_3–F_4$ $F_3–F_z$		$T_4–C_4$	$C_4–C_2$
$T_6–O_2$	$F_4–P_4$ $F_4–F_8$ $F_z–F_4$		$C_4–C_z$	
ECG	$P_4–C_4$ $F_4–F_8$		$B_1–B_2$	

B_1 and B_2 are equivalent to A_1 and A_2 or T_1 and T_2 for routine EEG laboratory tests and sphenoidal electrodes for long-term recordings.
°Routine temporal montage is necessary for recognizing normal variants such as small sharp spikes and 14- and 6-Hz positive spikes. EGG is necessary for recognizing ECG and pulse artifact.
†Recommended for 12-channel machines only. $C_3–C_4$ can be used instead of $T_3–T_4$ to increase signal; the temporal-to-basal channel may be isoelectric.
‡More channels provide options of additional coverage and longer basal chains. Basal electrodes can be separated by recording across the nose (N_z). Using central and temporal electrodes together provides better localization than central or temporal alone. The $B_1–B_2$ channel may help detect the direction of interhemispheric spread.

anterior to the tragus of the ear (Pampiglione and Kerridge, 1956). Rapid insertion of the needle to its full length, and then withdrawal, leaves the wire in place and causes only minimal discomfort to the patient. The depth of the sphenoidal electrode and the relationship of the electrode tip to the foramen ovale do not appear to be critical parameters for accurate recording (Wilkus and Thompson, 1985). The needle is then slipped off the free end of the wire, which is soldered to an appropriate connector. The wire is coiled at its exit from the skin and fixed with collodion-soaked gauze and tape. There is initial discomfort with chewing, but this resolves completely during the first day, and patients are then unaware of the wires for the remainder of the evaluation. The only potentially serious complication would result from accidental penetration of the temporomandibular joint, which could cause aseptic inflammation. A finger placed at the correct insertion point should feel the joint capsule move into this space as the mouth is opened, and out again as the mouth is closed.

Minisphenoidals (Laxer, 1984) consisting of EEG needle electrodes inserted under the zygoma have been used, but the relative yield of this technique has not been compared with that of either standard sphenoidals, on the one hand, or true temporal electrodes, on the other.

Epileptiform EEG transients recorded by all basal electrodes reflect activity in mesial temporal and orbitofrontal regions. However, it can be difficult to distinguish abnormal transients recorded with basal electrode placements from normal variants such as *small sharp spikes* and *14- and 6-Hz positive spikes* (Chapter 13) unless the typical morphology of the latter can be recognized from simultaneously recorded routine scalp derivations. Consequently, montages must be used that display lateral temporal activity independently from activity recorded from basal electrodes (see Table 12–6). Basal electrode recordings require at least 10, and ideally 16 or more, channels to provide sufficient coverage for accurate diagnosis. Mesial temporal spikes should be considered epileptic only if they display a field over the appropriate temporal scalp that is not characteristic of 14- and 6-Hz positive spikes or small sharp spikes.

Physiological Activation Procedures

Hyperventilation should be performed during all routine EEG recordings unless medically contraindicated, in an attempt to activate interictal epileptiform spikes and focal slow waves. Hyperventilation also commonly activates absences, and prolonged hyperventilation can provoke focal seizures in some patients. Small

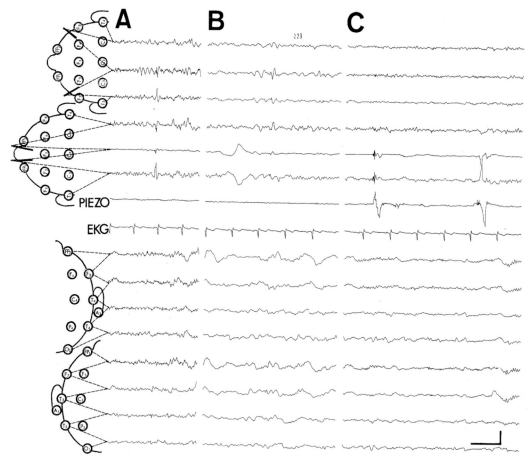

Figure 12–7. Simultaneous recordings from sphenoidal electrodes (*top three channels*), nasopharyngeal electrodes (*next three channels*), a piezoelectrode placed in one nasopharynx to record movements, ECG, and routine temporal surface EEG derivations. **A.** Left temporal spike is well localized by the sphenoidal derivation but might be considered a bilaterally synchronous event on the nasopharyngeal recording. **B.** Left sphenoidal sharp wave, which is poorly reflected but apparent over the anterior temporal surface, and therefore real, would not have been recognized on the nasopharyngeal record. **C.** At the left, an obvious pharyngeal movement artifact appears from the left nasopharyngeal electrode but not from the left sphenoidal. The second nasopharyngeal transient, which is also not seen from the sphenoidal derivation, might be mistaken for an interictal spike, but the piezoelectrode demonstrates that this is also a movement artifact. (From Engel, 1984a, with permission.)

children will usually hyperventilate when asked to blow on a pinwheel or to blow out an imaginary candle. Normal hyperventilation-induced high-voltage synchronous slowing occurs in children and some adults (particularly when blood sugar is low) and must be distinguished from EEG patterns that indicate an epileptic condition. Hyperventilation-induced *convulsive syncope* is not evidence for an epileptic condition (Chapter 13). This disorder should be treated as *syncope* and not with antiseizure drugs. Contraindications for hyperventilation usually include active coronary disease, *chronic obstructive pulmonary disease*, and unstable

cerebrovascular disease, including *acute stroke*, *intracranial hemorrhage*, *sickle cell anemia*, and *moyamoya disease*.

Sleep can activate interictal EEG spike activity, particularly frontotemporal spikes associated with limbic seizures. Unwarranted diagnoses of epilepsy, however, are most commonly due to overreading of sleep recordings, because many normal sharp transients of sleep can be confused with abnormal epileptiform spikes (Chapter 13). When there is doubt about transients seen during sleep, the recording should be continued on the same montage after the patient is aroused. Occurrence of the same transients during wakefulness rules out a normal sleep phenomenon.

Sufficient periods of sleep can usually be obtained naturally in the EEG laboratory when recordings are performed with the patient lying down in a quiet darkened room. The added advantages provided by sleep deprivation are not sufficient to justify its use on a routine basis, although it can be helpful in selected cases if other tests are negative (Ellingson et al., 1984). In situations where a waking EEG is normal, sleep could not be naturally obtained, and the appearance of epileptiform EEG spikes would alter management, or when patients will not cooperate for the EEG study, narcosis can be achieved by sedative drugs such as *secobarbital sodium* (100 or 200 mg in adults or 2–6 mg/kg up to 100 mg in children) or *chloral hydrate* (1.0–2.0 g in adults and 50 mg/kg up to 1.0 g in children), administered orally. Chloral hydrate is preferred in children and produces less fast activity than secobarbital, but barbiturate fast activity may also provide opportunities to note focal attenuation, as discussed later in this chapter. A sedative drug should not be administered prior to an initial EEG study unless absolutely necessary, because this can compromise recording of a waking EEG pattern.

Epileptic seizures that habitually occur during nighttime sleep (Chapters 7 and 9) are not necessarily provoked in the EEG laboratory by brief natural or sedated sleep recordings. All-night *polysomnography* (Broughton, 1982; Tassinari and Rubboli, 2008) with special channels to monitor eye movements, muscle activity, respiration, and occasionally other parameters is necessary for capturing these events and determining the sleep stages during which they occur. Polysomnography is particularly useful for distinguishing nocturnal epileptic seizures from other sleep disturbances (Chapter 13).

Specific stimulation can be used to activate reflex seizures in the EEG laboratory (Chapter 9). This technique is most helpful for diagnosing photosensitive epilepsy (Jeavons and Harding, 1975; Newmark and Penry, 1979; Takahashi, 1982; Zifkin et al., 2008), using intermittent flash or pattern photic stimulation. Photic stimulation is intended to induce an EEG epileptiform *photoparoxysmal (photoconvulsive) response* that may be associated with brief ictal behavior (see Fig. 13–17), but it should not be continued at the risk of producing a generalized convulsion. When a photoparoxysmal response is obtained, information about the effective frequency band and sensitivity to various colors may help the patient avoid provocative situations (Chapter 9). Photoparoxysmal responses must be distinguished from nonepileptic photic-induced EEG changes such as *photomyogenic (photomyoclonic) responses* and *occipital spike driving* (Chapter 13).

Other specific visual, auditory, or somatosensory stimuli may precipitate rarer forms of reflex epileptic seizures (Forster, 1977; Zifkin et al., 2008) (Chapter 9). Observing such responses can be useful in documenting an epilepsy condition and in planning behavioral treatment (Chapter 16).

Pharmacological Activation Procedures

Epileptic seizures can be provoked in the EEG laboratory by fractional intravenous injections of convulsant agents (Kaufman et al., 1947). Both *pentylenetetrazol* and *bemegride* have been used in the past in association with EEG and video monitoring in an attempt to observe habitual seizures (Wieser et al., 1979). Variations of this technique include measurements of pentylenetetrazol threshold for obtaining photic-induced myoclonic jerks in the diagnosis of genetic generalized epilepsy (Gastaut, 1950) and intracarotid injection of convulsant agents for unilateral hemispheric activation (Garretson et al., 1966). With the development of long-term monitoring, observation of spontaneous seizures has yielded much more reliable information than observation of pharmacologically induced seizures (Wieser et al., 1979), and these activation techniques are now used only rarely (Salinsky et al., 1987).

Fractional administration of intravenous *barbiturates* (*thiopental* and *methohexital*) induces narcosis and interictal spikes (Engel et al., 1975); however, interictal spikes during sleep and narcosis have less localizing value than those that occur during wakefulness (Lieb et al., 1980). While barbiturate narcosis for interictal spike induction has been abandoned, these drugs and *diazepam* were more commonly used to induce beta activity in the EEG, because attenuation of those rhythms is useful for localizing focal functional deficits at the site of ictal onset (Brazier et al., 1976; Engel et al., 1975; Kennedy and Hill, 1958). A standard approach is to give *thiopental* at a rate of 25 mg every 30 seconds until beta activity is prominent and the corneal reflex is absent. This is best performed with the aid of an anesthesiologist, because there is a risk of respiratory arrest or laryngospasm. Computer analysis (Gotman et al., 1982) in association with visual analysis (Lieb et al., 1986b) provides the best interpretation of these data. With the advent of functional neuroimaging, particularly *positron emission tomography (PET)*, this approach is now rarely necessary to demonstrate a focal functional deficit.

Barbiturate suppression of EEG activity has been used in evaluating surgical candidates who have bilateral or multifocal interictal epileptiform discharges to determine whether a primary EEG focus exists and where it might be. Fractional *methohexital* is usually given (Lombroso and Erba, 1970; Morrell, 1978) until only a single EEG spike focus remains. It is then assumed that this focus is the site of the primary epileptogenic region. This technique should also be carried out with an anesthesiologist present. Intracarotid *amobarbital* (Rovit et al., 1961b) has been used in a similar fashion to suppress epileptiform activity in one hemisphere when there are bilateral EEG spike foci, to determine which focus might be primary and which secondary. The value of these suppression tests in the evaluation of patients for surgical therapy has not been definitively determined (Quesney, 1987) (Chapter 16).

Video-EEG Monitoring

When clinical doubt persists after all other reasonable studies have been performed, video-EEG monitoring (VEM, also called *long-term monitoring* or *intensive neurodiagnostic monitoring*) may be indicated for determining whether a patient has epilepsy, diagnosing the seizure types, quantifying and characterizing patterns of seizure occurrence, or localizing a surgically removable epileptogenic zone (Fig. 12–8). There are many techniques available for VEM (Engel et al., 1985a; Fisch, 2010; Sperling and Clancy, 2008; Legatt and Ebersole, 2008; Sirven and Stern, 2011; Stern and Engel, 2011) (Table 12–7), and practice guidelines have been published by the American Clinical Neurophysiology Society (2008).

The simplest VEM procedure uses direct connection between the patient and a standard EEG machine either in a modified EEG laboratory setting or with an ambulatory unit in a hospital room. This allows digital EEG records to be obtained with constant observation by a technologist or nurse for periods of 8–10 hours (Engel et al., 1985a; American Clinical Neurophysiology Society, 2008; Sirven and Stern, 2011; Stern and Engel, 2012). This procedure is supplemented by video recording of clinical behaviors (Ives, 1987; Porter et al., 1985; Sirven and Stern, 2011) and can be repeated daily until a sufficient number of seizures are captured to permit a diagnosis.

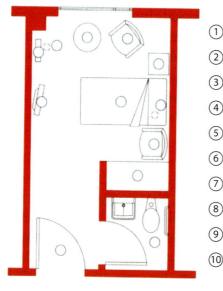

① Wall mounted E.E.G. station
② Ceiling mounted video camera with infrared light
③ Wall mounted TV
④ Ceiling mounted microphone
⑤ Chair
⑥ Bed
⑦ Bathroom
⑧ Entry
⑨ Table
⑩ Closet

Figure 12–8. Schematic diagram of a typical video-EEG monitoring unit bed, showing the camera with infrared light, and microphone locations in the patient's living area. In this room, the patient spends most of his or her time in the bed or the chair next to the window. Both of these locations are well covered by the video camera mounted near the opposite wall and by the microphone mounted above the bed. The small size of the room makes it easier to keep the patient on camera as often as possible while allowing for privacy in the bathroom area. (From Schevon et al., 2011, with permission.)

Table 12–7 **Commonly Used VEM System Configurations**

Monitoring with Paper Printout Only
EEG transmission: "hard wire" (standard cable) or telemetry (cable or radio)
EEG recording/storage: continuous paper printout
EEG review/analysis: complete manual review
Behavior monitoring: self, observer, and video
Monitoring with Continuous Storage
EEG transmission: cable or radio telemetry
EEG recording/storage: analog or videotape, digital media (hard disk, server, CD/DVD)
EEG review/analysis: selective review of clinical ictal events, random sampling review for subclinical ictal and interictal events
Behavior monitoring: self, observer, and video
Computer-Assisted Selective Monitoring
EEG transmission: cable or radio telemetry
EEG recording/storage: digital tape/disk, computer-assisted selective storage
EEG review/analysis: selective review of clinical and computer-recognized ictal and interictal events on high-resolution monitor
Behavior monitoring: self, observer, and video
Ambulatory Cassette Selective Event Recording/Epoch Sampling
EEG transmission: ambulatory flash memory or hard disk (16-or 24-channel)
EEG recording/storage: flash memory, hard disk, or digital media (CD/DVD); event recording/epoch sampling (periodic or after trigger)
EEG review/analysis: epoch review
Behavior monitoring: self, observer

From Stern and Engel, 2012, with permission.

The most commonly employed VEM technique makes use of *cable telemetry*, although *radiotelemetry* is also available. These systems usually employ 32, 64, or more channels. EEG signals are amplified in a telemetry pack attached to the patient's head or body, multiplexed, and transmitted over wires or through the air to an antenna and a storage device, where they are decoded (Ives, 1985; Nuwer et al., 1985). Most systems use analog-to-digital conversion methods and store data on computer hard drives, servers, or compact disk or DVD media (American Clinical Neurophysiology Society, 2008; Stern and Engel, 2012; Bergey and Nordli, 2008). Telemetry has several advantages over direct EEG recording. Patients can move around the room or ward if necessary, depending on the length of the cable or the limit of the radio signal. They are practically confined to a bed or chair in most cases, however, by the need for simultaneous video recording. Specialized systems with multiple cameras or tracking devices exist that permit the patient more freedom of movement. Movement artifact is minimal, because EEG signals must travel only a very short distance before amplification. Typically, patients are continuously monitored by telemetry 24 hours a day for days or weeks until sufficient information is obtained, although daily 8- to 10-hour sessions in a special telemetry laboratory provide an alternative approach. Activation procedures such as antiseizure drug withdrawal and sleep deprivation are commonly performed to induce seizures (So and Fisch, 2008). Ictal events can be identified by the patient, observers, and automatic detection devices, so only the relevant EEG correlates need be stored and analyzed. Interictal EEG activity can also be stored for review as required. VEM is usually performed in association with synchronized video recording to allow precise correlation of EEG and behavior. Although VEM recording does not require the continuous attention of an EEG technologist, a nurse or monitoring technologist should be readily available at all times to observe the patient either directly or via a video monitor and to interact with the patient for assessment of clinical status during ictal events. Patients on VEM units with multiple beds are typically observed continuously by one or more monitoring technologists at a central station with individual video monitors and two-way audio contact as well as facilities for video camera pan, tilt, and zoom, to optimize the video image during seizures.

A third type of long-term monitoring uses an *ambulatory recorder* (Ebersole, 1987; Ebersole and Leroy, 1983a; Ebersole and Leroy, 1983b; American Clinical Neurophysiology Society, 2008). EEG signals are amplified on the patient's head and transmitted directly over wires to a small digital storage unit carried on the belt or in a pocket. This device accommodates up to 32 channels of EEG. There is complete freedom of movement, electrodes can be hidden by hair or a hat, and EEG recordings can be obtained while the patient goes about normal daily activities at home, work, or school. Whereas ambulatory recording originally stored analog data continuously, the current digital systems use spike and seizure detection programs and a button press when a patient or an observer identifies an ictal event, so that only epochs containing potential interictal and ictal epileptiform events are captured, along with occasional runs of baseline activity. Depending on the frequency of ictal and interictal events, this approach can permit continuous recording for several days, although patients usually need to return every 48 hours to have the electrodes regelled. In selected patients, particularly those with easily recognizable generalized EEG discharges, this technique can be used for identifying an episode as epileptic and determining the frequency or pattern of occurrence of such episodes. However, the high incidence of difficult-to-interpret artifacts and the absence of video-recorded behavioral data limit the usefulness of this technique for characterizing ictal events. Ambulatory recording, at the present level of technology, is also not appropriate for presurgical evaluation (American Clinical Neurophysiology Society, 2008). Without automatic detection, the long-term selected-event approach (Ives, 1985) relies on the ability of the patient or an observer to trigger the recording. This restricts its application to situations where the onset of a seizure can be easily and reliably recognized. Ambulatory recorders can be used in the hospital in association with video monitoring for presurgical evaluation.

Approximately one-third of patients admitted to VEM units are evaluated for differential diagnosis between epilepsy and nonepileptic seizures. VEM with scalp and basal electrodes provides important information that can lead to a definitive diagnosis of epilepsy. On the other hand, there are situations where it is impossible, even with the most sophisticated techniques, to determine with certainty that an ictal event is *not* epileptic (Chapter 13). Inpatient VEM is also used to characterize seizure types and, most commonly, to localize epileptogenic regions in patients who are candidates for resective surgical therapy. Specialized intracranial telemetry recording techniques, as well as intraoperative *electrocorticography (ECoG)*, used for presurgical evaluation, are described in Chapter 16.

Computer-Enhanced EEG

Computerized EEG techniques have greatly enhanced epilepsy diagnosis (LeVan and Gotman, 2008). The tremendous amount of data accumulated during long-term EEG monitoring requires computer-assisted data reduction techniques such as *compressed spectral arrays (CSAs)* to display the occurrence of epileptic seizures and interictal spikes over hours or days (Fig. 12–9). Computerized approaches can help in selecting EEG segments for review (Gotman, 1985a;b), identifying and quantifying interictal spike and seizure occurrence in space or time (Gotman, 1985a;b), and determining the sites of ictal onset (Darcey and Williamson, 1985; Gotman, 1985b; 1983) and spread (Lieb et al., 1986a). The ability to alter montages and filter settings post hoc often permits clarification of equivocal signals. Computer analysis of interictal spike morphology can have value for assessing the efficacy of antiseizure drug treatment, because parameters of spike morphology may change when seizures become controlled (Frost et al., 1986). Many brain-mapping programs are available for displaying topographic distributions of EEG activity, such as power of individual frequency bands, occurrence of epileptiform discharges, and features of evoked potentials (Duffy, 1986; Nuwer, 1988a;b;c; Ebersole et al., 2008).

Electroencephalographic *source modeling* can be used to localize interictal spikes and ictal EEG activity when this is required for surgical treatment (Ebersole et al., 2008; Ebersole and Ebersole, 2010) (Fig. 12–10). Predicting the deep source of electrical activity recorded at the scalp, referred to as the *inverse solution*, remains a relatively inexact science. Not only can more than one dipole model fit any given topographic EEG spike distribution, but there are multiple approaches to analysis as well as confounding factors related to the choice and categorization of spikes to analyze, the numbers and placements of electrodes, multiple dipoles, and moving dipoles. Alternatives to dipole localization, including *current density distribution* (Fig. 12–11) and the use of a *dipole patch* composed of several different dipoles, have not added accuracy. Nevertheless, promising results are being obtained (Coutin-Churchman et al. 2012), and it is likely that further experience, especially involving standardized methodologies, mapping EEG activity onto the patient's own MRI, and combined use of EEG and *magnetoencephalography (MEG)*, will result in the replacement of routine EEG analysis with computerized approaches for presurgical localization.

An entirely different application of computerized EEG analysis is *seizure prediction* (Lehnertz et al., 2008). Most approaches have

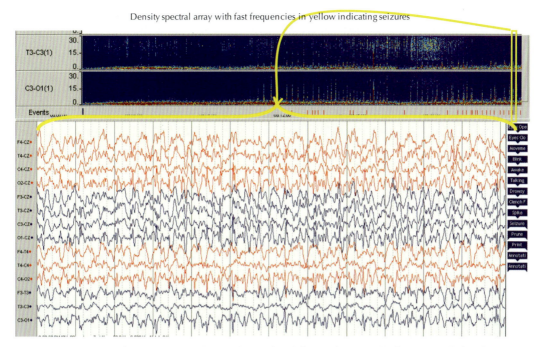

Figure 12–9. *Top*: Dot density compressed spectral array (CSA) for a 12-hour epoch of EEG recorded in the intensive care unit from a patient with severe head trauma. Frequency is along the ordinate, time along the abscissa, and color intensity indicates relative power, with *yellow* indicating high power. Each yellow peak represents fast frequencies indicating an occurrence of seizure activity. *Bottom*: Expanded view of the raw EEG segment representative of the seizure occurring at the defined time along the CSA trend on top. Generalized spike-and-wave activity is seen. (Courtesy of Dr. Paul Vespa.)

use nonlinear EEG analysis techniques in an effort to identify alterations occurring many minutes prior to ictal onset. Such changes would provide sufficient warning of an imminent seizure to permit patients to protect themselves from injury or embarrassment and to greatly reduce the disability caused by the unpredictable nature of most epileptic seizures (Chapter 11). Seizure prediction could also form the basis of feedback mechanisms designed to abort seizures before they occur. To date, this approach remains of considerable research interest, but practical applications have yet to emerge. Seizure prediction has yet to find a place in clinical diagnosis, but results of these studies may provide insights into basic mechanisms of ictogenesis (Bragin and Engel, 2008).

Evoked Potentials

Demonstration of impaired sensory function can be used to document the existence and location of specific lesions in the brain. *Visual field testing* is occasionally helpful in patients

with epilepsy who have posterior temporal and occipital epileptogenic regions, and *averaged evoked potentials* can be used to identify disruption of visual, auditory, and somatosensory pathways. Computerized mapping of evoked-potential data has been used to improve visualization of focal cerebral dysfunction, and this approach may find application to epilepsy (Nuwer, 1988a). These techniques have not revealed abnormalities peculiar to specific epileptogenic abnormalities or epilepsy disorders, with the following exceptions: *visual evoked potentials (VEPs)* are altered in some patients with photosensitive seizures (Broughton et al., 1969; Faught and Lee, 1984); enhanced *somatosensory evoked potentials (SEPs)* are seen in certain forms of myoclonus (Halliday, 1967); photic stimulation at slow frequencies (<3 Hz) produces large visual evoked potentials visible on the EEG in *late infantile ceroid lipofuscinosis (Jansky-Bielschowsky disease)* (Pampiglione and Harden, 1973); and the combination of a grossly enlarged VEP and an absent *electroretinogram (ERG)* is said to be unique to that disorder (Harden et al., 1973).

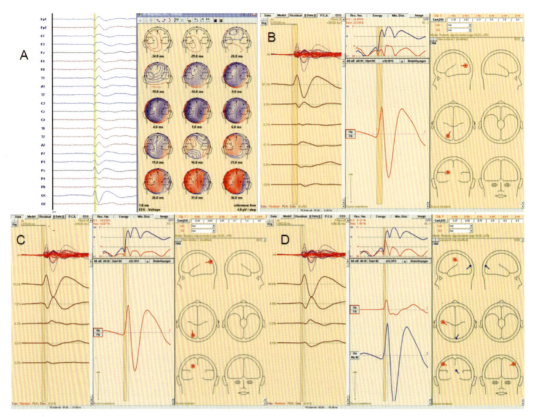

Figure 12–10. Dipole adjustment process for an averaged spike. **A.** The highest amplitude at the spike peak was over O_1. However, inspection of the sequential topographic map shows that the negativity first appeared between P_3 and Pz around 25 msec before the peak, then shifted to O_1. **B.** A single-dipole model was adjusted over the interval from the start of the first deflection to the peak of the highest spike (-35 to 0 msec). The solution yielded a source over the left occipital lobe with a very high residual variance (RV) of 24%. The principal component analysis (*first column*) during the onset-to-peak interval shows a strong first and a second weaker component. **C.** The end of the fitting interval was shifted 15 msec to the left (−35 to −15 msec) to exclude the second component, but the RV of the single-dipole model was still high, at 18%. **D.** A second dipole was then added to the model. A dramatic decrease in RV (down to 6%) was then achieved. The new solution shows a first, weaker dipole source at the left postrolandic region, peaking a few milliseconds before the second, stronger, but likely propagated dipole source at the right occipital pole. Patient had a left postrolandic lesion (dysplasia), which was resected, and is now seizure-free. (From Coutin-Churchman et al., 2012, with permission.)

Magnetoencephalography

Magnetoencephalography uses a *superconducting quantum interference device (SQUID)* to record magnetic fields induced by current flow in the brain (Williamson and Kaufman, 1981). MEG transients such as epileptiform spikes can be measured by averaging techniques, the source of these transients can in theory be localized in three dimensions, and the direction of current flow can be determined (Barth et al., 1984a;b; Barth et al., 1982; Ebersole et al., 2008). Although similar computerized approaches to source localization

are possible with EEG, MEG offers certain advantages, because the depth of a generator can be more easily determined and signals are not distorted by the skull (Ebersole et al., 2008; Ebersole and Ebersole, 2010). MEG and EEG are complementary techniques: MEG preferentially measures current flowing tangential to the surface of the brain, whereas EEG measures tangential and radial current flow but is better suited to detect the latter. Consequently, use of these two techniques together theoretically should make it possible to distinguish activity generated along the banks of sulci from activity generated at the tops of gyri.

Interval: −35 to 0 ms

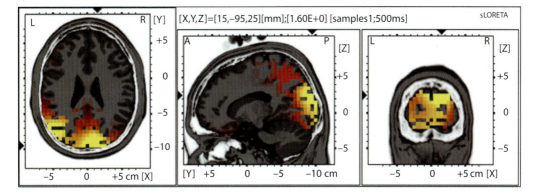

Interval: −35 to −15 ms

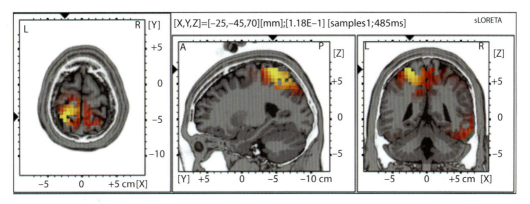

Figure 12–11. *Top: Standardized low resolution brain electromagnetic tomography (sLORETA)* solution maps for the onset-to-peak interval of the same spike as in Figure 12–10. The "lighted" areas represent voxels above 90% of the maximum value. An extended active area with maxima over the right mesial and left lateral occipital lobe is seen. *Bottom:* During the restricted interval the occipital contribution is suppressed, and a previously overshadowed left parietal focus comprising the postrolandic region is now apparent. (From Coutin-Churchman et al., 2012, with permission.)

Technology using over 100 probes as well as the ability to measure ongoing activity confidently without averaging has greatly enhanced the potential for MEG to become clinically useful (Knowlton et al., 2008). MEG studies of patients with focal epilepsy have demonstrated that interictal EEG epileptiform spike transients can have multiple current sources deep within the brain (Fig. 12–12; see also Fig. 12–18). This test can also provide information about the location of ictal discharges (Barth et al., 1984a;b; Sutherling et al., 1987; Eliashiv et al., 2002). A variety of MEG approaches are used, and clinical practice guidelines have recently been published by the American Clinical Magnetoencephalography Society (Bagic et al., 2011a;b;c; Burgess et al., 2011).

Transcranial Magnetic Stimulation

Transcranial magnetic stimulation (TMS) provides a noninvasive method of stimulating the brain by depolarizing neuronal elements directly under a magnetic coil (Epstein et al., 2008). Different shapes of coils are used to stimulate large or relatively small areas of brain for mapping cortical function, but this technique can also measure cortical excitability. Responses to single pulses can assess, for instance, effects

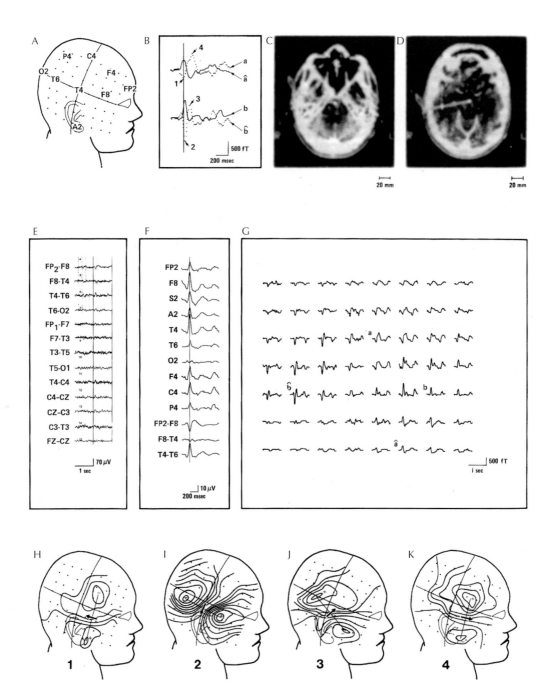

Figure 12–12. Demonstration of mapping of magnetic signals from the brain with MEG. **A.** Rectangular MEG measurement matrix (2-cm spacing) oriented along the temporal axis. All EEG electrodes are marked except the sphenoidal electrode (S₂). **B.** Enlargements of averaged magnetic spikes from separate, complementary regions (*a* and *b*) of the scalp show four components; the opposing polarities reflect the magnetic field simultaneously emerging from (*upward*) and reentering (*downward*) the cranium. **C, D.** CT sections at the levels of sources *a* and *b*, respectively, show the depth of the source (*cross*) located along a line connecting the surface location of the source marked with a washer (*arrow*) to the center of the cranium. **E.** Spike in the raw EEG recorded from both hemispheres. **F.** Averaged EEG spike from three bipolar channels (*lower three traces*). **G.** Averaged magnetic spikes recorded from the MEG matrix exhibit two distinct, complementary regions of differing morphology marked *a* and *b*. **H–K.** Isocontour maps displaying the magnetic fields for each of the four temporal components of the magnetic spike complex shown in **B.** *fT*, femtotesla. (From Barth et al., 1984b, with permission.)

428

of antiseizure drugs, while repetitive stimulation, similar to paired pulse stimulation used in experimental animals (Chapter 4), can provide information regarding inhibitory tone. In one recent study, motor threshold and cortical excitability predicted seizure control with antiseizure medication (Badawy et al., 2010). TMS remains a research tool but has promise for clinical application in the future.

Structural Neuroimaging

Demonstration of some lesions may indicate the need for specific therapy, whereas other findings are useful in distinguishing structural from genetic epilepsy disorders (Chapter 7). For confirmation of diagnosis or to reduce the possibility that some treatable cause has been overlooked, structural neuroimaging, preferably *magnetic resonance imaging (MRI)*, is generally recommended for almost all patients presenting with chronic recurrent epileptic seizures. Exceptions may include some children (through late adolescence) whose history and other examinations indicate a genetic epilepsy disorder or a nonprogressive lesion (Gaillard et al., 2009), as well as patients with indwelling pacemakers and other metallic objects that are not MRI-compatible. The current generation of *vagus nerve stimulators* are MRI-compatible, but the stimulator should be set to zero for the duration of the study, because the device could be accidentally activated by the scanner. The study must be done with a receiver-transmitter head coil, in order to avoid inclusion of the VNS device.

MAGNETIC RESONANCE IMAGING

MRI produces three-dimensional images of brain structure with excellent spatial resolution (Kressel, 1987; Wong et al., 1987; Jackson and Kuzniecky, 2008). *T1-weighted* images (made with short *repetition time [TR]* and *echo time [TE]*) provide detailed views of cerebral anatomy in which gray matter is gray, white matter is bright, and CSF is black. *T2-weighted* images (long TR and TE), where gray matter has a higher signal intensity than white matter and CSF is white, assess tissue abnormality. For *hippocampal sclerosis*, the most common lesion associated with limbic seizures (Chapter 5),

the sclerotic hippocampus typically appears smaller on the T1-weighted image, shows increased signal on the T2-weighted image, and has blurred cytoarchitecture with both techniques. In some cases increased signal is the only evidence of hippocampal abnormality and false negatives occur. *Fluid-attenuated inversion recovery (FLAIR)* images are manipulations of T2-weighted images that suppress the water signal. On FLAIR images, CSF appears black rather than white, reducing the partial-volume effects that make it difficult to assess lesions in periventricular and subpial structures (Fig. 12–13).

Routine MRI scans are often read as normal in patients with typical epileptogenic abnormalities such as hippocampal sclerosis and many types of *malformations of cortical development (MCDs)*. MRI evaluations for epilepsy are best carried out by neuroradiologists who are knowledgeable about lesions that are common causes of epilepsy, and an epileptologist needs to be part of the imaging team. An *epilepsy protocol* should be used, with thin sections displayed at the proper angle (for instance, parallel and perpendicular to the long axis of the hippocampus) that maximize signal-to-noise ratio and reduce partial-volume effects (Jackson and Kuzniecky, 2008). The epilepsy protocol typically includes T1-weighted imaging to define brain anatomy, T2-weighted images, and FLAIR. High-resolution three-dimensional volume acquisition of contiguous slices is important in determining the spatial extent of anatomical structures and gray matter lesions such as heterotopias.

Additional MRI manipulations include *cortical reconstruction* and *curvilinear surface images*, which are useful for identifying abnormalities of gyral patterns (Fig. 12–14), and quantitative analyses using *voxel-based morphometry* and *statistical parametric mapping*, which can display areas of cortical thinning and patterns of hippocampal atrophy (Fig. 12–15 see also Figs. 4–23; 5–16; and 7–7). *Diffusion-weighted imaging (DWI)* is used to distinguish *anisotropic diffusion*, in which molecular motion is restricted in tissues with linear arrangement, such as white matter, from *isotropic diffusion*, where molecular motion is not restricted. Whereas DWI is commonly used to identify cerebral ischemia, such as occurs in early cerebrovascular infarcts, and can localize postictal changes after *status epilepticus*,

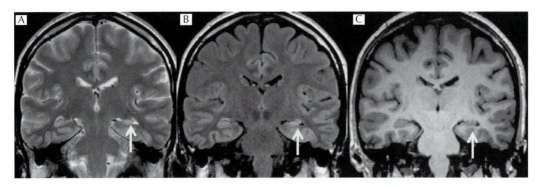

Figure 12–13. Example of same pathology in three different imaging sequences (T2, fluid-attenuated inversion recovery [FLAIR], and T1). **A.** Coronal T2. T2-weighted image shows high signal in the CSF space (i.e., ventricles). Neoplasm, gliosis, and edema stroke, for instance, demonstrate high signal in T2-weighted sequence. Gray matter is higher intensity than white matter. This case shows small left hippocampus and high signal intensity within the hippocampus (*arrow*). **B.** Coronal FLAIR. In FLAIR, the water signal is suppressed; therefore, the CSF space is dark. The lesion (e.g., gliosis) stays hyperintense; therefore, lesions adjacent to the ventricle become more conspicuous. In this case, the hyperintense focus in the left hippocampus is better seen on FLAIR than on T2-weighted image. Normal gray matter signal is higher than that of white matter. **C.** Coronal T1. T1-weighted image shows the CSF signal as dark, and gray matter signal is lower than that of the white matter. T1 images can be used for structural assessment. In this case, left hippocampal atrophy is well demonstrated. (Courtesy of Dr. Noriko Salamon.)

diffusion tensor imaging (DTI) is increasingly used in epilepsy to create detailed images of cerebral white matter tracts (*tractography*) (Fig. 12–16). Epileptogenic gray matter lesions are commonly associated with reduction in associated white matter tracts, and these abnormalities on DTI can help confirm the presence of gray matter abnormalities or point to areas that could be reexamined. *Magnetic resonance arteriography (MRA)* and *venography (MRV)*

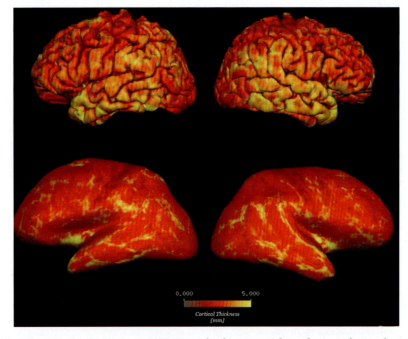

Figure 12–14. Using isometric 1 × 1 × 1-mm MRI T1-weighted images, surface volume rendering of a patient with epilepsy was obtained. *Top:* Right and left hemisphere of the same patient. Gray matter thickness is shown with color-coded scale (from yellow, 5 mm, to gray, 0 mm). *Bottom:* Smooth surface rendering images. No significant area of cortical thinning or thickening is observed in this case. (Courtesy of Dr. Noriko Salamon.)

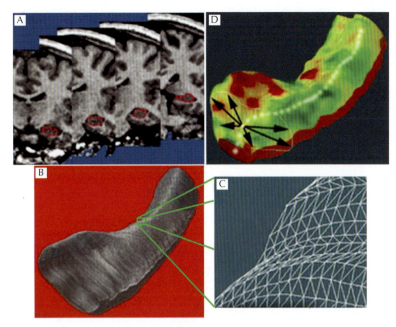

Figure 12–15. Methods for generating three-dimensional hippocampal contour maps. **A.** Outlined hippocampal formation on consecutive coronal MRI scans. **B.** Neuroimaging algorithms convert hippocampal tracing into a lattice-like three-dimensional parametric model (**C**) for each subject that can then be used to generate an averaged surface contour map. **D.** Hippocampal radial size (depicted as *black arrows*) is computed as the distance between each point of intersection on the surface and underlying medial curve that derives from the centers of mass along the length of hippocampus (*white dots* inside the hippocampus). (Figure modified from Thompson et al., 2004 with permission.)

are helpful when vascular abnormalities are suspected. MRA without contrast shows flow voids, while postcontrast MRI reveals both arteries and veins. Although most centers still use 1.5-tesla MRI equipment, many now also have 3-tesla capability. A 3-tesla field provides higher anatomical resolution but also increases susceptibility artifacts and is not necessarily better for identifying lesions commonly associated with epilepsy.

MRI is the structural imaging test of choice for epilepsy and has become the most important

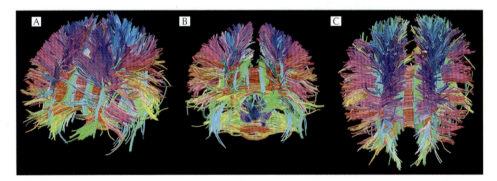

Figure 12–16. DTI fiber tractography. Whole brain fiber tractography can be computed by placing seed regions in a uniform distribution covering the brain—then performing tractography across them. Similarly oriented fibers are similarly colored for easier visualization. It is useful to bear in mind that these reconstructions carry no information about which of these are afferent versus efferent projections; also, the spatial resolution of these tracts is much larger than the size of the individual axons. Mapping of white matter tracts can identify localized aberrant connectivity in epilepsy for diagnosis and research and, in surgical candidates, will help neurosurgeons to avoid postsurgical deficit. (Reproduced with the authors' permission from Thomason ME and Thompson PM (2011). Diffusion Imaging, White Matter and Psychopathology, Annual Review of Clinical Psychology 2011 Apr;7:63–85.)

diagnostic test for patients with medically intractable seizures who are candidates for surgical treatment, although EEG is still required to demonstrate that a structural lesion is epileptogenic (Chapter 16). Sedation is necessary for performing MRI on small children; however, MRI-compatible incubators now make it possible to scan neonates without sedation.

X-RAY COMPUTED TOMOGRAPHY

When MRI is not available, or not possible because of incompatible metallic implants, *X-ray computed tomography (CT)* can reveal a variety of intracerebral pathological processes responsible for epileptic seizures (Adams et al., 1987; Engel and Henry, 1990; Gastaut and Gastaut, 1976). CT is also useful for identifying cerebral calcifications that are not readily visible on MRI (Fig. 12–17); however, subtle calcifications and microhemosiderin deposits are better visualized on MRI using gradient echo sequences. *CT arteriography (CTA)* and *venography (CTV)* display static images, while postcontrast MRA and MRV provide dynamic information and are superior in most situations. As with MRI, anatomical structures involved in status epilepticus can be visualized with

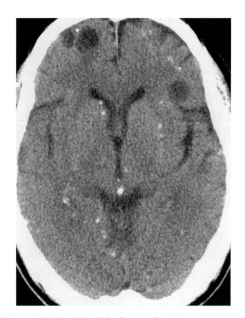

Figure 12–17. CT of the brain of cysticercosis patient shows multiple foci of calcifications in the basal ganglia and subcortical white matter. There are some cysts in the right and left frontal lobes. (Courtesy of Dr. Noriko Salamon.)

perfusion imaging using CT (Gelfand et al., 2010; Hauf et al., 2009).

RADIOGRAPHS

Radiographs of the skull are useful when neither CT nor MRI is available, particularly when bony defects, rather than intraparenchymal lesions, are suspected. Focal seizures can be due to cortical irritation from the skull in conditions such as old depressed skull fractures or *Paget's disease*. The classical patterns of calcification seen in disorders such as Sturge-Weber syndrome and tuberous sclerosis are readily apparent on skull X-rays. Cerebral angiography is generally reserved for preoperative evaluations to better characterize neoplasms, arteriovenous malformations, and aneurysms and to outline important vessels that must be avoided during surgical intervention. *Angiographic stains* have been reported in the area of the epileptogenic lesion when cerebral angiograms are done at the time of a seizure (Lee and Goldberg, 1977), but this observation is not applicable to routine diagnosis.

Functional Neuroimaging

Positron emission tomography (PET) and *single-photon emission computed tomography (SPECT)* are standard diagnostic tests, and *functional magnetic resonance imaging (fMRI)* is rapidly gaining credibility for diagnosis in epilepsy. *Magnetic resonance spectroscopy (MRS)* has more limited clinical application, and *rectilinear radionuclide brain scanning* is rarely of value in epilepsy diagnosis today. Two research tools not discussed here include *optical imaging* of seizure activity (Haglund et al., 2008), which currently has only been clinically applied intraoperatively, and *cellular imaging* (Trevelyan and Yuste, 2008), which remains a basic research tool.

POSITRON EMISSION TOMOGRAPHY

PET produces three-dimensional functional images of the brain (Phelps et al., 1986). The latest generation of PET scanners are approaching 4-mm resolution, capable of identifying structures of great interest in epilepsy, such as the amygdala, hippocampus, and substantia nigra. Various aspects of cerebral function can be measured, depending on the positron-labeled tracer used. A number of positron-labeled biologically active compounds are available, and many others are being developed for study of a great variety of biochemical processes in the brain (Table 12–8). The most commonly used tracers are ^{18}F-*fluorodeoxyglucose (FDG)*, for measuring glucose metabolism; $^{15}O_2$, for measuring oxygen metabolism; and $C^{15}O_2$ and $H_2^{15}O$, for measuring blood flow.

Focal areas of epileptic dysfunction appear interictally on PET scans as zones of hypometabolism and decreased blood flow (Bernardi et al., 1983; Engel, 1985; Engel, 1984b; Engel et al., 1982a;c;d; Theodore et al., 1984; Yamamoto et al., 1983; Henry and Chugani, 2008), whereas areas involved in focal seizure onset and spread appear on ictal PET scans as both increased and decreased metabolism and blood flow, in part as a result of measurements of both ictal and postictal effects (Engel et al., 1982b; Engel et al., 1983; Theodore et al., 1984; Henry and Chugani, 2008). The interictal zone of hypometabolism correlates highly with the site of the epileptogenic region (Engel et al., 1982a;c;d; Henry and Chugani, 2008), but ictal scans show propagation and can be unreliable indicators of the site of ictal onset (Engel et al., 1982b; Engel et al., 1983; Henry and Chugani, 2008).

FDG-PET is now a standard part of the presurgical evaluation for patients with medically refractory epileptic seizures (Henry and Chugani, 2008) (Chapter 16). The yield of positive FDG-PET scans is greater for mesial temporal lobe than for neocortical epileptogenic lesions and remains slightly higher than that of positive MRI scans for mesial temporal lobe lesions and *focal cortical dysplasia* (Knowlton et al., 2008; Lerner et al., 2009; Hogan et al., 2008). Coregistration of FDG-PET with MRI improves the diagnostic yield, particularly for the identification of focal cortical dysplasia (Salamon et al., 2008) (Fig. 12–18).

Many disorders of cerebral structure and function cause zones of hypometabolism and hypoperfusion on PET. This finding alone, therefore, can help in localizing an epileptogenic region but is insufficient for a diagnosis of epilepsy (Engel and Henry, 1990). Demonstration that a zone of decreased function becomes hypermetabolic or hyperperfused during ictus, however, should be pathognomonic for an epileptic condition. Unfortunately, ictal PET scans are difficult to obtain and not practical as routine studies because of the short half-life of positron-emitting isotopes.

FDG-PET also localizes abnormalities in neonatal seizures (Chugani et al., 1990) and focal or lateralized areas of hypometabolism

Table 12–8 Positron-Emitting Radiopharmaceuticals Used in PET Studies of Epilepsy

Function	Radiopharmaceuticals
Glucose metabolism	2-[^{18}F]fluoro-2-deoxyglucose (FDG)
Oxygen metabolism and oxygen extraction ratio	[^{15}O]O_2
Cerebral blood flow	[^{15}O]O_2, [^{15}O]H_2O, [^{15}O]CO_2, [^{13}N]NH_3
Central benzodiazepine receptor distribution	[^{11}C]flumazenil (formerly [^{11}C]RO15-1788)
Muscarinic cholinergic receptor distribution	[^{11}C]N-methyl piperidyl benzilate
Opiate receptor distribution	[^{11}C]carfentanil (μ-receptors)
	[^{18}F]cyclofoxy (μ-*lk*-receptors)
	[^{11}C]Diprenorphine (μ-*lk*-1δ-receptors)
Serotonin synthesis	[^{11}C]α-methyl-tryptophan
Serotonin 1A receptor distribution	[^{11}C]WAY100635, [^{18}F]FCWAY, [^{18}F]MPPF
Drug distribution	[^{11}C]phenytoin
	[^{11}C]valproic acid
Monoamine oxidase B distribution	[^{11}C]deuterium-deprenyl

[^{11}C]WAY100635 = [O-*methyl*-^{11}C]N-(2(4(2-methoxyphenyl)-1-piperazinyl)ethyl)N-(2-piridinyl)cyclohexanecarboxamide trihydrochloride; [^{18}F]FCWAY = [^{18}F]*trans*-4-fluoro-N-2[4-(2-methoxyphenyl)piperazin-1-yl)ethyl]-*N*-(2-pyridyl) cyclohexanecarboxamide; [^{18}F]MPPF = 2'-methoxyphenyl-(N-2'-pyridinyl)-*p*-[^{18}F]fluoro-benzamidoethylpiperazine. Adapted from Henry and Chugani, 2008, with permission.

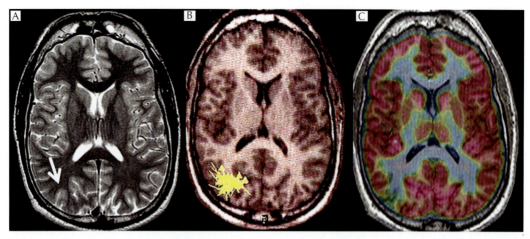

Figure 12–18. Occipital focal cortical dysplasia Type IIa, which would be easily missed on MRI without PET fusion. MEG confirmed the location. **A.** Axial T2-weighted image shows very subtle gray matter thickening at the depth of the right occipital sulcus (*arrow*). **B.** MEG demonstrates cluster of spikes in the right occipital region, corresponding to the thickened gray matter. **C.** FDG-PET and MRI coregistration image demonstrates hypometabolism (*green*) in the right occipital lesion. The patient had surgery, and the pathology showed cortical dysplasia Type IIA. (Courtesy of Dr. Noriko Salamon.)

in infants and young children with *infantile spasms* and other severe seizure disorders (Chugani and Engel, 1986; Chugani et al., 1987; Engel et al., 1982b). FDG-PET, therefore, became important in identifying diffuse lateralized epileptogenic lesions that were not seen on earlier MRIs in children who had apparent generalized seizures but were candidates for hemispherectomy and large multilobar resections (Chugani et al., 1990; 1988). In most cases, the epileptogenic lesions were MCDs, which are now for the most part visible on high-resolution MRI.

FDG-PET has also been used in studying patients with absence seizures and could be useful in differentiating typical childhood absences from atypical absence conditions associated with generalized spike-and-wave discharges. The former demonstrate marked diffuse ictal hypermetabolism (Engel et al., 1985b), whereas the latter may not (Ochs et al., 1987; Theodore et al., 1985).

Other PET tracers have been used for epilepsy. The most common is ^{11}C-*flumazenil*, which measures reduced *benzodiazepine* receptor binding in the epileptogenic region (Savic et al., 1988). Uptake of ^{11}C-*carfentanil*, a μ-opiate receptor ligand, is increased in lateral temporal cortex of patients with temporal lobe epilepsy (Frost et al., 1988), an observation that may have relevance to mechanisms of interictal behavioral disturbances in epilepsy

(Engel et al., 1986) (Chapter 11). ^{11}C-α-*methyl-tryptophan (AMT)* concentrates in the epileptogenic tubers of patients with tuberous sclerosis who have epileptic seizures and multiple tubers on MRI (Chugani et al., 1998; Kagawa et al., 2005; Chugani, 2011; Kumar et al., 2011), and there is evidence that this ligand might identify epileptogenic tissue in other epilepsies as well (Natsume et al., 2003) (Fig. 12–19).

Other potential uses for PET in epilepsy may come from pharmacological studies. PET can detect global hypometabolism during treatment with *phenobarbital* (Theodore et al., 1986a) and *phenytoin* (Theodore et al., 1986b) and could provide a means of assessing toxic effects of drugs. Studies of in vivo cerebral pharmacokinetics are theoretically possible with positron-labeled antiseizure drugs (Baron et al., 1983; Ramsay, 1983).

SINGLE-PHOTON EMISSION COMPUTED TOMOGRAPHY

SPECT uses tracers labeled with single-photon-emitting isotopes to produce images of cerebral function (Bonte et al., 1983; Kuhl et al., 1982; Lee et al., 1987; Lee et al., 1986; Lee et al., 1988; Sanabria et al., 1983; Kazemi et al., 2008) that are similar to those of PET. The major advantage of SPECT over PET derives from the fact that single-photon-emitting isotopes have

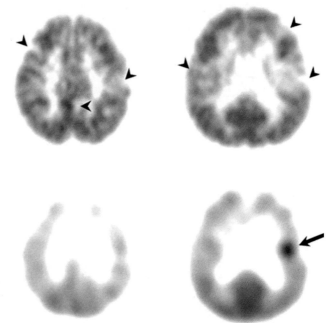

Figure 12–19 Interictal 2-deoxy-2[^{18}F] fluoro-D-glucose ([^{18}F]FDG) PET and [^{11}C]α-methyl-tryptophan ([^{11}C]AMT) PET images of a patient with tuberous sclerosis. These transaxially oriented images show multiple foci of glucose hypometabolism (*arrowheads*) and a single site of increased [^{11}C]AMT activity (*arrow*) in a patient with refractory seizures. The image planes are coregistered at higher (*left*) and lower levels (*right*). Resection of cortex at the site of increased AMT uptake resulted in improved seizure control. (From Henry and Chugani, 2008, with permission.)

relatively long half-lives and an on-site medical cyclotron is unnecessary. SPECT tracers can be purchased commercially. The disadvantages of SPECT, however, are a much decreased resolution of the image, a higher radiation exposure for the patient, and only a few opportunities for incorporation of available isotopes into biologically active compounds (Engel and Henry, 1990; Kazemi et al., 2008). SPECT is used principally to measure cerebral blood flow, blood volume, and blood-brain barrier permeability. The two most commonly used tracers are *(99m)Tc-hexamethylpropyleneamine oxime (HM-PAO)* and *(99m)Tc-ethylcysteinate dimer (ECD)* to measure blood flow. Interictal blood flow studies with SPECT in patients with focal epilepsy are less reliable than interictal studies with FDG-PET; however, because SPECT tracers can be easily prepared at the bedside, this technique is well suited for ictal studies. Focal hyperperfusion occurs when tracer is injected during and at variable intervals after focal seizures, even if they secondarily generalize (Lee et al., 1986; Lee et al., 1988). The epileptogenic region is identified by subtracting the ictal SPECT scan from the interictal scan; the accuracy of this technique has been improved by coregistration with MRI, a method referred to as *subtraction ictal*

SPECT with coregistration on MRI (SISCOM) (O'Brien et al., 1998) (Fig. 12–20). SPECT, therefore, can help in identifying focal brain pathology as well as in locating the epileptogenic lesion when resective surgical therapy is being considered.

FUNCTIONAL MAGNETIC RESONANCE IMAGING

Blood oxygenation level–dependent (BOLD) fMRI takes advantage of the fact that oxyhemoglobin is paramagnetic, while deoxyhemoglobin is diamagnetic. Neuronal activity in the brain increases capillary perfusion, resulting in a localized increase in oxygenated hemoglobin, which produces an increased MRI signal. The changes are small, on the order of 1–2%, but by averaging repeated acquisitions, and subtracting baseline from experimental conditions, patterns of blood flow can be detected that identify the anatomical substrates of specific cerebral functions (Krakow et al., 1999; Goldman et al., 2002; Cohen and Bookheimer, 2008). Functional MRI is useful for mapping cortical function in patients with epilepsy who are candidates for surgical treatment. It is particularly useful for localizing motor and sensory cortices and lateralizing language functions;

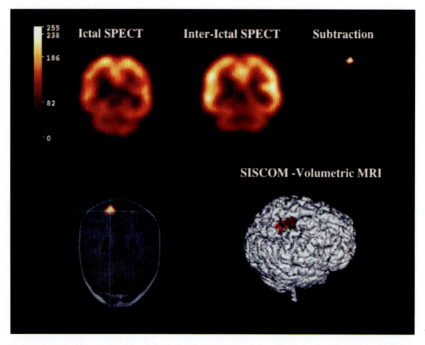

Figure 12–20 Steps to obtaining subtraction ictal SPECT coregistered to MRI (SISCOM) image. Ictal (*upper left*) and interictal (*upper middle*) SPECT images are obtained. After normalization of their mean intensities and coregistration with each other, subtraction is performed to obtain a "difference" image (*upper right*). The difference image is then coregistered with MRI at specific planes (*lower left*) or on the surface of a three-dimensional MRI (*lower right*). (From So, 2002, with permission.)

however, results of fMRI memory testing have not yet been sufficiently validated to warrant replacing the *intracarotid amobarbital procedure (IAP)* (Cohen and Bookheimer, 2008) (see below).

A more direct application of fMRI to research and clinical diagnosis in epilepsy is the recent development of *simultaneous EEG and fMRI (SEM)* techniques. The challenge posed by reciprocal artifacts that occur when these two techniques are combined has now been overcome. Analysis employs a statistical comparison of periods with and without either interictal or ictal epileptiform EEG activity and creates images depicting the neuronal substrates responsible for generating these epileptiform events (Lemieux et al., 2001; Gotman et al., 2006; Gotman and Pittau, 2011) (Fig. 12–21). When seizures occur in the magnet, SEM can identify the site of onset and propagation of epileptic discharge (Fig. 12–22). Although this remains a research application, the field is moving rapidly, and SEM has a tremendous potential for delineating epileptogenic brain

tissue by identifying sites of interictal EEG spike origin and propagation as well as their relationships to sites of ictal onset. A goal of SEM would be to distinguish between interictal EEG spikes that are generated by, and thus localize, the epileptogenic region and those that are either propagated by, or originate in, areas that are not capable of generating spontaneous seizures. Given that interictal EEG spikes that localize the epileptogenic region are preferentially associated with *pathological high-frequency oscillations (pHFOs)* (Chapter 4), it is likely that these events reflect unique neuronal events with metabolic signatures that could be identified with fMRI.

Functional MRI carried out on normal subjects in the resting state (i.e., without behavioral or stimulation paradigms) have demonstrated a characteristic pattern of connectivity involving frontal, parietal, and temporal lobe structures, referred to as the *default mode network (DMN)* (Smith et al., 2009) (Chapter 3). The DMN may be identified with either *independent component analysis (ICA)* or seed-based (*region of*

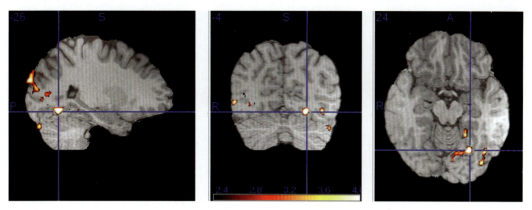

Figure 12–21. Functional MRI of occipital lobe interictal epileptiform discharges mapped onto structural MRI. Analysis included a combination of six O_1 spikes and was thresholded at Z > 2. The center of the identified region colocalizes with a malformation of cortical development. (From Stern et al., 2010, with permission.)

interest) analysis. ICA produces collections of anatomical regions that have shared characteristics in spontaneous fMRI signal fluctuation. Seed-based analysis identifies which regions have fMRI signal that shares characteristics with a selected region, so it identifies a network using a region within the network. Whereas seed-based analysis requires some preliminary working hypothesis, ICA does not. The DMN is of considerable interest to neuroscientists concerned with understanding neuronal network connectivity during behavior, and there is increasing evidence that these networks are disrupted in characteristic ways in patients with both focal onset and generalized onset seizures (Meador, 2011) (Fig. 12–23). Not only may such studies be useful for lateralizing and localizing epileptogenic abnormalities in patients with epilepsy who are surgical candidates, but they may also identify specific disturbances in

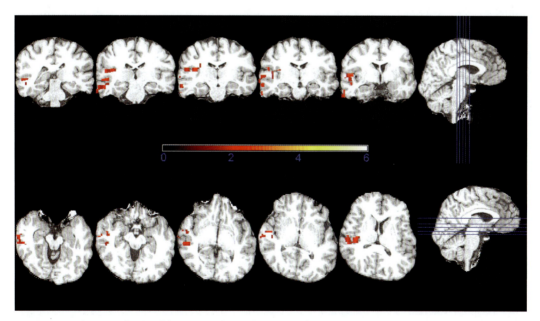

Figure 12–22. Functional MRI of first 10 sec after ictal onset based on EEG. The patient had musicogenic dyscognitive focal seizures and experienced a habitual seizure during fMRI when stimulated with music. A tailored anterior temporal lobe resection produced seizure freedom. (From Stern et al., 2006, with permission.)

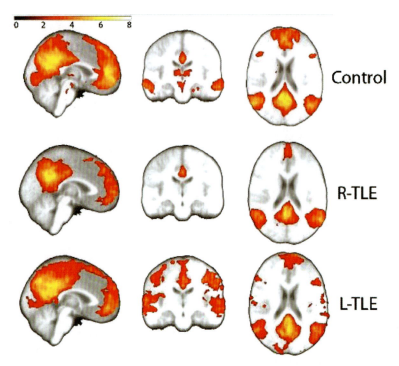

Figure 12–23. Resting-state fMRI depicting default mode network (DMN) for three subject groups. Region-of-interest analysis used a seed in posterior medial cortex. DMN from control group of 13 subjects demonstrates greater frontal connectivity than is seen in either 11 subjects with right temporal lobe epilepsy (TLE) or 12 subjects with left TLE. (From Haneef et al., 2012, with permission.)

neuronal network connectivity that underlie interictal behavioral disturbances associated with epilepsy, information that could be useful for diagnosis, treatment, and prevention of these disabling disorders.

MAGNETIC RESONANCE SPECTROSCOPY

MRS measures minute-to-minute changes in phosphorous compounds in the brain and allows functional information to be derived about dynamic changes in cerebral energy metabolism and pH (Petroff and Duncan, 2008). Initial MRS studies on patients with epilepsy identified low levels of N-*acetyl-aspartate (NAA)* and *phosphocreatine (PCr)*, which could be used to lateralize the epileptogenic hemisphere (Petroff et al., 1984; 1986). With the development of *multivoxel MRS*, which can sample multiple bilateral areas and can be tailored to specific anatomical structures, such as the hippocampus, localized interictal metabolic disturbances can be identified, providing

useful information in patients who are candidates for surgical treatment (Chapter 16). High-field (3 tesla and greater) spectrometers now permit measurements of *glutamate, glutamine, GABA, homocarnosine, glutathione,* and N-*acetyl-aspartylglutamate*, which could provide additional information for diagnosis of, and research on, patients with epilepsy during the interictal and postictal periods (Petroff and Duncan, 2008). Although MRS is no longer considered purely a research tool, the importance of its role in the diagnosis of epilepsy remains to be established.

RECTILINEAR RADIONUCLIDE BRAIN SCANNING

Rectilinear radionuclide brain scanning has been supplanted, for the most part, by CT and MRI in the diagnosis of structural epileptogenic lesions, but there are situations in which this test may provide additional useful functional information. These scans are likely to reveal focal disturbance of the blood-brain barrier in areas of infection, vascular compromise, and trauma that can give rise to epileptic seizures. They can also occasionally identify localized increases in blood flow and blood-brain barrier permeability following focal seizures (Prensky et al., 1973). Rectilinear radionuclide brain scanning offers no advantages, however, over SPECT and PET.

PSYCHOLOGICAL EVALUATION

Psychometric testing is of particular value in assessing attention, performance and verbal IQ, memory, language, executive function, and personality (Filskov and Boll, 1981; Rausch, 1987; Loring et al., 2008; Rankin and Vargha-Khadem, 2008; Wilson and Engel, 2010; Jones-Gotman et al., 2010). These tests can yield important information about the nature and location of a focal functional disturbance, particularly for presurgical evaluation (Chapter 16), and serial studies can document deterioration in progressive disorders or evaluate the effects of therapeutic intervention. Many test batteries are used, and there is no standardized protocol. Table 12–9 lists the neurocognitive domains that are usually evaluated and some of the tests that are commonly used, especially for patients who are candidates for surgical treatment of epilepsy.

In addition, psychometric testing of patients with epilepsy and impaired mental function is essential for determining realistic goals and instituting special programs for education and vocational training (Chapter 17). Psychologists can also provide services that are useful for characterizing a patient's particular problems and for planning means of dealing with them. These may involve specific tests of personality, mood, or psychosocial adaptation and could suggest the need for formal counseling or psychiatric intervention (Chapter 11).

The *intracarotid amobarbital procedure (IAP)*, or *Wada test* (Wada, 1949; Wada and Rasmussen, 1960) was initially introduced to identify the language-dominant hemisphere. This test was subsequently modified for use in assessing memory function independently in both hemispheres to assure that removal of one mesial temporal lobe would not result in global amnesia (Klove et al., 1969; Milner et al., 1962). Memory disturbance with injection of amobarbital into one carotid artery can also be considered evidence for focal dysfunction of contralateral mesial temporal structures (Engel et al., 1981; Sirven at al., 1997). Despite the inconsistency of techniques used and controversies over interpretation of results (Rausch, 1987; Jones-Gotman et al., 2008), the use of the IAP to evaluate memory function is an essential part of the diagnostic armamentarium at most centers performing mesial temporal lobe resections for epilepsy. There is considerable variation from center to center, however, regarding which patients require an IAP and when bilateral IAPs are necessary. *Topiramate* and *zonisamide* can antagonize the

Table 12–9 **Neurological Tests for Use in Evaluating Patients with Epilepsy**

Domain	Common Tests
Visual attention	Trail Making Test, parts A & B (TMT)
Auditory attention	WAIS-IV or WISC-IV Digit Span
Motor speed/dexterity	Grooved Pegboard
General verbal ability	WAIS-IV or WISC-IV Vocabulary
General visuospatial ability	WAIS-IV or WISC-IV Block Design
Verbal memory	Rey Auditory Verbal Learning Test (RAVLT), WMS-IV: Logical Memory (immediate and delayed), Paired Associate Learning (immediate and delayed)
Visuospatial memory	Brief Visuospatial Memory Test—Revised (BVMT-R), WMS-IV Visual Reproduction
Word retrieval	Boston Naming Test (60 item) (BNT)
	Controlled Oral Word Association Test (COWAT)
Executive function	Wisconsin Card Sorting Test, Delis-Kaplan Executive Function Test

WAIS = Wechsler Adult Intelligence Scale; WISC = Wechsler Intelligence Scale for Children; WMS = Wechsler Memory Scale.
Courtesy of Dr. Susan Bookheimer

effect of amobarbital and should be discontinued several weeks before an IAP (Bookheimer et al., 2005). Because of intermittent shortages of amobarbital and the fact that this drug is not available in some countries, other drugs have been proposed, including *methohexital* and *propofol*, but perhaps the most promising alternative technique is the *etomidate speech and memory test (eSAM)*, because the level of anesthesia can be maintained with infusion for as long as is necessary to complete testing (Jones-Gotman et al., 2005).

BIOMARKERS

Biomarkers are biological changes that indicate the presence and severity of a disease process, such as *blood sugar levels* for *diabetes* and *prostate-specific antigen (PSA)* for *prostate cancer* (Engel, 2011a;b). Biomarkers are more specific than *risk factors* (Chapter 2). *Surrogate markers* are also measures of a disease process and are often used as *outcome measures*, but are not necessarily biological. As the name implies, surrogate markers substitute for more important clinical outcomes. Biomarkers can be surrogate markers; for instance, biomarkers of epilepsy could substitute for epileptic seizures to facilitate clinical trials of antiseizure or antiepileptogenic interventions. There currently are no reliable surrogate epilepsy biomarkers, but this is an area of intensive basic research (Engel, 2011a;b).

Epilepsy is a chronic disorder resulting from an enduring epileptogenic abnormality of the brain, and the primary biomarker of this disorder is the occurrence of epileptic seizures. Epileptic seizures, however, are transient and occur intermittently; there are no reliable biomarkers of *epileptogenesis* (the development of an epilepsy condition before seizures begin) or of *epileptogenicity* (the presence or severity of an epilepsy condition during the interictal state). Interictal EEG spikes are helpful, but neither their presence nor their absence is sufficient for ruling an epilepsy condition in or out (Chapter 13); their frequency does not correlate with severity of the epilepsy disorder, except for genetic absence epilepsies, and they don't accurately delineate the epileptogenic region for surgery (Chapter 16). Interictal neuroimaging can identify structural and functional abnormalities but does not determine whether they are epileptogenic.

A reliable biomarker of epileptogenesis that could identify which patients are developing epilepsy following an epileptogenic insult would be important for devising and testing antiepileptogenic interventions and for applying them once they become available. A reliable biomarker of epileptogenicity would permit diagnosis of epilepsy after a single seizure, so that treatment could be instituted before a second seizure. A reliable biomarker of epileptogenicity that measured the severity of an epilepsy condition could be used to assess the efficacy of antiseizure treatment without the need to wait for another seizure. In both situations, considerable risk of morbidity and mortality associated with another seizure might be avoided. A reliable biomarker of epileptogenicity that identified progressive and pharmacoresistant epilepsy conditions would permit early referral for surgical treatment, and a biomarker that reliably localized epileptogenic brain tissue might obviate the need for expensive and invasive presurgical evaluation.

Several possible epilepsy biomarkers are under investigation, and others might evolve from research into fundamental mechanisms of epileptogenesis and ictogenesis (Engel, 2011a;b). The most promising to date is 80- to 600-Hz EEG pHFOs (Chapter 4), which, when recorded directly from the brain, appear to localize epileptogenic tissue in experimental animals and in patients (Staba and Bragin, 2011; Worrell and Gotman, 2011). These pHFOs may also predict the development of epilepsy following an epileptogenic insult (Chapter 4). When recorded with stereotactically implanted depth electrodes or subdural grids, pHFOs will likely be useful for delineating the epileptogenic region for surgical treatment. Recent studies indicate that some HFOs can be identified with scalp EEG (Andrade-Valenca et al., 2011); however, it is not certain whether these are the same as epileptiform pHFOs recorded intracranially. If so, these transients might be excellent candidates for much wider application as biomarkers of epileptogenesis and epileptogenicity. Further studies with AMT-PET may identify situations when this tracer can act as a reliable biomarker (Chugani, 2011; Kumar et al., 2011). There is evidence that signal changes in hippocampus revealed by MRI following prolonged febrile seizures identifies children who will subsequently experience spontaneous seizures (Gomes and Shinnar, 2011) and that similar MRI findings might become reliable biomarkers of epileptogenesis. The many molecular mechanisms involved in the early stages of epileptogenesis, in particular activation of inflammatory systems (Chapter 4) and alterations in gene expression, could ultimately serve as biomarkers for epileptogenesis, epileptogenicity, or both (Vezzani and Friedman, 2011; Pitkänen and Lukasiuk, 2011). These might be measured in the brain with specific PET tracers or perhaps even identified in peripheral blood; for instance, specific gene expression profiles derived from white blood cells could indicate an epileptogenic process.

SUMMARY AND CONCLUSIONS

Diagnosis of the patient with suspected epilepsy is directed at five aspects of the problem: (1) the existence of an epileptic condition, (2) a treatable underlying cause, if present, (3) the seizure type(s), (4) the epilepsy syndrome, if present, and (5) the psychosocial predicament. Most diagnoses of epilepsy are made by history, and it is often essential that the interview include a close relative or friend who has witnessed ictal events. The history should always include complete descriptions of habitual seizures, possible predisposing factors, epilepsy and other neurological disorders among family members, and psychosocial factors that contribute to the patient's disability.

A general physical examination and routine laboratory studies are useful when systemic diseases are responsible for the seizure disorder. A neurological examination is most helpful in eliciting focal features that suggest a localized, rather than generalized, underlying cause. Lumbar puncture is not necessary unless the expected results would clearly alter management or provide new information about prognosis.

The most important diagnostic laboratory test remains the EEG, which can often establish the existence of an epilepsy condition, distinguish between focal and generalized epileptic abnormalities, and reveal patterns characteristic of specific epileptic seizures and epilepsy syndromes. The most common cause of an unwarranted diagnosis of epilepsy, however, is overinterpretation of the EEG. Epilepsy is a clinical, not an EEG, diagnosis, and EEGs should be read by specialists familiar with normal transients that might be mistaken for epileptiform phenomena. An initial routine EEG is recommended for all patients with suspected epilepsy for diagnostic purposes and also to provide baseline information in the event that progression occurs. Repeat EEGs are not necessary, however, unless findings would alter management or result in a reevaluation of prognosis.

An MRI scan is appropriate for all adults presenting with a recent onset of seizures, to identify structural lesions that might require specific treatment. CT can be useful when a disorder associated with intracranial calcification is suspected. Structural imaging can be avoided in some children (up to late adolescence) when the history and other examinations indicate a genetic epilepsy disorder or a nonprogressive lesion.

Psychometric testing can identify focal or diffuse disturbances of cerebral function that can be of diagnostic value, may be useful for documenting deterioration or beneficial effects of therapy, and may yield information essential for planning realistic goals and instituting special programs. Psychological evaluation may also suggest the need for formal counseling or psychiatric intervention.

If clinical doubt persists concerning the nature of the condition, the patient should be referred to an epilepsy center where epileptologists have specialized expertise in diagnosis. It may be necessary to use inpatient VEM or outpatient ambulatory recording. Both are useful for documentation and quantification of ictal events, but inpatient VEM is more appropriate for diagnosis of seizure type and pseudoseizures. Only inpatient VEM can be used for localizing an epileptogenic zone for surgical resection.

Additional electrophysiological procedures, sensory testing, and PET or SPECT are indicated for specific conditions and are most useful for evaluation of candidates for surgical treatment. MEG, fMRI, and MRS can also be helpful in localizing an epileptogenic region when surgery is an option.

Research on diagnosis in epilepsy has focused primarily on improving identification of a treatable underlying cause and defining epileptic seizure types and epilepsy syndromes that have prognostic and therapeutic implications. There is now a great need for reliable biomarkers of epileptogenesis and epileptogenicity to identify patients at risk for developing epilepsy, identify and validate antiepileptogenic interventions, diagnose the presence of epilepsy, assess the effectiveness of antiseizure treatments, and localize the epileptogenic region for surgery.

As diagnosis in epilepsy moves from history, physical examination, and paper-and-pencil psychometric testing to the sophisticated technologies of computerized EEG, MRI, and PET, it is necessary to evaluate the relative contributions of these new tests to patient management. Diagnostic procedures that increase the cost of medical care or compromise patients' convenience and safety are justified only if new, otherwise unobtainable information leads to an improved quality of life.

REFERENCES

Adams, CBT, Anslow, P, Molyneux, A, and Oxbury, J (1987). Radiological detection of surgically treatable pathology. In Surgical Treatment of the Epilepsies. Edited by J Engel, Jr. New York: Raven Press, pp. 213–234.

Aicardi, J, and Taylor, DC (2008). History and physical examination. In Epilepsy: A Comprehensive Textbook, 2nd ed. Edited by J Engel, Jr, and TA Pedley. Philadelphia: Lippincott Williams & Wilkins, pp. 785–789.

Ajmone-Marsan, C, and Zivin, LS (1970). Factors related to the occurrence of typical paroxysmal abnormalities in the EEG records of epileptic patients. Epilepsia 11:361–381.

American Clinical Neurophysiology Society (2008). Guideline 12: Guidelines for long-term monitoring for epilepsy. J Clin Neurophysiol 25:170–180.

Andrade-Valenca, LP, Dubeau, F, Mari, F, Zelmann, R, and Gotman, J (2011). Interictal scalp fast oscillations as a marker of the seizure onset zone. Neurology 77:524–531.

Badawy, RAB, Macdonell, RAL, Berkovic, SF, Newton, MR, and Jackson, GD (2010). Predicting seizure control: Cortical excitability and antiepileptic medication. Ann Neurol 67:64–73.

Bagic, AI, Barkley, GL, Rose, DF, and Ebersole, JS, for the ACMEGS Clinical Practice Guideline (CPG) Committee (2011a). American Clinical Magnetoencephalography Society Clinical Practice Guideline 4: Qualifications of MEG-EEG Personnel. J Clin Neurophysiol 28:364–365.

Bagic, AI, Knowlton, RC, Rose, DF, and Ebersole, JS, for the ACMEGS Clinical Practice Guideline (CPG) Committee (2011b). American Clinical Magnetoencephalography Society Clinical Practice Guideline 1: Recording and Analysis of Spontaneous Cerebral Activity. J Clin Neurophysiol 28:348–354.

Bagic, AI, Knowlton, RC, Rose, DF, and Ebersole, JS, for the ACMEGS Clinical Practice Guideline (CPG) Committee (2011c). American Clinical Magnetoencephalography Society Clinical Practice Guideline 3: MEG-EEG Reporting. J Clin Neurophysiol 28:362–363.

Baron, JC, Roeda, D, Munari, C, Crouzel, C, Chodkiewicz, JP, and Comar, D (1983). Brain regional pharmacokinetics of (11)C-labeled diphenylhydantoin: Positron emission tomography in humans. Neurology 33:580–585.

Barth, DS, Sutherling, W, Engel, J, Jr, and Beatty, J (1982). Neuromagnetic localization of epileptiform spike activity in the human brain. Science 218:891–894.

Barth, DS, Sutherling, W, and Beatty, J (1984a). Fast and slow magnetic phenomena in focal epileptic seizures. Science 226:855–857.

Barth, DS, Sutherling, W, Engel, J, Jr, and Beatty, J (1984b). Neuromagnetic evidence of spatially distributed sources underlying epileptiform spikes in the human brain. Science 223:293–296.

Bergey, GK, and Nordli, DR, Jr (2008). The epilepsy monitoring unit. In Epilepsy: A Comprehensive Textbook, 2nd ed. Edited by J Engel, Jr, and TA Pedley. Philadelphia: Lippincott Williams & Wilkins, pp. 1085–1090.

Bernardi, S, Trimble, MR, Frackowiak, RSJ, Wise, RJS, and Jones, T (1983). An interictal study of partial epilepsy using positron emission tomography and the oxygen-15 inhalation technique. J Neurol Neurosurg Psychiatry 46:473–477.

Bonte, FJ, Stokely, EM, Devous, MD, Sr, and Homan, RW (1983). Single-photon tomographic study of regional cerebral blood flow in epilepsy: A preliminary report. Arch Neurol 40:267–270.

Bookheimer, S, Schrader, LM, Rausch, R, Sankar, R and Engel, J, Jr (2005). Reduced anesthetization during the intracarotid amobarbital (Wada) test in patients taking carbonic anhydrase-inhibiting medications. Epilepsia 46:236–243.

Bragin, A, and Engel, J, Jr (2008). Is prediction of the time of a seizure onset the only value of seizure-prediction studies? In Seizure Prediction in Epilepsy: From Basic Mechanisms to Clinical Applications. Edited by B Schelter, J Timmer, and A Schulze-Bonhage. Berlin: Wiley-VCH, pp. 163–168.

Brazier, MAB, Crandall, PH, and Walsh, GO (1976). Enhancement of EEG lateralizing signs in temporal lobe epilepsy: A trial of diazepam. Exp Neurol 51:241–258.

Broughton, R (1982). Polygraphic recordings of sleep and sleep disorders. In Electroencephalography: Basic Principles, Clinical Applications and Related Fields. Edited by E Niedermeyer and F Lopes da Silva. Baltimore: Urban and Schwarzenberg, pp. 571–598.

Broughton, R, Meier-Ewert, KH, and Ebe, M (1969). Evoked visual, somatosensory and retinal potentials in photosensitive epilepsy. Electroencephalogr Clin Neurophysiol 27:373–386.

Burgess, RC, Funke, ME, Bowyer, SM, Lewine, JD, Kirsch, HE, and Bagic, AI, for the ACMEGS Clinical Practice Guideline (CPG) Committee (2011). American Clinical Magnetoencephalography Society Clinical Practice Guideline 2: Presurgical Functional

Brain Mapping Using Magnetic Evoked Fields. J Clin Neurophysiol 28:355–361.

Cavazzuti, GB, Capella, L, and Nalin, A (1980). Longitudinal study of epileptiform EEG patterns in normal children. Epilepsia, 21:43–55.

Chugani, DC (2011). α-Methyl-L-tryptophan: Mechanisms for tracer localization of epileptogenic brain regions. Biomark Med 5:567–575.

Chugani, DC, Chugani, HT, Muzik, O, Shah, JR, Shah, AK, Canady, A, Mangner, TJ, and Chakraborty, PK (1998). Imaging epileptogenic tubers in children with tuberous sclerosis complex using alpha-[11C] methyl-L-tryptophan positron emission tomography. Ann Neurol 44:858–866.

Chugani, HT, and Engel, J, Jr (1986). PET in intractable epilepsy. In Workshop on Intractable Epilepsy: Experimental and Clinical Aspects. Edited by PL Morselli and D Schmidt. New York: Raven Press, pp. 119–128.

Chugani, HT, Mazziotta, JC, Engel, J, Jr, and Phelps, ME (1987). The Lennox-Gastaut syndrome: Metabolic subtypes determined by 2-deoxy-2[(18)F]fluoro-D-glucose positron emission tomography. Ann Neurol 21:4–13.

Chugani, HT, Shewmon, DA, Peacock, WJ, Shields, WD, Mazziotta, JC, and Phelps, ME (1988). Surgical treatment of intractable neonatal seizures: The role of positron emission tomography. Neurology 38:1178–1188.

Chugani, HT, Phelps, ME, Shewmon, DA, and Barnes, D (1990). Cerebral glucose utilization in intractable neonatal seizure in the developing brain. In Neonatal Seizures: Pathophysiology and Pharmacologic Management. Edited by P Vert and CG Wasterlain. New York: Raven Press, pp. 171–181.

Cohen, MS, Bookheimer, SY (2008). Functional magnetic resonance imaging. In Epilepsy: A Comprehensive Textbook, 2nd ed. Edited by J Engel, Jr, and TA Pedley. Philadelphia: Lippincott Williams & Wilkins, pp. 989–998.

Cooper, R, Osselton, JW, and Shaw, JC (1980). EEG Technology, 3rd ed. London: Butterworths.

Coutin-Churchman, P, Chen, LLK, Wu, JY, Shattuck, K, Dewar, S, Nuwer, MR (2012). Quantification and localization of EEG interictal spike activity in patients with surgically removed epileptogenic foci. Clin Neurophysiol123:471–485.

Darcey, TM, and Williamson, PD (1985). Spatio-temporal EEG measures and their application to human intracranially recorded epileptic seizures. Electroencephalogr Clin Neurophysiol 61:573–587.

Duffy, FH (1986). Topographic Mapping of Brain Electrical Activity. Boston: Butterworths.

Ebersole, JS (1987). Ambulatory EEG: Telemetered and cassette-recorded. Adv Neurol 46:139–155.

Ebersole, JS, and Ebersole, SM (2010). Combining MEG and EEG source modeling in epilepsy evaluations. J Clin Neurophysiol 27:360–371.

Ebersole, JS, and Leroy, RF (1983a). An evaluation of ambulatory, cassette EEG monitoring. II. Detection of interictal abnormalities. Neurology 33:8–18.

Ebersole, JS, and Leroy, RF (1983b). An evaluation of ambulatory cassette EEG monitoring. III. Diagnostic accuracy compared to intensive inpatient EEG monitoring. Neurology 33:853–860.

Ebersole, JS, and Pedley, TA (eds) (2003). Current Practice of Clinical Electroencephalography, 3rd ed. Philadelphia: Lippincott Williams & Wilkins.

Ebersole, JS, Stefan, H, and Baumgartner, C (2008). Electroencephalographic and magnetoencephalographic source modeling. In Epilepsy: A Comprehensive Textbook, 2nd ed. Edited by J Engel, Jr, and TA Pedley. Philadelphia: Lippincott Williams & Wilkins, pp. 895–916.

Eliashiv, DS, Elsas, SM, Squires, K, Fried, I, and Engel, J, Jr (2002). Ictal magnetic source imaging as a localizing tool in partial epilepsy. Neurology 59:1600–1610.

Ellingson, RJ, Wilken, K, and Bennett, DR (1984). Efficacy of sleep deprivation as an activation procedure in epileptic patients. J Clin Neurophysiol 1:83–101.

Elmslie, F (2008). Genetic counseling. In Epilepsy: A Comprehensive Textbook, 2nd ed. Edited by J Engel, Jr, and TA Pedley. Philadelphia: Lippincott Williams & Wilkins, pp. 211–215.

Engel, J, Jr (1984a). A practical guide for routine EEG studies in epilepsy. J Clin Neurophysiol 1:109–142.

Engel, J, Jr (1984b). The use of positron emission tomographic scanning in epilepsy. Ann Neurol 15(suppl 1):S180–S191.

Engel, J, Jr (1985). Positron emission tomography (PET) in the diagnosis of epilepsy. In The Epilepsies. Edited by RJ Porter and PL Morselli. London: Butterworths, pp. 242–266.

Engel, J, Jr (ed) (2011a). Biomarkers in epilepsy. Biomark Med 5:529–664.

Engel, J, Jr (2011b). Biomarkers in epilepsy—Introduction. Biomark Med5:537–544.

Engel, J, Jr, and Henry, TR (1990). Neuroimaging and EEG. In EEG Handbook, Vol 4. Edited by JA Wada and RJ Ellingson. Amsterdam: Elsevier, pp. 207–234.

Engel, J, Jr, Driver, MV, and Falconer, MA (1975). Electrophysiological correlates of pathology and surgical results in temporal lobe epilepsy. Brain 98:129–156.

Engel, J, Jr, Rausch, R, Lieb, JP, Kuhl, DE, and Crandall, PH (1981). Correlation of criteria used for localizing epileptic foci in patients considered for surgical therapy of epilepsy. Ann Neurol 9:215–224.

Engel, J, Jr, Brown, WJ, Kuhl, DE, Phelps, ME, Mazziotta, JC, and Crandall, PH (1982a). Pathological findings underlying focal temporal lobe hypometabolism in partial epilepsy. Ann Neurol 12:518–528.

Engel, J, Jr, Kuhl, DE, and Phelps, ME (1982b). Patterns of human local cerebral glucose metabolism during epileptic seizures. Science 218:64–66.

Engel, J, Jr, Kuhl, DE, Phelps, ME, and Crandall, PH (1982c). Comparative localization of epileptic foci in partial epilepsy by PCT and EEG. Ann Neurol 12:529–537.

Engel, J, Jr, Kuhl, DE, Phelps, ME, and Mazziotta, JC (1982d). Interictal cerebral glucose metabolism in partial epilepsy and its relation to EEG changes. Ann Neurol 12:510–517.

Engel, J, Jr, Kuhl, DE, Phelps, ME, Rausch, R, and Nuwer, M (1983). Local cerebral metabolism during partial seizures. Neurology 33:400–413.

Engel, J, Jr, Ebersole, JS, Burchfiel, JL, Gates, JR, Gotman, J, Homan, RW, Ives, JR, King, DW, Sato, S, and Wilkus, RJ (1985a). American Electroencephalographic Society guidelines for long-term neurodiagnostic monitoring in epilepsy. J Clin Neurophysiol 2:419–452.

Engel, J, Jr, Lubens, P, Kuhl, DE, and Phelps, M (1985b). Local cerebral metabolic rate for glucose during petit mal absences. Ann Neurol 17:121–128.

Engel, J, Jr, Caldecott-Hazard, S, and Bandler, R (1986). Neurobiology of behavior: Anatomic and physiologic implications related to epilepsy. Epilepsia 27(suppl 2): S3–S11.

Epstein, CM, Michelucci, R, and Hallett, M (2008). Transcranial magnetic stimulation. In Epilepsy: A Comprehensive Textbook, 2nd ed. Edited by J Engel, Jr, and TA Pedley. Philadelphia: Lippincott Williams & Wilkins, pp. 1041–1050.

Faught, E, and Lee, SI (1984). Pattern-reversal visual evoked potentials in photosensitive epilepsy. Electroencephalogr Clin Neurophysiol 59:125–133.

Filskov, SB, and Boll, TJ (eds) (1981). Handbook of Clinical Neuropsychology. New York: Wiley Intersciences.

Fisch, BJ (ed) (2010). Epilepsy and Intensive Care Monitoring. New York: Demos.

Fisch, BJ, and Spehlmann, R (1999). EEG Primer, 3rd ed. Amsterdam: Elsevier/North-Holland Biomedical Press.

Forster, FM (1977). Reflex Epilepsy, Behavioral Therapy and Conditional Reflexes. Springfield, IL: Charles C Thomas.

Frost, JD, Jr, Kellaway, P, Hrachovy, RA, Glaze, DG, and Mizrahi, EM (1986). Changes in epileptic spike configuration associated with attainment of seizure control. Ann Neurol 20:723–731.

Frost, JJ, Mayberg, HS, Fisher, RS, Douglass, KH, Dannals, RF, Links, JM, Wilson, AA, Ravert, HT, Rosenbaum, AE, Snyder, SH, and Wagner, HN (1988). Mu-opiate receptors measured by positron emission tomography are increased in temporal lobe epilepsy. Ann Neurol 23:231–237.

Gaillard, WD, Chiron, C, Cross, H, Harvey, AS, Kuzniecky, R, Hertz-Pannier, L, and Vezina, LG, for the ILAE Committee for Neuroimaging, Subcommittee for Pediatric Neuroimaging (2009). Guidelines for imaging infants and children with recent-onset epilepsy. Epilepsia 50:2147–2153.

Garretson, H, Gloor, P, and Rasmussen, T (1966). Intracarotid amobarbital and Metrazol test for the study of epileptiform discharges in man: A note on its technique. Electroencephalogr Clin Neurophysiol 21:607–610.

Gastaut, H (1950). Combined photic and Metrazol activation of the brain. Electroencephalogr Clin Neurophysiol 2:249–261.

Gastaut, H, and Gastaut, JL (1976). Computerized transverse axial tomography in epilepsy. Epilepsia 17:325–336.

Gelfand, JM, Wintermark, M, and Josephson, SA (2010). Cerebral perfusion-CT patterns following seizure. Eur J Neurol 17:594–601.

Glauser, TA (2011). Biomarkers for antiepileptic drug response. Biomark Med 5:635–644.

Goldensohn, ES, Legatt, AD, Koszer, S, and Wolf, SM (1999). Goldensohn's EEG Interpretation: Problems of Overreading and Underreading, 2nd ed. Mount Kisco, NY: Futura.

Goldman, RI, Stern, JM, Engel, J, Jr, and Cohen, MS (2002). Simultaneous EEG and fMRI of the alpha rhythm. Neuro Report 13:2487–2492.

Gomes, WA, and Shinnar, S (2011). Prospects for imaging-related biomarkers of human epileptogenesis: Acritical review. Biomark Med 5:599–606.

Gotman, J (1983). Measurement of small time differences between EEG channels: Method and application to epileptic seizure propagation. Electroencephalogr Clin Neurophysiol 56:501–514.

Gotman, J (1985a). Automatic recognition of interictal spikes. Electroencephalogr Clin Neurophysiol Suppl 37: 93–114.

Gotman, J (1985b). Seizure recognition and analysis. Electroencephalogr Clin Neurophysiol Suppl 37: 133–145.

Gotman, J (1985c). Practical use of computer-assisted EEG interpretation in epilepsy. J Clin Neurophysiol 2:251–265.

Gotman, J, and Pittau, F (2011). Combining EEG and fMRI in the study of epileptic discharges. Epilepsia 52(suppl 4): 38–42.

Gotman, J, Gloor, P, Quesney, LF, and Olivier, A (1982). Correlations between EEG changes induced by diazepam and the localization of epileptic spikes and seizures. Electroencephalogr Clin Neurophysiol 54:614–621.

Gotman, J, Kobayashi, E, Bagshaw, AP, Benar, CG, and Dubeau, F (2006). Combining EEG and fMRI: Amultimodal tool for epilepsy research. J Magn Reson Imaging 23:906–920.

Haglund, MM, Hochman, D, and Toga, AW (2008). Optical imaging of seizure activity. In Epilepsy: A Comprehensive Textbook, 2nd ed. Edited by J Engel, Jr, and TA Pedley. Philadelphia: Lippincott Williams & Wilkins, pp. 1025–1030.

Halliday, AM (1967). The electrophysiological study of myoclonus in man. Brain 90:241–284.

Haneef, Z, Lenartowicz, A, Engel, J, Jr, Yeh, SJ, and Stern, J: Functional connectivity MRI asymmetries in lateralized temporal lobe epilepsy. Epilepsy Behav (in press)

Harden, A, Pampiglione, G, and Picton-Robinson, N (1973). Electroretinogram and visual evoked response in a form of "neuronal lipidosis" with diagnostic EEG features. J Neurol Neurosurg Psychiatry 36:61–67.

Hauf, M, Slotboom, J, Nirkko, A, von Bredow, F, Ozdoba, C, and Wiest, R (2009). Cortical regional hyperperfusion in nonconvulsive status epilepticus measured by dynamic brain perfusion CT. AJNR Am J Neuroradiol 30:693–698.

Henry, TR, and Chugani, HT (2008). Positron emission tomography. In Epilepsy: A Comprehensive Textbook, 2nd ed. Edited by J Engel, Jr, and TA Pedley. Philadelphia: Lippincott Williams & Wilkins, pp. 945–964.

Hogan, RE, Carne, RP, Kilpatrick, CJ, Cook, MJ, Patel, A, King, L, and O'Brien, TJ (2008). Hippocampal deformation mapping in MRI negative PET positive temporal lobe epilepsy. J Neurol Neurosurg Psychiatry 79:636–640.

Ives, JR (1985). Recording media for the EEG. Electroencephalogr Clin Neurophysiol Suppl 37:61–72.

Ives, JR (1987). Video recording during long-term EEG monitoring of epileptic patients. Adv Neurol 46:1–11.

Jackson, GD, and Kuzniecky, RI (2008). Structural neuroimaging. In Epilepsy: A Comprehensive Textbook, 2nd ed. Edited by J Engel, Jr, and TA Pedley. Philadelphia: Lippincott Williams & Wilkins, pp. 917–944.

Jeavons, PM, and Harding, GFA (1975). Photosensitive Epilepsy: A Review of the Literature and a Study of 460 Patients (Clinics in Developmental Medicine, No 56). Philadelphia: JB Lippincott.

Jennett, B (1975). Epilepsy After Non-missile Head Injuries, 2nd ed. Chicago: William Heinemann.

Jones-Gotman, M, Sziklas, V, Djordjevic, J, et al. (2005). Etomidate speech and memory test (*e*SAM): Anew drug and improved intracarotid procedure. Neurology 65:1723–1729.

Jones-Gotman, M, Smith, ML, and Wieser, HG (2008). Intraarterial amobarbital procedures. In Epilepsy: A Comprehensive Textbook, 2nd ed. Edited by J Engel, Jr, and TA Pedley. Philadelphia: Lippincott Williams & Wilkins, pp. 1833–1841.

Jones-Gotman, M, Smith, ML, Risse, GL, Westerveld, M, Swanson, SJ, Giovagnoli, AR, Lee, T, Mader-Joaquim, MJ, and Piazzini, A (2010). The contribution of neuropsychology to diagnostic assessment in epilepsy. Epilepsy Behav 18:3–12.

Kagawa, K, Chugani, DC, Asano, E, Juhasz, C, Muzik, O, Shah, A, Shah, J, Sood, S, Kupsky, WJ, Mangner, TJ, Chakraborty, PK, and Chugani, HT (2005). Epilepsy surgery outcome in children with tuberous sclerosis complex evaluated with alpha-[11C] methyl-L-tryptophan positron emission tomography (PET). J Child Neurol 20:429–438.

Kaufman, IC, Marshall, C, and Walker, AE (1947). Activated electroencephalography. Arch Neurol Psychiatry 58:533–549.

Kazemi, NJ, O'Brien, TJ, Cascino, GD, and So, EL (2008). Single photon emission computed tomography. In Epilepsy: A Comprehensive Textbook, 2nd ed. Edited by J Engel, Jr, and TA Pedley. Philadelphia: Lippincott Williams & Wilkins, pp. 965–973.

Kellaway, P (1980). The incidence, significance and natural history of spike foci in children. In Current Clinical Neurophysiology: Update on EEG and Evoked Potentials. Edited by RE Henry. Amsterdam: Elsevier/North Holland, pp. 151–175.

Kellaway, P, Saltzberg, B, Frost, JD, Jr, and Crawley, JW (1979). Relationship between clinical state, ictal and interictal EEG discharges, and serum drug levels: Generalized epilepsy/ethosuximide [abstract]. Neurology 29:559.

Kennedy, WA, and Hill, D (1958). The surgical prognostic significance of the electroencephalographic prediction of Ammon's horn sclerosis in epileptics. J Neurol Neurosurg Psychiatry 21:24–30.

Kiloh, LG, McComas, AJ, Osselton, JW, and Upton, ARM (1981). Clinical Electroencephalography, 4th ed. London: Butterworths.

King, DW, So, EL, Marius, R, and Gallagher, BB (1986). Techniques and applications of sphenoidal recording. J Clin Neurophysiol 3:51–65.

Klove, H, Trites, RL, and Grabow, JD (1969). Evaluation of memory functions with intracarotid sodium amytal. Trans Am Neurol Assoc 94:76–80.

Knowlton, RC, Elgavish, RA, Bartolucci, A, et al. (2008). Functional imaging: II. Prediction of epilepsy surgery outcome. Ann Neurol 64:35–41.

Krakow, K, Woermann, FG, Symms, MR, Allen, PJ, Lemieux, L, Barker, GJ, Duncan, JS, and Fish, DR (1999). EEG-triggered functional MRI of interictal epileptiform activity in patients with partial seizures. Brain 122:1679–1688.

Krauss, GL, and Fisher, RS (eds) (2006). The Johns Hopkins Atlas of Digital EEG. Baltimore: Johns Hopkins University Press.

Kressel, HY (ed) (1987). Magnetic Resonance Annual. New York: Raven Press.

Kuhl, DE, Barrio, JR, Huang, SC, Selin, C, Ackermann, RF, Lear, JL, Wu, JL, Lin, TH, and Phelps, ME (1982). Quantifying local cerebral blood flow by N-isopropyl-p(123)iodoamphetamine (IMP) tomography. J Nucl Med 23:196–203.

Kumar, A, Asano, E, and Chugani, HT (2011). α-[11C]-methyl-L-tryptophan PET for tracer localization of epilepto- genic brain regions: Clinical studies. BiomarkMed 5:577–584.

Laxer, KD (1984). Mini-sphenoidal electrodes in the investigation of seizures. Electroencephalogr Clin Neurophysiol 58:127–129.

Lee, BI, Markand, ON, Siddiqui, AR, Park, HM, Mock, B, Wellman, HN, Worth, RM, and Edwards, MK (1986). Single photon emission computed tomography (SPECT) brain imaging using N,N,N′-trimethyl-N′-(2hydroxy-3-methyl-5-(123)I-iodobenzyl)-1,3-propanediamine 2 HCl (HIPDM): Intractable complex partial seizures. Neurology 36:1471–1477.

Lee, BI, Markand, ON, Wellman, HN, Siddiqui, AR, Mock, B, Krepshaw, J, and Kung, H (1987). HIPDM single photon emission computed tomography brain imaging in partial onset secondarily generalized tonic-clonic seizures. Epilepsia 28:305–311.

Lee, BI, Markand, ON, Wellman, HN, Siddiqui, AR, Park, HM, Mock, B, Worth, RM, Edwards, MK, and Krepshaw, J (1988). HIPDM-SPECT in patients with medically intractable complex partial seizures. Arch Neurol 45:397–402.

Lee, SH, and Goldberg, HI (1977). Hypervascular pattern associated with idiopathic focal status epilepticus. Radiology 125:159–163.

Legatt, AD, and Ebersole, JS (2008). Options for long-term monitoring. In Epilepsy: A Comprehensive Textbook, 2nd ed. Edited by J Engel, Jr, and TA Pedley. Philadelphia: Lippincott Williams & Wilkins, pp. 1077–1084.

Lehnertz, K, Le Van Quyen, M, and Litt, B (2008). Seizure prediction. In Epilepsy: A Comprehensive Textbook, 2nd ed. Edited by J Engel, Jr, and TA Pedley. Philadelphia: Lippincott Williams & Wilkins, pp. 1011–1024.

Lemieux, L, Krakow, K, and Fish, DR (2001). Comparison of spike-triggered functional MRI BOLD activation and EEG dipole model localization. Neuroimage 14:1097–1104.

Leppik, IE (2008). Laboratory tests. In Epilepsy: A Comprehensive Textbook, 2nd ed. Edited by J Engel, Jr, and TA Pedley. Philadelphia: Lippincott Williams & Wilkins, pp. 791–796.

Lerner, JT, Salamon, N, Hauptman, JS, et al. (2009). Assessment and surgical outcomes for mild type I and severe type II cortical dysplasia: Acritical review and the UCLA experience. Epilepsia 50:1310–1335.

LeVan, P, and Gotman, J (2008). Computer-assisted data collection and analysis. In Epilepsy: A Comprehensive Textbook, 2nd ed. Edited by J Engel, Jr, and TA Pedley. Philadelphia: Lippincott Williams & Wilkins, pp. 1099–1115.

Lieb, JP, Joseph, JP, Engel, J, Jr, Walker, J, and Crandall, PH (1980). Sleep state and seizure foci related to depth spike activity in patients with temporal lobe epilepsy. Electroencephalogr Clin Neurophysiol 49:538–557.

Lieb, JP, Engel, J, Jr, and Babb, TL (1986a). Interhemispheric propagation time of human hippocampal seizures. I. Relationship to surgical outcome. Epilepsia 27(3):286–293.

Lieb, JP, Sperling, MR, Mendius, JR, Skomer, CE, and Engel, J, Jr (1986b). Visual versus computer evaluation of thiopental-induced EEG changes in temporal lobe epilepsy. Electroencephalogr Clin Neurophysiol 63:395–407.

Lieb, JP, Hoque, K, Skomer, CE, and Song, X (1987). Inter-hemispheric propagation of human mesial temporal lobe seizures: A coherence/phase analysis. Electroencephalogr Clin Neurophysiol 67:101–119.

Lombroso, CT, and Erba, G (1970). Primary and secondary bilateral synchrony in epilepsy: A clinical and electroencephalographic study. Arch Neurol 22:321–334.

Loring, DW, Barr, WB, Hamberger, M, and Helmstaedter, C (2008). Neuropsychology evaluation—Adults. In Epilepsy: A Comprehensive Textbook, 2nd ed. Edited by J Engel, Jr, and TA Pedley. Philadelphia: Lippincott Williams & Wilkins, pp. 1057–1065.

Mavor, H, and Hellen, MK (1964). Nasopharyngeal electrode recording. Am J EEG Technol 4:43–50.

Meador, KJ (2011). Networks, cognition, and epilepsy. Neurology 77:930–931.

Milner, B, Branch, C, and Rasmussen, T (1962). Study of short-term memory after intracarotid injection of sodium amytal. Trans Am Neurol Assoc 87:224–226.

Mintzer, S, Nicholl, JS, Stern, JM, and Engel, J, Jr (2002). Relative utility of sphenoidal and temporal surface electrodes for localization of ictal onset in temporal lobe epilepsy. Clin Neurophysiol 113:911–916.

Morrell, F (1978). Aspects of experimental epilepsy. In Modern Perspectives in Epilepsy: Proceedings of the Inaugural Symposium of the Canadian League Against Epilepsy. Edited by JA Wada. Montreal: Eden Press, pp. 24–75.

Natsume, J, Kumakura, Y, Bernasconi, N, Soucy, JP, Nakai, A, Rosa, P, Fedi, M, Dubeau, F, Andermann, F, Lisbona, R, Bernasconi, A, and Diksic, M (2003). Alpha-[11C]methyl-L-tryptophan and glucose metabolism in patients with temporal lobe epilepsy. Neurology 60:756–761.

Newmark, ME, and Penry, JK (1979). Photosensitivity and Epilepsy: A Review. New York: Raven Press.

Nuwer, MR (1988a). Frequency analysis and topographic mapping of EEG and evoked potentials in epilepsy. Electroencephalogr Clin Neurophysiol 69:118–126.

Nuwer, MR (1988b). Quantitative EEG: I. Techniques and problems of frequency analysis and topographic mapping. J Clin Neurophysiol 5:1–43.

Nuwer, MR (1988). Quantitative EEG: II. Frequency analysis and topographic mapping in clinical settings. J Clin Neurophysiol 5:45–85.

Nuwer, MR, Engel, J, Jr, Sutherling, WW, and Babb, TL (1985). Monitoring at the University of California, Los Angeles. Electroencephalogr Clin Neurophysiol Suppl 37:385–401.

O'Brien, T, O'Connor, M, Mullan, B, et al. (1998). Subtraction ictal SPECT co-registered to MRI in partial epilepsy: Description and technical validation of the method with phantom and patient studies. Nucl Med Commun 19:31–45.

Ochs, RF, Gloor, P, Tyler, JL, Wolfson, T, Worsley, K, Andermann, F, Diksic, M, Meyer, E, and Evans, A (1987). Effect of generalized spike-and-wave discharge on glucose metabolism measured by positron emission tomography. Ann Neurol 21:458–464.

Ottman, R, Hirose, S, Jain, S, Lerche, H, Lopes-Cendes, I, Noebels JL, Serratosa J, Zara F, and Scheffer, IE (2010). Genetic testing in the epilepsies—Report of the ILAE Genetics Commission. Epilepsia 51:655–670.

Pampiglione, G, and Kerridge, J (1956). EEG abnormalities from the temporal lobe studied with sphenoidal electrodes. J Neurol Neurosurg Psychiatry 19:117–129.

Pampiglione, G, and Harden, A (1973). Neurophysiological identification of a late infantile form of neuronal lipidosis. J Neurol Neurosurg Psychiatry 36:68–74.

Petroff, OA, and Duncan, JS (2008). Magnetic resonance spectroscopy. In Epilepsy: A Comprehensive Textbook, 2nd ed. Edited by J Engel, Jr, and TA Pedley. Philadelphia: Lippincott Williams & Wilkins, pp. 975–988.

Petroff, OA, Prichard, JW, Behar, KL, Alger, JR, and Shulman, RG (1984). In vivo phosphorus nuclear magnetic resonance spectroscopy in status epilepticus. Ann Neurol 16:169–177.

Petroff, OAC, Prichard, JW, Ogino, T, Avison, M, Alger, JR, and Shulman, RG (1986). Combined (1)H and (31)P nuclear magnetic spectroscopic studies of bicuculline-induced seizures in vivo. Ann Neurol 20:185–193.

Phelps, ME, Mazziotta, JC, and Schelbert, HR (1986). Positron Emission Tomography and Autoradiography: Principles and Applications for the Brain and Heart. New York: Raven Press.

Pitkänen, A, and Lukasiuk, K (2011). Molecular biomarkers of epileptogenesis. Biomark Med 5:629–633.

Porter, RJ, Penry, JK, and Lacy, JR (1977). Diagnostic and therapeutic reevaluation of patients with intractable epilepsy. Neurology 27:1006–1011.

Porter, RJ, Sato, S, and Long, RL (1985). Video recording. Electroencephalogr Clin Neurophysiol Suppl 37:73–82.

Prensky, AL, Swisher, CN, and De Vivo, DC (1973). Positive brain scans in children with idiopathic focal epileptic seizures. Neurology 23:798–807.

Pritchard, PB, III, Wannamaker, BB, Sagel, J, and Daniel, CM (1985). Serum prolactin and cortisol levels in evaluation of pseudoepileptic seizures. Ann Neurol 18:87–89.

Quesney, LF (1987). Extracranial EEG evaluation. In Surgical Treatment of the Epilepsies. Edited by J Engel, Jr. New York: Raven Press, pp. 129–166.

Ramsay, RE (1983). Valproate brain tissue kinetics determined by PETT [abstract]. Neurology 33(suppl 2):147.

Rankin, PM, and Vargha-Khadem, F (2008). Neuropsychological evaluation—Children. In Epilepsy: A Comprehensive Textbook, 2nd ed. Edited by J Engel, Jr, and TA Pedley. Philadelphia: Lippincott Williams & Wilkins, pp. 1067–1076.

Rausch, R (1987). Neurophysiological evaluation. In Surgical Treatment of the Epilepsies. Edited by J Engel, Jr. New York: Raven Press, pp. 181–196.

Rausch, R, and Crandall, PH (1982). Psychological status related to surgical control of temporal lobe seizures. Epilepsia 23:191–202.

Remillard, GM, Andermann, F, Rhi-Sausi, A, and Robbins, NM (1977). Facial asymmetry in patients with temporal lobe epilepsy: A clinical sign useful in the lateralization of temporal epileptogenic foci. Neurology 27:109–114.

Rovit, RL, Gloor, P, and Rasmussen, T (1961). Sphenoidal electrodes in the electrographic study of patients with temporal lobe epilepsy: An evaluation. J Neurosurg 18:151–158.

Rovit, RL, Gloor, P, and Rasmussen, T (1961b). Intracarotid amobarbital in epileptic patients. Arch Neurol 5:606–626.

Salamon, N, Kung, J, Shaw, SJ, Koo, J, Koh, S, Wu, JY, Lerner, JT, Sankar, R, Shields, WD, Engel, J, Jr, Fried, I, Miyata, H, Yong, WH, Vinters, HV, and Mathern, GW (2008). FDG-PET/MRI coregistration improves detection of cortical dysplasia in patients with epilepsy. Neurology 71:1594–1601.

Salinsky, M, Kanter, R, and Dasheiff, M (1987). Effectiveness of multiple EEGs in supporting the diagnosis of epilepsy: An operational curve. Epilepsia 28:331–334.

Sanabria, E, Chauvel, P, Askienazy, S, Vignal, JP, Trottier, S, Chodkiewicz, JP, and Bancaud, J (1983). Single photon emission computed tomography (SPECT) using (123)I-isopropyl-iodo-amphetamine (IAMP) in partial epilepsy. In Current Problems in Epilepsy 1: Cerebral Blood Flow, Metabolism and Epilepsy. Edited by M Baldy-Moulinier, D-H Ingvar, and BS Meldrum. London: John Libbey, pp. 82–87.

Satz, P, Orsini, DL, Saslow, E, and Henry, R (1985). Early brain injury and pathological left-handedness: Clues to a syndrome. In The Dual Brain: Hemispheric Specialization in Humans. Edited by DF Benson and E Zaidel. New York: Guilford Press, pp. 117–125.

Savic, I, Persson, A, Roland, P, et al. (1988). In-vivo demonstration of reduced benzodiazepine receptor binding in human epileptic foci. Lancet 8616:863–866.

Scheffer, IE (2011). Genetic testing in epilepsy: What should you be doing? Epilepsy Curr 11:107–111.

Schevon, CA, Toro, ER, Karceski, SC (2011). Fundamentals of digital video recording. In Atlas of Video-EEG Monitoring. Edited by JI Sirven, and JM Stern. New York: McGraw-Hill, pp. 85–95.

Schomer, DL, and Lopes da Silva, F (eds) (2011). Niedermeyer's Electroencephalography: Basic Principles, Clinical Applications, and Related Fields, 6thed. Philadelphia: Wolters Kluwer.

Silverman, D (1960). The anterior temporal electrode and the ten-twenty system. Electroencephalogr Clin Neurophysiol 12:735–737.

Sirven, JI, and Stern, JM (2011). Atlas of Video-EEG Monitoring. New York: McGraw-Hill.

Sirven, JI, Malamut, BL, Liporace, JD, O'Connor, MJ, and Sperling, MR (1997). Outcome after temporal lobectomy in bilateral temporal lobe epilepsy. Ann Neurol 42:873–878.

Smith, SM, Fox, PT, Miller, KL, Glahn, DC, Fox, PM, Mackay, CE, Filippini, N, Watkins, KE, Toro, R, Laird, AR, and Beckmann, CF (2009). Correspondence of the brain's functional architecture during activation and rest. Proc Natl Acad Sci USA 106:13040–13045.

So, E (2002). Role of neuroimaging in the management of seizure disorders. Mayo Clin Proc 77:1251–1264.

So, EL, and Fisch, BJ (2008). Drug withdrawal and other activating techniques. In Epilepsy: A Comprehensive Textbook, 2nd ed. Edited by J Engel, Jr, and TA Pedley. Philadelphia: Lippincott Williams & Wilkins, pp. 1091–1097.

Sperling, MR, and Clancy, RR (2008). Ictal electroencephalogram. In Epilepsy: A Comprehensive Textbook, 2nd ed. Edited by J Engel, Jr, and TA Pedley. Philadelphia: Lippincott Williams & Wilkins, pp. 825–854.

Sperling, MR, and Engel, J, Jr (1985). Electroencephalographic recording from the temporal lobes: A comparison of ear, anterior temporal, and nasopharyngeal electrodes. Ann Neurol 17:510–513.

Sperling, MR, and Engel, J, Jr (1986). Sphenoidal electrodes. J Clin Neurophysiol 3:67–73.

Sperling, MR, Pritchard, PB, III, Engel, J, Jr, Daniel, C, and Sagel, J (1986a). Prolactin in partial epilepsy: An indicator of limbic seizures. Ann Neurol 20:716–722.

Sperling, MR, Mendius, JR, and Engel, J, Jr (1986b). Mesial temporal spikes: A simultaneous comparison of sphenoidal, nasopharyngeal, and ear electrodes. Epilepsia 27:81–86.

Staba, RJ, and Bragin, A (2011). High-frequency oscillations and other electrophysiological biomarkers of epilepsy: Underlying mechanisms. Biomark Med 5:545–556.

Stern, J, and Engel, J, Jr (2005). Atlas of EEG Patterns. Philadelphia: Lippincott, Williams & Wilkins.

Stern, JM, and Engel, J, Jr (2012). Video-EEG monitoring for epilepsy. In Aminoff's Electrodiagnosis in Clinical Neurology, 6thed. Edited by J Aminoff, J. San Diego: Elsevier, pp. 143–163.

Stern, JM, Tripathi, M, Akhtari, M, Korb A, Engel, J, Jr, and Cohen, MS (2006). Musicogenic seizure localization with simultaneous EEG and functional MRI (SEM). Neurology 66(suppl 2):90.

Stern, JM, Haneef, Z, Yeh, H, Okamoto, Y, Akai, L, Parvizi, J, and Homma, I (2010). Comparison of dipole analysis and functional MRI in localization of epileptiform discharges. Clin Neurophysiol 121(suppl 1):S136.

Sutherling, WW, Crandall, PH, Engel, J, Jr, Darcey, TM, Cahan, LD, and Barth, DS (1987). The magnetic field of complex partial seizures agrees with intracranial localization. Ann Neurol 21:548–558.

Takahashi, T (1982). Activation methods. In Electroencephalography: Basic Principles, Clinical Applications and Related Fields. Edited by E Niedermeyer and F Lopes da Silva. Baltimore: Urban & Schwarzenberg, pp. 179–195.

Tassinari, CA, and Rubboli, G (2008). Polygraphic recordings. In Epilepsy: A Comprehensive Textbook, 2nd ed. Edited by J Engel, Jr, and TA Pedley. Philadelphia: Lippincott Williams & Wilkins, pp. 873–894.

Theodore, H, Brooks, R, Margolin, R, Patronas, N, Sato, S, Porter, RJ, Mansi, L, Bairamian, D, and DiChiro, G (1985). Positron emission tomography in generalized seizures. Neurology 35:684–690.

Theodore, WH, Newmark, ME, Sato, S, De LaPaz, R, DiChiro, G, Brooks, R, Patronas, N, Kessler, RM, Manning, R, Margolin, R, Channing, M, and Porter, RJ (1984). (18)F-fluorodeoxyglucose positron emission tomography in refractory complex partial seizures. Ann Neurol 14:429–437.

Theodore, WH, DiChiro, G, Margolin, R, Fishbein, D, Porter, RJ, and Brooks, RA (1986a). Barbiturates reduce human cerebral glucose metabolism. Neurology 36:60–64.

Theodore, WH, Vairamian, D, Newmark, ME, DiChiro, G, Porter, RJ, Larson, S, and Fishbein, D (1986b). Effect of phenytoin on human cerebral glucose metabolism. J Cereb Blood Flow Metab 6:315–320.

Thomason, ME, and Thompson PM (2011). Diffusion imaging, white matter and psychopathology. Annu Rev Clin Psychol 7:63–85.

Thompson, PM, Hayashi, KM, de Zubicaray, GI, Janke, AL, Rose, SE, Semple, J, Hong, MS, Herman, DH, Gravano, D, Doddrell, DM, and Toga, AW (2004). Mapping hippocampal and ventricular change in Alzheimer disease. Neuroimage 22:1754–1766.

Trevelyan, AJ, and Yuste, RM (2008). Cellular imaging of epilepsy. In Epilepsy: A Comprehensive Textbook, 2nd ed. Edited by J Engel, Jr, and TA Pedley. Philadelphia: Lippincott Williams & Wilkins, pp. 1051–1056.

Vezzani, A, and Friedman, A (2011). Brain inflammation as a biomarker in epilepsy. Biomark Med 5:607–614.

Vossler, DG, Wilensky, AJ, Cawthon, DF, Abson Kraemer, DL, Ojemann, LM, Caylor, LM, and Morgan, JD (2002). Serum glutamine levels in valproate-related hyperammonemic encephalopathy. Epilepsia 43: 154–158.

Wada, J (1949). A new method for determination of the side of cerebral speech dominance. A preliminary report on the intra-carotid injection of sodium amytal in man. Igaku to Seibutsugaku (Medicine and Biology) 14:221–222. (In Japanese)

Wada, J, and Rasmussen, T (1960). Intracarotid injection of sodium amytal for the lateralization of cerebral speech dominance: Experimental and clinical observations. J Neurosurg 17:266–282.

Walczak, TS, Jayakar, P, and Mizrahi, EM (2008). Interictal electroencephalography. In Epilepsy: A Comprehensive Textbook, 2nd ed. Edited by J Engel, Jr, and TA Pedley. Philadelphia: Lippincott Williams & Wilkins, pp. 809–823.

Wieser, HG, Bancaud, J, Talairach, J, Bonis, A, and Szikla, G (1979). Comparative value of spontaneous and chemically and electrically induced seizures in establishing the lateralization of temporal lobe seizures. Epilepsia 20:47–59.

Wilkus, RJ, and Thompson, PM (1985). Sphenoidal electrode positions and basal EEG during long term monitoring. Epilepsia 26:137–142.

Williamson, PD, Wieser, HG, and Delgado-Escueta, AV (1987). Clinical characteristics of partial seizures. In Surgical Treatment of the Epilepsies. Edited by J Engel, Jr. New York: Raven Press, pp. 101–123.

Williamson, SJ, and Kaufman, L (1981). Biomagnetism: Topical review. J Magn Mater 22:129–201.

Wilson, SJ, and Engel, J, Jr (2010). Diverse perspectives on developments in epilepsy surgery. Seizure 19:659–668.

Wong, W, Tsuruda, S, Kortman, KE, and Bradley, WG (1987). Practical Magnetic Resonance Imaging: A Case Study Approach. Rockville, MD: Aspen.

Worrell, G, and Gotman, J (2011). High-frequency oscillations and other electrophysiological biomarkers of epilepsy: Clinical studies. Biomark Med 5:557–566.

Yamamoto, YL, Ochs, R, Gloor, P, Ammann, W, Meyer, E, Evans, AC, Cooke, B, Sako, K, Gotman, J, Feindel, WH, Diksic, M, Thompson, CJ, and Robitaille, Y (1983). Patterns of rCBF and focal energy metabolic changes in relation to electroencephalographic abnormality in the inter-ictal phase of partial epilepsy. In Current Problems in Epilepsy 1: Cerebral Blood Flow, Metabolism and Epilepsy. Edited by M Baldy-Moulinier, D-H Ingvar, and BS Meldrum. London: John Libbey, pp. 51–62.

Zifkin, BG, Guerrini, R, and Plouin, P (2008). Reflex seizures. In Epilepsy: A Comprehensive Textbook, 2nd ed. Edited by J Engel, Jr, and TA Pedley. Philadelphia: Lippincott Williams & Wilkins, pp. 2559–2572.

Zivin, L, and Ajmone-Marsan, C (1968). Incidence and prognostic significance of "epileptiform" activity in the EEG of non-epileptic subjects. Brain 91:751–778.

Chapter 13

Differential Diagnosis

DIFFERENTIAL DIAGNOSIS OF NONEPILEPTIC PAROXYSMAL EVENTS
Systemic Disturbances
Neurological Disturbances
Psychogenic Disturbances

DIFFERENTIAL DIAGNOSIS OF REACTIVE (ACUTE SYMPTOMATIC, PROVOKED) EPILEPTIC SEIZURES
Alcohol Withdrawal Seizures
Recurrent Reactive Seizures

DIFFERENTIAL DIAGNOSIS OF CHRONIC EPILEPSY

USE OF THE EEG IN THE DIFFERENTIAL DIAGNOSIS OF EPILEPSY
Avoiding an Inappropriate Diagnosis of Epilepsy
EEG Contributions to a Positive Diagnosis of Epilepsy
EEG Contributions to Diagnosis of the Type of Epilepsy

USE OF FUNCTIONAL IMAGING IN THE DIFFERENTIAL DIAGNOSIS OF EPILEPSY

SUMMARY AND CONCLUSIONS

There are a number of well-defined, hierarchical stages in the differential diagnosis of one or more paroxysmal events (Fig. 13–1). First, it is necessary to determine whether any events are epileptic seizures. Nonepileptic paroxysmal phenomena that can be confused with epileptic seizures may be induced by *systemic*, *neurological*, or *psychogenic* disorders (Hirsch et al., 2008; Crompton and Berkovic, 2009) (Table 13–1). If it appears an event in question is epileptic, it is then necessary to determine

whether this reflects a chronic epilepsy condition or a reactive seizure due to some transient reversible insult (Chapters 5 and 7). When a chronic epilepsy condition does exist, it becomes important to search for a treatable underlying cause (Chapter 5). If this underlying cause is subsequently removed (e.g., surgical excision of a brain tumor) with abolition of epileptic seizures, a patient should no longer be considered to have epilepsy. If chronic recurrent epileptic seizures continue with or

449

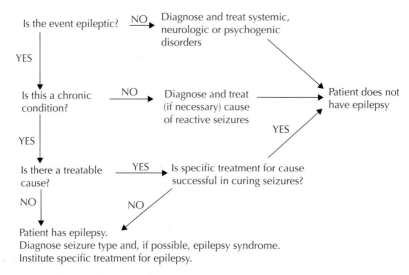

Figure 13–1. Steps in evaluation of paroxysmal events.

without therapy for an underlying cause, treatment and prognosis depend on the type of epileptic seizures the patient is having (Chapter 6) and whether the clinical picture fits that of a specific epilepsy syndrome (Chapter 7).

The importance of recognizing nonepilepsy conditions that produce transient symptoms cannot be overemphasized. A mistaken diagnosis of epilepsy not only deprives the patient of appropriate therapy if the actual condition is treatable but also creates additional disability as a result of the diagnosis itself. Applying the label of *epilepsy* can have irreversible adverse psychosocial consequences; for instance, loss of a driver's license, a job, independence, and self-esteem. Furthermore, patients misdiagnosed as having epilepsy are generally exposed unnecessarily to the risks and inconveniences of antiseizure medications. Consequently, a physician often does more harm by making this diagnosis when it is unwarranted than by reserving judgment until the true nature of the disorder has been adequately demonstrated. When doubt exists, it is usually sufficient to delay diagnosis and merely warn the patient to avoid conditions that might have precipitated the event as well as situations that could be dangerous should another event occur. Overreading of an interictal EEG is the most common cause of a mistaken diagnosis of epilepsy. This diagnosis should always be based on clinical judgment, taking into account history, descriptions of the ictal events, and careful documentation of

precipitating factors, as well as EEG findings and other test results (Chapter 12).

DIFFERENTIAL DIAGNOSIS OF NONEPILEPTIC PAROXYSMAL EVENTS

Systemic Disturbances

SYNCOPE

The most common paroxysmal disturbance of systemic origin that is confused with epilepsy is syncope (Quigg and Bleck, 2008). In one series, almost one-third of patients who were initially diagnosed as having epilepsy eventually were found to have syncope (Gastaut and Gastaut, 1958). The ultimate basis of syncope is cerebral hypoxia, which has a variety of causes (Engel, 1962; Gastaut, 1974; Riley, 1982; Quigg and Bleck, 2008). *Vasovagal* or *vasodepressor syncope* can be psychogenic or neurogenic or can be induced by carotid sinus disturbances, urination (*micturition syncope*), coughing (*tussive syncope*), and *Valsalva maneuvers*. Cardiac causes of syncope include arrhythmias such as *Stokes-Adams syndrome, paroxysmal ventricular* and *atrial tachycardia*, and *asystole*, as well as a variety of congenital and acquired heart diseases. The function of the heart, like that of the brain, is dependent on excitable

Table 13–1 Nonepileptic Paroxysmal Phenomena

Systemic Disturbances
- Syncope
  - Vasovagal
  - Cardiogenic
  - Orthogenic hypotension (Shy-Drager, familial dysautonomia, hypovolemia, Parkinson's disease, diabetes, porphyria, amyloidosis, vasoactive drugs)
- Breath holding
- Hyperventilation
- Toxic and metabolic disturbances
  - Alcoholic blackouts
  - Delirium tremens
  - Porphyria
  - Hypoglycemia
  - Pheochromocytoma
  - Asterixis with hepatic and renal failure
  - Tetanus
  - Rabies
  - Psychomimetic drugs
  - Toxic spasm with camphor and strychnine
  - Jitteriness in newborns

Neurological Disturbances
- Cardiovascular disorders
  - Transient ischemic attacks (TIAs)
  - Vertebral basilar insufficiency
  - Moyamoya disease
  - Migraine
  - Transient global amnesia
- Sleep disorders
  - Narcolepsy (catalepsy, sleep paralysis, hypnogogic or hypnopompic hallucinations)
  - Neutral-state syndrome (microsleeps)
  - Encephalitis lethargica
  - Kleine-Levin syndrome
  - Pickwickian syndrome
- REM behavioral disorder
- Parasomnias (non-REM dysomnia)
  - Incubus
  - Pavor nocturna
  - Somnambulism
  - Sleep talking
  - Bruxism
  - Jactatio capitis nocturna
  - Adult parasomnias (nocturnal wandering and night terrors)
- Motor disorders
  - Myoclonus
  - Infantile spasms
  - Dystonia
  - Chorea
  - Athetosis
  - Hemiballismus

(continued)

Table 13–1 (Continued)

  - Tremors
  - Paroxysmal dyskinesias
    - Familial paroxysmal kinesigenic choreoathetosis
    - Familial paroxysmal dystonic choreoathetosis
    - Acquired paroxysmal dyskinesias
    - Nocturnal paroxysmal dystonias
  - Startle disease (hyperekplexia)
  - Gilles de la Tourette syndrome
  - Alternating hemiplegia in childhood
  - Hemifacial spasms
  - Cerebellar fits
- Sensory disorders
  - Paroxysmal vertigo
  - Trigeminal neuralgia
  - Peduncular hallucinosis
- Neonatal disorders
  - Some neonatal seizures
  - Intraventricular hemorrhage

Psychogenic Disturbances
- Psychogenic nonepileptic seizures (PNES)
- Episodic dyscontrol
- Dissociative states (dissociative hysterical neuroses)
  - Psychogenic fugue
  - Multiple personality disorder
  - Psychogenic amnesia
  - Depersonalization disorder
- Daydreaming (vs. absence seizures)
- Obsessive-compulsive behavior
- Panic attacks
- Schizophrenia (hallucinations)

membranes, which are influenced by genetic mutations that affect voltage-gated ion channels. A number of mutations have been identified for *long* and *short QT syndromes*, the *Brugada syndrome*, and *progressive cardiac conduction disease*, and there may be commonalities among these genetic defects and those that cause epilepsy and perhaps *sudden unexplained death of epilepsy (SUDEP)* (Hartmann et al., 1999; Crompton and Berkovic, 2009; Goldman et al., 2009) (Chapter 9). Noncardiac causes of syncope include *orthostatic hypotension* and *shock*. Orthostatic hypotension may be due to *hypovolemia*; to central autonomic disturbances such as *familial dysautonomia*, *Shy-Drager syndrome*, and *Parkinson's disease*; to peripheral autonomic neuropathies like those that occur with *diabetes*, *porphyria*, and *amyloidosis*; and to vasoactive drugs such as antihypertensives, *tricyclic antidepressants*, *phenothiazines*, and *levodopa*.

Syncopal disorders are characterized by stereotyped recurrent attacks of impaired consciousness with loss of motor tone. In episodes of syncope where cerebral hypoxia occurs slowly, there is classically a prodromal malaise or light-headedness. This presyncopal state can be associated with sensory disturbances such as blurred vision, vertigo, tinnitus or other auditory disturbances, and, rarely, hallucinations. The patient then loses consciousness and slides to the ground. Tonic spasms, multifocal myoclonic movements, dystonic posturing, and, rarely, automatisms can be seen after the fall but are more likely to occur if the patient is held up or left sitting. Incontinence of urine and even feces may occur. The entire episode usually lasts less than a few seconds, and afterward the patient is immediately alert but occasionally complains of nausea. Longer episodes of up to 10 seconds may be followed by brief confusion. There may be a postictal urge to urinate, but because of an increase in release of antidiuretic hormone, this can be followed by prolonged oliguria.

The EEG during the prodromal period shows diffuse high-amplitude 3- to 5-Hz slowing, which reduces to 1–3 Hz when consciousness is lost. When tonic or myoclonic movements occur, the EEG is isoelectric (Gastaut, 1974). The tonic and myoclonic movements reflect decerebrate rigidity and have been referred to as *convulsive syncope*, (Gastaut, 1974) although syncope might also rarely give rise to a true generalized tonic-clonic seizure in a susceptible individual. In either case, the disorder is due to syncope and should be treated as such.

With syncope, the pattern of sliding to the ground followed by tonic rigidity can easily be distinguished from generalized tonic-clonic seizures, where the tonic component begins first and causes the fall, and from ictal drop attacks due to atonic or focal seizures, which consist of sudden collapse or retropulsion (Chapter 6). For this reason, patients frequently hurt themselves when falling as a result of such epileptic events and are less likely to hurt themselves as a result of syncopal episodes. Focal dyscognitive seizures that are associated with a more gradual loss of tone can usually be identified by their longer duration and postictal confusion.

Table 13–2 shows specific points that are important in the differential diagnosis between syncope and generalized tonic-clonic epileptic seizures. The history is the most revealing part of the evaluation, and a detailed account of each individual event should be obtained. The physical examination should include blood pressure in both arms and legs, lying down and standing for 3 minutes, and careful auscultation for bruits. *Catecholamines* measured while the patient is lying down and on standing can also be helpful, because the usual rise in plasma catecholamines on standing will be absent with certain autonomic disturbances. Cardiac evaluation, including an electrocardiogram, is important. *Holter monitoring* as well as ambulatory EEG monitoring or EEG telemetry with video recording can be used to document cardiac arrhythmias associated with loss of consciousness. Cardiac arrhythmias can also be associated with epileptic seizures, however, and misdiagnosis might occur in these situations. When the disturbance in cardiac rhythm is considered sufficient to impair consciousness, it must be determined whether these electrocardiogram (ECG) changes precede ictal symptoms or are a consequence of the ictal event (Chapter 9). Other specific tests for autonomic neuropathy may be appropriate (Low, 1987).

Syncope is likely when a hyperreactive parasympathetic response is demonstrated by the *oculocephalic reflex* (Gastaut, 1974). Strong pressure on both closed eyelids for 4–8 seconds can induce bradycardia or asystole associated with syncope in susceptible individuals. This test is uncomfortable and potentially dangerous and therefore not recommended unless absolutely necessary. ECG monitoring must always be carried out. Similar results may be obtained by compression of the *carotid sinus* or a simple *Valsalva maneuver* (Gastaut, 1974).

BREATH HOLDING

Breath holding occurs from the neonatal period to 6 years of age but is most common between 6 and 18 months. It is considered to be a form of syncope affecting 4–5% of infants and has been referred to as *infantile syncope* (Lombroso and Lerman, 1967). There is often a positive family history. Breath-holding spells are classically precipitated by surprise, fright, frustration, or mild injuries. Most patients have a *cyanotic form* that commonly begins with a long cry or a gasp, followed by autonomic signs, including cyanosis and a cold sweat, before loss of consciousness. The child then becomes limp but can have a

Table 13–2 Differential Diagnosis of Generalized Convulsions, Syncope, Breath Holding, and Hyperventilation

	Convulsive Epileptic Seizures	Syncope	Breath Holding	Hyperventilation
Age of onset	Rare in infancy	Rare in infancy	Often in infancy	Adolescence and young adult
Family history	Positive or negative	Often positive	Often positive	Positive or negative
Precipitating factors	Variable or absent; can occur during sleep	Emotional, Valsalva, other specific causes	Emotional	Emotional
Heart rate	Increased	Irregular or decreased	Decreased	Can be irregular or increased
Posture	Unrelated	Usually erect	Usually erect	Unrelated
Ictal symptoms	Tonic and clonic movements	Loss of tone, falling; may have clonic jerks or tonic spasms	Cyanosis, clonic jerks, opisthotonos	Paresthesias, dizziness, carpopedal spasms, tetany, gradual loss of consciousness
Duration	Usually 1 minute or less	Usually less than 3 seconds	Usually 1 minute or less	Prolonged symptoms, brief loss of consciousness
Postictal symptoms	Confusion, sleep	Alert, or brief confusion with longer spells	Alert, tired	Alert, anxious
Interictal EEG	May have epileptiform transients	Normal	Normal	Normal
Ictal EEG	Ictal epileptiform patterns	Slow or isoelectric	Slow or isoelectric	Normal or slow
Other diagnostic tests	May be evidence of focal deficit or structural lesion; postictal elevated prolactin	Oculocephalic reflex may be positive; may have cardiac arrhythmias or other autonomic disturbances	Oculocephalic reflex may be positive	Relieved by rebreathing exhaled air

few clonic jerks and opisthotonic posturing. The event lasts for less than a minute. EEG recordings resemble those of syncope. Diffuse high-amplitude delta waves are seen as consciousness is lost, and the tracing becomes isoelectric during the clonic and opisthotonic phase, again suggesting decorticate rigidity. Postictally, there is immediate return of consciousness without symptoms. A less common, *pallid form* of infantile syncope is an abnormal reflex not actually due to breath holding. Consciousness may be lost more quickly, without crying; there is pallor rather than cyanosis; and tonic or clonic movements at the termination of the attack are more common than with the cyanotic form (King et al., 1982). The prognosis for both

forms is excellent, but other types of syncope often develop later. The differential diagnosis of infantile syncope and generalized tonic-clonic seizures is shown in Table 13–2. Infants with the pallid form demonstrate an oculocephalic reflex with prolonged asystole, high-amplitude delta activity on EEG, and loss of consciousness (Lombroso and Lerman, 1967).

HYPERVENTILATION

Hyperventilation is most common in adolescents and young adults (Ettinger et al., 2008). Transient hyperventilation is usually induced by stress, anxiety, and other emotional stimuli. Some individuals have *chronic hyperventilation syndrome*, characterized by continuous asymptomatic overbreathing. Repeated attacks occur when slight increases in respiration that are difficult to detect bring about symptoms. Symptoms do not accompany the hyperventilation that normally results from exercise, drugs, and other conditions causing acidosis, because increased respiration in these situations corrects an acid-base imbalance.

Hyperventilation can produce neurological, cardiovascular, respiratory, gastrointestinal, and musculoskeletal symptoms (Riley, 1982; Ettinger et al., 2008). Central nervous system (CNS) symptoms due to decreased cerebral perfusion include light-headedness, depersonalization, blurred vision, anxiety, and loss of consciousness. Peripheral nerve symptoms due to the induced hypocalcemia include paresthesias, tetany, and muscle spasms. Cardiovascular and respiratory symptoms include palpitations, tachycardia, precordial pain, *Raynaud's phenomenon*, and shortness of breath. Patients may also complain of heartburn, epigastric pain, nausea, muscle cramps, weakness, and easy fatigability.

The typical hyperventilation episode begins with a sensation of shortness of breath, perioral paresthesias, and tingling of the fingers. There can be twitching of eyelids and facial muscles, carpopedal spasms, or frank tetany. Some patients may lose consciousness, but the loss comes on gradually, beginning with a sense of unreality. The respiratory rate is not necessarily increased at the time of the initial symptoms; rather, breathing is deeper, with a peculiar heaving of the sternum, as with sighing. Sobbing in infants can also give rise to the hyperventilation syndrome. The symptoms are not stereotyped, and parts or all of the symptom complex may be present at any given time. Hyperventilation can also cause a generalized tonic-clonic seizure in susceptible individuals or any type of seizure in patients with epilepsy. The EEG at the time nonepileptic symptoms occur shows diffuse high-amplitude delta activity.

Historical information is usually sufficient to distinguish hyperventilation-induced transient neurological symptoms from epilepsy (see Table 13–2). Also, in the former, symptoms are relieved by rebreathing exhaled air. Focal dyscognitive seizures associated with increased breathing might be mistaken for the hyperventilation syndrome, but in the former the breathing does not have the typical deep sternal heaving of hyperventilation, consciousness is impaired before hyperventilation begins, and automatisms may also occur at that time. When doubt remains, the diagnosis may be confirmed if hyperventilation in the EEG laboratory produces the typical symptoms and high-amplitude EEG slowing. However, it is often not possible to induce symptoms in a laboratory setting, where hyperventilation is dissociated from the emotional stimuli that precipitate the syndrome naturally.

TOXIC AND METABOLIC DISTURBANCES

The most common exogenous toxin causing nonepileptic intermittent symptoms is alcohol, which produces *alcoholic blackouts* and, on alcohol withdrawal, *delirium tremens* (Brust, 2008). Alcoholic blackouts consist of episodes of amnesia lasting for hours or sometimes days (the "lost weekend" phenomenon) during periods of heavy drinking (Goodwin et al., 1969). The amnesic episode can begin suddenly and be complete or can begin gradually, with only incomplete loss of recall. Short-term recall is also lost during the time of the episode. Alcoholic blackouts occur during the period of drinking, whereas the tremor, irritability, confusion, and hallucinations of delirium tremens, as well as alcohol withdrawal seizures (described later in this chapter), occur within 48 hours after drinking is terminated.

Sudden onset of confusion with hallucinations can be seen as a first symptom of acute intermittent *porphyria*. To further confound the differential diagnosis between this disorder and epilepsy, convulsions also occur in 10–20% of patients with porphyria during an acute attack (Waldenstrom, 1957). All of the older antiseizure medications and many new ones exacerbate symptoms of porphyria (Chapter 14).

Transient or intermittent neurological dysfunction can be produced by a variety of other toxic and metabolic disturbances induced by disease states or exogenous agents (Kaplan and Basaria, 2008). These include autonomic, psychic, and sensory symptoms with *hypoglycemia* and *pheochromocytoma*; *asterixis* with *hepatic* and *renal failure*; tonic spasms with *tetanus*; and bizarre behavior with *rabies*. *Psychomimetic drugs* can cause acute symptoms and *flashbacks* at a later date, and *strychnine* and *camphor* produce tonic spasms of brain stem origin. The differential diagnosis between these various conditions and epilepsy can usually be made by history, physical examination, and specific laboratory tests. However, asking the appropriate questions and obtaining the appropriate studies require a certain degree of suspicion.

Coma due to toxic and metabolic encephalopathies can be mistaken for status epilepticus, particularly when the EEG shows a *triphasic* or *burst suppression* pattern or when coma is superimposed on some focal or diffuse structural damage associated with *pseudoperiodic* EEG discharges and *myoclonic jerks* (Chapter 10). Muscle artifacts during coma can resemble epileptiform EEG potentials, and paralyzing agents such as *pancuronium bromide* may be necessary to rule them out. This diagnostic issue arises most commonly in comatose patients after hypoxic or ischemic brain injury. In contradistinction to focal epileptic motor symptoms, the myoclonic phenomena of acute postanoxic coma do not tend to involve body parts in proportion to the size of their representation on the precentral gyrus; whereas epileptic seizures preferentially involve face or hand, myoclonic jerks might involve poorly represented muscle groups such as the *rectus abdominis* or *sternocleidomastoid*. Postanoxic myoclonus is very refractory to anticonvulsant drugs. The end stage of generalized tonic-clonic status epilepticus may be associated with pseudoperiodic EEG discharges and muscle jerks with similar focal features but usually is recognized by the more obvious status preceding this clinical picture (Chapter 10). Because generalized tonic-clonic status epilepticus can result in permanent brain damage, treatment for status is appropriate when this diagnosis cannot be ruled out.

Jitteriness in the neonatal period results from hypoxic or ischemic insults, drug withdrawal, toxic states, and metabolic conditions such as hypocalcemia and hypoglycemia (Scher and Vigevano, 2008) (Chapter 6). Typical features of jitteriness help to distinguish it from epileptic seizures: it is usually stimulus sensitive, consists of more rapid movements of all four extremities, and does not include abnormal eye movements. The flexion and extension phases of jitteriness are equal, and movements can be abolished by passive flexion or restraint of the limbs (Holmes, 1985). There are no EEG correlates of jitteriness, and the condition does not respond to antiseizure medication. In severely asphyxiated infants, spontaneous and stretch-induced clonus, hypertonia, and hyperreflexia can also be confused with epileptic seizures.

ABDOMINAL EPILEPSY

The term *abdominal epilepsy* has been inappropriately used to describe brief episodes of abdominal pain, nausea, and occasionally vomiting, unassociated with apparent gastrointestinal insult. These symptoms in childhood were once believed to be manifestations of epileptic conditions and referred to as *epileptic equivalents*. It is now believed that these phenomena are due only rarely to epileptic mechanisms, but they may presage the development of *migraine*. In the infrequent instances where such symptoms in children are focal seizures (Chapter 6), the interictal EEG may show a temporal spike focus. The ictal EEG, however, is almost always normal. In most children with these symptoms it is inappropriate to consider the condition an epileptic disorder. Gastrointestinal evaluation and treatment of an underlying cause, if found, are indicated. *Paroxysmal extreme pain disorder* is a rare autosomal dominant disorder of infancy in which certain local triggers produce severe rectal pain or occasionally pain in the eyes or jaw caused by a gain-of-function sodium channel mutation in the dorsal root ganglion and sympathetic neurons (Dib-Hajj et al., 2007).

Neurological Disturbances

CEREBROVASCULAR DISORDERS

Transient ischemic attacks (TIAs) produce intermittent focal neurological symptoms that may be stereotyped and can be confused with epilepsy (Wright et al., 2008). These usually occur in the elderly and consist of negative symptoms such as paresis, somatosensory or visual deficits, and dysphasia. Sudden falls in clear consciousness are almost never epileptic in older people and are most often due to *vertebral basilar insufficiency*. Strokes can cause reactive focal epileptic seizures, and scars from old cerebral vascular insults can give rise to a chronic epilepsy disorder (Chapter 5). Because TIAs, reactive seizures, and epilepsy secondary to old strokes all occur in the setting of cerebrovascular disease or an extracranial source of embolization, the differential diagnosis can be difficult by history and neurological examination alone. TIAs are much less likely to have positive symptoms than seizures; however, atypical TIAs involving the anterior circulation can occasionally produce limb shaking, speech arrest, *anosognosia*, and *akinetic mutism*; involvement of the vertebral basilar system can produce *asterixis*, visual disturbances, auditory hallucinations, and drop attacks; and both anterior and posterior circulation TIAs can produce *dyskinesias* and pure sensory deficits. All of these signs and symptoms mimic epileptic seizures (Wright et al., 2008). Distinction between a TIA and a single reactive seizure induced by a cerebral embolus is not necessarily important, because management and prognosis are the same (Lesser et al., 1985). Differential diagnosis of recurrent TIAs and recurrent seizures, however, is essential, because further evaluation and treatment are quite specific. A chronic seizure disorder caused by a scar from an old stroke may be diagnosed by an interictal EEG spike focus.

Many pathological processes affect the cerebrovascular system. Paroxysmal symptoms presenting at any age, therefore, can be due to transient cerebral ischemia. Although *moyamoya disease* is rare, it is of particular interest to electroencephalographers, because it is associated with an unusual EEG finding, the reappearance of diffuse slow waves 20–60 seconds after termination of hyperventilation (*rebuildup*) (Kodama et al., 1979). However, if the diagnosis of moyamoya is strongly suspected, hyperventilation is contraindicated (Chapter 12).

Classical migraine beginning with focal neurological symptoms can be mistaken for a focal epileptic seizure followed by postictal headache (Silberstein et al., 2008). There is no impairment of consciousness during most migraine attacks, however, and postictal headaches are uncommon after focal seizures without clouding of consciousness. Consequently, this diagnosis is usually apparent from history. In rare instances, migraine-induced focal neurological symptoms occur in the absence of headache (*acephalgic migraine*). Migraine symptoms can still usually be distinguished from epilepsy by their characteristically slow march, which takes minutes, as opposed to seconds for an epileptic Jacksonian march. Transient confusion and amnesia can occur during migraine attacks (*confusional migraine*), particularly with *basilar artery migraine* in children (Golden and French, 1975). These attacks can also be associated with agitation, lethargy, depersonalization, and hallucinations. The distinction between these unusual forms of migraine and epilepsy can be difficult, particularly because of the increased incidence of epileptiform EEG abnormalities in patients with migraine (Hockaday and Whitty, 1969). A family history of migraine, the occurrence of the migrainous headache, and the characteristic slow march are useful differential diagnostic features (Panayiotopoulos, 1987). Migraine is a common comorbidity of epilepsy and vice versa, suggesting shared mechanisms. It has been estimated that 8–15% of patients with epilepsy have migraine, and up to 17% of migraineurs have epilepsy (Andermann and Andermann, 1987). A high degree of suspicion is often necessary for recognizing some migraine conditions as nonepileptic, particularly in children, in whom symptoms of migraine may be controlled by maintenance antiseizure medications.

If the differential diagnosis of epilepsy and migraine can be difficult, the pathophysiological distinction between these disorders also is not always clear (Andermann and Lugaresi, 1987). Epileptic seizures can be precipitated by migraine, and chronic epilepsy can be caused by migraine-induced cerebral lesions (Andermann, 1987; Camfield et al., 1978). Epileptic seizures cause postictal headaches that can be migrainous, the genetic occipital epilepsies are classically associated with migraine headaches, and some diseases produce both epilepsy and migraine (e.g., *mitochondrial disorders*, *arteriovenous malformations of the occipital lobe*, *neurofibromatosis*, and *Sturge-Weber syndrome*) (Silberstein et al., 2008). Mutations of several genes (*CACNA1A*, *ATP1A2*, and *SCN1A*) are known causes of the rare autosomal dominant trait *familial hemiplegic migraine*, and these mutations can also cause epilepsy (Crompton and Berkovic, 2009).

Transient global amnesia (Fisher and Adams, 1964) is a syndrome of sudden loss of memory lasting minutes to hours. Although usually confused and concerned about memory impairment during the episode, the patient may appear to be functioning adequately. Afterward, however, memory is permanently lost for that period of time. Otherwise, recovery is almost always complete, and the condition is usually benign. Transient global amnesia occurs most often in older patients but only rarely recurs, and then at widely spaced, irregular intervals. Although transient global amnesia is generally believed to reflect cerebral vascular compromise of the hippocampi bilaterally, there are probably several causes for this phenomenon. Cerebrovascular disease (Kushner and Hauser, 1985) and migraine (Hinge et al., 1986) have been implicated, whereas reports that some cases may be epileptic (Caplan, 1985) have been unconvincing. Isolated epileptic amnesia should be considered a distinctly different phenomenon (Miller et al., 1987). Usually, these epileptic episodes are brief and recurrent, probably reflecting postictal dysfunction following undetected focal dyscognitive seizures (Simos and Papanicolau, 2005).

SLEEP DISORDERS

Narcolepsy is believed to be due to a presumably autoimmune hypothalamic deficiency in *hypocretin* (also called *orexin*), a neuropeptide that mediates wakefulness (Dauvilliers et al., 2007). It is characterized by the occurrence of inappropriate and irresistible excessive daytime sleepiness (*hypersomnia*), often in association with *rapid eye movement (REM)* intrusion phenomena: *cataplexy, sleep paralysis*, and *hypnagogic* or *hypnopompic hallucinations* (Mahowald and Schenck, 2008). The sleep attacks are sudden. Cataplexy consists of drop attacks due to paralysis of voluntary movement and loss of muscle tone, often triggered by surprise or by a sudden emotional response such as laughing (*Lachschlag*). Consciousness is preserved. Muscle control may return immediately, or the patient may remain in flaccid paralysis for several minutes. Sleep paralysis affects voluntary movement and respiration and occurs on awakening. Hypnagogic and hypnopompic hallucinations are extremely vivid dreamlike phenomena that occur on going to sleep and on waking, respectively. All four components of the syndrome may be present in 10% of patients; hypersomnia, cataplexy, and one other associated symptom occur in 20–30%; and hypersomnia occurs with cataplexy in approximately 50% (Gastaut and Broughton, 1972; Parkes, 1982).

Narcolepsy may be familial or sporadic and can also occur as a result of a variety of cerebral disorders (Guilleminault and Dement, 1986). When all or most of the features of the narcoleptic syndrome are present, it can be easily distinguished from epilepsy. At times, however, narcoleptic sleep attacks and cataplexy may be difficult to distinguish historically from epileptic lapses of consciousness and atonic seizures. Sleep attacks differ from epileptic events in their longer duration, sometimes as much as an hour, the absence of any motor phenomena, the lack of postictal symptoms, and the characteristic occurrence of non-REM or REM EEG sleep patterns during the episode. Cataplexy, unlike atonic epileptic seizures, is characteristically precipitated by laughter or surprising or strong emotional situations. Narcolepsy without cataplexy is treated with wake-promoting agents (*modafinil, armodafinil*, and *sodium oxybate*) as well as sympathomimetic stimulants (*amphetamines* and *methylphenidate*), whereas narcolepsy with cataplexy can be treated with *sodium oxybate, imipramine*, and other *tricyclic compounds*.

Narcolepsy also can manifest as prolonged daytime periods of altered consciousness consisting of wakefulness with frequent *microsleep* episodes, previously referred to as the *neutral-state syndrome*. These episodes are associated with automatic, sometimes complex behavior superficially similar to that seen with focal dyscognitive seizures; for instance, a patient might drive an automobile but arrive some distance from the intended destination with no memory of what happened. In narcolepsy, however, the alteration in consciousness occurs slowly. This syndrome may occur in as many as 60% of patients with narcolepsy and also can be a consequence of sleep apnea (Guilleminault et al., 1975).

As opposed to the excessive periods of daytime sleepiness seen in narcolepsy, hypersomnia of *encephalitis lethargica* and disorders of diencephalic structures involved in sleep and of the brain stem are characterized by long periods of deep sleep with only brief or no episodes of full wakefulness. The *Kleine-Levin syndrome*, occurring almost exclusively in adolescent boys, consists of behavioral disturbances, hyperphagia, hypersexuality, and severe, prolonged, episodic hypersomnia. Patients with this syndrome have disturbed nighttime sleep and bouts of recurrent hypersomnia lasting days or weeks. In the *Pickwickian syndrome*, obese patients are continuously sleepy because of hypoxia from inadequate respiratory function. Routine EEG for all of these conditions shows rhythms of normal sleep or abnormal diffuse slowing but no epileptiform interictal or ictal disturbances. When *polysomnography* is performed, the pattern of sleep stages is abnormal (Broughton, 1982).

A number of paroxysmal motor disorders occurring during light and slow-wave non-REM sleep (*NREM parasomnias*) and during REM sleep (*REM parasomnias*) (Table 13–3) were erroneously considered to be epileptic equivalents in the past (Mahowald and Schenck, 2008; Derry et al., 2006; Avidan and

Table 13–3 The Major Paroxysmal Motor Disorders of Sleep

I. Parasomnias
  a. NREM arousal disorders
    i. Confusional arousals
    ii. Sleepwalking
    iii. Sleep terrors
  b. Parasomnias usually associated with REM sleep
    i. REM sleep behavior disorder
    ii. Parasomnia overlap disorder
    iii. Sleep paralysis
  c. Other parasomnias
    i. Catathrenia (nocturnal groaning)
II. Sleep-related movement disorders
  a. Periodic limb movements of sleep
  b. Sleep bruxism
  c. Normal leg cramps
  d. Rhythmic movement disorder (jactatio capitis nocturna)
III. Other (nonparasomnia, nonmovement disorder) paroxysmal nocturnal events
  a. Sleep starts
  b. Somniloquy
  c. Benign sleep myoclonus of infancy
  d. Nocturnal psychogenic nonepileptic seizures (PNES, pseudoseizures)
  e. Nocturnal panic attacks
  f. Sleep-related breathing disorders
  g. Gastroesophageal reflux
  h. Newly recognized conditions
    i. Excessive fragmentary myoclonus
    ii. Propriospinal myoclonus at sleep onset
    iii. Rhythmic feet movements while falling asleep
    iv. Alternating leg muscle activation during sleep and arousals

From Derry et al., 2006, with permission.

Kaplis, 2010). Night terrors (*pavor nocturnus*), in which the patient awakens screaming and fearful, with increased sympathetic activity, and may require several minutes to console, vivid nightmares (*incubus*), confusion (*confusional arousals*), sleepwalking (*somnambulism*), and sleep talking (*somniloquy*) occur during stage N3 non-REM sleep. There is amnesia for these episodes, the EEG shows generalized slowing, and a family history of the problem often can be elicited. Movement disorders of sleep include grinding of the teeth (*bruxism*), seen in young children during stage N3 non-REM sleep, usually during the first half of the night (Gastaut and Broughton, 1965; Guilleminault and Silvestri, 1982), and head banging (*jactatio capitis nocturna*), rhythmic head and sometimes body movements at a frequency of 1–3 Hz during transition from wakefulness to stage N1 non-REM sleep, which is common before the age of 5 but after this may indicate a behavioral disturbance. Occasionally, head banging is preceded by an arousal pattern on the EEG. Nocturnal enuresis (*nocturia*) can occur at any stage of sleep. These sleep disorders are distinguished from seizures by their characteristic history and confirmed, when necessary, by polysomnography. All of these behaviors could also occur as the only clinical manifestation of a nocturnal epileptic seizure, in which case they would respond to antiseizure medication (Guilleminault and Silvestri, 1982). Therefore, polysomnography is warranted when symptoms are disturbing or the clinical picture is unclear.

Sleep and wakefulness are not mutually exclusive states, and parasomnias result from intrusion of wakefulness into REM and non-REM sleep (Avidan and Kaplis, 2010). The second edition of the *International Classification of Sleep Disorders (ICSD-II)* (American Academy of Sleep Medicine, 2005) categorizes parasomnias into three groups: NREM, REM, and other conditions that are not confined to non-REM or REM sleep. NREM parasomnias are further categorized as *confusional arousals*, *sleepwalking*, and *night terrors*, and REM parasomnias as *nightmares*, *recurrent isolated sleep paralysis*, and *REM sleep behavior disorder (RBD)*. Conditions that can occur during either NREM or REM include *nocturia*, *groaning*, *eating disorder*, *dissociative disorders*, and *hallucinations*. Nocturnal yelling, screaming, confusion, disorientation, and sleepwalking in adults can also occur as a result of hypoxia due to repetitive *obstructive sleep apnea*, rather than as parasomnias. The term *secondary parasomnia* is used when there are specific medical or pharmacological causes for the sleep phenomena. This is usually a condition of adults.

Confusional arousals have an abrupt onset with behavior that is more violent than in other NREM parasomnias, associated at times with screaming, yelling, mumbling, or hypersexual behavior. Amnesia is complete, and there is no recollection of dreamlike events. Interictal EEGs in some patients of this group have demonstrated epileptiform transients. Although nocturnal EEGs have not confirmed that these events are epileptic, some patients have responded to antiseizure medications (Pedley and Guilleminault, 1977). Nocturnal wanderings are common in children and usually begin in the first or second sleep cycle. They are preceded by bursts of hypersynchronous delta waves on the EEG. Patients are amnesic for these events and may not know they had an episode if there are no witnesses. When questioned in depth, however, patients often will produce a story of concern about some imminent dreamlike disaster that required them to escape. At times their behavior during these wanderings is appropriate for a perceived threat, and they may even attempt to remove others from the room. Night terrors are also most common in children, and when they occur in adults there may also be a history of emotional or psychiatric disturbances. They typically begin with a scream and involve the sympathetic activation associated with fear. Episodes last from 30 seconds to five minutes, and some memory for dream fragments can persist.

Nightmares and sleep paralysis are easily distinguished from epileptic seizures. RBD, however, is one of the most interesting parasomnias and can easily be mistaken for epilepsy, particularly *autosomal dominant nocturnal frontal lobe epilepsy (ADNFLE)* (Chapter 7). The behaviors during REM sleep are often violent, as patients appear to "act out their dreams" because the normal atonia of this sleep stage is absent. This highly disturbing disorder, which can occur nightly, is distinguished from epilepsy by the absence of epileptiform EEG activity on polysomnography and responds to *clonazepam* or *melatonin* (Schenck and Mahowald, 2005). RBD is currently the only parasomnia requiring formal polysomnography to establish the

diagnosis (Avidan and Kaplis, 2010). It is seen primarily in older men, is often predictive of an evolving *synucleinopathy* or other dementing neurodegenerative disease, and occurs in about one-quarter of men with *Parkinson's disease*.

At times, myoclonic and dystonic movements during sleep can be so severe as to cause arousal (Chapter 7). A bed partner or observer may be concerned that these are epileptic events. The differential diagnosis usually is made easily by history, but if necessary, polysomnography will demonstrate characteristic sleep patterns and the absence of associated epileptiform EEG transients.

MOTOR DISORDERS

In addition to the *dystonia, chorea, athetosis, hemiballismus*, and *tremors* that occur intermittently with neurological disorders of the extrapyramidal systems, focal tonic spasms from spinal cord lesions seen, for instance, with *multiple sclerosis*, (Matthews, 1975) and *myoclonus*, which has already been discussed in Chapters 6 and 7, there are a number of other paroxysmal disturbances of motor function that can be confused with epilepsy.

The *paroxysmal dyskinesias* (Goodenough et al., 1978; Lance, 1977; Fahn and Frucht, 2008; Crompton and Berkovic, 2009) have been divided into four types: (1) *Familial paroxysmal kinesigenic choreoathetosis (paroxysmal kinesigenic dyskinesia)* has autosomal dominant or recessive patterns of inheritance, and the genetic basis is unknown. This disorder begins in childhood and is characterized by brief dystonic or choreoathetotic posturing lasting less than five minutes. The abnormal posturing is precipitated by sudden movement and can occur up to 100 times a day. The EEG shows no evidence of interictal or ictal epileptiform activity, but the motor symptoms respond well to antiseizure medication. (2) *Familial paroxysmal dystonic choreoathetosis (paroxysmal nonkinesigenic dyskinesia)* has an autosomal dominant pattern of inheritance and also begins in childhood; approximately half of those affected have a mutation in the *myofibrillogenesis regulator* gene, *PNKD*. Attacks are precipitated by alcohol, tea, coffee, fatigue, excitement, relaxation, heat, and cold; often are preceded by a prodrome of paresthesias or a tightening sensation in a limb; and are followed by prolonged dystonic posturing lasting from five minutes to four hours. They occur no more than three times a day. The EEG in this condition also shows no epileptic abnormalities. The episodes are not responsive to antiseizure medication, although benzodiazepines may be effective. (3) *Paroxysmal exertional dyskinesia* is a rare intermediate form with attacks that are briefer than in the other nonkinesigenic condition and are precipitated by prolonged exercise. This has been associated with a mutation in the *SLC2A1* gene, leading to *GLUT1 deficiency*, and patients respond to the *ketogenic diet*. (4) There are many varieties of *acquired paroxysmal dyskinesias*, including the painful tonic spasms that occur with *multiple sclerosis* and kinesigenic choreoathetosis associated with *cerebral palsy*, *hypoparathyroidism*, and *thyrotoxicosis*. Some of these acquired dyskinesias respond to antiseizure medication as well as specific treatment for the underlying disorder. The EEG is often abnormal interictally, but no interictal or ictal epileptiform discharges are seen unless the patient also has epilepsy. All these events can be distinguished from movement-induced and tonic epileptic seizures, because only the latter are associated with epileptiform ictal discharges on the EEG. *Nocturnal paroxysmal dystonias* occurring during sleep (Lugaresi et al., 1986) were originally felt to be movement disorders but are now recognized as epileptic events due to ADNFLE (Chapter 7).

In *startle disease (hyperekplexia)*, a startling stimulus precipitates sudden loss of voluntary postural control and falling, without attempts at protective movements (Andermann and Andermann, 1986; Kirstein and Silfveskiold, 1958). Nocturnal or diurnal spontaneous clonus without impaired consciousness can also occur in these conditions. Hyperekplexia is inherited as an autosomal dominant or recessive trait with incomplete penetrance, attributed in most cases to a genetic *glycine receptor* malfunction (Crompton and Berkovic, 2009). Stiffness in infancy (*stiff baby syndrome*) (Lingam et al., 1981) that disappears during sleep is characteristic and can result in fatal apnea during birth. There may be associated mild mental retardation and epileptic seizures. Patients with hyperekplexia have enhanced sensory evoked potentials, and this disorder is believed by some workers to be related to *cortical* and *reticular reflex myoclonus* (Wilkins et al., 1986). Other electrophysiological features, such as shorter electromyographic discharges, differentiate the hyperekplectic event from exaggerated startle responses that occur in some normal individuals (Wilkins et al., 1986). Hyperekplexia should be distinguished from startle epilepsy (Chapter 9). The latter usually is due to diffuse or lateralized cerebral insults from disorders such as *infantile storage diseases, anoxic encephalopathy, encephalitis*, and *Down's syndrome* (Saenz-Lope et al., 1984; Wilkins et al., 1986). Startle epilepsy is nonfamilial, and patients usually demonstrate epileptic interictal and ictal EEG abnormalities. There are a number of other, culturally determined nonepileptic behavioral disorders characterized by *excessive startle, echolalia, echopraxia*, and *forced obedience*, such as the *jumping Frenchmen of Maine, Malay latah, Burmese jauns, Thai bah-tsche, Philippine mali-mali, Ainu imu, Siberian ikota*, and *Lapp panic* (Andermann and Andermann, 1986). Although psychosocial factors influence the manifestations of these disorders, the suggestion that they are learned behaviors (Saint-Hilaire et al., 1986) is not generally accepted.

Gilles de la Tourette syndrome consists of multiple tics and, at times, utterances, which may be of a scatological or profane nature (*coprolalia*). These tics initially appear in children as uncontrolled snorting or sniffing and often become more elaborate with age. There are no associated EEG or structural abnormalities. Although initially considered psychogenic, this condition is now believed to be an extrapyramidal movement disorder and responds to neuroleptic, but not antiseizure, medication (Shapiro et al., 1988).

Alternating hemiplegia in childhood (Dalla Bernardina et al., 1987; Andermann et al., 1995) is a rare disorder usually occurring during the first year of life. Bilaterally independent or, at times, simultaneous (*double hemiplegia*) attacks occur with monocular nystagmus or other ocular movements, crying, head turning, and sudden tonic or dystonic posturing of one side of the body followed by flaccid hemiplegia lasting minutes to days. Consciousness is almost always retained. Attacks are initially frequent and gradually decrease with age, but children often develop progressive *hypotonia, dystonia, dyskinesia*, or *spasticity*. The EEG contains no paroxysmal abnormalities, and alternating hemiplegia in childhood is not believed to be an epileptic phenomenon; however, seizures occur in half of affected children. Etiologies similar to those of *migraine, benign paroxysmal vertigo*, and *paroxysmal dyskinesias* have been proposed. Although calcium channel blockers have been beneficial in some patients, there is no accepted treatment.

Hemifacial spasms are the motor equivalent of *trigeminal neuralgia* and consist of rhythmic twitching of facial muscles, including blinking; a characteristic electromyographic (EMG) pattern (rhythmic bursts at 5–20 Hz and individual discharges at 150–250 Hz with complete synchronization of all involved muscles); and a normal EEG (Apfelbaum, 1983). This disorder usually results from irritation of the seventh cranial nerve by mass lesions or aberrant blood vessels. Drugs are ineffective, but surgical treatment is often successful (Jannetta, 1977). Variants of this typical clinical picture could be focal motor epileptic seizures without EEG correlates.

Intermittent muscle spasms that occur in comatose patients with intracranial mass lesions, usually of the posterior fossa, were once referred to as *cerebellar fits* and believed to be epileptic. They are now known to reflect brief episodes of decerebrate posturing due to fluctuating increased intracranial pressure (Ingvar and Lundberg, 1961). Similarly, *diencephalic autonomic seizures* (Penfield and Jasper, 1954), at times associated with decerebrate posturing, appear to be release phenomena mediated by the upper brain stem and not epileptic (Bullard, 1987).

SENSORY DISORDERS

Intermittent sensory symptoms occur in all modalities and can be misdiagnosed as epileptic (Bazil, 2008). *Paroxysmal vertigo* occurs as a result of a number of central and peripheral neurological disturbances. It can be distinguished from vertiginous seizures when it is position sensitive or displays the clear directional components of true vertigo. Vertigo due to epileptic discharges in the parietal or lateral temporal lobe usually does not have a well-defined directional component and is not provoked by positional changes. Epilepsy and vertigo can coincide in the monogenic *episodic ataxias* due to mutations in the *KCNA1* and *CACNA1A* genes, the latter of which is also associated with familial hemiplegic migraine (Crompton and Berkovic, 2009). Focal sensory

symptoms such as trigeminal neuralgia, like the motor symptoms of hemifacial spasms, are usually due to nerve root irritation (Jannetta, 1977), but *carbamazepine* or *phenytoin* may be effective treatments. *Peduncular hallucinosis* (Caplan, 1980; Van Bogaert, 1927), which consists of vivid visual hallucinations and occasionally other sensory hallucinations, can be caused by brain stem and diencephalic lesions. Patients with this disorder often experience altered behavior resembling a dreamlike state while awake. Hallucinations of the *Charles Bonnet syndrome* (Rovner, 2006) are due to damage of the retina or optic pathways and often take the form of small characters or objects *(liliput hallucinations)*. The exact mechanisms of these types of hallucinatory symptoms are unknown, and antiseizure medication is ineffective. The EEGs in all of these conditions are free of epileptiform abnormalities.

Psychogenic Disturbances

PSYCHOGENIC NONEPILEPTIC SEIZURES

Psychogenic nonepileptic seizures (PNES) are involuntary, intermittent episodes that resemble epileptic seizures but are psychogenically induced (Kanner et al., 2008; Schachter and LaFrance, 2010). The older terms *pseudoseizures* and *hysteroepilepsy* for this condition are discouraged, because they have a pejorative connotation. The qualifying term *psychogenic* is important because there are many other types of nonepileptic seizures, that is paroxysmal disorders that mimic epilepsy, as noted above. Some epileptic seizures can be provoked by psychogenic factors, and these ictal events are referred to as *psychogenic epileptic seizures*. PNES must be differentiated, on the one hand, from psychogenic epileptic seizures and, on the other, from voluntary simulation or induction of epileptic attacks (*malingering* and *factitious disorder*) (American Psychiatric Association, 2000).

Distinguishing between PNES and epileptic seizures can be one of the most challenging tasks in epileptology. It is particularly problematic when patients with PNES have epileptic seizures as well. Diagnosis of PNES and discontinuation of antiseizure medication can cause status epilepticus when patients also have epilepsy. In other patients, antiseizure medications may be increased to toxic levels for prolonged periods of time, because PNES continue after epileptic seizures are controlled with much lower doses of drugs. For these reasons, it is essential to obtain a careful description of all the seizure types that occur and their individual responses to therapeutic intervention.

There is considerable controversy concerning the prevalence of epilepsy among patients who have PNES. Conflicting experiences appear to reflect differences in referral patterns, which suggest that patients with severe medically refractory epileptic seizures are more likely to also have PNES than the epilepsy population as a whole. The vast majority of patients with PNES referred to general neurology practices do not appear to have epileptic seizures (Lesser, 1985; Ramsay et al., 1993), while some tertiary referral epilepsy centers have estimated that two-thirds of their patients with PNES also have epilepsy (Mattson, 1980). A study that used stringent criteria to identify epileptiform discharges revealed that 10% of patients with PNES also have epilepsy (Benbadis et al., 2001).

PNES have been reported in patients from 4 to 73 years old but occur most often in young adults and are three times more common in women than in men (Lesser, 1985; Kanner et al., 2008). The classical behavior pattern of these ictal events, initially described by Charcot (1886), consists of uncoordinated nonsynchronous thrashing of the limbs, quivering, pelvic thrusting, side-to-side movements of the head, and opisthotonic posturing, occasionally with screaming or talking. The belief that these behaviors are characteristic of and unique to PNES has resulted in the erroneous and dangerous assumption that PNES can be diagnosed by merely observing an episode or even hearing a description of it. This is emphatically not the case, and even experienced epileptologists are incorrect in 20–30% of cases when attempting to differentiate psychogenic from epileptic disorders on the basis of ictal behavior alone (King et al., 1982). Although some psychogenic events have features that can help to distinguish them from epileptic seizures (Syed et al., 2011), these are merely factors that must be taken into account along with all other clinical information when one is making a diagnosis. A good general rule is that any transient behavior can be an epileptic seizure.

Features often encountered with psychogenic events but by no means exclusive of epilepsy include the occurrence of seizures only when other people are around, particularly at home; eye flutter; eye closure; precipitation by emotional factors; manifestations, including those described in the previous paragraph, that are different from one episode to another, rather than stereotyped; screaming and talking throughout the ictal episode; prolongation for many minutes or even hours; abrupt termination without postictal confusion; and evidence of some recall during the ictal event. On the other hand, PNES may include features that are generally thought to be evidence for epilepsy, such as pupillary dilatation, depressed corneal reflexes, Babinski responses, autonomic cardiorespiratory changes, urinary and fecal incontinence, and self-injury. Patients with PNES do on occasion fall and hurt themselves and may also bite the lips and tip of the tongue during seizures. In contrast, mouth lacerations with epileptic seizures typically involve the buccal mucosa and sides of the tongue. The onset of a psychogenic event can be gradual, and warnings can occur. Habitual attacks may include signs and symptoms of typical epileptic seizures learned in the course of neurological consultations.

As a group, patients with PNES are more likely than the general population to have increased scores on the *hypochondriasis, hysteria*, and *schizophrenia* scales of the *Minnesota Multiphasic Inventory (MMPI)* (Wilkus et al., 1984). It may be possible to elicit a history of secondary gain and a template of a close relative or friend with epilepsy. The template could also be the patient's own seizures, and in patients with both PNES and epilepsy, the epilepsy invariably begins first. In patients with known epilepsy, behavioral features of the seizure might change after what should have been effective therapeutic intervention. This change could reflect replacement of epileptic seizures with psychogenic events. In general, a diagnosis of PNES is aided by knowledge of existing psychopathology and of a relationship between this behavioral disturbance and the occurrence of seizures.

Although the interictal EEG can be helpful in this differential diagnosis, there are many hazards in drawing conclusions from interictal EEG studies alone. Interictal epileptiform events are not seen on routine EEGs of many patients with epilepsy, whereas interictal EEG spikes can be seen in patients without epilepsy (Chapter 12) as well as in patients with epilepsy who also have PNES. EEG recordings during an ictal event provide the most useful information but still are not always definitive. In many instances, ictal EEG correlates recorded in the routine EEG laboratory are obscured by muscle and movement artifacts. Often, however, it is still possible to recognize characteristic ictal epileptiform patterns, a focal EEG change, asymmetry, or postictal disturbances despite movement-induced baseline shifts and muscle potentials. Conversely, these artifacts can create changes on the EEG that simulate spike-and-wave discharges. Experienced observers, such as nurses and EEG technologists, will often recognize characteristic behavioral features of attacks that help in the differential diagnosis, even if the EEG is not revealing. As noted previously, however, these clinical observations are never diagnostic by themselves.

Ambulatory recording (Chapter 12) offers an option for obtaining ictal EEGs when seizures are more likely to occur outside the hospital. While ictal EEG changes can be recognized with this technique in many patients, the absence of an ictal EEG pattern is usually of no diagnostic value (Ebersole, 1986; Engel et al., 1985).

Inpatient video-EEG monitoring (VEM) (Chapter 12) provides the best opportunity to obtain an artifact-free ictal EEG and to observe associated clinical behavior of the episode in question (Engel et al., 1985; Ramani, 1987). An ictal epileptiform EEG pattern recorded during a typical seizure is sufficient to identify that event as epileptic but does not rule out the existence of PNES as well. By the same token, evidence that an ictal event is psychogenic does not rule out an epileptic condition. Definitive diagnosis requires recorded examples of all seizure types experienced by the patient.

If the ictal event in question involves impaired consciousness, either a focal dyscognitive seizure or a generalized tonic-clonic seizure, there should be ictal EEG changes (although these may not always include spike discharges) and postictal depression. The EEG is likely to be normal, however, during focal seizures without impaired consciousness and in certain forms of nonepileptic myoclonus (Chapter 6). Consequently, when the ictal EEG is normal during events occurring in full consciousness, the diagnosis must depend on other clinical information.

Often the most useful information obtained during inpatient VEM is observation of the behavioral seizure with an opportunity to interact with the patient during the event. Not only are clinical features discussed above useful, but PNES is suspected when patients resist efforts to open their eyes during ictal events, prevent a limp extremity from being dropped on their face, or otherwise respond in ways that demonstrate that they are cognitively intact despite their involuntary appearance of unconsciousness.

Postictal *prolactin* measurements have been advocated as a means of distinguishing PNES from epileptic events (Pritchard et al., 1985) (Chapter 12). This test can be helpful in the diagnosis of focal dyscognitive and generalized tonic-clonic seizures, but prolactin is not consistently elevated when epileptiform discharges involve mesial temporal structures unilaterally, and prolactin is normal when focal seizures do not involve mesial temporal structures (Sperling et al., 1986) (Chapter 11). In these latter situations, therefore, negative results have no diagnostic value.

Because PNES can be precipitated in many cases by suggestion, a test was devised that involves two intravenous saline injections during EEG monitoring with the suggestion that the first will induce a seizure and the second will stop it (Cohen and Suter, 1982). This approach is not recommended for several reasons. From a procedural point of view, epileptic seizures can also be induced by suggestion. The risk of misdiagnosis is great when EEG monitoring is not used, when epileptic seizures occur without EEG changes, and when ictal EEG discharges are obscured by artifact. Ethical considerations are of even more concern (Lesser, 1985). Despite careful phrasing, the use of suggestion in this manner might be perceived as deception or entrapment and could adversely influence the doctor-patient relationship. The *American Medical Association Council on Ethical and Judicial Affairs* has published a practice report on the clinical use of *placebo* (Bostick et al., 2008) stating that the use of placebo infusion to precipitate PNES is unethical unless the patient is fully informed, in which case the test is likely to be ineffective (Bernat, 2010).

The diagnosis of PNES and decisions about treatment depend on recognition of conditions that predispose to psychogenic ictal events. Although it is generally well recognized that mechanisms of classical *conversion reactions* (*hysteria*) cannot account for all PNES, there has been little attempt to identify and define the various types of PNES. According to one approach that defines five types of PNES (Gates, 1987), the majority of patients have psychological distress and emotional conflict. Secondary gain may be present in this group. Approximately half of these patients have epileptic seizures as well, and insight psychotherapy is the treatment of choice. The next most common group have inappropriate coping mechanisms. Most of these patients also have epilepsy, and many are mentally retarded. Insight psychotherapy is useful in those with normal or above-normal intelligence, whereas behavior modification is effective in those with subnormal intelligence. A third group of patients misinterpret or elaborate normal physiological phenomena. Many of these patients also have epilepsy. Patients in this group are the most readily treated and respond to reassurance, relaxation therapy, or stress management. The fourth subgroup, which may be a variation of the third, consists of patients who have brief epileptic seizures that then precipitate PNES (*highlighting* or *embellishing*). Reassurance and stress management also are effective in this group. The final group consists of psychotic patients, who respond to appropriate antipsychotic medications.

It is inaccurate and counterproductive to imply that patients with PNES are voluntarily responsible for their condition. Conversely, the ictal events are voluntary for patients who are *malingering* or who have *factitious* seizures. Malingering can usually be distinguished from psychogenic disorders by history, but the diagnosis depends on the patient's admission that he or she has consciously contrived ictal events for secondary gain. Factitious seizures are diagnosed by evidence that the patient has been self-administering an epileptogenic agent or has been feigning seizures purely to achieve patient status (Savard et al., 1988). A tragically malicious form of factitious disorder (*Munchausen syndrome*) manifesting as seizures is *factitious seizures by proxy* (*Munchausen syndrome by proxy*), a condition in which parents induce seizures in their children or, occasionally, caretakers induce seizures in their charges so that the "afflicted" individual will be admitted to the hospital.

Care must be taken when discussing the diagnosis of PNES with patients and their families. It is important to emphasize that PNES is an involuntary condition that is as disabling as epileptic seizures but that the cause and treatment are different. It helps to introduce this diagnosis as "good news," indicating that the patient has nothing seriously wrong with the brain and does not need to take antiseizure medications, which are expensive and associated with some risk. The patient and family need to be assured that the psychogenic nature of the condition does not mean that the patient is "crazy" but that emotional issues can sometimes lead to medical disturbances, such as ulcers or skin rashes, that can be resolved when a psychiatrist or psychologist uncovers the emotional conflicts involved. It also is useful sometimes to add that it is typically stronger people who do not like to complain who internalize these problems so that they emerge as medical conditions. With proper bedside manner, patients and family are often relieved to learn the diagnosis of PNES and are willing to proceed with treatment by a psychiatrist or psychologist.

INTERMITTENT EXPLOSIVE DISORDERS

Intermittent explosive disorder, formerly referred to as *episodic dyscontrol*, is diagnosed when (1) there have been several discrete episodes of loss of control or aggressive impulses resulting in serious assault or destruction of property; (2) this behavior is grossly out of proportion to any precipitating psychosocial stressor; (3) there are no signs of generalized impulsivity or aggressiveness between episodes; and (4) acting out is not due to schizophrenia, antisocial personality disorder, or conduct disorder (Tebartz van Elst and Trimble, 2008; American Psychiatric Association, 2000).

The manifestation of intermittent explosive disorder (Monroe, 1978; Rickler, 1982; Tebartz van Elst and Trimble, 2008) has sufficiently variable features to indicate that it is not a well-defined, homogeneous entity; rather, it is a variety of episodically or impulsively violent behaviors that occur as a result of numerous disorders. Patients with a diagnosis of intermittent explosive disorder often have features of minimal brain dysfunction or a history of head injury with loss of consciousness. Distinction between this condition and epilepsy is complicated by the common occurrence of epileptic seizures in this patient population (Elliot, 1978). Although some investigators have reported epileptiform EEG discharges in limbic structures of patients with intermittent explosive disorder and suggested an epileptic etiology (Mark and Ervin, 1970), this view is not generally accepted. Epileptic ictal aggressive behavior is currently believed to be rare and to involve stereotyped automatic behaviors easily distinguished from the directed attacks of intermittent explosive disorder (Delgado-Escueta et al., 1981; Saint-Hilaire et al., 1981), and the occasional more directed postictal combativeness is preceded by an obvious seizure with motor and dyscognitive features (Chapters 9 and 11).

Cultural and environmental influences on the manifestations of intermittent explosive behaviors are evident from the fact that most who suffer from this disorder are large men. Typically, patients experience sudden anger out of proportion to any provocative stimulus and act violently in either a directed or nondirected fashion. Episodes last many minutes, but rarely more than an hour. They usually consist only of verbal abuse and threats but can result in damaged property and injury to others as well as to the patient. There are often prominent autonomic features, such as tachycardia, flushing, sweating, and hypertension. Patients appear to be conscious, although unreasonable, and may later have complete or partial amnesia regarding the events. The explosive outburst is inconsistent with baseline behavior, and the patient is always deeply sorry afterward. In some cases, there is a premonition for many hours that an attack will occur. In these situations, the patient may warn others of impending danger and then take steps to protect people and property.

Some patients with intermittent explosive behaviors benefit from antiseizure medications, most commonly *carbamazepine*; for others, *anxiolytic benzodiazepines*, *antidepressants*, *lithium*, and *propranolol* have been effective (Rickler, 1982; Tebartz van Elst and Trimble, 2008). In those few patients for whom a toxic or metabolic cause can be identified, such as an *endocrinopathy* or *hypoglycemia*, corrective therapy can abolish the explosive behaviors. Studies that have attempted to characterize the features of this condition, its association with a variety of neurological and systemic disorders (Elliot, 1978), and responses of symptoms to various treatments have not identified specific pathophysiological mechanisms for this behavior. The effectiveness of carbamazepine and occasionally other antiseizure drugs in some patients may be due to psychotropic actions of these agents; the possibility that some forms of this syndrome are epileptic remains conjecture. Epileptiform discharges in limbic structures could conceivably induce such behaviors via projections into hypothalamic structures without producing surface EEG correlates (Griffith et al., 1987), but there is no evidence for such a mechanism in humans. For medicolegal purposes, directed aggressive behavior in clear consciousness cannot be considered an epileptic seizure, even in a patient who is known to have chronic epilepsy. Epilepsy is not a valid defense for premeditated or directed violent acts (Chapter 11 and 17).

DISSOCIATIVE STATES

Dissociative disorders, or *dissociative hysterical neuroses*, include *psychogenic fugue*, *multiple personality disorders*, *psychogenic amnesia*, and *depersonalization disorders* (American Psychiatric Association, 2000; Brown and Trimble, 2008). Fugue states consist of prolonged periods of compulsive aimless wandering with amnesia concerning the event. Typically, patients find themselves in strange surroundings, sometimes many hundreds of miles from home, with no knowledge of what transpired. In the rare multiple personality disorders, patients take on different names and personalities for varying periods. This disorder also includes *possession states*, in which patients feel their minds and bodies have been taken over by other beings. In psychogenic amnesia there may be indifference to the memory loss. The depersonalization state involves an alteration in the perception or experience of self while reality testing remains intact. These disorders can occur singly or repetitively. They are believed to have a psychogenic etiology and can occur in patients who are depressed. Fugue states in patients with epilepsy have been referred to as *poriomania*, and some workers believe these occasionally can be epilepsy-related behaviors (Mayeux et al., 1979). Multiple personality states and possession states have also been reported to occur as ictal or periictal phenomena in epilepsy (Benson et al., 1986; Mesulam, 1981), although they must be rare (Chapter 17). Prolonged memory loss can occur after focal dyscognitive status epilepticus (Engel et al., 1978a), and depersonalization can be the only symptom of a prolonged focal seizure with psychic symptoms, as discussed later in this chapter. The absence of an interictal epileptiform EEG pattern does not rule out epilepsy. Conversely, the presence of such a pattern or the known existence of an epilepsy condition does not indicate whether such dissociative states are ictal or postictal events or interictal psychogenic behaviors unrelated to epilepsy. Definitive diagnosis requires EEG recording during the dissociative state. Even then, the EEG is usually normal for focal seizures in clear consciousness, and postictal behavioral symptoms can outlast EEG slowing.

DAYDREAMING

Daydreaming in children may occasionally be mistaken for epilepsy. More often, however, children with epileptic seizures characterized only by brief lapses of consciousness (Chapter 6) are accused of misbehavior by teachers and parents, who may punish them for not responding during ictal inattention. History and EEG are usually diagnostic when concerned parents seek medical help, but too often the true condition is overlooked until a more obvious seizure occurs. Teachers and other professionals who regularly deal with children should be taught to recognize absences and focal dyscognitive seizures.

PSYCHOSES AND NONPSYCHOTIC PSYCHIATRIC CONDITIONS

A variety of other nonpsychotic psychiatric disturbances, such as *panic attacks* (Ettinger et al., 2008) and certain forms of *obsessive-compulsive behavior (OCD)* (George and Mula, 2008) can be intermittent and mistaken for epilepsy. A careful history is usually sufficient for the diagnosis. Panic attacks occur with anxiety disorders and consist of unexpected periods of intense fear or discomfort. Symptoms include dyspnea, dizziness, palpitations, trembling, sweating, choking, nausea, depersonalization, paresthesias, flushes, chest pain, and a sensation of impending doom (American Psychiatric Association, 2000). Panic attacks can be induced by intravenous injection of *lactic acid* in about half of patients with this disorder. *Obsessions* are intrusive, senseless, and insuppressible ideas, thoughts, impulses, or images, whereas *compulsions* are repetitive intentional behaviors performed in response to obsessions according to certain rules or in a stereotyped fashion (American Psychiatric Association, 2000). Patients are aware that their obsessions and compulsions are excessive or unreasonable and, in contrast to epilepsy, recognize them as a product of their own mind.

Focal seizures (Chapter 6) can mimic symptoms seen with *schizophrenia* (Trimble and Schmitz, 2008). Epileptic hallucinations tend to be stereotyped and are likely to contain visual components, often accompanied by hallucinations in other modalities. Some formed visual, auditory, or mixed-modality epileptic hallucinations may be misinterpreted, however, when the events lend themselves to psychoanalytic interpretation. Hallucinations that occur with schizophrenia are usually auditory and commonly consist of voices saying different things at different times. Somatosensory hallucinations can occur in schizophrenia and typically include sensations of tingling, burning, or snakes crawling in the abdomen. Visual, gustatory, or olfactory hallucinations in the absence of auditory hallucinations are rare and raise suspicion of an organic disorder such as epilepsy (American Psychiatric Association, 2000).

Ictal epileptic psychic or autonomic symptoms such as forced thinking, depersonalization, or anxiety can usually be distinguished from psychiatric disturbances when they are brief and intermittent and interictal behavior is normal. However, prolonged focal seizures with psychic or autonomic symptoms, clear consciousness, and a normal EEG (*aura continua*) might be mistaken for psychotic, affective, or neurotic disorders (Chapters 10 and 11). Focal status should be readily suspected in patients known to have epilepsy, particularly if the persistent disturbance resembles their habitual auras. Otherwise, a diagnosis of epilepsy is usually unwarranted, because it is extremely rare for this form of aura continua to appear de novo. If clinical doubt persists, it may be useful to try to abort symptoms with intravenous diazepam, but this drug also occasionally blocks psychogenic symptoms. A positive response, therefore, is not necessarily diagnostic of epilepsy.

DIFFERENTIAL DIAGNOSIS OF REACTIVE (ACUTE SYMPTOMATIC, PROVOKED) EPILEPTIC SEIZURES

Epileptic seizures are a natural response of the normal brain to transient insult and can be provoked in susceptible individuals by psychological stress, certain external stimuli, and vascular, traumatic, infectious, toxic, and metabolic disturbances. When these occur singly or transiently as a result of some reversible or remediable cause, they can be considered reactive and not an indication of an epilepsy condition (Chapters 1 and 7).

Recognition of reactive epileptic seizures depends on a careful history to elucidate precipitating factors (Chapters 5 and 9) as well as physical and laboratory examinations aimed at identifying biological causes. This is not a difficult diagnosis when the cause of the epileptic seizure is apparent and the ictal event has the characteristic appearance of a generalized tonic-clonic seizure. In some situations, however, diagnosis can be complicated because of the coexistence of precipitating factors with a latent epileptic condition or a localized brain disturbance that causes a reactive epileptic event to have focal features. Alcohol withdrawal seizures and recurrent reactive seizures exemplify most of the phenomena encountered in such focal ictal events. Drug-induced reactive absence and myoclonic seizures can also occur (Chapter 5). Seizures occurring up to a week after trauma or stroke, referred to as *early seizures*, are considered to be reactive (Beghi et al., 2010) and not an indication of chronic epilepsy. *Late seizures*, occurring after this period, are more likely to indicate epileptogenicity, but posttraumatic seizures usually begin months or even years after injury (Chapter 8).

Alcohol Withdrawal Seizures

Generalized tonic-clonic seizures can occur during the first 48 hours of withdrawal from alcohol intoxication (*rum fits*) and are most common 13–24 hours after binge drinking (Mattson, 1983; Brust, 2008). The interictal EEG is usually normal, but 50% of patients will show a *photomyogenic response*, described later in this chapter. In this situation, the epileptic seizures can be controlled with diazepam,

paraldehyde, or alcohol replacement. Focal epileptic seizures occurring in alcoholics during the withdrawal period are usually the result of cerebral scars from previous head trauma or CNS infection. In this situation, the interictal EEG may also show focal abnormalities. The treatment of these focal seizures is the same as the treatment of rum fits. It is not necessary to consider either of these conditions epilepsy disorders, and subsequent antiseizure medication need not be instituted. In fact, antiseizure medication for people with recurrent alcohol withdrawal seizures might be unwise, because they often will stop taking the medication when they binge drink, and drug withdrawal could compound alcohol withdrawal effects.

In some patients with a benign predisposition to epilepsy, alcohol withdrawal seizures do not require binge drinking or intoxication but occur following only a few drinks (Mattson, 1983). This condition is not epilepsy if seizures do not occur at other times. Such patients should be counseled to avoid all alcohol, and antiseizure medication is not necessary.

Reactive seizures also occur in chronic alcoholics as a result of superimposed metabolic or cerebral insults such as electrolyte disturbance, *hypoglycemia*, or *meningitis*. The interictal EEG activity is slow, photosensitivity is usually absent, and specific treatment for the underlying cerebral disturbance is indicated. If these insults cause cerebral lesions early, reactive seizures do not predict the later onset of chronic epilepsy, and prophylactic antiseizure medication is unnecessary (Chapter 8).

Alcohol withdrawal may precipitate the first focal or generalized epileptic seizure of a chronic epilepsy condition. It is impossible to differentiate the initial seizure in this situation from reactive focal or generalized seizures due solely to alcohol withdrawal, because the behavioral and EEG features are the same. However, a second seizure occurring more than one week following abstinence indicates a chronic epilepsy condition, and the patient should be placed on antiseizure medication.

Finally, patients with a chronic epilepsy condition may find that their epileptic seizures are exacerbated after alcohol use. This is not likely to occur after one or two drinks, but 85% of patients with epilepsy experience epileptic seizures after moderate to heavy alcohol consumption (five or six drinks) (Mattson, 1983). In this situation, the patient has a condition already diagnosed as an epilepsy disorder, and antiseizure medication has presumably been prescribed. Such episodes should then serve as a warning for the patient to take alcohol only in moderation.

Recurrent Reactive Seizures

Recurrent epileptic events due to reversible or remediable causes constitute a special category of reactive seizures. Such seizures can be induced by infectious, toxic, and metabolic cerebral processes or acute trauma as well as by certain structural lesions of the brain, such as tumors or vascular malformations, which can be surgically removed. *Benign febrile seizures*, the most common reactive seizures, can recur widely spaced in time (Chapter 7). Although all of these epileptic events are recurrent and may require antiseizure medication for acute control, they cease when the underlying insult resolves or is removed. Patients with recurrent reactive seizures should not be considered to have epilepsy unless their seizures continue despite adequate treatment of the suspected cause.

DIFFERENTIAL DIAGNOSIS OF CHRONIC EPILEPSY

When a chronic epilepsy condition exists, treatment and prognosis depend on identification of specific epileptic seizure types and, where possible, diagnosis of an epilepsy syndrome. In most cases, this can be accomplished on the basis of historical information, careful description of the epileptic events, and a routine EEG, as discussed in Chapters 6 and 7. If doubt persists, epileptiform abnormalities may be physiologically induced in the EEG laboratory (e.g., with photic stimulation or hyperventilation), or patients with sufficiently frequent seizures can be admitted to the hospital for VEM (Chapter 12). In patients who have more than one seizure type, it is best to capture and review each one.

USE OF THE EEG IN THE DIFFERENTIAL DIAGNOSIS OF EPILEPSY

Despite the importance of neuroimaging in identifying underlying causes of epilepsy, the EEG remains the most important laboratory test for differential diagnosis. Because of the reliance most clinicians put on the EEG in this situation, referring physicians and practicing electroencephalographers must be aware of EEG patterns that can result in an unwarranted diagnosis of epilepsy as well as those that help distinguish one form of epilepsy from another. With the almost universal adaptation of digital EEG, it is imperative to manipulate the recording by altering filter settings, montages, and time scale when necessary to eliminate artifacts and maximize the display of cerebral events of interest (Stern and Engel, 2005).

Avoiding an Inappropriate Diagnosis of Epilepsy

Sharp artifacts such as electrode pops and potentials produced by muscle activity, eye movements, intravenous drips, and electrocardiographic signals can usually be recognized by their characteristic patterns and field distribution. Comments written on the tracing by an alert informed technician are essential. As a general rule, when the origins of sharp EEG transients are in doubt, they should be considered artifacts. Respiration-linked spindle patterns obtained from nasopharyngeal, and occasionally sphenoidal and even intracranial, leads are vibration artifacts (Engel, 1980; Engel et al., 1978b).

Normal EEG phenomena that can be confused with epileptic potentials occur during sleep, such as *vertex sharp waves*, *positive occipital sharp transients of sleep (POSTS)*, posterior *cone waves* in small children, and *frontal mitten patterns* (Fig. 13–2), and during wakefulness, such as sharp *mu rhythms*, *lambda waves* (including the large occipital *shut-eye waves* of children), and *occipital delta waves* (also called *posterior slow waves of youth, youth waves*, and *delta de la jeunesse*) (Fig. 13–3) (Cooper et al., 1980; Ebersole and Pedley, 2003; Fisch and Spehlmann, 1999; Kiloh et al., 1981; Klass and Daly, 1990; Remond, 1978; Schomer and Lopes da Silva 2011; Stern and Engel, 2005). *Vertex sharp waves* in young children and *hypnagogic hypersynchrony* during feeding in infants can have very sharp spike-and-wave configurations (Tharp, 1980) (Fig. 13–4). EEG spikes that grow out of ongoing baseline rhythms or recur with a regular frequency, such as unusually sharp *sleep spindles* as well as

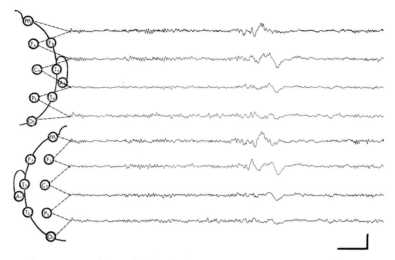

Figure 13–2. Frontal mittens, seen bilaterally, should not be mistaken for pathological sharp-and-slow-wave complexes; they are normal sleep phenomena. Calibration in this and all subsequent figures in this chapter: 1 second, 100 µV. (From Engel, 1984, with permission.)

sleep spindle harmonics, *beta harmonics*, and *alpha harmonics* (Fig. 13–5), should not be confused with epileptic ictal or interictal patterns. Regular rhythmicity is a clue that a prolonged pattern represents a normal variant and not an ictal epileptic EEG discharge. The latter should demonstrate a frequency and amplitude progression, usually beginning with low-voltage fast activity or irregular spikes and evolving to higher-amplitude, slower sharp waves. Notable exceptions are the neonatal ictal discharge, which may assume extremely

regular focal rhythmic patterns, and the 3-Hz spike-and-wave of typical absence seizures (Chapter 6). Bilaterally synchronous, isolated focal sharp waves that are not clearly defined spike-and-wave discharges must be interpreted with caution, because these events, particularly in posterior temporal regions, are often normal (Fig. 13–6).

A number of well-documented *sharp transients of dubious significance* are now recognized as normal variants (Chatrian, 1976; Engel, 1984; PeBenito and Cracco, 1979;

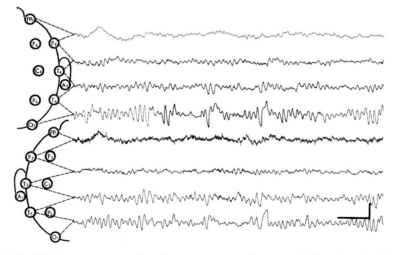

Figure 13–3. Delta de la jeunesse, or occipital youth waves, are normally seen in children through adolescence and may even appear occasionally in adults. They are often asymmetrical but have a characteristic pattern that should not be confused with pathological sharp-and-slow-wave complexes. (From Engel, 1984, with permission.)

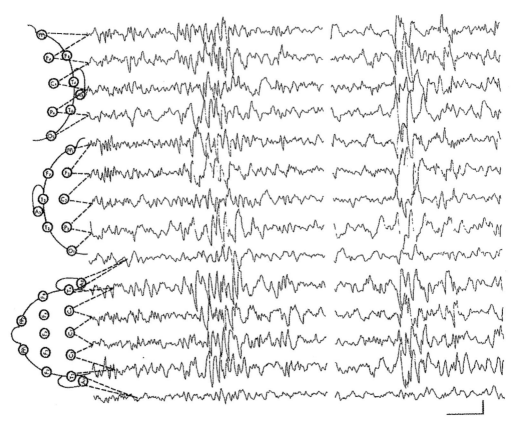

Figure 13–4. Examples of normal vertex sharp waves, recorded from a 4-year-old boy, that have taken on a spike-and-wave-like pattern due to admixture with normal faster sleep rhythms. This EEG pattern resulted in an erroneous diagnosis of epilepsy in this child, who was then unnecessarily placed on phenobarbital.

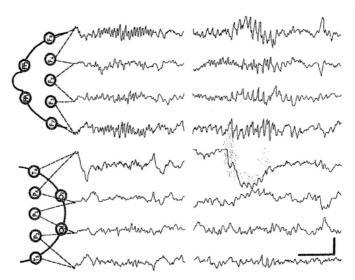

Figure 13–5. *Right side* shows a run of 7-Hz vertex sharp waves with a topographical distribution that exactly matches that of the 14-Hz sleep spindles recorded from the same patient and shown on the *left*. This is a sleep spindle subharmonic and should not be confused with pathological vertex spikes that have more irregular frequencies and different topography. (From Engel, 1984, with permission.)

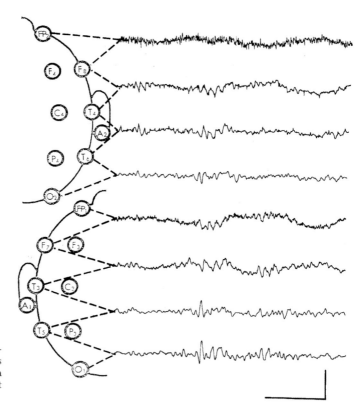

Figure 13–6. Isolated, bilaterally synchronous, sharply contoured slow waves such as these are more likely to be a normal pattern reflecting intermittent drowsiness than an epileptiform event.

Fisch and Spehlmann, 1999; Stern and Engel, 2005; Schomer and Lopes da Silva, 2011; Ebersole and Pedley, 2003). These patterns include the sleep phenomena of *14- and 6-Hz positive spikes (ctenoids)* (Eeg-Olofsson, 1971; Lombroso et al., 1966; Reiher and Klass, 1968) (Fig. 13–7) and *small sharp spikes (SSS)* (Reiher and Klass, 1968), also called *benign epileptiform transients of sleep (BETS)* (White et al., 1977), which have a characteristic low-amplitude, extremely fast, and occasionally polyphasic morphology (Fig. 13–8), as well as phenomena that occur during wakefulness, such as *wicket spikes* (Reiher and Lebel, 1977) (Fig. 13–9), which take on the appearance of mu rhythms in the midtemporal areas, and the *psychomotor variant* or *rhythmic midtemporal discharge (RMTD)* (Eeg-Olofsson et al., 1971) (Fig. 13–10), which often has a characteristic posterior temporal square or flat-top pattern. The *6-Hz spike-and-wave* pattern (Eeg-Olofsson et al., 1971; Thomas and Klass, 1968) (Fig. 13–11), also called *phantom* or *larval spike-and-wave*, is usually maximal in posterior midline derivations, but this pattern has some increased association with epilepsy when

paroxysms are predominantly anterior and of high amplitude (Hughes, 1980). The benign form occurs more often in females, is predominantly occipital or parietal, of lower amplitude, and prominent during drowsiness (*FOLD pattern*), while the more epileptogenic form occurs during waking and is high amplitude, anterior, and more frequent in males (*WHAM pattern*). A *midline theta rhythm (Cigánek rhythm)* (Cigánek, 1961; Westmoreland and Klass, 1986) (Fig. 13–12) is considered to be a nonspecific finding, although it does have a greater-than-expected association with epilepsy.

Normal variants such as 14- and 6-Hz spikes and SSS can lose their characteristic features and look like pathological transients when recorded from special basal electrodes (Figs. 13–8 and 13–13). Therefore, to recognize such spikes as normal variants and not consider them evidence of an epileptic condition, it is essential to use these electrodes in association with independently recorded standard scalp derivations (Chapter 12).

Pathological spikes may not be epileptic. *Pseudoperiodic lateralized epileptiform discharges (PLEDs)* (Chatrian et al., 1964; Cobb,

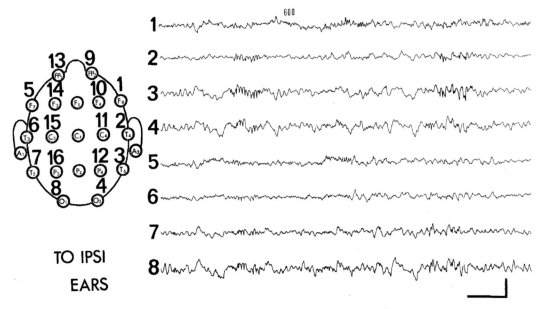

Figure 13–7. Fourteen- and 6-Hz positive spikes are seen during sleep in normal children and are best recorded by common reference montages. They should not be considered evidence of an epilepsy disorder. (From Engel, 1984, with permission.)

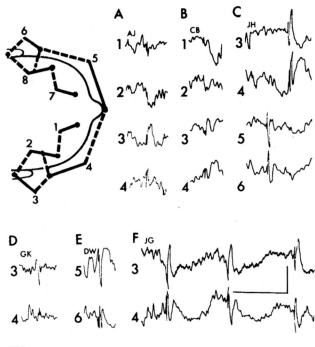

Figure 13–8. Examples of small sharp spikes (SSS) recorded from temporal (*1, 2, 7, 8*) and sphenoidal (*3, 4, 5, 6*) derivations. SSS may be unilateral or bilateral and most commonly occur over the temporal areas during light sleep in nonepileptic individuals. They have a characteristic rapid single or polyspike appearance when recorded from the scalp but appear as much larger spikes when recorded from sphenoidal derivations. These latter basilar transients are often indistinguishable from the spikes of temporal lobe epilepsy. (From Engel et al., 1975, with permission.)

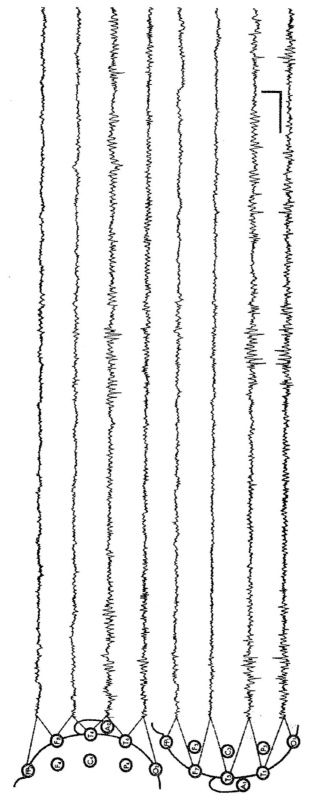

Figure 13–9. Trains of sharp temporal wicket spikes can easily be recognized as normal variants based on their mu-like pattern and regular rhythm. However, isolated transients, like that seen to the far right at T_6, could be mistaken for epileptic spikes. The fact that this transient grows out of the background frequency, even though the ongoing rhythms are not sharp, identifies it as a wicket spike. (From Engel, 1984, with permission.)

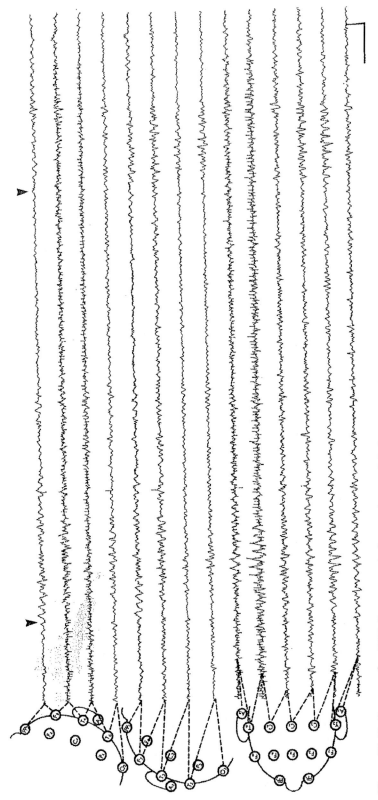

Figure 13–10. Segment of an EEG illustrating a rhythmic midtemporal discharge, or psychomotor variant pattern, that has no clinical correlate. The *first arrow* indicates the beginning of a bilateral event, and the *second arrow* indicates the beginning of an event seen only on the left side. Notice the characteristic flat-topped rhythmic theta waves.

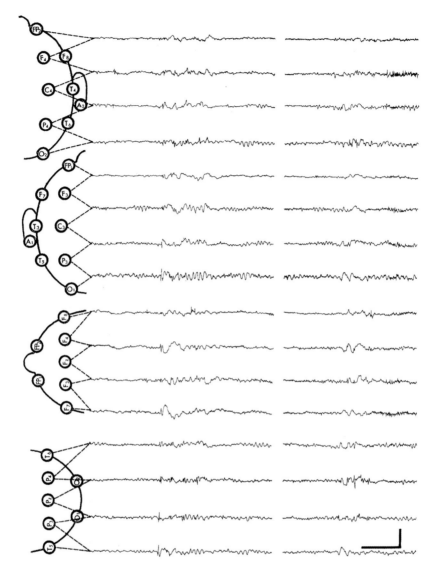

Figure 13–11. Characteristic low-amplitude spike or polyspike discharges followed by a slow wave, repeated at 5–7 Hz, and maximal at P_2, constitute the normal variant known as 6-Hz, phantom, or larval spike-and-wave. This may be mixed at times with bilaterally synchronous theta or delta waves and is not indicative of an epileptic condition. There is evidence, however, that frontal forms with higher amplitude predominating during wakefulness may be associated with epilepsy. (From Engel, 1984, with permission.)

1979; PeBenito and Cracco, 1979) (Fig. 13–14) reflect focal cortical dysfunction that is often but not always associated with epileptic seizures. Bilateral *pseudoperiodic* and true *periodic complexes* as well as *triphasic patterns* are characteristic EEG features of specific cerebral disorders and should not be considered evidence of an epileptic condition (Cooper et al., 1980; Kiloh et al., 1981; Klass and Daly, 1990; Schomer and Lopes da Silva, 2011; Remond,

1978; Fisch and Spehlmann, 1999; Stern and Engel, 2005; Ebersole and Pedley, 2003). Focal EEG spikes occur independently over the occipital lobes in patients with impaired vision due to peripheral lesions (Stillerman et al., 1952) (Fig. 13–15). Spikes, particularly in the centroparietal area (*CP spikes*) (Perlstein et al., 1947) (Fig. 13–16), can be seen in nonepileptic children with *cerebral palsy*, *Rett syndrome* (Robertson et al., 1988), and other diffuse brain

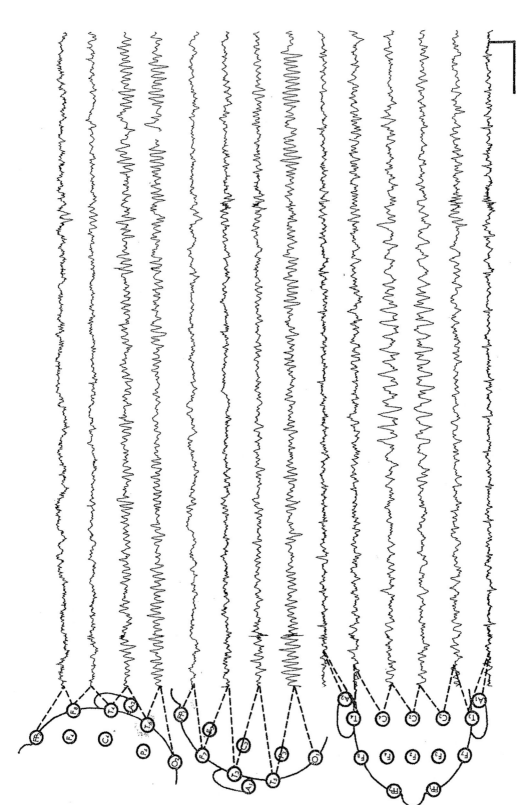

Figure 13–12. Vertex theta activity referred to as the Cigánek rhythm. This normal variant may be notched, as here, resembling spike-and-wave discharge pattern.

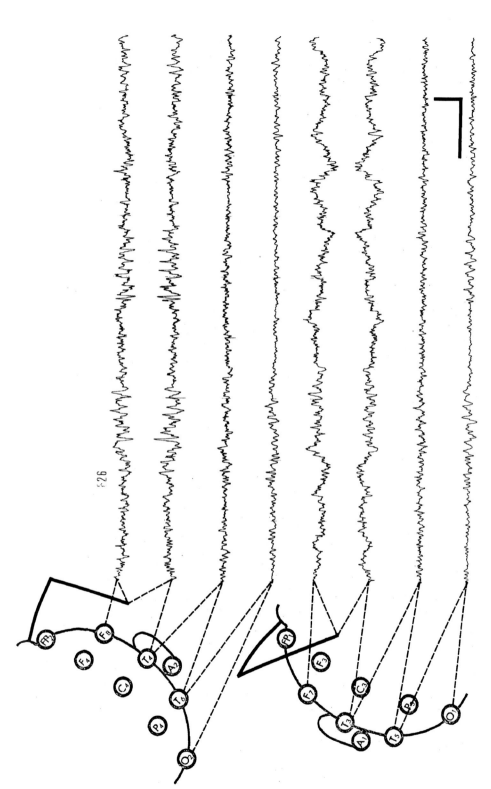

Figure 13–13. Sharp negative transients appear to arise from the right nasopharyngeal electrode. These are actually positive sharp waves coming from the lateral derivations and represent a normal variant, 6-Hz positive spikes. It may be impossible to differentiate between negative mesial temporal and positive lateral temporal transients with the usual nasopharyngeal or sphenoidal montage arrangement unless simultaneous recordings can be obtained from adequate independent lateral temporal derivations, as discussed in Chapter 12. (From Engel, 1984, with permission.)

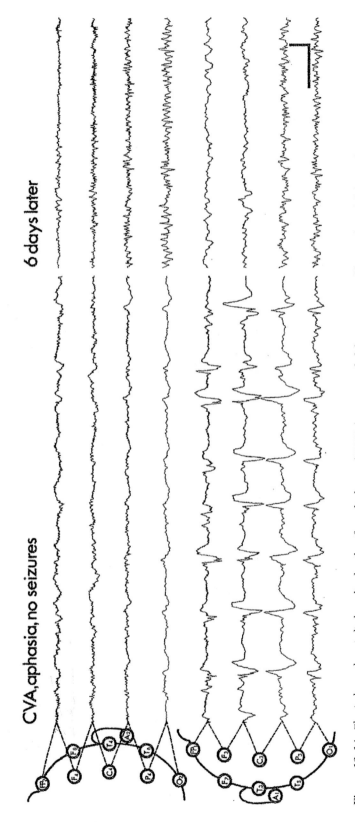

Figure 13–14. Classical pseudoperiodic lateralized epileptiform discharges (PLEDs) were recorded from a 69-year-old man after a left hemisphere cerebral vascular accident (CVA) that produced hemiparesis and aphasia but no seizures. Six days later the PLEDs were no longer seen.

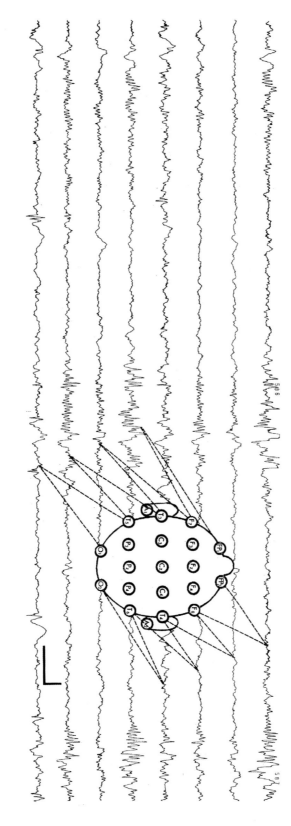

Figure 13–15. Bilaterally independent interictal occipital spikes are seen in a blind child with retrolental fibroplasia. These transients are not evidence of an epilepsy disorder. (From Engel, 1984, with permission.)

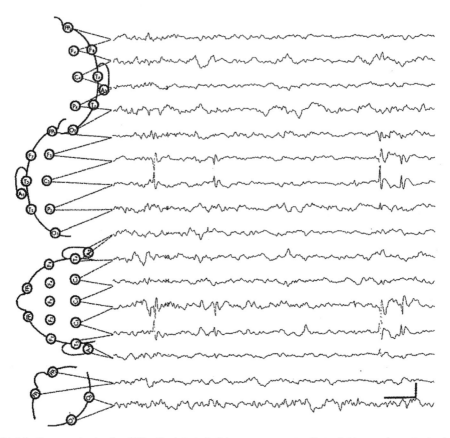

Figure 13–16. Centroparietal spikes (CP spikes) typical of those seen occasionally in children with cerebral palsy. These transients usually do not indicate the presence of an epilepsy disorder.

damage and behavioral disturbances (Kellaway, 1980; Torres, 1981).

In addition to the phenomena mentioned above, any interictal epileptiform EEG pattern may occur in individuals who will never manifest clinical epileptic seizures (Chatrian, 1976; Kellaway, 1980; Zivin and Ajmone-Marsan, 1968). This is particularly true with the characteristic EEG patterns of certain genetic conditions, such as the *absence epilepsies* and *benign childhood epilepsy with centrotemporal spikes*, where the EEG trait is common in relatives who do not have epilepsy (Chapter 7). Consequently, interictal epileptiform EEG transients of any type can never, by themselves, justify a definitive diagnosis of epilepsy. The incidence of epilepsy in children with specific focal EEG spike localizations is shown in Table 8–4. These EEG abnormalities must always be considered in light of all available clinical information.

Photic stimulation can evoke paroxysmal EEG patterns that must be interpreted with

caution. An epileptic *photoparoxysmal (photoconvulsive) response* (Fig. 13–17) consists of clear spike-and-wave or polyspike-and-wave activity recorded over central and frontal as well as occipital regions (Chapter 9). It is not absolutely time-locked to the stimulus frequency, usually continues after the stimulation is terminated, and may be associated with altered consciousness. This response must be distinguished from electroretinal potentials that can be recorded from frontal electrode placements, photochemical responses of silver electrodes, artifacts induced by the stimulator, and two physiological responses that are not indicative of epilepsy: the *photomyogenic response* and *occipital spike driving*.

The photomyogenic *(photomyoclonic)* response (Bickford et al., 1952) (Fig. 13–18) consists of muscular twitching of the eyes, face, and sometimes extremities. EEG-recorded movement and muscle artifacts can resemble frontopolar spread of spike-and-wave

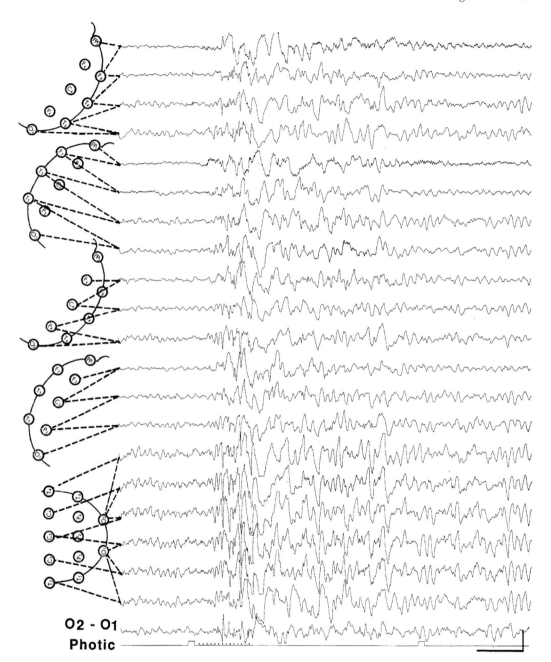

O2 - O1

Photic

Figure 13–17. A photoparoxysmal (photoconvulsive) response to photic stimulation is characterized by high-amplitude sharp and slow transients that are not time-locked to the stimulus and continue after the stimulus train is terminated. This response can be seen in patients with epilepsy, as discussed in Chapter 9.

discharges, but they are time-locked to the stimulation frequency or a subharmonic of it and stop when the stimulus is discontinued. This response is never associated with altered consciousness. A photomyogenic response is commonly seen with sedative drug or alcohol withdrawal and also appears spontaneously in some apparently normal individuals.

Occipital spike driving consists of high-amplitude spike or spike-and-wave discharges that remain limited to the occipital region, are time-locked to the stimulus, and stop when

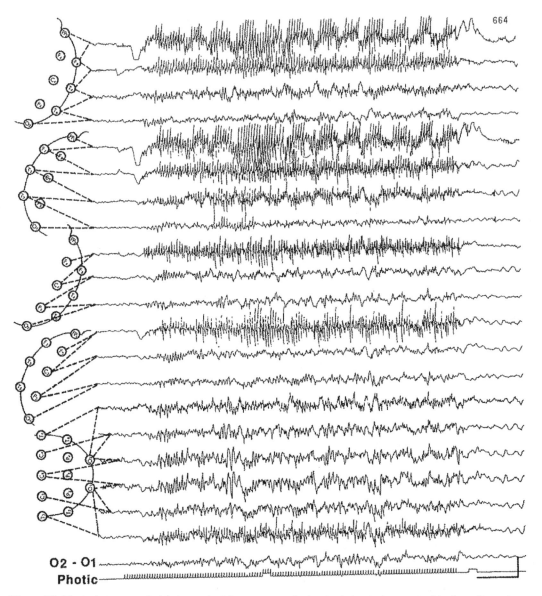

664

O2 - O1
Photic

Figure 13–18. A photomyogenic (photomyoclonic) response to photic stimulation is characterized by frontally predominant sharp transients that are time-locked to the stimulus and end abruptly when the stimulus train is terminated. This response can be seen in certain hyperirritable states, such as sedative drug or alcohol withdrawal, and in normal individuals. It is not indicative of an epilepsy condition.

the stimulus is discontinued (Fig. 13–19). This is an exaggerated but normal visual evoked potential. Normal occipital spike driving must also be distinguished from the enhanced photic driving that occurs only at slow frequencies and is characteristic of *late infantile ceroid lipofuscinosis* (Pampiglione and Harden, 1973) (Chapters 4 and 12).

When ictal EEG patterns are associated with clinical behavior suggestive of an epileptic seizure, a positive diagnosis of epilepsy can be made. When no behavioral correlate of the ictal EEG discharge can be demonstrated, however, such a conclusion is not justified. *Subclinical rhythmic EEG discharges of adults (SREDA)* (Fig. 13–20) resemble ictal EEG patterns

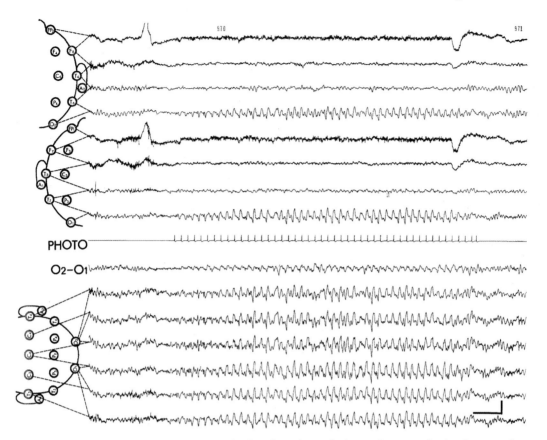

Figure 13–19. Photic stimulation drives high-amplitude spike-and-wave discharges that are confined to the occipital area and time-locked to the stimulation. This occipital spike driving represents enhanced visual evoked potentials and is not indicative of an epilepsy condition. (From Engel, 1984, with permission.)

but occur in individuals who are not epileptic (Westmoreland and Klass, 1981).

EEG Contributions to a Positive Diagnosis of Epilepsy

Characteristic interictal epileptiform EEG transients may provide sufficient information, in combination with seizure description, neuroimaging, and available clinical data, to make a diagnosis of epilepsy with a high degree of confidence. The diagnosis can be made definitively, however, if an ictal event occurs in the EEG laboratory and clear epileptiform ictal EEG discharges can be correlated with clinical behavior typical of the episodes in question.

Any focal or diffuse change in ongoing EEG baseline activity that is inconsistent with normal alterations in consciousness or normal variant patterns may be an ictal discharge. The patient's clinical behavior state must be assessed at this point and abnormalities noted by the EEG technologist during the EEG recording. EEG technologists, therefore, must be trained to recognize EEG and clinical manifestations of seizures (Chapter 6) and be able to provide clear descriptions of ictal events. Each laboratory should have a standard evaluation for technologists to perform in the event a seizure occurs during routine recording (Chapter 12).

Difficulties arise when the patient's habitual seizure occurs during an EEG recording but no clear epileptiform electrical abnormality is seen or the recording is obscured by movement and muscle artifacts. In the latter situation, it may still be possible with appropriate filter settings to recognize underlying ictal EEG patterns that (1) have a different topographic distribution than would be expected from muscle, (2) show a consistent relationship between spikes and waves, (3) demonstrate

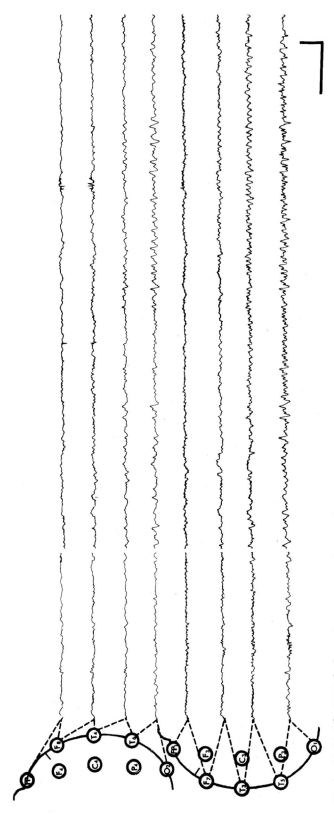

Figure 13–20. This EEG discharge demonstrates evolution with a pattern suggestive of an epileptiform ictal event, although no clinical seizure occurred. Because the patient is an adult without epilepsy, the EEG event should be considered a subclinical rhythmic EEG discharge of adults (SREDA) and not an epileptic seizure. (From Engel, 1984, with permission.)

clear evolution, or (4) are followed by postictal attenuation of preictal rhythms. The last should be expected after generalized tonic-clonic and prolonged focal dyscognitive seizures; however, bilaterally synchronous myoclonic jerking can mimic generalized tonic-clonic seizures without postictal EEG changes and without an associated alteration in consciousness. Focal seizures in clear consciousness and typical absence seizures are usually not associated with postictal EEG suppression.

Lack of epileptiform EEG discharges during a clinical seizure does not necessarily rule out an epilepsy condition. Focal seizures in clear consciousness, particularly those without motor phenomena, usually have no EEG correlates, whereas *epilepsia partialis continua*, focal dyscognitive seizures, and some generalized seizures may be associated with abnormally slow asymmetrical or unusually rhythmic EEG patterns that are not clearly epileptiform (Chapter 6). Furthermore, patients with PNES also may have epileptic seizures.

Additional studies are indicated when routine EEG evaluations yield negative or equivocal results and definitive diagnosis would alter management. Special electrode placements might clarify interictal or ictal EEG transients; interictal and ictal phenomena can be provoked by a variety of activation procedures; and outpatient ambulatory EEG monitoring or inpatient video-EEG monitoring can be undertaken. However, all of these procedures also provide additional opportunities for misdiagnosis, as discussed in Chapter 12.

EEG Contributions to Diagnosis of the Type of Epilepsy

The electrographic features of specific epileptic seizures and epilepsy syndromes are discussed in Chapters 6, 7, and 10. Important diagnostic information can be obtained from EEG-recorded interictal epileptiform transients and baseline rhythmic activity. Most importantly, focal interictal epileptiform or nonepileptiform EEG abnormalities help determine whether a patient has a localized or bilaterally diffuse epileptogenic abnormality. Characteristic interictal epileptiform EEG patterns, as well as the integrity of baseline rhythms, can often distinguish genetic from structural or metabolic epilepsy disorders. In particular, *slow spike-and-wave discharges, independent multifocal spike discharges (IMSD)*, and *generalized paroxysmal fast activity (GPFA)* indicate diffuse brain damage; other EEG patterns suggest epileptic encephalopathies such as *West, Ohtahara*, and *Dravet syndromes* as well as *continuous spike-and-wave during sleep (CSWS)*, including *Landau-Kleffner syndrome*; and specific EEG phenomena are characteristic of certain genetic syndromes, such as the *absence epilepsies* and *benign childhood epilepsy with centrotemporal spikes* (Chapter 7). These EEG findings all contribute greatly to making a definitive diagnosis with prognostic and therapeutic implications.

When and how bilaterally synchronous interictal epileptiform EEG discharges occur with focal cerebral disturbances is of considerable clinical interest. The term *secondary bilateral synchrony* is used to imply that a bilateral EEG discharge actually results from a focal epileptogenic abnormality. The EEG diagnosis of secondary bilateral synchrony is usually made when focal and bilaterally synchronous epileptiform abnormalities coexist in the same tracing or when the bilaterally synchronous discharges appear to have a consistent focal onset. These EEG patterns can reflect a focal abnormality, most often in the frontal lobe (Blume and Pillay, 1985), that rapidly generalizes. However, three other conditions can give rise to the same EEG patterns: (1) diffuse but irregularly distributed structural epileptogenic brain disturbances can cause both focal and generalized epileptiform EEG discharges as well as generalized discharges with focal features (Chapter 7), (2) patients with genetic epilepsies and generalized seizures can occasionally acquire focal epileptogenic lesions and have two diseases (Chapter 5), and (3) the genetic epilepsies associated with generalized spike-and-wave patterns can also exhibit focal frontal interictal spikes or focal frontal ictal onsets that occur with equal frequency from either side (Chapter 7). A discrete EEG focus can occasionally be identified in patients with secondary bilateral synchrony by suppressing the generalized EEG discharges with deep *barbiturate* or *benzodiazepine* anesthesia (Lombroso and Erba, 1970; Morrell, 1978) (Chapter 12); however, these four diagnostic alternatives are usually distinguished on the basis of additional, nonelectrophysiological information.

When a definitive diagnosis cannot be made from clinical data plus an interictal EEG, and further information would alter management, repeat EEGs with sleep may be helpful, but decreasing yield does not justify more than four studies (Salinsky et al., 1987). More often, it is appropriate to obtain an EEG recording during one or several ictal events. If spontaneous seizures occur frequently or can easily be provoked (Chapter 9), it may be possible to obtain ictal recordings in the routine EEG laboratory. In many cases, however, it is necessary or more expedient to use inpatient VEM for this purpose (Chapter 12). Ambulatory recording is usually inadequate for characterizing the type of epileptic seizure, and in-hospital direct or telemetry EEG with video monitoring is recommended in most situations (Engel et al., 1985; Gotman et al., 1985; American Clinical Neurophysiology Society, 2008).

A definitive diagnosis of seizure type and epilepsy syndrome can usually be made with inpatient VEM, and often this diagnosis results in an alteration in treatment plan and reevaluation of prognosis (Porter et al., 1977). Although it is best to evaluate spontaneous ictal events while patients are taking their usual antiseizure medications, seizures may not occur naturally in the hospital (Riley et al., 1981). In this case, antiseizure medications can be tapered; however, in rare instances, doing so precipitates atypical epileptic seizures that confound diagnosis when their reactive nature is not recognized (Engel and Crandall, 1983; Gotman and Marciani, 1985; Spencer et al., 1981). It is then useful for family members or others close to the patient to review the video of the ictal behavior and determine whether it resembles seizures that occur at home.

That ictal events consistently begin focally is sufficient evidence for diagnosis of a localized epileptogenic abnormality. Impairment of consciousness during a focal seizure suggests bilateral limbic involvement. Seizures that appear to be generalized from the start, on the other hand, do not necessarily indicate a generalized epileptogenic disturbance, because the focal onset of a secondarily generalized seizure may not be seen from scalp recording. The focal nature of these seizures can sometimes be revealed by focal or unilateral postictal depression or slow activity on the EEG, as well as by focal postictal signs or symptoms.

The recording of ictal events is of particular clinical value in distinguishing among brief lapses of consciousness in childhood that reflect the typical absences of genetic absence epilepsies, atypical absences that occur with diffuse brain dysfunction, as seen in the Lennox-Gastaut syndrome, and focal dyscognitive seizures without motor signs that indicate a localized abnormality of the brain (see Table 7–1). Inpatient VEM is also useful for distinguishing between typical focal dyscognitive seizures with a discrete focal onset and atypical events that are due to multifocal or diffuse cerebral lesions (Chapter 6). The former are more amenable to surgical therapy (Chapter 16). Of less interest, but still worthwhile in some patients, is the use of ictal recording to diagnose recently recognized epilepsy syndromes that represent subtypes of broader categories (Chapter 7). In general, a definitive diagnosis allows more accurate prognoses, suggests different approaches to management, indicates a need for genetic counseling, and accumulates data for more accurate classification and categorization of epilepsy syndromes (Berg et al., 2010).

USE OF FUNCTIONAL IMAGING IN THE DIFFERENTIAL DIAGNOSIS OF EPILEPSY

Theoretically, it is possible to distinguish epileptic seizures from PNES without EEG by using functional neuroimaging. When an area of inactivity (hypometabolism on *positron emission tomography* [PET] or hypoperfusion on *single-photon emission computed tomography* [SPECT] and *functional magnetic resonance imaging* [fMRI]) becomes hyperactive (hypermetabolism on PET or hyperperfusion on SPECT and fMRI), this could be pathognomonic of an epileptic condition. Although ictal SPECT is now commonly used to help localize the epileptogenic region for surgical treatment (Chapters 12 and 16), ictal PET is very difficult to obtain because of the short half-life of positron-emitting tracers, and ictal fMRI remains a research tool at present (Engel et al., 1982; 1983; 1985; Jackson et al., 1994; Kazemi et al., 2008). These approaches have not yet found usefulness in differential diagnosis per se. If comparison of interictal and ictal functional neuroimaging is used to determine whether subtle behaviors represent epileptic seizures or PNES, it is also necessary to perform a scan with the patient mimicking the behavior voluntarily to ensure that any changes on the "ictal" study do not merely reflect patterns of normal activation.

SUMMARY AND CONCLUSIONS

It is exceedingly important to recognize nonepileptic events that can be mistaken for epilepsy. An unwarranted diagnosis of epilepsy can cause a patient to be denied appropriate therapy and create additional disabilities due to the stigma and other psychosocial consequences of being labeled epileptic. In general, when the diagnosis is in doubt, it is prudent to wait until subsequent events clarify the issue while warning the patient to avoid precipitating factors and potentially dangerous situations.

The most common cause of an erroneous diagnosis of epilepsy is overreading of the EEG. Many normal and pathological EEG transients resemble interictal spikes but are not indicative of an epilepsy condition. Furthermore, epileptiform interictal and even ictal events can occur, under special circumstances, in patients who do not and never will have epilepsy. A diagnosis of epilepsy should always be based on clinical judgment that takes into account all available information. The EEG can be definitively diagnostic, however, if an epileptic seizure is recorded and ictal EEG changes are associated with behavior characteristic of the habitual episode in question.

Differential diagnosis of epilepsy requires an awareness of the great number of systemic, neurological, and psychogenic disturbances that give rise to transient symptoms mimicking epilepsy. Conversely, familiarity with the many manifestations of epilepsy reduces the risk of misdiagnosis when epileptic symptoms resemble those of other disorders. Of particular concern in the distinction between epileptic and nonepileptic paroxysmal events is the recognition of PNES. PNES can occur in patients with epilepsy, and their demonstration does not rule out the concurrent existence of a chronic epilepsy condition.

Reactive epileptic seizures should not be mistaken for a chronic epilepsy condition, because these symptoms do not recur once the transient provocative stress or cerebral insult is removed. Provoked generalized tonic-clonic seizures that occur in isolation (e.g., febrile seizures and seizures induced by sleep deprivation, alcohol or sedative drug withdrawal, use of convulsant drugs, and acute head trauma), as well as recurrent seizures that occur in association with reversible infectious, toxic, or metabolic processes and are limited to the period of systemic illness, need not be considered evidence of an epilepsy disorder. When seizures result from a remediable structural lesion, such as a brain tumor, and stop when the lesion is adequately treated or removed, the patient does not have epilepsy.

Differential diagnosis of epileptic seizure type and an epilepsy syndrome, if present, determines treatment and prognosis. Incorrect diagnosis is a common cause of uncontrolled seizures. When description of the habitual ictal events, interictal EEG, neuroimaging, and additional clinical information are insufficient, referral to an epilepsy center for VEM can result in definitive diagnostic information. Inpatient VEM is recommended when the diagnosis is in doubt and seizures do not respond to treatment.

Clinical research could do much to better define conditions that are frequently confused with epilepsy, particularly those that respond to antiseizure drugs, often coexist with epilepsy, and share genetic substrates. The various forms of PNES should be characterized and their relationship to epilepsy clarified. Reactive seizures will always pose a challenge to diagnosticians, but the risk factors for choosing to treat or not to treat under different circumstances could be more clearly established. Management and prognosis will necessarily improve as differential diagnosis becomes based more on neurobiological than on phenomenological grounds.

REFERENCES

American Academy of Sleep Medicine (2005). The International Classification of Sleep Disorders: Diagnostic and Coding Manual, 2nd ed. Westchester, IL: American Academy of Sleep Medicine, pp. 139–147.

American Clinical Neurophysiology Society (2008). Guideline 12: Guidelines for long-term monitoring for epilepsy. J Clin Neurophysiol 25:170–180.

American Psychiatric Association (2000). Diagnostic and Statistical Manual of Mental Disorders, 4th ed, with text revision (DSM– IV-TR). Washington, DC: American Psychiatric Association.

Andermann, E, and Andermann, F (1987). Migraine-epilepsy relationships: Epidemiological and genetic aspects. In Migraine and Epilepsy. Edited by F Andermann and E Lugaresi. Boston: Butterworths, pp. 281–291.

Andermann, F (1987). Clinical features of migraine-epilepsy syndromes. In Migraine and Epilepsy. Edited by F Andermann and E Lugaresi. Boston: Butterworths, pp. 3–30.

Andermann, F, and Andermann, E (1986). Excessive startle syndromes: Startle disease, jumping and startle epilepsy. Adv Neurol 43:321–338.

Andermann, F, and Lugaresi, E (eds) (1987). Migraine and Epilepsy. Boston: Butterworths.

Andermann, F, Aicardi, J, and Vigevano, F (eds) (1995). Alternating Hemiplegia of Childhood. New York: Raven Press.

Apfelbaum, RI (1983). Trigeminal and glossopharyngeal neuralgia and hemifacial spasm. In The Clinical Neurosciences. Edited by RN Rosenberg, RG Grossman, SS Schochet, Jr, ER Heinz, and WD Willis, Jr. New York: Churchill Livingstone, pp. 1251–1267.

Avidan, AY, and Kaplis, N (2010). The parasomnias: Epidemiology, clinical features, and diagnostic approach. Clin Chest Med 31:353–370.

Bazil, CW (2008). Sensory disorders. In Epilepsy: A Comprehensive Textbook, 2nd ed. Edited by J Engel, Jr, and TA Pedley. Philadelphia: Lippincott Williams & Wilkins, pp. 2779–2782.

Beghi, E, Carpio, A, Forsgren, L, Hesdorffer, DC, Malmgren, K, Sander, JW, Tomson, T, and Hauser, WA (2010). Recommendation for a definition of acute symptomatic seizure. Epilepsia 51:671–675.

Benbadis, SR, Agrawal, V, Tatu, WO 4th (2011). How many patients with psychogenic nonepileptic seizures also have epilepsy? Neurology 57:915–917.

Benson, DF, Miller, BL, and Signer, SF (1986). Dual personality associated with epilepsy. Arch Neurol 43:471–474.

Berg, AT, Berkovic, SF, Brodie, MJ, Buchhalter, J, Cross, JH, van Emde Boas, W, Engel, J, Jr, French, J, Glauser, TA, Mathern, GW, Moshé, SL, Nordli, D, Jr, Plouin, P, and Scheffer, IE (2010). Revised terminology and concepts for organization of seizures and epilepsies: Report of the ILAE Commission on Classification and Terminology, 2005–2009. Epilepsia 51:676–685.

Bernat, JL (2010). The ethics of diagnosing nonepileptic seizures with placebo infusion. Virtual Mentor 12:854–859.

Bickford, RG, Sem-Jacobsen, CW, White, PT, and Daly, D (1952). Some observations on the mechanism of photic and photo-Metrazol activation. Electroencephalogr Clin Neurophysiol 4:275–282.

Blume, WT, and Pillay, N (1985). Electrographic and clinical correlates of secondary, bilateral synchrony. Epilepsia 26:636–641.

Bostick, NA, Sade, R, Levine, MA, and Stewart, DM, Jr (2008). Placebo use in clinical practice: Report of the American Medical Association Council on Ethical and Judicial Affairs. J Clin Ethics 19:58–61.

Broughton, R (1982). Polygraphic recordings of sleep and sleep disorders. In Electroencephalography: Basic Principles, Clinical Applications and Related Fields Edited by E Niedermeyer and F Lopes da Silva. Baltimore: Urban & Schwarzenberg, pp. 571–598.

Brown, RJ, and Trimble, MR (2008). Dissociative disorders. In Epilepsy: A Comprehensive Textbook, 2nd ed. Edited by J Engel, Jr, and TA Pedley. Philadelphia: Lippincott Williams & Wilkins, pp. 2819–2827.

Brust, JCM (2008). Alcohol and drug abuse. In Epilepsy: A Comprehensive Textbook, 2nd ed. Edited by J Engel, Jr, and TA Pedley. Philadelphia: Lippincott Williams & Wilkins, pp. 2683–2687.

Bullard, DE (1987). Diencephalic seizures: Responsiveness to bromocriptine and morphine. Ann Neurol 21:609–611.

Camfield, PR, Metrakos, K, and Andermann, F (1978). Basilar migraine, seizures and severe epileptiform EEG abnormalities. Neurology 28:584–588.

Caplan, LR (1980). "Top of the basilar" syndrome. Neurology 30:72–79.

Caplan, LR (1985). Transient global amnesia. In Clinical Neuropsychology (Handbook of Clinical Neurology, Vol 45). Edited by PJ Vinken, GW Bruyn, and HL Klawans. Amsterdam: Elsevier, pp. 205–218.

Charcot, JM (1886). Leçonssur les Maladies du Système Nerveux, Recueillieset Publiéespar Bourneville, Tome I. Paris. [Oeuvres Complètes, I]

Chatrian, GE (1976). Paroxysmal patterns in "normal" subjects. In The Normal EEG Throughout Life: The EEG of the Waking Adult (Handbook of Electroencephalography and Clinical Neurophysiology, Vol 6A). Edited by GE Chatrian and GC Lairy. Edited by A Rémond., pp. 114–122.

Chatrian, GE, Shaw, CM, and Leffman, H (1964). The significance of periodic lateralized epileptiform discharges in EEG: An electrographic clinical and pathological study. Electroencephalogr Clin Neurophysiol 17:177–193.

Cigánek, L (1961). Theta-discharges in the middle-line: EEG symptom of temporal lobe epilepsy. Electroencephalogr Clin Neurophysiol 13:669–672.

Cobb, WA (1979). Evidence on the periodic mechanism in herpes simplex encephalitis. Electroencephalogr Clin Neurophysiol 46:345–350.

Cohen, RJ, and Suter, C (1982). Hysterical seizures—Suggestion as a provocative EEG test. Ann Neurol 11:391–395.

Cooper, R, Osselton, JW, and Shaw, JC (1980). EEG Technology, 3rd ed. London: Butterworths.

Crompton, DE, and Berkovic, SF (2009). The borderland of epilepsy: Clinical and molecular features of phenomena that mimic epileptic seizures. Lancet Neurol 8:370–381.

Dalla Bernardina, B, Capovilla, G, Trevisan, E, Colamaria, V, Andrighetto, G, Fontana, E, and Tassinari, CA (1987). Alternating hemiplegia in childhood. In Migraine and Epilepsy. Edited by F Andermann and E Lugaresi. Boston: Butterworths, pp. 189–201.

Dauvilliers, Y, Arnulf, I, and Mignot, E (2007). Narcolepsy with cataplexy. Lancet 369:499–511.

Delgado-Escueta, AV, Mattson, RH, King, L, Goldensohn, ES, Spiegel, H, Madsen, J, Crandall, P, Dreifuss, F, and Porter, RJ (1981). Special report: The nature of aggression during epileptic seizures. N Engl J Med 305:711–716.

Derry, CP, Duncan, JS, and Berkovic, SF (2006). Paroxysmal motor disorders of sleep: The clinical spectrum and differentiation from epilepsy. Epilepsia 47:1775–1791.

Dib-Hajj, SD, Cummins, TR, Black, JA, and Waxman, SG (2007). From genes to pain: Na 1.7 and human pain disorders. Trends Neurosci 30:555–563.

Ebersole, JS (1986). Ambulatory EEG: Telemetered and cassette-recorded. Adv Neurol 46:139–155.

Ebersole, JS, and Pedley, TA (eds) (2003). Current Practice of Clinical Electroencephalography, 3rd ed. Philadelphia: Lippincott Williams & Wilkins.

Eeg-Olofsson, O (1971). The development of the electro-encephalogram in normal children from the age of 1 through 15 years: 14 and 6 Hz positive spike phenomenon. Neuropaediatrie 2:405–427.

Eeg-Olofsson, O, Petersen, I, and Sellden, U (1971). The development of the electroencephalogram in normal children from the age of 1 through 15 years: Paroxysmal activity. Neuropaediatrie 2:375–404.

Elliot, FA (1978). Neurological aspects of antisocial behavior. In The Psychopath: A Comprehensive Study of Antisocial Disorders and Behaviors. Edited by WH Reid. New York: Brunner/Mazel, pp. 146–189.

Engel, GL (1962). Fainting. Springfield, IL: Charles C Thomas.

Engel, J, Jr (1980). Respiration-linked "limbic spindles": Vibration artifact recorded from nasopharyngeal and intracerebral electrodes. Electroencephalogr Clin Neurophysiol 49:366–372.

Engel, J, Jr (1984). A practical guide for routine EEG studies in epilepsy. J Clin Neurophysiol 1:109–142.

Engel, J, Jr, and Crandall, PH (1983). Falsely localizing ictal onsets with depth EEG telemetry during anticonvulsant withdrawal. Epilepsia 24:344–355.

Engel, J, Jr, Driver, MV, and Falconer, MA (1975). Electrophysiological correlates of pathology and surgical results in temporal lobe epilepsy. Brain 98:129–156.

Engel, J, Jr, Ludwig, BI, and Fetell, M (1978a). Prolonged partial complex status epilepticus: EEG and behavioral observations. Neurology 28:863–869.

Engel, J, Jr, Jerrett, S, Niedermeyer, E, Schenk, G, Gucer, G, and Burnite, R (1978b). "Limbic spindles": A re-appraisal. Electroencephalogr Clin Neurophysiol 44:389–392.

Engel, J, Jr, Kuhl, DE, and Phelps, ME (1982). Patterns of human local cerebral glucose metabolism during epileptic seizures. Science 218:64–66.

Engel, J, Jr, Kuhl, DE, Phelps, ME, Rausch, R, and Nuwer, M (1983). Local cerebral metabolism during partial seizures. Neurology 33:400–413.

Engel, J, Jr, Ebersole, JS, Burchfiel, JL, Gates, JR, Gotman, J, Homan, RW, Ives, JR, King,DW, Sato, S, and Wilkus, RJ (1985). American Electroencephalographic Society guidelines for long-term neurodiagnostic monitoring in epilepsy. J Clin Neurophysiol 2:419–452.

Ettinger, AB, Bird, JM, and Kanner, AM (2008). Panic disorder and hyperventilation syndrome. In Epilepsy: A Comprehensive Textbook, 2nd ed. Edited by J Engel, Jr, and TA Pedley. Philadelphia: Lippincott Williams & Wilkins, pp. 2829–2836.

Fahn, S, and Frucht, SJ (2008). Movement disorders. In Epilepsy: A Comprehensive Textbook, 2nd ed. Edited by J Engel, Jr, and TA Pedley. Philadelphia: Lippincott Williams & Wilkins, pp. 2771–2778.

Fisch, BJ, and Spehlmann, R (1999). EEG Primer, 3rd ed. Amsterdam: Elsevier/North-Holland Biomedical Press.

Fisher, CM, and Adams, RD (1964). Transient global amnesia. Acta Neurol Scand 40(suppl 9): 1–83.

Gastaut, H (1974). Syncopes: Generalized anoxic cerebral seizures. In The Epilepsies (Handbook of Clinical Neurology, Vol 5). Edited by O Magnus and AM Lorentz de Haas. Amsterdam: North Holland, pp. 815–835.

Gastaut, H, and Broughton, R (1965). A clinical and polygraphic study of episodic phenomena during sleep: Academic address. Recent Adv Biol Psychiatry 7:198–221.

Gastaut, H, and Broughton, R (1972). Epileptic Seizures: Clinical and Electrographic Features, Diagnosis and Treatment. Springfield, IL: Charles C Thomas.

Gastaut, H, and Gastaut, Y (1958). Electroencephalographic and clinical study of anoxic convulsions in children: Their location within the group of infantile convulsions and their differentiation from epilepsy. Electroencephalogr Clin Neurophysiol 10:607–620.

Gates, JR (1987). Psychogenic seizures. MerrittPutnam Q4(1): 3–13.

George, MS, and Mula, M (2008). Obsessive-compulsive behavior. In Epilepsy: A Comprehensive Textbook, 2nd ed. Edited by J Engel, Jr, and TA Pedley. Philadelphia: Lippincott Williams & Wilkins, pp. 2837–2840.

Golden, GS, and French, JH (1975). Basilar artery migraine in young children. Pediatrics 56:722–726.

Goldman, AM, Glasscock, E, Yoo, J, Chen, TT, Klassen, TL, and Noebels, JL (2009). Arrhythmia in heart and brain: KCNQ1 mutations link epilepsy and sudden unexplained death. Sci Transl Med 14:1–11.

Goodenough, DJ, Fariello, RG, Annis, BL, and Chun, RW (1978). Familial and acquired paroxysmal dyskinesias: A proposed clarification with delineation of clinical features. Arch Neurol 35:827–831.

Goodwin, DW, Crane, JB, and Guze, SB (1969). Alcoholic "blackouts": A review and clinical study of 100 alcoholics. Am J Psychiatry 126:191–198.

Gotman, J, and Marciani, MG (1985). Electroencephalographic spiking activity, drug levels, and seizure occurrence in epileptic patients. Ann Neurol 17:597–603.

Gotman, J, Ives, JR, and Gloor, P (eds) (1985). Long-term monitoring in epilepsy. Electroencephalogr Clin Neurophysiol Suppl 37.

Griffith, N, Engel, J, Jr, and Bandler, R (1987). Ictal and enduring interictal disturbances in emotional behaviour in an animal model of temporal lobe epilepsy. Brain Res 400:360–364.

Guilleminault, C, and Dement, WC (eds) (1986). Narcolepsy. Sleep9:99–291.

Guilleminault, C, and Silvestri, R (1982). Disorders of arousal and epilepsy during sleep. In Sleep and Epilepsy. Edited by MB Sterman, MN Shouse, and P Passouant. New York: Academic Press, pp. 513–531.

Guilleminault, C, Phillips, R, and Dement, WC (1975). A syndrome of hypersomnia with automatic behavior. Electroencephalogr Clin Neurophysiol 38:403–413.

Hartmann, HA, Colom, LV, Sutherland, ML, and Noebels, JL (1999). Selective localization of cardiac SCN5A sodium channels in limbic regions of rat brain. Nat Neurosci 2:593–595.

Hinge, HH, Jensen, TS, Kjaer, M, Marquardsen, J, and Olivarius, BdF (1986). The prognosis of transient cerebral ischemia. Acta Neurol Scand 43:673–676.

Hirsch, LJ, Andermann, F, and Pedley, TA (2008). Differential diagnosis. In Epilepsy: A Comprehensive Textbook, 2nd ed. Edited by J Engel, Jr, and TA Pedley. Philadelphia: Lippincott Williams & Wilkins, pp. 773–782.

Hockaday, JM, and Whitty, CWM (1969). Factors determining the electroencephalogram in migraine: A study of 560 patients according to the clinical type of migraine. Brain 92:769–788.

Holmes, GL (1985). Neonatal seizures. In Recent Advances in Epilepsy 2. Edited by TA Pedley and BS Meldrum. New York: Churchill Livingstone, pp. 207–235.

Hughes, JR (1980). Two forms of the 6/sec spike and wave complex. Electroencephalogr Clin Neurophysiol 48:535–550.

Ingvar, DH, and Lundberg, N (1961). Paroxysmal symptoms in intracranial hypertension, studied with ventricular fluid pressure recording and electroencephalography. Brain 84:446–459.

Jackson, GD, Connelly, A, Cross, JH, Gordon, I, and Gadian, DG (1994). Functional magnetic resonance imaging of focal seizures. Neurology 44:850–856.

Jannetta, PJ (1977). Observations on the etiology of trigeminal neuralgia, hemifacial spasm, acoustic nerve dysfunction and glossopharyngeal neuralgia: Definitive microsurgical treatment and results in 117 patients. Neurochirurgia 20:145–154.

Kanner, AM, LaFrance,WC, Jr, and Betts, T (2008). Psychogenic non-epileptic seizures. In Epilepsy: A Comprehensive Textbook, 2nd ed. Edited by J Engel, Jr, and TA Pedley. Philadelphia: Lippincott Williams & Wilkins, pp. 2795–2810.

Kaplan, PW, and Basaria, S (2008). Metabolic and endocrine disorders resembling seizures. In Epilepsy: A Comprehensive Textbook, 2nd ed. Edited by J Engel, Jr, and TA Pedley. Philadelphia: Lippincott Williams & Wilkins, pp. 2713–2721.

Kazemi, NJ, O'Brien, TJ, Cascino, GD, and So, EL (2008). Single photon emission computed tomography. In Epilepsy: A Comprehensive Textbook, 2nd ed. Edited by J Engel, Jr, and TA Pedley. Philadelphia: Lippincott Williams & Wilkins, pp. 965–973.

Kellaway, P (1980). The incidence, significance and natural history of spike foci in children. In Current Clinical Neurophysiology: Update on EEG and Evoked Potentials. Edited by RE Henry. Amsterdam: Elsevier/North Holland, pp. 151–175.

Kiloh, LG, McComas, AJ, Osselton, JW, and Upton, ARM (1981). Clinical Electroencephalography, 4th ed. London: Butterworths.

King, DW, Gallagher, BB, Murvin, AJ, Smith, DB, Marcus, DJ, Hartlage, LC, and Ward, LC, III (1982). Pseudoseizures: Diagnostic evaluation. Neurology 32:18–23.

Kirstein, L, and Silfveskiold, BP (1958). A family with emotionally precipitated "drop seizures." Acta Psychiatr Neurol Scand 33:471–476.

Klass, DW, and Daly, DD (eds) (1990). Current Practice of Clinical Electroencephalography. New York: Raven Press, 1979. See also Daly, DD, and Pedley, TA (eds): Current Practice of Clinical Electroencephalography, 2nd ed. New York: Raven Press.

Kodama, N, Aoki, Y, Hiraga, H, Wada, T, and Suzuki, J (1979). Electroencephalographic findings in children with moyamoya disease. Arch Neurol 36:16–19.

Kushner, MJ, and Hauser, WA (1985). Transient global amnesia: A case-control study. Ann Neurol 18:684–691.

Lance, JW (1977). Familial paroxysmal dystonic choreoathetosis and its differentiation from related syndromes. Ann Neurol 2:285–293.

Lesser, RP (1985). Psychogenic seizures. In Recent Advances in Epilepsy 2. Edited by TA Pedley and BS Meldrum. New York: Churchill Livingstone, pp. 273–296.

Lesser, RP, Lüders, H, Dinner, DS, and Morris, HH (1985). Epileptic seizures due to thrombotic and embolic cerebrovascular disease in older patients. Epilepsia 26:622–630.

Lingam, S, Wilson, J, and Hart, EW (1981). Hereditary stiff-baby syndrome. Am J Dis Child 135:909–911.

Lombroso, CT, and Lerman, P (1967). Breathholding spells (cyanotic and pallid infantile syncope). Pediatrics 39:565–581.

Lombroso, CT, and Erba, G (1970). Primary and secondary bilateral synchrony in epilepsy: A clinical and electroencephalographic study. Arch Neurol 22:321–334.

Lombroso, CT, Schwartz, IH, Clark, DM, Muench, H, and Barry, J (1966). Ctenoids in healthy youths: Controlled study of 14-and6-per-second positive spiking. Neurology 16:1152–1158.

Low, PA (1987). Autonomic neuropathy. Semin Neurol 7:49–57.

Lugaresi, E, Cirignotta, F, Coccagna, G, and Montagna, P (1986). Nocturnal myoclonus and restless legs syndrome. Adv Neurol 43:295–307.

Mahowald, MW, and Schenck, CH (2008). Sleep disorders. In Epilepsy: A Comprehensive Textbook, 2nd ed. Edited by J Engel, Jr, and TA Pedley. Philadelphia: Lippincott Williams & Wilkins, pp. 2757–2764.

Mark, VH, and Ervin, FR (1970). Violence and the Brain. New York: Harper & Row.

Matthews, WB (1975). Paroxysmal symptoms in multiple sclerosis. J Neurol Neurosurg Psychiatry 38:619–623.

Mattson, RH (1980). Value of intensive monitoring. In Advances in Epileptology: Xth Epilepsy International Symposium. Edited by JA Wada and JK Penry. New York: Raven Press, pp. 43–51.

Mattson, RH (1983). Seizures associated with alcohol use and alcohol withdrawal. In Epilepsy: Diagnosis and Management. Edited by TR Browne and RG Feldman. Boston: Little, Brown & Co, pp. 325–332.

Mayeux, R, Alexander, MD, Benson, DF, Brandt, J, and Rosen, J (1979). Poriomania. Neurology 29:1616–1619.

Mesulam, MM (1981). Dissociative states with abnormal temporal lobe EEG: Multiple personality and the illusion of possession. Arch Neurol 38:176–181.

Miller, JW, Yanagihara, T, Petersen, RC, and Klass, DW (1987). Transient global amnesia and epilepsy: Electroencephalographic distinction. Arch Neurol 44:629–633.

Monroe, RR (1978). Brain Dysfunction in Aggressive Criminals. Lexington, MA: Lexington Books.

Morrell, F (1978). Aspects of experimental epilepsy. 1977. In Modern Perspectives in Epilepsy: Proceedings of the Inaugural Symposium of the Canadian League Against Epilepsy. Edited by JA Wada. Montreal: Eden Press, pp. 24–75.

Pampiglione, G, and Harden, A (1973). Neurophysiological identification of a late infantile form of neuronal lipidosis. J Neurol Neurosurg Psychiatry 36:68–74.

Panayiotopoulos, CP (1987). Difficulties in differentiating migraine and epilepsy based on clinical and EEG findings. In Migraine and Epilepsy. Edited by F Andermann and E Lugaresi. Boston: Butterworths, pp. 31–46.

Parkes, JD (1982). Narcolepsy. In Pseudoseizures. Edited by TL Riley and A Roy. Baltimore: Williams & Wilkins, pp. 62–82.

PeBenito, R, and Cracco, J (1979). Periodic lateralized epileptiform discharges in infants and children. Ann Neurol 6:47–50.

Pedley, TA, and Guilleminault, C (1977). Episodic nocturnal wanderings responsive to anticonvulsant drug therapy. Ann Neurol 2:30–35.

Penfield, W, and Jasper, H (1954). Epilepsy and the Functional Anatomy of the Human Brain. Boston: Little, Brown & Co.

Perlstein, MA, Gibbs, EL, and Gibbs, FA (1947). The electroencephalogram in infantile cerebral palsy. In Epilepsy (Proceedings of the Association for Research in Nervous and Mental Disease, Research Publications, Vol 26). Edited by WG Lennox, HH Merritt, and TE Bamford. Baltimore: Williams & Wilkins, pp. 377–384.

Porter, RJ, Penry, JK, and Lacy, JR (1977). Diagnostic and therapeutic reevaluation of patients with intractable epilepsy. Neurology 27:1006–1011.

Pritchard, PB, III, Wannamaker, BB, Sagel, J, and Daniel, CM (1985). Serum prolactin and cortisol levels in evaluation of pseudoepileptic seizures. Ann Neurol 18:87–89.

Quigg, MS, and Bleck, TP (2008). Syncope. In Epilepsy: A Comprehensive Textbook, 2nd ed. Edited by J Engel, Jr, and TA Pedley. Philadelphia: Lippincott Williams & Wilkins, pp. 2699–2711.

Ramani, V (1987). Intensive monitoring of psychogenic seizures, aggression, and dyscontrol syndromes. Adv Neurol 46:203–217.

Ramsay, RE, Cohen, A, and Brown, MC (1993). Coexisting epilepsy and non-epileptic seizures. In Non-epileptic Seizures, 1st ed. Edited by AJ Rowan and JR Gates. Stoneham, MA: Butterworth-Heinemann, pp. 47–54.

Reiher, J, and Klass, DW (1968). Two common EEG patterns of doubtful clinical significance. Med Clin N Am 52:933–940.

Reiher, J, and Lebel, M (1977). Wicket spikes: Clinical correlates of a previously undescribed EEG pattern. Can J Neurosci 4:39–47.

Remond, A (ed) (1978). Handbook of Electroencephalography and Clinical Neurophysiology, Vols 1–16. Amsterdam: Elsevier/North Holland.

Rickler, KC (1982). Episodic dyscontrol. In Psychiatric Aspects of Neurological Disease, Vol II. Edited by DF Benson and D Blumer. New York: Grune & Stratton, pp. 49–73.

Riley, TL (1982). Syncope and hyperventilation. In Pseudoseizures. Edited by TL Riley and A Roy. Baltimore: Williams & Wilkins, pp. 34–61.

Riley, TL, Porter, RJ, White, BG, and Penry, JK (1981). The hospital experience and seizure control. Neurology 31:921–915.

Robertson, R, Langill, L, Wong, PKH, and Ho, HH (1988). Rett syndrome: EEG presentation. Electroencephalogr Clin Neurophysiol 70:388–395.

Rovner, BW (2006). The Charles Bonnet syndrome: A review of recent research. Curr Opin Ophthalmol 17:275–277.

Saenz-Lope, E, Herranz, FJ, and Masdeu, JC (1984). Startle epilepsy: A clinical study. Ann Neurol 16:78–81.

Saint-Hilaire, H, Saint-Hilaire, JM, and Granger, L (1986). Jumping Frenchmen of Maine. Neurology 36:1269–1271.

Saint-Hilaire, JM, Gilbert, M, Bouvier, G, and Barbeau, A (1981). Epilepsie avec manifestations agressives. Deux cas etudes avec electrodes en profondeur. Rev Neurol 3:161–179.

Salinsky, M, Kanter, R, and Dasheiff, M (1987). Effectiveness of multiple EEGs in supporting the diagnosis of epilepsy: An operational curve. Epilepsia 28:331–334.

Savard, G, Andermann, F, Teitelbaum, J, and Lehmann, H (1988). Epileptic Munchausen's syndrome: A form of pseudoseizures distinct from hysteria and malingering. Neurology 38:1628–1630.

Schachter, SC, and LaFrance, WC, Jr (eds) (2010). Gates and Rowan's Nonepileptic Seizures. Cambridge, UK: Cambridge University Press.

Schenck, CH, and Mahowald, MW (2005). REM sleep parasomnias. Neurol Clin 23:1107–1126.

Scher, MS, and Vigevano, F (2008). Systemic nonepileptic paroxysmal disorders from neonatal to childhood periods. In Epilepsy: A Comprehensive Textbook, 2nd ed. Edited by J Engel, Jr, and TA Pedley. Philadelphia: Lippincott Williams & Wilkins, pp. 2723–2732.

Schomer, DL, and Lopes da Silva, F (eds) (2011). Niedermeyer's Electroencephalography: Basic Principles, Clinical Applications, and Related Fields, 6th ed. Philadelphia: Wolters Kluwer.

Shapiro, AK, Shapiro, ES, Young, JG, and Feinberg, TE (1988). Gilles de la Tourette Syndrome. New York: Raven Press.

Silberstein, SD, Lipton, RB, and Haut, S (2008). Migraine. In Epilepsy: A Comprehensive Textbook, 2nd ed. Edited by J Engel, Jr, and TA Pedley. Philadelphia: Lippincott Williams & Wilkins, pp. 2733–2743.

Simos, P, and Papanicolau, AC (2005). Transient global amnesia. In The Amnesias: A Clinical Textbook of Memory Disorders. Edited by AC Papanicolau. Amsterdam: Elsevier, pp. 171–189.

Spencer, SS, Spencer, DD, Williamson, PD, and Mattson, RH (1981). Ictal effects of anticonvulsant medication withdrawal in epileptic patients. Epilepsia 22:297–307.

Sperling, MR, Pritchard, PB, III, Engel, J, Jr, Daniel, C, and Sagel, J (1986). Prolactin in partial epilepsy: An indicator of limbic seizures. Ann Neurol 20:716–722.

Stern, J, and Engel, J, Jr (2005). Atlas of EEG Patterns. Philadelphia: Lippincott, Williams & Wilkins.

Stillerman, ML, Gibbs, EL, and Perlstein, MA (1952). Electroencephalographic changes in strabismus. Am J Ophthalmol 35:54–63.

Syed, TU, LaFrance, WC, Jr, Kahriman, ES, et al. (2011). Can semiology predict psychogenic nonepileptic seizures? A prospective study. Ann Neurol 69:997–1004.

Tebartz van Elst, L, and Trimble, MR (2008). Episodic dyscontrol. In Epilepsy: A Comprehensive Textbook, 2nd ed. Edited by J Engel, Jr, and TA Pedley. Philadelphia: Lippincott Williams & Wilkins, pp. 2811–2818.

Tharp, B (1980). Neonatal and pediatric electroencephalography. In Electrodiagnosis in Clinical Neurology. Edited by MJ Aminoff. New York: Churchill Livingstone, pp. 67–117.

Thomas, JE, and Klass, DW (1968). Six-per-second spike-and-wave pattern in the electroencephalogram. Neurology 18:587–593.

Torres, F (1981). Epilepsy-electroclinical correlations as a function of age. In Current Clinical Neurophysiology. Edited by CE Henry. Amsterdam: Elsevier/North Holland, pp. 177–233.

Trimble, MR, and Schmitz, B (2008). Nonaffective psychoses, schizophrenia, and schizophrenia-like psychoses. In Epilepsy: A Comprehensive Textbook, 2nd ed. Edited by J Engel, Jr, and TA Pedley. Philadelphia: Lippincott Williams & Wilkins, pp. 2841–2844.

Van Bogaert, L (1927). L'hallucinoscepedonculaire. Rev Neurol (Paris) 43:608–617.

Waldenstrom, J (1957). The porphyrias as inborn errors of metabolism. Am Med 22:758–773.

Westmoreland, BF, and Klass, DW (1981). A distinctive rhythmic EEG discharge of adults. Electroencephalogr Clin Neurophysiol 51:186–191.

Westmoreland, BF, and Klass, DW (1986). Midline theta rhythm. Arch Neurol 43:139–141.

Chapter 14

General Principles of Treatment

PHARMACOLOGICAL TREATMENT

Pharmacological Principles
Adverse Side Effects
Drug Monitoring
Choosing the Appropriate Drug
Discontinuation of Medication
Special Considerations

MEDICALLY REFRACTORY SEIZURES

ALTERNATIVE THERAPY

PSYCHOSOCIAL CONSIDERATIONS

USE OF EEG IN ASSESSING TREATMENT

MANAGEMENT AFTER A SINGLE SEIZURE

EMERGENCY TREATMENT

SUMMARY AND CONCLUSIONS

The ideal objective of treatment for epilepsy is *no seizures, no side effects, as soon as possible*; however, this is too often not a realistic goal. Studies on prognosis have yielded variable results, but overall prognosis has not changed appreciably over many decades; perhaps only half of patients with epilepsy seen in hospitals and specialty clinics can expect medical therapy to render them seizure-free without additional unacceptable side effects (Elwes et al., 1984; Mattson et al., 1985; Rodin, 1968, Kwan and Brodie, 2000, Luciano and Shorvon, 2007). Although these discouraging statistics are not as grim for the epilepsy population as a whole,

it is all too common for adverse side effects of drugs to appear before seizures are completely abolished. When this is unavoidable, the most effective treatment plan does not necessarily require replacement of all ictal symptoms with iatrogenically induced interictal discomfort and disability. The most beneficial balance between epileptic seizure control and drug-related adverse side effects can usually be achieved when patients are able to complain about their medications. In small children, however, reversible drug-induced psychomotor retardation is often misinterpreted by the physician, the patient, and the family as an unavoidable

493

consequence of the underlying disease process when dysfunction might not occur with a different drug regimen.

Several general rules guide the aggressiveness of treatment of epilepsy:

1) Pharmacological treatment of *generalized tonic-clonic seizures* and *dyscognitive focal seizures* should aim for complete control of ictal events as soon as possible, because these can result in serious injury, death, structural damage to the brain, and irreversible social and psychological disability (Chapter 10).

2) There is no need to abolish all minor focal motor seizures, auras, or brief generalized myoclonic and absence seizures that do not interfere with work, school, interpersonal relations, or other routine activities if doing so requires medication regimens that introduce additional discomfort or disability (Chapter 8).

3) In patients with mental impairment and multiple seizure types who require constant supervision, an occasional more severe ictal event may be preferable to levels of antiseizure drugs that further compromise cognitive function or otherwise decrease quality of life. If drop attacks contribute to disability, vagus nerve stimulation or corpus callosum section should be considered (Chapter 16).

4) If disabling seizures continue after trials of two appropriate antiseizure drugs at maximum doses, either alone or in combination, the patient is considered to have drug-resistant epilepsy (Kwan et al., 2010) and should be referred to an *epilepsy center*. Patients with drug-resistant epilepsy are not well served by the common practice of referral back and forth among many physicians when definitive decisions might be made at an epilepsy center. Seizure freedom is unlikely to occur with further attempts at medical management (Dreifuss, 1987; Elwes et al., 1984; Mattson et al., 1985; Kwan and Brodie, 2000). Even though some patients do respond after prolonged multiple drug trials (Luciano and Shorvon, 2007; Bauer et al., 2008; Liimatainen et al., 2008), this is often not sustained (Callaghan et al., 2011), and early referral for definitive treatment, such as surgery (Chapter 16), could prevent the irreversible adverse social and psychological consequences of long-standing, repetitive, and disabling ictal events.

5) Primary care physicians and general neurologists must be able to identify conditions that require surgery, such as brain tumors; however, they need not determine whether a patient might be a surgical candidate before referral to an epilepsy center. Rather, all patients with drug-resistant epilepsy should be referred as soon as two appropriate antiseizure trials fail, because epilepsy specialists at epilepsy centers are best qualified to identify potential surgical candidates (Chapter 16). Early surgical intervention for drug-resistant seizures provides the best opportunity to avoid irreversible disabling psychological and social consequences of recurrent seizures. Furthermore, epilepsy specialists at epilepsy centers are trained to consider and apply alternative treatments for patients with drug-resistant epilepsy who are not surgical candidates or in whom surgery has failed to abolish disabling seizures. Vagus nerve and direct brain stimulation, experimental drug trials, the ketogenic diet, and a variety of other approaches can be beneficial in selected patients (Chapter 16).

6) The appropriate balance between seizure occurrence and undesirable side effects of antiseizure drugs must be tailored to each patient's need and preferences. It may be beneficial to slowly taper and, very rarely, even discontinue medication, which in some patients can actually improve the seizure condition (Taylor and McKinlay, 1984). If antiseizure medications offer no benefit, freedom from the bother of taking pills and from unpleasant side effects can be gratifying, particularly when patients and their families do not recognize toxic symptoms until medication is decreased or discontinued.

The American Academy of Neurology (AAN) has published evidence-based performance measures that can be used to measure quality of care for epilepsy (Fountain et al., 2011). These eight measures (Table 14–1) also serve as guidelines to physicians for diagnosis and treatment of their patients with epilepsy.

PHARMACOLOGICAL TREATMENT

Pharmacological Principles

The use of antiseizure drugs requires knowledge of *physicochemical* and *physiological* processes that influence their uptake and elimination as well as of the *pharmacokinetic* principles that predict their *bioavailability* (Wilder and Bruni,

1981; Woodbury et al., 1989; Perucca, 2008; 2009a) (Fig. 14–1). Dose schedules are determined by (1) the unique behavior of specific pharmacological agents in the body, which can be calculated from their known pharmacokinetic values (Table 14–2), and (2) individual patient variation, which can be determined by monitoring serum antiseizure drug levels.

ABSORPTION

The absorption of antiseizure drugs into the blood following oral, rectal, or intramuscular administration depends on (1) *water solubility*, which determines the degree to which the drug is in solution and available to be transported, and (2) *lipid solubility*, which determines the degree to which it crosses membranes. Formulation of a drug influences solubility; for example, medications such as *phenytoin* are absorbed more readily from suspensions than from capsules (Neuvonen, 1979). In addition, absorption rates can be different with different generic formulations of drugs (Melikian et al., 1977; MacDonald, 1987; Wyllie et al., 1987; Koch and Allen, 1987; Gidal, 2009). Lipid solubility depends on ionization, which in turn depends on pH of the body fluids. Changes in pH will affect absorption of different medications in different ways. Consequently, presence of food in the stomach retards absorption of oral *valproic acid* (Levy et al., 1980), but increases absorption of oral *carbamazepine* (Melander, 1978). The presence of other drugs, as well as disease states that influence gastric function and splanchnic blood flow, also affects absorption of antiseizure medication following oral doses. *Phenytoin* precipitates at the pH of muscle and is absorbed poorly from intramuscular injection. *Diazepam* is also not recommended for intramuscular injection, whereas *phenobarbital* is readily solubilized and absorbed at this pH. Dosage regimens for intramuscular *phenytoin* and diazepam must take into account delayed

Table 14–1 Final Eight Epilepsy Measures Approved by the American Academy of Neurology and Physician Consortium for Performance Improvement

Measure title and description

No. 1: Seizure type and current seizure frequency
  All visits with the type(s) of seizure(s) and current seizure frequency for each seizure type documented in the medical record.
No. 2: Documentation of etiology of epilepsy or epilepsy syndrome
  All visits with the etiology of epilepsy or epilepsy syndrome reviewed and documented if known, or documented as unknown or cryptogenic.
No. 3. EEG results reviewed, requested, or test ordered.
  All initial evaluations with the results of at least one EEG reviewed or requested, or if EEG was not performed previously, then an EEG ordered.
No. 4: MRI/CT scan reviewed, requested, or scan ordered
  All initial evaluations with the results of at least one MRI or CT scan reviewed or requested or, if a MRI or CT scan was not obtained previously, then a MRI or CT scan ordered (MRI preferred).
No. 5: Querying and counseling about antiepileptic drug side effects
  All visits where patients were queried and counseled about antiepileptic drug side effects and the querying and counseling was documented in the medical record.
No. 6: Surgical therapy referral consideration for intractable epilepsy
  All patients with a diagnosis of intractable epilepsy who were considered for referral for a neurologic evaluation of appropriateness for surgical therapy and the consideration was documented in the medical record within the past 3 years.
No. 7: Counseling about epilepsy-specific safety issues
  All patients who were counseled about context-specific safety issues, appropriate to the patient's age, seizure type(s) and frequency(ies), occupation and leisure activities, etc. (e.g., injury prevention, burns, appropriate drug restrictions, or bathing) at least once per year.
No. 8: Counseling for women of childbearing potential with epilepsy
  All female patients of childbearing potential (12–44 years old) diagnosed with epilepsy who were counseled about epilepsy and how its treatment may affect contraception and pregnancy at least once per year.

From Fountain et al., 2011, with permission.

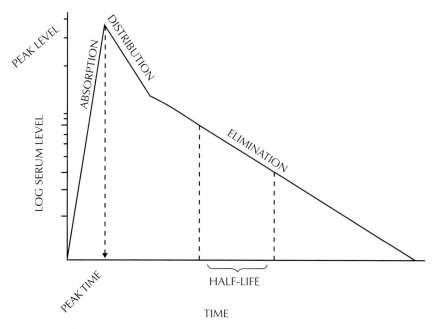

Figure 14–1. Serum level of a drug following a single oral dose increases rapidly because of absorption from the gut until it reaches peak level. It then decreases in two phases: a rapid phase due to distribution into several body compartments and a slower phase due to metabolism and clearance (elimination). *Peak time* is the time at which the peak level is attained, and *half-life* is the time it takes the level to be reduced by one-half after absorption and distribution are complete. Note that serum level is shown on a log scale.

absorption if this route is unavoidable (Wilder et al., 1974). Rapid, complete bioavailability is achieved by intravenous administration.

PROTEIN BINDING

Most antiseizure drugs are partially bound in the serum by protein (Table 14–2). Whereas routine clinical measurements of serum drug concentration include both protein-bound and unbound (or *free*) fractions, only the free fraction diffuses into the brain to produce a therapeutic or toxic effect. Consequently, when serum albumin concentration is decreased, as happens in a variety of medical conditions, the free fraction of a drug can be greater than expected, and therapeutic or toxic effects will occur at lower total serum drug levels (Fig. 14–2). This is of clinical importance only for drugs that are more than 90% protein-bound, specifically *phenytoin* and, perhaps, *valproic acid*. In situations involving *hypoalbuminemia* and administration of displacing agents such as *aspirin*, decisions regarding dose

schedules may require measurement of the free fraction of drug in the serum. Although this cannot be done directly by all clinical chemistry laboratories, a measure of free levels of most antiseizure drugs can be obtained from fluid samples that do not contain a protein-bound fraction, such as saliva, tears, and cerebrospinal fluid. If protein binding decreases during the course of chronic administration of a drug, the increase in free fraction also causes increased elimination. Consequently, with the same dose rate and clearance, the actual amount of free drug is usually unchanged. Protein binding is an important consideration for patients on dialysis and for treatment of drug overdose, because dialysis can remove only the unbound fraction.

DISTRIBUTION

After the administration of an antiseizure drug, there is a rise in the serum concentration due to absorption, followed by a fall resulting from elimination and from distribution into various

Table 14–2 Pharmacokinetics of Commonly Used Antiseizure Drugs

	Oral Bioavailability (%)	Effect of food	Peak time (hrs)	Time to steady state (days)	Volume of distribution l/kg	Pharmacokinetics Linear	Protein binding (%)	Metabolism Liver	Other	Active Metabolites	Urinary excretion (% unchanged)	Half-life (hrs)	
CBZ	75–85		4–8	2–4	0.8–2	No	75	CYP3A4		Yes	<5	10–20	CBZ
CLB	>95		0.5–2	2–7	0.9–1.8	Yes	85	CYP2C19/3A4		Yes		10–30 / 36–46°	CLB
CLN	>85		1–2	2–10	1.5–4.4	Yes	80	CYP3A4		No	2	24–48	CLN
ESL			2–3	4–5	2.7	Yes	30			Yes	67	20–40°	ESL
ESM	>90		1–5	8–12	0.7	Yes	10	CYP3A		No	10–20	25–70	ESM
EZG			1–2		2–3	Yes	80		Gluc	No		7–11	EZG
FBM	>90		1–6	3–5	0.8	Yes	20–25	CYP3A4/2E1		No	50	16–22	FBM
GBP	<60	Delays	2–3	1–2	0.65–1.04	No	0	No		No	100	5–9	GBP
LCM	100		1–2	2–3	0.6–0.7	Yes	15	CYP2C19		No	40	12–16	LCM
LTG	>95	Delays	1–3	3–7	0.9–1.3	Yes	55	Gluc		No	10	15–35†	LTG
LEV	>95	Delays	0.5–2	1–2	0.5–0.7	Yes	0	No	Hyd	No	60	6–8	LEV
OXC	100		4–6°	2–3	0.7–0.8°	Yes	40°	Gluc		Yes	28	8–15°	OXC
PB	>90	Delays	0.5–4	15–29	0.5	Yes	40–60	CYP2C9/2C19		No	20–40	70–130	PB
PHT	>80	Delays	4–12	6–21	0.5–0.8	No	90	CYP2C9		No	<5	20	PHT
PGN	>90	Delays	1–2	1–2	0.57	Yes	0	No		No	98	5–7	PGN
PRM	>90		2–4	2–4	0.5–0.8	Yes	10	CYP2C9		Yes	40	12 / 10–130°	PRM
RUF	>85	Increases	4–6	1–2	0.71–1.14	No	35		Hyd	No	4	6–10	RUF
TGB	>90	Delays	0.5–2	1–2	1.0	Yes	96	CYP3A4		No	<1	5–9	TGB
TPM	>80		2–4	4–5	0.6–1.0	Yes	15	CYP3A4/2C19		No	60–100	10–30	TPM
VPA	>90	Delays	1–4	2–4	0.1–0.4	No	70–90	Multiple		No	<5	8–16	VPA
VGB	60–80	Delays	1–2	1–2	0.8	Yes	0	No		No	95	~5–8	VGB
ZON	>90	Delays	2–5	10–15	1.0–1.9	Yes	40	CYP3A4		No	35	50–70	ZON

° For active metabolite.
† As monotherapy.
Desm = desmethylation; Gluc = glucuronidation; Hyd = hydroxylation.
For key to drug name abbreviations, see Table 15–1.

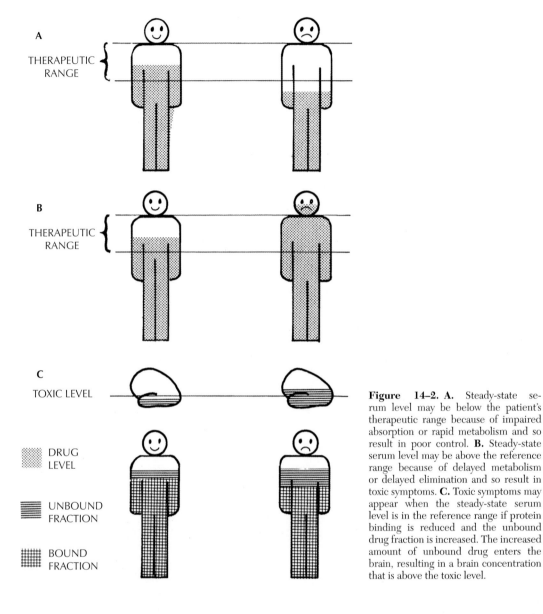

Figure 14–2. A. Steady-state serum level may be below the patient's therapeutic range because of impaired absorption or rapid metabolism and so result in poor control. **B.** Steady-state serum level may be above the reference range because of delayed metabolism or delayed elimination and so result in toxic symptoms. **C.** Toxic symptoms may appear when the steady-state serum level is in the reference range if protein binding is reduced and the unbound drug fraction is increased. The increased amount of unbound drug enters the brain, resulting in a brain concentration that is above the toxic level.

theoretical body compartments. The total volume of body compartments within which a given drug appears to be distributed is referred to as its *volume of distribution (Vd)*. Because a drug may be unevenly distributed throughout the body, Vd does not represent an actual physiological volume, but rather the fluid volume that would be required if the drug were evenly distributed. The magnitude of Vd influences the half-life of a drug and, together with redistribution among tissues, contributes to its duration of action. Drug distribution depends on factors that influence blood flow and transfer of the drug across membranes. Protein binding (see Table 14–2) in the plasma prevents the bound fraction from leaving the vascular compartment, whereas protein binding in other tissue holds the drug in that compartment and can result in a higher concentration of the drug in that tissue than in the blood. There is evidence of an *active transport* system for brain uptake of *valproic acid* (Frey and Loscher, 1978; Levy et al., 2002), *gabapentin*, and *pregabalin* (Del Amo et al., 2008).

ELIMINATION

Elimination refers to the removal of the active antiseizure drug from the blood, which occurs by *clearance* and *metabolism*. Most antiseizure drugs or their metabolites (or both) are excreted through the kidneys (see Table 14–2), a mechanism that, like absorption, can be pH- dependent. Alkalinization of the urine can increase the rate of clearance of some drugs, whereas impaired renal function reduces clearance. Antiseizure drugs can also be excreted in bile and the small intestine. *Paraldehyde* is eliminated predominantly through the lungs, which could make it a useful medication for patients with severe renal and hepatic disease. Excretion of antiseizure drugs in breast milk and saliva does not influence pharmacokinetic determinations but may be an important consideration for other reasons discussed later in this chapter.

Elimination of most antiseizure drugs depends to a great extent on *biotransformation* by the liver (see Table 14–2). Most drugs are converted into inactive metabolites, but some, such as *primidone, carbamazepine, oxcarbazepine, fosphenytoin, diazepam, eslicarbazepine acetate,* and *clobazam*, have metabolites with antiseizure properties. In these situations, pharmacokinetic analyses of the primary drug do not accurately predict the degree and duration of antiseizure effect; pharmacokinetic analysis of metabolites is also necessary. Elimination of an active antiseizure drug is altered by hepatic dysfunction. Also, the antiseizure drug itself or other drugs can inhibit or induce liver enzymes responsible for drug metabolism. Elimination is reduced by *enzyme inhibition* (Fig. 14–3), which leads to increased serum drug levels and adverse side effects. Elimination is facilitated by *enzyme induction* (activation) (Fig. 14–4), which leads to decreased serum drug levels and recurrence of epileptic seizures. Enzyme inhibition and induction can account for delayed changes in drug effectiveness for drug interactions that occur with *polypharmacy* (use of multiple drugs), as discussed later in this chapter.

Biotransformations in the liver involve oxidation, reduction, and hydrolysis (*Phase I reactions*) and conjugation (*Phase II reactions*). Oxidation, the most important metabolic reaction for detoxifying antiseizure drugs, is catalyzed by a group of microsomal isozymes that utilize *cytochrome P450*. Knowledge of the specific families of cytochrome P450 isozymes responsible for metabolizing different drugs is important for understanding drug-drug interactions as well as genetic predisposition to aberrant drug metabolism (Perucca, 2008). Most metabolites of antiseizure drugs are conjugated as glucuronides prior to renal clearance (Chapter 15).

HALF-LIFE

As previously noted, the time required for a single dose of an antiseizure drug to reach peak serum concentration (*peak time*) (see Table 14–2) depends on the route of administration and the rate of absorption. In some

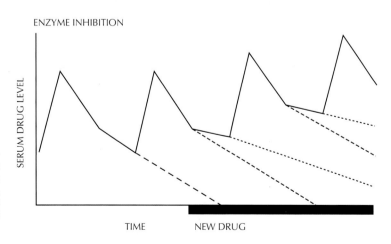

Figure 14–3. Enzyme inhibition, in this case due to addition of a new drug, retards elimination due to metabolism (*dotted line*), resulting in a progressive increase in serum drug level with repeated doses.

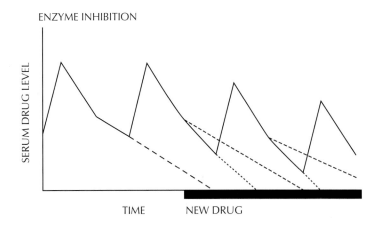

ENZYME INHIBITION

SERUM DRUG LEVEL

TIME   NEW DRUG

Figure 14–4. Enzyme induction, in this case due to addition of a new drug, enhances elimination due to metabolism (*dotted line*), resulting in a progressive decrease of serum drug level with repeated doses.

instances, an early, rapid decrease in concentration is due to drug distribution as well as elimination, but the subsequent slower decrease represents elimination (metabolism and clearance) (see Fig. 14–1). The *half-life* of a drug refers to the time it takes for the drug concentration to decrease by 50% after absorption and distribution are complete. The half-life of a drug is the most important pharmacokinetic parameter for determining dose schedules. The half-life values shown in Table 14–2 are determined after a single oral dose and can be altered by enzyme inhibition and induction as well as by factors that influence clearance. For some drugs, Vd is the most important factor in determining half-life; if body stores of a drug are large, elimination processes will require a longer time to produce a decline in plasma drug levels. Individual differences in metabolism may also cause an unusually short or unusually long half-life in some patients. When dose schedules determined on the basis of the expected half-life of an antiseizure drug do not produce anticipated results, fluctuations in plasma drug level can be directly measured for individual patients, as discussed in the section below on drug monitoring.

ZERO-ORDER KINETICS

In most circumstances, antiseizure drugs are metabolized according to first-order enzyme kinetics, in which the rate of metabolism is directly proportional to drug concentration. Consequently, a straight-line relationship exists between the dose and serum concentration of a drug (Fig. 14–5). With zero-order kinetics, the enzyme responsible for drug metabolism becomes saturated after a certain concentration is reached, metabolism is not proportionately increased with further increments in dose, the half-life becomes prolonged, and serum drug levels increase by a disproportionately greater magnitude than the increase in dose (see Fig. 14–5). Zero-order kinetics are particularly important in the metabolism of *phenytoin*, for which adverse side effects can occur following very small increases above a dose of 4–7 mg/kg in most patients.

PHARMACODYNAMIC ACTIONS

Pharmacodynamic mechanisms account for drug actions at the neuronal level (Macdonald and Rogawski, 2008). Antiseizure medications presumably all act at receptor sites on neuronal membranes to influence neurotransmitters, neuromodulator function, or membrane permeability to various ions (Chapter 3) (Table 14–3). Alterations in drug effect may result from changes in drug-receptor interactions. *Tolerance*, or reduced efficacy with continued drug use, is common, is influenced by many factors including genetics, and consists of two major types (Löscher and Schmidt, 2006). *Pharmacokinetic (metabolic) tolerance* results from enzyme induction and is discussed later. *Pharmacodynamic (functional) tolerance* reflects adaptation of the drug targets such as downregulation of receptors, diminished binding capacity, and interference with binding by

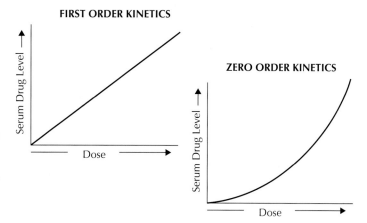

FIRST ORDER KINETICS

Serum Drug Level →

Dose →

ZERO ORDER KINETICS

Serum Drug Level →

Dose →

Figure 14–5. With first-order kinetics, serum drug level increases proportionately with dose. With zero-order kinetics, because of saturation of the enzyme necessary for drug metabolism, serum drug level increases exponentially with increasing dose; and after a certain point very small changes in dose result in very large changes in serum drug level.

drug metabolites. Development of tolerance to unwanted adverse side effects is a useful phenomenon, but tolerance to antiseizure effects decreases therapeutic value (Meldrum, 1986). Tolerance to antiseizure effects has been well documented and in most situations can be attributed to downregulation of receptors or receptor sensitivity (Poisbeau et al., 1997; Löscher and Schmidt, 2006). Such tolerance is most commonly observed clinically for the *benzodiazepines* and *acetazolamide* but exists to some degree for all drugs. *Physical dependence* develops as a result of similar receptor modulation and is responsible for *withdrawal* reactions. This is most often seen with antiseizure drugs that have sedative or hypnotic effects, such as the *benzodiazepines* and *barbiturates*, and may not occur with *phenytoin*, *carbamazepine*, *valproic acid*, and the newer drugs. *Drug interactions* at the receptor level account for some problems encountered with polypharmacy, and *cross-tolerance* between drugs exists.

DOSE PLANNING

To institute chronic antiseizure drug treatment, it is necessary to achieve a *steady-state* condition, where the appropriate dose of the drug given at the appropriate intervals results in serum concentrations that fluctuate within the *reference range* (Fig. 14–6; Table 14–4) (Patsalos et al., 2008). The bottom of the reference range is that serum concentration above which most patients will be expected to experience improvement in epileptic seizure control.

The top of the reference range is that serum concentration above which most patients will be expected to experience dose-related adverse side-effects. The reference range, therefore, is a statistical concept derived from a large population of patients and should be used as a guide only. For individual patients, the serum concentrations between efficacy and intolerance can be referred to as the *therapeutic range*. The therapeutic range can be determined only on an individual basis. If epileptic seizures are controlled with serum levels below the reference range, there is no need to increase the dose, whereas serum levels can be increased above the reference range if necessary for full beneficial effects if there are no unacceptable toxic side effects.

At the institution of chronic antiseizure drug treatment, the steady-state level is reached roughly within five half-lives of the drug (see Fig. 14–6). From a practical point of view, the dose schedule for beginning a new drug requires balancing the need for rapid protection against epileptic seizures, on the one hand, and avoidance of side effects, on the other. If the patient has been warned about the possibility of another seizure and if appropriate precautions will be taken, there is usually no need to build a serum level of drug rapidly at the risk of producing severe side effects; "*Start low, go slow*," is a popular mantra for instituting antiseizure drugs.

When the danger of repeated seizures requires that therapeutic serum levels be achieved rapidly, a *loading dose* can be given, although dose-related side effects make this

Table 14–3 Mechanisms of Action of Commonly Used Antiseizure Drugs

| | Voltage-Gated Channels | | | | Ligand-Gated Channels | | Other GABA potentiation | Sv2a | Carbonic Anhydrase Inhibitor | |
	Na⁺	K⁺	Ca²⁺ T-type	Ca²⁺ Other	Glutamate	GABA				
CBZ	xxx	–	–	x	–	–	–	–	–	CBZ
CLB	–	–	–	–	–	xxx	–	–	–	CLB
CLN	–	–	–	–	–	xxx	–	–	–	CLN
ESL	xxx	–	–	–	–	–	–	–	–	ESL
ESM	–	–	xxx	–	–	–	–	–	–	ESM
EZG	–	xxx	–	–	–	–	–	–	–	EZG
FBM	–	–	–	xxx	xx	–	xx	–	–	FBM
GBP	–	–	–	xxx	–	–	x	–	–	GBP
LCM	xxx	–	–	–	–	–	–	–	–	LCM
LTG	xx	x	–	xx	x	–	xx	–	–	LTG
LEV	–	–	–	–	–	–	–	xxx	–	LEV
OXC	xxx	x	–	x	–	–	–	–	–	OXC
PB	x	–	–	x	–	xxx	–	–	–	PB
PHT	xxx	–	–	x	–	x	–	–	–	PHT
PGN	–	–	–	xxx	–	–	x	–	–	PGN
PRM	x	–	–	x	–	xxx	–	–	–	PRM
RUF	xx	–	–	–	–	–	–	–	–	RUF
TGB	–	–	–	–	–	–	xxx	–	–	TGB
TPM	xx	x	–	xx	xx	xx	xx	–	xx	TPM
VPA	x	–	xx	x	–	–	xx	–	–	VPA
VGB	–	–	–	–	–	–	xxx	–	–	VGB
ZON	xx	–	xx	–	–	–	xx	–	xx	ZON

For key to drug name abbreviations, see Table 15–1.

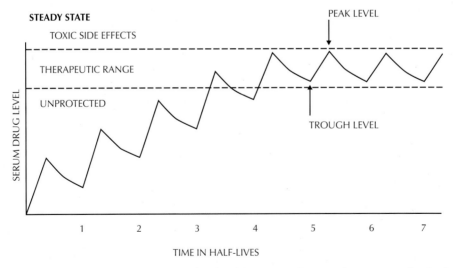

Figure 14–6. Repeated doses of a drug at intervals of one half-life or less result in a steady-state serum drug level after five half-lives. The objective of dose planning is to maintain the serum drug level within each patient's therapeutic range, so that the peak level does not cause toxic side effects and the trough level is sufficient to maintain protection against seizures.

practically difficult except for *phenytoin* and *phenobarbital*. Avoidance of titration, rather than a loading dose, is possible with *levetiracetam,* if necessary. Although theoretically the loading dose (in milligrams per kilogram) required to institute or raise drug levels is equivalent to the increment level $[(\mu g/ml) \times Vd\ (L/kg)]$, it is always advisable to consult the manufacturer's information.

To maintain a steady-state level, the ideal time between doses of the older drugs should not exceed one half-life. When the patient is instructed to divide the total daily dose using the maximal permissible interdose interval, serum levels are likely to fall below the protective range if a single dose is missed (Fig. 14–7). On the other hand, a schedule that requires a patient to take drugs too frequently may be inconvenient and reduce compliance. The ideal approach is to use an interdose interval of 0.5 half-life (see Fig. 14–7). This rule, however does not necessarily pertain to some of the newer drugs with relatively short half-lives. The actual dose schedule depends on other practical considerations as well as the tolerability of high plasma drug levels. Whereas a short half-life in a drug with a narrow reference range requires more frequent dosing, because greater fluctuations in peaks and troughs can cause transient adverse dose-related side effects, this is not the case for a drug with a wide reference range, such as *levetiracetam* (Perucca, 2009a). Many extended-release formulations are now available for drugs with relatively short half-lives to smooth out the serum levels, reduce dose-related side effects, and permit more convenient dosing schedules. Table 14–4 shows basic information for administration of the commonly used antiseizure drugs.

Therapeutic failure with recommended dose schedules in some patients can be due to aberrant absorption, metabolism, or clearance, which causes lower- or higher-than-expected serum concentrations of the drug. In these patients, dose schedules must be individually determined for best results. Furthermore, serum drug levels do not necessarily predict the pharmacodynamic action of a drug in the brain. For instance, the antiseizure efficacy of valproate and *levetiracetam* can lag hours or days behind increases and decreases in serum drug levels (Chapter 15).

APPROACH TO MONOTHERAPY AND POLYTHERAPY

An essential goal of modern pharmacological treatment of epilepsy is to control epileptic seizures, preferably with one medication; however, the few studies that have compared monotherapy to polytherapy have found no significant differences (Beghi et al., 2003; Deckers et al., 2001). After adequate seizure control is achieved with a constant dose of drug over some period of time, seizures may recur. This usually reflects functional tolerance, but for *carbamazepine*, it may be due to enzyme induction, which can be demonstrated by reduced serum drug levels. The proper response is then to increase the amount of drug and not to begin a second drug. Under these circumstances, the original drug can be given at higher doses than those that might have caused adverse symptoms initially, without producing these problems. Inappropriate institution of a second drug at this time can further increase enzyme induction and result in subtherapeutic levels of both drugs (Fig. 14–8). The antiseizure effects of the two drugs are not necessarily cumulative in this situation, but side effects can be. Consequently, the patient may experience increases in both seizures and adverse symptoms. The current strategy for instituting pharmacological management is to choose the best drug for the seizure type or epilepsy syndrome (or both) and for the patient and to gradually increase the dose of that drug until either adequate control of seizures or intolerable side effects occur. When dose-related adverse symptoms develop, backing off or slowing down may allow the patient to be coaxed into achieving higher levels with better therapeutic results. It is necessary to wait until a steady-state condition has been reached (and for *valproic acid,* somewhat longer) before drawing any conclusions concerning the effectiveness of an antiseizure drug regimen.

Whereas the prevalent teaching on the approach to monotherapy when seizures are not controlled is to increase the dose of the antiseizure drug until unacceptable side effects appear, this is not necessarily the most effective approach today, with so many new antiseizure medications available. Indeed, most patients with pharmacosensitive seizures respond to relatively low drug doses, and high-dose treatment is often not necessary to demonstrate

Table 14–4 Administration Parameters for Commonly Used Antiseizure Drugs

	Adults					Children[†]					
	Maintenance Dose (mg/day)	Dose Interval (per day)	Starting Dose (mg/day)	Incremental Dose (mg/day)	Increment Interval (days)	Maintenance Dose (mg/kg/day)	Dose Interval (per day)	Starting Dose (mg/kg/day)	Incremental Dose (mg/kg/day)	Increment Interval (days)	
CBZ	800–1200	3–4	200–400	200	7	<35	3–4	10–20	5–10	7	CBZ
CLB	20–40	2	10	10	7	0.4–0.8	2	0.1–0.2	0.1	7	CLB
CLN	4–10	2	1.5	0.5–1	3–7	0.1–0.2	2	0.01–0.02	0.01–0.02	3–7	CLN
ESL	800–1200	1	400	400	14						ESL
ESM	500–1500	2–3	250	250	4–7	20–30	2–3	5–10	5–10	5–7	ESM
EZG	300–600	3	300	150	7						EZG
FBM	1200–3600	2–4	1200	600	14	45	2–4	15	15	7	FBM
GBP	900–3600	3	300	300	1	25–40	3	10–15	10	1	GBP
LCM	200–400	2	100	100	7						LCM
LTGm	100–400	2	25	25	14	1–5	2	0.15	0.3	14	LTGm
LTGv	100–250	2	25 qod	25	14	1–5	2	0.15	0.3	14	LTGv
LTGei	200–600	2	50–100	100	14	5–15	2	0.6	1.2	14	LTGei
LEV	1000–3000	2	500–1000	500–1000	7–14	30–40	2–3	20	20	7–14	LEV
OXC	600–2400	2	300	150	2	35–45	2	5–10	5	7	OXC
PB	100–300	1–2	100–300			3–6	1–2	3–6			PB
PHT	200–400	1–2	150–300	50–100	14–28	5–10	1–2	5	5	14–28	PHT
PGN	150–600	2–3	150	150	7						PGN
PRM	750–1500	3–4	125	125	3	10–20	3–4	5	5	3	PRM
RUF	1800–3200	2	400–800	400–800	2	45	2	10	10	2	RUF
TGB	16–56	2–4	4–5	4–5	7–14	0.4–0.7	2–4	0.1	0.1	7	TGB
TPM	200–600	2	25–50	25–50	7–14	3–9	2	0.5–1	0.5–1	7–14	TPM
VPA	1000–2500	2–3	1000	500	5–7	20–40	2–3	15	15	5–7	VPA
VGB	1000–3000	1–2	500	500	7	50–150	1–2	50	25–50	7	VGB
ZON	100–600	1–2	100	100	14	8	1–2	1–2	1–2	14	ZON

Table 14–4 (Continued)

	Decreased by Enzyme inducers	Increased by Valproate	Reference Range (µg/ml)	IV Formulation	Syrup	Extended Release	Generic Formulation	
CBZ	+	+	8–12	No	Yes	Yes	Yes	CBZ
CLB	+		0.03–0.3°	No	No	No	Yes	CLB
CLN	+		0.01–0.07°	No	Yes	No	Yes	CLN
ESL	+			No	Yes	No	No	ESL
ESM	+	+	40–100	No	Yes	No	Yes	ESM
EZG	+			No	No	No	No	EZG
FBM	+	+	30–60	No	Yes	No	No	FBM
GBP			2–20	No	Yes	No	Yes	GBP
LCM			10–20	Yes	Yes	No	No	LCM
LTGm	+	+	3–15	No	Yes	No	Yes	LTGm
LTGv	+	+	3–15	No	Yes	No	Yes	LTGv
LTGei	+	+	3–15	No	Yes	No	Yes	LTGei
LEV			12–46	Yes	Yes	Yes	Yes	LEV
OXC	+	+	3–35	No	Yes	No	Yes	OXC
PB	+		10–40	Yes	Yes	No	Yes	PB
PHT	+	+	10–20	Yes	Yes	Yes	Yes	PHT
PGN				No	No	No	No	PGN
PRM	+		3–12	No	Yes	No	Yes	PRM
RUF	+	+	10–25	No	No	No	No	RUF
TGB	+	+	0.02–0.2°	No	No	No	No	TGB
TPM	+		5–20	No	No	No	Yes	TPM
VPA	+		50–100	Yes	Yes	Yes	Yes	VPA
VGB			50–100°	No	Yes	No	No	VGB
ZON	+		10–40	No	No	No	Yes	ZON

°Serum levels only useful for monitoring compliance.
°Children's doses may not apply to infants.
LTGm = lamotragine as monotherapy, LTGv = lamotragine with valproate, LTGm = lamotragine with enzyme inducing drugs. For key to other drug name abbreviations, see Table 15–1.

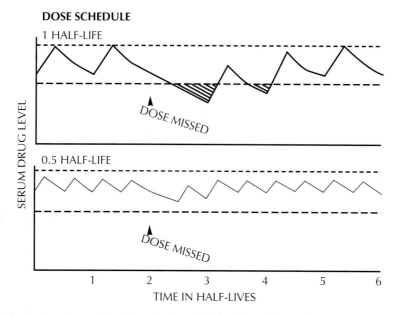

DOSE SCHEDULE

Figure 14–7. If a drug dose is repeated at intervals of one half-life, it is usually possible to maintain the serum drug level within the patient's therapeutic range, but a single missed dose causes the serum drug level to fall into the unprotected range. With a dose interval of 0.5 half-life, fluctuation of serum drug level is decreased, and a missed dose is less likely to cause inadequate protection.

that a given drug is not effective (Brodie et al., 2007). Once a drug trial has failed at a reasonably high dose, chances of obtaining complete seizure control may be considerably greater with another medication that has a different mechanism of action than with a higher dose of the current medication, which would cause the discomfort of dose-related side effects (Brodie et al., 2011; Perucca, 2011). There is, therefore, no general guideline for moving from one antiseizure drug trial to the next; however, in any event, after failure of two

appropriate trials, referral to an epilepsy center is recommended.

When the first-choice drug is clearly ineffective, the second-choice drug should be instituted. Institution of the second drug should follow the same procedures as for the first; however, substitution may take longer if the problem is intolerance rather than inefficacy. Adverse side effects, if they occur, may be due to enzyme inhibition by the second drug, which increases the serum concentration of the first drug (see Fig. 14–9). When serum drug levels

ENZYME INDUCTION

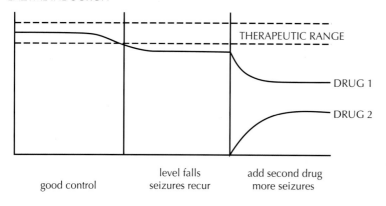

Figure 14–8. Self-induction of enzymes or enzyme induction caused by other pharmacological agents can lower the steady-state serum drug level below the patient's therapeutic range and decrease seizure control. The proper response is to increase the dose of the first drug and not to add a second. Addition of a second drug can lead to further enzyme induction and an even greater lowering of the steady-state serum level of the first drug.

ENZYME INHIBITION

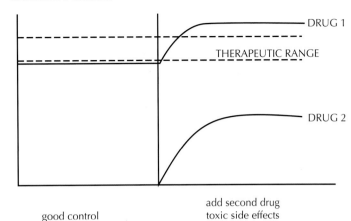

Figure 14–9. Addition of a second drug can cause enzyme inhibition, raising the serum level of the first drug above the patient's therapeutic range. In this situation, the appearance of toxic symptoms is likely to be due to the first drug and not the second. The appropriate response is to lower the dose of the first drug and not to abandon attempts to institute the second.

indicate that this is the case, it is appropriate to reduce the dose of the first drug and not to discontinue attempts to institute the second. Should steady-state levels of the second drug be effective in controlling epileptic seizures, the first drug can then be tapered and discontinued. The objective of drug substitution is to avoid seizures without causing intolerable side effects. Discontinuing the first drug abruptly will result in a complete disappearance from the blood in five half-lives. This is not recommended, however, because of the risk of withdrawal exacerbation of seizures. Although a general rule for tapering medication in this condition is to remove 20% of the total daily dose every five half-lives, slower tapering is often more appropriate when there is no pressing need to hurry. Withdrawal exacerbation of seizures is particularly prominent with *barbiturates, primidone,* and *benzodiazepines,* and does not indicate that the drug was necessary for maintenance of control. When epileptic seizures recur during withdrawal of the first drug, the tapering process can be delayed but does not necessarily need to be discontinued. Withdrawal seizures with *phenobarbital* or *primidone,* however, are reported to occur when serum *phenobarbital* levels pass between 20 and 15 µg/ml and may not depend on the rate of drug withdrawal (Theodore et al., 1987). The patient should always be warned during tapering that withdrawal seizures may occur but that this effect is likely to be transient.

In some situations, when the second-choice drug has pharmacokinetic properties that are similar to those of the first choice, it is possible to decrease one while increasing the other. This process, referred to as *crossover,* is not generally recommended, because introducing multiple variables makes it more difficult to determine the cause of a particular effect. For instance, the apparent failure to control seizures may not be due to ineffectiveness of the second drug but, rather, may be a withdrawal response to the first. Crossover is justified, however, when side effects of two drugs are intolerable or there is a need to change from one drug to another quickly. Protocols have been developed for rapid substitution between some of the older antiseizure drugs, which can be accomplished in approximately five days and often is best carried out in the hospital (Bourgeois, 2008); however, similar protocols have not yet been developed for the newer drugs, and some, such as *lamotrigine,* should not be instituted quickly.

Although ease of administration and perhaps lower risk of teratogenicity (see below) remain advantages of monotherapy, many physicians (and patients) prefer not to make changes when seizures are controlled and to continue with two drugs. There is no strict rule in this regard; some studies have found that more than one drug is rarely effective when a single drug is not (Mattson et al., 1985; Kwan and Brodie, 2000), unless the patient has multiple seizure types that respond individually to different antiseizure medications, while others have found no difference in effectiveness between monotherapy and polytherapy (Beghi et al., 2003; Deckers et al., 2001). In practice, therefore, adjunctive and combination therapy is common in patients with difficult-to-control seizures. In this situation, it is important to take into consideration pharmacokinetic and pharmacodynamic interactions, cumulative toxicity, and higher costs (Bourgeois and Gilliam, 2008). Table 14–5 shows pharmacological interactions for the commonly used antiseizure drugs. Given that synergistic drug combinations have become essential in treating other medical conditions, such as infectious diseases and cancer, it is likely that rational polypharmacy will eventually offer important therapeutic advantages for epilepsy. Evidence is accumulating that some drug combinations are better than others (Brodie et al., 2011; Perucca, 2011).

CLINICAL FACTORS INFLUENCING DRUG EFFICACY

Intercurrent illness can affect pharmacokinetic processes. Decreased antiseizure drug clearance with the appearance of adverse side effects is most commonly seen in acute hepatic and renal failure. Febrile illness, on the other hand, can accelerate drug metabolism and cause a fall in serum levels (Leppik et al., 1986). Serum levels can also be lowered by enhanced elimination in chronic well-compensated liver disease, such as alcohol-induced cirrhosis, and in chronic uremia. *Pregnancy* is associated with reduced protein binding of some and enhanced elimination of many antiseizure drugs (Philbert and Dam, 1982; Tomson, 2009), causing a decrease in serum levels. The unbound fraction that reaches the brain, however, may not always be decreased, so this is not necessarily an indication to increase the dosage if seizures remain controlled.

Drug interactions complicate the pharmacokinetics of antiseizure drugs (Levy et al., 2008; Spina, 2009). In addition to enzyme inhibition and induction, there may be competition for protein binding, resulting in an increase in the free fraction and decrease in serum level of a particular drug (Fig. 14–10), as well as pharmacodynamic interactions at the drug receptor site. Antiseizure drugs affect each other, are affected by other medications, and also influence the serum levels of other medications. Polypharmacy involving the use of more than one antiseizure drug or the use of a single antiseizure drug in association with other medications can therefore account for unexpected failure of therapeutic effect or the appearance of adverse side effects. These interactions occur not only when a second drug is added, as shown in Figures 14–8, 14–9, and 14–10, but also when a second drug is withdrawn (Fig. 14–11).

As a general rule, *phenobarbital, phenytoin, and carbamazepine* tend to be enzyme inducers and decrease the levels of other antiseizure drugs, whereas *valproic acid* is primarily an enzyme inhibitor and increases the level of *phenobarbital* and *lamotrigine*, among other drugs. Chapter 15 discusses drugs that interact with each of the available antiseizure medications, and Table 14–5 shows interactions among antiseizure drugs. Of common practical concern are the reduced efficacy of *oral contraceptives* in women taking enzyme-inducing antiseizure drugs (Mattson et al., 1986) (breakthrough bleeding can be a warning that there is a risk of unwanted pregnancy) and the enhancement of *carbamazepine* levels by the commonly used analgesic *propoxyphene* and the antibiotic *erythromycin*.

Adverse Side Effects

The clinical *effectiveness* of an antiseizure drug depends not only on its *efficacy*, defined as its ability to reduce or eliminate epileptic seizures, but also by its *tolerability*, as determined by the presence or absence of adverse effects (Dodson and Brodie, 2008; Zaccara et al., 2009) (Table 14–6). Adverse side effects of antiseizure drugs can be acute, occurring shortly after the institution of treatment, or chronic, occurring months or years later. They are usually divided into four types (Glauser, 2000): Type A, directly related to the pharmacological effects of the drug, predictable, and reversible with drug removal (*dose dependent*); Type B, unrelated to the pharmacological effects of the drug and unpredictable (*idiosyncratic, hypersensitive, allergic*), which can be life threatening; Type C, cumulative effects of long-term therapy; and Type D, delayed consequences such as carcinogenic and teratogenic effects. Hematological and hepatic side effects are of the highest concern. Consequently, preliminary evaluation before beginning antiseizure drug treatment should include a complete blood count, including platelets, and

Table 14–5 Drug Interactions for Commonly Used Antiseizure Drugs (effect of drugs listed across the top on serum levels of drugs listed to the left)

	CBZ	CLB	CLN	ESL	ESM	EZG	FBM	GBP	LCM	LTG	LEV	OXC	PB	PHT	PGN	PRM	RUF	TGB	TPM	VPA	VGB	ZON
CBZ	–	–	–	–	–	–	↓*	–	–	–	–	↓*	↓	↓	–	↓	↓	–	–	↑	–	–
CLB	↓*	–	–	–	–	–	–	–	–	–	–	–	↓*	↓*	–	↓*	–	–	–	–	–	–
CLN	↓	–	–	–	–	–	–	–	–	–	–	–	↓	↓	–	–	–	–	–	–	–	–
ESL	↓	–	–	–	–	–	–	–	–	–	–	–	↓	↓	–	↓	–	–	–	–	–	–
ESM	↓	–	–	–	–	–	–	–	–	–	–	–	↓	↓	–	–	–	–	–	↑	–	–
EZG	↓	–	–	–	–	–	–	–	–	–	–	–	–	↓	–	–	–	–	–	–	–	–
FBM	↓	–	–	–	–	–	–	–	–	–	–	–	↓	↓	–	↓	–	–	–	↑	–	–
GBP	–	–	–	–	–	–	–	–	–	–	–	–	–	–	–	–	–	–	–	–	–	–
LCM	–	–	–	–	–	–	–	–	–	–	–	–	–	–	–	–	–	–	–	–	–	–
LTG	↓	–	–	–	–	–	–	–	–	–	–	↑	↓	↓	–	↓	↓	–	–	↑	–	–
LEV	–	–	–	–	–	–	–	–	–	–	–	–	–	–	–	–	–	–	–	–	–	–
OXC	↓	–	–	–	–	–	–	–	–	–	–	–	↓	↓	–	↓	↑	–	–	–	–	–
PB	–	–	–	–	–	–	↑	–	–	–	–	↑	–	↑	–	↑	↑	–	–	↑	–	–
PHT	↓	–	–	–	–	–	↑	–	–	–	–	↑	↑	–	–	–	↑	–	↑	↑	↓	–
PGN	–	–	–	–	–	–	–	–	–	–	–	–	–	–	–	–	–	–	–	–	–	–
PRM	↓	–	–	–	–	–	↑	–	–	–	–	–	↓	↓	–	–	↑	–	–	↑	–	–
RUF	↓	–	–	–	–	–	–	–	–	–	–	–	↓	↓	–	↓	–	–	–	↑	–	–
TGB	↓	–	–	–	–	–	–	–	–	–	–	–	↓	↓	–	↓	–	–	–	–	–	–
TPM	↓	–	–	–	–	–	–	–	–	–	–	–	↓	↓	–	↓	–	–	–	↓	–	–
VPA	↓	–	–	–	–	–	–	–	–	–	–	–	↓	↓	–	↓	–	↓	↓	–	–	–
VGB	–	–	–	–	–	–	–	–	–	–	–	–	–	–	–	–	–	–	–	–	–	–
ZON	↓	–	–	–	–	–	–	–	–	–	–	–	↓	↓	–	↓	–	–	–	↓	–	–

*Increases active metabolite.
For key to other drug name abbreviations, see Table 15–1.

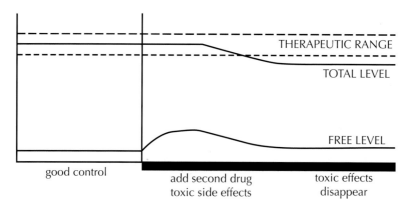

Figure 14–10. For a drug that is largely protein-bound, the free level responsible for seizure control represents a small percentage of the total level in the serum. When a second medication that competes with protein binding is added, the free fraction of the first drug may increase without altering total serum level. Toxic side effects in this situation can reflect increased access of the first drug to the brain rather than an action of the newly added second drug. With chronic administration, however, increased clearance of the first drug usually occurs, causing the total serum level to fall while the free level returns to its original value. In this situation, the decreased total serum level is not a reason to increase drug dose.

routine liver function tests. Although these tests should be repeated intermittently as long as treatment continues, frequent repetition is usually not necessary; alerting patients to warning signs and symptoms can be far more important. Recommendations for the specific tests and their frequency depend on the medications, as discussed in Chapter 15. Drug effects on interictal behavior are discussed in Chapter 11. Carcinogenic effects are not a concern with antiseizure drugs and teratogenicity is discussed later in this chapter.

DOSE-DEPENDENT ADVERSE SIDE EFFECTS

The most common adverse effects caused by antiseizure drugs are dose-related (Schmidt and Schachter, 2008). They occur when a *toxic level* of drug is reached and generally disappear when the drug concentration is subsequently lowered. Although dose-related side effects can appear at any time during the course of chronic treatment, as a result of the many pharmacokinetic factors that transiently effect serum level, they are usually encountered when antiseizure

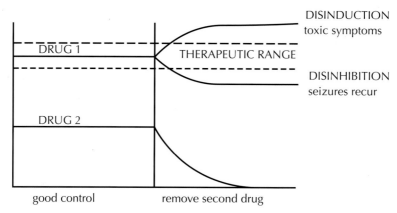

Figure 14–11. When two or more drugs are prescribed, the steady-state serum level of one drug may be dependent on enzyme induction or enzyme inhibition by a second drug. Withdrawal of the second drug, therefore, removes these drug interactions. Removal of enzyme induction (disinduction) would elevate the serum level of the first drug and could cause toxic symptoms, whereas removal of enzyme inhibition (disinhibition) would reduce the serum level of the first drug and could cause seizures to recur. In the latter situation, seizure recurrence might be erroneously attributed to removal of the second drug. The appropriate response in this instance is to increase the dose of the first drug and attempt to reestablish seizure control with monotherapy.

Table 14–6 Adverse Effects of Commonly Used Antiseizure Drugs

	Dose-Related				Idiosyncratic						
	CNS Movement	CNS Cognitive	CNS Psychiatric	Other	Withdrawal Effects	Aplastic Anemia	Hepatotoxicity	StevensJohnson	Renal stones	Other	
CBZ	+	++	–	GI	–	+	+	+	–	–	CBZ
CLB	+	++	+	GI	+	–	–	–	–	–	CLB
CLN	+	++	–	GI	+	–	–	–	–	–	CLN
ESL	+	+	–	GI, HA	–	–	+	–	–	–	ESL
ESM	–	+	+	GI, HA	–	+	–	+	–	SLE	ESM
EZG	+	+	–		–	–	–	–	–	UTR	EZG
FBM	+	+	–	GI, HA	–	++	++	–	–	–	FBM
GBP	+	+	–	GI, I	–	–	–	–	–	AP	GBP
LCM	+	+	+	GI	–	–	–	–	–	–	LCM
LTG	+	+	–	GI, R, HA	–	+	+	++	–	–	LTG
LEV	+	+	+		–	+	+	–	–	–	LEV
OXC	+	++	–	GI, R	–	+	+	+	–	AP	OXC
PB	+	++	+	I	+	+	+	+	–	–	PB
PHT	+	++	+	GI	–	+	+	+	–	PL	PHT
PGN	+	+	–	GI, I	–	+	–	–	–	AE	PGN
PRM	+	++	+	I	+	–	+	+	–	–	PRM
RUF	+	+	–	GI	–	–	+	–	–	–	RUF
TGB	+	+	+	GI, E	–	–	–	–	–	–	TGB
TPM	–	+++	–	GI, E	–	–	–	–	+	MA, H	TPM
VPA	+	+	–	GI, MA, H, GL	–	+	+	–	–	A, HY, AP	VPA
VGB	+	+	+	GI, HA	–	–	–	–	–	VF	VGB
ZON	+	+	+	GI, MA, H	–	+	+	+	+	–	ZON

(continued)

Table 14–6 (Continued)

	Long Term					Seizure Aggravation				
	Osteoporosis	Connective Tissue	Cardiac Arrhythmia	SIADH	Weight (↑ gain, ↓ loss)	Absence	Lennox-Gastaut/West	Generalized Tonic-Clonic	Myoclonic	
CBZ	+	–	+	+	–	+	+	–	+	CBZ
CLB	–	–	–	–	–	–	–	–	–	CLB
CLN	–	–	–	–	–	–	–	+	–	CLN
ESL	–	–	–	–	–	–	–	–	–	ESL
ESM	–	–	–	–	–	–	+	+	–	ESM
EZG	–	–	–	–	–	–	–	–	–	EZG
FBM	–	–	–	–	↓	–	–	–	–	FBM
GBP	–	–	–	–	↑↑	+	+	+	+	GBP
LCM	–	–	+	–	–	–	–	–	–	LCM
LTG	–	–	+	–	↔	–	–	–	+	LTG
LEV	–	–	–	–	↔	–	–	–	–	LEV
OXC	–	–	+	+	↔	+	+	–	+	OXC
PB	+	+	–	–	–	+	–	–	–	PB
PHT	–	+	+	–	–	+	+	–	+	PHT
PGN	–	–	–	–	↑↑	–	+	–	+	PGN
PRM	+	+	+	–	–	+	–	–	–	PRM
RUF	–	–	–	–	↔	–	–	–	–	RUF
TGB	–	–	–	–	↔	+	–	–	–	TGB
TPM	–	–	–	–	↓↓↓	–	–	–	–	TPM
VPA	+	–	–	–	↑↑	–	–	–	–	VPA
VGB	–	–	–	–	↑↑	+	–	–	+	VGB
ZON	–	–	–	–	↓	–	–	–	–	ZON

A = alopecia; AE = angioedema with airway obstruction; AP = acute pancreatitis; E = ecchymosis; GI = gastrointestinal; GL = glaucoma; H = hyperthermia; HA = headache; HY = hyperammonemia; I = impotence, decreased libido; MA = metabolic acidosis; R = rash; SIADH = syndrome of inappropriate antidiuretic hormone hypersecretion; SLE = systemic lupus erythematosus; UTR = Urinary tract retention; VF = visual field defect. For key to drug name abbreviations, see Table 15–1.

drug treatment is being instituted. Patients will commonly develop a tolerance to these initial effects. Consequently, if the drug dose is unchanged or lowered only slightly, the side effects often disappear over a week or two, and a higher level of drug can then be ultimately achieved. This phenomenon is of great clinical importance, because it means that early occurrence of dose-related side effects is not a reason to discontinue the drug of choice. Pushing a drug too quickly risks the occurrence of severe dose-related side effects that can cause a patient to refuse to continue a drug that might have been beneficial. Hence the *"Start low, go slow"* philosophy.

There is concern that some acute dose-related side effects may be irreversible. Whether permanent cerebellar damage can result from a single severe episode of *phenytoin* intoxication is a controversial issue discussed later in this chapter. On the other hand, there is no evidence that even a brief exposure to major toxic levels of any antiseizure drug is harmless, and avoidance of such acute dose-dependent adverse effects may be one means of preventing chronic side effects (Reynolds, 1983a). Nevertheless, fears of minor, transient discomfort from dose-related side effects should not prevent the prescribing physician from maximizing the therapeutic potential of a given agent.

The most common acute dose-related side effects of antiseizure medication are gastrointestinal and neurological (Chapter 15). Nausea, gastric distress, and occasionally vomiting, diarrhea, and constipation are typical, particularly of the older drugs. These symptoms often disappear with time without a change in dosage and invariably respond to a decrease or discontinuation of the medication. Sedation and impairment of cognitive function occur with *barbiturates*, *benzodiazepines*, *topiramate*, and, to a certain extent, other antiseizure drugs such as *phenytoin*, *carbamazepine*, and *oxcarbazepine*. These effects are less likely with *valproic acid* and the newer drugs. Nystagmus, slurred speech, ataxia, and diplopia are most commonly encountered with *phenytoin* and *carbamazepine*; a postural tremor can develop with *valproic acid*. Behavioral side effects are often of great clinical concern, such as the hyperkinetic activity seen in children on *barbiturates* and, to a lesser degree, *benzodiazepines*; the progressive encephalopathy

that occurs with *phenytoin* and *valproic acid*; irritability with *levetiracetam*; cognitive dysfunction with *topiramate*; and the depression and psychosis that are induced by a number of drugs (Chapter 11). The sedative effects of *barbiturates* and *benzodiazepines* are a particular problem in the elderly. Impotence is a disturbing and avoidable dose-related side effect of some antiseizure medications. Because this effect is not always spontaneously reported, the physician should ask the patient relevant questions.

All of the antiseizure drugs are capable of producing a dose-related skin rash, but the rash is less likely to appear if the dose is started at a low level and increased gradually. These skin rashes are usually benign and can often be adequately treated with antiallergenic agents such as *diphenhydramine*. A bullous dermatitis, mucosal involvement, fever, lymphadenopathy, or malaise, however, suggest the development of a potentially life-threatening allergic reaction such as *erythema multiforme*, *exfoliative dermatitis*, the *Stevens-Johnson syndrome*, or other serious idiosyncratic reactions, requiring immediate termination of the drug (Booker, 1975).

One peculiar dose-related side effect of antiseizure drugs is a paradoxical increase in epileptic seizure frequency. Although this has been reported most often with *phenytoin* at levels above 40 μg/ml (Troupin and Ojemann, 1975), it can be seen with other medications as well (Perucca et al., 1998). In some cases the antiseizure drugs that produce sedation increase the likelihood of seizures that are precipitated by drowsiness; in other cases there may be a direct agonistic effect of the drug on ictogenic mechanisms.

HYPERSENSITIVE AND CHRONIC ADVERSE SIDE EFFECTS

Epilepsy, perhaps more than any other medical disorder, often requires prolonged treatment with a variety of pharmacological agents. Chronic and other non-dose-dependent toxicity of these agents has manifested as disturbances in almost every system of the body, but several such effects of antiseizure drugs are particularly common and require some mention here (Pirmohamed and Arroyo, 2008; Pack and Gidal, 2008; Zaccara et al., 2009). The serious hypersensitive adverse dermatological side effects have already been discussed, and a genetic susceptibility for these allergic reactions is presumed. It is likely that most, perhaps all, adverse reactions are genetically mediated and that pharmacogenetics will eventually help identify patients at risk for specific serious toxic effects, leading to personalized medicine (Glauser, 2000). The identification of the *HLA-B°1502* allele as a marker of high risk for *Stevens-Johnson syndrome* in Han Chinese and other South Asian ethnic groups taking *carbamazepine* is the first example of the promise of this approach (Chung et al., 2004; Chen et al., 2011).

Of the numerous *hematological* disorders that have been attributed to chronic treatment with antiseizure drugs, the most serious is bone marrow suppression, which can result in *aplastic anemia*. This has been a particular concern with *carbamazepine, phenytoin*, and *felbamate*. There is controversy concerning the role of *phenytoin* and *carbamazepine* in producing this effect, however, because most patients who were reported with aplastic anemia on these drugs had additional disease processes and were taking other drugs that could also account for the blood dyscrasia (Reynolds, 1983b). There were several reports of aplastic anemia when *carbamazepine* was given in older patients for trigeminal neuralgia, but this experience has not been repeated with the use of *carbamazepine* for the treatment of epilepsy (Chapter 15). Benign depression of leukocytes commonly occurs with *carbamazepine* treatment. A white count even as low as 3,000/mm^3 does not necessarily require termination of treatment, as long as the total neutrophil count is not allowed to descend below 1,000/mm^3 (Bourgeois et al., 1987). Whereas *carbamazepine* may be associated with a five to eight times greater incidence of aplastic anemia than the general population, the risk with *felbamate* is estimated to be 1 per 4,000–10,000 exposed patients, several hundred times that in the general population (Pirmohamed and Arroyo, 2008). *Agranulocytosis, leukopenia*, and *thrombocytopenia* can occur as allergic reactions with *phenytoin* and other antiseizure drugs (Reynolds, 1983b; Zaccara et al., 2009). Bleeding disturbances due to abnormalities in platelet aggregation and other clotting factors occur with *valproic acid. Megaloblastic anemia* is seen with many antiseizure drugs, particularly *phenytoin, primidone*, and *phenobarbital*, and is attributed to the *folic acid* depression

commonly encountered in patients taking these drugs.

Hepatotoxicity (Jeavons, 1983; Pirmohamed and Arroyo, 2008) can occur as a hypersensitivity reaction in association with fever, rash, eosinophilia, lymphangiopathy, and jaundice or as an idiosyncratic response. Hepatotoxocity is most commonly seen with *phenytoin, carbamazepine, and phenobarbital* and appears one to six weeks after initiation of treatment. Idiosyncratic reactions are also seen with these drugs, as well as with several others, including *valproic acid*. The defect predisposing to hepatotoxicity may be genetic, and symptoms can appear acutely or up to a year after treatment begins. Additional medications and enzyme induction are believed to be facilitating factors in some hepatotoxic reactions. Although a persistent moderate elevation of liver enzymes occurs in a high percentage of patients who are taking antiseizure drugs, this is usually benign and does not require termination of medication. On the other hand, serious toxic effects are not always preceded by alterations in liver function tests. Overt hepatic toxicity is reported in 0.1–1.0% of patients on antiseizure medication. Fatal hepatic dysfunction associated with *valproic acid* therapy is more similar to *Reye's syndrome* than to hepatotoxicity seen with other antiseizure drugs (Dreifuss and Langer, 1987). Deaths from this disorder have occurred in 1 in 30,000 patients taking *valproic acid*. However, the risk may be as high as 1 in 500 for children under the age of 2 on polytherapy, particularly those with inborn errors of metabolism, whereas no deaths of patients over the age of 10 on monotherapy have been noted (Dreifuss et al., 1987). Symptoms of *valproic acid*–induced hepatotoxicity include malaise, lethargy, anorexia, vomiting, jaundice, and recurrence of seizures, usually within 18–180 days after initiation of treatment, although one patient developed hepatotoxicity after two years of treatment. It has been recommended that (1) *valproic acid* be avoided as polytherapy in children under 3 years of age and in children with a congenital metabolic defect, preexisting liver disease, or a family history of liver disease, (2) this drug be administered at the lowest effective dose, (3) children taking *valproic acid* not be given *salicylates* or fasted, and (4) *valproic acid* be discontinued if symptoms of *valproic acid* hepatotoxicity occur (Dreifuss and Langer, 1987). The mechanisms by which *felbamate* causes hepatic failure are unknown, but the risk is estimated to be 1 per 18,500–25,000 exposed individuals, with females being more susceptible than males (Pirmohamed and Arroyo, 2008). *Felbamate*-induced hepatotoxicity usually presents within 25–181 days after institution of the treatment. *Pancreatitis* is a potentially serious complication of *valproic acid* treatment and is not readily predicted by routine amylase levels.

Chronic effects of antiseizure drugs on the *nervous system* can be central or peripheral. There is concern that *cerebellar degeneration* can result from *phenytoin* administration, and sporadic reports have suggested it may occur after a single episode of intoxication or with continued treatment at therapeutic levels. No unequivocal data have been presented to support this notion, however (Pack and Gidal, 2008), and cerebellar atrophy is relatively common in patients with epilepsy who have not taken *phenytoin* (Oyegbile et al., 2011). Cerebellar atrophy in patients with epilepsy might result from seizures or be related to epileptogenic predisposing factors, and *phenytoin* does not cause cerebellar damage in laboratory animals (Dam, 1983). Whether antiseizure drugs can produce irreversible or progressive *dementia*, perhaps due to folate deficiency (Reynolds, 1983c), remains controversial (Chapter 11). *Dyskinesias* have been seen with *phenytoin* and *carbamazepine* (Davies-Jones, 1985). The occurrence of *peripheral neuropathy* with *phenytoin* treatment is well documented, but this is rarely symptomatic. This effect may be transient because of acute toxicity or permanent with long-term therapy (Chadwick, 1985). A specific relationship with *phenytoin*, however, is unclear (Taylor et al., 1985). A *myasthenia gravis–like* syndrome has also been reported in association with *phenytoin* treatment (Norris et al., 1964), as have sporadic cases of other neurological disturbances (Oxley et al., 1983; Wilder and Bruni, 1981). Irreversible visual field constriction with *vigabatrin* is well documented (Eke et al., 1997) and has greatly limited the use of this drug.

Reversible asymptomatic changes that can be seen on *magnetic resonance imaging (MRI)* with antiseizure dug treatment include increased T2 signal intensity of *thalamus, globus pallidus, dentate, brain stem*, and the *splenium* of the *corpus callosum* with *vigabatrin* (Pearl et al., 2009); similar changes in

the *corpus callosum* with *phenytoin* and perhaps other drugs (Kim et al., 1999); and the well-known shrinkage effect of *adrenocorticotropic hormone (ACTH)* (Fig. 14–12).

Connective tissue disturbances (Schmidt, 1983) are common with *phenytoin, phenobarbital*, and *primidone* treatment. *Gingival hyperplasia* is present in one-third of patients on chronic *phenytoin* therapy and can be minimized by careful gum hygiene. Other cosmetic side effects, such as coarsening of facial features and hirsutism, are also commonly encountered with long-term use of *phenytoin* (Falconer and Davidson, 1973). *Dupuytren's contractures* develop from three months to 20 years after beginning treatment in one-quarter to one-third of patients taking *phenobarbital* and *primidone* and may be associated with fibromas of the mouth and of the plantar fascia of the foot (*lederhosen syndrome*). A complex genetic susceptibility to Dupuytren's contracture has been reported (Dolmans et al., 2011). *Frozen shoulder syndrome*, which is reversible when treatment is discontinued without undue delay, and fibrous induration of the penis (*Peyronie's disease*) (Schmidt, 1983) have also been reported with *barbiturates*.

Disorders of *mineral metabolism* (Offermann, 1983; Pack and Gidal, 2008) lead to *osteoporosis* and *rickets* in 5–10% of patients after long-term treatment with some antiseizure drugs, most often including high doses of *phenytoin, primidone*, and *carbonic anhydrase inhibitors*. These bone disorders are associated with a mild *vitamin D* deficiency, and a disturbance in calcium metabolism can be treated with calcium and vitamin D. *Dual-energy X-ray absorptiometry (DEXA)* scans should be performed routinely in patients after long-term chronic treatment with antiseizure drugs. *Alopecia* with *valproic acid* results from deficiencies in zinc, selenium, and manganese, which are important for free-radical scavenging. This condition might respond to zinc and selenium replacement.

Antiseizure drugs can affect *endocrine metabolism* in many ways, although this usually does not result in symptoms (Davies-Jones, 1985; Wilder and Bruni, 1981, Pack and Gidal, 2008). *Phenytoin, carbamazepine*, and *phenobarbital*, being enzyme inducers, can cause failure of a low-dose *dexamethasone suppression test* and a subnormal *metyrapone test*. *Phenytoin* can decrease the insulin response to

516 Seizures and Epilepsy

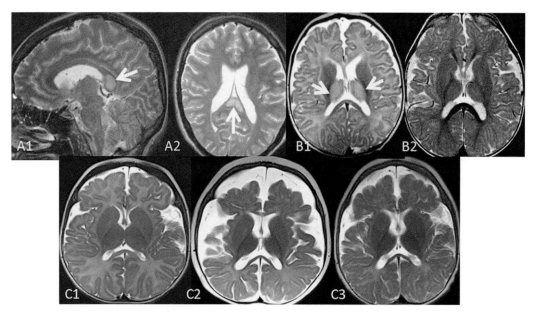

Figure 14–12. Toxic metabolic change of the brain related to the antiseizure medication. **A.** Sagittal T2-weighted image (*A1*) and axial T2-weighted image (*A2*) show a well-defined focus of high signal within the splenium of the corpus callosum (*arrow*). This finding usually indicates reversible edema within the corpus callosum, which is most commonly seen in the splenium; here it is thought to be due to phenytoin toxicity. **B.** Axial T2-weighted image (*B1*) demonstrates high signal within the thalamus bilaterally (*arrows*), which is nonspecific but in this case is due to vigabatrin toxicity–related edema. The treatment was discontinued and an MRI six weeks later (*B2*) demonstrates reversal of signal abnormality within the thalamus. **C.** *C1:* Pretreatment axial T2-weighted image in a patient with infantile spasm. The brain is symmetric and normal in size. *C2:* After months of ACTH treatment, there is significant atrophy of the cerebrum with enlarged lateral ventricles. *C3:* Four months after ACTH was discontinued, MRI shows recovery of brain size and slightly smaller ventricles. (Courtesy of Dr. Noriko Salamon.)

glucose and produces hyperglycemia as well as an abnormal glucose tolerance test. Thyroxine binding is decreased by *phenytoin, valproic acid*, and *carbamazepine*, which usually results in abnormally low values for protein-bound iodine, although thyroid function remains normal. A number of disturbances in sex hormones have been reported with various antiseizure medications (Toone, 1987). Polycystic ovaries and hyperandrogenism can occur with valproate. Elevated cholesterol with *phenytoin* and *phenobarbital* treatment may be due to increased high-density lipoproteins. *Phenytoin* can inhibit secretion of antidiuretic hormone, whereas *carbamazepine* and *oxcarbazepine* cause water intoxication. Whether the often disturbing weight gain seen with *valproic acid, gabapentin, pregabalin*, and *vigabatrin* and the weight loss seen with *topiramate, felbamate*, and *zonisamide* are due to endocrinological disturbances is not known.

Immunological side effects of antiseizure medications also occur (Cereghino, 1983;

Zaccara et al., 2009). Patients on *phenytoin* develop depressed cellular and humoral immunity, and an IgA deficiency may be related to an *HLA-A* histocompatibility antigen. *Pseudolymphoma* can occur with chronic *phenytoin* treatment and has been seen with *primidone* and *phensuximide*. The relationship of this phenomenon to immune depression and malignant lymphoma is not clear. Autoimmune disorders also develop with a variety of antiseizure medications, and *lupoid drug reactions* as well as *lupus erythematosus* have been associated with *phenytoin, carbamazepine, primidone, mephenytoin, trimethadione*, and *ethosuximide*. The importance of genetic factors in these chronic drug-induced immunological disturbances remains to be determined.

The appearance of chronic adverse symptoms is influenced by the age at which treatment was begun, duration of treatment, polypharmacy, occurrence of acute toxicity, and vulnerability factors such as institutionalization, poor nutrition, pregnancy, intercurrent illness, and chronic disabilities (Reynolds, 1983a). Recommendations for avoiding chronic toxicity include (1) establishment of the correct diagnosis, (2) early institution of effective treatment, (3) use of the appropriate drug as monotherapy at doses that do not produce acute toxicity, (4) recognition by family members and the physician as soon as dose-related side effects occur, particularly in children who have been treated over a long period, and (5) prevention of unnecessary use of antiseizure drugs in patients who have been given incorrect diagnoses of epilepsy (Reynolds, 1983a). The potential for withdrawing antiseizure medication after the patient has been seizure-free for several years should be realized, as discussed later in this chapter. The risk presented by the possible transient recurrence of seizures during withdrawal may not outweigh the opportunity to prevent potential chronic toxicity from long-term medication.

Drug Monitoring

The introduction of techniques for easy measurement of serum concentrations of antiseizure drugs has greatly improved the effectiveness of pharmacological treatment (Johannessen et al., 2008; Patsalos et al., 2008). Table 14–7 lists important uses of antiseizure drug monitoring. Serum drug level determinations are

Table 14–7 Uses of Antiseizure Drug Monitoring

1. Evaluate degree of compliance.
2. Determine whether initial failure of a drug to control seizures or appearance of toxic symptoms is due to:
   a. Pharmacokinetic factors that require changing drug dose and/or schedule.
   b. Pharmacodynamic factors that require changing to another drug.
3. Determine effective drug level when initiation of treatment is successful in controlling seizures.
4. Determine whether seizure recurrence after control, or late appearance of side effects, is due to changes in serum drug levels.
5. Determine whether appearance of behavioral disturbances might represent toxic side effects of a drug.
6. Determine which drug is responsible for toxic side effects when more than one drug is used.

specifically indicated (1) when initiating treatment while seizures remain uncontrolled or when seizures ordinarily occur infrequently, (2) to establish the therapeutic concentration in the individual patient once seizures are controlled, (3) when seizures become uncontrolled or adverse side effects appear due to intercurrent illness, addition of other drugs, or state changes such as pregnancy or puberty, and (4) when unexplained behavioral changes or other neurological symptoms occur that may be evidence of drug toxicity (Patsalos et al., 2008). Establishing the therapeutic concentration for individual patients is especially useful to guide clinical management should the patient later show a change in drug response or be exposed to conditions modifying drug disposition, such as pregnancy, concurrent disease, or interacting medications.

For direct comparison of successive values of serum drug concentrations, each sample must be drawn at the same time with respect to the dose schedule. Although many workers recommend routinely obtaining a *trough level* just before the morning dose, when the serum concentration is the lowest, others maintain that any convenient sampling point is equally appropriate for most patients as long as it is used consistently. Trough levels are necessary, however, when drug monitoring is used for diagnosis and correction of an aberrant drug response. This is particularly true for drugs that have short half-lives. Measurements must take into account pharmacokinetic factors, compliance, meals, the time of sampling, genetic influences, and drug formulation. When an abnormally shortened half-life is suspected, it is helpful to obtain both peak and trough levels, as well as levels at other points on the curve, for two or more cycles, to determine whether more frequent dosing is needed. Interindividual variability in pharmacokinetics is most pronounced for *clobazam, clonazepam, carbamazepine, felbamate, gabapentin, lamotrigine, phenytoin, tiagabine, topiramate, valproic acid*, and *zonisamide* (Johannessen et al., 2008).

A variety of analytical techniques are available for measuring antiseizure drug levels in the plasma (Johannessen et al., 2008). Commercial reagents are available for measurements of older drugs such as *carbamazepine, phenytoin, phenobarbital, primidone, ethosuximide*, and *valproic acid* and for some of the newer drugs, such as *lamotrigine, topiramate*, and *zonisamide*. Measurements of *benzodiazepines*, their metabolites, and most of the newer anti-seizure drugs require specialized equipment, most often *high-performance liquid chromatography*, and some drugs, such as *vigabatrin*, *gabapentin*, and *pregabalin*, require more difficult techniques such as *fluorescence*. It is important to ensure that quality control has been established for laboratories to be used for determining antiseizure drug levels.

Choosing the Appropriate Drug

The choice of drug is dictated to some degree by each patient's seizure types and epilepsy syndrome if present (see Table 14–8) but remains in most cases a matter of individual preference, based largely on the side effects profile and dosing schedule. Cost and insurance limitations also often place restrictions on drug choice. The recommended drugs for specific epilepsy syndromes are discussed with the treatment of these syndromes in Chapters 7

and 10. Chapter 15 gives further information on individual drugs. The older concept of first- and second-line drugs no longer applies, and there can be good reason to initiate treatment with newer drugs; however, *tiagabine* is generally considered less effective than other commonly used medications, and serious adverse side effects limit the use of *felbamate* and *vigabatrin* to last-resort status.

An early study comparing the older antiseizure drugs *carbamazepine, phenytoin, phenobarbital*, and *primidone* found no significant difference in efficacy for focal and generalized tonic-clonic seizures; however, failure of treatment due to unacceptable side effects was less frequent with *carbamazepine* than with the other medications (Mattson et al., 1985).

More recent practice parameters published by the AAN and the American Epilepsy Society (AES) (French et al., 2004a) considered efficacy and tolerability of the new antiseizure drugs for treatment of new-onset epilepsy. The report concluded: "*Gabapentin, lamotrigine, topiramate, and oxcarbazepine have efficacy as*

Table 14–8 Indications for Commonly Used Antiseizure Drugs

	Focal Seizures	Generalized Tonic-Clonic Seizures	Absence Seizures	Myoclonic Seizures	Lennox-Gastaut	West Syndrome	Myoclonus	
CBZ	xxx	xxx						CBZ
CLB	xxx	xxx		xxx	xxx		xxx	CLB
CLN	xx	xx	x	xxx	xx	x	xxx	CLN
ESL	xxx	xxx						ESL
ESM			xxx	x				ESM
EZG	xxx	xxx						EZG
FBM	xxx	xxx	x	x	xxx	x		FBM
GBP	xxx	xxx						GBP
LCM	xxx	xxx						LCM
LTG	xxx	xxx	xx	xx	x	x		LTG
LEV	xxx	xxx	xx	xx	xx	x	xx	LEV
OXC	xxx	xxx						OXC
PB	xxx	xxx		x	x			PB
PHT	xxx	xxx						PHT
PGN	xxx	xxx						PGN
PRM	xxx	xxx		x	x			PRM
RUF	x	x	x	x	xxx			RUF
TGB	xx	xx						TGB
TPM	xxx	xxx	x	xx	xx	x		TPM
VPA	xx	xx	xx	xxx	xx	x	xx	VPA
VGB	xxx	xxx			xxx			VGB
ZON	xxx	xxx	xx	xx	xx	xx		ZON

For key to drug name abbreviations, see Table 15–1.

monotherapy in newly diagnosed adolescents and adults with either partial or mixed seizure disorders. There is also evidence that *lamotrigine* is effective for newly diagnosed absence seizures in children." An accompanying report for refractory seizures (French et al., 2004b) concluded that "all new AEDs [antiepileptic drugs] were found to be appropriate for adjunctive treatment of refractory partial seizures in adults. *Gabapentin* can be effective for the treatment of mixed seizure disorders, and *gabapentin, lamotrigine, oxcarbazepine, and topiramate* for the treatment of refractory partial seizures in children. Limited evidence suggests that *lamotrigine* and *topiramate* are also effective for adjunctive treatment of idiopathic generalized epilepsy in adults and children, as well as treatment of the Lennox-Gastaut syndrome." The term *mixed seizure disorders* in these reports, however, can be misleading, as some of these drugs, such as *gabapentin* and *oxcarbazepine*, can make absence and myoclonic seizures worse (see Table 14–6) (Chapter 15).

The International League Against Epilepsy (ILAE) subsequently published treatment guidelines for new-onset epilepsy based on a systematic review of controlled studies and found specific drugs to be effective with level A (established as efficacious as initial monotherapy) or level B (probably efficacious as initial monotherapy) for only three seizure conditions: *carbamazepine* and *phenytoin* were level A and *valproic acid* level B for focal seizures in adults, *oxcarbazepine* was level A for focal seizures in children, and *gabapentin* and *lamotrigine* were level A for focal seizures in elderly adults (Glauser et al., 2006). Insufficient evidence was available to permit conclusions regarding other antiseizure drugs. However, it should be stressed that the authors of the ILAE guidelines rated antiseizure drugs purely on the basis of clinical trials that met a predefined set of strict quality criteria, including double blinding, and emphasized that drugs with the best evidence for efficacy based on the quality of those trials are not necessarily the most efficacious for the indicated conditions.

The *Standard and New Antiepileptic Drug (SANAD)* study compared new drugs with older ones in unblinded randomized controlled trials. Based on time to treatment failure and time to 12-month remission, *lamotrigine* fared best for focal epilepsy, slightly better than *carbamazepine* and *oxcarbazepine*

and clearly better than *gabapentin* and *topiramate* (Marson et al., 2007a), and *valproic acid* fared best for treatment of generalized seizures and unclassifiable epilepsy, where it was better tolerated than *topiramate* and more efficacious than *lamotrigine* (Marson et al., 2007b). *Levetiracetam* and other newer drugs were not included in these studies. It is clear, however, from all investigations that clinical effectiveness of antiseizure drugs depends more on tolerability than on efficacy, and the superiority of *valproic acid* in the second SANAD trial must be balanced against the increased teratogenic risk of this drug in women of childbearing age (see below).

A randomized controlled trial found that *ethosuximide* and *valproic acid* were more effective than *lamotrigine* for childhood absence seizures and that *ethosuximide* had fewer adverse attentional effects (Glauser et al., 2010). *Felbamate* is particularly effective against drop attacks associated with the *Lennox-Gastaut syndrome* but is a drug of last resort, because of the high risk of aplastic anemia and hepatotoxicity. In randomized controlled trials, *lamotrigine, rufinamide,* and *clobazam* have also been found to be effective against drop attacks in patients with the Lennox-Gastaut syndrome. *Benzodiazepines, valproic acid, levetiracetam,* and *zonisamide* can be used to treat myoclonus associated with epilepsy in *progressive myoclonus epilepsy.*

When mixed seizures cannot be controlled with a single medication, it is useful to use two drugs that are effective against the different seizure types. Except for these situations, there are no specific guidelines for attempting to treat a seizure disorder with two drugs when monotherapy fails (Perucca, 2011). A commonly stated general rule is to avoid combining drugs with similar mechanisms of action, e.g., *phenytoin* and *carbamazepine* or *phenobarbital* and *primidone* (see Table 14–3). Although there is no justification for the latter combination, because *phenobarbital* is the major metabolite of *primidone,* some patients do appear to respond better to the combination of *carbamazepine* and *phenytoin* than to either drug alone. If epileptic seizures are not adequately controlled after trials of two appropriate medications have failed, the chance that seizure control will be achieved by adding a second drug is extremely small (Kwan and Brodie, 2000; Elwes et al., 1984; Mattson et al., 1985;

Schmidt, 1982; Kwan et al., 2010), although a few studies suggest a better response than previously believed (Luciano and Shorvon, 2007; Bauer et al., 2008; Liimatainen et al., 2008).

Other pharmacological agents are also occasionally useful as therapy for seizures. *Acetazolamide* before and during menses and *oral contraceptives* can be of benefit for women with *catamenial* exacerbation of epileptic seizures (Chapter 9). *Infantile spasms* are commonly treated with *ACTH, corticosteroids,* or *vigabatrin* (Chapter 7).

Generic preparations of antiseizure drugs, where available, usually are cheaper than brand-name drugs; however, there is considerable controversy concerning the advisability of their use for epilepsy. Formulations differ, and it is likely that any given generic will not have exactly the same bioavailability as a brand-name drug or another generic. The US Food and Drug Administration (FDA) requires *bioequivalence* between generic and brand-name antiseizure drugs, but this is not the same as *therapeutic equivalence* when differences in pharmacokinetics result in different efficacy and tolerability (Privitera, 2008). Although a meta-analysis of randomized controlled trials did not reveal a loss of seizure control with generic substitution (Kesselheim et al., 2010), there remain numerous convincing case reports in the literature of problems occurring with generic substitution (Jain, 1993; Andermann et al., 2007; Fitzgerald and Jacobson, 2011). Acknowledged problems with these uncontrolled studies, however, are the *nocebo effect*, that is, the possibility that breakthrough seizures occur when patients know that they have been placed on generic drugs that could have an inferior efficacy, and the increased tendency of physicians and patients to report deterioration. Higher peaks and lower troughs occur with more rapid absorption of some generic preparations, and there is always the risk that raised or lowered serum levels, with consequent adverse side effects or seizure relapse, will occur if one preparation is substituted for another.

Beginning a patient on a generic formulation rather than a brand-name drug does not necessarily avoid this risk, because pharmacies tend to switch from one generic preparation to another as availability and wholesale prices change, and even the same generic company may switch from one manufacturer to another, with accompanying differences in formulation.

Whereas the FDA mandates that the bioavailability of a generic drug be between 0.80 and 1.25 of the brand-name formulation, the difference between two generic drugs can be twice this amount, which could have a significant effect on seizure control and toxic side effects for individual patients. Most studies have considered effects of changing from brand name to generic; however, changing from one generic to another presents a much greater danger for patients (Krauss et al., 2011). Because of the psychological and social consequences of a breakthrough seizure in individuals whose seizures are under control, until an appropriate large-scale randomized controlled trial can be performed the AAN and the AES do not recommend generic substitution without physician approval (Liow et al., 2007). Given the increased importance of cost in health care delivery, a reasonable solution would be for hospitals or pharmacies to contract with manufacturers of generic antiseizure drugs to ensure consistent formulation, as the *Veterans Administration* has done.

With so many antiseizure drugs to choose from, all with very similar therapeutic efficacies, the choice of medication usually depends largely on the side effect profile. For instance, drugs that cause weight gain or cosmetic changes would be unacceptable to many patients, drugs that have few or no interactions with other drugs may be preferable in the elderly or any patients with other chronic diseases that require drug treatment, and *carbamazepine* and *oxcarbazepine* can cause water retention and should not be used in patients at risk for congestive heart failure. Those antiseizure drugs that also have beneficial effects in other conditions, such as migraine headaches, neuropathic pain, and bipolar disorder, would be good choices for patients who also have these conditions (Table 14–9). *Carbamazepine* should be avoided in Han Chinese and anyone with the *HLA-B*1502* allele. Future pharmacogenetic studies should lead to the identification of patients with genetic susceptibility to other serious allergic drug reactions.

Discontinuation of Medication

The decision to stop medication is as important as the decision to begin it (Dulac et al., 2008). Adult patients who have been seizure-free on

Table 14–9 Nonepilepsy Uses for Commonly Used Antiseizure Drugs

	Bipolar Disorder		Anxiety	Psychosis	Migraine	Neuropathic Pain	Trigeminal Neuralgia	Obesity	Sedation Drug Withdrawal	Tremor	
	Mania	Disorder									
CBZ	x	x	–	–	–	x	x	–	–	x	CBZ
CLB	–	–	x	–	–	–	–	–	–	–	CLB
CLN	–	–	x	–	–	–	–	–	–	–	CLN
GBP	–	x	x	x	–	x	x	–	–	–	GBP
LTG	–	x	–	–	x	x	x	–	–	–	LTG
LEV	x	–	–	–	–	–	–	–	–	–	LEV
OXC	–	x	–	–	–	x	x	–	–	–	OXC
PB	–	–	–	–	–	–	–	–	x	–	PB
PHT	–	–	–	–	–	–	x	–	–	–	PHT
PGN	–	–	x	–	–	x	–	–	–	–	PGN
PRM	–	–	–	–	–	–	–	–	–	x	PRM
TGB	–	–	x	–	–	x	–	–	–	–	TGB
TPM	–	x	x	–	x	x	–	x	–	–	TPM
VPA	x	x	–	x	x	–	–	–	–	–	VPA
VGB	–	–	–	–	–	–	–	–	–	–	VGB
ZON	–	x	–	–	x	x	–	x	–	x	ZON

For key to drug name abbreviations, see Table 15–1.

medication for many years often either are no longer under the care of a specialist or have very low serum blood levels as a result of an increasing degree of noncompliance. Also, many patients in remission terminate their own medication. Although spontaneous remission is quite common in some chronic epilepsy disorders, particularly the benign genetic epilepsies of childhood (Chapter 7), very few studies have systematically analyzed the factors that lead to relapse following drug withdrawal in seizure-free adult patients (Dulac et al., 2008). Furthermore, those studies that have examined relapse under these conditions have not taken into account that after many years some patients also experience relapse while on medication.

Reported remission rates in epilepsy vary considerably and depend on the type of seizures and epilepsy syndromes (Chadwick, 1985). The remission rate for generalized tonic-clonic seizures may be as high as 80%, whereas the rate for focal dyscognitive seizures may be as low as 20%. For most studies, remission rates are higher for children than for adults, as would be expected because of the benign genetic epilepsy disorders that begin in childhood (Chapter 7). That actual figures have not changed appreciably throughout the past century suggests that remission rates reflect the natural history of epilepsy and not the influence of antiseizure drugs (Chadwick, 1985; Dulac et al., 2008). Therefore, an important issue when one is attempting to analyze the effect of medication withdrawal in seizure-free patients is whether relapse would have occurred even if medication had not been withdrawn. Studies that have examined relapse rates following drug withdrawal after a seizure-free interval, usually two to four years, have variously indicated that 17–65% of adults and 6–39% of children experience recurrence of seizures, half of these during the withdrawal period (Chadwick, 1985; Specchio and Beghi, 2004). The risk of relapse on drugs is variously reported to be 1.6–12.8% per year; and in patients who experience immediate remission on institution of medication, the risk of relapse is approximately 8% per year (Chadwick, 1985; Berg and Shinnar, 1994). In the only double-blind randomized controlled trial of drug withdrawal, of 160 participants who had been seizure-free on medication for two to five years, 15% of those randomized to

the withdrawal condition and 7% of those who continued on medication experienced relapse (Lossius et al., 2008). There remains concern about whether seizures that relapse as a result of withdrawal will respond to reintroduction of treatment. Failure to regain control does occur in a minority of patients, most often adults with focal seizures due to structural or metabolic causes (Perucca and Thomson, 2011).

When deciding whether medication should be withdrawn from a seizure-free patient, an important factor is the diagnosis. As discussed in Chapter 7, identification of an epilepsy syndrome often implies prognosis. Thus, for instance, *benign childhood epilepsy with centrotemporal spikes* almost invariably resolves by age 15, and medication can then be discontinued with only rare exceptions (Lüders et al., 1987). The seizures of *juvenile myoclonic epilepsy*, on the other hand, are usually controlled by medication, but relapse on withdrawal is high, and most patients must remain on medication (Janz et al., 1983). Seizures beginning in the first year of life and those associated with the *West* and *Lennox-Gastaut syndromes* have a high rate of relapse. Seizure type also predicts relapse: recurrence of seizures with drug withdrawal is rare for typical absences consisting of impaired consciousness only, slightly more likely if clonic or myoclonic features are present, moderately more likely for generalized tonic-clonic seizures, and very likely for focal seizures (Chadwick, 1985).

Several older studies of children have attempted to identify additional factors that might influence the decision to withdraw medication. In one series of 148 children followed for 15–23 years (Holowach et al., 1972; Holowach-Thurston et al., 1982), the risk of relapse after four seizure-free years was most closely correlated with seizure type: 14% for generalized tonic-clonic seizures, 12% for febrile seizures and petit mal absences, 31% for focal dyscognitive seizures, 43% for multiple seizure types, and 58% for Jacksonian seizures. Relapse was more likely in patients with neurological dysfunction and with a long duration of seizures before control, whereas EEG findings and age of onset were not risk factors. Eighty-five percent of patients with relapses had them within five years after drug withdrawal. In another study (Todt, 1984), more than half of relapses occurred during or within three months of drug withdrawal, and 86% occurred within one year after discontinuation of medication. Although some children exhibited no relapse with rapid withdrawal of medication after only one or two seizure-free years, the best results were obtained when medication was tapered over a 12-month period after the child had been seizure-free on medication for four years. A third study (Shinnar et al., 1985) suggests that drug withdrawal after only two years might be acceptable. Both these latter studies found the presence of paroxysmal activity on the EEG to be a significant risk factor. A study of 92 adults and children withdrawn from medication after two seizure-free years found no correlation between relapse rate and age; an abnormal EEG prior to treatment that persisted until the time of withdrawal was a sign of a poor prognosis (Callaghan et al., 1988). Other risk factors identified in more recent studies include having had more than 10 seizures before seizure control, age of onset after 12 years, a family history of seizures, EEG slowing prior to medication withdrawal, atypical febrile seizures, and mental retardation (Dulac et al., 2008). Studies of drug withdrawal continue to be confounded by pooling of data from patients with different epilepsy conditions. Drug withdrawal following successful surgical treatment remains an additional topic of particular interest (Schiller et al., 2000) (Chapter 16).

Patients who begin treatment with antiseizure drugs at an early age are at the greatest risk for the development of chronic side effects (Reynolds, 1983a) and therefore stand to gain the most from medication withdrawal. If antiseizure drugs are to be withdrawn in childhood onset epilepsy, this is best carried out early enough that any transient recurrence of seizures would not result in loss of a driver's license or other serious psychosocial consequences. A primary consideration should be the likelihood of relapse based on a diagnosis of seizure type and, if possible, epilepsy syndrome (Chapter 7). An abnormal EEG may indicate an increased risk of relapse but is not necessarily a contraindication to withdrawal attempts. When to begin to withdraw antiseizure medication is important when it is necessary to complete the process during adolescence; whereas a meta-analysis suggests that at least two seizure-free years are necessary in children, there are no data to support the timing of withdrawal in seizure-free

adults (Sirven et al., 2010). Although the occurrence of withdrawal seizures may not necessarily be related to rate of withdrawal of a drug (Theodore et al., 1987), there is usually no reason to rush, and a conservative approach would be to take 6 to 12 months. A withdrawal seizure complicates management and could result in a decision to continue drug treatment in a child who might not need the medication.

With adult onset epilepsy the psychosocial consequences of seizure recurrence after two to four years of seizure control may be relatively greater than in children when compared with the risk of chronic drug toxicity. Driving restrictions during withdrawal add an additional inconvenience (Chapter 17). The patient and the physician together must, therefore, carefully weigh the risks and benefits of withdrawing medication, and decisions ultimately depend on the individual situation. When patients have been noncompliant and serum drug levels are already low, withdrawal can be accomplished more quickly. It is a mistake, however, to assume that a small amount of a drug is not exerting a necessary antiseizure effect. Consequently, a chronically low serum drug level is not an indication for abruptly terminating medication.

Phenobarbital, primidone, and *benzodiazepine* withdrawal are most likely to precipitate seizures; little is known concerning whether withdrawal seizures ever occur with other antiseizure medications. When a generalized tonic-clonic seizure occurs during withdrawal of one of the former agents and is not typical of the patient's habitual seizure type, it is likely to be a withdrawal seizure and not necessarily a contraindication to complete removal of the drug at a slower rate or at a later time.

Special Considerations

AGE

The rate of metabolism is slower, renal clearance is decreased, and protein binding is less in *neonates* and in the *elderly* compared with children and adults (Leppik and Birnbaum, 2008; Arif et al., 2009; Mizrahi and Scher, 2008; Chiron, 2009). Consequently, the half-life of drugs will be greater at the extremes of age, and the amount of free drug in the serum will be greater for a given serum concentration. In contrast, *children* have a higher rate of metabolism than adults, and the half-life in this age group may be shorter than anticipated, requiring more frequent doses to minimize fluctuations in serum drug levels at steady state (Morselli et al., 1983; Pellock et al., 2008). Therapy in neonates, infants, and children is discussed in the sections dealing with seizures and syndromes common in there age groups (Chapters 6, 7, and 10). In the very young there is an overriding concern to protect the brain from long-term sequelae of recurrent seizures, although there is very little evidence that relates seizure cessation to prognosis. It is important to reassure parents with realistic information about the causes and consequences of these very frightening events. In general, *infants* have slower absorption, higher volumes of distribution, and faster metabolism and clearance than adults, so doses of most antiseizure drugs need to be higher and dose intervals shorter. Toxicity is also increased for some drugs in this age group, most importantly the susceptibility to hepatotoxicity with *valproic acid* in children under the age of 3, and the paradoxical hyperexcitation induced by *barbiturates* and *benzodiazepines*.

The elderly are the fastest-growing segment of the population in the industrialized world, and there is an increasing incidence of epilepsy in this group (Leppik and Birnbaum, 2008; Arif et al., 2009). Although the elderly have been divided into the *young old* (65–74 years old), *middle old* (75–84), and *old old* (85 and older), treatment considerations are based on overall health and living conditions. The primary concerns are the effects of aging on organ systems that influence pharmacokinetics of antiseizure drugs, increased comorbidity, and drug side effects. Absorption decreases, serum albumin levels are often reduced, and hepatic metabolism and renal clearance decline with age. There may be increased fluctuations in drug serum levels that complicate decisions regarding dosing. The status of these functions will influence the choice of drugs. Not only can other medical conditions common in the elderly affect brain excitability and seizure occurrence, but they are also treated with medications that can interact with antiseizure drugs. Consequently, the newer antiseizure drugs that do not have significant drug-drug interactions are preferred. Side effect profiles are also important

depending in part on comorbidity; for instance, the *hyponatremia* caused by *carbamazepine* and *oxcarbazepine* make these drugs a poor choice for patients at risk for congestive heart failure. In one study, *levetiracetam* was the best tolerated and *oxcarbazepine* consistently the worst tolerated in patients over the age of 55 (Arif et al., 2010). Diagnosis and treatment of osteoporosis is important in the elderly, particularly when this can be exacerbated by antiseizure drugs. Finally, compliance is a problem, especially for elderly patients living alone, and must be considered as a cause of apparent pharmacoresistance.

PREGNANCY

Antiseizure drug treatment in pregnant women presents a number of important problems (Janz et al., 1982; Yerby et al., 2008; Sabers and Harden, 2008; Tomson, 2009) (Table 14–10). Although reports in the literature are inconsistent, perhaps one-third of pregnant women with epilepsy experience an increase, one-third a decrease, and one-third no change in seizure frequency during pregnancy. Hormonal and metabolic factors, respiratory changes, psychological problems, noncompliance, and altered disposition of antiseizure drugs are responsible for these new patterns of seizure occurrence. Noncompliance and increased clearance of antiseizure drugs are the first and second most important causes, respectively, of lowered serum drug levels and increased seizure frequency. Postpartum alterations of drug metabolism can also create problems. Measurement of serum drug levels monthly for *lamotrigine* and the active metabolite of *oxcarbazepine* and at less frequent intervals for other drugs has been recommended during pregnancy and at weekly levels after delivery until drug clearance has returned to prepregnancy values (Philbert and Dam, 1982; Patsalos et al., 2008). However, a decrease in serum level of the highly protein-bound drugs *phenytoin* and *valproic acid* during pregnancy does not reflect the level in the brain and need not be corrected unless it is accompanied by an exacerbation of seizures. Ideally, free levels should be obtained.

There is no increased incidence in the onset of new epileptic seizures or of status epilepticus during uncomplicated pregnancy. The neurological consequences of *eclampsia*, including convulsions, reflect hypertensive

Table 14–10 **Use of Antiseizure Drugs in Pregnancy**

	FDA Rating for Teratogenicity	Vitamin K Deficiency	Breast Milk %	Serum Levels (% of mother's level)	
CBZ	D	+	10–30°	10–20	CBZ
CLB	D		13–36	No data	CLB
CLN	D		13–33	No data	CLN
ESL	No data		No data	No data	ESL
ESM	C		50–80	30–50	ESM
EZG	No data		No data	No data	EZG
FBM	C		No data	No data	FBM
GBP	C		70–130	4–12	GBP
LCM	C		No data	No data	LCM
LTG	C		40–80	25–50	LTG
LEV	C		80–130	<20	LEV
OXC	C		50–80†	7–12†	OXC
PB	D	+	30–50	50–100	PB
PHT	D	+	10–60	<10	PHT
PGN	C		No data	No data	PGN
PRM	D	+	40–96	30–50	PRM
RUF	C		No data	No data	RUF
TGB	C		No data	No data	TGB
TPM	D		70–110	9–17	TPM
VPA	D	+	4–20	4–12	VPA
VGB	C		4–20	No data	VGB
ZON	C		90	100	ZON

° Epoxide 50%.
† Active metabolite.
For key to drug name abbreviations, see Table 15–1.

encephalopathy and generally respond to control of blood pressure or delivery. The common practice of treating seizures in preeclamptic and eclamptic women with *magnesium sulfate* is controversial. Although preferred by many obstetricians because of concern for the fetus, there is evidence from animal models of epilepsy (Koontz and Reid, 1985) and from clinical studies (Sibai et al., 1984) that this intervention has little or no effect on central epileptogenic mechanisms. Indeed, it can be argued that this treatment is contraindicated, because magnesium sulfate causes neuromuscular blockade, which could mask continuing cerebral epileptic activity, a particular danger if seizures are not actually due to eclampsia. Short-term administration of appropriate antiseizure agents during late pregnancy poses little or no risk to the fetus; however, a recent meta-analyses suggest that magnesium sulfate may still be the best treatment for convulsions in eclamptic women (Duley et al., 2010a;b).

Although stillbirth and decreased head circumference of the neonate appear to be related to treatment with antiseizure drugs to some extent, the specific effects of these pharmacological agents on fetal development can be difficult to assess (Yerby et al., 2008). The risk of major and minor malformations in children born of parents with epilepsy is approximately double that of the general population. However, some evidence suggests that the risk is also increased in children of fathers with epilepsy, suggesting genetic factors related to the epilepsy condition. Malformations are twice as common in children of mothers with epilepsy on antiseizure medication as in children of untreated mothers with epilepsy, but this may relate as much to the severity of the disorder as to the presence of medication (Yerby et al., 2008). The FDA has rated all antiseizure drugs with respect to teratogenicity as risk category C (some animal studies show adverse effects; no controlled studies in humans) or D (positive evidence of risk to the human fetus) (Table 14–10). In general, the class D risk drugs are the older drugs that have been around long enough to determine human teratogenicity potential.

Many of the drugs in risk category C may be determined to have a significant risk as results of pregnancy registries become available.

There is little doubt that chronic antiseizure drug treatment during the first trimester of pregnancy increases the risk of minor and major malformations in the child, but there is continuing controversy about the correlation between specific drugs or dosages and patterns of abnormalities (Yerby et al., 2008). Several pregnancy registries have been developed and have been collecting data for over 10 years (Tomson et al., 2010), but results are only now beginning to emerge. Because there undoubtedly will be more definitive information on teratogenic effects of specific antiseizure drugs in the near future as a result of these ongoing studies, any detailed discussion here will be out of date by the time this text is published. Broadly speaking, reported enhanced teratogenic effects of *phenytoin* (*fetal hydantoin syndrome*) have not been substantiated, but those for the *barbiturates* have (Holmes et al., 2004). *Valproic acid* significantly increases the risk of neural tube defects and other congenital malformations (Gomez, 1981; Jentink et al., 2010). Serum *γ-fetoprotein* determinations, ultrasound, or amniocentesis (or some combination thereof) may be indicated for women taking these drugs during their first trimester. A teratogenic effect of *trimethadione* has also been fairly well established (Zackai et al., 1975), and *topiramate* is also now believed to impart a higher-than-average risk, but not as great as that of *valproic acid* (Hunt et al., 2008). More recently, it has become clear that in utero exposure to antiseizure drugs can have a negative effect on cognitive function many years later. This has been most clearly demonstrated for *valproic acid* (Meador et al., 2009; Nadebaum et al., 2011).

Experience with other drugs has not been sufficient for concluding which, if any, are better than others (Yerby et al., 2008). Although *trimethadione, valproic acid*, and *topiramate* are not recommended for use in women of childbearing age, dose is as important as drug type (Tomson et al., 2011a). A low dose of a known teratogenic drug could be safer than a high dose of another drug. There is evidence suggesting that the risk of major birth defects with most newer-generation antiseizure drugs is minimal (Mølgaard-Nielsen and Hviid, 2011), but these results have been questioned (Tomson et al. 2011b). The most common malformations seen in children of mothers with epilepsy include cleft palate and lip; congenital heart diseases; facial dysplasias; hypoplasia of fingers and toes; and skeletal, *central nervous system* (CNS), gastrointestinal, and urogenital malformations. Polypharmacy and unnecessarily high drug levels increase the potential for problems during pregnancy and should definitely be avoided in these patients. The incidence of malformed infants born to mothers with epilepsy has decreased in areas where monotherapy and routine serum drug level determinations have reduced the risk of overmedication.

Women of childbearing age who are taking antiseizure medications should also take *folic acid* daily, because folic acid can reduce the risk of neural tube defects and other congenital malformations in the general population of women (MRC, 1991); however, this protective effect has not been definitively demonstrated in women taking antiseizure medications. No dosage has been established, but 2–4 mg per day is usually recommended. Attempts might be made to discontinue medication in women who wish to become pregnant and who have been seizure-free for many years. Discontinuing medication in women with active epilepsy or changing medication in women who are already pregnant is not recommended, because uncontrolled seizures or status may present a greater risk to the fetus than drugs. Genetic factors most likely determine abnormal drug metabolism responsible for an increased incidence of fetal malformation, suggesting that only a small number of women are at high risk for drug-induced teratogenicity and that pharmacogenetics will permit this at-risk population to be identified in the future (Strickler et al., 1985; Glauser, 2011).

Coagulation defects in newborns of treated mothers with epilepsy occur most often with enzyme-inducing antiseizure drugs, are potentially life threatening, and should be anticipated. Giving small doses of *vitamin K* to the mother before delivery has been recommended (Bossi, 1982), but the necessity of this practice has been challenged in favor of routine intramuscular vitamin K in the newborn (Kaaja et al., 2002).

Babies born to mothers with epilepsy, who are taking sedative antiseizure medications such as *barbiturates* or *benzodiazepines*, may be lethargic or jittery after delivery, but drug withdrawal is usually not a problem. Maternal medication need not be altered, but careful observation of the neonate is warranted. There is no relationship between the occurrence of neonatal seizures and either epilepsy or antiseizure drug treatment in the mother.

Antiseizure drugs are excreted through breast milk, which presents a theoretical risk to the baby of serious allergic or idiosyncratic side effects from nursing (Table 14–10); however, this has not been a practical problem, because drug levels are relatively low (Philbert and Dam, 1982). Of more concern is that sedative drugs can cause continued minor dose-related sedation, poor sucking, and reduced weight gain in nursing babies (Kaneko et al., 1982). It is not necessary to discourage nursing for mothers taking antiseizure drugs (Sabers and Tomson, 2009). However, plasma drug levels should be obtained from the baby if toxic symptoms appear, and breastfeeding should be discontinued when indicated (Philbert and Dam, 1982). This problem is most likely to occur with *barbiturates, benzodiazepines, primidone, ethosuximide*, and *lamotrigine*.

Three recent AAN/AES practice parameters have been published regarding management issues for women with epilepsy. The first recommends "avoidance of valproate and antiepileptic drug polytherapy during the first trimester of pregnancy...avoidance of valproate and antiepileptic drug polytherapy throughout pregnancy to prevent reduced cognitive outcomes...[and] avoidance of *phenytoin* and phenobarbital during pregnancy to prevent reduced cognitive outcomes" and notes that "offspring of women with epilepsy taking antiepileptic drugs are probably at increased risk for being small for gestational age" (Harden et al., 2009a). A second states that "seizure freedom for at least nine months prior to pregnancy is probably associated with a high rate of remaining seizure free during pregnancy" but points out that women with epilepsy who smoke have an increased risk of premature contractions and labor (Harden et al., 2009b). A third recommends supplemental folic acid before becoming pregnant and monitoring of

lamotrigine, carbamazepine, phenytoin, levetiracetam, and *oxcarbazepine* levels during pregnancy (Harden et al., 2009c).

COMORBIDITY

Diseases most likely to influence medical treatment of epilepsy are those that affect liver and kidney function (Singh, 2009). Practical considerations for pharmacotherapy in patients with hepatic dysfunction include avoidance of *valproic acid, felbamate*, and possibly *carbamazepine, phenytoin*, and *lamotrigine* as chronic therapy; avoidance of *benzodiazepines* (except possibly *midazolam*) for acute seizures; slow titration; and monitoring of free serum drug concentrations because of decreased albumin in these conditions. Dosages of drugs that are cleared by the kidneys must be appropriately adjusted in patients with kidney disease. Renal dysfunction does not affect loading dose, but the effect on chronic maintenance therapy is complex and unpredictable. Not only is clearance in the urine compromised, but uremia displaces protein binding, gastric absorption is impaired, and for drugs that are also metabolized in the liver this metabolism will be enhanced. Dosage of antiseizure medication should be reduced or interdose interval should be increased (or both) based on creatinine clearance. For patients on dialysis, a dialysis-related drug may require immediate postdialysis supplementation.

Treatment of infections in patients with epilepsy must consider the interactions between antibiotic and antiseizure medications. A particularly problematic issue is selecting antiseizure drugs for people being treated with *antiretroviral agents* for HIV/AIDS, 55% of whom are also being treated for epileptic seizures (Birbeck et al., 2012). Recent AAN guidelines recommend that *lopinavir/ritonavir* dosage may require a 50% increase when given with *phenytoin*, that *zidovudine* may need to be reduced when given with *valproic acid*, and that *lamotrigine* may require a 50% increase when given with *ritonavir/atazanavir* (Birbeck et al., 2012).

Seizures occasionally occur with *acute porphyria* and can create a particular problem, because most of the older antiseizure drugs exacerbate the porphyric state. That effect appears to be related to some extent to the ability of antiseizure drugs to induce liver enzymes.

Consequently, the *benzodiazepines*, which are not potent enzyme inducers, are least likely to create problems in patients with porphyria. It has been stated that among the older drugs, *diazepam* and *paraldehyde* are safe to use for the treatment of status epilepticus in porphyria (Reynolds and Miska, 1981), but this has been contested, and *clonazepam* has been proposed as an alternative (Shedlofsky and Bonkowsky, 1984). Among the newer drugs, *gabapentin* and *levetiracetam* are believed to be safe treatments for seizures with porphyria. *Bromide*, however, may be the only entirely safe medication for the chronic treatment of patients with acute porphyria and epileptic seizures.

SURGERY

Surgical treatment and general anesthesia present no special problems for patients with epilepsy as long as the risks for seizures are appreciated and taken into account. Postoperative seizures can cause wound dehiscence or complicate management in other ways, and appropriate precautions are necessary. Drugs that must be given orally should be replaced by intravenous medications during the time oral intake is contraindicated. A common practice is to deliver a loading dose of *fosphenytoin* intravenously, with *electrocardiograph (ECG)* monitoring, after the patient is anesthetized, although other intravenous formulations are now available. Crossover back to the original drug must be carried out with attention to differences in half-life, so that one drug is at therapeutic levels at all times during the postoperative period. Sedative drugs should be withdrawn slowly, and potentially convulsant drugs (Chapter 5), particularly *tramadol* and *meperidine*, should be avoided. *Propoxyphene* should not be used by inpatients taking *carbamazepine* and *oxcarbazepine*, because it increases the serum level of these drugs and causes acute toxicity

PSYCHIATRIC CONDITIONS

Concern is often raised about the treatment of patients with epilepsy with *phenothiazines* and certain antidepressant medications that lower the seizure threshold (Chapter 5). In fact, most antidepressant drugs, including the selective serotonin reuptake inhibitors, are generally regarded as safe in people with epilepsy. Under routine circumstances, there is no reason to deprive patients with epilepsy of these drugs as long as antiseizure pharmacotherapy is effective. Precautions must be taken, however, if the occurrence of a seizure would cause serious difficulties (e.g., postoperatively or during antiseizure drug withdrawal).

Patients at high risk for suicide require special consideration, because many antiseizure drugs could provide a convenient mechanism for suicide attempts. In addition to considering the potentially lethal consequences of overdose with CNS depressant drugs such as *phenobarbital*, it is necessary to recognize that drugs with high protein binding, such as *phenytoin* and *diazepam* (see Table 14–2), cannot easily be removed by dialysis. The best approach is to dispense medication frequently, in small amounts.

As a result of a meta-analysis of placebo-controlled clinical trials that revealed an increased risk of suicidality in patients treated with antiseizure drugs, the FDA issued a safety warning (Katz, 2008) that generated considerable concern and criticism. Suicidality, however, is not the same as suicide risk. Subsequently, a large observational study concluded that the use of antiseizure drugs was not associated with an increased risk of suicide-related events among patients with epilepsy but was associated with increased risk both for patients with depression and for those who did not have epilepsy, depression, or bipolar disorder (Arana et al., 2010). The topic remains controversial (Mula and Hesdorffer, 2011)

ALCOHOL AND SEDATIVE DRUG WITHDRAWAL

Treatment of seizures caused by inadvertent withdrawal from a drug that has been appropriately used for therapeutic purposes usually consists of drug replacement. When the initial agent is a substance of abuse, such as alcohol, replacement with a drug having cross-tolerance is recommended, in most cases *diazepam* or *paraldehyde*. *Diazepam* is given intravenously in doses of 5–10 mg, repeated every 15 minutes to every several hours, depending on recurrence of symptoms (Chapter 10). It can then be tapered over a few days to a week, because the period of the withdrawal effect is short. *Paraldehyde* is usually given in doses of 0.1–0.2 ml/kg orally, in fruit juice, every two to four hours and tapered over several days. Although *paralde-hyde* can be given intravenously or rectally, as for status epilepticus (Chapter 10), parenteral formulations are no longer available in the United States. Other *benzodiazepines*, particularly *chlordiazepoxide, lorazepam*, and *clorazepate*, may be as effective as *diazepam* and *paraldehyde*.

Sedative and depressant medications, such as sleeping pills, must be prescribed with care for patients with epilepsy and should not be given p.r.n. if there is any potential for abuse. Intermittent overmedication or persistent use followed by sudden discontinuation increases the potential for withdrawal seizures in patients who are otherwise well controlled.

MEDICALLY REFRACTORY SEIZURES

There are two hypotheses to explain pharmacoresistance in epilepsy: the *target hypothesis*, which postulates that the epileptogenic tissue itself is not responsive to the actions of the antiseizure agent, and the *transport hypothesis*, which postulates enhanced *efflux transporter* activity in the epileptogenic region (Sisodiya et al., 2008; Löscher and Schmidt, 2009; Kwan et al., 2011). Antiseizure drugs have limited potency against certain types of epileptic seizures or epilepsy syndromes from the outset (Löscher and Schmidt, 2011), but a pharmacosensitive target may become pharmacoresistant over time as a result of tolerance or other pharmacodynamic mechanisms. Considerable animal research is focused on identifying irreversible causes of target insensitivity. Pharmacokinetic mechanisms can also underlie decreasing responsivity to antiseizure drugs when enzyme induction results in subtherapeutic plasma levels, a problem that can easily be corrected by increasing the drug dose. There is evidence suggesting that overactivity of drug efflux transporters may limit antiseizure drug levels in epileptogenic tissue and account for some types of pharmacoresistance (Sisodiya et al., 2008; Löscher and Schmidt, 2006). Upregulation of efflux transporters such as the *multidrug resistance protein 1 (MDR1)*, also known as *P-glycoprotein (P-gp)*, in epileptogenic brain areas has been reported, but

this hypothesis remains controversial. It is important to note that this mechanism would not explain all drug resistance, as not all antiseizure drugs are substrates for drug efflux transporters.

Fortunately, there are many remediable causes of failed medical management, the most common of which include noncompliance, inadequate drug dosage, drug interactions, use of an inappropriate drug (usually due to an incorrect diagnosis), precipitating factors in the environment, lifestyle issues, the presence of a progressive neurological disorder, and drug toxicity (Kwan et al., 2011). Careful monitoring of antiseizure drug levels should reveal noncompliance, inadequate dosage, and drug interactions as reasons for failure to control epileptic seizures. Inpatient video-EEG monitoring (VEM) may be necessary to verify the diagnosis of seizure type and epilepsy syndrome, if possible, and appropriate changes in medication can be made if this evaluation reveals a different epilepsy condition from that previously suspected. Precipitating factors (Chapter 9) may be elucidated by more careful questioning and verified by VEM if necessary. In some situations these factors can be avoided by simple alterations in behavior patterns or lifestyle, although these changes are not always acceptable to the patient. Control may be impossible in patients who refuse to alter dangerous habits such as drug and alcohol abuse. Evaluation of a patient with progressive symptoms may reveal a localized lesion, such as a brain tumor, that can be surgically removed. Adverse side effects of drugs may be reversed by adjusting dose schedules (e.g., more frequent administration to reduce peak levels or taking the largest dose at bedtime) or by changing the medication. In some unfortunate patients, idiosyncratic adverse side effects occur with all effective antiseizure medications, and pharmacological treatment is not possible.

If a patient does not obtain adequate benefit from standard approaches to medical management after failure of two drug trials, the patient should be referred to a specialized epilepsy center to determine whether there is a correctable cause of medical failure or whether surgery or some alternative treatment is an option. VEM is often indicated. With subsequent treatment intervention based on results of testing at an epilepsy center, over half of patients who are not surgical candidates can expect a marked reduction in seizure frequency and in medication toxicity, resulting in improved psychosocial adjustment in most of these (Theodore and Porter, 1983). Patients for whom the seizure diagnosis is changed as a result of VEM have the most favorable outcome; the least favorable outcome occurs in patients with focal dyscognitive seizures who are not surgical candidates and those with impaired mental status.

ALTERNATIVE THERAPY

The most effective alternative therapy for epilepsy is surgery (Chapter 16). There has been a progressive increase in the use of surgery for seizures due to localized epileptogenic lesions, but this approach remains an extremely under-utilized modality. Surgical treatment of epilepsy has been proven safe and beneficial and is the only therapy capable of actually curing a chronic epilepsy condition. The best results are obtained with *anteromesial temporal lobectomy*, the most common resective procedure performed. *Neocortical resection* for an identifiable lesion and *hemispherectomy* are also associated with a high success rate. *Corpus callosum section* is of value for controlling drop attacks, but *vagus nerve stimulation (VNS)* is now preferred for most patients with these seizures. It has been estimated that in the United States alone 100,000–200,000 patients may be candidates for resective surgery, but only about 2,000 of these surgical procedures are performed annually (Engel and Shewmon, 1993; Engel, 2008). Similar discrepancies exist for most other industrialized countries.

VNS is now widely performed as a palliative treatment (Schachter and Boon, 2008). The efficacy in patients with medically refractory seizures is about the same as demonstrated with new drug trials, and few patients become seizure-free; however, the side effect profile is different from that of pharmacotherapy, and there is evidence that benefits increase over time (Chapter 16). VNS should not be used in patients who are candidates for surgical therapy and have an excellent opportunity to become seizure-free. *Deep-brain stimulation* may be superior to VNS and has been

approved in Europe but, as of this writing, is not yet approved in the United States (Fisher et al., 2010) (Chapter 16). *Responsive brain stimulation* is also under study as an alternative surgical treatment (Fisher et al., 2008) (Chapter 16).

Other alternative treatment approaches include dietary manipulations such as the *ketogenic diet* (Stafstrom et al., 2008); behavioral manipulations such as operant conditioning (biofeedback), desensitization, relaxation, and meditation; and herbal and folk remedies (Schachter et al., 2008; Wolf, 2008) (Chapter 16). The last may be effective in certain cultural contexts or may have actual antiseizure effects.

PSYCHOSOCIAL CONSIDERATIONS

The occurrence of epileptic seizures, perhaps more than any other neurological symptom, is markedly influenced by internal and external influences that are under the control of the patient and others (Taylor, 2008). Common examples of avoidable precipitating factors are emotional stress, sleep deprivation, and withdrawal of alcohol or sedative drugs (Chapter 9). In addition, patients with epilepsy are often disabled by the psychosocial consequences of their condition or other interictal behavioral disturbances that may or may not be related to their epilepsy (Chapter 11). For this reason, treatment of the patient with epilepsy requires much more than the manipulation of antiseizure drugs, and prognosis does not depend on seizure control alone. Dealing with these environmental and psychosocial problems is an essential part of the management of the patient with epilepsy (Chapters 11 and 17).

USE OF EEG IN ASSESSING TREATMENT

Single or sequential routine EEGs may be useful in determining whether behavioral deterioration in a patient with epilepsy is due to an increase in subclinical seizures, an increase in antiseizure drug side effects, or a progressive underlying lesion. Increased generalized slow waves or slowing of baseline rhythmic activity may substantiate overmedication; however, these findings can also reflect a postictal state or indicate a progressive encephalopathy (Chapters 12 and 13).

An increase or decrease in the frequency of interictal EEG spike activity does not correlate with a change in seizure frequency, except in absence epilepsy (Kellaway et al., 1979). Consequently, in most epilepsy conditions, repeated interictal EEGs are not useful for routine assessment of the efficacy of treatment. Documentation of the frequency and severity of ictal events, however, does provide a clear measure of therapeutic effect. When such information may be historically unreliable, it can be obtained for some patients on an outpatient basis by the use of *ambulatory monitoring* (Chapter 12). Inpatient VEM is less useful for this purpose, because admission to the hospital commonly alters the frequency of seizure occurrence (Riley et al., 1981); however, inpatient VEM can be combined with frequent measurements of antiseizure drug levels for assessing the effects of medical therapy over days and making appropriate adjustments in drug doses (Porter et al., 1977). Correlation between ictal events and serum drug concentrations helps in planning a dose schedule that provides maximum protection when a patient is at greatest risk for seizures. EEG monitoring can be an essential component in the treatment of *status epilepticus* (Chapter 10).

Computerized analysis of interictal EEG features (Frost, 1985; Frost et al., 1986; Worrell and Gotman, 2011) may someday provide more definitive information about the effect of medical intervention on certain epilepsy conditions (Chapter 12). It would be ideal to have a means of determining whether therapy is appropriate without waiting to see if another seizure occurs. At present, however, it is necessary to observe patients clinically by means of serum drug levels and self-reports. Repeat EEGs are indicated only when the clinical picture changes and specific EEG findings (e.g., increased paroxysms in a child with absence epilepsy or patterns diagnostic of absence status or focal dyscognitive status) would influence clinical management. As discussed previously, there remains some controversy concerning

the role of the EEG when considering drug withdrawal in seizure-free patients; however, an EEG should be obtained at this time, at least to serve as a baseline for assessing any subsequent changes. Long-term monitoring is used for evaluating therapeutic effect in only the most difficult situations.

MANAGEMENT AFTER A SINGLE SEIZURE

The approach to a patient who has had only one seizure requires special consideration. A single seizure raises the diagnostic question of whether this seizure was a reactive event or an indication of a chronic epilepsy condition (Chapter 12). If there is sufficient evidence for a precipitating factor (Chapter 9), features of the episode in question are consistent with those of a reactive ictal event (Chapter 7), and diagnostic evaluation does not produce evidence of a chronic cerebral disorder (Krumholz et al., 2007; Hirtz et al., 2003) (Chapter 12), it is usually in the patient's best interest not to make a diagnosis of epilepsy and not to give the patient antiseizure medication. In this instance, it is sufficient to warn the patient that a second seizure might occur, recommend avoidance of suspected precipitating factors (Chapter 9), and render advice about potential risks should another seizure occur (Chapter 17).

There has been controversy over the probability of recurrent epileptic seizures in a patient who has suffered a single, unprovoked ictal event (Elwes et al., 1985; Hachinski, 1986; Hart and Easton, 1986; Hauser et al., 1986; Hauser et al., 1982; Hauser et al., 1983; Perucca and Thomson, 2011). Data vary depending on whether the study was prospective or retrospective, the time between seizure occurrence and entrance into the study, and the commitment of the physician to obtaining an accurate history. Most patients with epilepsy present with recurrent seizures, and one study found a history of at least one previous unrecognized unprovoked ictal event in 20% of patients presenting with what was purported by treating physicians to be a first unprovoked seizure (Hauser et al., 1986). Risk factors for recurrence after a single unprovoked seizure include a presumptive underlying neurological disturbance, a generalized spike-and-wave pattern on EEG, a sibling with epilepsy, a postictal Todd paralysis, and a prior reactive seizure (Hauser et al., 1986). These findings might lead to a diagnosis of epilepsy and therefore treatment after a single unprovoked seizure (Fisher et al. 2005). The risk of recurrence over five years without these factors was reported to be as low as 25% and with a combination of these factors may be over 70% (Hauser et al., 1986).

When balancing the risks and benefits of treatment for a single unprovoked seizure, most epileptologists agree that the adverse psychosocial consequences of a diagnosis of epilepsy and the potential discomfort and hazards of chronic antiseizure medication are more damaging for most persons than a second epileptic seizure (Hauser, 1986). Furthermore, there is no evidence to support concern that treatment will be less effective after two or three seizures than after one (Leone et al., 2006; Kim et al., 2006). Whether to treat a single unprovoked epileptic seizure, therefore, becomes a matter of individual decision for each patient, dependent on the potential detrimental effect of antiseizure drugs on the one hand and the risk and consequences of a second seizure on the other. If antiseizure therapy is begun and a second seizure never occurs, it is impossible to know whether the drug was necessary. At some point, then, drug discontinuation must be considered, and if it is decided to discontinue, the risk of a second seizure reappears. Decision to treat the patient for a finite period of time, therefore, merely delays rather than abolishes this risk. Unless there is an overriding reason why a second seizure now would be more disabling than one several years later, these arguments are sufficient for opting against treatment.

EMERGENCY TREATMENT

Epileptic seizures are generally self-limiting, and first aid for an epileptic seizure usually requires ensuring a safe environment for the event to run its course. For generalized tonic-clonic seizures this consists of protecting the patient from self-injury by removing sharp objects from the area and cushioning the patient's head from impact if necessary. Hard instruments or fingers must not be inserted into the patient's mouth during the ictal episode. When the seizure is over, the patient's head should be turned to one side to drain all secretions, and the airway can be cleared if necessary. Attempts should not be made to restrain patients forcibly during or after focal dyscognitive seizures, but they should be protected from surrounding hazards until ictal and postictal symptoms cease. For both generalized tonic-clonic and dyscognitive focal seizures, someone should stay with the patient until full consciousness has returned. It is generally not necessary to call an ambulance unless the patient has never had a seizure before, the seizure lasts longer than five minutes, another attack occurs before consciousness is regained, the seizure occurred in water, or there is evidence of serious injury, respiratory distress, or pregnancy. Patients are often able to go about their business in a relatively short time after a seizure. Unnecessary imposition of rest periods or hospital visits further compounds the disability caused by the ictal event.

Generalized tonic-clonic status epilepticus is a medical emergency requiring immediate intervention, not only to stop seizures but also to identify and treat any potentially life-threatening underlying cause (Chapter 10). Some forms of *neonatal seizures* also reflect reversible cerebral disturbances that require prompt intervention (Chapter 7).

SUMMARY AND CONCLUSIONS

The objective of treatment for epilepsy is to maximize the useful functional capacity of the patient. Although complete eradication of seizures as soon as possible without introduction of unwanted side effects is the ideal, too many patients treated for chronic epilepsy cannot expect to become seizure-free indefinitely. For some patients, the disability caused by continuation of seizures may be less than the disability induced by aggressive therapy.

The standard strategy for pharmacological management of epilepsy has been to choose the best drug for the seizure disorder and to continue to increase the dose of that drug until adequate therapeutic effects or intolerable side effects occur; however, with many drugs to choose from, it may be reasonable today to switch to another drug sooner than in the past. Usually treatment should be instituted slowly, to avoid side effects. If dose-related adverse symptoms appear before seizure control is achieved, backing off or slowing down may allow the patient to be coaxed into achieving higher levels with better therapeutic effects. If seizures are controlled on a lower dose, there is no need to push until adverse symptoms develop. If a toxic level is reached before seizure control is achieved, and the patient does not become tolerant to these symptoms, it is necessary to try a second drug. If the second drug is effective, the first can then be tapered and discontinued; however, physicians and patients may prefer not to change medications once control has been achieved. Consequently, although monotherapy, or treatment with one drug, is the preferred pharmacological approach to the treatment of epilepsy, use of two drugs is acceptable. It is best, however, to avoid polytherapy with more than two drugs if possible. The recommended dose is that required to control seizures without producing intolerable side effects.

Pharmacokinetic principles are important in choosing dose schedules and in understanding problems that arise during drug treatment. The efficacy of a drug cannot be determined until a steady state exists. For older drugs it is usually safest to give medication at intervals of 0.5 half-life, but doses may be divided at intervals of 1 half-life or longer if the reference range is wide and if this will improve compliance. Serum drug level measurements are used in determining the causes of alterations in response to medication and in treating them specifically. When changing from one drug to another, withdrawal seizures do not necessarily indicate that the drug being withdrawn is necessary. Rejection of the drug of choice because of dose-related side effects may be avoided when treatment is instituted slowly and drug doses are transiently reduced if adverse symptoms occur. Mild elevation of liver enzymes and leukopenia are not necessarily causes for discontinuing a drug. Correct diagnosis, early treatment with the appropriate drug, monotherapy, and attention to unnecessary dose-related adverse symptoms are the best means of preventing chronic side effects.

Discontinuation of medication after a two- to four-year seizure-free interval is recommended for most children. This should be accomplished over a 12-month period, ideally before the child reaches driving age. Discontinuation of medication in seizure-free adults is an individual decision, because the psychosocial risk of seizure recurrence may be greater than the risk of chronic side effects with continued therapy.

Birth defects occur twice as often in babies of mothers with epilepsy than in the general population, although this difference may not be due entirely to antiseizure medications. The use of trimethadione, *valproic acid*, or *topiramate* is not recommended in women of childbearing age who might become pregnant. There is no clearly best alternative drug in this situation, but because teratogenic effects are dose-related, a low dose of one of these agents may be safer than a high dose of another drug. Folic acid is believed to reduce the risk of teratogenicity and should be taken by all women of childbearing age who are using antiseizure medications. A single drug at the lowest effective dose is the safest regimen for a patient who is considering becoming pregnant. There is no reason to alter medication in women who are being appropriately treated for their seizures after they have become pregnant, and on no account should medication be discontinued. Increased seizure frequency during pregnancy is usually due to noncompliance or increased drug elimination, both of which can be determined by serum drug levels. Mothers taking antiseizure drugs need not be discouraged from nursing, but breastfeeding should be discontinued if babies feed poorly because of high serum drug levels.

Patients should be referred to a specialized epilepsy center if seizures are not controlled with two appropriate medication trials. Epilepsy centers have more to offer than just surgery. Delaying a definitive consultation can adversely affect outcome. Patients who continue to have disabling focal seizures and infants and small children who continue to have any type of seizure associated with a lateralized structural lesion should be considered for resective surgical therapy after failure of two appropriate medication trials. Patients with frequent drop attacks may be candidates for corpus callosum section or VNS. VNS can be a useful palliative adjunctive therapy, but it should not be a first choice for patients who are potential surgical candidates and could become seizure-free with a more definitive treatment. Dietary, behavioral, and various folk therapies may be useful under certain circumstances. Patients with epilepsy often have psychosocial problems that require special attention; improving psychosocial adjustment can improve seizure control.

Management of the patient who has had a single seizure requires distinguishing a reactive seizure from a potentially chronic epilepsy condition. If this diagnosis remains in doubt, it must be kept in mind that the psychosocial consequences of a diagnosis of epilepsy are often more damaging than the risk of a second seizure. Whether to treat a patient remains an individual decision; however, medication is usually not prescribed until a chronic epilepsy disorder is apparent. Treatment of a single seizure does not resolve, but merely delays, the problem.

Epileptic seizures are self-limited and require no specific first aid other than protection from hazards in the environment. For someone with established epilepsy, it is not necessary to seek medical attention at a hospital unless a seizure lasts longer than five minutes, a second attack occurs before consciousness is regained, or there is evidence of serious injury, respiratory distress, or pregnancy. Forced rest or emergency room visits following seizures constitute avoidable causes of disability and expense for patients with epilepsy.

Basic and clinical research has appropriately focused on improving pharmacological and surgical treatment as well as finding alternative treatment modalities. Important areas of research that deserve active attention concern approaches for (1) determining that pharmacological treatment is ineffective without needing to wait for another seizure to occur and (2) identifying genetic susceptibility for adverse reactions to specific antiseizure drugs before these drugs are prescribed.

REFERENCES

Andermann, F, Duh, MS, Gosselin, A, and Paradis, PE (2007). Compulsory generic switching of antiepileptic drugs: High switchback rates to branded compounds compared with other drug classes. Epilepsia 48:464–469.

Arana, A, Wentworth, CE, Ayuso-Mateos, JL, and Arellano, FM (2010). Suicide-related events in patients treated with antiepileptic drugs. N Engl J Med 363:542–551.

Arif, H, Mendiratta, A, and Hirsch, HJ (2009). Management of epilepsy in the elderly. In The Treatment of Epilepsy, 3rd ed. Edited by S Shorvon, E Perucca, and J Engel, Jr. West Sussex, UK: Wiley-Blackwell, pp. 203–217.

Arif, H, Buchsbaum, R, Pierro, J, Whalen, M, Sims, J, Resor, R, Jr, Bazil, C, and Hirsch, LJ (2010). Comparative effectiveness of 10 antiepileptic drugs in older adults with epilepsy. Arch Neurol 67:408–415.

Bauer, J, Buchmüller, L, Reuber, M, and Burr, W (2008). Which patients become seizure free with antiepileptic drugs? An observational study in 821 patients with epilepsy. Acta Neurol Scand 117:55–59.

Beghi, E, Gatti, G, Tonini, C, Ben-Menachem, E, Chadwick, DW, Nikanorova, M, Gromov, SA, Smith, PE, Specchio, LM, and Perucca, E; BASE Study Group (2003). Adjunctive therapy versus alternative monotherapy in patients with partial epilepsy failing on a single drug: A multicentre, randomised, pragmatic controlled trial. Epilepsy Res 57:1–13.

Berg, AT, and Shinnar, S (1994). Relapse following discontinuation of antiepileptic drugs: A meta-analysis. Neurology 44:601–608.

Birbeck, GL, French, JA, Perucca, E, Simpson, DM, Fraimow, H, George, JM, Okulicz, JF, Clifford, DB, Hachad, H, and Levy, RH (2012). Evidence-based guideline: Antiepileptic drug selection for people with HIV/AIDS. Neurology 78:139–145.

Booker, HE (1975). Idiosyncratic reactions to the antiepileptic drugs. Epilepsia 16:171–181.

Bossi, L (1982). Neonatal period including drug disposition in newborns: Review of the literature. In Epilepsy, Pregnancy and the Child. Edited by D Janz, M Dam, A Richens, L Bossi, H Helge, and D Schmidt. New York: Raven Press, pp. 327–341.

Bourgeois, BFD (2008). Rapid substitution of antiepileptic drugs. In Epilepsy: A Comprehensive Textbook, 2nd ed. Edited by J Engel, Jr, and TA Pedley. Philadelphia: Lippincott Williams & Wilkins, pp. 1317–1319.

Bourgeois, BFD, and Gilliam, F (2008). Adjunctive and combination therapy. In Epilepsy: A Comprehensive Textbook, 2nd ed. Edited by J Engel, Jr, and TA Pedley. Philadelphia: Lippincott Williams & Wilkins, pp. 1321–1325.

Bourgeois, B, Beaumanoir, A, Blajev, B, de la Cruz, N, Despland, PA, Egli, M, Geudelin, B, Kaspar, U, Ketz, E, Kronauer, C, Meyer, C, Scollo-Lavizzari, G, Tosi, C, Vassella, F, and Zagury, S (1987). Monotherapy with valproate in primary generalized epilepsies. Epilepsia 28(suppl 2):S8–S11.

Brodie, MJ, Perucca, E, Ryvlin, P, Ben-Menachem, E, and Meencke, HJ; Levetiracetam Monotherapy Study Group (2007). Comparison of levetiracetam and controlled-release carbamazepine in newly diagnosed epilepsy. Neurology 68:402–408.

Brodie, MJ, Covanis, A, Gil-Nagel, A, Lerche, H, Perucca, E, Sills, GJ, and White, HS (2011). Antiepileptic drug therapy: Does mechanism of action matter? Epilepsy Behav 21:331–341.

Callaghan, B, Schlesinger, M, Rodemer, W, Pollard, J, Hesdorffer, D, Hauser, WA, and French, J (2011). Remission and relapse in a drug-resistant epilepsy population followed prospectively. Epilepsia 52:619–626.

Callaghan, N, Garrett, A, and Goggin, T (1988). Withdrawal of anticonvulsant drugs in patients free of seizures for two years. N Engl J Med 318:942–946.

Cereghino, JJ (1983). Immunological aspects of epilepsy and antiepileptic drugs. In Chronic Toxicity of Antiepileptic Drugs. Edited by J Oxley, D Janz, and H Meinardi. New York: Raven Press, pp. 251–259.

Chadwick, D (1985). The discontinuation of antiepileptic therapy. In Recent Advances in Epilepsy 2. Edited by TA Pedley and BS Meldrum. New York: Churchill Livingstone, pp. 111–124.

Chen, P, Linn, J-J, Lu, C-S, et al. (2011). Carbamazepine-induced toxic effects and HLA-B*1502 screening in Taiwan. N Engl J Med 364:1126–1133.

Chiron, C (2009). Management of epilepsy in infants. In The Treatment of Epilepsy, 3rd ed. Edited by S Shorvon, E Perucca, and J Engel, Jr. West Sussex, UK: Wiley-Blackwell, pp. 171–178

Chung, WH, Hung, SI, Hong, HS, et al. (2004). Medical genetics: A marker for Stevens-Johnson syndrome. Nature 428:486.

Dam, M (1983). Chronic toxicity of antiepileptic drugs with respect to cerebellar and motor function. In Chronic Toxicity of Antiepileptic Drugs. Edited by J Oxley, D Janz, and H Meinardi. New York: Raven Press, pp. 223–228.

Davies-Jones, GAB (1985). Anticonvulsant drugs. In Side Effects of Drugs Annual 9. Edited by MNG Dukes. New York: Elsevier Science, pp. 55–62.

Deckers, CL, Hekster, YA, Keyser, A, van Lier, HJ, Meinard, H, and Renier, WO (2001). Monotherapy versus polytherapy for epilepsy: A multicenter double-blind randomized study. Epilepsia 42:1387–1394.

Del Amo, EM, Urtti, A, and Yliperttula, M (2008). Pharmacokinetic role of L-type amino acid transporters LAT1 and LAT2. Eur J Pharm Sci 35:161–174.

Dodson, WE, and Brodie, MJ (2008). Efficacy of antiepileptic drugs. In Epilepsy: A Comprehensive Textbook, 2nd ed. Edited by J Engel, Jr, and TA Pedley. Philadelphia: Lippincott Williams & Wilkins, pp. 1185–1192.

Dolmans, GH, Werker, PM, Hennies, HC, et al. (2011). Wnt signaling and Dupuytren's disease. N Engl J Med 365:307–317.

Dreifuss, FE (1987). Goals of surgery for epilepsy. In Surgical Treatment of the Epilepsies. Edited by J Engel, Jr. New York: Raven Press, pp. 31–50.

Dreifuss, FE, and Langer, DH (1987). Hepatic considerations in the use of antiepileptic drugs. Epilepsia 28(suppl 3): S23–S29.

Dreifuss, FE, Santilli, N, Langer, DH, Sweeney, KP, Moline, KA, and Menander, KB (1987). Valproic acid hepatic fatalities: A retrospective review. Neurology 37:379–385.

Dulac, O, Leppik, IE, Chadwick, DW, and Specchio, L (2008). Starting and stopping treatment. In Epilepsy: A Comprehensive Textbook, 2nd ed. Edited by J Engel, Jr, and TA Pedley. Philadelphia: Lippincott Williams & Wilkins, pp. 1301–1309.

Duley, L, Henderson-Smart, DJ, and Chou, D (2010a). Magnesium sulphate versus phenytoin for eclampsia. Cochrane Database Syst Rev Oct 6(10):CD000128.

Duley, L, Henderson-Smart, DJ, Walker, GJ, and Chou, D (2010b). Magnesium sulphate versus diazepam for eclampsia. Cochrane Database Syst Rev Dec 8(12):CD000127.

Eke, T, Talbot, JF, and Lawden, MC (1997). Severe persistent visual field constriction associated with vigabatrin. Br Med J 314:180–181.

Elwes, RD, Johnson, AL, Shorvon, SD, and Reynolds, EH (1984). The prognosis for seizure control in newly diagnosed epilepsy. N Engl J Med 311:944–947.

Elwes, RDC, Chesterman, P, and Reynolds, EH (1985). Prognosis after a first untreated tonic-clonic seizure. Lancet 2:752–753.

Engel, J, Jr (2008). Surgical treatment for epilepsy: Too little too late? JAMA 300:2548–2550.

Engel, J, Jr, and Shewmon, DA (1993). Overview: Who should be considered a surgical candidate? In Surgical Treatment of the epilepsies, 2nd ed. Edited by J Engel, Jr. New York: Raven Press, pp. 23–34.

Falconer, MA, and Davidson, S (1973). Coarse features in epilepsy as a consequence of anticonvulsant therapy. Lancet 2:1112–1114.

Fisher, RS, van Emde Boas, W, Blume, W, Elger, C, Engel, J, Jr, Genton, P, and Lee, P (2005). Epileptic seizures and epilepsy: Definitions proposed by the International League against Epilepsy (ILAE) and the International Bureau for Epilepsy (IBE). Epilepsia 46:470–472.

Fisher, RS, McKhann, GM, II, Stern, JM, et al. (2008). New therapeutic directions in Epilepsy: A Comprehensive Textbook, 2nd ed. Edited by J Engel, Jr, and TA Pedley. Philadelphia: Lippincott Williams & Wilkins, pp. 1415–1430.

Fisher, R, Salanova, V, Witt, T, et al. (2010). Electrical stimulation of the anterior nucleus of thalamus for treatment of refractory epilepsy. Epilepsia 51:899–908.

Fitzgerald, CL, and Jacobson, MP (2011). Generic substitution of levetiracetam resulting in increased incidence of breakthrough seizures [published online ahead of print May 11, 2011]. Ann Pharmacother 45(5):e27. doi:10.1345/aph.1P765

Fountain, NB, Van Ness, PC, Swain-Eng, R, et al. (2011). Quality improvement in neurology: AAN epilepsy quality measures. Report of the Quality Measurement and Reporting Subcommittee of the American Academy of Neurology. Neurology 76:94–99.

French, JA, Kanner, AM, Bautista, J, et al. (2004a). Efficacy and tolerability of the new antiepileptic drugs I: Treatment of new onset epilepsy. Report of the Therapeutics and Technology Assessment Subcommittee and Quality Standards Subcommittee of the American Academy of Neurology and the American Epilepsy Society. Neurology 62:1252–1260.

French, JA, Kanner, AM, Bautista, J, et al. (2004b). Efficacy and tolerability of the new antiepileptic drugs II: Treatment of refractory epilepsy. Report of the Therapeutics and Technology Assessment Subcommittee and Quality Standards Subcommittee of the American Academy of Neurology and the American Epilepsy Society. Neurology 62:1261–1273.

Frey, HH, and Löscher, W (1978). Distribution of valproate across the interface between blood and cerebrospinal fluid. Neuropharmacology 17:637–642.

Frost, JD (1985). Automatic recognition and characterization of epileptiform discharges in the human EEG. J Clin Neurophysiol 2:231–249.

Frost, JD, Jr, Kellaway, P, Hrachovy, RA, Glaze, DG, and Mizrahi, EM (1986). Changes in epileptic spike configuration associated with attainment of seizure control. Ann Neurol 20:723–731.

Gidal, BE (2009). Bioequivalence of antiepileptic drugs: How close is close enough? Curr Neurol Neurosci Rep 9:333–337.

Glauser, T (2000). Idiosyncratic reactions: New methods of identifying high risk patients. Epilepsia 41(suppl 8): S16–S29.

Glauser, T (2011). Biomarkers for antiepileptic drug response. Biomark Med 5:635–641.

Glauser, T, Ben-Menachem, E, Bourgeois, B, et al. (2006). ILAE treatment guidelines: Evidence-based analysis of antiepileptic drug efficacy and effectiveness as initial monotherapy for epileptic seizures and syndromes. Epilepsia 47:1094–1120.

Glauser, TA, Cnaan, A, Shinnar, S, et al. (2010). Ethosuximide, valproic acid, and lamotrigine in childhood absence epilepsy. N Engl J Med 362:790–799.

Gomez, MR (1981). Possible teratogenicity of valproic acid. J Pediatr 98:508–509.

Hachinski, V (1986). Management of a first seizure. Arch Neurol 43:1290.

Harden, CL, Meador, KJ, Pennell, PB, et al. (2009a). Practice parameter update: Management issues for women with epilepsy—Focus on pregnancy (an evidence-based review): Teratogenesis and perinatal outcomes. Report of the Quality Standards Subcommittee and Therapeutics and Technology Subcommittee of the American Academy of Neurology and the American Epilepsy Society. Neurology 50:1237–1246.

Harden, CL, Hopp, J, Ting, TY, et al. (2009b). Practice parameter update: Management issues for women with epilepsy—Focus on pregnancy (an evidence-based review): Obstetrical complications and change in seizure frequency. Report of the Quality Standards Subcommittee and Therapeutics and Technology Assessment Subcommittee of the American Academy of Neurology and the American Epilepsy Society. Neurology 50:1229–1236.

Harden, CL, Pennell, PB, Koppel, BS, et al. (2009c). Practice parameter update: Management issues for women with epilepsy—Focus on pregnancy (an evidence-based review): Vitamin K, folic acid, blood levels, and breastfeeding. Report of the Quality Standards Subcommittee and Therapeutics and Technology Assessment Subcommittee of the American Academy of Neurology and the American Epilepsy Society. Neurology 50:1247–1255.

Hart, RG, and Easton, JO (1986). Seizure recurrence after a first, unprovoked seizure. Arch Neurol 43:1289–1290.

Hauser, WA (1986). Should people be treated after a first seizure? Arch Neurol 43:1287–1288.

Hauser, WA, Anderson, VE, Loewenson, RB, and McRoberts, SM (1982). Seizure recurrence after a first unprovoked seizure. N Engl J Med 307:522–528.

Hauser, WA, Rich, SS, Jacobs, MP, and Anderson, VE (1983). Patterns of seizure occurrence and recurrence risks in patients with newly diagnosed epilepsy. Epilepsia 24:516–517.

Hauser, WA, Rich, S, and Anderson, VE (1986). Seizure recurrence after the first unprovoked seizure: An extended follow-up [abstract]. Epilepsia 27:617.

Hirtz, D, Berg, A, Bettis, D, et al. (2003). Practice parameter: Treatment of the child with a first unprovoked seizure. Report of the Quality Standards Subcommittee of the American Academy of Neurology and the Practice Committee of the Child Neurology Society. Neurology 60:166–175.

Holmes, LB, Wyszynski, DF, and Lieberman, E (2004). The AED (antiepileptic drug) pregnancy registry: A 6-year experience. Arch Neurol 61:673–678.

Holowach, J, Thurston, DL, and O'Leary, J (1972). Prognosis in childhood epilepsy. N Engl J Med 286:169–174.

Holowach-Thurston, J, Thurston, DL, Hixon, BB, and Keller, A (1982). Prognosis in childhood epilepsy. Additional follow-up of 148 children 15 to 23 years after withdrawal of anticonvulsant therapy. N Engl J Med 306:831–836.

Hunt S, Russell, A, Smithson, WH, Parsons, L, Robertson, I, Waddell, R, Irwin, B, Morrison, PJ, Morrow, J, and Craig, J (2008). Topiramate in pregnancy: Preliminary experience from the UK Epilepsy and Pregnancy Register. Neurology 22;71:272–276.

Jain, KK (1993). Investigation and management of loss of efficacy of an antiepileptic medication using carbamazepine as an example. J R Soc Med 86:133–136.

Janz, D, Dam, M, Richens, A, Bossi, L, Helge, H, and Schmidt, D (eds) (1982). Epilepsy, Pregnancy and the Child. New York: Raven Press.

Janz, D, Kern, A, Mossinger, HJ, and Puhlmann, HU (1983). Ruckfallprognose wahrend und nach Reduktion der Medikamente bei Epilepsiebehandlung. In Epilepsie 1981: Verlauf und Prognose, Neuropsychologische und Psychologische Aspekte. Edited by H Remschmidt, R Rentz, and J Jungmann. Stuttgart: Thieme, pp. 17–24.

Jeavons, PM (1983). Hepatotoxicity of antiepileptic drugs. In Antiepileptic Therapy: Chronic Toxicity of Antiepileptic Drugs. Edited by J Oxley, D Janz, and H Meinardi. New York: Raven Press, pp. 1–45.

Jentink, J, Loane, MA, Dolk, H, et al. (2010). Valproic acid monotherapy in pregnancy and major congenital malformations. N Engl J Med 362:2185–2193.

Johannessen, SI, Patsalos, PN, Tomson, T, and Perucca, E (2008). Therapeutic drug monitoring. In Epilepsy: A Comprehensive Textbook, 2nd ed. Edited by J Engel, Jr, and TA Pedley. Philadelphia: Lippincott Williams & Wilkins, pp. 1171–1183.

Kaaja, E, Kaaja, R, Matila, R, and Hiilesmaa, V (2002). Enzyme-inducing antiepileptic drugs in pregnancy and the risk of bleeding in the neonate. Neurology 58:549–553.

Kaneko, S, Suzuki, S, Sato, T, Ogawa, Y, and Nomura, Y (1982). The problems of antiepileptic medication in the neonatal period: Is breast-feeding advisable? In Epilepsy, Pregnancy and the Child. Edited by D Janz, M Dam, A Richens, L Bossi, H Helge, and D Schmidt. New York: Raven Press, pp. 343–348.

Katz, R (2008). Briefing document for the July 10 advisory committee meeting to discuss antiepileptic drugs (AEDs) and suicidality [memorandum]. (Accessed July 9, 2010, at http://www.fda.gov/ohrms/dockets/ac/08/briefing/2008–4372b1–01-FDA-Katz.pdf)

Kellaway, P, Saltzberg, B, Frost, JD, Jr, and Crawley, JW (1979). Relationship between clinical state, ictal and interictal EEG discharges, and serum drug levels: Generalized epilepsy/ethosuximide [abstract]. Neurology 29:559.

Kesselheim, AS, Stedman, MR, Bubrick, EJ, et al. (2010). Seizure outcomes following use of generic vs. brand-name antiepileptic drugs: A systematic review and meta-analysis. Drugs 70(5):605–621.

Kim, LG, Johnson, TL, Marson, AG, and Chadwick, DW; MRC MESS Study Group (2006). Prediction of risk of seizure recurrence after a single seizure and early epilepsy: Further results from the MESS trial. Lancet Neurol 5:317–322.

Kim, SS, Chang, KH, Kim, ST, Suh, DC, Cheon, JE, Jeong, SW, Han, MH, and Lee, SK (1999). Focal lesion in the splenium of the corpus callosum in epileptic patients: Antiepileptic drug toxicity? AJNR Am J Neuroradiol 20:125–129.

Koch, G, and Allen, J (1987). Untoward effects of generic carbamazepine therapy [abstract]. Arch Neurol 44:578–579.

Koontz, WL, and Reid, KH (1985). Effect of parenteral magnesium sulfate on penicillin-induced seizure foci in anesthetized cats. Am J Obstet Gynecol 153:96–99.

Krauss, GL, Caffo, B, Chang, Y-T, Hendrix, GW, and Chuang, K (2011). Assessing bioequivalence of generic antiepilepsy drugs. Ann Neurol 70:221–228.

Krumholz, A, Wiebe, S, Gronseth, G, et al. (2007). Practice parameter: Evaluating an apparent unprovoked Kutt first seizure in adults (an evidence-based review). Report of the Quality Standards Subcommittee of the American Academy of Neurology and the American Epilepsy Society. Neurology 69:1996–2007.

Kwan, P, and Brodie, MJ (2000). Early identification of refractory epilepsy. New Engl J Med 342:314–319.

Kwan, P, Arzimanoglou, A, Berg, AT, Brodie, MJ, Hauser, WA, Mathern, G, Moshé, SL, Perucca, E, Wiebe, S, and French, J (2010). Definition of drug resistant epilepsy: Consensus proposal by the ad hoc Task Force of the ILAE Commission on Therapeutic Strategies. Epilepsia 51:1069–1077.

Kwan, P, Schachter, SC, and Brodie, MJ (2011). Drug-resistant epilepsy. N Engl J Med 365:919–926.

Leone, MA, Solari, A, and Beghi, E; FIRST Group (2006). Treatment of the first tonic-clonic seizure does not affect long-term remission of epilepsy. Neurology 67:2227–2229.

Leppik, IE, Fisher, J, Kriel, R, and Sawchuck, RJ (1986). Altered phenytoin clearance with febrile illness. Neurology 36:1367–1370.

Leppik, IE, and Birnbaum, AK (2008). Drug treatment in the elderly. In Epilepsy: A Comprehensive Textbook, 2nd ed. Edited by J Engel, Jr, and TA Pedley. Philadelphia: Lippincott Williams & Wilkins, pp. 1269–1277.

Levy, RH, Cenraud, B, Loiseau, P, Akbaraly, R, Brachet-Lierman, A, Guyot, M, Gomeni, R, and Morselli, PL (1980). Meal-dependent absorption of enteric-coated sodium valproate. Epilepsia 21:273–280.

Levy, RH, Shen, DD, Abbott, FS, Riggs, KW, and Hachad, H (2002). Chemistry, biotransformation, and pharmacokinetics. In Antiepileptic Drugs, 5th ed. Edited by RH Levy, RH Mattson, BS Meldrum, and E Perucca. Philadelphia: Lippincott Williams & Wilkins, pp. 780–800.

Levy, RH, Bourgeois, BFD, and Hachad, H (2008). Drug-drug interactions. In Epilepsy: A Comprehensive Textbook, 2nd ed. Edited by J Engel, Jr, and TA Pedley. Philadelphia: Lippincott Williams & Wilkins, pp. 1235–1248.

Liimatainen, SP, Raitanen, JA, Ylinen, AM, Peltola, MA, and Peltola, JT (2008). The benefit of active drug trials is dependent on the aetiology in refractory focal epilepsy. J Neurol Neurosurg Psychiatry 79:808–812.

Liow, K, Barkley, GL, Pollard, JR, Harden, CL, and Bazil, CW (2007). Position statement on the coverage of anticonvulsant drugs for the treatment of epilepsy. Neurology 68:1249–1250.

Löscher, W, and Schmidt, D (2006). Experimental and clinical evidence for loss of effect (tolerance) during prolonged treatment with antiepileptic drugs. Epilepsia 47:1253–1284.

Löscher, W, and Schmidt, D (2011). Modern antiepileptic drug development has failed to deliver: Ways out of the current dilemma. Epilepsia 52:657–678.

Lossius, MI, Hessen, E, Mowinckel, P, et al. (2008). Consequences of antiepileptic drug withdrawal: A randomized, double-blind study (Akershius study). Epilepsia 49:455–463.

Luciano, AL, and Shorvon, SD (2007). Results of treatment changes in patients with apparently drug-resistant chronic epilepsy. Ann Neurol 62:375–381.

Lüders, H, Lesser, RP, Dinner, DS, and Morris, HH, III (1987). Benign focal epilepsy of childhood. In Epilepsy: Electroclinical Syndromes. Edited by H Lüders and RP Lesser. London: Springer-Verlag, pp. 303–346.

MacDonald, JT (1987). Breakthrough seizures following substitution of Depakene capsules (Abbott) with a generic product. Neurology 37:1885.

Macdonald RL, and Rogawski, MA (2008). Cellular effects of antiepileptic drugs. In Epilepsy: A Comprehensive Textbook, 2nd ed. Edited by J Engel, Jr, and TA Pedley. Philadelphia: Lippincott Williams & Wilkins, pp. 1433–1445.

Marson, AG, Al-Kharusi, AM, Alwaidh, M, et al. (2007a). The SANAD study of effectiveness of carbamazepine, gabapentin, lamotrigine, oxcarbazepine, or topiramate for treatment of partial epilepsy: An unblinded randomised controlled trial. Lancet 369:1000–1015.

Marson, AG, Al-Kharusi, AM, Alwaidh, M, et al. (2007b). The SANAD study of effectiveness of valproate, lamotrigine, or topiramate for generalised and unclassifiable epilepsy: An unblinded randomised controlled trial. Lancet 369:1016–1026.

Mattson, RH, Cramer, JA, Collins, JF, Smith, DB, Delgado-Escueta, A, Brown, TR, Williamson, PD, Treiman, DM, McNamara, JO, McCutchen, DB, Homan, RW, Crill, WE, Lubozynski, MF, Rosenthal, NP and Mayerdorf, A (1985). Comparison of carbamazepine, phenobarbital, phenytoin and primidone in partial and secondarily generalized tonic-clonic seizures. N Engl J Med 313:145–151.

Mattson, RH, Cramer, JA, Darney, PD, and Naftolin, F (1986). Use of oral contraceptives by women with epilepsy. JAMA 256:238–240.

Meador, KJ, Baker, GA, Browning, N, et al. (2009). Cognitive function at 3 years of age after fetal exposure to antiepileptic drugs. N Engl J Med 360:1597–1605.

Melander, A (1978). Influence of food on the bioavailability of drugs. Clin Pharmacokinet 3:337–351.

Meldrum, BS (1986). Pharmacological approaches to the treatment of epilepsy. In New Anticonvulsant Drugs. Edited by BS Meldrum and RJ Porter. London: John Libbey, pp. 17–30.

Melikian, AP, Straughn, AB, Slywka, GWA, Whyatt, PL, and Meyer, MC (1977). Bioavailability of 11 phenytoin products. J Pharmacokinet Biopharm 5:133–146.

Mizrahi, EM, and Scher, MS (2008). Treatment of neonatal seizures. In Epilepsy: A Comprehensive Textbook, 2nd ed. Edited by J Engel, Jr, and TA Pedley. Philadelphia: Lippincott Williams & Wilkins, pp. 1335–1343.

Mølgaard-Nielsen, D, and Hviid, A (2011). Newer-generation antiepileptic drugs and the risk of major birth defects. JAMA 305:1996–2002.

Morselli, PL, Pippenger, CE, and Penry, JK (eds) (1983). Antiepileptic Drug Therapy in Pediatrics. New York: Raven Press.

MRC Vitamin Study Research Group (1991). Prevention of neural tube defects: Results of the Medical Research Council Vitamin Study. Lancet 338:131–137.

Mula, M, and Hesdorffer, DC (2011). Suicidal behavior and antiepileptic drugs in epilepsy: Analysis of the emerging evidence. Drug Healthc Patient Saf 3:15–20.

Nadebaum, C, Anderson, VA, Vajda, F, Reutens, DC, Barton, S, and Wood, AG (2011). Language skills of school-aged children prenatally exposed to antiepileptic drugs. Neurology 76:719–726.

Neuvonen, PJ (1979). Bioavailability of phenytoin: Clinical pharmacokinetic and therapeutic implications. Clin Pharmacokinet 4:91–103.

Norris, FH, Jr, Colella, JAB, and McFarlin, D (1964). Effect of diphenylhydantoin on neuromuscular synapse. Neurology 14:869–876.

Offermann, G (1983). Chronic antiepileptic drug treatment and disorders of mineral metabolism. In Chronic Toxicity of Antiepileptic Drugs. Edited by J Oxley, D Janz, and H Meinardi. New York: Raven Press, pp. 175–184.

Oxley, J, Janz, D, and Meinardi, H (eds) (1983). Chronic Toxicity of Antiepileptic Drugs. New York: Raven Press.

Oyegbile, TO, Bayless, K, Dabbs, K, et al. (2011). The nature and extent of cerebellar atrophy in chronic temporal lobe epilepsy. 52:698–706.

Pack, AM, and Gidal, BE (2008). Long-term adverse events. In Epilepsy: A Comprehensive Textbook, 2nd ed. Edited by J Engel, Jr, and TA Pedley. Philadelphia: Lippincott Williams & Wilkins, pp. 1209–1212.

Patsalos, PN, Berry, DJ, Bourgeois, BFD, et al. (2008). Antiepileptic drugs—Best practice guidelines for therapeutic drug monitoring: A position paper by the Subcommission on Therapeutic Drug Monitoring, ILAE Commission on Therapeutic Strategies. Epilepsia 49:1239–1276.

Pearl, PL, Vezina, LG, Saneto, RP, McCarter, R, Molloy-Wells, E, Heffron, A, Trzcinski, S, McClintock, WM, Conry, JA, Elling, NJ, Goodkin, HP, de Menezes, MS, Ferri, R, Gilles, E, Kadom, N, and Gaillard, WD (2009). Cerebral MRI abnormalities associated with vigabatrin therapy. Epilepsia 50:184–194.

Pellock, JM, Nordli Jr, DR, and Dulac, O (2008). Drug treatment in children. In Epilepsy: A Comprehensive Textbook, 2nd ed. Edited by J Engel, Jr, and TA

Pedley. Philadelphia: Lippincott Williams & Wilkins, pp. 1249–1257

Perucca, E (2008). Pharmacokinetics. In Epilepsy: A Comprehensive Textbook, 2nd ed. Edited by J Engel, Jr, and TA Pedley. Philadelphia: Lippincott Williams & Wilkins, pp. 1151–1169.

Perucca, E (2009a). General principles of medical management. In The Treatment of Epilepsy, 3rd ed. Edited by S Shorvon, E Perucca, and J Engel, Jr. West Sussex, UK: Wiley-Blackwell, pp. 121–139.

Perucca, E (2009b). Extended-release formulations of antiepileptic drugs: Rationale and comparative value. Epilepsy Curr 9:153–157.

Perucca, E (2011). The pharmacology of new antiepileptic drugs: Does a novel mechanism of action really matter? CNS Drugs 25:1–6.

Perucca, E, and Tomson, T (2011). The pharmacological treatment of epilepsy in adults. Lancet Neurol 10:446–456.

Perucca, E, Gram, L, Avanzini, G, and Dulac, O (1998). Antiepileptic drugs as a cause of worsening seizures. Epilepsia 39:5–17.

Philbert, A, and Dam, M (1982). The epileptic mother and her child. Epilepsia 23:85–99.

Pirmohamed, M, and Arroyo, S (2008). Idiosyncratic adverse reactions. In Epilepsy: A Comprehensive Textbook, 2nd ed. Edited by J Engel, Jr, and TA Pedley. Philadelphia: Lippincott Williams & Wilkins, pp. 1201–1208.

Poisbeau, P, Williams, SR, and Mody, I (1997). Silent GABA$_A$ synapses during flurazepam withdrawal are region-specific in the hippocampal formation. J Neurosci 17: 3467–3475.

Porter, RJ, Penry, JK, and Lacy, JR (1977). Diagnostic and therapeutic reevaluation of patients with intractable epilepsy. Neurology 27:1006–1011.

Privitera, MD (2008). Generic antiepileptic drugs: Current controversies and future directions. Curr Rev Clin Sci 8:113–117.

Reynolds, EH (1983a). How to avoid chronic toxicity. In Chronic Toxicity of Antiepileptic Drugs. Edited by J Oxley, D Janz, and H Meinardi. New York: Raven Press, pp. 285–291.

Reynolds, EH (1983b). Adverse haemotological effects of antiepileptic drugs. In Chronic Toxicity of Antiepileptic Drugs. Edited by J Oxley, D Janz, and H Meinardi. New York: Raven Press, pp. 91–100.

Reynolds, EH (1983c). Mental effects of antiepileptic medication: A review. Epilepsia 24(suppl 2):S85–S95.

Reynolds, NC, Jr, and Miska, RM (1981). Safety of anticonvulsants in hepatic porphyrias. Neurology 31:480–484.

Riley, TL, Porter, RJ, White, BG, and Penry, JK (1981). The hospital experience and seizure control. Neurology 31:912–915.

Rodin, EA (1968). The Prognosis of Patients with Epilepsy. Springfield, IL: Charles C Thomas.

Sabers, A, and Harden, CL (2008). Gender issues for drug treatment. In Epilepsy: A Comprehensive Textbook, 2nd ed. Edited by J Engel, Jr, and TA Pedley. Philadelphia: Lippincott Williams & Wilkins, pp. 1263–1268.

Sabers, A, and Tomson, T (2009). Managing antiepileptic drugs during pregnancy and lactation. Curr Opin Neurol 22:157–161.

Schachter, SC, and Boon, P (2008). Vagus nerve stimulation. In Epilepsy: A Comprehensive Textbook, 2nd ed. Edited by J Engel, Jr, and TA Pedley. Philadelphia: Lippincott Williams & Wilkins, pp. 1395–1399.

Schachter, SC, Acevedo, C, Acevedo, KA, Lai, C-W, and Diop, AG (2008). Complementary and alternative medical therapies. In Epilepsy: A Comprehensive Textbook, 2nd ed. Edited by J Engel, Jr, and TA Pedley. Philadelphia: Lippincott Williams & Wilkins, pp. 1407–1414.

Schiller, Y, Cascino, GD, So, EL, et al. (2000). Discontinuation of antiepileptic drugs after successful epilepsy surgery. Neurology 54:346–349.

Schmidt, D (1982). Two antiepileptic drugs for intractable epilepsy with complex-partial seizures. J Neurol Neurosurg Psychiatry 45:1119–1124.

Schmidt, D (1983). Connective tissue disorders induced by antiepileptic drugs. In Chronic Toxicity of Antiepileptic Drugs. Edited by J Oxley, D Janz, and H Meinardi. New York: Raven Press, pp. 115–124.

Schmidt, D, and Schachter, SC (2008). Dose-related side effects. In Epilepsy: A Comprehensive Textbook, 2nd ed. Edited by J Engel, Jr, and TA Pedley. Philadelphia: Lippincott Williams & Wilkins, pp. 1193–1200.

Shedlofsky, SI, and Bonkowsky, HL (1984). Seizure management in the hepatic porphyrias: Results from a cell-culture model of porphyria [letter]. Neurology 34:399.

Shinnar, S, Vining, EPG, Mellits, ED, DiSouza, BJ, Holden, K, Baumgardner, RA, and Freeman, JM (1985). Discontinuing antiepileptic medication in children with epilepsy after two years without seizures: A prospective study. N Engl J Med 313:976–980.

Sibai, BM, Spinnato, JA, Watson, DL, Lewis, JA, and Anderson, GD (1984). Effect of magnesium sulfate on electroencephalographic findings in preeclampsia-eclampsia. Obstet Gynecol 64:261–266.

Singh, G (2009). Management of medical co-morbidity associated with epilepsy: In The Treatment of Epilepsy, 3rd ed. Edited by S Shorvon, E Perucca, and J Engel, Jr. West Sussex, UK: Wiley-Blackwell, pp. 259–272.

Sirven, J, Sperling, MR, and Wingerchuk, DM (2010). Early versus late antiepileptic drug withdrawal for people with epilepsy in remission. The Cochrane Collaboration. Chichester, UK: Wiley.

Sisodiya, SM, Beck, H, Löscher, W, and Vezzani, A (2008). Mechanisms of drug resistance. In Epilepsy: A Comprehensive Textbook, 2nd ed. Edited by J Engel, Jr, and TA Pedley. Philadelphia: Lippincott Williams & Wilkins, pp. 1279–1289.

Specchio, LM, and Beghi, E (2004). Should antiepileptic drugs be withdrawn in seizure-free patients? CNS Drugs 18:201–212.

Spina, E (2009). Drug interactions. In The Treatment of Epilepsy, 3rd ed. Edited by S Shorvon, E Perucca, and J Engel, Jr. West Sussex, UK: Wiley-Blackwell, pp. 361–377.

Stafstrom, CE, Vining, EPG, and Rho, JM (2008). Ketogenic diet. In Epilepsy: A Comprehensive Textbook, 2nd ed. Edited by J Engel, Jr, and TA Pedley. Philadelphia: Lippincott Williams & Wilkins, pp. 1377–1385.

Strickler, SM, Miller, MA, Andermann, E, Dansky, LV, Seni, MH, and Spielberg, SP (1985). Genetic predisposition to phenytoin-induced birth defects. Lancet 2:746–749.

Taylor, DC (2008). Broader aspects of treatment. In Epilepsy: A Comprehensive Textbook, 2nd ed. Edited by J Engel, Jr, and TA Pedley. Philadelphia: Lippincott Williams & Wilkins, pp. 1129–1132.

Taylor, DC, and McKinlay, I (1984). When not to treat epilepsy with drugs. Dev Med Child Neurol 26:822–833.

Taylor, JW, Murphy, MJ, and Rivey, MP (1985). Clinical and electrophysiologic evaluation of peripheral nerve function in chronic phenytoin therapy. Epilepsia 26:416–420.

Theodore, WH, and Porter, RJ (1983). Removal of sedative-hypnotic antiepileptic drugs from the regimens of patients with intractable epilepsy. Ann Neurol 13:320–324.

Theodore, WH, Porter, RJ, and Raubertas, RF (1987). Seizures during barbiturate withdrawal: Relation to blood level. Ann Neurol 22:644–647.

Todt, H (1984). The late prognosis of epilepsy in childhood: Results of a prospective follow-up study. Epilepsia 25:137–144.

Tomson, T (2009). Reproductive aspects of epilepsy treatment. In The Treatment of Epilepsy, 3rd ed. Edited by S Shorvon, E Perucca, and J Engel, Jr. West Sussex, UK: Wiley-Blackwell, pp. 323–333.

Tomson, T, Battino, D, Craig, J, et al. (2010). Pregnancy registries: Differences, similarities, and possible harmonization. Epilepsia 51:909–915.

Tomson, T, Battino, D, Bonizzoni, E, Craig, J, Lindhout, D, Sabers, A, Perucca, E, and Vajda, F, for the EURAP study group (2011a). Dose-dependent risk of malformations with antiepileptic drugs: An analysis of data from the EURAP epilepsy and pregnancy registry. Lancet Neurol 10:609–617.

Tomson, T, Battino, D, and Perucca, E (2011b). Major birth defects after exposure to newer-generation antiepileptic drugs. JAMA 306:826–827.

Toone, B (1987). Sexual disorders in epilepsy. In Recent Advances in Epilepsy 3. Edited by TA Pedley and BS Meldrum. New York, Churchill Livingstone, pp. 233–259.

Troupin, AS, and Ojemann, LM (1975). Paradoxical intoxication: A complication of anticonvulsant administration. Epilepsia 16:753–758.

Wilder, BJ, and Bruni, J (1981). Seizure Disorders: A Pharmacological Approach to Treatment. New York: Raven Press.

Wilder, BJ, Serrano, EE, Ramsay, RE, and Buchanan, RA (1974). A method for shifting from oral to intramuscular diphenylhydantoin administration. Clin Pharmacol Ther 16:507–513.

Wolf, P (2008). Behavioral therapies. In Epilepsy: A Comprehensive Textbook, 2nd ed. Edited by J Engel, Jr, and TA Pedley. Philadelphia: Lippincott Williams & Wilkins, pp. 1401–1405.

Woodbury, DM, Penry, JK, and Pippenger, CE (eds) (1989). Antiepileptic Drugs, 2nd ed. New York: Raven Press, 1982. See also Levy, RH, Dreifuss, FE, Mattson, RH, Meldrum, BS, and Penry, JK (eds): Antiepileptic Drugs, 3rd ed. New York: Raven Press.

Worrell, G, and Gotman, J (2011). High-frequency oscillations and other electrophysiological biomarkers of of epilepsy: Clinical studies. Biomark Med 5:557–566.

Wyllie, E, Pippenger, CE, and Rothner, D (1987). Increased seizure frequency with generic primidone. JAMA 258:1216–1217.

Yerby, MS, Battino, D, and Montouris, GD (2008). General principles: Teratogenicity of antiepileptic drugs. In Epilepsy: A Comprehensive Textbook, 2nd ed. Edited by J Engel, Jr, and TA Pedley. Philadelphia: Lippincott Williams & Wilkins, pp. 1213–1224.

Zaccara, G, Balestrieri, F, and Ragazzoni, A (2009). Management of side-effects of antiepileptic drugs. In The Treatment of Epilepsy, 3rd ed. Edited by S Shorvon, E Perucca, and J Engel, Jr. West Sussex, UK: Wiley-Blackwell, pp. 289–299.

Chapter 15

Antiseizure Drugs

STANDARD OLDER DRUGS
Phenobarbital (PB)
Phenytoin (PHT)
Primidone (PRM)
Ethosuximide (ESM)
Benzodiazepines
Carbamazepine (CBZ)
Valproic Acid (VPA)

NEWER DRUGS
Eslicarbazepine Acetate (ESL)
Ezogabine (EZG)
Felbamate (FBM)
Gabapentin (GBP)
Lacosamide (LCM)
Lamotrigine (LTG)
Levetiracetam (LEV)
Oxcarbazepine (OXC)
Pregabalin (PGN)
Rufinamide (RUF)
Tiagabine (TGB)
Topiramate (TPM)
Vigabatrin (VGB)
Zonisamide (ZON)

SPECIAL AND RARELY USED DRUGS
Acetazolamide
ACTH and Adrenocorticosteroids
Barbiturates
Benzodiazepines
Bromides
Hydantoins
Oxazolidinediones
Paraldehyde
Phenacemide
Piracetam
Progabide
Propofol
Stiripentol
Succinimides
Sulthiame

NEW-DRUG DEVELOPMENT
Identification of New Compounds
Preclinical Evaluation
Clinical Evaluation

DRUGS UNDER INVESTIGATION
Drugs in Phase III Trials
Drugs in Preclinical Development

SUMMARY AND CONCLUSIONS

Pharmacological intervention is required for most patients with epilepsy disorders. Therefore, antiseizure drugs are discussed throughout this book. For additional information related to mechanisms of action, the reader should turn to Chapters 3 and 4. Pharmacological treatment of specific epileptic seizures and epilepsy syndromes is presented in Chapters 6, 7, and 10, and side effects of antiseizure drugs are dealt with in Chapters 11 and 14. Chapter 14 also contains basic data on each of the commonly used antiseizure drugs needed to formulate a general pharmacotherapy approach to the management of most patients with epilepsy and reviews of studies on comparative effectiveness. This chapter provides further details about individual drugs.

For convenience and completeness, this chapter contains (1) a pharmacological description of all drugs currently available for the treatment of epilepsy and (2) brief mention of some compounds currently under investigation. The data provided here have been largely condensed from the *Physician's Desk Reference* (Physician's Desk Reference, 2011), several books and monographs dealing specifically with antiseizure drugs (Glaser et al., 1980; Wilder and Bruni, 1981; Woodbury et al., 1982; Morselli et al., 1983; Frey and Janz, 1985; Levy et al., 2002, 2010; Asadi-Pooya and Sperling, 2009; Patsalos and Bourgeois, 2010), and recent epilepsy textbooks (Engel and Pedley, 2008; Shorvon et al., 2009).

Rational pharmacological therapy for epilepsy began in 1857 when Locock (1857) used *potassium bromide* to treat *catamenial seizures*; the modern era, however, dates from the introduction of *phenobarbital* as an antiseizure drug by Hauptmann (1912) (Chapter 2). Over a quarter of a century passed before Merritt and Putnam (1938) used electroconvulsive shock in cats to test a large number of drugs with chemical structures resembling *phenobarbital*. This approach led to discovery of the *anticonvulsant* properties of *phenytoin*. Subsequent reliance on such *structure-activity relationships* and *screening procedures* predictably resulted in identification of many new drugs similar in action to phenytoin but curiously also yielded *trimethadione* (Everett and Richards, 1944; Richards and Everett, 1944) and a new line of compounds, including the *succinimides*,

with selective *antiabsence* activity. It was more than 50 years after the introduction of *phenobarbital* that a first-line antiseizure drug with a completely different chemical structure, *carbamazepine*, was identified (Theobald and Kunz, 1963). At approximately the same time, the *benzodiazepines* (Gastaut et al., 1965; Swinyard and Castellion, 1966) and *valproic acid* (Carraz et al., 1964; Meunier et al., 1963), each with a distinctive chemical structure, were also undergoing evaluation as potential antiseizure agents. Compounds were all screened against two acute mouse seizure models, *maximal electroshock (MES)* for anticonvulsant properties and *subcutaneous pentylenetetrazol (PTZ)* for antiabsence properties (Meldrum, 1986b; White et al., 2008a). Of note is that all antiseizure drugs approved for use in the United States through the 1980s were discovered by trial and error. Advances in our understanding of the basic mechanisms of epilepsy (Chapters 3 and 4) eventually stimulated the development of compounds designed to correct specific epileptogenic neuronal abnormalities. Since 1989, a large number of second- and third-generation antiseizure drugs have entered the market (Fig. 15–1). Many of these have targeted molecular substrates of epileptogenicity; however, the majority appear to have principal mechanisms of action different from those initially intended or multiple mechanisms of action (Löscher and Schmidt, 2011).

Most antiseizure agents are sold under a variety of brand names in different countries, and some are known by more than one nonproprietary (*generic*) name as well. This chapter will specify brand names used in the United States (Fig. 15–2) and some of the more common names used elsewhere, but it would be impossible to list all the available brands and formulations here. That information is available, however, from the Worldwide AED (antiepileptic drug) Database at http://www.ilae.org/Visitors/Centre/AEDs/index.cfm. Table 15–1 shows nonproprietary names and abbreviations, corresponding US brand names, and other common names. The units used to express plasma levels of antiseizure drugs also vary from one country to another. The present system in the United States uses *micrograms per milliliter* (μg/ml) but most other countries now prefer *SI units (Système*

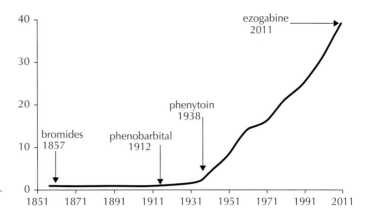

Figure 15–1. Introduction of antiseizure medications into the market.

International d'Unités), which are expressed as
micromoles per liter (µmol/1) (Young, 1987).
Molecular weights and conversion factors for
converting µg/ml to µmol/1 are also shown in
Table 15–1.

For historical purposes, the standard older
drugs will be discussed in order of their introduction in the United States. The newer drugs,
special and rarely used drugs, and compounds
under investigation are organized in alphabeti-
cal order.

STANDARD OLDER DRUGS

Phenobarbital (PB)

The chemical structure of barbiturate compounds determines whether they are more
effective as antiseizure or anesthetic agents.
Barbiturates commercially available for the
treatment of chronic epilepsy are *phenobarbital*, *methylphenobarbital*, and *metharbital*.

Some anesthetic barbiturates, such as *pentobarbital* and *thiopental*, are useful for the treatment of refractory status epilepticus (Chapter
10); others, with short durations of action, such
as *thiopental* and *methohexital*, have been
used to activate interictal EEG spike activity
(Chapter 12). Still other barbiturates are convulsants (Wilder and Bruni, 1981). Research
on how different barbiturates exert their anticonvulsant, proconvulsant, or anesthetic properties (Gallagher and Freer, 1985; Macdonald
and McLean, 1982; Olsen, 1982; Schafer, 1985;
Eadie and Kwan, 2008; Michelucci et al., 2009)
may lead to the development of more effective
drugs. Methylphenobarbital and metharbital
are discussed later in the section on Special
and Rarely Used Drugs.

The chemical name for *phenobarbital* is
5-ethyl-5-phenylbarbituric acid or *phenyleth-
ylmalonylurea*. The phenyl group at position
5 is important for the anticonvulsant activity
(Rall and Schleifer, 1985; Eadie and Kwan,
2008; Michelucci et al., 2009). *Phenobarbital*
was originally marketed in the United States in
1912 under the trade name of *Luminal* but is
now sold in a variety of generic forms. Names
elsewhere include *Phenobarbiton*, *Phenemal*,
Eskabarb, and *Gardenal*.

MECHANISMS OF ACTION

Phenobarbital acts on the *γ-aminobutyric
acid* (GABA) receptor–chloride ionophore
complex to prolong its opening (Olsen, 1982).
Phenobarbital also depresses normal excitatory
synaptic transmission, perhaps by interference

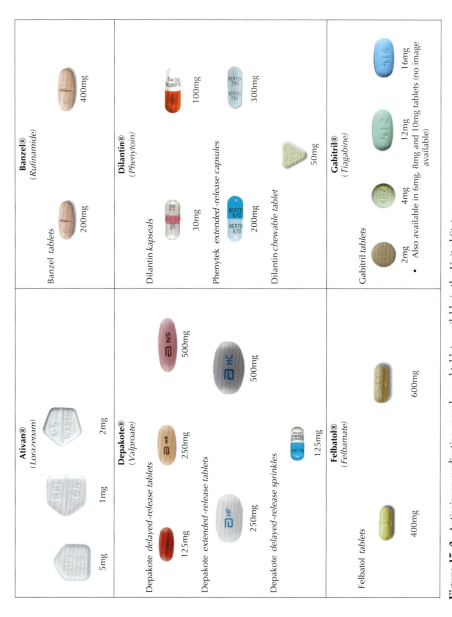

Figure 15–2. Antiseizure medication capsules and tablets available in the United States.

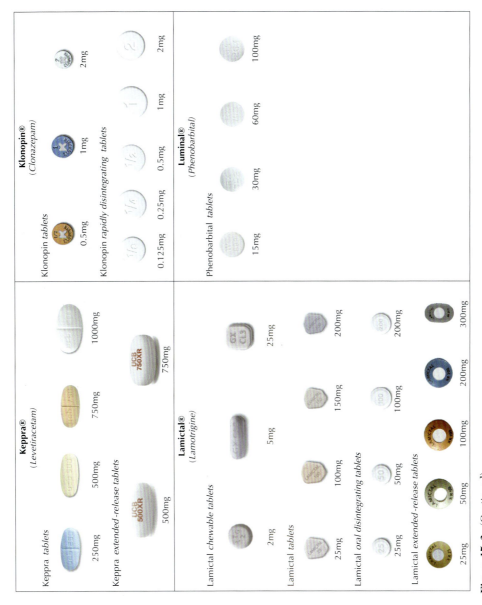

Figure 15–2. (Continued)

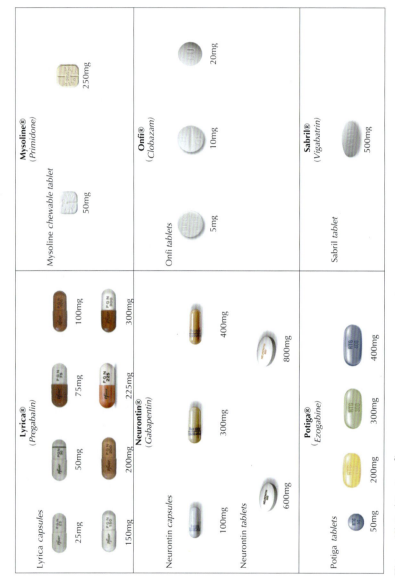

Figure 15–2. (Continued)

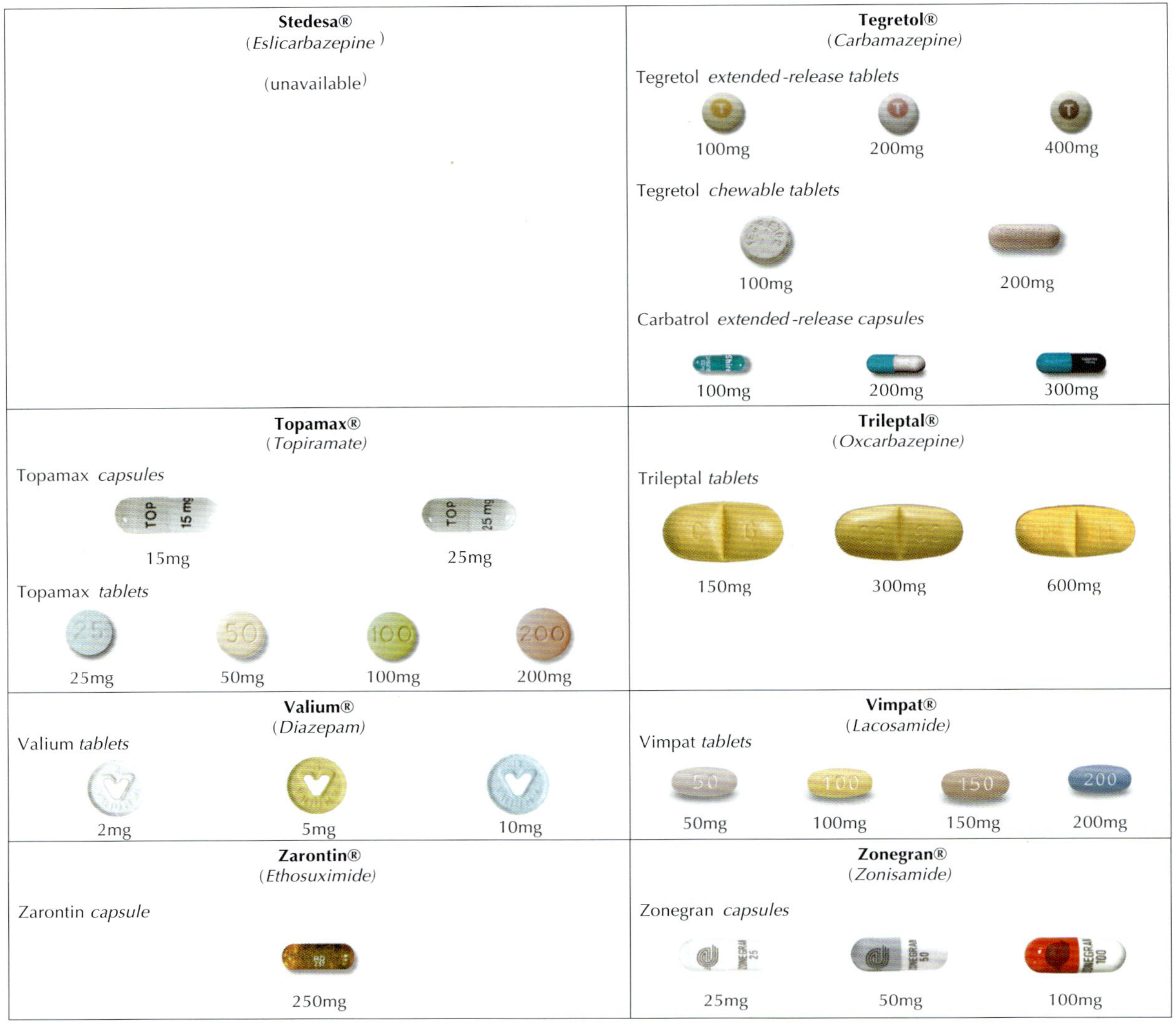

Stedesa®
(*Eslicarbazepine*)

(unavailable)

Tegretol®
(*Carbamazepine*)

Tegretol *extended-release tablets*

100mg   200mg   400mg

Tegretol *chewable tablets*

100mg   200mg

Carbatrol *extended-release capsules*

100mg   200mg   300mg

Topamax®
(*Topiramate*)

Topamax *capsules*

15mg   25mg

Topamax *tablets*

25mg   50mg   100mg   200mg

Trileptal®
(*Oxcarbazepine*)

Trileptal *tablets*

150mg   300mg   600mg

Valium®
(*Diazepam*)

Valium *tablets*

2mg   5mg   10mg

Vimpat®
(*Lacosamide*)

Vimpat *tablets*

50mg   100mg   150mg   200mg

Zarontin®
(*Ethosuximide*)

Zarontin *capsule*

250mg

Zonegran®
(*Zonisamide*)

Zonegran *capsules*

25mg   50mg   100mg

Figure 15–2. (Continued)

with the action of excitatory amino acids (Jurna, 1985) and Na$^+$, K$^+$, and Ca^{2+} conductances (McLean and Macdonald, 1988). Sedative effects occur because phenobarbital interferes with normal synaptic mechanisms and does not act selectively against those abnormal events that cause epileptogenic hyperexcitability, hypersynchronization, or both.

PHARMACOKINETICS

Phenobarbital is almost completely absorbed after oral administration, and peak concentration in plasma is achieved after 0.5 to 4 hours. The ratio of brain to plasma concentration varies considerably from one individual to another. The drug is 40–60% bound to plasma proteins. The volume of distribution (Vd) is 0.5 l/kg. Phenobarbital is 20–40% eliminated by pH-dependent renal excretion, whereas the remainder is metabolized in the liver, largely by CYP2C9, to two inactive metabolites. Plasma half-life is 70–130 hours in adults but can be longer in neonates and shorter in young children (Gallagher and Freer, 1985; Rall and Schleifer, 1985).

TOXICITY

The most common dose-related side effects of phenobarbital are sedation in adults, irritability and hyperactivity in children, and agitation and confusion in the elderly. Depression can be a subtle but serious emotional side effect. Phenobarbital impairs mental function at therapeutic levels and can cause nystagmus and ataxia at toxic concentrations. Although the drug is safer than most antiseizure agents, it interferes with vitamin D and calcium metabolism, can cause vitamin K deficiency in neonates, can sufficiently reduce folate levels to cause megaloblastic anemia, is commonly associated with *Dupuytren's contractures* and other chronic toxic effects on connective tissues, and is capable of inducing all the typical allergic reactions (Chapter 14). According to the most recent pregnancy registry data, the risk of teratogenicity with phenobarbital administration to pregnant women is not significantly different from that of other antiseizure drugs (Holmes et al., 2004); however, it is classified as risk category D (positive evidence of risk to the human fetus) by the *US Food and Drug Administration (FDA)*.

DRUG INTERACTIONS

Phenobarbital is an active hepatic microsomal enzyme inducer (Chapter 14) and therefore reduces serum concentrations of many drugs, including *alprenolol, antipyrine, bishydroxycoumarin, carbamazepine, clonazepam, digitoxin, dipyrone, griseofulvin, isoniazid, metoprolol, phenylbutazone, phenytoin, propranolol,* and *warfarin*. Phenobarbital metabolism is inhibited by valproic acid (Gallagher and Freer, 1985) and coadministration can result in severe sedation and coma. Interaction between phenobarbital and phenytoin is unpredictable.

INDICATIONS

Phenobarbital is an effective agent for generalized tonic-clonic and focal seizures, but the appearance of sedation in adults and hyperkinetic activity in children makes it less useful than other, equally effective antiseizure drugs that do not induce these side effects. Both functional and metabolic tolerance develop over time to phenobarbital-induced sedation (Gallagher and Freer, 1985). Although most physicians in the industrialized world generally reserve phenobarbital for patients who are unable to take the more commonly used agents, it remains the drug of choice in developing countries, where cost is often the most important adverse side effect. Many patients can benefit from low doses that produce few or no side effects. There is evidence to suggest that efficacy is better and side effects less problematic for phenobarbital than currently believed and that the role of this drug in the pharmacological treatment of epilepsy should be reevaluated (Kwan and Brodie, 2004). Intravenous phenobarbital is one of the standard treatments for status epilepticus (Chapter 10).

ADMINISTRATION

Generic phenobarbital and phenobarbital sodium are available for oral use in tablet and elixir form and also in vials of sterile solution for parenteral use. The usual daily dose is 100–300 mg in adults and 3–6 mg/kg in

Table 15–1 **Antiseizure Medications: Trade Names, Common Abbreviations, and Conversion Factors**

Antiseizure Medication	Trade Name (United States)	Common Trade Name Elsewhere	Abbreviation	Molecular Weight (g)	Conversion Factor (µg/ml to µmol/l)
Carbamazepine	Tegretol, Carbatrol		CBZ	236.27	4.23
Clobazam	Onfi	Frisium	CLB	300.70	3.33
Clonazepam	Klonopin	Rivotril, Ravotril, Iktoril	CLN	315.72	3.17
Diazepam	Valium	Alupram, Atensin, Dialar, Rimapam, Solis	DZP	284.74	3.51
Eslicarbazepine acetate	Stedesa	Zebenix, Exalief	ESL	296.32	3.37
Ethosuximide	Zarontin	Suxinutin, Zartalin	ESM	141.17	7.06
Ezogabine (retigabine)	Potiga	Trobalt	EZG (RTG)	303.30	3.30
Felbamate	Felbatol	Felbamyl, Taloxa	FBM	238.24	4.20
Gabapentin	Neurontin		GBP	171.24	5.84
Lacosamide	Vimpat		LCM	250.30	4.00
Lamotrigine	Lamictal		LTG	256.09	3.90
Levetiracetam	Keppra		LEV	170.21	5.88
Lorazepam	Ativan	Almazine, Intensol, Temesta	LZP	321.16	3.11
Oxcarbazepine	Trileptal		OXC	252.27	3.96
Phenobarbital	Luminal	Eskabarb, Phenemal, Phenobarbiton, Gardenal, Lumina	PB	232.24	4.31
Phenytoin	Dilantin, Phenytek	Epanutin, Epamin	PHT	275.25	3.63
Pregabalin	Lyrica		PGN	159.23	6.28
Primidone	Mysoline	Majsolin, Mylepsinum, Prysolin	PRM	218.25	4.58
Rufinamide	Banzel	Inovelon	RUF	238.2	4.20
Tiagabine	Gabitril		TGB	412.0	2.43
Topiramate	Topamax		TPM	339.36	2.95
Valproic acid	Depakote, Depakene, Depacon	Epilim, Ergenyl	VPA	166.2	6.02
Vigabatrin	Sabril		VGB	129.16	7.74
Zonisamide	Zonegran		ZON	212.23	4.71

children. It can be given once a day or twice daily. Because of the long half-life, steady-state levels are generally not reached for two to three weeks, and treatment can begin with the maintenance dose. Although giving twice the daily amount provides an effective loading dose, this is not recommended as a routine procedure, because of the excessive sedation induced. The usual therapeutic range is 10–40 µg/ml, dose-related side effects are commonly minimal below 30 µg/ml, and some patients, particularly children, may tolerate serum drug levels well above 40 µg/ml. Dose-related side effects of phenobarbital develop insidiously, however, and the full impact on mental function is often not appreciated, especially in children, unless the drug is reduced or removed.

Phenytoin (PHT)

Discovery of the anticonvulsant properties of *phenytoin* by Merritt and Putnam (1938) demonstrated that this effect could be dissociated from sedation. Their work heralded the beginning of an organized search for new drugs with selective antiseizure activity. *Phenytoin* not only was a successful anticonvulsant but also was a more potent agent than *phenobarbital* against psychomotor seizures. After subsequent screening of a large number of hydantoins, however, only *mephenytoin* and *ethotoin* made it to general usage in the United States, as infrequently prescribed second-line drugs. *Phenytoin*, on the other hand, remains, over 70 years after its initial introduction, one of the more important pharmacological agents used in the treatment of epilepsy, and *fosphenytoin* is a valuable alternative for intravenous use (Stern et al., 2008; Eadie, 2009). Studies of structure-activity relationships have yet to reveal why other hydantoins with at least equal effectiveness have not emerged (Jones and Wimbish, 1985). Fosphenytoin, mephenytoin, and ethotoin are discussed later in the section on Special and Rarely Used Drugs.

Phenytoin is also known as *diphenylhydantoin* and *5,5-diphenylhydantoin* (Eadie, 2009; Stern et al., 2008). It has been marketed in the United States as *Dilantin* since 1938, but many generic versions are now available. The drug is sold elsewhere under many other names, the most common being *Epanutin, Epamin,* and *Phenytek.* Generic formulations are available.

MECHANISMS OF ACTION

Phenytoin is commonly viewed as having a stabilizing effect on the membrane by interfering with ionic currents (Chapter 3). In contradistinction to the barbiturates, which strongly influence normal neuronal activity and greatly elevate the threshold for electroshock seizures, phenytoin acts primarily on excessive neuronal firing; it has less of an effect on the threshold for electroshock seizures but suppresses epileptogenic spread (Macdonald and McLean, 1982). These properties of phenytoin are similar in some ways to those of local anesthetic agents (Rall and Schleifer, 1985). Specific actions of phenytoin that have been identified include stimulation of the Na$^+$ pump; inhibition of passive Na$^+$ influx; prolongation of *inhibitory postsynaptic potentials (IPSPs)*; attenuation of *excitatory postsynaptic potentials (EPSPs)*; inhibition of Ca^{2+} influx and the effect of the *Ca^{2+}-calmodulin complex* on protein phosphorylation; and multiple effects on neurotransmitter metabolism, disposition, and dynamics, including enhancement of GABA concentrations (Jones and Wimbish, 1985). Phenytoin has no effect on *T-type Ca^{2+} conductances* in the thalamus (Macdonald, 1999). It has been postulated that the excitation of cerebellar Purkinje cells by phenytoin contributes to its antiseizure effect (Laxer et al., 1980), but this concept has not been substantiated. Undoubtedly many other mechanisms of phenytoin action on the brain have yet to be identified.

PHARMACOKINETICS

Phenytoin has variable and incomplete absorption following oral and intramuscular administration. Peak concentrations in the plasma occur 4–12 hours after ingestion (Rall and Schleifer, 1985). Ninety percent of phenytoin is bound to plasma proteins, which complicates its use in certain clinical situations (Chapter 14). Distribution to all tissues, including brain, is rapid after absorption, and concentrations in serum and brain are equal within minutes after intravenous injection. Vd is about 0.5–0.8 l/kg (Woodbury, 1982).

Phenytoin is 95% metabolized by the liver, predominantly by CYP2C9 to an inactive *para-hydroxyphenyl derivative.* Other metabolites also appear to be inactive. *Arene oxide* intermediates are believed to be responsible for some toxic and teratogenic effects of phenytoin, and their accumulation may reflect an inherited defect (Spielberg et al., 1981; Strickler et al.,

1985). Metabolism of phenytoin is *first order* at very low plasma concentrations and *zero order* at high concentrations (Chapter 14), which makes it impossible to adequately define the half-life of this drug. Although the half-life at steady state is usually given as 20 hours, a very small increment in phenytoin dose can result in a very large increment in serum concentration. In addition, there is considerable individual variation in the ability to metabolize phenytoin, greatly complicating the management of some patients. Dependence on metabolism for elimination means that phenytoin levels are markedly influenced by liver disease, pregnancy, age, and administration of other medications that alter hepatic enzyme activity.

TOXICITY

Common dose-related toxic side effects of phenytoin include ataxia, dizziness, nystagmus, diplopia, and tremor. Reports of irreversible cerebellar damage due to phenytoin administration at therapeutic levels are controversial (Chapter 14). Some patients may experience hyperactivity, confusion, sedation, and cognitive impairment. Nausea and epigastric pain can be avoided by taking the drug with food.

Approximately 20% of patients on chronic phenytoin therapy experience gingival hyperplasia, and this symptom, together with hirsutism and general coarsening of features, is a significant deterrent to the use of phenytoin in children and women. Almost one-third of patients develop electrophysiological evidence of peripheral neuropathy, but this is only rarely symptomatic (Rall and Schleifer, 1985), usually as a sensory polyneuropathy (Dam, 1982).

Effects of phenytoin on the endocrine system include hyperglycemia and glycosuria due to inhibition of insulin secretion; altered metabolism and absorption of vitamin D and calcium, resulting in osteomalacia, hypocalcemia, and elevated alkaline phosphatase activity; and increased metabolism of vitamin K. Phenytoin can also increase steroid excretion, causing failure of the low-dose *dexamethasone suppression test* and a subnormal *metyrapone test*. Although concentrations of protein-bound iodine, total thyroxine, and free thyroxine can be significantly reduced in patients taking phenytoin, they remain euthyroid (Chapter 14).

Phenytoin is capable of causing any of the drug-induced allergic reactions, including life-threatening dermatological and hematological conditions (Chapter 14). It can interfere with immunoglobulin A production, and both pseudolymphoma and malignant lymphoma have occurred (Chapter 14). Although the FDA has classified phenytoin as risk category D with respect to teratogenicity, the actual risk of serious malformations may be no greater than that of other drugs and is less than that of *carbamazepine* and *valproic acid* (Eadie, 2008). The existence of a specific *fetal hydantoin syndrome* (Hanson and Smith, 1975) remains controversial.

DRUG INTERACTIONS

Because the effectiveness, toxicity, and elimination of phenytoin depend on the relatively small fraction of unbound drug (Chapter 14), interference with protein binding can initially enhance activity but ultimately lowers total plasma concentration. Drugs that compete for protein-binding sites, such as *sulfisoxazole*, *phenylbutazone*, *salicylates*, and *valproic acid*, increase free phenytoin levels and may produce toxic symptoms on acute administration. Chronic administration, however, facilitates elimination of phenytoin, causing a reduction in total levels, whereas free phenytoin and the antiseizure effect remain essentially unchanged.

Drugs that act as enzyme inhibitors and increase phenytoin plasma concentration include *chloramphenicol*, *cimetidine*, *dicumarol*, *disulfiram*, *isoniazid*, *fluconazole*, *metronidazole*, *stiripentol*, and some *sulfonamides*. *Ethosuximide*, *methsuximide*, *felbamate*, and *oxcarbazepine* can also increase phenytoin plasma levels. *Carbamazepine*, *phenobarbital*, and *vigabatrin* have unpredictable effects on phenytoin. Enzyme inducers reduce phenytoin plasma levels, but *phenobarbital* is also capable of elevating phenytoin levels by competitive inhibition of enzymes and reduction of oral absorption, whereas *carbamazepine* competes for protein-binding sites. Valproic acid can inhibit phenytoin metabolism but also competes for protein binding. The effects of *ethanol* on phenytoin pharmacokinetics are similar to those of phenobarbital. Calcium-containing products such as antacids, *molindone hydrochloride*, nutritional supplements, and tube feeding delay phenytoin absorption from the stomach.

Phenytoin is an enzyme inducer and reduces levels of antiseizure drugs that are metabolized by the *cytochrome P450 system* and other hepatic enzymes, but it can increase or decrease phenobarbital levels. Phenytoin increases the rate of clearance of *theophylline*, enhances *corticosteroid* metabolism, and has been reported to decrease the effectiveness of *oral contraceptives* (Mattson et al., 1986; Rall and Schleifer, 1985).

INDICATIONS

Phenytoin is used primarily for the treatment of focal and generalized tonic-clonic seizures (Chapter 14). Intravenous phenytoin is effective therapy for status epilepticus (Chapter 10); however, the solvent required for parenteral formulation causes tissue damage if extravasated, and fosphenytoin is now a safer alternative for intravenous use when a central line is not available (Stern et al., 2008). The antiseizure potency of phenytoin is equivalent to that of carbamazepine, but side effects of phenytoin are somewhat more troublesome (Mattson et al., 1985). Phenytoin is no longer considered a first-line drug by many physicians because of the disturbing cosmetic side effects and the zero-order kinetics that make dosing difficult. The use of phenytoin for prophylactic therapy appears unwarranted (Chapter 8).

ADMINISTRATION

Dilantin is available in many forms, including 50-mg chewable tablets, 30-, 100-, 200-, and 300-mg extended-release capsules, 25- and 125-mg/5 ml oral suspension, and 50-mg/ml injection solution. Generic preparations differ in bioavailability (Chapter 14).

The recommended daily dose for phenytoin is 200–400 mg for adults and 5–10 mg/kg for children, divided into two portions. Treatment can begin at half the daily dose and gradually be increased over two to four weeks, but a loading dose of one-and-a-half times the daily dose can be administered when necessary (Chapter 14). The therapeutic range is 10–20 μg/ml. A paradoxical increase in seizures may occur at serum concentrations above 40 μg/ml (Chapter 14). The use of intravenous phenytoin for the treatment of status epilepticus is discussed in Chapter 10.

Primidone (PRM)

Primidone is a *deoxybarbiturate* in which the carbonyl oxygen of the urea moiety of phenobarbital has been replaced by two hydrogen atoms. It is chemically known as *5-ethyldi hydro-5-phenyl-4,6(1H,5H)-pyrimidinedione* (Bourgeois, 2008a; Michelucci et al., 2009). Primidone has been marketed in the United States under the trade name *Mysoline* since 1954. It is sold elsewhere under a variety of trade names, including *Majsolin, Mylepsinum,* and *Prysolin.* Other generic names for primidone include *hexamidine, primaclone,* and *desoxyphenobarbital.*

MECHANISMS OF ACTION

It is uncertain whether the antiseizure action of primidone is attributable solely to its metabolism to phenobarbital or whether primidone itself and its other major metabolite, *phenylethylmalonamide (PEMA)*, also account for its antiseizure effect (Bourgeois, 2008a). Primidone may account for only 11% and PEMA for only 2% of the total antiseizure effect (Frey, 1985). The sites of antiseizure action of primidone and PEMA are unknown. Because of the relatively short half-lives of these compounds, which lead to considerable fluctuation in plasma levels, for practical purposes primidone can be considered a phenobarbital prodrug unless the primidone-to-phenobarbital serum ratio remains high.

PHARMACOKINETICS

Primidone is almost completely absorbed after oral administration and reaches a peak concentration in the serum within two to four hours. Vd is 0.5–0.8 l/kg, and protein binding is 10%.

Plasma half-life of primidone averages 12 hours but is quite variable. Approximately 60% of the drug is metabolized in the liver to phenobarbital and PEMA, and the remainder is excreted unchanged in the urine. PEMA has a half-life of approximately 16 hours. Primidone and PEMA are less protein bound than phenobarbital, but brain-to-plasma ratios are less than for phenobarbital (Frey, 1985).

TOXICITY

Dose-related side effects of primidone are similar to those of phenobarbital but are more likely to include vertigo, dizziness, nausea, vomiting, ataxia, and diplopia. It is unclear to what extent the parent drug or its metabolites contribute to creating these side effects, particularly since tolerance develops as *phenobarbital* reaches a steady state. Idiosyncratic, allergic, and chronic side effects are also similar to those of phenobarbital, but higher incidences of personality change and acute psychotic reactions have been reported with primidone (Laxer et al., 1980). Primidone is classified by the FDA as a category D risk for teratogenicity.

DRUG INTERACTIONS

Drug interactions are the same as those for phenobarbital except in instances where other medications influence the pharmacokinetics of primidone itself. *Acetazolamide* may reduce absorption of primidone. *Carbamazepine* and *phenytoin* have been reported to increase the conversion of primidone to phenobarbital, while *isoniazid* decreases it (Frey, 1985).

INDICATIONS

Primidone is effective against generalized tonic-clonic and focal seizures but is tolerated less well than other first-line antiseizure drugs because of its unpleasant side effects (Mattson et al., 1985). It is useful in some patients as an adjunctive medication or when given alone because other drugs cannot be tolerated. It is inappropriate to use primidone and phenobarbital together because primidone is metabolized to phenobarbital. If primidone is prescribed because it is believed to be effective apart from its phenobarbital metabolite, then it should not be given with enzyme-inducing drugs like phenytoin and carbamazepine, which

lower the primidone-phenobarbital serum ratio (Bourgeois, 2008a).

As with phenobarbital, the sedative and other behavioral side effects of primidone may develop insidiously and not be fully appreciated. Disturbances in psychosocial adaptation that may be attributed to seizures or taken for granted, particularly in children, are often reversed by replacing primidone with another medication.

ADMINISTRATION

Mysoline comes in 50- and 250-mg tablets and in a suspension of 250 mg/5 ml for oral administration only. Generic preparations differ in bioavailability (Chapter 14). The usual maintenance dose is 750–1,500 mg per day for adults and children, divided into four portions. Dosing and dose schedules are determined by monitoring serum levels of both primidone and phenobarbital. The therapeutic range for the former is 3–12 µg/kg. Treatment with primidone is usually instituted with 125 mg in adults and 5 mg/kg in children and increased gradually to minimize unpleasant side effects.

Ethosuximide (ESM)

The succinimides were introduced specifically for the treatment of absence seizures. *Phensuximide* appeared first, followed by *methsuximide* and finally by *ethosuximide*, which has proven the most effective. Phensuximide and methsuximide are discussed in the section on Special and Rarely Used Drugs.

The chemical name for ethosuximide is α-*ethyl*-α-*methylsuccinimide*; 3-*ethyl*-3-*methylpyrrolidone*-2,5-*dione* is also used (Bromfield, 2008; Glauser and Perucca, 2009). It has been marketed in the United States under the trade name *Zarontin* since 1960. The drug is sold under this name in many other countries but also has other names, including *Suxinutin* and *Zartalin*. Generic preparations are available.

MECHANISMS OF ACTION

Ethosuximide is effective against *PTZ seizures* as well as other experimental models of human absence epilepsy, including the *generalized feline penicillin* model, the *γ-hydroxybutyrate model*, and the *intracerebroventricular enkephalin model* (Chapter 4), but it is generally ineffective against *MES* and *kindling models* of generalized tonic-clonic and focal seizures (Teschendorf and Kretzschmar, 1985). Ethosuximide is presumed to block low-threshold Ca^{2+} channels in the thalamus responsible for mediating the characteristic 3-Hz spike-and-wave discharge of absence seizures (Coulter et al., 1989) (Chapter 4). Catecholamines may be involved in the activity of ethosuximide; the anticonvulsant effect of this drug in some cases may depend on intact dopaminergic function (Ferrendelli and Klunk, 1982); dopaminergic mechanisms have been postulated in some forms of human generalized epilepsy (Quesney and Reader, 1984); and ethosuximide is effective against seizures in the *tottering mouse model* (Heller et al., 1983), which may be due to the result of abnormally increased norepinephrine (Noebels, 1986).

PHARMACOKINETICS

Ethosuximide is completely absorbed after oral administration and reaches peak concentration in the plasma within one to five hours. It is evenly distributed in all tissues except fat, Vd is 0.7 l/kg, it is less than 10% protein bound, and it achieves a concentration in the *cerebrospinal fluid (CSF)* that is similar to that in plasma. Seventy percent to 90% of ethosuximide is metabolized in the liver to inactive hydroxylated products, primarily by *CYP3A*, and the remainder is predominantly excreted in the urine. Half-life is 25–70 hours.

TOXICITY

Ethosuximide is notable for its relatively low toxicity. Dose-related gastrointestinal and central nervous system (CNS) symptoms are similar to those induced by other antiseizure drugs but include photophobia. Patients usually develop tolerance to these effects. Behavioral symptoms, such as paranoid psychosis, depression, sleep disturbances, night terrors, inability to concentrate, and aggressiveness, are rare and usually limited to patients with a history of psychiatric problems. Idiosyncratic and allergic reactions can involve the skin and hemopoietic system, and fatal bone marrow depressions have occurred. With this drug, unlike the other succinimides, serious hepatic and renal toxicity have not been reported. The FDA has classified the teratogenic potential of ethosuximide as category C (some animal studies show adverse effects, there are no available data in humans).

DRUG INTERACTIONS

Although ethosuximide serum levels can be affected by enzyme-inducing and enzyme-inhibiting drugs, it is uncommon for it to be involved in clinically significant drug interactions. In theory, however, drugs that increase or decrease catecholamine activity could potentiate or depress ethosuximide potency (Strickler et al., 1985).

INDICATIONS

Ethosuximide is a first-line drug when only absence seizures occur, because of its potent action against these ictal events and its relatively low risk of serious toxic side effects. When used alone in patients with mixed seizures, there is some evidence that ethosuximide may exacerbate generalized tonic-clonic seizures.

ADMINISTRATION

Zarontin is available as 250-mg capsules and 250-mg/5 ml syrup for oral administration. The manufacturer advises that the syrup be protected from freezing and light. The recommended daily dose of ethosuximide is 500–1,500 mg, or 20–30 mg/kg in children under the age of 6 divided into two or three portions, to achieve a therapeutic range of 40–100 μg/ml. Adverse dose-related side effects are best avoided when the dose is initially 250 mg and is increased by 250 mg every four to seven days or, in children under the age of 6, is initially 5–10 mg/kg, and is increased by that amount every five to seven days until seizure control is achieved.

Benzodiazepines

As a class, the benzodiazepines are used clinically for their sedative-hypnotic, muscle relaxant, and anxiolytic, as well as antiseizure, properties. Some benzodiazepine analogs, such as β-*carboline*, act as *inverse agonists* and cause seizures (Morin, 1984; Schmidt and Wilensky, 2008; Camfield and Camfield, 2008). The antiseizure benzodiazepines are the most potent drugs against PTZ-induced seizures but are also effective against MES and most other experimental models of epilepsy. Their antiseizure properties are due primarily to suppression of the spread of ictal discharge. Intensive research has been carried out on the action of these drugs on *benzodiazepine receptors* associated with the GABA$_A$ receptor–chloride ionophore complex (Olsen, 1982; Macdonald, 2002; Macdonald and Mody, 2008) (Chapter 3). More than facilitation of GABA$_A$-mediated inhibition appears to be necessary to explain all the antiseizure properties of benzodiazepines. Furthermore, it is not entirely clear what pharmacodynamic mechanisms differentiate antiseizure properties from sedative and anxiolytic effects as well as convulsant effects of benzodiazepines (Trimble and Thompson, 1983; Macdonald and Mody, 2008) (Chapters 3 and 4).

Clobazam, clonazepam, clorazepate, and nitrazepam are used for the chronic treatment of epilepsy. *Diazepam, lorazepam*, and *midazolam* are principal drugs for the treatment of status epilepticus (Chapter 10). Clorazepate, midazolam, and nitrazepam are discussed later in the section on Special and Rarely Used Drugs.

DIAZEPAM (DZP)

The chemical name for *diazepam* is *7-chloro-1,3-dihydro-1-methyl-5-phenyl-2H1,4-benzodiazepine-2-one*. It is marketed in the United States under the trade name *Valium* and was approved for treatment of epilepsy in 1968. Outside the United States the drug is sold as Valium but also under many other names. Generic formulations are available.

Diazepam is classified as a long-acting benzodiazepine. It is completely absorbed after oral administration, reaching peak plasma concentrations in 0.5 to 3 hours. Absorption after intramuscular injection is slow and erratic, but there is good absorption from the rectum (Wilder and Bruni, 1981). Ninety percent to 95% of the drug is bound to plasma proteins. The Vd is 1–2 l/kg, with initial accumulation in brain but later accumulation in adipose tissue. Diazepam is metabolized in the liver, primarily by *CYP2C19* to its active metabolite *nordiazepam*, which is also metabolized by the same enzyme. The half-life of diazepam is represented as a biphasic decay curve, the first phase reflecting distribution and the second elimination. Following oral administration, the first phase is 2–10 hours, and the second phase 27–48 hours. With chronic administration, plasma concentrations of diazepam and nordiazepam are essentially equal. Although nordiazepam may achieve stable therapeutic plasma levels, there are superimposed peaks of diazepam that produce disturbing side effects. Diazepam, therefore, is not an effective oral agent for the treatment of chronic epilepsy; however, this drug has a major role in the treatment of status epilepticus (Chapter 10).

Valium is available as 2-, 5-, and 10-mg tablets, 5-mg/5 ml liquid and emulsion for injection, 10-mg rectal suppositories, and various gel preparations for rectal administration, including preloaded syringes (*Diastat*). Buccal and nasal preparations are under investigation. Administration of diazepam for the treatment of status epilepticus is discussed in Chapter 10.

CLONAZEPAM (CLN)

The chemical name for *clonazepam* is *5-(2-chlorophenyl)-1,3-dihydro-7-nitro-2H1, 4-benzodiazepine-2-one* (Schmidt and Wilensky, 2008; Camfield and Camfield, 2008). It has been approved for treatment of epilepsy in the United States since 1975 and is marketed under the trade name *Klonopin*. Names in other countries include *Rivotril*, *Ravotril*, and *Iktoril*. Generic formulations of clonazepam are available.

Clonazepam is rapidly absorbed, reaching peak plasma concentration within one to two hours. It is 80% protein bound but readily distributed in all body tissues. Vd is 1.5–4.4 1/kg. Clonazepam is classified as an intermediate-acting benzodiazepine with a half-life of 24–48 hours. It is 95% metabolized in the liver by *CYP3A4* and has no known active metabolites (Caccia and Garattini, 1985).

The major dose-related side effects of clonazepam are sedation, muscular incoordination, and ataxia. Tolerance to these symptoms can develop with chronic administration. Behavioral disturbances also occur, most often in children and the elderly. They commonly appear as hyperactivity in the former and depression or difficulty concentrating in the latter. Hypotonia, dysarthria, dizziness, anorexia, hyperphagia, and increased bronchial and salivary secretions can be seen. The last can result in troublesome drooling. Hematological, hepatic, and renal toxicity are relatively rare. Because animal studies have suggested that the benzodiazepines exert some anticholinergic effects, the FDA has required manufacturers to cite acute narrow-angle glaucoma as a contraindication to use of these agents. There are, however, no clinical reports of problems with the use of benzodiazepines in patients being treated for glaucoma. Clonazepam is classified as teratogenic risk factor D by the FDA.

Clonazepam may potentiate the sedative action of other hypnotic-sedative drugs such as *ethanol* and *barbiturates* as well as *antihistaminics*, *tricyclic antidepressants*, *phenothiazines*, and *analgesics*. Coadministration of *valproic acid* and clonazepam can result in absence status (Jeavons et al., 1977). Clonazepam plasma levels may be reduced by *phenobarbital* and *phenytoin*.

Clonazepam is a first-line drug for myoclonic seizures and is generally preferred for non-epileptic myoclonic phenomena. It is used as a second-line drug for absence seizures and because of its relatively broad spectrum of action may be useful in mixed seizure disorders. However, tolerance to antiseizure effects develops in approximately one-third of patients on clonazepam within three months of initiation of treatment and is a major problem with its use. Clonazepam must be withdrawn slowly, because withdrawal seizures can occur.

Klonopin is available as 0.5-, 1-, and 2-mg tablets and 0.125-, 0.25-, 0.5-, 1-, and 2-mg disintegrating wafers. The usual daily dose is 0.1–0.2 mg/kg in children and 4–10 mg in adolescents and adults, given in two equal portions. Initiation of treatment should be gradual, so that drowsiness will be minimized. The initial recommended dose is 1.5 mg per day for adults and 0.01–0.02 mg/kg per day for children, with increases of 0.5–1 mg per day in adults and 0.01–0.02 mg/kg per day in children every three to seven days. The therapeutic range of plasma concentration for clonazepam has not been well studied. It is usually given as 0.01–0.07 µg/ml but is probably higher and is not a clinically useful measure except for monitoring compliance.

LORAZEPAM (LZP)

The chemical name for *lorazepam* is *7-chloro-5-(o-chlorophenyl)-1,3-dihydro-3-hydroxy-2H-1,4-benzodiazepine-2-one*. It is marketed in the United States under the trade name *Ativan* as a sedative and anxiolytic agent. Generic preparations are available. Because lorazepam is not rapidly redistributed, it has a much longer duration of action than *diazepam*, but it is actually classified as a short-acting benzodiazepine with a half-life of approximately 24 hours. Unlike diazepam, lorazepam is converted in the liver by glucuronidation to inactive metabolites.

Because of a high incidence of behavioral side effects, lorazepam is difficult to administer in sufficiently high doses to treat chronic epilepsy. However, it is the first choice of most epileptologists for the treatment of status epilepticus (Chapter 10). Ativan is available as 0.5-, 1-, and 2-mg tablets and at strengths of 2 and 4 mg/ml in sterile solutions for injection. The use of lorazepam in the treatment of status epilepticus is discussed in Chapter 10.

CLOBAZAM (CLB)

The chemical name for *clobazam* is *7-chloro-1-methyl-5-phenyl-1,5-benzodiazepine-2,4-dione* (Schmidt and Wilensky, 2008; Camfield and Camfield, 2008). It has been approved for treatment in Europe under the trade name *Frisium* since 1975 but has only recently become available in the United States, under the trade name *Onfi*. Generic formulations of clobazam are available.

Clobazam is rapidly absorbed, reaching peak plasma levels within 0.5 to 2 hours. It is 85% protein bound but readily distributed in all body tissues. Vd is 0.9–1.8 l/kg. Clobazam is metabolized in the liver by desmethylation primarily to *N-desmethylclobazam*, which is pharmacologically active. Elimination half-life for clobazam in adults is 10–30 hours, and that for *N-desmethylclobazam*, which contributes importantly to efficacy, is 36–46 hours.

Adverse effects and drug interactions of clobazam are similar to those of *clonazepam*, but this drug may be better tolerated than other benzodiazepines. Side effects are also due to its active metabolite.

Clobazam is used alone or as adjunctive therapy for focal and generalized tonic-clonic seizures but has also been useful for *catamenial*

epilepsy, *startle epilepsy*, alcohol withdrawal seizures, and the *Lennox-Gastaut syndrome (LGS)*. Tolerance occurs in one-third to one-half of patients on clobazam. As with other benzodiazepines, clobazam must be withdrawn slowly, because withdrawal seizures can occur and sudden termination can result in status epilepticus.

Onfi is available as 5-, 10-, and 20-mg tablets. The usual daily dose, given in two equal portions, is 0.4–0.8 mg/kg for children under 30 kg and 20–40 mg for children over 30 kg and adults. Initial recommended treatment for children under 30 kg is 0.1–0.2 mg/kg per day, doubled after the first week and again after the second. Over 30 kg, the initial recommended dose is 10 mg per day increased to 20 mg per day in one week and 40 mg per day in two weeks. The therapeutic range of plasma concentration for clobazam is 0.03–0.3 μg/ml and is the same for *N*-desmethylclobazam; however, these values are not clinically useful except for monitoring compliance.

Carbamazepine (CBZ)

Carbamazepine is an *iminostilbene derivative* related chemically to the *tricyclic antidepressants*. Its chemical name is *5H-dibenz[b,f]azepine-5-carboxamide* or *5-carbamoyl-5H-dibenz[b,f]azepine* (Fertig and Mattson, 2008; Sillanpää et al., 2009). The drug was synthesized in the late 1950s, its anticonvulsant properties were recognized shortly afterward (Theobald and Kunz, 1963), and it was approved as an antiseizure drug in Europe in 1965. However, it was initially used in the United States for other purposes and was not approved for treatment of epilepsy until 1974. Carbamazepine is marketed under the trade name *Tegretol* in most countries of the world and remains one of the most important antiseizure agents (Fertig and Mattson, 2008; Sillanpää et al., 2009). *Carbatrol* is a brand name extended-release capsule. Many generic preparations are available.

MECHANISMS OF ACTION

Carbamazepine has a spectrum of action in the animal laboratory similar to that of phenytoin, although it may be more effective than phenytoin against amygdala-kindled seizures (Albright, 1983). Carbamazepine is considered to have a membrane-stabilizing effect due to influences on ionic conductances, as described earlier for *phenytoin* (McLean and Macdonald, 1986). In addition, however, carbamazepine may act as an adenosine receptor agonist (Skerritt et al., 1983) and may also increase the firing rate of noradrenergic locus coeruleus neurons (Olpe and Jones, 1983). Adenosine is postulated to play a role in suppressing seizure spread and terminating seizures, whereas noradrenergic systems seem to decrease epileptogenicity (Chapters 3 and 4). Sporadic reports have suggested that carbamazepine alters the activities of other neurotransmitters, but it is difficult to differentiate drug effects from the effects of seizure control. As with phenytoin, carbamazepine undoubtedly has numerous mechanisms of action, many of which have yet to be elucidated (Schmutz, 1985).

PHARMACOKINETICS

Carbamazepine is slowly absorbed after oral administration, and times of peak concentration in plasma vary considerably from individual to individual. The peak time is usually four to eight hours but may be as long as 24 hours. The drug is rapidly and uniformly distributed in all body tissues and is 75% protein bound. Vd is 0.8–2 1/kg. Pharmacokinetics is nonlinear because of autoinduction.

Less than 5% of carbamazepine is excreted unchanged in the urine, most being metabolized by four main pathways (Schmutz, 1985), primarily by CYP3A4. The most important metabolite is the *10,11-epoxide*, which also possesses antiseizure properties. The half-life of carbamazepine is greatly influenced by drugs that induce liver enzymes. Because it is itself an enzyme inducer, its own half-life is shortened by chronic administration. The average half-life is 10–20 hours on chronic therapy, but it is much longer after a single dose of the drug and may be even shorter after long-term treatment or when given in combination with *phenobarbital*, phenytoin, or enzyme inducers. The half-life of the epoxide is shorter than that of carbamazepine, and plasma concentrations of the latter are usually used for determining dosing regimens.

TOXICITY

The common dose-related side effects of carbamazepine are similar to those of phenytoin, although gastrointestinal disturbances are somewhat more prominent. Taking the drug with meals can reduced these bothersome symptoms. Tolerance to dose-related side effects develops, and patients can generally be coaxed to therapeutic doses of carbamazepine by beginning gradually, with small divided doses at mealtimes, and backing down temporarily when unwanted symptoms occur. This drug has fewer sedative effects than phenytoin, *primidone*, and phenobarbital. Therefore, cognitive function generally improves when carbamazepine is substituted for these other antiseizure drugs (Trimble and Robertson, 1986). All of the common allergic and idiosyncratic toxic effects have been seen with carbamazepine. Original reports of increased incidence of aplastic anemia and agranulocytosis when carbamazepine is compared with other antiseizure drugs have not been substantiated (Chapter 14). Persistent leukopenia is common with chronic carbamazepine administration but is usually of no clinical concern (Chapter 14). The risk of toxic *epidermal necrolysis* and *Stevens-Johnson syndrome* is significantly increased in Han Chinese with the *HLA-B*1502* allele (Chung et al., 2004; Chen et al., 2011), and there may be similar genetic markers for persons of Northern European ancestry (McCormack et al., 2011). Carbamazepine augments the effect of antidiuretic hormone, resulting in water retention. For this reason it has been used for treatment against diabetes insipidus but is not recommended in patients at risk for congestive heart failure. Although recent data from prospective registries suggest a relatively low teratogenic potential for carbamazepine and a risk of major congenital malformations on monotherapy of 2–3% (Tomson et al., 2007), the FDA classifies it as risk category D.

DRUG INTERACTIONS

Plasma levels of carbamazepine are decreased by enzyme-inducing drugs such as phenobarbital and phenytoin and increased by a variety of medications, most notably *propoxyphene* and *erythromycin*. Carbamazepine competes with *valproic acid* and phenytoin for protein-binding sites, resulting in increased free but decreased total plasma levels of these drugs. Valproic acid also inhibits metabolism of the 10,11-epoxide, increasing the serum level of this active metabolite. The conversion of primidone to phenobarbital is enhanced by carbamazepine.

INDICATIONS

Carbamazepine has been a first-line drug for most patients with focal seizures, with or without secondarily generalized tonic-clonic seizures. It is particularly preferred over phenytoin in patients for whom cosmetic side effects should be avoided. Because carbamazepine is reported to have psychotropic effects in bipolar affective illness, benefiting the hypomanic more than the depressive phase (Post et al., 1984) (Chapter 11), it is at least theoretically appropriate for patients with epilepsy who have interictal affective symptoms. Carbamazepine is not effective against absence, myoclonic, and atonic seizures or epileptic spasms and can make these seizures worse. For this reason, it is not appropriate in children with LGS, *West syndrome,* or other conditions where these seizure types occur. The drug is not recommended for patients who are at risk for congestive heart failure, have a history of previous bone marrow depression, or are taking *monoamine oxidase inhibitors*.

ADMINISTRATION

Carbamazepine is available as Tegretol in 200- mg tablets, 100-mg chewable tablets, and a 100-mg/5 ml suspension. Generic preparations differ in bioavailability (Chapter 14). Slow-release preparations of carbamazepine are also available as Tegretol XR tablets (100, 200, and 400 mg) and Carbatrol XR capsules (100, 200 and 300 mg). Maintenance dose is 800–1,200 mg per day in adults, 400–800 mg per day in children over the age of 6, and less than 35 mg/kg per day in children below the age of 6. Treatment is initiated with 200–400 mg per day in adolescents and adults and 10–20 mg/kg per day in children under the age of 6 and is increased by half this amount at weekly intervals. Doses are divided three or four times a day for regular carbamazepine and twice a day for extended-release tablets and capsules. Therapeutic range is generally given as 8–12 μg/ml, although patients with temporal lobe epilepsy may benefit from higher plasma concentrations (Schmidt et al., 1986). The drug should be given with meals to minimize gastrointestinal side effects. Success with carbamazepine often depends on the patient's ability to tolerate dosing increments. It is no longer considered necessary to monitor hematological functions more frequently than for other antiseizure drugs (Chapter 14). Although white blood cell counts may fall below 4,000/mm (Bartholini et al., 1985), this is not an absolute reason to discontinue therapy unless the neutrophil count drops below 1,000/mm (Bartholini et al., 1985). Carbamazepine potency is reduced by 50% in humid conditions, and the drug should be stored in a cool, dry place. Individually foil-wrapped tablets are available in some tropical countries where storage is difficult.

Valproic acid (VPA)

Valproic acid is a simple branched-chain carboxylic acid known as *di-n-propylacetic acid,* *2-propylpentanoic acid,* and *2-propylvaleric acid* among other names. It was first synthesized at the end of the 19th century, and its antiseizure properties were discovered in the early 1960s (Meunier et al., 1963; Carraz et al., 1964). Sodium valproic acid was an important antiseizure drug in Europe for over a decade before it was approved for use in the United States in 1978. Since that date valproic acid and sodium valproate have been marketed in the United States under the trade name *Depakene.* Forms of this drug are sold in other countries under this name and variations of this name as well as others, including *Epilim* and *Ergenyl*. The enteric-coated tablet, *Depakote*, consisting of a stable 1:1 molar compound of the acid and the sodium salt (*divalproex sodium*), is now more commonly used than Depakene (Beydoun et al., 2008b; Bourgeois, 2008b; 2009). Generic formulations are available.

MECHANISMS OF ACTION

Valproic acid has a broad spectrum of action, being particularly effective against generalized tonic-clonic, absence, and myoclonic seizures and less effective against focal seizures. Valproic acid increases GABA concentrations in the brain, which is believed to account for at least part of its antiseizure action. This effect is not sufficient, however, to explain the antiseizure effect that lags behind and outlasts measured increases and decreases in GABA levels (Chapman et al., 1982). Valproic acid is believed to enhance GABA concentrations in axon terminals by interfering with GABA metabolism, but the exact mechanism is unknown (Löscher, 1985). Evidence that valproic acid enhances GABA synthesis is controversial. Several other mechanisms of action for valproic acid have been suggested, including (1) inhibition of formation of the epileptogenic GABA metabolite γ-*hydroxybutyrate* (Chapter 4), (2) alteration of presynaptic release, postsynaptic receptor binding, reuptake of GABA, or some combination, (3) direct agonist effects on postsynaptic GABA receptors, (4) blockade of T-type Ca^{2+} currents in the thalamus responsible for 3-Hz spike-and-wave generation, and (5) other non-GABA mechanisms including effects on glycine, aspartate, biogenic amines, cyclic nucleotides, Na^+ channels, and Ca^{2+}-dependent K^+ currents (Löscher, 1985; Beydoun et al., 2008b; Bourgeois, 2008b; 2009).

PHARMACOKINETICS

Valproic acid is rapidly absorbed after oral administration. Plasma concentrations reach peak levels within one to four hours with regular tablets and several hours later with enteric-coated tablets. Absorption decreases with increasing pH (Levy et al., 1980). *Probenecid-sensitive* transport of valproic acid from intestine to blood is suspected (Löscher, 1985). The Vd is between 0.1 and 0.4 l/kg.

Valproic acid is 70–90% protein bound in plasma, and brain concentrations equilibrate with free drug levels in the blood. There is evidence for carrier-mediated active transport of valproic acid into brain tissue (Löscher, 1985; Levy et al., 2002). Pharmacokinetics is nonlinear due to saturable protein binding.

Over 95% of valproic acid is metabolized in the liver by complex mechanisms involving many CYP isoenzymes, glucuronidation, and other processes. Its half-life ranges from 8 to 16 hours but in the same individual does not appear to be affected by chronic administration. Several metabolites of valproic acid also have antiseizure activity. Some of these appear to enter the brain and may account for the persistence of the antiseizure effect after valproic acid has disappeared from the blood.

TOXICITY

Dose-related gastrointestinal side effects of valproic acid, including anorexia, nausea, and vomiting, occur in about 16% of patients (Rall and Schleifer, 1985). Dose-related CNS side effects, such as sedation and ataxia, are uncommon compared with those of most other antiseizure drugs, but tremor is more common. Valproic acid presents no unusual risk for most idiosyncratic and allergic toxic reactions but is more likely to produce alopecia and appetite stimulation than other antiseizure drugs. Alopecia can respond to zinc and selenium replacement. Weight gain is a particular problem and a major reason for discontinuation. The occurrence of fatal hepatotoxicity with valproic acid has created some fear regarding the use of this drug. Such concern seems justified only in children under 10 years of age, particularly those under the age of 2 on polytherapy, in whom the risk may be as high as 1 in 500 (Dreifuss et al., 1987) (Chapter 14). A valproic acid–induced encephalopathy can occur with hyperammonemia, without evidence of hepatic dysfunction (Zaret et al., 1982). Valproic acid inhibits the second phase of platelet aggregation, and its administration increases the risk of cerebral hemorrhage with closed head intracranial procedures such as depth electrode implantation (Chapter 16). The incidence of *polycystic ovary syndrome* is higher in women with epilepsy than in the general population, and this effect may be exacerbated by valproic acid (Sabers and Harden, 2008). Valproic acid is associated with a greater risk of cognitive impairment and serious teratogenicity, particularly neural tube defects, in offspring of treated mothers than other antiseizure drugs and should be avoided, if possible, in women of childbearing age (Meador et al., 2009) (Chapter 14). FDA has classified valproic acid as risk category D.

DRUG INTERACTIONS

Valproic acid does not appear to have enzyme-inducing effects. Free valproic acid levels in plasma are increased by drugs that compete for protein-binding sites such as *phenytoin, carbamazepine, salicylates,* and *phenylbutazone,* whereas valproic acid inhibits *cytochrome P450, glucuronyl transferase,* and *epoxide hydrolase* systems, increasing levels of coadministered drugs that utilize these forms of hepatic metabolism. Plasma levels of *phenobarbital* are commonly, and often markedly, elevated when valproic acid is added to a regimen of barbiturates or *primidone.* CNS depression has been reported with this drug combination in the absence of elevated phenobarbital plasma levels. Valproic acid also greatly prolongs the half-life of *lamotrigine,* requiring a lower initial dose and a slower titration of lamotrigine when this drug is added to a regimen of valproic acid, as well as an increased lamotrigine dose when valproic acid is withdrawn from combination therapy with this drug. Valproic acid can also increase serum levels of *ethosuximide, rufinamide, felbamate,* and the *10,11-epoxide* of *carbamazepine,* as well as *tricyclic antidepressants, zidovudine,* and *nimodipine.* Valproic acid inhibits metabolism of phenytoin but also competes with it for protein binding. There is some evidence for pharmacodynamic synergy between valproic acid and both lamotrigine and ethosuximide. Coadministration of valproic acid and *clonazepam* is infrequently associated with the development of absence status epilepticus (Jeavons et al., 1977). Valproic acid interferes with the measurement of ketone bodies and prevents quantitative monitoring of children on the *ketogenic diet* (Chapter 16).

INDICATIONS

Valproic acid remains the most effective drug for mixed seizure disorders, because of its broad spectrum of action, and for *juvenile myoclonic*

epilepsy (Marson et al., 2007b) (Chapters 7 and 14). However, its teratogenic risk is problematic in women of childbearing age, and the risk of hepatotoxicity has dampened enthusiasm for its use in infants and young children.

ADMINISTRATION

A variety of preparations of Depakene and Depakote are available in the United States as enteric-coated tablets, crushable tablets, sustained-release tablets, sprinkles, solution, syrup, and sterile solution for injection. The most commonly used Depakote delayed-release capsules come in 125 mg; delayed-release tablets in 125, 250, and 500 mg; and extended-release tablets in 250- and 500-mg strengths. The usual daily dose is 1,000–2,500 mg in adults and 20–40 mg/kg in children, given in three equal portions to achieve a plasma drug concentration of 50–100 μg/ml. The extended-release formulation, Depakote ER, is intended to be used once or twice daily. Treatment is usually begun with 500 mg twice a day in adults and 15 mg/kg twice a day in children and is increased by 500 mg or 15 mg per day, respectively, at five- to seven-day intervals. Antiseizure effects often lag behind achievement of steady-state plasma drug levels (Bourgeois et al., 1987) and persist after levels have disappeared from the blood (Lockard and Levy, 1976). Side effects are less likely when therapy is begun gradually. Gastrointestinal side effects may be less problematic with use of Depakote than with Depakene.

NEWER DRUGS

Eslicarbazepine Acetate (ESL)

Eslicarbazepine acetate was designed to be structurally similar to carbamazepine and oxcarbazepine but is metabolized differently, in that eslicarbazepine acetate is a prodrug of only eslicarbazepine, which is responsible for its pharmaceutical action (Almeida et al., 2009; Falcão et al., 2012). The chemical name is *(S)-10-acetoxy-10,11-dihydro-5H-dibenz[b,f] azepine-5-carboxamide*. It was authorized in Europe in 2009, where it is marketed under the trade names of *Zebenix* and *Exalief*, and has since been approved in the United States under the trade name *Stedesa*.

MECHANISMS OF ACTION

Eslicarbazepine is a use-dependent voltage-gated sodium channel blocker with a spectrum of action similar to that of carbamazepine.

PHARMACOKINETICS

Eslicarbazepine acetate has a peak time after oral administration of two to three hours, is 30% protein bound, and has a Vd 2.7 l/kg. The pharmacokinetics is linear. The drug is rapidly hydrolyzed in the liver to its pharmacologically active metabolite eslicarbazepine, also known as *S-licarbazepine*. Other pharmacologically active metabolites include R-licarbazepine and oxcarbazepine. Autoinduction does not occur. The half-life of the prodrug is less than two hours, but the half-life of the active metabolite is 20–24 hours. Eslicarbazepine is excreted in the urine, approximately two-thirds unchanged and two-thirds as a glucuronide conjugate, along with other metabolites of eslicarbazepine acetate.

TOXICITY

Eslicarbazepine acetate is usually well tolerated. Common dose-related adverse side effects include dizziness, blurred vision, diplopia, nausea and vomiting, fatigue, incoordination, headache, and somnolence. More serious side effects include increased PR interval, which may cause a heart block in at-risk patients, as well as rare allergic and idiosyncratic reactions. No data on teratogenicity are available.

DRUG INTERACTIONS

Although eslicarbazepine acetate and its metabolites do not utilize the P450 isoenzymes, they do have interactions with other drugs. *Carbamazepine* and *phenytoin* decrease eslicarbazepine plasma levels, while eslicarbazepine can increase plasma levels of phenytoin and decrease plasma levels of *lamotrigine*, *topiramate*, and *warfarin*.

INDICATIONS

Eslicarbazepine acetate is a narrow-spectrum drug approved for adjunctive therapy of focal seizures with or without secondarily generalized seizures in patients over the age of 16. Advantages over carbamazepine include that it is not metabolized to the more toxic epoxide, and advantages over oxcarbazepine as well as carbamazepine include that it does not have the same propensity to cause hyponatremia. It also does not cause autoinduction. A possibility of once-a-day dosing is another advantage.

ADMINISTRATION

Various brand name eslicarbazepine acetate compounds are available as 400- and 800-mg tablets and a 60-mg/ml suspension. Recommended adult dose is 800–1,200 mg per day, which can be given once daily. Treatment should begin with 400 mg daily for one to two weeks, then increased by 400 mg per day at biweekly intervals to a maximum dose of 1,200 mg per day. The therapeutic range has not been established.

Ezogabine (EZG)

Ezogabine, also known as *retigabine (RTG)*, is *N-[2-amino-4-(4-fluorobenzylamino)-phenyl] carbamic acid ethyl ester* and is the first antiseizure drug to exert its effect on K$^+$ channels (Brodie et al., 2010). It was approved in 2011 for marketing in the United States under the trade name *Potiga* and in the United Kingdom as *Trobalt* (French et al., 2011).

MECHANISMS OF ACTION

Ezogabine's novel mechanism of action stabilizes a group of voltage-gated K$^+$ channels in open conformation. The *Kv7.2* and *Kv7.3* channels, corresponding to genes *KCNQ2* and *KCNQ3*, give rise to the M-current, important for regulating subthreshold neuronal firing. Ezogabine attenuates neuronal hyperexcitability by enhancing the M-current, which appears to be an important target for treating epileptic seizures.

PHARMACOKINETICS

Ezogabine is rapidly absorbed, with peak plasma concentration achieved within one to two hours. Vd is 2–3 l/kg, and protein binding is less than 80%. It is metabolized in the liver by glucuronidation to form two inactive *n-glucuronide* metabolites, as well as by acetylation, and these processes do not involve cytochrome P450 isoenzymes. Elimination half-life is approximately 7–11 hours.

TOXICITY

Ezogabine is well tolerated, the most common dose-related side effects being dizziness, headache, somnolence, tremor, fatigue, cognitive disturbances, and insomnia. Urinary retention is also reported in some patients. The complete adverse effects profile has yet to be determined.

DRUG INTERACTIONS

Ezogabine does not alter the pharmacokinetics of *carbamazepine, phenytoin, valproic acid*, or *topiramate*; however, carbamazepine and phenytoin increase ezogabine clearance by 40%, resulting in reduced plasma levels.

INDICATIONS

Ezogabine is approved for adjunctive treatment of focal seizures in adults. Effectiveness against other seizure types and epilepsy syndromes has not yet been determined.

ADMINISTRATION

Potiga is available in strengths of 50, 200, 300, 400 mg. Maintenance dose is 300–600 mg per day in three divided doses. Potiga can be initiated with a dose of 100 mg three times a day and increased by 50 mg three times a day at weekly intervals. Therapeutic range has not yet been established.

Felbamate (FBM)

Felbamate is chemically related to the antianxiety drug *meprobamate* and its chemical name is *2-phenyl-1,3-propanediol dicarbamate* (Leppik and White, 2009; Theodore, 2008). Initially synthesized in 1954, its antiseizure potential was identified by the Antiepileptic Drug Development program of the National Institutes of Health in the 1980s, and it was approved for adjunctive and monotherapy of focal seizures in adults and as adjunctive therapy for children with LGS under the trade name *Felbatol* in 1993. Although the drug was highly effective, postmarketing surveillance revealed an unacceptably high rate of aplastic anemia and hepatic failure, which has now relegated felbamate to use as a drug of last resort in patients with the most serious forms of epilepsy who are not surgical candidates. Felbamate is also sold under the names *Felbamyl* and *Taloxa*.

MECHANISMS OF ACTION

Felbamate most likely has multiple mechanisms of action, none of which have been definitively demonstrated. One most likely effect, demonstrated in mice, is action on a high-affinity glycine site on the *N-methyl-D-aspartate (NMDA)* receptor to antagonize intracellular Ca^{2+} currents (White et al., 1992; Kuo et al., 2004). Felbamate also appears to potentiate $GABA_A$-mediated inhibition at a novel receptor site (Ticku et al., 1991; Rho et al., 1994).

PHARMACOKINETICS

Felbamate is rapidly absorbed after oral administration and peak plasma concentration is obtained within one to six hours. It is distributed to a number of tissues, including the brain, and is 20–25% protein bound. Vd is approximately 0.8 l/kg. Fifty percent of felbamate is metabolized in the liver by CYP3A4 and *CYP2E1* to form several metabolites that do not have antiseizure properties but some of which may be cytotoxic. The other 50% is excreted unchanged in the urine. The half-life of felbamate is 16–22 hours, and this can be substantially reduced by coadministration of enzyme-inducing drugs.

TOXICITY

Common dose-related adverse effects of felbamate include nausea, anorexia, insomnia, irritability, dizziness, somnolence, diplopia, and headache. Although felbamate was relatively well tolerated during clinical trials, postmarketing surveillance revealed an unacceptably high rate of aplastic anemia, more than 100 times that for the general population, with a 30–40% fatality rate (Leppik and White, 2009). Also observed was a rate of hepatic toxicity similar to that seen with valproic acid. Females are at a 67% greater risk than males for aplastic anemia, and a 78% greater risk for hepatotoxicity. Risk factors for aplastic anemia include a prior history of allergy to antiseizure drugs, a history of prior cytopenia, and evidence of an immune disease, especially lupus erythematosus. These serious adverse events usually have occurred within the first six months after treatment, but they can appear later, although none have been reported after 18 months of treatment. There are no human data regarding the teratogenic risk of felbamate, and it is classified by the FDA as risk category C.

DRUG INTERACTIONS

Felbamate plasma levels are decreased by enzyme-inducing drugs such as *carbamazepine*, *phenobarbital*, *phenytoin*, and *primidone*, and clearance is also increased by *gabapentin*. *Valproic acid* increases felbamate plasma levels. Felbamate can act as both an enzyme inducer and inhibitor, but most often it inhibits metabolism and can increase plasma levels of *carbamazepine-10,11-epoxide*, *N-desmethylclobazam*, *methsuximide*, phenytoin, phenobarbital, and *valproic acid*. Felbamate decreases plasma levels of *warfarin* and contraceptive steroids (Leppik and White, 2009).

INDICATIONS

Clinical trials of felbamate as an add-on medication and also with the use of low-dose valproic acid as an *active placebo* demonstrated its efficacy against dyscognitive focal seizures with or without secondarily generalized seizures, and it subsequently was found to be effective in children with LGS. Felbamate, therefore, was the first new drug to significantly reduce the frequency of atonic seizures, one of the most medically refractory seizure types. There is also evidence of its effectiveness against *myoclonic seizures* and *infantile spasms*. The use of felbamate, however, has been seriously compromised by the high incidence of life-threatening aplastic anemia and hepatotoxicity, and its use is now reserved for patients with severe medically refractory seizures who are not surgical candidates; informed consent is required at most institutions. Felbamate should not be prescribed in patients with a history of cytopenia, drug allergies, or immune disorders.

ADMINISTRATION

Felbatol is available as 400- and 600-mg tablets and 600-mg/5 ml syrup. The usual daily dosage is 45 mg/kg per day in children and 1200–3600 mg per day in adults. Treatment usually begins with 600 mg per day dose in two to four divided doses and is increased by this amount at 14 days intervals as monotherapy, or 1200 mg per day increased at weekly intervals as adjunctive therapy. The therapeutic range of plasma felbamate is 30–60 μg/ml, and serum level monitoring can be useful in some cases. Complete blood count and liver function tests at baseline, at one month after initiation of treatment, and then at three-month intervals are recommended; however, there is no evidence that such testing will detect toxic effects before symptoms occur. In any event, felbamate must be discontinued immediately if signs or symptoms of blood dyscrasia or hepatic toxicity appear.

Gabapentin (GBP)

Gabapentin is *1-aminomethyl-cyclohexyl-acetic acid* and was originally synthesized as a GABA-mimetic agent that could cross the blood-brain barrier. There is no evidence, however, that gabapentin exerts its antiseizure effect via GABAergic mechanisms. Gabapentin was approved as an antiseizure drug in 1993 under the trade name *Neurontin* (Chadwick and Browne, 2008; Somerville and Mitchell, 2009). Generic formulations of gabapentin are available.

MECHANISMS OF ACTION

Gabapentin does not act on $GABA_A$ or $GABA_B$ receptors, nor is it converted to GABA or a GABA agonist. Although there is some evidence that gabapentin increases GABA synthesis and inhibits GABA metabolism, it is unlikely this modest effect has any relevance to its antiseizure potency. Gabapentin does, however, have a unique binding site in neocortex and hippocampus, identified as the $\alpha_2\gamma$ subunit of the voltage-gated Ca^{2+} channel (Gee et al., 1996), and this is currently assumed to be its primary site of action.

PHARMACOKINETICS

Gabapentin is rapidly absorbed via a saturable transport system, *system L*, from gut to blood and also across the blood-brain barrier. Pharmacokinetics, therefore, is nonlinear. There is evidence for carrier-mediated active transport of gabapentin into brain tissue (Del Amo et al., 2008). Peak time is two to three hours, and Vd is 0.65–1.04 l/kg. Gabapentin is not metabolized in the liver and is excreted unchanged in the urine. Elimination half-life is five to nine hours. Gabapentin is not protein-bound.

TOXICITY

Gabapentin is generally well tolerated compared with other antiseizure drugs, but the more common dose-related side effects include drowsiness, dizziness, cognitive dysfunction, ataxia, headache, tremor, diplopia, nausea, rhinitis, leg and facial edema, and weight gain. Gabapentin can cause aggressive and hyperkinetic behavior in children under the age of 12. Serious idiosyncratic reactions with gabapentin are extremely rare and may include rash, leukopenia, pancreatitis, and angina. The teratogenic potential of gabapentin has not yet been determined, and it is classified by the FDA as risk category C.

DRUG INTERACTIONS

Since gabapentin is not metabolized in the liver, it does not induce or inhibit cytochrome P450 or other enzyme systems and has no interactions with other drugs. Gabapentin absorption is reduced by 20%, however, when given within two hours of antacids containing aluminum or magnesium hydroxide.

INDICATIONS

Gabapentin is a narrow-spectrum antiseizure drug used specifically for focal seizures. It may aggravate generalized seizures. Its major advantage is that it is tolerated somewhat better than other antiseizure drugs, but clinical trials have shown it to be somewhat less effective (Chapter 14). Another advantage is its lack of drug-drug interactions, making it particularly useful in elderly patients on multiple other medications. Gabapentin is an effective treatment for *neuropathic pain*, particularly *postherpetic neuralgia, diabetic neuropathy*, and *trigeminal neuralgia*. There is also evidence that gabapentin can be used to treat *movement disorders, migraine, cocaine dependence*, and *anxiety*.

ADMINISTRATION

Neurontin is available in capsules of 100, 300, and 400 mg; tablets of 600 and 800 mg; and an oral solution of 250 mg/5 ml. The usual dose is 900–3,600 mg per day for adults and 25–40 mg/kg per day for children ages 3–12, to achieve a plasma level of 2–20 µg/ml. Treatment in adults usually begins with 300 mg per day, increased to 300 mg twice a day on the second day, and 300 mg three times a day on the third day, then further increased as necessary. In children, treatment can begin with 10–15 mg/kg daily and increase by 10 mg/kg per day in three divided doses. Precautions need to be taken in patients with renal impairment, and capsules should not be given to patients with lactose intolerance. Therapeutic range is 2–20 µg/ml.

Lacosamide (LCM)

Lacosamide is *(R)-2-acetamido-M-benzyl-3-m ethoxypropramide*, formally known as *harkoseride*. It was approved in the United States in 2008 under the trade name *Vimpat* (White et al., 2008b; Sachdeo, 2009).

MECHANISMS OF ACTION

Lacosamide has a unique mechanism of action, stabilizing hyperexcitable neuronal membranes by selectively enhancing slow inactivation of voltage-gated Na^+ channels without affecting fast inactivation.

PHARMACOKINETICS

Lacosamide is rapidly and completely absorbed after oral administration, with a peak time of one to two hours. Pharmacokinetics is linear. The drug is less than 15% protein bound, and the Vd is 0.6–0.7 l/kg. Lacosamide is partially metabolized in the liver, primarily by isoenzyme CYP2C19 to an inactive *O-desmethyl* metabolite, *SPM12809*, which is not pharmacologically active; approximately 40% of lacosamide is excreted unchanged in the urine. The half-life of lacosamide is 12–16 hours and is not affected by dose, duration of treatment, or oral versus intravenous administration.

TOXICITY

Common dose-related side effects of lacosamide include dizziness, headache, diplopia, nausea, pruritis, and depression. Somnolence and cognitive disturbances appear to be less common with lacosamide than with most other antiseizure drugs. Lacosamide can increase the PR interval, an effect that only rarely is symptomatic; however, caution is advised in elderly patients and those with known second- or third-degree atrial ventricular block. Life-threatening idiosyncratic adverse events have not been reported. No data are available on teratogenicity, but the FDA has indicated lacosamide as risk category C.

DRUG INTERACTIONS

Although lacosamide is metabolized by the liver, using the cytochrome P450 system, no significant drug-drug interactions have been identified.

INDICATIONS

Lacosamide is licensed for adjunctive treatment of focal seizures with or without secondarily generalized seizures in patients over

16 years of age. Its major advantages include predictable and linear pharmacokinetics, low potential for drug-drug interactions, and a relatively long half-life, permitting twice-daily dosing. Like *gabapentin*, lacosamide appears to be effective treatment for neuropathic pain.

ADMINISTRATION

Vimpat is available in 50-, 100-, 150-, and 200-mg tablets, 10-mg/ml syrup, and 10-mg/ml solution. The recommended adult dose is 200–400 mg per day in two divided doses. Treatment should begin with 50 mg twice a day for one week and increased by 100 mg per day in divided doses at weekly intervals. The infusion solution and tablets are bioequivalent and can be used interchangeably. The intravenous infusion should be administered over 15–30 minutes. Therapeutic range is 10–20 µg/ml.

Lamotrigine (LTG)

Lamotrigine is *3,5-diamino-6-[2,3-dichlorophenyl]-1,2,4-triazine*. It was initially synthesized as a folic acid antagonist, but the view that antifolate drugs may have antiseizure properties was subsequently discredited. Lamotrigine was approved as adjunctive treatment for focal seizures in the United Kingdom in 1991 and in the United States in 1994 under the trade name *Lamictal* (Tomson et al., 2008; Matsuo and Riaz, 2009). Generic formulations of lamotrigine are available.

MECHANISMS OF ACTION

Lamotrigine's primary mechanism of action is by use- and voltage-dependent blockade of voltage-activated Na^+ channels, similar to the action of phenytoin and carbamazepine. Lamotrigine also appears to alter release of a number of neurotransmitters, including glutamate, GABA, dopamine, serotonin, and noradrenaline, and modulates K^+ and Ca^{2+} currents. It is unclear whether any of these actions contribute to lamotrigine's antiseizure effects, but there is also a suggestion that some of these mechanisms could be neuroprotective.

PHARMACOKINETICS

Lamotrigine is rapidly absorbed after oral administration, peak level is achieved at one to three hours, and pharmacokinetics is linear. Vd is 0.9–1.3 l/kg, and protein binding is 55%. Lamotrigine is metabolized in the liver by conjugation with *glucuronic acid* to various inactive metabolites. Most of the lamotrigine is converted to *N-2-* and *N-5-glucuronides* (80% and 10%, respectively) by different isoforms of *UDP-glucuronosyltransferase*. The elimination half-life of lamotrigine is 15–35 hours, but it undergoes autoinduction, which increases clearance by 17–37%. Comedication with valproic acid increases the half-life of lamotrigine to 30–90 hours, while comedication with enzyme-inducing drugs reduces the half-life to 8–20 hours. Ninety percent of metabolites and 10% of lamotrigine are excreted in the urine.

TOXICITY

Common dose-related side effects include dizziness, diplopia, headache, tremor, anxiety, drowsiness, insomnia, and nausea. Although benign rash also occurs as a dose-dependent effect, the most serious idiosyncratic adverse effect is a rash leading to *Stevens-Johnson syndrome* and *toxic epidermal necrolysis*. This adverse effect can occur within eight weeks of initiation on lamotrigine or when the medication is suddenly stopped and then resumed at the usual dose. The risk is increased with rapid initiation and with valproic acid comedication. The incidence of serious rash is 1 in 1,000 in adults and children over 12, but it may be as high as 1 in 100 in children under the age of 12. Blood dyscrasias, hepatic dysfunction, and cardiac arrhythmias have also been reported with lamotrigine, and the last could increase the risk of *sudden unexpected death in epilepsy (SUDEP)*. Extrapyramidal effects, including choreoathetosis, ticks, and exacerbation of Parkinson's symptoms, occur rarely. The teratogenic risk of lamotrigine remains to be determined; however, the FDA has classified lamotrigine as risk category C.

DRUG INTERACTIONS

As noted previously, enzyme-inducing drugs have a profound effect on the clearance of lamotrigine, and because this drug is often given as adjunctive therapy, lamotrigine dosing needs to be adjusted when coadministered with enzyme-inducing antiseizure drugs such as *phenobarbital, primidone, phenytoin, carbamazepine, oxcarbazepine, ethosuximide*, and possibly *topiramate*. *Valproic acid* decreases the clearance of lamotrigine and increases lamotrigine plasma levels, also requiring appropriate dosage adjustment. *Sertraline* increases lamotrigine plasma levels, and oral contraceptives, *acetaminophen, olanzapine, rifampicin*, and *ritonavir* can decrease lamotrigine plasma levels. Conversely, lamotrigine has very little effect on coadministered medications, with the exception that it can decrease plasma levels of clonazepam and valproic acid. There is evidence for pharmacodynamic synergistic therapeutic effects between lamotrigine and valproic acid and possibly an adverse synergistic effect between these two drugs and between lamotrigine and carbamazepine, resulting in increased incidence of dose-related side effects.

INDICATIONS

Lamotrigine is a broad-spectrum antiseizure drug effective against all seizure types except myoclonus. It is contraindicated in syndromes with predominant myoclonic seizures, including *Dravet syndrome* and *progressive myoclonus epilepsy*, but it may not exacerbate the myoclonic jerks of *juvenile myoclonic epilepsy* and can be an alternative treatment for this condition. The major advantages of lamotrigine are that it is efficacious for most epilepsy syndromes and well tolerated. The major disadvantages are its significant pharmacokinetic interactions with other antiseizure drugs and the need for slow titration. Lamotrigine also

has a mood-elevating effect and is used for the treatment of bipolar disorder, particularly bipolar depression (Hahn et al., 2004).

ADMINISTRATION

Lamictal is available in 25-, 100-, 150-, and 200-mg tablets; 2-, 5-, and 25-mg chewable tablets; and 25-, 50-, 100-, and 200-mg disintegrating tablets. Extended-release Lamictal XR is available in 25-, 50-, 100-, 200-, 250-, and 300-mg tablets. Initiation of therapy and maintenance dosage depend on whether lamotrigine is prescribed alone, with enzyme-inducing medications, or with valproic acid. For adults and children over the age of 12, the recommended maintenance dose as monotherapy varies from 100 to 400 mg per day in two divided doses for adults and children over the age of 12 and from 1 to 5 mg/kg per day in two divided doses for children ages 2–12 years. When lamotrigine is given with valproic acid, the maintenance dose in adults is 100–250 mg per day in two divided doses, and in children it is the same as with monotherapy. When lamotrigine is given with an enzyme-inducing drug, the recommended maintenance dose varies from 200 to 600 mg per day for adults and 5 to 15 mg/kg per day in children. Titration for adults and children over the age of 12 for monotherapy begins with 25 mg per day for two weeks, and is then increased by 25 mg per day every one to two weeks; in children an initial dose of 0.15 mg/kg per day is given for two weeks and increased by 0.3 mg/kg per day at two-week intervals thereafter. With valproic acid, in adults the initial treatment is 25 mg every other day for two weeks, then increased by 25 mg per day at two-week intervals thereafter; in children titration can be the same as with monotherapy. With enzyme-inducing drugs, in adults treatment is initiated with 50–100 mg per day for two weeks, then increased by 100 mg per day at two-week intervals; in children treatment begins with 0.6 mg/kg per day for two weeks and then is increased by 1.2 mg/kg per day at two-week intervals thereafter. If the patient, for any reason, stops taking the medication for five days or more, it should not be restarted at the prior dose but titrated again from the beginning. Care must be taken when valproic acid or an enzyme-inducing drug is added to an established regimen of lamotrigine and when these drugs are discontinued, as these will alter the lamotrigine plasma concentration. Therapeutic range is 3–15 µg/ml.

Levetiracetam (LEV)

Levetiracetam is *(−)(S)-α-ethyl-2-oxo-1-pyrro-lidine-acetamide*, which was first approved in the United States in 1999 and is marketed under the brand name *Keppra* (Privitera and Cavitt, 2008; French and Tonner, 2009). Generic formulations are available.

MECHANISMS OF ACTION

The screening history of levetiracetam is unique, in that this compound was not found to be effective against *MES* or *subcutaneous PTZ seizures* in mice but was then tested and found to be effective against *amygdala-kindled seizures* in rats as well as other models of *mesial temporal lobe epilepsy (MTLE)* following status induced by *pilocarpine* and *kainic acid* in rats (Klitgaard et al., 1998; Löscher et al., 2000). Levetiracetam subsequently became one of the most effective drugs for the treatment of MTLE; it also has broad-spectrum efficacy against all seizure types. Levetiracetam selectively binds to *synaptic vesicle protein 2a (Sv2a)*, which is involved in synaptic vesicle trafficking; however, the exact mechanism by which this exerts its antiseizure effect is unknown. Levetiracetam has no effect on Na^+ and T-type Ca^{2+} channels or GABAergic inhibition. Its effect on neurotransmitter release inhibits burst firing without affecting normal neuronal excitability.

PHARMACOKINETICS

Levetiracetam is rapidly absorbed after oral administration, it demonstrates linear pharmacokinetics, and peak plasma concentrations are reached in 0.5–2 hours. Solutions for intravenous injection are available, and intravenous infusion is bioequivalent to the oral formulation. The Vd for levetiracetam is 0.5–0.7 l/kg, and it is not protein bound. Sixty-six percent of orally administered levetiracetam is excreted unchanged in the urine, and the remainder is hydrolyzed to a carboxylic acid in various body tissues independent of the cytochrome P450 system. The elimination half-life of levetiracetam is 6–8 hours, but the functional half-life may be much longer. The metabolites have no antiseizure properties.

TOXICITY

Levetiracetam is well tolerated; the most common dose-related side effects include somnolence and dizziness as well as adverse behavioral symptoms, particularly agitation, anxiety, emotional lability, and depression. Serious idiosyncratic side effects are rare, although cases of Stevens-Johnson syndrome and toxic epidermal necrolysis have been reported to occur between two weeks and four months after drug initiation, resulting in a recommendation that levetiracetam be discontinued at the first sign of a rash unless it is clearly not drug related. Teratogenicity has not yet been well established, but levetiracetam is classified by the FDA as risk category C.

DRUG INTERACTIONS

Levetiracetam has no effects on the pharmacokinetics of other drugs, nor do other drugs have effects on the pharmacokinetics of levetiracetam. There is evidence, however, that *valproic encephalopathy* can be induced by the addition of levetiracetam and that levetiracetam can exacerbate the toxic side effects of *carbamazepine* and *topiramate*. The depressant effects of levetiracetam will be enhanced by CNS depressants such as alcohol, other antiseizure drugs, and *monoamine oxidase inhibitors*.

INDICATIONS

Levetiracetam is highly effective against all seizure types in adults and children. It was too new to be compared with other second-generation antiseizure drugs in the *Standard* and New Antiepileptic Drug (SANAD) trials (Marson et al., 2007a, 2007b) (Chapter 14); however, it would appear to be at least as good as *lamotrigine*, carbamazepine, and *oxcarbazepine* for focal seizures and in many instances as good as valproic acid for mixed seizure disorders. The most important potential disadvantage of levetiracetam is the behavioral and psychiatric adverse effects, which could limit its use in patients with a history of behavioral disorder.

ADMINISTRATION

Keppra is available in 250-, 500-, 750-, and 1,000-mg tablets, as Keppra XR in 500 and 750-mg extended-release tablets, as 100-mg/ml oral solution, and as 500-mg/5ml solution for intravenous injection. The maintenance dose of levetiracetam for adults is 1,000–3,000 mg per day and for children 30–40 mg/kg per day in two divided doses. Treatment in adults and children over the age of 12 can begin with 250–500 mg twice a day and in children under 12 years, 20 mg/kg per day twice or three times daily. This dose is usually increased by this amount at one- to two-week intervals but can be titrated more rapidly if needed. Appropriate intravenous loading dose has not yet been determined for levetiracetam. The therapeutic range for levetiracetam is 12–46 μg/ml.

Oxcarbazepine (OXC)

Oxcarbazepine is *10,11-dihydro-10-oxo-5H-dibenz[b,f]azepine-5-carboxamide*, a 10-keto analog of carbamazepine (Faught and Limdi, 2009; Beydoun et al., 2008a). It was first

marketed in Denmark in 1990 and has been available in the rest of Europe since 1999 and in the United States since 2000 under the trade name *Trileptal*. Generic formulations of oxcarbazepine are available.

MECHANISMS OF ACTION

Oxcarbazepine and its primary active metabolite, the *10-monohydroxy derivative (MHD)*, block Na^+ channels in a use-dependent manner similar to the action of *carbamazepine* and *phenytoin*, but MHD has a greater affinity for the inactivated state of the channel and inhibits M- and P-type Ca^{2+} currents. Evidence also suggests that oxcarbazepine and its metabolite increase K^+ conductance and elevate hippocampal dopamine and serotonin levels.

PHARMACOKINETICS

Oxcarbazepine is rapidly and completely absorbed and reaches peak concentration within one hour; however, it is rapidly converted to MHD, which is primarily responsible for the antiseizure efficacy. MHD reaches peak concentration within four to six hours, has a Vd of 0.7–0.8 l/kg, and is 40% protein bound, while oxcarbazepine is 60% protein bound. Pharmacokinetics is linear. Whereas carbamazepine is metabolized to an epoxide intermediate by the cytochrome P450 system, oxcarbazepine is metabolized to the active metabolite MHD by *cytosolic aldoketoreductase enzymes* in the liver, and has a half-life of 1–2.5 hours. MHD is partially glucuronidated in the liver, with 28% excreted unchanged in the urine, and has a half-life of 8–15 hours. Oxcarbazepine and MHD are enzyme inhibitors and increase phenytoin, phenobarbital, and carbamazepine epoxide levels but decrease carbamazepine levels, while MHD levels are decreased by enzyme-inducing drugs. Oxcarbazepine also reduces serum levels of steroids, oral contraceptives, and *felodipine*. Adverse pharmacodynamic synergy has occurred on coadministration of oxcarbazepine with lamotrigine and lithium.

TOXICITY

Dose-related and idiosyncratic adverse effects are similar to those of carbamazepine, although oxcarbazepine is in general better tolerated than carbamazepine. Hyponatremia, however, is more common with oxcarbazepine than with carbamazepine and, therefore, should be avoided in patients at risk for congestive heart failure. Oxcarbazepine is poorly tolerated in the elderly for other reasons as well (Arif et al., 2010). Approximately 25–30% of patients who experience skin rash with carbamazepine will also experience skin rash with oxcarbazepine. Oxcarbazepine is classified by the FDA as risk category C.

DRUG INTERACTIONS

Drug interactions of oxcarbazepine are similar to those of carbamazepine. Plasma levels are decreased by enzyme-inducing drugs and increased by *valproic acid*. Oxcarbazepine decreases plasma levels of carbamazepine, *lamotrigine*, and *topiramate*, but unlike carbamazepine, it can increase plasma levels of *phenobarbital* and phenytoin. Oxcarbazepine also lowers plasma levels of hormonal contraceptives and can enhance the neurotoxicity of lithium.

INDICATIONS

Although the metabolic pathways and, to some degree, the mechanisms of action of oxcarbazepine and MHD are different from those of carbamazepine, they have the same spectrum of effectiveness, specifically for focal seizures with and without secondarily generalized seizures. The major advantage of oxcarbazepine over carbamazepine is a better-tolerated side effect profile and fewer drug-drug interactions, although hyponatremia and interaction with oral contraceptives remain problematic, and side effects are common in the elderly (Arif et al., 2010). Oxcarbazepine has also been used to treat *bipolar depression*, *acute mania*, and *neuropathic pain*.

ADMINISTRATION

Trileptal is available as 150-, 300-, and 600-mg tablets and 300-mg/5 ml oral suspension. Maintenance dose is 600–2,400 mg per day for adults and 35–45 mg/kg per day for children, in two divided doses. Tolerance is best with a low starting dose for adults of 300 mg

per day increased by half this amount every two days and for children of 5–10 mg/kg per day increased by half this amount weekly. Carbamazepine and oxcarbazepine are not bioequivalent. Doses of oxcarbazepine need to be approximately one-third higher than those of carbamazepine. The therapeutic range for oxcarbazepine is 3–35 µg/ml.

Pregabalin (PGN)

Pregabalin is *(S)-3-(aminomethyl)-5-methyl-hexanoic acid* and was approved for marketing in Europe in 2004 and the United States in 2005 under the trade name *Lyrica* (Bergey, 2008; Rheims and Ryvlin, 2009). It is a congener of gabapentin with important similarities and differences.

MECHANISMS OF ACTION

Although pregabalin, like *gabapentin*, is structurally related to GABA, also like gabapentin it does not appear to act on GABA or its receptors. Both drugs bind to the $\alpha_2\gamma$ *subunit* of the voltage-gated Ca^{2+} P, Q, and N presynaptic calcium channels, reducing Ca^{2+} influx in a use-dependent manner. The effect is to decrease presynaptic release of neurotransmitters including *glutamate*, *noradrenaline*, and *substance P*.

PHARMACOKINETICS

Pregabalin is rapidly absorbed, with a peak time of one to two hours. Absorption is delayed by two to three hours when it is ingested with food. Pharmacokinetics is linear. The Vd is 0.57 l/kg, and pregabalin is not protein bound.

There is evidence for carrier-mediated active transport of pregabalin into brain tissue (Del Amo et al., 2008). Pregabalin is 98% excreted unchanged in the urine, and elimination half-life is five to seven hours.

TOXICITY

Like gabapentin, pregabalin is well tolerated with minimal dose-related side effects at low doses; however, side effects are twice as common at the higher dose range. The most common include somnolence, dizziness, diplopia, memory impairment, dry mouth, peripheral edema, and decreased libido. Weight gain is common. Serious idiosyncratic adverse effects are rare. There are as yet inadequate data on the teratogenic risk of pregabalin, but it is classified by the FDA as risk category C.

DRUG INTERACTIONS

Like gabapentin, pregabalin has no known pharmacokinetic drug-drug interactions, but pharmacodynamic interactions may potentiate effects of sedative, respiratory depressant, and cognitive-impairing medications.

INDICATIONS

Pregabalin is a narrow-spectrum agent approved as adjunctive therapy for focal seizures with and without secondarily generalized seizures. Its spectrum of efficacy is similar to that of gabapentin, but it appears to be more potent and better tolerated. A major advantage, as with gabapentin, is the lack of drug-drug interactions. Weight gain is an important disadvantage. Like gabapentin, pregabalin is also used to treat neuropathic pain and anxiety.

ADMINISTRATION

Lyrica is available in 25-, 50-, 75-, 100-, 150-, 200-, 225-, and 300-mg capsules. Maintenance dose is 150–600 mg in two or three equally divided doses for adults. Treatment should be initiated at 75 mg twice daily and increased by this amount at weekly intervals. Therapeutic range for pregabalin has not yet been determined.

Rufinamide (RUF)

Rufinamide is *1-(2–6-difluorophenyl)methyl-1-H-1,2,3-triazole-4-carboxamide*, a novel compound structurally unrelated to any other antiseizure drug. It was first approved for marketing in Europe in 2008, specifically in children over the age of 4 with LGS but subsequently was approved in Europe and the United States for wider use (Glauser and Bialer, 2008; Biton, 2009). It is marketed under the trade names *Banzel* and *Inovelon.*

MECHANISMS OF ACTION

The exact mechanisms by which rufinamide exerts its antiseizure effects are unknown; however, they appear to involve modulation of voltage-gated Na^+ channels and perhaps inhibition of the glutamate receptor subtype *mGluR5.*

PHARMACOKINETICS

Rufinamide is slowly absorbed, with peak levels attained within four to six hours. This time is substantially increased by coingestion with food. Pharmacokinetics is linear up to 1600 mg per day and nonlinear above this amount due to reduced oral bioavailability. The Vd of rufinamide is 0.71–1.14 l/kg, and it is 35% protein bound. Rufinamide is metabolized in the liver primarily by hydrolysis to *CGP 47292*, a process that is not P450-dependent. Metabolites are inactive and excreted primarily in the urine. Elimination half-life in adults is 6–10 hours and is 50% longer in children.

TOXICITY

Rufinamide is well tolerated, with common dose-related adverse effects including dizziness, diplopia, somnolence, nausea, and fatigue. Hypersensitivity reactions have been reported. Rufinamide also decreases QTc interval and may increase the risk of status epilepticus. Teratogenic effects of rufinamide have not been determined, and it is classified by the FDA as risk category C.

DRUG INTERACTIONS

Enzyme-inducing drugs increase clearance of rufinamide and decrease plasma levels, while valproic acid decreases clearance and increases rufinamide plasma levels. Although rufinamide does not appear to affect the cytochrome P450 system, it can decrease plasma levels of carbamazepine and lamotrigine and increase plasma levels of phenobarbital and phenytoin.

INDICATIONS

Rufinamide is the first new antiseizure drug since felbamate to show effectiveness against atonic seizures, and its efficacy has been clearly demonstrated for LGS. Efficacy for other seizure types and syndromes has not been well established. It is, therefore, currently approved for this specific indication.

ADMINISTRATION

Banzel is available as 200- and 400-mg tablets and 40-mg/ml oral suspension. Recommended maintenance dose is based on age. For children age 4 years or older, the maintenance dose is 45 mg/kg per day, and for adults it is 1,800–3,200 mg per day, both in two divided doses. Treatment is initiated in children at 10 mg/kg per day and in adults at 400–800 mg per day, in two divided doses,

and increased every other day by the same amount. Therapeutic range for rufinamide is 10–25 µg/ml.

Tiagabine (TGB)

Tiagabine is (−)-(R)-1-[4,4-bis(3-methyl-2-th ienyl)-3-butenyl]-3-nipecotic acid hydrochloride (Kälviäinen, 2008, 2009). It was approved in the United States in 1997 and is marketed under the trade name *Gabitril.*

MECHANISMS OF ACTION

Tiagabine enhances inhibition by blocking glial and neuronal GABA uptake by *GABA transporter-1 (GAT-1)*, thereby temporarily prolonging the presence of endogenously released GABA in the synapse. The potential advantage of this effect is that the pattern of GABA enhancement is physiological and limited by the amount of GABA released. Inhibition of the glial uptake is 2.5 times greater than that for neuronal uptake.

PHARMACOKINETICS

Tiagabine is rapidly absorbed, with a peak time of 0.5–2 hours. Pharmacokinetics is linear. The Vd is 1.0 l/kg, and 96% of tiagabine is protein-bound. The drug is 60% metabolized in the liver, 60% by CYP3A4 to two inactive *5-oxo-tiagabine isomers*. Metabolites of the other 40% have not been identified. Elimination half-life is five to nine hours but is decreased by coadministration with enzyme-inducing drugs.

TOXICITY

Common dose-related side effects of tiagabine include dizziness, depression, nausea, and bruising. There is an increased incidence of psychosis, particularly with rapid titration, but somnolence and cognitive side effects are not as great as with other GABA agonist drugs. As with other GABA agonists, however, tiagabine can aggravate absence seizures and increase the risk of *nonconvulsive status epilepticus*. The visual field deficits seen with vigabatrin have not been found with tiagabine. Teratogenic risk for tiagabine has not been determined, but it is classified by the FDA as risk category C.

DRUG INTERACTIONS

Carbamazepine, phenobarbital, phenytoin, primidone, and other enzyme-inducing drugs increase clearance of tiagabine and decrease plasma levels. *Valproic acid, naproxen*, and *salicylic acid* increase free tiagabine by competing for protein binding. Tiagabine, on the other hand, can decrease valproic acid plasma levels.

INDICATIONS

Tiagabine is a narrow-spectrum drug with efficacy limited to focal seizures with or without secondarily generalized seizures. Its potency is somewhat less than that of other available antiseizure drugs, and it is used primarily as an adjunctive medication in severe forms of focal seizures or when the patient cannot tolerate any other medication. There is some suggestion that tiagabine may also be effective for epileptic spasms.

ADMINISTRATION

Gabitril is available as 2-, 4-, 6-, 8-, 10-, 12-, and 16-mg tablets. The recommended maintenance dose is 16–32 mg per day, or 32–56 mg per day with enzyme-inducing drugs, in two to four divided doses. The usual starting dose is 4–5 mg per day, which can be increased weekly by 4–5 mg per day. For older children the initial dose is 0.1 mg/kg per day increased by 0.1 to 0.2 mg/kg per week to a maintenance dose of 0.4 mg/kg per day with enyme-inducing drugs and 0.7 mg/kg per day without enzyme inducers. Therapeutic range is 0.02–0.2 µg/ml but is clinically useful only for monitoring compliance.

Topiramate (TPM)

Topiramate is *2,3:4,5-di-O-isopropylidene-β-D-fructopyranose sulfamate* (Faught and Glauser, 2008; Cross and Riney, 2009). It was originally developed as a fructose-related compound with hypoglycemic activity but was then discovered to have antiseizure properties in animal models. Topiramate was approved initially in the United States in 1996 with the brand name *Topamax*. Generic formulations are available.

MECHANISMS OF ACTION

Topiramate is of particular interest because it has at least five mechanisms of action and the relative importance of each is not entirely clear. Topiramate inhibits *voltage-activated Na^+ channels* in a dose-dependent manner, similar to the actions of *phenytoin* and *carbamazepine*. It decreases *glutamate-mediated* excitatory neurotransmission by action on the *GluR5* subtype of the *kainate receptor* and also by action on the *α-amino-3-hydroxy-5-methyl-4-isoxazole propionic acid (AMPA) receptor*. Glutamate receptor effects also modulate Ca^{2+} currents, and topiramate had a direct effect on *L-type voltage-sensitive Ca^{2+}*

currents. Like the benzodiazepines, topiramate enhances inhibition by increasing the opening of GABA-mediated Cl⁻ channels, but it does not bind to the *benzodiazepine receptor* site and appears to increase GABA content in the brain. Topiramate may also enhance inhibitory function by facilitating *K⁺ channel* conduction. Finally, topiramate, like *acetazolamide*, inhibits the enzyme *carbonic anhydrase (CA)*, but this is a weak effect and more likely to contribute to toxicity such as *renal stones* and paresthesias than to its antiseizure potency.

PHARMACOKINETICS

Topiramate is rapidly absorbed, with a peak time of two to four hours. Pharmacokinetics is linear. It is widely distributed in all tissues, with a Vd of 0.6–1.0 l/kg. Fifteen percent of topiramate is protein bound. Topiramate is mostly excreted unchanged in the urine, but the 30% that is metabolized in the liver, by CYP3A4 and 2C19 isoenzymes, is increased when it is coadministered with enzyme-inducing drugs. At least 12 inactive metabolites have been identified, but the actual metabolic pathways have not been fully elucidated. Elimination half-life is 10–30 hours depending on the presence of enzyme-inducing drugs.

TOXICITY

Troublesome CNS-related adverse effects, particularly cognitive impairment, were reported early after the introduction of topiramate, but these dose-related effects are now less problematic, because the recommended dose ranges have been reduced. Other than the cognitive changes, dose-related side effects can include fatigue, anorexia, nausea, metabolic acidosis, hypohidrosis, dizziness, double vision, and tremor. Weight loss is common, usually seen within three months and with the greatest effect between 12 and 18 months. Renal stones occur in 1–2% of patients. Paresthesias, metabolic acidosis, oligohidrosis with hyperthermia, and acute bilateral secondary narrow angle-closure glaucoma are more serious adverse effects. The chronic metabolic acidosis can also cause osteoporosis and reduced growth in children. Recent registry data have revealed an increased risk of teratogenicity with topiramate,

which is higher than that of carbamazepine but not as high as that of valproic acid (Hunt et al., 2008). The FDA classifies topiramate as risk category D.

DRUG INTERACTIONS

Enzyme-inducing drugs such as carbamazepine, *oxcarbazepine, phenobarbital, phenytoin*, and *primidone* increase topiramate clearance and decrease plasma levels, as does *valproic acid*. Topiramate decreases clearance of phenytoin, increasing its plasma levels, and increases clearance of valproic acid, decreasing its plasma levels. *Amitriptyline, lithium, metformin, propranolol*, and *sumatriptan* increase topiramate plasma levels, and topiramate increases clearance of *digoxin, glibenclamide, pioglitazone, risperidone, sumatriptan*, and *oral contraceptives*. It decreases clearance and increases plasma levels of *amitriptyline, haloperidol, hydrochlorothiazide, lithium*, and *metformin*. Pharmacodynamic interactions account for an increased risk of hyperammonemia and encephalopathy when topiramate is administered with valproic acid and of weight loss and nervousness when administered with levetiracetam. Coadministration with other CA inhibitors increases the risk of renal stones. Topiramate can invalidate the results of the *intracarotid amobarbital procedure* (Bookheimer et al., 2005) (Chapters 12 and 16).

INDICATIONS

Topiramate is an effective broad-spectrum antiseizure drug as monotherapy or adjunctive therapy for almost all seizure types. It is used primarily to treat difficult focal seizures with or without secondarily generalized seizures but is also useful in conditions with mixed seizures, such as LGS. Efficacy against absence and myoclonic seizures and epileptic spasms has not been adequately demonstrated, but topiramate does not appear to exacerbate any seizure types and is not contraindicated in any epilepsy syndromes. Topiramate is also used as prophylactic treatment for migraine, and is useful in a variety of psychiatric conditions, as therapy for neuropathic pain, and as treatment for obesity.

ADMINISTRATION

Topamax is available as 25-, 50-, 100-, and 200-mg tablets and 15- and 25-mg sprinkle capsules. Maintenance dose in adults is 200–400 mg per day or, when coadministered with enzyme-inducing drugs, 400–600 mg per day, in two divided doses. In children, the dose is 3 mg/kg per day as monotherapy and 6–9 mg/kg per day with enzyme-inducing drugs. Initial dose in adults and children over the age of 12 is 25–50 mg per day, increased by this amount at one- to two-week intervals. For children under the age of 12 and infants, the dose is initially 0.5–1 mg/kg in two to three divided doses and is increased by this amount at one- to two-week intervals. Therapeutic range is 5–20 μg/ml.

Vigabatrin (VGB)

Vigabatrin, (±)-aminohex-5-enoic acid, was identified through a systematic search for molecules that increase brain GABA levels by inhibiting *GABA transaminase* (Ben-Menachem et al., 2008; Krämer and Wohlrab, 2009). It was approved in Europe and many other countries under the brand name *Sabril,* but approval in the United States was delayed until 2009, because of the postmarketing discovery of serious retinal toxicity.

MECHANISMS OF ACTION

Vigabatrin is an analog of GABA that binds irreversibly and covalently to GABA-transaminase, permanently inactivating the breakdown of GABA to *succinic acid semialdehyde* in neurons and glia. It is, therefore, referred to as an *irreversible suicide inhibitor* of GABA transaminase. The result is prolonged elevation of brain GABA levels within synapses, and the duration and pharmacological effect are determined by the time needed to resynthesize

GABA transaminase rather than by the half-life of vigabatrin. Restoration of normal enzyme activity after withdrawal of vigabatrin takes several days.

PHARMACOKINETICS

Vigabatrin is rapidly absorbed and reaches peak levels in one to two hours. Pharmacokinetics is linear, Vd is 0.8 l/kg, and the drug is not protein bound. Vigabatrin is eliminated unchanged in the urine. Although the elimination half-life is five to eight hours, the functional effect can last days until normal GABA transaminase activity is restored.

TOXICITY

The most serious common adverse effect of vigabatrin is retinal toxicity manifested as concentric visual field constriction, which is irreversible. Prevalence in adults may be as high as one-third, although this effect is symptomatic in a much smaller number of patients. The risk is higher in males than in females, depends on the duration of treatment, and is lower in children, particularly under the age of 2. Dose-related sedation, dizziness, headache, cognitive defects, psychosis, paresthesias, nausea, and fatigue can also occur. More serious idiosyncratic adverse effects include angioedema, rash, and hallucinations. Weight gain is common, and as with other GABAergic drugs, there can be exacerbation of absence seizures and a risk of nonconvulsive status epilepticus. Reversible asymptomatic T_2 *magnetic resonance imaging (MRI) hyperintensities* can be seen in diencephalic and brain stem structures (Pearl et al., 2009) (see Fig. 14–12). Teratogenic risk is undetermined, but vigabatrin is classified by the FDA as risk category C.

DRUG INTERACTIONS

Vigabatrin can decrease plasma levels of *phenytoin* but has no other known pharmacodynamic or pharmacokinetic drug interactions.

INDICATIONS

Vigabatrin is a narrow-spectrum antiseizure drug originally found to be highly effective against focal seizures with or without secondarily generalized seizures, but it is contraindicated for absence and myoclonic seizures, which it can exacerbate. It is now indicated almost entirely for treatment of infantile spasms and is considered the drug of choice for this condition by some physicians, not only because it is highly effective against these seizures but because long-term treatment is not necessary and the risk of retinal toxicity is relatively low in infants (Chapter 7). Guidelines have been published favoring vigabatrin and *adrenocorticotropic hormone (ACTH)* for the treatment of infantile spasms (Pellock et al., 2010; Go et al., 2012).

ADMINISTRATION

Sabril is available as 500-mg tablets and 500-mg sachets. The maintenance dose is 1,000–3,000 mg per day in adults, 50–150 mg/kg per day in children, and 150–200 mg/kg per day as monotherapy for infantile spasms in infants, given as a single dose or in two divided doses. Treatment in adults is initiated with 500 mg per day and increased by this amount weekly, in children with 50 mg/kg per day and increased by 25–50 mg/kg weekly, and in infants with 50 mg/kg per day and increased by this amount weekly. It is recommended that vigabatrin be withdrawn if the desired effect is not achieved within three months, to avoid visual field toxicity. Therapeutic range is 50–100 µg/ml but is clinically useful only for monitoring compliance.

Zonisamide (ZON)

Zonisamide is *1,2-benzisoxazole-3-methanesulfonamide* (Wroe, 2009; Seino and Leppik, 2009). Zonisamide was widely used in Japan and Korea for several decades, but approval in Europe and the United States was delayed for many years, because of concern about serious adverse side effects. It was approved as add-on therapy for focal seizures in the United States in 2000 and in Europe in 2005 under the brand name *Zonegran*. Generic formulations of zonisamide are available.

MECHANISMS OF ACTION

Zonisamide has multiple mechanisms of action. Like carbamazepine and phenytoin, it blocks voltage-gated Na^+ channels in a use-dependent manner, but it also blocks T-type calcium channels in the thalamus, which makes it effective against generalized absence seizures as well as focal onset seizures. Zonisamide also inhibits K^+-mediated glutamate release, increases extracellular levels of dopamine and serotonin, upregulates the *excitatory amino acid carrier-1 (EAAC-1)*, downregulates expression of GAT-1, and is a CA inhibitor, although, as with topiramate, this effect is much weaker than it is for acetazolamide. The relative importance of these mechanisms in the broad-spectrum antiseizure potency of zonisamide is not entirely clear.

PHARMACOKINETICS

Zonisamide is rapidly absorbed, with a peak time of two to five hours, which can be delayed an hour or so by administration with food. Pharmacokinetics is linear, the Vd is 1.0–1.9 l/kg, and zonisamide is 40% protein-bound. Zonisamide is metabolized in the liver to *2-sulphamoylacetyl-phenol (SMAP)* by CYP3A4, to *N-acetylzonisamide* by acetylation, and by glucuronidation. Metabolites are inactive. Elimination half-life is 50–70 hours but decreases to 25–35 hours when zonisamide is coadministered with enzyme-inducing drugs. Thirty-five percent of zonisamide is excreted unchanged in the urine.

TOXICITY

Dose-related side effects of zonisamide include somnolence, dizziness, ataxia, headache, cognitive disturbances, irritability, diplopia, and nausea, and weight loss is common. As a CA inhibitor, zonisamide also has a 4% risk of renal stones and can produce hypohidrosis with hyperthermia. The risk of allergic rash and Stevens-Johnson syndrome is less than with the sulfonamide antibacterials and is reported to be 4.6 cases per 100,000 patient-years of exposure. There is also a risk of other serious idiosyncratic adverse effects such as hepatic necrosis and aplastic anemia. The teratogenicity risk of zonisamide has not been determined, but the FDA classifies it as risk category C.

DRUG INTERACTIONS

Enzyme-inducing drugs such as *carbamazepine, phenobarbital, phenytoin*, and *primidone* increase zonisamide clearance, as does *valproic acid*, and decrease plasma levels, while there is no evidence that zonisamide affects serum levels of other drugs. *Risperidone* can decrease zonisamide plasma levels. Zonisamide also interferes with the intracarotid amobarbital procedure (Chapters 12 and 16).

INDICATIONS

Zonisamide is an effective broad-spectrum antiseizure drug and is approved for focal seizures with and without secondarily generalized seizures, generalized tonic-clonic and absence seizures, epileptic spasms of West syndrome, other epileptic encephalopathies in infants and children, mixed seizure types seen in LGS, and myoclonic epilepsies. It remains a second-line drug, however, because of a high incidence of adverse CNS side effects as well as the risk of renal stones. It does not exacerbate any seizure types. Zonisamide should not be prescribed in patients with a known allergy to sulfonamide drugs, but this is not an absolute contraindication.

ADMINISTRATION

Zonegran is available in 25-, 50-, and 100-mg capsules. Maintenance dose is 100–600 mg per day in adults and 8 mg/kg per day in children under the age of 12; dosages may need to be higher when zonisamide is coadministered with enzyme-inducing drugs. It can be taken once a day but usually is given in two divided doses. In adults and children over the age of 12 treatment is initiated with 100 mg per day and increased at two-week intervals, and in children under the age of 12 the dose is initially 1–2 mg/kg per day and is increased at two-week intervals. Therapeutic range is 10–40 μg/ml.

SPECIAL AND RARELY USED DRUGS

Acetazolamide

Acetazolamide, known chemically as *5-acetamido-1,3,4-thiadiazole-2-sulfonamide*, is a CA inhibitor (Browne et al., 2008; Neufeld, 2009). It is marketed in the United States and many other countries under the trade name *Diamox* for the treatment of fluid retention but is also useful as adjunctive therapy for epilepsy.

Acetazolamide suppresses MES in the laboratory, and this effect is directly related to its ability to inhibit CA. CA in the brain is located primarily in glia and functions to maintain pH by catalyzing the hydration and dehydration of carbon dioxide. CA inhibition leads to carbon dioxide retention, which reduces neuronal excitability (Chapter 3). Chronic administration of acetazolamide induces CA synthesis and glial proliferation, causing tolerance to the drug's effect (Woodbury and Kemp, 1982; Neufeld, 2009). Because CSF production in the choroid plexus results from CA-dependent transport of Cl^- and *bicarbonate* (HCO_3^-) across the blood-brain barrier, this process is decreased by acetazolamide. High doses of acetazolamide can enhance epileptogenic excitability by blocking CA-dependent glial uptake of Cl^- and HCO_3^- (Woodbury and Kemp, 1982; Neufeld, 2009).

Acetazolamide is completely absorbed in the stomach and upper intestine, reaching peak concentration in the plasma within one to three hours after oral administration. Ninety percent of the drug is protein bound, and the free portion is distributed throughout body water. Penetration into the brain and CSF occurs slowly and is dependent on CSF flow, blood-brain barrier permeability, and rate of transport of drug from the CSF. Acetazolamide is bound to CA, and within 24 hours most of the drug exists as this *enzyme-inhibitor complex*. Brain and CSF concentrations remain lower than the plasma concentration, and the highest concentration of bound drug is in erythrocytes. Acetazolamide is not metabolized by the liver, and most of the drug is slowly excreted in the urine by tubular reabsorption and secretion. The half-life of acetazolamide is 10–15 hours but can be reduced by increasing urinary pH.

Acetazolamide is one of the least toxic antiseizure drugs, with a side effect profile similar to that of other sulfonamides. Drowsiness and paresthesias occur; allergic and idiosyncratic toxic effects are rare. With continuous administration, the incidence of renal stones may be as high as 12%. Teratogenicity has been reported in animals, and acetazolamide is classified by the FDA as risk category C. Although the effects of acetazolamide on gastrointestinal pH, CSF production, urinary alkalinization, and protein binding may influence the pharmacokinetics of other drugs, these interactions do not appear to have much clinical importance. Acetazolamide should be discontinued one to two weeks before beginning the ketogenic diet, because serious metabolic acidosis can occur (Chapter 16).

Diamox is sold as 125-mg and 250-mg tablets, 500-mg sustained-release capsules, and a powder form for parenteral administration. Generic acetazolamide is also available. This drug is effective against most types of seizures and has been used in the past primarily for absence attacks. The development of tolerance, however, has limited its general application. Acetazolamide is more effective when given intermittently and is used today more specifically for conditions in which water retention may contribute to epileptic manifestations. In particular, adjunctive therapy with acetazolamide can help control catamenial seizures (Chapter 14). In this case, it is usually given 10 days before anticipated menses and continued through the termination of bleeding. The recommended daily dose is 250–750 mg per day in two or three divided doses to achieve a plasma drug level of 10–14 µg/ml.

ACTH and Adrenocorticosteroids

ACTH and adrenocorticosteroid hormones have been proven effective against a variety of seizure types in children (Wilder and Bruni, 1981) but are now used almost exclusively in the short-term treatment of West syndrome and other epileptic encephalopathies (Kutt

and Paris-Kutt, 1982; Browne et al., 2008; Hrachovy and Frost, 2008; Vigevano and Cilio, 2009; Pellock et al., 2010) (Chapter 7). The exact mechanisms by which ACTH and corticosteroids reduce epileptic excitability are unknown. There is evidence that ACTH may have direct actions on the brain independent of its ability to release corticosteroids from the adrenal cortex (Kendell et al., 1982). Although the relative merits of ACTH versus corticosteroids were debated in the past (Hrachovy et al., 1983), clinical evidence indicates that the former is more effective (Snead et al., 1983), and it is now generally preferred (Pellock et al., 2010). ACTH is inactivated in the gastrointestinal tract and must be given parenterally. The hormone is rapidly metabolized after intramuscular, subcutaneous, or intravenous administration and has a half-life of only 15 minutes, but sustained-release preparations permit adequate plasma levels for hours. Corticosteroids are readily absorbed after oral administration but can also be given parenterally; they are 90% protein bound in plasma but are rapidly metabolized by the liver, giving a half-life of approximately one to four hours. Phenytoin can initially elevate plasma ACTH and corticosteroids, but chronic administration of phenytoin or phenobarbital increases excretion of corticosteroids (Wilder and Bruni, 1981). Adverse reactions to ACTH and corticosteroids result from the known physiological effects of corticosteroid hormones, and reversible brain shrinkage is commonly seen on MRI (see Fig. 14–12). Serious idiosyncratic and allergic reactions are rare.

ACTH is available in gel form for subcutaneous or intramuscular administration and also in sterile aqueous suspension. Dose and duration of treatment for epileptic encephalopathies are controversial and are discussed in Chapter 7. The adrenocorticosteroids *prednisolone*, *prednisone*, *methylprednisolone*, and *dexamethasone* are available in a variety of oral and injectable preparations. There is no general agreement for treatment regimens with these agents, but consensus reports have been published for treatment of infantile spasms (Pellock et al., 2010; Go et al., 2012) ACTH and corticosteroids are intended only for short-term use over several weeks (DeVivo, 1983; Mackay et al., 2004; Vigevano and Cilio, 2009). Commonly used daily doses are 2 mg/kg for the first three of these corticosteroids and

0.3 mg/kg for dexamethasone, divided into four portions. Some workers advocate switching patients from ACTH injections to oral corticosteroids during the course of therapy. There are now other, newer drugs that are also effective against epileptic encephalopathies, particularly vigabatrin, and that offer the potential for longer-term treatment (Chapter 7).

Barbiturates

METHYLPHENOBARBITAL

Methylphenobarbital, or *N-methylphenobarbital*, is also known as *mephobarbital*. Its chemical name is *5-ethyl-1-methyl-5-phenylbarbituric acid* or *methyl-ethyl-phenyl-malonyl urea* (Eadie and Kwan, 2008; Michelucci et al., 2009). The drug was first marketed in the United States in 1935 under the trade name *Mebaral*, and it continues to be sold under this name in several countries. Other generic names include *mephobarbitone* and *enphenemalum*. It is sold outside the United States under many other trade names, the most common being *Prominal*.

Mephobarbital is metabolized in the liver to *phenobarbital*, which is believed to account for its major pharmacodynamic effects. The mechanism of action, toxicity, interactions with other drugs, and indications for usage, therefore, are the same as for phenobarbital. The pharmacokinetics, however, is somewhat different, resulting in a more linear relationship between drug dose and plasma phenobarbital levels (Eadie, 1982). Mephobarbital is only approximately 50% absorbed from the gut and is less protein-bound than phenobarbital but enters the brain more readily (Eadie, 1982). The recommended adult daily dose of mephobarbital is 4–10 mg/kg administered in one or two portions. Dosing is regulated by monitoring the plasma concentration of phenobarbital. Mebaral is available as 32-, 50-, and 100-mg tablets for oral administration only.

METHARBITAL

Metharbital is an *N*-methylated derivative of phenobarbital known as *1-methyl-5,5-diethylbarbituric acid*. This drug has been marketed in the United States under the trade name *Gemonil* since 1952, but is rarely used today (Michelucci et al., 2009). Other generic names for metharbital are *metharbitone* and *endiemalum*. Gemonil is available under this name in several other countries. Whether metharbital's antiseizure and toxic effects are due to its metabolism by the liver to *phenobarbital* is unknown. There are no specific advantages of metharbital over *phenobarbital* (Eadie, 1982) and it is rarely prescribed in the United States. Gemonil is available as 100-mg tablets for oral administration only. The usual daily dose is 5–15 mg/kg divided into three portions.

Benzodiazepines

CLORAZEPATE

Clorazepate is used as a potassium salt of *7-chloro-2,3-dihydro-2-oxo-5-phenyl-1H-1,4-benzodiazepine-3-carboxylic acid*. Clorazepate dipotassium has been marketed in the United States under the trade name *Tranxene* as a minor tranquilizer and was approved for use as an antiseizure agent in 1981.

Clorazepate is rapidly hydrolyzed to *N-desmethyldiazepam (nordiazepam)* in the acidic pH of the stomach prior to absorption. This active metabolite reaches peak concentration in the blood within one hour after oral administration of clorazepate. Clorazepate is classified as a long-acting benzodiazepine (Caccia and Garattini, 1985), but autoinduction of liver enzymes with chronic administration reduces the half-life of the active metabolite to about 30 hours. Drug interactions are similar to those of clonazepam, but toxicity may be somewhat less severe. Clorazepate presumably acts on a class of benzodiazepine receptors different from those acted on by *clonazepam*, because its spectrum of clinical effectiveness resembles that of *carbamazepine*. It is used as an adjunctive drug primarily for the treatment of dyscognitive focal and generalized tonic-clonic seizures (Troupin et al., 1979).

Tranxene is available as 3.75-, 7.5-, and 15-mg capsules; 3.75-, 7.5-, and 15-mg tablets; and 11.5- and 22.5-mg sustained-release tablets. The usual daily dose is 0.7–1.0 mg/kg divided into two or three portions. Treatment should begin slowly so that drowsiness is minimized. The recommended initial dose for children 9–12 years old is 7.5 mg twice a day, and that for adults is 7.5 mg three times a day, with an increase of 7.5 mg weekly in both cases. The therapeutic range for plasma concentration of nordiazepam is 1–2 µg/ml. Clorazepate is not currently recommended for children under the age of 9.

MIDAZOLAM

The chemical name for *midazolam* is *8-chloro-6-(2-fluorophenyl)-1-methyl-4H-imidazo[1,5-a][1,4]benzodiazepine*. Midazolam is marketed in the United States under the trade name *Versed*. Midazolam is not an effective treatment for chronic epilepsy, but its rapid onset of action makes it a useful second-line treatment for early status epilepticus, where it can be given intramuscularly as well as intravenously, and also by the nasal, buccal, and rectal routes. Versed is available as 2-mg/ml syrup and various sterile liquids for intravenous, intramuscular, and, in some countries, buccal, nasal, or rectal administration. The use of midazolam in the treatment of status epilepticus is discussed in Chapter 10.

NITRAZEPAM

Nitrazepam is *7-nitro-5-phenyl-1,3-dihydro-1,4-benzodiazepine-2–1*, a broad-spectrum benzodiazepine used specifically as a second- or third-line treatment for West syndrome (Camfield and Camfield, 2008). The most common trade name is *Mogadon*. It is rapidly absorbed, with a peak time of 1.3–2.5 hours and a Vd of 2.5–2.9 l/kg. Nitrazepam is 85–88% protein bound. It is metabolized in the liver, with no active metabolites, and the elimination half-life is 20–40 hours. The most important side effect is bulbar dysfunction, causing drooling, coughing, gagging, and difficulty swallowing, with occasional mortality in children due to swallowing problems. Other common side effects of benzodiazepines are seen. Nitrazepam clearance is increased by enzyme-inducing drugs, and its adverse effects are enhanced by coadministration with other CNS depressants. It is available as 5-mg tablets, with dosing beginning at 0.25 mg/kg per day and gradually increasing to a maintenance dose of 5–20 mg per day in adults and 1.5 mg/kg per day in children. Plasma levels are not useful.

Bromides

The discovery by Locock (1857) that *potassium bromide* was effective against catamenial seizures marked the beginning of rational antiseizure drug therapy (Chapter 2). Bromides have been used effectively to treat all seizure types, but their usefulness is limited by the common appearance of toxic side effects at therapeutic levels. These usually consist of sedation and psychic disturbances (Browne et al., 2008; Meierkord and Holtkamp, 2009). Bromides are rarely used today for treating seizure disorders but until recently were considered the only safe antiseizure medication for patients with *acute intermittent porphyria* (Chapter 14).

Bromide is a simple inorganic ion that is rapidly absorbed after oral administration and has a Vd essentially the same as that of Cl⁻. CSF and brain concentrations are approximately one-third that in plasma. Elimination is achieved by renal excretion in competition with Cl⁻. The plasma half-life of bromide is approximately 12 days.

The exact mechanisms of bromide's antiseizure action are unknown. The ion inhibits CA and may also influence passive movements of other ions across cell membranes (Woodbury and Pippenger, 1982). Bromide rapidly traverses Cl⁻ channels, which might enhance the hyperpolarizing effect of GABA-mediated inhibition.

Bromides are commercially available in various salt forms but may be difficult to obtain from pharmacies. The recommended daily dose is 3 g per day, divided into three portions, increased slowly to a maximum of 6 g per day. Therapeutic effects are usually achieved between 10 and 20 mEq/l (1,000–2,000 mg/ml sodium bromide), but toxic symptoms often appear above 15 mEq/l (Woodbury and Pippenger, 1982). Consequently, daily bromide administration must be carefully adjusted to achieve seizure control without unwanted side effects, and allowances must be made for factors that may affect plasma bromide levels, such as food and salt intake, dehydration, vomiting, diarrhea, and impaired renal function

(Woodbury and Pippenger, 1982). Bromide intoxication, known as *bromism*, can develop gradually over weeks. Characteristic features of bromism include rash, anorexia, constipation, gastric distress, conjunctivitis, and mental disturbances consisting of delirium, hallucinations, mania, and coma. Bromism is one of the few causes of dissociation between EEG and behavior; high-voltage delta activity occurs while the patient remains awake and alert, although seriously disturbed (Greenblatt et al., 1945).

Hydantoins

FOSPHENYTOIN

Fosphenytoin, a disodium phosphate ester of phenytoin, is a water-soluble formulation of phenytoin developed specifically as a prodrug for intravenous injection. Whereas injectable phenytoin is formulated with 40% *propylene glycol* and 10% *ethanol* and has a pH of 13, which can cause severe tissue damage if extravasated, fosphenytoin is formulated as a simple aqueous solution in *tromethamine (tris) buffer* at pH 8.8 (Stern et al., 2008). Fosphenytoin was approved in 1996 and has been marketed in the United States since 2004 under the trade name *Cerebyx*.

Fosphenytoin is metabolized to *phenytoin*, which accounts for its mechanism of action. Peak levels are achieved from 0.5 to 1 hour following intravenous infusion and 1.5 to 4 hours following intramuscular administration.

Half-life for conversion of fosphenytoin to phenytoin is 8–15 minutes, after which metabolism is the same as for phenytoin. A 1.5-mg dose of fosphenytoin releases 1 mg of phenytoin, so fosphenytoin doses are often converted to *phenytoin-equivalent doses* (phenytoin dose multiplied by 1.5). Fosphenytoin is preferred when intravenous or intramuscular administration is necessary, because the patient cannot take oral doses of phenytoin for medical or surgical reasons, and when treating serial seizures or status epilepticus, as discussed in Chapter 10.

MEPHENYTOIN

Mephenytoin is *3-methyl-5-ethyl-5phenyl-hydantoin*. It has been marketed in the United States under the trade name *Mesantoin* since 1947 (Stern et al., 2008). Mephenytoin is sold elsewhere under a few other trade names, one common one being *Sedantoinal*.

Mephenytoin is metabolized in the liver by hydroxylation and *N-demethylation* to *5-ethyl-5-phenylhydantoin*, which also has antiseizure properties. Because the half-life of this compound is close to 100 hours and that of mephenytoin is approximately 7 hours, chronic administration of mephenytoin produces plasma concentrations that are 90% active metabolite (Jones and Wimbish, 1985). Antiseizure properties and side effects of mephenytoin, therefore, can be essentially attributed to this desmethyl derivative, which was briefly marketed as an antiseizure agent (*Nirvanol*) but was associated with an unacceptable incidence of serious toxic side effects.

The mechanisms of action of mephenytoin are presumed to be similar to those of phenytoin, although mephenytoin antagonizes PTZ-induced seizures and elevates seizure threshold to a much greater extent than phenytoin. Mephenytoin also has more of a sedative effect than *phenytoin*.

Metabolism of mephenytoin is zero order, as with phenytoin. Toxic side effects are believed to be due to the accumulation of this metabolite and the formation of *arene oxide* intermediates. Serious toxicity is common, with morbilliform rash seen in 10% of patients (Rall and Schleifer, 1985). Other toxic reactions include fever, blood dyscrasias, hepatotoxicity, *periarteritis nodosa*, and *lupus erythematosus*. On the other hand, dose-related cognitive impairment, cerebellar symptoms, gastric distress, and cosmetic side effects are less common with mephenytoin than with phenytoin.

Mesantoin is available in 100-mg tablets and can be administered once a day at a dose of 2–20 mg/kg. The therapeutic range for plasma concentration of the desmethyl derivative is considered to be 10–40 μg/ml. Because of its serious toxicity, mephenytoin should be used only in patients who are unable to tolerate other antiseizure agents. Careful medical supervision is indicated during chronic administration.

ETHOTOIN

Ethotoin is *3-ethyl-5-phenylhydantoin*. It has been marketed in the United States under the trade name *Peganone* since 1957 (Stern et al., 2008; Meierkord and Holtkamp, 2009). The drug is available in several other countries under this trade name and also as *Accenon*. Metabolism of ethotoin is complex, but the antiseizure properties appear to be due entirely to the parent compound. Because ethotoin has a half-life of approximately five hours, it must be administered at least four times a day. Both the antiseizure properties and toxic side effects are considerably less than for phenytoin and mephenytoin. The spectrum of action is the same as for phenytoin.

Ethotoin is rarely used, and then usually as an adjunct. It is available as Peganone in 250- and 500-mg tablets. The usual daily dose is 2–3 g for adults and 500 mg to 1 g for children, divided in four to six parts and taken after food. The therapeutic range has not been extensively studied but is considered to be 15–50 μg/ml. Skin rash, gastrointestinal distress, and drowsiness are the most common side effects, and lymphadenopathy can occur.

Oxazolidinediones

The oxazolidinediones, *trimethadione* and *paramethadione*, are rarely used second-line drugs for the treatment of absence seizures but are of considerable historical interest. Trimethadione was reported to suppress PTZ-induced seizures in the laboratory in 1944 (Everett and Richards, 1944; Richards and Everett, 1944) and two years later was found to have specific clinical effectiveness against absence seizures (Perlstein and Andelman, 1946). Phenytoin, which antagonizes MES- but not PTZ-induced seizures, was known to be clinically effective against generalized tonic-clonic and some focal seizures but ineffective against absences. This difference between the two compounds, therefore, clearly demonstrated that pharmacological compounds could have selective antiseizure properties and suggested that MES- and PTZ-induced seizures would be useful for screening agents for anticonvulsant and anti-absence activity, respectively. Trimethadione and paramethadione were replaced as primary antiabsence agents in the 1960s by the more effective and less toxic *ethosuximide* and more recently have receded further into the background with the advent of *clonazepam, valproic acid*, and the newer broad-spectrum agents (Browne et al., 2008; Meierkord and Holtkamp, 2009).

TRIMETHADIONE

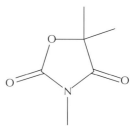

Trimethadione is *3,5,5-trimethyloxazoli-dine-2,4-dione*. It has been marketed in the United States under the trade name *Tridione* since 1946. It is sold in many countries under this name but is known as *Trimedone* in Canada (Browne et al., 2008; Meierkord and Holtkamp, 2009).

The mechanisms of action of trimethadione are unknown, but it is presumed to block thalamic T-type Ca^{2+} currents. It is rapidly absorbed after oral administration and reaches a peak plasma concentration in 0.5–2 hours. Protein binding is negligible, and 95% of the drug is metabolized in the liver. The primary metabolite, *dimethadione*, accumulates with chronic administration and is largely responsible for the antiseizure effect. *Dimethadione* reaches a peak concentration in plasma 120–240 hours after oral administration of trimethadione and has a half-life of 6–13 days.

Dose-related side effects include sedation and blurred vision in bright light (*hemeralopia*). The latter may require the use of tinted glasses. Other, more serious idiosyncratic and allergic toxic effects involving skin, blood, and kidney occur, and a myasthenic syndrome has been reported (Booker, 1982). Trimethadione has a clear teratogenic effect and should not be given to women of childbearing age (Chapter 14). There are no clinically relevant drug interactions reported for trimethadione. Trimethadione can be considered for treatment of patients with absence seizures who are unable to take other antiabsence medication. Tridione is available as 300-mg capsules, 150-mg chewable tablets, and a 40-mg/ml solution. The usual daily dose is 20–40 mg/kg, given once a day to achieve a therapeutic range of 500–1200 μg/ml. Close medical supervision during trimethadione therapy is advised. The maximum therapeutic response may not be seen for two or more weeks.

PARAMETHADIONE

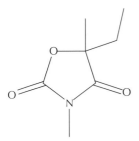

Paramethadione is known chemically as *3,5-dimethyl-5-ethyloxazolidine-2,4-dione*. It has been marketed in the United States under the trade name *Paradione* since 1949 and is sold in many other countries under this name. Paramethadione is somewhat more potent against PTZ seizures than *trimethadione* and has a half-life of approximately 16 hours. It is almost entirely converted by the liver to an *N-demethylated* metabolite that may also have antiseizure effectiveness. The half-life of this metabolite is two or more weeks, and it may take more than two months after initiation of chronic administration for steady-state levels to be achieved. Therapeutic and toxic effects of paramethadione are similar to those of trimethadione. Patients who are unable to tolerate trimethadione may do well with paramethadione, because cross-sensitivity between the two drugs does not necessarily occur. As with trimethadione, close medical supervision is advised, and administration to women of childbearing age is not recommended. Paradione is available as 150-mg and 300-mg capsules and in 300-mg/ml solution. Twenty to 40 mg/kg is usually administered daily in three or four divided doses. Therapeutic ranges for plasma levels of paramethadione and its metabolite have not been determined.

Paraldehyde

Paraldehyde is chemically known as *2,4,6-trimethyl-1,3,5-trioxane*, a cyclic trimer of acetaldehyde (Browne et al., 2008; Meierkord and Holtkamp, 2009). This hypnotic drug has been used primarily for the treatment of withdrawal seizures (Chapter 14) and status epilepticus (Chapter 10). Production of sterile solution for parenteral administration has recently been discontinued in the United States, but it is available and often used in developing countries, particularly for intramuscular administration when intravenous routes are not available. Generic preparations for oral and rectal administration continue to be sold.

The mechanisms of action of paraldehyde are unknown. The drug is rapidly absorbed and reaches a peak concentration in the plasma within 20–60 minutes after intramuscular, 30 minutes after oral, and one to two hours after rectal administration. Twenty percent to 30% is eliminated via the lungs; most of the remainder is metabolized in the liver to *acetaldehyde*. Elimination half-life is 3.5–9.5 hours in adults and 10–25 hours in neonates.

Paraldehyde decomposes to acetaldehyde and *acetic acid* on exposure to air and light and should be stored in airtight, dark glass containers. Toxicity results largely from administration of decomposed solutions, producing acidosis and pulmonary edema. Direct contact can also cause irritation and corrosion of oral and rectal mucosa. *Disulfiram* interferes with paraldehyde metabolism, resulting in accumulation of paraldehyde and acetaldehyde in the blood (Wilder and Bruni, 1981).

Paraldehyde is currently available in the United States only as a solution for oral or rectal administration, but intravenous preparations are still available elsewhere. The usual initial dose for treatment of acute withdrawal seizures is 0.1–0.2 ml/kg repeated as necessary at two- to four-hour intervals. For long-term treatment, 0.05–0.1 ml/kg can be repeated every four to six hours over several days. Patient cooperation is essential for oral administration because aspiration can result in pulmonary edema. Paraldehyde is usually mixed with fruit juice; however, even then awake and alert patients are often unwilling to take the drug because of its unpleasant taste and odor. The latter remains on the breath as the drug is exhaled. Administration by nasogastric tube is contraindicated unless an endotracheal tube with inflated cuff is in place to prevent aspiration. Paraldehyde can be safely and effectively administered rectally as a 2:1 dilution in mineral oil or in 200 ml of 0.9% NaCl. Where available, parenteral paraldehyde preparations can be administered intravenously as a 4% solution diluted in normal saline or intramuscularly at full strength, 5 ml per injection site (Chapter 10). Plastic syringes decompose on contact with the drug and should not be used, but modern plastic intravenous infusion sets are believed to be safe (Treiman, 1987).

Phenacemide

Phenacemide is *phenylacetylurea*, a compound structurally related to the hydantoins. It has been marketed in the United States under the trade name *Phenurone* since 1951 (Browne et al., 2008; Meierkord and Holtkamp, 2009). Phenacemide is available in a few other countries under various trade names but has been used only rarely, because of its potential for serious toxicity and what has been perceived to be inferior antiseizure potency.

Phenacemide has a broad spectrum of antiseizure actions. Clinical reports have not supported the early claim for particular effectiveness against temporal lobe seizures (Swinyard, 1985). Little is known about the specific mechanisms of action of phenacemide. It is rapidly absorbed after oral administration, and peak plasma concentrations are reached within three to five hours. The drug is essentially completely metabolized by the liver to a *glucuronic acid conjugate* and has a half-life of approximately 40 hours with chronic administration (Swinyard, 1985).

Chronic administration of phenacemide has been associated with a risk of potentially fatal side effects, including bone marrow depression and hepatic and renal toxicity. However, these problems are less responsible for phenacemide's unpopularity than are the more commonly encountered psychotic reactions, disorders of affect, and other behavioral changes, as well as anorexia, weight loss, sedation, insomnia, paresthesia, vertigo, and headaches (Wilder and Bruni, 1981). Depressed mood is a particularly frequent consequence of phenacemide therapy.

Phenurone is available as 500-mg tablets. This drug is used primarily for temporal lobe and mixed seizure disorders and has been considered as a last resort, if used at all (Coatsworth and Penry, 1972). The effective daily dose is 20–40 mg/kg divided into three equal portions. It is recommended that treatment in adults begin with 500 mg three times a day and increase by 500 mg per week as needed. In children the recommendations are 250 mg three times a day, increased by 250 mg per week as needed. Effective plasma drug levels have been reported in the range of 16–75 µg/ml (Coker et al., 1987). Close medical supervision is required, with monitoring of blood counts and hepatic and renal function at least monthly.

Piracetam

Piracetam is *2-oxo-1-pyrrolidine acetamide*, a compound structurally related to *levetiracetam* (Shorvon, 2009). Pyrrolidine compounds have been developed over many decades for a variety of purposes, including psychoactive and neuroprotective effects, and piracetam was demonstrated to have antiseizure and antimyoclonic potency as early as 1978. It is marketed for this purpose under many names, predominantly in developing countries. Mechanisms of piracetam's antiseizure and antimyoclonic actions are unknown, but it does have anticholinergic effects, enhances oxidative glycolysis, increases cerebral blood flow, reduces platelet aggregation, and improves erythrocyte function. It is rapidly absorbed, with a peak time of 0.5 to 1.5 hours. Pharmacokinetics is linear, Vd is 0.6 l/kg, and it is not protein-bound. Piracetam is excreted unchanged in the urine. It is well tolerated, with rarely reported dizziness, insomnia, nausea, weight gain, and agitation. No serious idiosyncratic side effects have been reported. Piracetam does not interact with other drugs. Therapeutic range has not been determined.

Piracetam is available as 800- and 1,200-mg tablets and 200-mg/ml or 333.3-mg/ml solutions. Initial doses between 4.8 and 8 g per day are progressively increased to 24 g per day in two to three divided doses as needed. Daily doses up to 32 g are used.

Progabide

Progabide, 4-{[(4-chlorophenyl)[(1E)-3-fluoro-6-oxocyclohexa-2,4-dien-1-ylidene]methyl] amino]butanamide, a prodrug of GABA, was initially demonstrated to have broad-spectrum efficacy in animal models (Worms et al., 1982). The mechanism of action of progabide is uncertain and cannot be attributed entirely to its effect on GABA receptors.

Progabide was licensed in France in 1985 under the trade name *Gabrene* but was subsequently found to be inferior to *valproic acid* at a dose of 30–40 mg/kg per day, and concern was raised about liver toxicity (Crawford and Chadwick, 1986). Progabide is well absorbed, with a bioavailability of 60%. It is 95% protein-bound and metabolized in the liver. Half-life is four hours. Gabrene remains available only in France, where it is used for monotherapy and adjunctive therapy of generalized tonic-clonic, myoclonic, and focal seizures, and for LGS in children and adults.

Propofol

Propofol, 2,6-diisopropylphenol, is an intravenous anesthetic used in the management of refractory status epilepticus (Meierkord and Holtkamp, 2009). Propofol has a direct effect on inward hyperpolarizing Cl^- currents, which differs from the effects of barbiturates and benzodiazepines, and it also enhances $GABA_A$ receptor–mediated activity. Other propofol actions that might contribute to its antiseizure potency include inhibition of *pro-inflammatory cytokine secretion*, modulation of *nitric oxide* expression, impairment of monocyte and neutrophil functions, radical-scavenging activity, and effects on Ca^{2+} channels (Vanlersberghe and Camu, 2008). Propofol is active within two to four minutes of intravenous injection and has a half-life of 30–60 minutes; however, the clinical effects after intravenous administration last only four to eight minutes, which is an advantage for an intravenous anesthetic. Propofol is 98% protein bound and is metabolized primarily in the liver, using the cytochrome P450 system and glucuronidation. Seizure-like behavior reported with propofol administration and withdrawal may not be epileptic (Zubair et al., 2011). A more serious adverse effect is the *propofol infusion syndrome*, characterized by cardiac failure, severe metabolic acidosis, rhabdomyolysis, hyperkalemia, and renal failure, which is often fatal. Although this syndrome is rare, risk is increased with infusions lasting longer than four days at doses higher than 4 mg/kg per hour. The use of propofol in the treatment of status epilepticus is discussed in Chapter 10.

Stiripentol

Stiripentol is *4,4-dimethyl-1[(3,4-methylene-dioxy)phenyl]-1-penten-3-ol*, an aromatic *allyl alcohol* (Eriksson and Keränen, 2009). Conditional marketing authorization under the brand name *Diacomit* was granted by the European Union in 2007 as the first orphaned antiseizure drug in children, specifically for adjunctive treatment of Dravet syndrome. Stiripentol is believed to act by enhancing GABA effects; it reduces synaptosomal uptake of GABA, resulting in small increases in brain GABA concentration, and may also modulate GABAergic function at the barbiturate binding site.

Stiripentol is rapidly absorbed, with a peak time of one to two hours. Stiripentol is rapidly degraded in the acidic environment of the stomach, so effective bioavailability requires that it be taken with food. It is 99% protein-bound, so distribution is slow, and pharmacokinetics is nonlinear as a result of saturation of enzyme systems responsible for drug metabolism. It is primarily metabolized in the liver by desmethylation and glucuronidation to 13 different inactive metabolites. Elimination half-life varies from 4 to 13 hours, increasing with increasing dose.

Dose-dependent adverse side effects of stiripentol include drowsiness, ataxia, tremor, hypotonia, dystonia, hyperactivity, behavior disorders, insomnia, nausea, anorexia, weight loss, and vomiting. Potentially serious adverse effects include cutaneous photosensitivity, rash, and urticaria, as well as neutropenia and thrombocytopenia. In general, however, stiripentol is well tolerated, and some of these adverse side effects may be attributed to coadministered medications.

Stiripentol has numerous drug interactions. Enzyme-inducing drugs, including *carbamazepine, phenobarbital, phenytoin*, and *primidone*, increase stiripentol clearance and decrease plasma levels, while stiripentol inhibits metabolism of phenytoin, carbamazepine, *phenobarbital, valproic acid*, and *clobazam* and its active metabolite.

Stiripentol is licensed specifically for adjunctive treatment of young children aged three years and older, particularly those with Dravet syndrome. Diacomit is available as 250- and 500-mg capsules and sachets. Treatment is initiated at 50 mg/kg per day in two or three divided doses and increased every three days by 100 mg/kg per day to a total maximum dose of 4 g. It is usually administered in combination with clobazam, valproic acid, or both. Therapeutic serum levels have not been determined; however, levels of coadministered drugs that might be affected by enzyme inducers should be monitored.

Succinimides

METHSUXIMIDE

The chemical name for *methsuximide* is *N,2-dimethyl-2-phenylsuccinimide* (Browne et al., 2008). This compound differs from ethosuximide in the substitution of a phenyl for an alkyl moiety. Methsuximide has been marketed in the United States under the trade name *Celontin* since 1957. It is also known in some countries as *Petinutin*.

The mechanisms of action of methsuximide are less well understood than those of *ethosuximide*. Some differences are clearly apparent in the greater activity of the former against experimental models of generalized tonic-clonic and focal seizures, including amygdaloid kindling (Teschendorf and Kretzschmar, 1985). This broader spectrum of action is presumably due to the phenyl substituent. Approximately two-thirds of methsuximide is metabolized by the liver. The primary metabolite is an *N-demethylated* product, *2-methyl-2-phenylsuccinimide*, which also possess antiseizure potency. Whereas the half-life of methsuximide is one to four hours, the half-life of the active metabolite is approximately 40 hours. Methsuximide and its metabolite are widely distributed throughout the body, including the brain, and protein binding is 45–60%.

Side effects are somewhat more problematic with methsuximide than with ethosuximide. Serious toxic reactions include severe depression, fever, periorbital edema, skin rash, blood dyscrasias, nephropathy, and hepatic dysfunction. Methsuximide can elevate plasma levels of phenytoin and phenobarbital.

Methsuximide has been used as a second-line drug against absence seizures but is actually more useful as adjunctive treatment for generalized tonic-clonic and focal seizures, particularly temporal lobe seizures. Celontin is available in 150- and 300-mg capsules. The usual daily dose is 10–25 mg/kg divided into two portions. Therapy is begun gradually and monitored by plasma concentration of the *N-desmethyl* metabolite, which is usually kept between 20–40 µg/ml. Methsuximide melts at 124°F and should not be stored near heat sources.

PHENSUXIMIDE

The chemical name for *phensuximide* is *N-methyl-2-phenylsuccinimide*. Like methsuximide, this compound has a phenyl substituent.

It has been marketed in the United States under the trade name *Milontin* since 1953 and is known by this name in most other countries. Like *methsuximide*, phensuximide is metabolized to an active *N-desmethyl* derivative, *2-phenylsuccinimide*. Consequently, the spectrum of action and toxicity of phensuximide are similar to those of methsuximide. The parent compound has a half-life of about eight hours, and the active metabolite is rapidly converted to an inactive product. The ratio of plasma concentration of phensuximide to active metabolite at steady state is approximately 3:1.

Phensuximide is less effective than methsuximide, because neither the drug nor its active metabolite accumulates in plasma. Therefore, phensuximide is used infrequently. Milontin is available as 500-mg capsules, and the recommended daily dose is 20–40 mg/kg divided into three or four portions. The therapeutic ranges for plasma concentration of the parent drug and its metabolite have not been determined.

Sulthiame

Sulthiame is *tetrahydro-2-p-sulfamoylphenyl-2H-1,2-thiazine-1–1-dioxide*, which has been marketed in Europe and Australia since the 1960s under the trade name *Ospolot*, among others, but has never been marketed in the United States. It is chemically related to *acetazolamide* and is about 1/16 as potent a CA inhibitor. Antiseizure properties appear also to be related to its effect on voltage-gated Na^+ channels and inhibition of glutamate release (Browne et al., 2008).

Sulthiame is rapidly absorbed, with peak time of one to five hours, and pharmacokinetics is linear. Protein binding is 29%. Twenty-five percent to 50% of sulthiame is metabolized in the liver to an inactive hydroxylated derivative, and the remainder is excreted unchanged in the urine. Elimination half-life is 8–15 hours in adults and 5–7 hours in children.

Side effects of CA inhibition are common, including hyperpnea and exertional dyspnea, which can be frightening when severe, paresthesias, and renal stones. Other side effects include headache, somnolence, ataxia, hypersalivation, dizziness, psychosis, catatonia, and weight loss. Serious idiosyncratic reactions, including Stevens-Johnson syndrome, occur rarely. Teratogenic risk is unknown.

Sulthiame inhibits the metabolism of phenytoin, and the increased levels of coadministered phenytoin were in part responsible for some of the positive antiseizure effects noted in early studies of sulthiame. Sulthiame also increases plasma levels of *lamotrigine* and *phenobarbital*. *Carbamazepine* and *primidone* increase clearance of sulthiame and decrease plasma levels. Pharmacodynamic interactions cause sulthiame to exacerbate adverse effects of primidone, administration with other CA inhibitors increases the risk of kidney stone formation, and enhanced toxicity can occur when patients taking sulthiame drink alcohol.

Sulthiame is particularly recommended by some workers for the treatment of the genetic focal epilepsies, such as *benign childhood epilepsy with centrotemporal spikes*, and also for juvenile myoclonic epilepsy. Ospolot is available in 50- and 200-mg tablets. The recommended maintenance dose is 200–600 mg per day in adults and 5–10 mg/kg per day for children in two divided doses. Treatment can begin with one-half of the minimum maintenance dose and be increased by this dose at weekly intervals to achieve a serum level of 2–10 μg/ml. Sulthiame should not be prescribed in patients with an allergy to sulfonamides.

NEW-DRUG DEVELOPMENT

In 1937, when Merritt and Putnam discovered the antiseizure properties of phenytoin (Merritt and Putnam, 1938), the US federal regulations were so lax that *Dilantin* was marketed in the United States within months. The *Food, Drug, and Cosmetic Act of 1938* subsequently established the requirement of proof of safety before new drugs could be sold for clinical purposes. The *Drug Amendment Act of 1962* (the *Kefauver-Harris Amendment*) required that standards of efficacy also be demonstrated. Such laws, in the United States and abroad, provided necessary protection for the consumer but greatly increased the cost to the pharmaceutical industry for the development of new medications. No new specific antiseizure agents were introduced in the United States between 1960 and 1974, presumably because the market potential was viewed as insufficient to justify the necessary corporate investment (Cereghino, 1988). During the late 1970s and 80s, the *Epilepsy Branch* of the *National Institute of Neurological Diseases and Stroke (NINDS)* facilitated new drug development with the *Antiepileptic Drug Development (ADD) Program* (Gladding et al., 1985), which screens promising new compounds and provides support and supervision for clinical trials (Porter et al., 1984; Cereghino, 1988). Approval of *carbamazepine, clonazepam, valproic acid*, and *clorazepate* for treatment of epilepsy in the United States resulted directly from these efforts. Subsequently, there was an increased interest on the part of the pharmaceutical industry to design new antiseizure drugs based on targets identified through basic research on epilepsy. Beginning with European approval of *vigabatrin* in 1989 and the FDA approval of *gabapentin* in 1993, 17 new antiseizure drugs have been marketed in the United States and Europe and are currently in general use. Despite this tremendous increase in available new antiseizure agents, the percentage of patients with pharmacoresistant seizures has not changed appreciably, suggesting that new drugs are effective against the same pharmacosensitive seizures as older drugs, most likely because the screening procedures for potential antiseizure compounds remain, for the most part, the same (Löscher and Schmidt, 2011). Consequently, the pharmaceutical industry has a reduced interest in pursuing production of new antiseizure drugs that have the same effectiveness as, and differ only in their side effect profiles from, older drugs. It remains a challenge for the epilepsy community to identify novel targets, more cost-effective screening methods, and biomarkers for pharmacoresistant seizures in order to restimulate the pharmaceutical industry's interest in epilepsy.

Development of new drugs for epilepsy begins with the synthesis of compounds that might possess antiseizure activity. Preclinical evaluation then requires screening these compounds in the animal laboratory for antiseizure and toxic properties (White et al., 2008a). Promising compounds are subsequently evaluated in controlled clinical trials (French et al., 2008).

Identification of New Compounds

New compounds come from the pharmaceutical industry and from academic medicinal chemists. They are recognized as potential antiseizure agents through essentially four routes of investigation:

1) Specific relationships between chemical structure and pharmacodynamic activity can be derived from previous experience with effective drugs. Knowledge of a desired *structure-activity relationship (SAR)* (Jones and Woodbury, 1982; Schafer, 1985; Weaver and Sankar, 2008) directs chemists to design compounds with a particular structural feature to achieve a particular pharmacological action. Because of reliance on this strategy, until 1968, all antiseizure drugs used in the United States had chemical structures resembling those of *phenytoin* and *phenobarbital*.

2) SARs also suggest ways in which chemists might modify the structure of existing antiseizure drugs to increase the potency and decrease the side effects of compounds. Thus a successful drug often gives rise to more successful analogs.

3) The antiseizure potency of a compound may be serendipitously discovered. For instance, *valproic acid* was synthesized in 1881, but was found to protect against seizures in 1963 only because it was used as a solvent for other experimental agents (Meunier et al., 1963).

4) As a result of advances in neuroscience, compounds can now be identified because they modify aspects of neuronal activity known to influence specific epileptic phenomena (Meldrum, 1986b, 2008). Some compounds that enhance GABA-mediated inhibition suppress seizures, but nonspecific depression of normal cerebral function also occurs. Drugs that appear to act only on excessive excitation by blocking NMDA receptors or Ca^{2+} entry into cells might cause hallucinations and disrupt important normal functions such as memory. Voltage-gated Na^+ channels remain an important target and a recently released drug, *ezogabine*, enhances the opening of K^+ channels. Other novel targets have been identified after the antiseizure properties have been demonstrated, such as the Sv2a site for *levetiracetam*, which appears to be involved in vesicle trafficking (Lynch et al., 2004). The challenge of the future will be to modify these compounds for more selective antiseizure activity.

Preclinical Evaluation

Because screening of new compounds for antiseizure activity is time-consuming, costly, and poorly standardized, most US potential antiseizure drugs have been evaluated by the ADD Program's *Anticonvulsant Screening Project (ASP)*. Well over 30,000 compounds have been tested, approximately one-third coming from the pharmaceutical industry and two-thirds from academic chemists (Cereghino, 1988; French and Ben Menachem, 2008). The screening procedure consists of several phases including: anticonvulsant identification, quantification and differentiation, assessment of proconvulsant potential, mechanisms-of-action studies, and determination of neurotoxicity (White et al., 2002). The first phase identifies specific antiseizure activity and is the most restrictive step along the road from synthesis to clinic. The objective of screening is to allow the drug sponsor to determine whether to pursue further studies of the compound, which would then require filing a full *investigational new drug (IND)* application with the FDA.

Most screening programs use the mouse MES model for assessing effects of the compound on convulsant activity and seizure spread and the mouse subcutaneous PTZ model for assessing effects of the drug on seizure threshold and myoclonic seizure–like activity (Chapter 4). As noted earlier, such limited procedures have been criticized for screening out only drugs with antiseizure properties similar to those of *phenytoin* and *ethosuximide*, which are already effective agents (Löscher and Schmidt, 2011). New compounds that might be ideal drugs for the treatment of epileptic phenomena that are pharmacoresistant, such as limbic and atonic seizures, may not have anticonvulsant or antiabsence potency and would not be identified by this screening process. Levetiracetam, for instance, failed MES and PTZ screening but was effective against amygdala kindling (Klitgaard et al., 1998; Löscher et al., 1998). Levetiracetam is now one of the most effective drugs for temporal lobe seizures. For this reason, the ASP and other screening programs have incorporated additional models, including the *6-Hz limbic seizure test* and the *amygdala-kindled model* (Chapter 4). When a potential therapy fails to block the seizure induced by MES or PTZ stimulation, it is subjected to one or both of these seizure tests. These two alternative tests help to avoid overlooking a potentially interesting antiseizure drug; for example, levetiracetam displays activity in both of these models and were it submitted to the ASP today, it would not likely be missed.

Although a great variety of alternative screening techniques are available, ranging from repetitive firing in dissociated neuronal cultures to limbic kindling (Meldrum, 1986b; White et al., 2008a; Löscher, 2011), they are often time-consuming and difficult to standardize. Furthermore, the relationships of these models to the various forms of human epilepsy have not been clarified (Chapter 4). Expansion of future drug-screening programs will improve the potential for identifying agents effective against clinical ictal events that are inadequately controlled by available antiseizure drugs. In addition to a continued search for more effective antiseizure drugs with fewer adverse side effects, there is also an urgent need for agents that will treat pharmacoresistant seizures, prevent epileptogenesis, and ameliorate disabling comorbidities. A concerted effort is being made to improve and standardize preclinical drug development (Galanopoulou et al., 2012; Simonato et al., 2012). Table 15–2 lists the rodent models currently in use for such preclinical studies.

Initial screening procedures identify neurotoxicity by the inability of a mouse to maintain its balance on a rotating rod. In later phases, other aspects of gait and station are tested, as well as sedative side effects and median lethal dose. Less than 1% of compounds entering the ASP successfully complete all phases of study. Those that do are then subjected to preclinical toxicology studies. Two weeks of drug administration in two species are required before single doses can be given to human volunteers. Complete biochemical, pathological, and teratological assessments after 6- to 12-month administration to animals are necessary before clinical trials can be carried out with patients. Simultaneous studies on mechanisms of action, pharmacokinetics, and dose determinations are also usually performed during this time.

Clinical Evaluation

When preclinical evaluation indicates that a new compound might be a clinically effective antiseizure agent, and required preclinical toxicology studies reveal no serious toxic risks, the drug sponsor can apply to the FDA for a *Notice of Claimed Investigational Exemption for a New Drug (IND)*. Clinical studies are then carried out in three phases (French et al., 2008). *Phase I* consists of administration of single and ascending doses to volunteer subjects to determine safety. *Phase II* involves pilot studies by clinical neuropharmacologists, who assess the efficacy of the drug in patients, further define pharmacokinetics, determine appropriate dose amounts and schedules, identify drug interactions, and obtain other information essential for designing the large controlled clinical trials that constitute the last phase. *Phase III* requires two independent controlled clinical trials or a multiple-center investigation in which data from at least three participating investigators can be independently evaluated. The road from preclinical compound identification to Phase III trials is long, expensive, and fraught with failure. Because so few drugs make it to this point, the process is referred to by the industry as the *"valley of death."* The government ADD program has made early antiseizure drug development possible by assuming much of this risk. This agency was also instrumental in organizing and supporting Phase II and Phase III clinical trials in collaboration with drug sponsors; however, budget restrictions in recent years have left these trials to the pharmaceutical industry, which will realize the profits when a successful drug is brought to market.

Identification of new effective antiseizure drugs ultimately depends on the appropriate design and performance of clinical trials. These trials require expensive and technically complex

Table 15–2 Representative Rodent Models of Seizures, Epileptogenesis, and Epilepsies in Preclinical Studies

Model of Seizures or Epilepsy	Seizure Type	NIH AED Screening Program	Used in Testing Effects in Drug-Resistant Seizures or Epilepsy	Used in Testing Antiepileptogenesis Effects	Used in Testing Effects on Comorbidities	Used in Early-Life AET Studies
Maximal electroshock seizures	Tonic-clonic	Yes	No	No	No	No
Pentylenetetrazol model	Clonic	Yes	No	No	No	No
Low-dose pentylenetetrazol model	Generalized absence	No	No	No	No	No
Bicuculline, picrotoxin models	Clonic	Yes	No	No	No	Yes
Flurothyl model	Clonic	No	No	No	No	Yes
Spike-wave discharge models	Generalized absence					
Genetic absence epilepsy rats of Strasbourg		No		Yes	Yes	No
WAG/Rij, γ-butyrolactone		No		Yes	Yes	No
Monogenic mouse models of absence epilepsy	Generalized absence					
Tetanus toxin	Focal	No	Yes	Yes	Yes	No
Audiogenic seizures	Wild running (focal onset); generalized tonic-clonic	Yes	No	No	Yes	No
Electrical kindling (corneal, hippocampal, amygdala)	Focal	Yes	Yes	Yes		Yes
Lamotrigine-resistant kindled rats	Focal	Yes	Yes	Yes		No
6-Hz electrical stimulation (32 and 44 mA)	Focal	Yes (32 mA)	Yes (44 mA)	No	No	No
Models of dysplasias						
Methylazoxymethanol-induced heterotopias (in two-hit models)	Focal	No	Yes	Yes		No
Post–status epilepticus spontaneous seizures						
Chemical induction (kainic acid, (lithium)–pilocarpine)	Focal onset, limbic	Yes	Yes	Yes	Yes	Yes
Stimulation (continuous hippocampal, perforant pathway, sustained amygdala stimulation)	Focal onset, limbic	No	Yes	Yes	Yes	No
Traumatic brain injury						
Cortical undercut	Focal onset	No				No
FeCl$_2$	Focal onset	No				No
Fluid percussion	Focal onset	No	Yes			No
Controlled cortical impact	Focal onset	No		Yes		No
Early-life epilepsy syndromes						
Hypoxia ± ischemia	Hypoxic ± ischemic	No	Yes	Yes		Yes
Febrile seizure/hyperthermia models	Febrile seizure	No				No
Infantile spasms models (i.e., multiple hit)	Infantile spasms	No	Yes	Yes	Yes	Yes
Transgenic rodent models	Genetic	No		Yes		No
In vitro models	Genetic	Yes	Yes	Yes	No	Yes

This table is largely based on the reported use of the models in the literature, not on the demonstrated suitability of these models for the indicated purposes of antiepilepsy drug testing.
AED = antiepilepsy drug; AET = antiepilepsy therapy; NIH = National Institutes of Health.
From Galanopoulou et al., 2012, with permission.

planning and management (Porter and White, 1986; French et al., 2008). Adequate numbers of patients with seizures that can be appropriately characterized and quantified must be recruited. The compound under study should be administered in a randomized, double-blind manner, taking into account confounding pharmacokinetic properties of the drug, drug interactions (because patients included in clinical trials are usually on other antiseizure medications as well), and ethical issues. Appropriate statistical approaches applied to a variety of experimental designs can determine whether a test compound is sufficiently effective and non-toxic to be marketed as an antiseizure drug. If this arduous task is successfully completed, the results are submitted to the FDA with a *New Drug Application (NDA)*.

Two particular problems with Phase III trials have limited the ability to bring potentially important new drugs to market. First, for a drug to be approved as monotherapy, FDA requires that it show efficacy versus a placebo; equivalent efficacy or noninferiority compared with an existing drug is not sufficient evidence. This requirement makes it difficult to design ethical monotherapy trials, and most new drugs are initially approved for adjunctive therapy only. Second, the vast majority of clinical trials are carried out on patients loosely defined as having "medically refractory complex partial seizures with or without secondarily generalized seizures". This is an amorphous group that undoubtedly includes multiple seizure types. Thus it may not be possible to recognize that a drug is highly effective against one specific seizure type if the effectiveness for other types is poor. Better classification of seizure types based on pathophysiological mechanisms would greatly facilitate clinical trial design (Engel, 2001, 2006; Berg et al., 2010) (Chapter 1).

The discovery of new drugs for epilepsy and their testing in clinical trials would be greatly facilitated if there were reliable *biomarkers* for specific types of epileptic seizures and epilepsy syndromes. High-throughput, cost-effective, animal models for screening tens of thousands of potential antiseizure compounds that might have efficacy against very specific but clinically important seizure mechanisms would be possible. Reliable biomarkers that could substitute for seizure recurrence as outcome measures for clinical trials would not only greatly reduce the expense of new studies but also reduce the risk to participants, particularly when the goal is to demonstrate effectiveness as monotherapy as compared with a placebo. The cost involved in identifying and validating potential antiepileptogenic interventions is currently prohibitive but could become practical with the development of reliable biomarkers of epileptogenesis for cost-effective, rapid-throughput screening, for identifying animals and patients at high risk for seizure development following a potential epileptogenic insult, and for monitoring effectiveness. For clinical trials of potential antiepileptogenic compounds, reliable biomarkers of epileptogenicity would also be necessary to document prevention and cure. The search for reliable biomarkers of epileptogenesis and epileptogenicity is a high-priority research effort (Engel, 2011a, 2011b) (Chapter 12).

DRUGS UNDER INVESTIGATION

At any given time, many compounds are under investigation as potential antiseizure drugs, and promising compounds are frequently entered into or withdrawn from investigation. Consequently, any list of potential antiseizure compounds currently undergoing clinical evaluation will undoubtedly be considerably out of date by the time this book is published. In the previous edition, published in 1989, 19 drugs were listed as undergoing clinical evaluation (Cereghino, 1988) and since then 17 have become commercially available: clobazam, ezogabine, felbamate, gabapentin, lacosamide, lamotrigine, levetiracetam, nitrazepam, oxcarbazepine, pregabalin, progabide, rufinamide, stiripentol, tiagabine, topiramate, vigabatrin, and zonisamide. This reflects the tremendous interest in new-drug development in the 1970s and 1980s, stimulated in large part by the ADD. Unfortunately, the pipeline is now somewhat reduced, as noted previously; however, several new drugs under investigation show particular promise and deserve brief mention here (White et al., 2008c; Patsalos and Sander, 2009; Bialer et al., 2010).

Drugs in Phase III Trials

BRIVARACETAM

When the site of action of *levetiracetam* was found to be the Sv2a, a search for an analog with a higher affinity for Sv2a than that of levetiracetam was conducted, which resulted in the identification of *brivaracetam, [2S]-2-[(4R)-2-oxo-4-propylpyrrolidinyl]butanamide* (von Rosenstiel and Perucca, 2009). Brivaracetam has a 10-fold-higher binding affinity for Sv2a than levetiracetam does and also inhibits voltage-dependent Na⁺ channels; it therefore has a higher antiseizure potency than levetiracetam. Efficacy profile is similar to levetiracetam.

GANAXOLONE

Ganaxolone is *3α-hydroxy-3β-methyl-5α-pregnan-20-one*, an analog of the endogenous steroid *allopregnanolone*, which exerts an agonistic effect on $GABA_A$ receptors. It is effective against focal and generalized tonic-clonic seizures, but continuous usage of ganaxolone, unlike the benzodiazepines, does not result in tolerance. Clinical trials suggest efficacy in infantile spasms.

PERAMPANEL

Perampanel is *5′-(2-cyanophenyl)-1′-phenyl-2,3′-vipyridinyl- 6′(1′)H-one*. It was formerly known as E2007 and is a first-in-class highly selective noncompetitive AMPA receptor antagonist. Clinical trials indicate efficacy against focal and generalized tonic-clonic seizures.

Drugs in Preclinical Development

2-DEOXY-D-GLUCOSE

2-Deoxyglucose is a chemical analog of glucose that is a substrate for the glucose transporter and is thus taken up into cells like glucose; however, it is not then further metabolized. For this reason, ¹⁸F-*fluorodeoxyglucose (FDG)* has been used for many years as a tracer for the measurement of glucose metabolism using *positron emission tomography (PET)*. It is, however, also an inhibitor of glycolysis and exerts an antiseizure effect. It is effective in the laboratory against a variety of models, including *MES, subcutaneous PTZ, kindling, status-induced*, and *audiogenic seizures*.

HUPERZINE A

Huperzine A is a *sesquiterpine lycopodium alkaloid* isolated from the Chinese club moss (*Huperzia serrata*), known as *Qian Ceng Ta* in Chinese medicine, where it is used to treat Alzheimer's disease. It is classified as a dietary supplement by the FDA. Huperzine A is a potent, specific, and reversible acetylcholinesterase inhibitor; reduces glutamate-induced toxicity, most likely as a noncompetitive NMDA antagonist; and elevates norepinephrine and dopamine levels in cortex.

ICA105665

ICA105665 is a molecule that opens KCNQ K⁺ ion channels and is believed to exert an antiseizure effect similar to that of *ezogabine*. It represents a continued effort to develop new antiseizure compounds that act on voltage-gated K⁺ channels.

T2000

T2000 is *1,3-dimethoxymethyl-5,5-diphenyl-barbituric acid*, a prodrug that has been developed for the treatment of essential tremor. It does, however, have a mechanism of action similar to that of *phenytoin* and the barbiturates. It is active against both MES- and subcutaneous PTZ–induced seizures in the laboratory and could find a place as a clinical treatment for epileptic seizures.

TONABERSAT

Tonabersat is a novel *benzoylamino-benzopyran* compound that is believed to act as an antiseizure agent by blocking gap junctions. It is effective in the laboratory against MES and the tonic but not myoclonic components of PTZ-induced seizures.

VALPROIC ACID DERIVATIVES

Several *valproic acid* derivatives, including *valnoctamide* and *valrocemide*, are under investigation as possible nonteratogenic and nonhepatotoxic compounds with antiseizure potency equal to or greater than that of the parent drug.

YKP3089

YKP3089 is a novel compound that is effective in the laboratory against a number of experimental models, including MES, subcutaneous PTZ, *picrotoxin-induced seizures*, and kindling.

VX-765

VX-765 is a novel *caspase-1 inhibitor* that decreases the production of *interleukin-1 beta (IL-1β)*, which is responsible for immune and inflammatory responses implicated in epileptogenicity. It has demonstrated efficacy against several animal models and in Phase II clinical trials for pharmacoresistant focal seizures.

SUMMARY AND CONCLUSIONS

At the time of publication of the first edition of this textbook, in 1989, 18 antiseizure drugs had been approved by the FDA, but only four were considered first-line drugs: phenytoin and carbamazepine for focal and generalized tonic-clonic seizures, ethosuximide for absence seizures, and valproic acid as the only broad-spectrum drug. In addition, diazepam was the treatment of choice for generalized tonic-clonic status epilepticus. Since then, the number of available drugs has almost doubled, with at least five new drugs in standard usage for focal and generalized tonic-clonic seizures (clobazam, gabapentin, lacosamide, oxcarbazepine, and pregabalin); four in general usage as broad-spectrum agents (lamotrigine, levetiracetam, topiramate, and zonisamide); and other, newer drugs that may have more specific benefits, such as rufinamide for LGS, vigabatrin for infantile spasms, stiripentol for Dravet syndrome, and a number of alternative treatments for generalized tonic status epilepticus, including lorazepam, midazolam, propofol, and fosphenytoin. This impressive development can be attributed largely to increased interest, on the part of the NINDS ADD as well as industry, during the 1970s and 80s in developing new antiseizure compounds. These drugs were frequently designed to act on specific targets responsible for seizure generation, such as voltage-gated ion channels, ligand-gated ion channels, and glutamate and GABA neurotransmission. Often, however, the mechanisms of action were different from those intended and new mechanisms have sometimes been identified, such as the vesicle trafficking modulation of Sv2a by levetiracetam.

A variety of comparison trials of early standard and second-generation antiseizure drugs have demonstrated relatively similar effectiveness against the intended seizure types but greatly different side effect profiles. In general, the newer drugs are better tolerated and commonly preferred for this reason; however, two highly effective drugs, felbamate and vigabatrin, are used only as a last resort, because of serious side effects that became apparent only with postmarketing surveys. Another advantage of some of the newer drugs, for instance, gabapentin, pregabalin, lacosimide, levetiracetam, and zonisamide, is relative lack of drug-drug interactions.

As discussed in Chapter 14, apart from narrow- versus broad-spectrum potency, the choice of antiseizure medication in individual patients depends more on the acceptability of the side effect profile and dosing intervals, as well as the need to be concerned about drug-drug interactions, than on effectiveness against seizures. Cost may also be an issue for some patients, and it remains a major concern in countries with limited resources, where it is often the most important adverse effect of pharmacotherapy. Extended-release formulations exist for many drugs with relatively short half-lives, permitting more convenient dosing regimens, and intravenous preparations are now available for several.

There were 19 potential antiseizure drugs under evaluation at the time the first edition of *Seizures and Epilepsy* was published in 1989. The pipeline has dwindled significantly, however, in part for economic reasons. There remains a great need for additional antiseizure drugs effective against specific seizure types that continue to exhibit a high degree of pharmacoresistance, such as limbic seizures, atonic seizures, and infantile spasms, as well as for antiepileptogenic drugs that might prevent or cure epilepsy. Interest on the part of the pharmaceutical industry has understandably waned with the reduction in profits resulting from new drugs that have the same effectiveness as the older drugs and differ only in their side effect profiles. It is now the responsibility of the epilepsy community to rekindle the interest of the pharmaceutical industry by finding novel targets, devising more cost-effective, rapid-throughput screening methodologies, and identifying reliable biomarkers of epileptogenicity, pharmacoresistance, and epileptogenesis for the purpose of discovering and validating new antiseizure and antiepileptogenic drugs.

Pharmacogenomics is only just beginning as an area of investigation that should eventually permit determination of drug effectiveness and toxicity in individual patients, leading to the ultimate goal of personalized pharmacotherapy.

REFERENCES

Albright, PS (1983). Effects of carbamazepine, clonazepam, and phenytoin on seizure threshold in amygdala and cortex. Exp Neurol 79:11–17.

Almeida, L, Nunes,T, Sicard, E, Rocha, JF, Falcão, A, Brunet, JS, Lefebvre, M, and Soares-da-Silva P (2010). Pharmacokinetic interaction study between eslicarbazepine acetate and lamotrigine in healthy subjects. Acta Neurol Scand 121:257–264.

Arif, H, Buchsbaum, R, Pierro, J, Whalen, M, Sims, J, Resor, R, Jr, Bazil, C, Hirsch, LJ (2010). Comparative effectiveness of 10 antiepileptic drugs in older adults with epilepsy. Arch Neurol 67:408–415.

Asadi-Pooya, AA, and Sperling, MR (2009). Antiepileptic Drugs: A Clinician's Manual. New York: Oxford University Press.

Bartholini, G, Bossi, L, Lloyd, KG, and Morselli, PL (eds) (1985). Epilepsy and GABA Receptor Agonists: Basic and Therapeutic Research. New York: Raven Press.

Ben-Menachem, E, Dulac, O, and Chiron, C (2008). Vigabatrin. In Epilepsy: A Comprehensive Textbook, 2nd ed. Edited by J Engel, Jr, and TA Pedley. Philadelphia: Lippincott Williams & Wilkins, pp. 1683–1693.

Berg, AT, Berkovic, SF, Brodie, MJ, Buchhalter, J, Cross, JH, van Emde Boas, W, Engel, J, Jr, French, J, Glauser, TA, Mathern, GW, Moshé, SL, Nordli D, Jr, Plouin, P, Scheffer, IE (2010). Revised terminology and concepts for organization of seizures and epilepsies: Report of the ILAE Commission on Classification and Terminology, 2005–2009. Epilepsia 51:676–685.

Bergey, GK (2008). Pregabalin. In Epilepsy: A Comprehensive Textbook, 2nd ed. Edited by J Engel, Jr, and TA Pedley. Philadelphia: Lippincott Williams & Wilkins, pp. 1629–1637.

Beydoun, A, Nasreddine, WM, and Albini, F (2008a). Oxcarbazepine. In Epilepsy: A Comprehensive Textbook, 2nd ed. Edited by J Engel, Jr, and TA Pedley. Philadelphia: Lippincott Williams & Wilkins, pp. 1593–1598.

Beydoun, AA, Farrell, K, and Nasreddine, WM (2008b). Valproate. In Epilepsy: A Comprehensive Textbook, 2nd ed. Edited by J Engel, Jr, and TA Pedley. Philadelphia: Lippincott Williams & Wilkins, pp. 1673–1681.

Bialer, M, Johannessen, SI, Levy, RH, Perucca, E, Tomson, T, and White, HS (2010). Progress report on new antiepileptic drugs: A summary of the Tenth Eilat Conference (EILAT X). Epilepsy Res 92:89–124.

Biton, V (2009). Rufinamide. In The Treatment of Epilepsy, 3rd ed. Edited by S Shorvon, E Perucca, and J Engel, Jr. West Sussex, UK: Wiley-Blackwell, pp. 647–655.

Booker, HE (1982). Trimethadione: Toxicity. In Antiepileptic Drugs, 2nd ed. Edited by DM Woodbury, JK Penry, and CE Pippenger. New York: Raven Press, pp. 701–703.

Bookheimer, S, Schrader, LM, Rausch, R., Sankar, R, and Engel, J, Jr (2005). Reduced anesthetization during the intracarotid amobarbital (Wada) test in patients taking carbonic anhydrase-inhibiting medications. Epilepsia 46:236–243.

Bourgeois, BFD (2008a). Primidone. In Epilepsy: A Comprehensive Textbook, Second Edition. Edited by J Engel Jr and TA Pedley. Philadelphia: Lippincott Williams & Wilkins, pp. 1639–1645.

Bourgeois, BFD (2008b). Valproate. In Epilepsy: A Comprehensive Textbook, 2nd ed. Edited by J Engel, Jr, and TA Pedley. Philadelphia: Lippincott Williams & Wilkins, pp. 685–697.

Bourgeois, BFD (2009). Valproate. In The Treatment of Epilepsy, 3rd ed. Edited by S Shorvon, E Perucca, and J Engel, Jr. West Sussex, UK: Wiley-Blackwell, pp. 685–697.

Bourgeois, B, Beaumanoir, A, Blajev, B, de la Cruz, N, Despland, PA, Egli, M, Geudelin, B, Kaspar, U, Ketz, E, Kronauer, C, Meyer, C, Scollo-Lavizzari, G, Tosi, C, Vassella, F, and Zagury, S (1987). Monotherapy with valproate in primary generalized epilepsies. Epilepsia 28(suppl 2):S8–S11.

Brodie, MJ, Lerche, H, Gil-Nagel, A, et al. (2010). Efficacy and safety of adjunctive ezogabine (retigabine) in refractory partial epilepsy. Neurology 75:1817–1824.

Bromfield, EB (2008). Ethosuximide. In Epilepsy: A Comprehensive Textbook, 2nd ed. Edited by J Engel, Jr, and TA Pedley. Philadelphia: Lippincott Williams & Wilkins, pp. 1557–1560.

Browne, TR, Leduc, BW, Kosta-Rokosz, MD, Bromfield, EB, Ramsay, RE, and de Toledo, J (2008). Trimethadione, paraldehyde, phenacemide, bromides, sulthiame, acetazolamide, and methsuximide. In Epilepsy: A Comprehensive Textbook, 2nd ed. Edited by J Engel, Jr, and TA Pedley. Philadelphia: Lippincott Williams & Wilkins, pp. 1703–1719.

Caccia, S, and Garattini, S (1985). Benzodiazepines. In Antiepileptic Drugs. Edited by H-H Frey and D Janz. New York: Springer-Verlag, pp. 575–593.

Camfield, P, and Camfield, C (2008). Benzodiazepines used primarily for chronic treatment (clobazam, clonazepam, clorazepate and nitrazepam). In Epilepsy: A Comprehensive Textbook, 2nd ed. Edited by J Engel, Jr, and TA Pedley. Philadelphia: Lippincott Williams & Wilkins, pp. 421–430.

Carraz, G, Fau, R, Chateau, R, and Bonnin, J (1964). Communication à propos des premiers essais cliniques sur l'activité anti-épileptique de l'acid n-dipropylacétique (sel de Na). Ann Med Psychol (Paris) 122:577–585.

Cereghino, JJ (1988). New and old antiepileptic drugs. In Mechanisms of Epileptogenesis: The Transition to Seizure. Edited by M Dichter. New York: Plenum Press., pp. 239–254.

Chadwick, DW, and Browne, TR (2008). Gabapentin. In Epilepsy: A Comprehensive Textbook, 2nd ed. Edited by J Engel, Jr, and TA Pedley. Philadelphia: Lippincott Williams & Wilkins, pp. 1569–1574.

Chapman, A, Keane, PE, Meldrum, BS, Simiand, J, and Vernieres, JC (1982). Mechanism of anticonvulsant action of valproate. Prog Neurobiol 19:315–359.

Chen, P, Lin, J-J, Lu, C-S, et al. (2011). Carbamazepine-induced toxic effects and HLA-B*1502 screening in Taiwan. N Engl J Med 364:1126–1133.

Chung, WH, Hung, SI, Hong, HS, et al. (2004). Medical genetics: A marker for Stevens-Johnson syndrome. Nature 428:486.

Coatsworth, JJ, and Penry, KJ (1972). General principles: Clinical efficacy and use. In Antiepileptic Drugs. Edited by DM Woodbury, JK Penry, and RP Schmidt. New York: Raven Press, pp. 87–96.

Coker, SB, Holmes, EW, Egel, RT (1987). Penacemide therapy of complex partial epilepsy in children: Determination of plasma drug concentrations. Neurology; 37:1861–1866.

Coulter, DA, Huguenard, JR, and Prince, DA (1989). Specific petit mal anticonvulsants reduce calcium currents in thalamic neurons. Neurosci Lett 98:74–78.

Crawford, P, Chadwick, D (1986). A comparative study of progabide, valproate, and placebo as add-on in patients with refractory epilepsy. J Neurol Neurosurg Psychiat 49:1251–1257.

Cross, JH, and Riney, CJ (2009). Topiramate. In The Treatment of Epilepsy, 3rd ed. Edited by S Shorvon, E Perucca, and J Engel, Jr. West Sussex, UK: Wiley-Blackwell, pp. 673–683.

Dam, M (1982). Phenytoin toxicity. In: Antiepileptic Drugs, 2nd ed. Edited by DM Woodbury, JK Penry, and CE Pippenger. New York: Raven Press, pp. 247–256.

Del Amo, EM, Urtti, A, and Yliperttula, M (2008). Pharmacokinetic role of L-type amino acid transporters LAT1 and LAT2. Eur J Pharm Sci 35:161–174.

DeVivo, DC (1983). How to use other drugs (steroids) and the ketogenic diet. In Antiepileptic Drug Therapy in Pediatrics. Edited by PL Morselli, CE Pippenger, and JK Penry. New York: Raven Press, pp. 283–292.

Dreifuss, FE, Santilli, N, Langer, DH, Sweeney, KP, Moline, KA, and Menander, KB (1987). Valproic acid hepatic fatalities: A retrospective review. Neurology 37:379–385.

Eadie, MJ (1982). Other barbiturates: Methylphenobarbital and metharbital. In Antiepileptic Drugs, 2nd ed. Edited by DM Woodbury, JK Penry, and CE Pippenger. New York: Raven Press, pp. 377–393.

Eadie, MJ (2008). Antiepileptic drugs as human teratogens. Exp Opin Drug Safety 7:195–209.

Eadie, MJ (2009). Phenytoin. In The Treatment of Epilepsy, Third Edition. Edited by S Shorvon, E Perucca, and J Engel Jr. West Sussex, UK, Wiley-Blackwell, pp. 605–618.

Eadie, MJ, and Kwan, P (2008). Phenobarbital and other barbiturates. In Epilepsy: A Comprehensive Textbook, 2nd ed. Edited by J Engel, Jr, and TA Pedley. Philadelphia: Lippincott Williams & Wilkins, pp. 1599–1607.

Engel, J Jr (2001). A proposed diagnostic scheme for people with epileptic seizures and with epilepsy: Report of the ILAE Task Force on Classification and Terminology. Epilepsia 42:796–803.

Engel, J, Jr (2006). Report of the ILAE Classification Core Group. Epilepsia 47:1558–1568.

Engel, J Jr (ed) (2011a). Biomarkers in Epilepsy. Biomarkers in Medicine (Special Issue) 5:529–664.

Engel, J Jr (2011b). Biomarkers in epilepsy—Introduction. Biomarkers in Medicine (Special Issue) 5:537–544.

Engel, J, Jr, and Pedley, TA (eds) (2008). Epilepsy: A Comprehensive Textbook, 2nd ed. Philadelphia: Lippincott Williams & Wilkins.

Eriksson, K, and Keränen, T (2009). Stiripentol. In The Treatment of Epilepsy, 3rd ed. Edited by S Shorvon, E Perucca, and J Engel, Jr. West Sussex, UK: Wiley-Blackwell, pp. 657–661.

Everett, GM, and Richards, RK (1944). Comparative anticonvulsant action of 3,5,5-trimethyloxazolidine-2, 4-dione (Tridone), Dilantin, and phenobarbital. J Pharmacol Exp Ther 1:402–407.

Falcão, A, Fuseau, E, Nunes, T, Almeida, L, and Soares-da-Silva,P (2012). Pharmacokinetics, drug interactions and exposure-response relationship of eslicarbazepine acetate in adult patients with partial-onset seizures: Population pharmacokinetic and pharmacokinetic/pharmacodynamic analyses. CNS Drugs 26:79–91.

Faught, E, and Glauser, TA (2008). Topiramate. In Epilepsy: A Comprehensive Textbook, 2nd ed. Edited by J Engel, Jr, and TA Pedley. Philadelphia: Lippincott Williams & Wilkins, pp. 1663–1671.

Faught, E, and Limdi, N (2009). Oxcarbazepine. In The Treatment of Epilepsy, 3rd ed. Edited by S Shorvon, E Perucca, and J Engel, Jr. West Sussex, UK: Wiley-Blackwell, pp. 575–584.

Ferrendelli, JA, and Klunk, WE (1982). Ethosuximide: Mechanisms of action. In Antiepileptic Drugs, 2nd ed. Edited by DM Woodbury, JK Penry, and CE Pippenger. New York: Raven Press, pp. 655–661.

Fertig, EJ, and Mattson, RH (2008). Carbamazepine. In Epilepsy: A Comprehensive Textbook, 2nd ed. Edited by J Engel, Jr, and TA Pedley. Philadelphia: Lippincott Williams & Wilkins, pp. 1543–1555.

French, JA, and Ben-Menachem, E (2008). Overview: antiepileptic drugs. In Epilepsy: A Comprehensive Textbook, 2nd ed. Edited by J Engel, Jr, and TA Pedley. Philadelphia: Lippincott Williams & Wilkins, pp. 1431–1432.

French, JA, and Tonner, F (2009). Levetiracetam. In The Treatment of Epilepsy, 3rd ed. Edited by S Shorvon, E Perucca, and J Engel, Jr. West Sussex, UK: Wiley-Blackwell, pp. 559–573.

French, JA, Glauser, TA, and Schmidt, B (2008). Clinical trials of antiepileptic drugs in adults and children. In Epilepsy: A Comprehensive Textbook, 2nd ed. Edited by J Engel, Jr, and TA Pedley. Philadelphia: Lippincott Williams & Wilkins, pp. 1487–1496.

French, JA, Abou-Khalil, BW, Leroy, RF, Yacubian, EM, Shin, P, Hall, S, Mansbach, H, Nohria, V (2011). Randomized double-blind placebo-controlled trial of ezogabine (retigabine) in partial epilepsy. Neurology 76:1555–1563

Frey, H-H (1985). Primidone. In Antiepileptic Drugs. Edited by H-H Frey and D Janz. New York: Springer-Verlag, pp. 449–477.

Frey, H-H, and Janz, D (eds) (1985). Antiepileptic Drugs. Berlin: Springer-Verlag.

Galanopoulou, AS, Buckmaster, P, Staley, K, Moshé, SL, Perucca, E, Engel, J, Jr, Löscher, W, Noebels, JL, Pitkänen, A, Stables, J, White, SH, O'Brien, TJ, and Simonato, M: Identification of new treatments for epilepsy: Issues in preclinical methodology. Epilepsia. (In press)

Gallagher, BB, and Freer, LS (1985). Barbituric acid derivatives. In Antiepileptic Drugs. Edited by H-H Frey and D Janz. New York: Springer-Verlag, pp. 421–447.

Gastaut, H, Roger, J, Soulayrol, R, Lob, H, and Tassinari, CA (1965). L'action du diazepam (Valium) dans le traitement des formes non convulsives de l'épilepsie généralisée. Rev Neurol 112:99–118.

Gee, NS, Brown, JP, Dissanayake, VU, et al. (1996). The novel anticonvulsant drug, gabapentin (Neurontin), binds to the alpha2delta subunit of a calcium channel. J Biol Chem 271:5768–5776.

Gladding, GD, Kupferberg, HJ, and Swinyard, EA (1985). Antiepileptic Drug Development Program. In Antiepileptic Drugs. Edited by H-H Frey and D Janz. New York: Springer-Verlag, pp. 341–347.

Glaser, GH, Penry, JK, and Woodbury, DM (eds) (1980). Antiepileptic Drugs: Mechanisms of Action. New York: Raven Press.

Glauser, TA, and Bialer, M (2008). Rufinamide. In Epilepsy: A Comprehensive Textbook, 2nd ed. Edited by J Engel, Jr, and TA Pedley. Philadelphia: Lippincott Williams & Wilkins, pp. 1647–1654.

Glauser, TA, and Perucca, E (2009). Ethosuximide. In The Treatment of Epilepsy, 3rd ed. Edited by S Shorvon, E Perucca, and J Engel, Jr. West Sussex, UK: Wiley-Blackwell, pp. 499–509.

Go, CY, Mackay, MT, Weiss, SK, Stephens, D, Adams-Webber, T, Ashwal, S, Snead III, OC (2012). Evidence-based guideline update: Medical treatment of infantile spasms. Neurology :78:1974–1980.

Greenblatt, M, Levin, S, and Schegloff, B (1945). Electroencephalographic findings in cases of bromide intoxication. Arch Neurol Psychiatry 53:431–436.

Hahn, CG, Gyulai, L, Baldassano, CE, et al.: The current understanding of lamotrigine as a mood stabilizer. J Clin Psychiatry 65:791–804.

Hanson, JW, and Smith, DW (1975). The fetal hydantoin syndrome. J Pediatr 87:285–290.

Hauptmann, A (1912). Luminal bei Epilepsie. Munch Med Wochenschr 59:1907–1909.

Heller, AH, Dichter, MA, and Sidman, RL (1983). Anticonvulsant sensitivity of absence seizures in the tottering mutant mouse. Epilepsia 24:25–33.

Holmes, LB, Wysznski, DF, and Lieberman, E (2004). The AED (antiepileptic drug) pregnancy registry: A 6-year experience. Arch Neurol 61:673–678.

Hrachovy, RA, and Frost, JD Jr (2008). Adrenocorticotropic hormone and steroids. In Epilepsy: A Comprehensive Textbook, 2nd ed. Edited by J Engel, Jr, and TA Pedley. Philadelphia: Lippincott Williams & Wilkins, pp. 1519–1529.

Hrachovy, RA, Frost, JD, Jr, Kellaway, P, and Zion, TE (1983). Double blind study of ACTH vs prednisone therapy in infantile spasms. J Pediatrics 103:641–645.

Hunt, S, Russell, A, Smithson, WH, Parsons, L, Robertson, I, Waddell, R, Irwin, B, Morrison, PJ, Morrow, J, and Craig, J (2008). Topiramate in pregnancy: Preliminary experience from the UK Epilepsy and Pregnancy Register. Neurology 71:272–276.

Jeavons, PM, Clark, JE, and Maheshwari, MD (1977). Treatment of generalized epilepsies of childhood and adolescence with sodium valproate (Epilim). Dev Med Child Neurol 19:9–25.

Jones, GL, and Wimbish, GH (1985). Hydantoins. In Antiepileptic Drugs. Edited by H-H Frey and D Janz. New York: Springer-Verlag, pp. 351–419.

Jones, GL, and Woodbury, DM (1982). Principles of drug action: Structure-activity relationships and mechanisms. In Antiepileptic Drugs, 2nd ed. Edited by DM Woodbury, JK Penry, and CE Pippenger. New York: Raven Press, pp. 83–109.

Jurna, I (1985). Electrophysiological effects of antiepileptic drugs. In Antiepileptic Drugs. Edited by H-H Frey and D Janz. New York: Springer-Verlag, pp. 611–658.

Kälviäinen, R: Tiagabine (2008). In Epilepsy: A Comprehensive Textbook, 2nd ed. Edited by J Engel, Jr, and TA Pedley. Philadelphia: Lippincott Williams & Wilkins, pp. 1655–1661.

Kälviäinen, R: Tiagabine (2009). In The Treatment of Epilepsy, 3rd ed. Edited by S Shorvon, E Perucca, and J Engel, Jr. West Sussex, UK: Wiley-Blackwell, pp. 663–672.

Kendell, DA, McEwen, BS, and Enna, SJ (1982). The influence of ACTH and corticosterone on [3H]GABA receptor binding in rat brain. Brain Res 236:365–374.

Klitgaard, H, Matagne, A, Gobert, J, et al. (1998). Evidence for a unique profile of levetiracetam in rodent models of seizures and epilepsy. Eur J Pharmacol 353:191–206.

Krämer, G, and Wohlrab, G (2009). Vigabatrin. In The Treatment of Epilepsy, 3rd ed. Edited by S Shorvon, E Perucca, and J Engel, Jr. West Sussex, UK: Wiley-Blackwell, pp. 699–712.

Kuo, CC, Lin, BJ, Chang HR, et al. (2004). Use-dependent inhibition of the N-methyl-D-aspartate currents by felbamate: A gating modifier with selective binding to the desensitized channels. Mol Pharmacol 65:370–380.

Kutt, H, and Paris-Kutt, H (1982). Phenobarbital: Interactions with other drugs. In Antiepileptic Drugs, 2nd ed. Edited by DM Woodbury, JK Penry, and CE Pippenger. New York: Raven Press, pp. 329–340.

Kwan, P, and Brodie, MJ (2004). Phenobarbital for the treatment of epilepsy in the 21st century: A critical review. Epilepsia 45:1141–1149.

Laxer, KD, Robertson, LT, Julien, RM, and Dow, RS (1980). Phenytoin: Relationship between cerebellar function and epileptic discharges. In Antiepileptic Drugs: Mechanisms of Action. Edited by GH Glaser, JK Penry, and DM Woodbury. New York: Raven Press, pp. 415–427.

Leppik, IE, and White, JR (2009). Felbamate. In The Treatment of Epilepsy, Third Edition. Edited by S Shorvon, E Perucca, and J Engel Jr. West Sussex, UK, Wiley-Blackwell, pp. 511–518.

Levy, RH, Cenraud, B, Loiseau, P, Akbaraly, R, Brachet-Liermain, A, Guyot, M, Gomeni, R, and Morselli, PL (1980). Meal-dependent absorption of enteric-coated sodium valproate. Epilepsia 21:273–280.

Levy, RH, Shen, DD, Abbott, FS, Riggs, KW, and Hachad, H (2002). Chemistry, biotransformation, and pharmacokinetics. In Antiepileptic Drugs, 5th Edition. Edited by RH Levy, RH Mattson, BS Meldrum, and E Perucca. Philadelphia: Lippincott Williams & Wilkins, pp. 780–800.

Levy, RH, Mattson, RH, Meldrum, BS, and Perucca, E (2010). Antiepileptic Drugs. Philadelphia: Lippincott Williams & Wilkins.

Lockard, JS, and Levy, RH (1976). Valproic acid: Reversibly acting drug? Epilepsia 17:477–479.

Locock, C (1857). Discussion of paper by EH Sieveking: Analysis of 52 cases of epilepsy observed by author. Lancet 1:527–528.

Löscher, W (1985). Valproic acid. In Antiepileptic Drugs. Edited by H-H Frey and D Janz. New York: Springer-Verlag, pp. 507–536.

Löscher ,W (2011). Critical review of current animal models of seizures and epilepsy used in the discovery and development of new antiepileptic drugs. Seizure. 20:359–368.

Löscher, W, Honack, D, and Rundtfeldt, C (1998). Antiepileptogenic effects of the novel anticonvulsant levetiracetam (ucb L059) in the kindling model of temporal lobe epilepsy. J Pharmacol Exp Ther 284:474–479.

Löscher, W, Reissmuller, E, and Ebert, U (2000). Anticonvulsant efficacy of gabapentin and levetiracetam in phenytoin-resistant kindled rats. Epilepsy Res 40:63–77.

Löscher, W, and Schmidt, D (2011). Modern antiepileptic drug development has failed to deliver: ways out of the current dilemma. Epilepsia 52:657–678.

Lynch, BA, Lambeng, N, Mocka, K, Kensel-Hammes, P, Bajjalieh, SM, Matagne, A, and Fuks, B (2004). The synaptic vesicle protein SV2A is the binding site for the antiepileptic drug levetiracetam. Proc Natl Acad Sci USA 101:9861–9866.

Macdonald, RL (1999). Cellular actions of antiepileptic drugs. In Antiepileptic Drugs: Pharmacology and Therapeutics. Edited by MJ Eadie and FJE Vajda. Berlin: Springer, pp. 123–150.

Macdonald, R (2002). Benzodiazepines. Mechanism of action. In Antiepileptic Drugs, 5th ed. Edited by R Levy, R Mattson, B Meldrum, et al. Philadelphia: Lippincott, Williams & Wilkins, pp. 179–186.

Macdonald, RL, and McLean, MJ (1982). Cellular bases of barbiturate and phenytoin anticonvulsant drug action. Epilepsia 23 (Suppl 1):7–18.

Macdonald, RL, and Mody, I (2008). GABA$_A$ and GABA$_B$ receptor-mediated inhibitory synaptic transmission. In Epilepsy: A Comprehensive Textbook, 2nd ed. Edited by J Engel, Jr, and TA Pedley. Philadelphia: Lippincott Williams & Wilkins, pp. 245–252.

Mackay, MT, Weiss, SK, Adams-Webber, T, Ashwal, S, Stephens, D, Ballaban-Gill, K, Baram, TZ, Duchowny, M, Hirtz, D, Pellock, JM, Shields, WD, Shinnar, S, Wyllie, E, and Snead, OC, 3rd (2004). Practice parameter: Medical treatment of infantile spasms: Report of the American Academy of Neurology and the Child Neurology Society. Neurology 62:1668–1681.

Marson, AG, Al-Kharusi, AM, Alwaidh, M, et al. (2007a). The SANAD study of effectiveness of carbamazepine, gabapentin, lamotrigine, oxcarbazepine, or topiramate for treatment of partial epilepsy: An unblinded randomised controlled trial. Lancet 369:1000–1015.

Marson, AG, Al-Kharusi, AM, Alwaidh, M, et al. (2007b). The SANAD study of effectiveness of valproate, lamotrigine, or topiramate for generalised and unclassifiable epilepsy: An unblinded randomised controlled trial. Lancet 369:1016–1026.

Matsuo, F, and Riaz, A (2009). Lamotrigine. In The Treatment of Epilepsy, 3rd ed. Edited by S Shorvon, E Perucca, and J Engel, Jr. West Sussex, UK: Wiley-Blackwell, pp. 535–558.

Mattson, RH, Cramer, JA, Collins, JF, Smith, DB, Delgado-Escueta, A, Brown, TR, Williamson, PD, Treiman, DM, McNamara, JO, McCutchen, DB, Homan, RW, Crill, WE, Lubozynski, MF, Rosenthal, NP, and Mayerdorf, A (1985). Comparison of carbamazepine, phenobarbital, phenytoin and primidone in partial and secondarily generalized tonic-clonic seizures. N Engl J Med 313:145–151.

Mattson, RH, Cramer, JA, Darney, PD, and Naftolin, F (1986). Use of oral contraceptives by women with epilepsy. JAMA 256:238–240.

McCormack, M, Alfirevic, A, Bourgeois, S, et al. (2011). HLA-A*3101 and carbamazepine-induced hypersensitivity reactions in Europeans. N Engl J Med 364:1134–1143.

McLean, MG, and Macdonald RL: (1988). Benzodiazepines, but not betacarbolines, limit high frequency repetitive firing of action potentials of mouse central neurons in cell culture. J Pharmacol Exp Ther 244:789–795.

McLean, MJ, and MacDonald, RL (1986). Carbamazepine and 10–11 epoxide produce use- and voltage-dependent limitation of rapidly firing action potentials of mouse central neurons in cell. J Pharmacol Exp Ther 238:727–738.

Meador, KJ, Baker, GA, Browning, N, et al. (2009). Cognitive function at 3 years of age after fetal exposure to antiepileptic drugs. N Engl J Med 360:1597–1605.

Meierkord, H, and Holtkamp, M (2009). Other drugs rarely used. In The Treatment of Epilepsy, 3rd ed. Edited by S Shorvon, E Perucca, and J Engel, Jr. West Sussex, UK: Wiley-Blackwell, pp. 721–731.

Meldrum, BS (1986a). Pharmacological approaches to the treatment of epilepsy. In Current Problems in Epilepsy, Vol 4: New Anticonvulsant Drugs. Edited by BS Meldrum and RJ Porter. London: John Libbey, pp. 17–30.

Meldrum, BS (1986b). Preclinical test systems for evaluation of novel compounds. In Current Problems in Epilepsy, Vol 4: New Anticonvulsant Drugs. Edited by BS Meldrum and RJ Porter. London: John Libbey, pp. 31–48.

Meldrum, BS (2008). Molecular targets for novel antiepileptic drugs. In Epilepsy: A Comprehensive Textbook, Second Edition. Edited by J Engel Jr and TA Pedley. Philadelphia: Lippincott Williams & Wilkins, pp. 1457–1468.

Merritt, HH, and Putnam, TJ (1938). A new series of anticonvulsant drugs tested by experiments on animals. Arch Neurol Psychiatry 39:1003–1015.

Meunier, H, Carraz, G, Meunier, Y, Eymard, P, and Aimard, M (1963). Propriétés pharmacodynamique de l'acide n-dipropylacétique. 1er memoire: Propriétés antiépileptiques. Thérapie 18:435–438.

Michelucci, R, Pasini, E, and Tassinari, CA (2009). Phenobarbital, primidone and other barbiturates. In The Treatment of Epilepsy, 3rd ed. Edited by S Shorvon, E Perucca, and J Engel, Jr. West Sussex, UK: Wiley-Blackwell, pp. 585–603.

Morin, A (1984). β-Carboline kindling of the benzodiazepine receptor. Brain Res 321:151–154.

Morselli, PL, Pippinger, CE, and Penry, JK (eds) (1983). Antiepileptic Drug Therapy in Pediatrics. New York: Raven Press.

Neufeld, MY (2009). Acetazolamide. In The Treatment of Epilepsy, 3rd ed. Edited by S Shorvon, E Perucca, and J Engel, Jr. West Sussex, UK: Wiley-Blackwell, pp. 399–410.

Noebels, JL (1986). Mutational analysis of inherited epilepsies. Adv Neurol 44:97–113.

Olpe, HR, and Jones, RSG (1983). The action of anticonvulsant drugs on the firing of locus coeruleus neurons: Selective, activating effect of carbamazepine. Eur J Pharmacol 91:107–110.

Olsen, RW (1982). Drug interactions at the GABA receptor-ionophore complex. Annu Rev Pharmacol Toxicol 22:245–277.

Patsalos, PN, and Bourgeois, BFD (2010). The epilepsy prescriber's guide to antiepileptic drugs. Cambridge: Cambridge Univrsity Press.

Patsalos, PN, and Sander, JW (2009). Antiepileptic drugs in early clinical development. In The Treatment of Epilepsy, Third Edition. Edited by S Shorvon, E Perucca, and J Engel Jr. West Sussex, UK, Wiley-Blackwell, pp. 733–740.

Pearl, PL, Vezina, LG, Saneto, RP, McCarter, R, Molloy-Wells, E, Heffron, A, Trzcinski, S, McClintock, WM, Conry, JA, Elling, NJ, Goodkin, HP, de Menezes, MS, Ferri, R, Gilles, E, Kadom, N, and Gaillard, WD (2009). Cerebral MRI abnormalities associated with vigabatrin therapy. Epilepsia 50:184–194.

Pellock, JM, Hrachovy, R, Shinnar, S, Baram, TZ, Bettis, D, Dlugos, DJ, Gaillard, WD, Gibson, PA, Holmes, GL, Nordl, DR, O'Dell, C, Shields, WD, Trevathan, E, and Wheless, JW (2010). Infantile spasms: A U.S. consensus report. Epilepsia 51:2175–2189.

Perlstein, MA, and Andelman, MB (1946). Tridione: Its use in convulsive and related disorders. J Pediatr 29:20–40.

Physician's Desk Reference, 65th ed. (2011). Montvale, NJ: PDR Network.

Porter, RJ, and White, BG (1986). Evaluation in man. In Current Problems in Epilepsy, Vol 4: New Anticonvulsant Drugs. Edited by BS Meldrum and RJ Porter. London: John Libbey, pp. 49–61.

Porter, RJ, Cereghino, JJ, Gladding, GD, Hessie, BJ, Kupferberg, HJ, Scoville, B, and White, BG (1984). Antiepileptic Drug Development Program. Cleve Clin Q 51:293–305.

Post, RM, Ballenger, JC, Uhde, TW, and Bunney, WE, Jr (1984). Efficacy of carbamazepine in manic-depressive illness: Implication for underlying mechanisms. In Neurobiology of Mood Disorders. Edited by RM Post and JC Ballenger. Baltimore: Williams & Wilkins, pp. 777–816.

Privitera, MD, and Cavitt, J (2008). Levetiracetam. In Epilepsy: A Comprehensive Textbook, 2nd ed. Edited by J Engel, Jr, and TA Pedley. Philadelphia: Lippincott Williams & Wilkins, pp. 1583–1591.

Quesney, LF, and Reader, T (1984). Role of cortical catecholamine depletion in the genesis of epileptic photosensitivity. In Neurotransmitters, Seizures, and Epilepsy II. Edited by RG Fariello, PL Morselli, KG Lloyd, LF Quesney, and J Engel, Jr. New York: Raven Press, pp. 11–21.

Rall, TW, and Schleifer, LS (1985). Drugs effective in the therapy of epilepsies. In Goodman and Gilman's The Pharmacological Basis of Therapeutics. Edited by AG Gilman, LS Goodman, TW Rall, and F Murad. New York: Macmillan, pp. 446–472.

Rheims, S, Ryvlin, P (2009). Pregabalin. In The Treatment of Epilepsy, 3rd ed. Edited by S Shorvon, E Perucca, and J Engel, Jr. West Sussex, UK: Wiley-Blackwell, pp. 627–635.

Rho, JM, Donevan, SD, and Rogawski, MA (1994). Mechanism of action of the anticonvulsant felbamate: Opposing effect on N-methyl-D-aspartate and gamma-aminobutyric acid A receptors. Ann Neurol 35:229–234.

Richards, RK, and Everett, GM (1944). Analgesic and anticonvulsive properties of 3,5,5-trimethyloxazolidine-2,4-dione (Tridione) [abstract]. Fed Proc 3:39.

Sabers, A, and Harden, CL (2008). Gender issues for drug treatment. In Epilepsy: A Comprehensive Textbook, Second Edition. Edited by J Engel Jr and TA Pedley. Philadelphia: Lippincott Williams & Wilkins, pp. 1263–1268.

Sachdeo, R (2009). Lacosamide. In The Treatment of Epilepsy, 3rd ed. Edited by S Shorvon, E Perucca, and J Engel, Jr. West Sussex, UK: Wiley-Blackwell, pp. 527–534.

Schafer, H (1985). Chemical constitution of pharmacological effect. In Antiepileptic Drugs. Edited by H-H Frey and D Janz. New York: Springer-Verlag, pp. 199–243.

Schmidt, D, and Wilensky, AJ (2008). Benzodiazepines. In Epilepsy: A Comprehensive Textbook, Second Edition. Edited by J Engel Jr and TA Pedley. Philadelphia: Lippincott Williams & Wilkins, pp. 1531–1541.

Schmidt, D, Einicke, I, and Haenel, F (1986). The influence of seizure type on the efficacy of plasma concentrations of phenytoin, phenobarbital and carbamazepine. Arch Neurol 43:263–265.

Schmutz, M (1985). Carbamazepine. In Antiepileptic Drugs. Edited by H-H Frey and D Janz. New York: Springer-Verlag, pp. 479–506.

Seino, M, and Leppik, IE (2008). Zonisamide. In Epilepsy: A Comprehensive Textbook, Second Edition. Edited by J Engel Jr and TA Pedley. Philadelphia: Lippincott Williams & Wilkins, pp. 1695–1701.

Shorvon, SD (2009). Piracetam. In The Treatment of Epilepsy, 3rd ed. Edited by S Shorvon, E Perucca, and J Engel, Jr. West Sussex, UK: Wiley-Blackwell, pp. 619–625.

Shorvon, S, Perucca, E, and Engel, J Jr (Eds.) (2009). The Treatment of Epilepsy, Third Edition. Oxford: Wiley-Blackwell.

Sillanpää, M, Haataja, L, Tomson, T, and Johannessen, SI (2009). Carbamazepine. In The Treatment of Epilepsy, 3rd ed. Edited by S Shorvon, E Perucca, and J Engel, Jr. West Sussex, UK: Wiley-Blackwell, pp. 459–474.

Simonato, M, Löscher, W, Cole, AJ, Dudek, FE, Engel, J, Jr, Kaminski, RM, Loeb, JA, Scharfman, H, Staley, KJ, Velisek, L, and Klitgaard, H: WONOEP XI Critical Appraisal: Preclinical screening strategies and experimental trial design for the development of new drugs for epilepsy. Epilepsia (in press).

Skerritt, JH, Johnston, GAR, and Chen Chow, S (1983). Interactions of the anticonvulsant carbamazepine with adenosine receptors. 2. Pharmacological studies. Epilepsia 24:643–650.

Snead, OC, Benton, JW, and Myers, GH (1983). ACTH and prednisone in childhood seizure disorders. Neurology 33:966–970.

Somerville, ER, and Mitchell, AW (2009). Gabapentin. In The Treatment of Epilepsy, 3rd ed. Edited by S Shorvon, E Perucca, and J Engel, Jr. West Sussex, UK: Wiley-Blackwell, pp. 519–526.

Spielberg, SP, Gordon, GB, Blake, DA, Goldstein, DA, and Herlong, HF (1981). Predisposition to phenytoin hepatotoxicity assessed in vitro. N Engl J Med 305:722–727.

Stern, JM, Perucca, E, and Browne, TR (2008). Phenytoin, fosphenytoin, and other hydantoins. In Epilepsy: A Comprehensive Textbook, 2nd ed. Edited by J Engel, Jr, and TA Pedley. Philadelphia: Lippincott Williams & Wilkins, pp. 1609–1627.

Strickler, SM, Miller, MA, Andermann, E, Dansky, LV, Seni, M-H, and Spielberg, SP (1985). Genetic predisposition to phenytoin-induced birth defects. Lancet 2:746–749.

Swinyard, EA (1985). Acetylurea derivatives. In Antiepileptic Drugs. Edited by H-H Frey and D Janz. New York: Springer-Verlag, pp. 601–610.

Swinyard, EA, and Castellion, AW (1966). Anticonvulsant properties of some benzodiazepines. J Pharmacol Exp Ther 151:369–375.

Teschendorf, HJ, and Kretzschmar, R (1985). Succinimides. In Antiepileptic Drugs. Edited by H-H Frey and D Janz. New York: Springer-Verlag, pp. 199–243.

Theobald, W, and Kunz, HA (1963). Zur pharmakologie des antiepileptikums 5-carbamyl5H-dibenzo(b,f)azepin. Arzneimittelforschung 13:122–125.

Theodore, WH: Felbamate (2008). In Epilepsy: A Comprehensive Textbook, Second Edition. Edited by J Engel Jr and TA Pedley. Philadelphia: Lippincott Williams & Wilkins, pp. 1561–1568.

Ticku, MK, Kamatchi, GL, and Sofia, RD (1991). Effect of anticonvulsant felbamate on GABA receptor system. Epilepsia 32:389–391.

Tomson, T, Battino, D, French, J, et al. (2007). Antiepileptic drug exposure and major congenital malformations: The role of pregnancy registries. Epilepsy Behav 11:277–282.

Tomson, T, Stephen, LJ, and Brodie, MJ (2008). Lamotrigine. In Epilepsy: A Comprehensive Textbook, 2nd ed. Edited by J Engel, Jr, and TA Pedley. Philadelphia: Lippincott Williams & Wilkins, pp. 1575–1582.

Treiman, DM (1987). Status epilepticus. In Current Therapy in Neurologic Disease, 2. Edited by RT Johnson. Philadelphia: CB Decker, pp. 38–42.

Trimble, MR, and Robertson, MM (1986). Clobazam. In Current Problems in Epilepsy, Vol 4: New Anticonvulsant Drugs. Edited by BS Meldrum and RJ Porter. London: John Libbey, pp. 65–84.

Trimble, MR, and Thompson, PJ (1983). Anticonvulsant drugs, cognitive function, and behavior. Epilepsia 24(Suppl 1): S55–S63.

Troupin, AS, Friel, P, Wilensky, AJ, Morretti-Ojemann, L, Levy, RH, and Fiegl, P (1979). Evaluation of clorazepate (Tranxene) as an anticonvulsant—A pilot study. Neurology 29:458–466.

Vanlersberghe, C, and Camu, F (2008). Propofol. Handb Exp Pharmacol 182:227–252.

Vigevano, F, and Cilio, MR (2009). Adrenocorticotropic hormone and corticosteroids. In The Treatment of Epilepsy, 3rd ed. Edited by S Shorvon, E Perucca, and J Engel, Jr. West Sussex, UK: Wiley-Blackwell, pp. 411–419.

von Rosenstiel P, and Perucca, E (2009). Brivaracetam: In The Treatment of Epilepsy, 3rd ed. Edited by S Shorvon, E Perucca, and J Engel, Jr. West Sussex, UK: Wiley-Blackwell, pp. 447–457.

Weaver, DF, and Sankar, R (2008). Basic principles of medicinal chemistry. In Epilepsy: A Comprehensive Textbook, 2nd ed. Edited by J Engel, Jr, and TA Pedley. Philadelphia: Lippincott Williams & Wilkins, pp. 1447–1455.

White, HS, Wolf, HH, Swinyard, EA, et al. (1992). A neuropharmacological evaluation of felbamate as a novel anticonvulsant. Epilepsia 33: 564–572.

White, HS, Woodhead, JH, Wilcox, KS, Stables, JP, Kupferberg, HJ, Wolf, HH (2002). General principles, discovery and prelinical development of antiepileptic drugs. In Antiepileptic Drugs, 5th Edition. Edited by RH Levy, RH Mattson, BS Meldrum, and E Perucca. Philadelphia: Lippincott Williams & Wilkins, pp. 36–48.

White, HS, Porter, RJ, and Kupferberg, HJ (2008a). Screening of new compounds and the role of the pharmaceutical industry. In Epilepsy: A Comprehensive Textbook, Second Edition. Edited by J Engel Jr and TA Pedley. Philadelphia: Lippincott Williams & Wilkins, pp. 1469–1485.

White, HS, Perucca, E, and Privitera, MD (2008b). Investigational drugs: Brivaracetam, carisbamate, eslicarbazepine, fluorofelbamate, ganaxolone, isovaleramide, lacosamide (harkoseride; SPM927), losigamine, retigabine, safinamide, seletracetam, stiripentol, talampanel, and valrocemide. In Epilepsy: A Comprehensive Textbook, 2nd ed. Edited by J Engel, Jr, and TA Pedley. Philadelphia: Lippincott Williams & Wilkins, pp. 1721–1740.

White, HS, Perucca, E, and Privitera, MD (2008c). Investigational drugs. In Epilepsy: A Comprehensive Textbook, 2nd ed. Edited by J Engel, Jr, and TA Pedley. Philadelphia: Lippincott Williams & Wilkins, pp. 1721–1740.

Wilder, BJ, and Bruni, J (1981). Seizure Disorders: A Pharmacological Approach to Treatment. New York: Raven Press.

Woodbury, DM (1982). Phenytoin absorption, distribution and excretion. In Antiepileptic Drugs. Edited by DM Woodbury, JK Penry, and CE Pippenger. New York: Raven Press, pp. 191–207.

Woodbury, DM, and Kemp, JW (1982). Other antiepileptic drugs: Sulfonamides and derivatives: Acetazolamide. In Antiepileptic Drugs, 2nd ed. Edited by DM Woodbury, JK Penry, and CE Pippenger. New York: Raven Press, pp. 771–789.

Woodbury, DM, and Pippenger, CE (1982). Other antiepileptic drugs: Bromides. In Antiepileptic Drugs, 2nd ed. Edited by DM Woodbury, JK Penry, and CE Pippenger. New York: Raven Press, pp. 791–801.

Woodbury, DM, Penry, JK, and Pippenger, CE (eds) (1982). Antiepileptic Drugs, ed 2. New York: Raven Press.

Worms, P, Depoorter, H, Durand, A, Morselli, PL, Lloyd, K, Bartholini, G (1982). Gamma-amino butyric acid (GABA) receptor stimulation. I. Neuropharmacological profiles of progabide (SL 76002) and SL 75102, with emphasis on their anticonvulsant spectra. J Pharmacol Exp Ther 220:660–671.

Wroe, SJ (2009). Zonisamide. In The Treatment of Epilepsy, 3rd ed. Edited by S Shorvon, E Perucca, and J Engel, Jr. West Sussex, UK: Wiley-Blackwell, pp. 713–720.

Young, DS (1987). Implementation of SI units for clinical laboratory medicine: Style specifi cations and conversion tables. Ann Intern Med 106:114–129.

Zaret, BS, Beckner, RR, Marini, AM, Wagle, W, and Passarelli, C (1982). Sodium valproate-induced hyperammonemia without clinical hepatic dysfunction. Neurology 32:206–208.

Zubair, S, Patton, T, Smithson, K, Sonmezturk, HH, Arain, A, and Abou-Khalil, B (2011). Propofol withdrawal seizures: Non-epileptic nature of seizures in a patient with recently controlled status epilepticus. Epileptic Disord 13:107–110.

Chapter 16

Nonpharmacological Therapy of Seizures

SURGICAL THERAPY
Historical Perspectives
Surgical Therapy Continues to Be
  Underutilized
Misconceptions about Surgical
  Candidates
Arguments for Early Surgical Intervention
Surgically Remediable Epilepsy
  Syndromes
Therapeutic Surgical Procedures
Surgical Protocols
Outcome
Development of New Centers

VAGUS NERVE STIMULATION

HORMONE THERAPY

IMMUNE THERAPY

**COMPLEMENTARY AND ALTERNATIVE
  MEDICINE**
Diet
Traditional and Folk Medicine
Behavioral Therapies
Physical Interventions
Nonallopathic Medical Systems

SUMMARY AND CONCLUSIONS

Although pharmacotherapy is sufficient to control seizures in most patients, many will benefit from other types of treatment. *Surgery* offers a safe and effective approach capable of eliminating disabling seizures in some pharmacoresistant epilepsy conditions (Engel, 1987a;b; Wieser and Elger, 1987; Engel, 1993; Engel et al., 2003; Lüders et al., 2008). This treatment is greatly underutilized (Engel, 2008). *Vagus nerve stimulation (VNS)* is a widely used palliative procedure (Schachter

and Boon, 2008; Schachter, 2009), and more invasive brain stimulation is now being offered (Fisher et al., 2008; Bergey, 2009; Morrell et al., 2011). *Hormonal* treatments and *immunotherapy* also have a place in the management of epilepsy (Herzog, 2008; Villani et al., 2008). *Complementary and alternative medicine (CAM)* is gaining credibility among Western physicians, and a great many approaches have been applied to epilepsy, including dietary and behavioral manipulations (Herzog, 2008;

603

Stafstrom et al., 2008; Wolf, 2008; Kossoff and Dorward, 2009), herbal and other traditional practices (Schachter et al., 2008; Whitmarsh, 2009), and novel interventions that deserve further investigation (Rogawski and Schwartzkroin, 2009).

SURGICAL THERAPY

Historical Perspectives

The modern era of epilepsy surgery began over 130 years ago when Macewen (1881) and Horsley (1886) successfully resected epileptogenic lesions localized by seizure semiology based on the clinical-pathological studies of Hughlings Jackson (Taylor, 1958) and confirmed with stimulation of monkey cortex by Ferrier (1874; Engel, 2005b) (Chapter 2). Subsequently, a variety of other surgical procedures were introduced. *Corpus callosotomy* (Van Wagenen and Herren, 1940) and *hemispherectomy* (Krynauw, 1950) are still in use, whereas various older stereotactic ablative techniques and cerebellar stimulation are no longer recommended by epileptologists. The most used surgical treatment for epilepsy continues to be localized resection of epileptogenic brain tissue (Penfield and Jasper, 1954; Purpura et al., 1975; Engel, 1987a; 1993; Engel et al., 2003; Spencer and Huh, 2008).

Initially, clinical information and ictal features provided localizing information, and the abnormal brain tissue was identified at surgery on the basis of a visible structural lesion, with or without induction of an aura or seizure by electrical stimulation of adjacent cortex (Foerster and Penfield, 1930). The advent of cerebral angiography (Moniz, 1934) and pneumoencephalography (Dandy, 1919) permitted preoperative identification of a structural lesion and increased the number of patients who could be considered surgical candidates (Penfield and Erickson, 1941; Penfield and Flanigin, 1950; Penfield and Jasper, 1954). Although Jasper was the first to use EEG to localize the origin of *psychomotor seizures* to the temporal lobe (Jasper and Kershman, 1941; Jasper et al., 1951), Bailey and Gibbs (1951) first reported surgical resection of epileptogenic brain tissue on

the basis of EEG findings alone. Following evidence that a unilateral temporal interictal EEG spike focus could identify an epileptogenic temporal lobe, many centers around the world began performing temporal lobe resection for what then became known as *temporal lobe epilepsy* (Engel, 2005b). Temporal lobe surgery became, and continues to be, the most commonly performed and generally successful surgical treatment available for epilepsy (Crandall, 1987; Engel, 1987a; 1993; Engel et al., 2003; Jensen, 1975; Spencer et al., 1984a; Spencer and Huh, 2008). Introduction of the modified *intracarotid amobarbital procedure (IAP)* to verify that the contralateral hemisphere could support memory added to the safety of mesial temporal lobe resection (Milner et al., 1962). The development of *stereotactic depth electrode electroencephalography (SEEG)* and other intracranial recording techniques greatly increased the number of patients who could benefit from this resective procedure (Talairach et al., 1958, 1974). The efficacy of epilepsy surgery was vastly improved by the ability to record spontaneous seizures (Crandall et al., 1963) and the advent of EEG telemetry (Dymond et al., 1971).

The previous chapter documents the tremendous increase in the number of available antiseizure medications since the first edition of this textbook was published in 1989. The past two decades have witnessed similar progress in the development of surgical treatment for epilepsy. At the time of the first *Palm Desert Conference* on *Surgical Treatment of the Epilepsies*, in 1986, there were approximately 50 epilepsy surgery centers worldwide (Engel, 1987a). By the time of the second Palm Desert conference, in 1992, there were 118 epilepsy surgery centers represented from North America, Europe, Asia, Latin America, and Australia (Engel, 1993). Not only did availability for surgical treatment more than double during that time, but major changes occurred in surgical approaches. In the 1980s there were two principal schools, each advocating its own diagnostic and surgical strategies. Those physicians following the teachings of Penfield at the Montreal Neurologic Institute tended to perform resections ultimately based on intraoperative *electrocorticography (ECoG)*; those deriving from the Bancaud and Talairach program at the Centre Sainte

Anne in Paris, modified by Crandall at the University of California, Los Angeles (UCLA), tended to perform resections based largely on results of chronic recordings from stereotactically implanted intracerebral electrodes. The Paris school used carefully constructed SEEG placements to localize the extent of the abnormal brain tissue and perform tailored resections. Falconer at the Maudsley Hospital in London introduced standardized en bloc anterior temporal lobe resections (Falconer, 1953), a surgical approach adapted by the UCLA school. Falconer's technique also made it possible to perform detailed histopathology of the resected tissue and to obtain electrocl inical-pathological correlations, which led to recognition of the importance of hippocampal sclerosis (Falconer, 1974; Engel et al., 1975). Somewhat later, with the development of chronic subdural grid and strip recordings, other centers used these exclusively to perform both tailored and standardized resections (Goldring and Gregorie, 1984; Lesser et al., 1987). In the interim between the first two Palm Desert conferences, with increased sharing of information among epilepsy surgery centers, it was agreed that the presurgical evaluation and ultimate surgical intervention depended on the seizure type and epilepsy syndrome. Today, as a result of the Palm Desert discussions and subsequent conferences, centers have tended to adopt a variety of approaches to use as most appropriate. Intracerebral depth electrodes are now usually reserved for seizures originating in the mesial temporal lobe or other areas deep to the lateral cortex, and subdural electrodes are used primarily for neocortical seizures where the extent as well as the location of the epileptogenic region needed to be defined in order to perform tailored resections.

With the development of modern neuroimaging, first *positron emission tomography (PET)* (Engel et al., 1982a, 1982b, 1982c), then high-resolution *magnetic resonance imaging (MRI)* (Jackson et al., 1990) and ictal *single-photon emission computed tomography (SPECT)* (Sanabria et al., 1983; Lee et al., 1988), the presumptive epileptogenic region could be localized in patients previously diagnosed with *cryptogenic focal epilepsy* who had hippocampal sclerosis or focal cortical dysplasia that could not be seen with older techniques.

Localization could then be confirmed noninvasively with ictal scalp video-EEG recordings (Engel et al., 1981), greatly reducing the need for invasive monitoring and enhancing cost-effectiveness and safety. *Functional MRI (fMRI)* and *magnetoencephalography (MEG)* also now play a role in presurgical evaluation (Chapter 12).

PET (Chugani et al., 1988, 1990) and, later, high-resolution MRI (Sankar et al., 1995) also helped to identify diffuse, usually dysplastic lesions limited to one hemisphere in infants and small children with catastrophic epileptic encephalopathies, who then became candidates for hemispherectomies and multilobar resections (Shields et al., 1990). The rapidly expanding field of pediatric epilepsy surgery is perhaps the most dramatic recent advance in surgical treatment, offering opportunities to arrest or reverse inevitable developmental delay and lifelong institutionalization in children whose conditions previously would have been considered hopeless (Duchowny et al., 2008; Hauptman and Mathern, 2009; Lerner et al., 2009; Hemb et al., 2010).

Improved understanding of the clinical presentations of various epilepsy conditions and their natural histories resulted in the concept of *surgically remediable syndromes* (Engel, 1996). The development of neurocognitive testing to localize lesions in the brain also contributed to an appreciation of the neuropsychological disabilities associated with epilepsy (Wilson and Engel, 2010) (Chapters 11 and 12). Subsequently, techniques for quantitative evaluation of *health-related quality of life (HRQOL)* following surgical treatment (Vickrey et al., 1992, 1995a, 1995b; Devinsky et al., 1995) helped to demonstrate that surgical intervention for pharmacoresistant epilepsy not only eliminated or reduced seizures but also had a positive impact on patients' lives. Surgery, therefore, was shown to provide the best opportunity to prevent or reverse adverse psychological and social consequences that lead to lifelong disability in patients with surgically remediable epilepsy syndromes. Finally, technological advances in MRI-based neuronavigation and microsurgery have reduced the risks of surgical complications. As a result of all these advances, many more patients are deemed candidates for surgical treatment today than two or three decades ago, presurgical evaluation is more accurate, surgical intervention is safer, and outcomes with respect to seizures and behavior are better.

Surgical Therapy Continues to Be Underutilized

Sadly, the tremendous progress in surgical treatment for the epilepsies discussed above has not been matched by a commensurate increase in the referral of patients for surgical therapy. In 1990, the last time a formal survey was taken, approximately 2,000 patients a year underwent surgical treatment in the United States for epilepsy (Engel, 1993). Data collected by the *US National Association of Epilepsy Centers (NAEC)* indicates that this number has not changed appreciably since (R. Gumnit, unpublished data; Engel, 2008). Furthermore, a large, multicenter study determined that the average delay from onset of epilepsy to surgery is 22 years (Berg et al., 2003), much too late for most patients to avoid irreversible disability. Despite a randomized controlled trial (RCT) demonstrating the superiority of surgery over continued pharmacotherapy for drug-resistant temporal lobe epilepsy (Engel, 2001a; Wiebe et al., 2001) and a practice parameter published by the *American Academy of Neurology (AAN)*, *American Epilepsy Society (AES)*, and *American Association of Neurological Surgeons (AANS)* declaring surgery to be the treatment of choice for pharmacoresistant temporal lobe epilepsy and advocating early surgical intervention (Engel et al., 2003), not only is surgical treatment still underused, but time to referral to surgery has not been reduced. Analysis of referral patterns at two centers before and after the RCT and publication of the practice parameter revealed no change in delay to surgery (Choi et al., 2009; Haneef et al., 2010), suggesting that these efforts have had little or no effect on attitudes of primary care physicians and general neurologists about the place of surgery in the treatment of epilepsy.

An estimated three million people in the United States have epilepsy, one-third of whom continue to have seizures despite medication (Chapter 2); perhaps 10–50% of these might conceivably be surgical candidates. Taking the lower figure and calculating the annual activity of the epilepsy centers in the United States, it would appear that less than 5% of the 100,000 patients who might be surgical candidates have been referred to an epilepsy center in any given year, and only 2% receive surgery annually. The reason for this is unclear. Undoubtedly, there is inadequate dissemination regarding the safety and efficacy of modern approaches to surgical treatment for epilepsy, although tens of thousands of papers on this subject have been published in recent years. At the time of the first Palm Desert conference, there were only two textbooks on epilepsy surgery (Penfield and Jasper, 1954; Purpura at el., 1975), but since then there have been over 20 (Engel, 1987a; Wieser and Elger, 1987; Dam et al., 1988; Duchowny et al., 1990; Pickard et al., 1990; Apuzzo, 1991; Spencer and Spencer, 1991; Lüders, 1992; Theodore, 1992; Engel, 1993; Silbergeld and Ojemann, 1993; Dam et al., 1994; Wyler and Hermann, 1994; Tuxhorn et al., 1997; Mathern, 1999; Lüders and Comair, 2001; Bingaman, 2002; Sutter and Schrottner, 2002; Zentner and Seeger, 2003; Miller and Silbergeld, 2006; Lüders et al., 2008; Baltuch and Villemure, 2009; Cataltepe and Jallo, 2010). Certainly the information is available. Fear of surgical treatment is understandable (Swarztrauber et al., 2003); however, persistent morbidity from complications of epilepsy surgery is approximately 3%, and mortality is less than 1% (Engel et al., 2003; Polkey, 2009), while pharmacoresistant epilepsy is associated with a mortality that is 5 to 10 times that of the general population (Sperling, 2004), and surgical treatment increases life span (Choi et al., 2008). While cost may also be a factor, the cost of surgery is considerably less than the cost of a lifetime of disability. Data have been compiled that demonstrate the cost-effectiveness of surgical intervention for pharmacoresistant epilepsy (Langfitt, 1997), and third-party payers are much more willing to approve epilepsy surgery today than they were a few decades ago.

In contrast to the stubbornly persistent underutilization of epilepsy surgery in virtually all industrialized countries of the world, there has in recent years been a successful effort to promote surgical treatment for epilepsy in countries with emerging economies and limited resources (Palmini, 2009). Whereas surgical therapy in the past had been considered an unaffordable luxury, it is now recognized as more cost-effective than pharmacotherapy for many patients with drug-resistant seizures. This shift was made possible in part by the concept of surgically remediable syndromes and by the advent of neuroimaging and other technological developments that have reduced the cost and increased the accuracy of presurgical evaluation in this population of patients. Consequently, excellent surgical centers now not only exist but are an important part of the national approach to people with epilepsy in countries such as Brazil, China, India, Israel, Korea, and Turkey, and surgical therapy for many is also becoming a reality in a number of other, smaller countries.

Misconceptions About Surgical Candidates

Undoubtedly, a major obstacle to surgical referral is the belief of most primary care physicians and general neurologists that it is their responsibility to determine whether patients might be surgical candidates before referring them to an epilepsy center (Engel, 2008; Engel and Wiebe, 2012). Because of misconceptions in the community about who is or is not a surgical candidate, many excellent candidates are never referred. Table 16–1 lists some of the most common misconceptions that prevent appropriate and timely referral.

The International League against Epilepsy (ILAE) has defined drug-resistant epilepsy as failure of two adequate antiseizure drug trials (Kwan et al., 2010), based on considerable evidence that very few patients will benefit from further drug trials. Although there are a few studies that might contradict this view (Callaghan et al., 2007; Luciano and Shorvon, 2007; Bauer et al., 2008), for the most part, when patients do eventually experience remission after multiple drug trials, this is after a prolonged period of continued seizures and does not persist. The resultant delay increases the risk of irreversible disability due to adverse psychological and social consequences of recurrent seizures, as well as of death.

Perhaps the most common erroneous belief is that patients with bilateral independent interictal spikes on EEG are not candidates for surgical treatment. Interictal EEG spikes do not always accurately localize the epileptogenic region, and many patients with unilateral ictal onsets, particularly those with *mesial temporal lobe epilepsy (MTLE)*, who are the best surgical candidates, have bilateral independent interictal EEG spikes.

The prevalent misconception that patients with normal MRIs cannot be treated surgically is likely responsible for failure to refer many excellent surgical candidates. Routine MRIs often do not reveal subtle structural abnormalities, including mild hippocampal

Table 16–1 Common Misconceptions About Epilepsy Surgery

Misconception	Fact
All drugs need to be tried.	Seizure freedom is unlikely after two drugs have failed.
Bilateral EEG spikes are a contraindication to surgery.	Patients with unilateral onset seizures usually have bilateral spikes.
Normal MRI is a contraindication to surgery.	Other techniques often detect a single epileptogenic zone in patients with normal MRIs.
Multiple or diffuse lesions on MRI are a contraindication to surgery.	The epileptogenic zone may involve only a part of the lesion.
Surgery is not possible if primary cortex is involved.	Essential functions can be localized and protected.
Surgery will make memory worse if there is an existing memory deficit.	Poor memory usually will not get worse and could get better.
Chronic psychosis is a contraindication to surgery.	Patients will still benefit if seizures are eliminated.
IQ less than 70 is a contraindication to surgery.	Outcome depends on the type of epilepsy and the type of surgery.
Patients with focal epilepsy and a focal lesion can have the lesion removed without detailed presurgical evaluation.	Focal lesions can be incidental findings unrelated to the epilepsy; epileptogenicity of a lesion always needs to be confirmed.

sclerosis and focal cortical dysplasia that can be seen with the special structural and functional imaging techniques available at epilepsy centers (Chapter 12). But even when detailed imaging reveals no structural abnormality, *video-EEG monitoring (VEM)* and invasive EEG approaches will often localize an epileptogenic region that can be resected with excellent results.

Patients with diffuse or multifocal lesions on MRI may still be candidates for localized resection if only a part of the structural abnormalities is epileptogenic. This is common for *tuberous sclerosis* when only one tuber is the site of ictal onset and for some malformations of cortical development such as *schizencephaly*, where the epileptogenic region is only a small part of the lesion. In these situations, a relatively limited resection can result in a seizure-free outcome. When all of the diffuse or multifocal abnormality is epileptogenic but it is limited to one hemisphere, multilobar resection or hemispherectomy might be considered.

Many physicians still believe that surgical resection is not possible for epileptogenic lesions in the language-dominant hemisphere or near essential cortical areas. Presurgical evaluation techniques are now extremely accurate in localizing essential cortex that must not be damaged during surgical resection. Even if the epileptogenic region involves essential cortex, it is often possible to do *selective lesionectomies* or other procedures, such as *multiple subpial transection*, that are capable of eliminating habitual seizures without inducing new neurological dysfunction.

Many patients with MTLE have memory deficits, which are usually material-specific: a verbal memory deficit if the epileptogenic region is in the language-dominant hemisphere and a visual-spatial memory deficit if the lesion is in the nondominant hemisphere. Sometimes, however, the memory deficit is more global. As discussed later in this chapter, if a memory deficit exists, it is rarely worsened by surgery and more often is improved if seizures become controlled, particularly when propagation to the contralateral temporal lobe is partially responsible for a more global memory deficit.

Patients with chronic psychosis and epilepsy may not experience improvement in their psychiatric condition but should not be deprived of the opportunity for freedom from epileptic seizures if they are good surgical candidates.

Furthermore, many psychiatric symptoms in patients with epilepsy are seizure-related, either ictally or postictally (Chapter 11), and these will remit if the surgery eliminates habitual seizures.

Patients with a low IQ generally have more diffuse epileptogenic abnormalities and are less likely to become completely seizure-free with localized resections, but many may benefit from larger resections. Low IQ is certainly not a contraindication to surgery for children who are candidates for hemispherectomy or multilobar resections.

The wide availability of high-resolution MRI in the community has resulted in the inappropriate surgical resection, in patients with pharmacoresistant epileptic seizures, of structural abnormalities that have nothing to do with the patient's epilepsy. *Venous angiomas* and *subarachnoid cysts* are not epileptogenic, and it is not uncommon for potentially epileptogenic lesions, such as those associated with *neurocysticercosis*, *cavernous angiomas*, and indeed any structural pathology, to be incidental findings. Unnecessary surgical removal of a nonepileptogenic lesion in patients with drug-resistant epileptic seizures not only introduces unwarranted additional risk and cost to the patient but also can make the epileptic seizures and any associated behavioral disturbances worse. Furthermore, resection of a structural lesion with incomplete removal of an adjacent epileptogenic region is a common cause of poor surgical outcome. A thorough presurgical evaluation by an experienced epilepsy surgery team at an epilepsy center is always necessary to confirm that any structural lesion seen on MRI is the cause of the patient's habitual seizures and to determine the extent of the epileptogenic region.

The principal point is that all patients with drug-resistant epilepsy should be referred to an epilepsy center. Specialists at epilepsy surgery centers are best equipped to determine whether a patient with drug-resistant epilepsy might be a surgical candidate, and *every* patient with drug-resistant epilepsy deserves the opportunity to be evaluated in this expert setting. Furthermore, when patients are referred to a comprehensive epilepsy center, those who are not found to be surgical candidates often benefit from the additional diagnostic and therapeutic expertise the center can provide. Patients might have the wrong diagnosis, might be candidates for experimental drug trials, or might benefit from alternative treatments such as VNS, a ketogenic diet, or a variety of investigational approaches that are available only at epilepsy centers.

Arguments for Early Surgical Intervention

Early surgery is important because of the considerable morbidity and mortality associated with persistent uncontrolled epileptic seizures (Sperling, 2004) (Chapter 9); the belief that some epilepsy disorders can be progressive also argues strongly for timely intervention. Epileptic encephalopathies are now recognized as conditions of infants and young children in which the epileptic activity itself is responsible for progression not only of the epilepsy condition but also of developmental delay, mental retardation, and other nonepileptic comorbidity (Engel, 2001b). This epilepsy-induced progressive process was recognized, in part, based on the observation that surgical treatment of infants and young children with severe, apparently generalized, epilepsy disorders who had localized lesions not only could render many seizure-free but, when seizures stopped, could interrupt or even reverse the progression of nonepileptic disturbances (Shields et al., 1990). Whereas early surgical intervention in infants and young children with these epileptic encephalopathies is now generally recognized as an urgent need if associated disability and mortality is to be avoided, the argument for early surgical intervention in adolescents and young adults with focal epilepsy is less apparent.

The progressive nature of focal epileptic activity has been definitively demonstrated in the animal laboratory using experimental animal models such as *kindling* (Goddard et al., 1969) and the *mirror focus* (Morrell, 1959/60) (Chapter 4). In these situations, recurrent epileptic discharges give rise to additional, distant areas of epileptogenicity that not only make the epilepsy condition worse but also can cause enduring disruption of brain function. Furthermore, homeostatic protective influences that develop in response to chronic epileptic activity not only account, in part, for postictal dysfunction but also may contribute to the development of interictal behavioral

disturbances (Engel et al., 2008) (Chapter 11). Some clinical reports support the existence of mirror foci in patients, suggesting that delayed surgical removal of the primary epileptogenic region can result in the development of an independent secondary epileptogenic region contralateral to the first or perhaps elsewhere in the brain (Morrell, 1985). Clinical evidence for kindling is difficult to obtain (Engel and Shewmon, 1991; Engel, 2005a), but it would seem reasonable to assume that processes that exist in lower vertebrates, including primates, would also exist in humans. The natural history of MTLE, which evolves over many years from pharmacosensitive to pharmacoresistant seizures (Berg et al., 2003), suggests a kindling-like mechanism (Chapters 4, 7, and 8). The progression of nonepileptic functional disturbances in MTLE is clearly demonstrated by the development of memory defects (Hermann et al., 2006), and MRI evidence shows progressive hippocampal atrophy (Cendes, 2005). Surgical series have also provided some evidence that earlier surgical intervention is more likely to result in a seizure-free outcome (Janszky et al., 2005). It would seem, therefore, that at least some forms of drug-resistant focal epilepsy in adolescents and young adults are progressive (Chapter 8). Whether or not this is the case, however, there is no doubt that the adverse psychological and social consequences of recurrent epileptic seizures during critical periods for acquisition of interpersonal and vocational skills can lead to irreversible disability that could be avoided with effective early surgical treatment.

Surgically Remediable Epilepsy Syndromes

At the time of publication of the first edition of this book in 1989, there were essentially three first-line antiseizure drugs: *phenytoin, carbamazepine,* and *valproic acid.* It was a relatively simple matter to determine when appropriate trials of these three medications were ineffective and so deem a patient's seizures pharmacoresistant. Today, however, there are so many antiseizure medications that it would literally take a lifetime to prove that all drugs, in every conceivable combination, are ineffective in controlling a given patient's seizures. Consequently, the concept of *surgically remediable epilepsy syndromes* was introduced in the mid-1990s (Engel, 1996) to define patients with conditions that are not likely to respond to further medication trials after two trials have failed but who are highly likely to benefit from surgical treatment (Table 16–2). These are patients whose epilepsy disorder has a known pathophysiology and a predictable natural history. This natural history has three features. First, the likelihood of seizure freedom occurring with continued pharmacotherapy after two appropriate antiseizure drug trials have failed is small, as indicated in the ILAE definition of drug-resistant seizures (Kwan et al., 2010). Second, there is a high likelihood of progressive adverse features, for instance, developmental delay in infants and small children, and of interictal behavioral disorders and psychosocial disturbances when seizures begin in adolescence or adulthood. Third, there is an excellent chance (60–80%) that surgery will eliminate disabling seizures. Surgical treatment is most cost-effective in patients with surgically remediable syndromes, because presurgical evaluation can usually be

Table 16–2 Surgically Remediable Epilepsy Syndromes

Characteristic features:
- Known pathophysiology
- Predictable natural history
- Unresponsive to pharmacotherapy
- Progressive features (e.g., developmental delay or interictal behavioral disorders)

Most cost-effective surgical candidates because:
- Presurgical evaluation can be performed noninvasively
- 70–90% chance of complete elimination of disabling seizures
- Disabling behavioral consequences can be avoided or reversed, but only if surgical intervention is early

Examples:
- Mesial temporal lobe epilepsy
- Epilepsies due to well-circumscribed resectable lesions
- Epilepsies in infants and young children due to large or diffuse lesions limited to one hemisphere (e.g., porencephalic cysts, Rasmussen's encephalitis, Sturge-Weber syndrome, hemimegalencephaly, and other large malformations of cortical development)

From Engel, 2009, with permission.

performed noninvasively and disabling behavioral consequences can be avoided or reversed, but only if surgical intervention is early.

MTLE is the prototype of a surgically remediable syndrome, but focal epilepsies due to well-circumscribed resectable neocortical lesions are also surgically remediable, as are epilepsies in infants and young children that are due to diffuse or multifocal lesions limited to one hemisphere, as occur, for instance, with widely distributed but unilateral *malformations of cortical development, hemimegalencephaly, Sturge-Weber syndrome, Rasmussen's encephalitis,* and *large porencephalic cysts.* MTLE, particularly with *hippocampal sclerosis* (Chapter 7), is the most common epilepsy syndrome in adolescents and adults and the most likely to be pharmacoresistant (Semah et al., 1998; Stephen et al., 2001). Anteromesial temporal resection for pharmacoresistant MTLE is not only the most common but also the most effective surgical procedure performed to treat epilepsy. Table 16–3 briefly describes the typical features of this surgically remediable syndrome. Refractory epilepsies due to well-circumscribed resectable structural lesions and severe epilepsies in infants and young children with structural lesions limited to one hemisphere can usually be easily identified today with routine MRI.

Patients with pharmacoresistant epilepsy who do not have surgically remediable epilepsy syndromes as defined here may still benefit from surgical treatment. If the epilepsy disorder has a more complicated etiology and the epileptogenic region cannot be easily identified noninvasively, but seizures are relatively stereotyped and there is a reasonable hypothesis regarding two or three possible epileptogenic regions, then more detailed evaluation, which may include invasive VEM with intracerebral depth or subdural electrodes, can still identify the source of habitual seizures in many patients who will benefit from surgery. Although the cost and risk of presurgical evaluation is greater in this population than in patients with the typical surgically remediable epilepsy syndromes, and the likelihood of a seizure-free outcome may be less, these patients still deserve surgical consideration if they are interested. This group includes not only patients who have normal MRI scans but also those who might have multiple lesions, as with tuberous sclerosis where only one tuber is epileptogenic or diffuse

Table 16–3 The Syndrome of Mesial Temporal Lobe Epilepsy

History
- Increased incidence of complicated febrile convulsions or other cerebral insults early in life
- Increased incidence of a family history of epilepsy
- Onset in latter half of first decade of life
- Auras common and occur in isolation
- Secondary generalized seizures occur infrequently
- Seizures often remit for several years until adolescence or early adulthood
- Seizures often become medically intractable
- Interictal behavioral disturbances can occur (most commonly depression)

Clinical seizure
- Aura is usually present. Most common is epigastric rising, often other autonomic or psychic symptoms, with emotion (e.g., fear), can be olfactory, gustatory, or nonspecific somatosensory sensations (several seconds)
- Complex partial seizure. Often begins with arrest and stare; oroalimentary automatisms and complex automatisms common. Posturing of one upper extremity may occur contralateral to the ictal discharge (1–2 min)
- Postictal phase. Usually includes disorientation, deficit in recent memory, amnesia for the event, and dysphasia if seizures begin in the language-dominant hemisphere (several minutes)

Neurological and laboratory evaluation
- Neurological examination usually normal except for memory deficit
- Unilateral or bilateral independent anterior temporal EEG spikes, maximum amplitude in basal electrodes
- Extracranial ictal EEG activity appears only with complex partial symptoms, usually initial or delayed focal onset pattern of 5–7-Hz rhythmic activity, maximum amplitude in one basal temporal derivation
- Usually temporal lobe hypometabolism on interictal FDG-PET, often involves ipsilateral thalamus and basal ganglia
- Usually temporal lobe hypoperfusion on interictal SPECT and characteristic pattern of hyper- and hypoperfusion on ictal SPECT
- Usually material-specific memory disturbances on neuropsychological testing and amnesia with contralateral intracarotid sodium amytal injection
- Hippocampal atrophy usually visible on MRI

EEG = electroencephalogram; FDG-PET = positron emission tomography with fluorodeoxyglucose; MRI = magnetic resonance imaging; SPECT = single-photon emission computed tomography.
Adapted from Engel, 1996, with permission.

lesions, such as schizencephaly, where only a small part of the malformation is epileptogenic. Experienced teams at epilepsy surgery centers are trained to determine the risks and benefits of pursuing surgery in such patients, and failure to refer them to an epilepsy center denies them a potential opportunity to benefit from this treatment. These patients represent the frontier for presurgical evaluation and considerable research is under way to identify more accurate techniques to localize the epileptogenic region and determine its extent, preferably noninvasively, as discussed later in this chapter.

Therapeutic Surgical Procedures

A list of surgical procedures commonly performed for the treatment of epilepsy is shown in Table 16–4. These can be divided into standardized resections, which are relatively the same for every patient; tailored resections, where the boundaries need to be individually determined; and disconnections, which do not remove brain tissue but interrupt epileptogenic pathways. Not shown in Table 16–4 are ablative approaches that are performed stereotactically; and stimulation.

STANDARDIZED RESECTIONS

Well over half of the surgical procedures performed for treatment of epilepsy today are temporal lobe resections for patients with pharmacoresistant MTLE. Initially, the amount of tissue removed was determined individually for each patient, based largely on ECoG (Penfield and Jasper, 1954; Crandall, 1987).

Table 16–4 **Common Surgical Procedures for Epilepsy and Numbers Performed Worldwide Between 1986 and 1990**

Procedure	Number of Patients (%)
Anterior temporal resections	4,862 (59)
Amygdalohippocampectomy	568 (7)
Extratemporal resection	1,073 (13)
Lesionectomy	440 (5)
Hemispherectomy and large multilobar resections	448 (5)
Corpus callosotomy	843 (10)
Total	8,234 (100)

From Engel and Shewmon, 1993, with permission.

A standard *anteromesial temporal resection* was eventually established, however, after years of extensive experience with chronic stereotactic depth electrode recording and pathological examination of resected tissue, which identified a relatively common pathophysiological and anatomical substrate for this condition involving hippocampus and parahippocampal structures (Falconer, 1953; Crandall et al., 1963; Spencer et al., 1984a; Vives et al., 2008; Leiphart and Fried, 2009). Typical anteromesial temporal resections today extend 3 cm posterior to the temporal pole laterally and as far back as possible mesially, to include most of the amygdala, the hippocampal pes, and most of the hippocampal tail (Fig. 16–1). Some

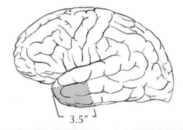

3.5"

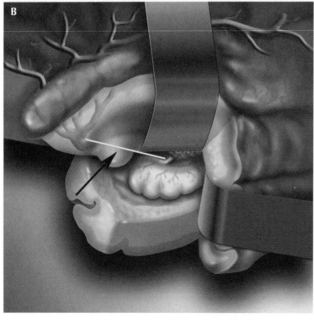

Figure 16–1. Anteromesial temporal resection. **A.** The lateral resection is invariant from dominant to nondominant side and consists of the anterior 2.5–3 cm of the middle and inferior temporal gyri. **B.** Diagram illustrating retractor placement and exposure of the medial temporal lobe structures as viewed from anterior to posterior. *Arrow* points to a line connecting the "knee" of the middle cerebral artery in the Sylvian fissure to the velum terminale or anterior choroidal point in the temporal horn of the lateral ventricle. This line is used as a guideline to the extent of the resection of the amygdala. (From Vives et al., 2008, with permission.)

centers, however, prefer to perform *selective amygdalohippocampectomies* (Yasargil et al., 1985; Wieser, 1986), which spare neocortex (except for some parahippocampal tissue), when it is clear that seizure generation is limited to the hippocampus.

Hemispherectomy is also a standardized resection, although it is performed differently in different centers. Hemispherectomy originally involved removal of most or all of one hemisphere, including the amygdala and hippocampus (Rasmussen, 1987). It was introduced as a treatment for infantile hemiplegia and seizures by Krynauw (1950) and is used for infants and young children with catastrophic epileptic encephalopathies due to diffuse or multifocal lesions limited to one hemisphere. Late complications, including *hemosiderosis,*

intracranial hemorrhage, and *hydrocephalus,* due to decreased absorption of cerebral spinal fluid and movement of the remaining hemisphere within the cranial vault, led to modifications of the original *anatomical hemispherectomy.* These problems were avoided by disconnecting but leaving in situ the frontal and occipital poles (Rasmussen, 1987). This *modified hemispherectomy* has now evolved into *hemispherotomies,* the most common procedures performed today, which involve removal of the minimum amount of brain tissue necessary to expose and sever the hemispheric connections, leaving most of the disconnected hemisphere in place (Binder and Schramm, 2008; Dorfmüller et al., 2009) (Fig. 16–2). Hemispherectomies and hemispherotomies are usually performed in patients who already

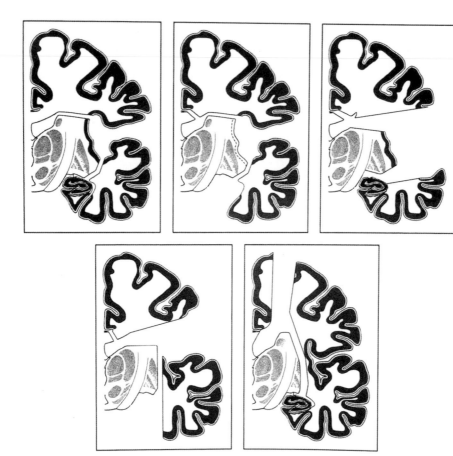

Figure 16–2. Modified functional hemispherectomy techniques. *Top left:* Transsylvian transsulcal keyhole approach to ventricle. *Top middle:* Second part in transsylvian keyhole approach: temporomesial resection, mesial disconnection, and insular cortex removal. *Top right:* Periinsular window technique. *Bottom left:* Variant of periinsular window technique. *Bottom right:* Dorsal transcortical subinsular hemispherotomy. (From Schramm, 2002, with permission.)

have hemiparesis and a useless hand, so no further neurological deficit is introduced, and contralateral motor function often improves postoperatively.

TAILORED RESECTIONS

Whereas it is only necessary to determine that habitual seizures originate somewhere within the boundaries of a standardized surgical resection, tailored resections are carried out when the extent of the epileptogenic region differs from patient to patient and needs to be individually determined. Neocortical resections are always tailored, because no standard procedures have been developed. Intracranial recordings, either intraoperative interictal spike mapping or extraoperative ictal recordings with chronic depth or subdural electrodes, are usually required to determine the extent of a tailored resection, but these tests are imperfect at delineating the epileptogenic brain tissue essential for seizure generation (Comair et al., 2008). Boundaries of essential primary cortex provide a practical limit to these resections. Whereas these boundaries were determined in the past by intraoperative functional brain mapping and later, in some cases, by functional mapping with extraoperative subdural grid recording (Jayakar and Lesser, 2008), noninvasive functional neuroimaging with fMRI, PET, and MEG now plays an important role as well. Tailored resections can be of any size, depending on the underlying pathological substrate, and in some patients large multilobar resections are performed as an alternative to hemispherectomy or hemispherotomy when it is clear that parts of the involved hemisphere are functioning normally and are not involved in the epileptogenic process.

Structural lesions visible on MRI or at surgery guide tailored resections, but it is usual practice to include *margins* of neocortex surrounding the region exhibiting epileptiform EEG abnormalities to ensure the best surgical outcome. When the lesion is within essential neocortex that cannot be damaged without inducing additional neurological deficit, *lesionectomies* are performed (Radhakrishnan et al., 2008). These operations, in which only the lesion is removed, without margins, often can reduce or even eliminate habitual seizures without producing residual neurological deficits. A unique form of lesionectomy is surgical

removal of *hypothalamic hamartomas*, which appear to generate some *gelastic seizures* (Munari et al., 1995) (Chapter 7).

DISCONNECTION SURGERY

The most common surgery performed to disconnect propagation of epileptic activity responsible for the clinical manifestation of ictal events is *corpus callosotomy*. Callosotomy was initially performed for the treatment of generalized tonic-clonic seizures (Van Wagenen and Herren, 1940; Bogen and Vogel, 1962) and involved complete section of the *corpus callosum, anterior commissure, hippocampal commissure,* and *fornix*. The results of this procedure were variable, with marked improvement in some patients but serious complications in others. An acute disconnection syndrome consisted of *mutism, apraxia* of the nondominant limbs, *agnosia, apathy, confusion, infantile behavior,* and *alternating focal motor seizures*. *Ventriculitis* was common, because of the need to enter the lateral and third ventricles, and damage often occurred to periventricular structures. Late complications included *hemorrhage* and *hydrocephalus*. Since the introduction of microsurgical techniques (Wilson et al., 1978, 1982; Roberts, 2008, 2009), serious postoperative complications can be avoided in most patients. The acute disconnection syndrome still occurs, however, perhaps in part as a result of traction on parasagittal structures of the nondominant hemisphere. Callosotomy is most effective in controlling the disabling tonic and atonic drop attacks that occur in many patients with severe medically refractory mixed seizure disorders, like the *Lennox-Gastaut syndrome*, but is considered only palliative, as other seizure types are usually not eliminated. The usual practice is to perform an anterior two-thirds callosotomy, which is less likely to be associated with disturbing disconnection symptoms, but complete callosotomy is indicated in patients with severe cognitive dysfunction who would not be impaired by those symptoms (Gates et al., 1987). The mechanism by which corpus callosum section alleviates epileptic seizures is not clear, particularly because callosal influences are often inhibitory rather than excitatory (Chapter 3). This fact may account for the observation that corpus callosum section in some patients can make frontal lobe seizures worse (Spencer et al., 1984b). Because VNS can be as effective for drop attacks as corpus callosotomy in many patients, this less invasive procedure is usually offered before callosotomy and has greatly reduced enthusiasm for surgery in the relevant patient population.

Predictors of good and poor outcome with corpus callosum section remain poorly defined. Results are reported to be best in patients who have drop attacks as the most disabling seizure type, only mild mental retardation, and lateralization of the primary dysfunction to one hemisphere. Disturbing behavioral sequelae are most likely to occur in patients with ipsilateral hand and hemispheric language dominance (Spencer et al., 1987).

Multiple subpial transection (MST) is designed to disconnect corticocortical fibers responsible for lateral spread of epileptic activity, leaving the cortical columns responsible for function intact (Morrell et al., 1989). This procedure has been carried out in primary motor and language cortices without producing significant neurological deficit and has been effective in eliminating or reducing spontaneous seizures. Most often, however, it is used in association with a tailored neocortical resection when the epileptogenic region is adjacent to and includes essential primary cortex that cannot be removed. Recent long-term follow-up studies, however, suggest that MST may not be as effective as originally presumed (Polkey and Smith, 2008; Smith et al., 2009).

ABLATIVE SURGERY

A number of stereotactic ablations have been used for treatment of epilepsy. Most attention early on was focused on *amygdalotomy* for temporal lobe seizures (Narabayashi and Mizutani, 1970) and *field of Forel lesions (Forel-H-otomy)* for unilateral and generalized motor seizures (Jinnai and Mukawa, 1970). Amygdalotomy was reported to be effective against seizures in some patients but more useful for controlling aggressive behavior. Because of association with psychosurgery and equivocal results with respect to seizures, these stereotactic ablations have fallen out of favor.

More recently, *stereotactic radiosurgery*, particularly *gamma knife surgery (GKS)*, has been used to produce localized ablation of epileptogenic tissue, including discrete lesions like *hypothalamic hamartomas* as well as more

diffuse hippocampal and amygdala abnormalities in *MTLE*. Some reports indicate results equivalent to those of open resection (Fisher et al., 2008; Yang et al., 2009; Chang et al., 2010). This process, however, induces edema, which can cause complications, and the tissue damage takes many months, usually over a year, to induce a beneficial effect. During this time, patients continue to have seizures, with associated morbidity and mortality. Laser ablation has a more immediate effect.

STIMULATION

Chronic intracranial stimulation has also been reported to control epileptic seizures. An early, actively advocated approach was cerebellar stimulation (Dow et al., 1962; Cooper et al., 1973). However, experience reported initially could not be reproduced (Wright et al., 1985), and cerebellar stimulation has been abandoned as a treatment for epileptic seizures.

More recently, recurrent deep-brain stimulation (device by *Medtronics*) has targeted various subcortical structures, and a large, multicenter controlled trial of stimulation of the *anterior thalamus* has yielded promising results (Fisher et al., 2010). Although the open-label phase of the study showed clear improvement with stimulation, results of the controlled trial itself were equivocal, because of an outlier in whom stimulation actually induced seizures until the stimulation parameters were changed. As a result, at the time of writing, the US Food and Drug Administration (FDA) has not approved deep-brain stimulation as a palliative treatment for epilepsy, although it is accepted in Europe.

Responsive stimulation (device by *Neuro-Pace*) refers to a stimulation paradigm designed to abort spontaneous seizures. This requires implantation of stimulating electrodes on or into a presumptive area of seizure generation that are connected to a small computer embedded in the skull. The computer detects the electrographic epileptiform abnormalities that might be ictal onsets and generates a stimulus that can prevent further development into a clinical seizure (Bergey, 2009; Morrell et al., 2011). Studies to date indicate not only that this approach is effective in reducing seizure frequency and severity but also that the device is triggered less often over time, suggesting that it might have an antiepileptogenic effect as well. Positive results from one Class 1 study have been published (Morrell et al., 2011), but at the time of writing, responsive stimulation as a palliative treatment remains investigational.

Surgical Protocols

STRATEGY

The presurgical evaluation for resective surgery is aimed at localizing the *epileptogenic zone* and, for tailored resections, determining its boundaries (Engel, 2009). There is, unfortunately, no specific test that reliably identifies epileptogenic tissue, so the epileptogenic zone is a theoretical concept defined as the area of brain necessary and sufficient for generating spontaneous seizures, which represents the minimal amount of tissue that must be removed or disconnected to eliminate habitual seizures. A number of diagnostic tests are used to approximate the volume of tissue included in the epileptogenic zone by identifying the *irritative zone*, the *ictal onset zone*, the *epileptogenic lesion*, the *symptomatogenic zone*, and the *functional deficit zone* (Lüders et al., 1993) (Table 16–5).

The *irritative zone* is the area of cortex that generates interictal spikes, usually recorded directly from the surface of the brain during

ECoG or extraoperatively with chronic subdural or depth electrodes. A single spike focus on scalp EEG may suffice to localize the irritative zone and confirm the epileptogenicity of a structural lesion but is not adequate to define the boundaries of the irritative zone when this is necessary for tailored resection. With direct brain recordings, the irritative zone is usually much larger than the epileptogenic zone and there may be multiple irritative zones; for instance, with MTLE it is common to record independent interictal spikes from both mesial temporal regions. Although the irritative zone indicates epileptogenicity, there are as yet no reliable features of interictal spikes that distinguish those generated within the epileptogenic zone (referred to as *red spikes*) from those that are propagated or represent tissue not capable of generating spontaneous seizures (referred to as *green spikes*). Techniques to distinguish red from green spikes are being investigated, as discussed later in this chapter. MEG, simultaneous EEG-fMRI, and EEG source localization can be used to better localize scalp-recorded interictal EEG spikes, but these techniques as yet do not selectively identify red spikes or reliably define critical boundaries of the epileptogenic zone.

The *ictal onset zone* is the area of cortex where initial ictal EEG discharges are recorded.

Table 16–5 Definition of Abnormal Brain Areas

	Definition	Measures
Epileptogenic zone	The area of brain that is necessary and sufficient for initiating seizures and whose removal or disconnection is necessary for abolition of seizures	Theoretical concept
Irritative zone	Area of cortex that generates interictal spikes	Electrophysiological (invasive and noninvasive)
Ictal onset zone	Area of cortex where seizures are generated (including areas of early propagation under certain circumstances)	Electrophysiological (invasive and noninvasive)
Epileptogenic lesion	Structural abnormality of the brain that is the direct cause of the epileptic seizures	Structural imaging and tissue pathology
Symptomatogenic zone	Portion of the brain that produces the initial clinical symptomatology	Behavioral observation and patient report
Functional deficit zone	Cortical area of nonepileptic dysfunction	Neurological examination, neuropsychological testing, EEG, PET, SPECT

EEG = electroencephalogram; PET = positron emission tomography; SPECT = single-photon emission computed tomography
From Lüders et al., 1993, with permission.

Although this can be inferred from ictal scalp recordings, particularly with a characteristic pattern recorded from basal electrodes in MTLE (Risinger et al., 1989) (see Fig. 6–6), more specific information regarding the location of the ictal onset zone is usually obtained from intracranial recordings. There is no standardized way to use information about the site of ictal onset and early propagation of ictal discharge to permit determination of the extent of the epileptogenic zone, but some workers feel that this zone must include sites of early propagation. Ictal SPECT and fMRI are now also used to delineate the ictal onset zone.

The *epileptogenic lesion* is the structural abnormality that is determined to be the cause of spontaneous seizures based on electrophysiological confirmation. As noted previously, patients with focal epilepsy can have structural lesions on MRI that are incidental findings and not epileptogenic. Hippocampal sclerosis is the most common epileptogenic lesion in adolescents and adults with surgically remediable epilepsy, and malformations of cortical development are the most common epileptogenic lesions in children but are also often seen in adolescents and adults, sometimes as dual pathology. Other frequently encountered lesions include scars, vascular malformations, cysts, neoplasms, and congenital defects, as discussed in Chapter 5. Seizures may begin within the epileptogenic lesion, as with hippocampal sclerosis and cortical dysplasia, or in brain adjacent to lesions, such as neoplasms and scars. As a rule, surgical results are not as good when the epileptogenic lesion is not completely removed, and in most patients the epileptogenic zone is likely to be larger than the structural lesion. However, in some cases, as discussed previously, only part of a large structural lesion or one of multiple lesions is epileptogenic and excellent results can be obtained by a limited resection. Most epileptogenic lesions are visible on high-resolution MRI, but occasionally when the MRI is normal and the epileptogenic region is defined primarily on the basis of electrophysiological information, structural abnormalities (usually hippocampal sclerosis or focal cortical dysplasia) can be seen on pathological evaluation of resected tissue.

The *symptomatogenic zone* is the area of brain responsible for generating the initial symptoms of the clinical seizure. These may consist of an aura or signs visible to an observer, as discussed in Chapter 6. Detailed description by patients and others of their habitual seizures and careful evaluation of video-recorded ictal events help to lateralize and occasionally localize an epileptogenic region, but often the symptomatogenic zone is distant from the site of ictal onset, which may be in a so-called silent area of the brain. For instance, behavioral signs and symptoms of mesial temporal lobe onset seizures occur only when the ictal discharge is propagated beyond hippocampus. Knowledge of typical propagation patterns, however, can be helpful in deriving localizing information from ictal behavior.

The *functional deficit zone* is identifiable when nonepileptic interictal disturbances are present and localize abnormal brain tissue. As with structural lesions, additional evidence is required to demonstrate that this dysfunctional area is epileptogenic. When the functional deficit zone involves essential cortex, it can manifest as deficits on the neurological or neurocognitive examination, but localized functional disturbances within the whole brain can be identified as areas of hypometabolism on PET with ^{18}F-fluorodeoxyglucose (FDG-PET) or hypoperfusion on SPECT as well as focal nonepileptic EEG abnormalities.

The protocol for diagnostic presurgical evaluation differs according to the type of epileptic seizures experienced by the patient and the anticipated surgical intervention. For MTLE, diagnostic testing is designed to lateralize the epileptogenic region, determine that it lies within the standard area for anteromesial temporal resection, and to establish that the contralateral hemisphere can support memory (Engel, 2009). For tailored neocortical resections, more detailed testing is required to determine the boundaries of the epileptogenic region as well as the boundaries of any adjacent essential primary cortical areas that should not be resected. Surgery can usually be planned based on results of noninvasive testing, although ECoG may be needed for some tailored neocortical resections. When noninvasive studies are equivocal but sufficient evidence is obtained to limit the potential epileptogenic zone to two or three areas, invasive studies can be performed, commonly involving depth electrodes when mesial temporal and other deeper structures are included in the hypothesis and subdural electrodes when the epileptogenic zone is presumed to involve lateral neocortex. Subdural grid placement requires craniotomy and therefore is usually only performed unilaterally, requiring the epileptogenic zone to be well lateralized. Subdural strips that can be introduced bilaterally through burr holes are preferred when lateralization has not been established. Typical problems that can be resolved by invasive VEM include questions of laterality when the hypothesis includes bilateral structures; questions that require examination of two potential epileptogenic regions, for instance, mesial versus lateral temporal or mesial temporal versus orbital frontal; and questions regarding the extent of the epileptogenic region.

Surgical treatment for infants and young children requires additional specialized skills and facilities (Duchowny et al., 2008; Hauptman and Mathern, 2009). It is difficult to localize the epileptogenic region in infants and young children, particularly those with epileptic encephalopathies and diffuse hemispheric lesions. Fortunately, at this stage of maturation, the brain is plastic and it is usually safer and more cost-effective to carry out larger resections than to perform detailed invasive studies to define the boundaries of a limited resection. Often, the most appropriate approach in infants and young children with diffuse hemispheric lesions is hemispherotomy, particularly when they already have hemiparesis and a useless hand. Multilobar resections can be performed, however, when unequivocally normal areas of ipsilateral brain tissue can be identified. Seizure and cognitive outcome of hemispheric resections are negatively affected by the presence of contralateral MRI abnormalities (Boshuisen et al., 2010). Whereas most surgical lesions in small children are static, a particularly problematic situation is *Rasmussen syndrome*, which is a progressive disorder in which frequent focal seizures or *epilepsia partialis continua* result from a hemispheric lesion that has not yet induced a hemiparesis with a useless hand (Chapter 7). When this occurs in the language-dominant hemisphere, often a decision needs to be made about whether or not to operate and introduce a new hemiparesis while the brain is still capable of transferring language to the opposite hemisphere, which is usually the case before the age of 7. In almost all cases, waiting would eventually produce a hemiparesis and language deficit, and opportunities for transfer of useful language could be lost.

Diagnostic evaluation for MST, ablative surgery, and response stimulation requires localization of the epileptogenic region; however, the diagnostic evaluation for corpus callosotomy and deep-brain stimulation, for the most part, is aimed at determining that the patient would not benefit from a more definitive resective procedure.

CANDIDATE SELECTION

For experienced clinicians, a detailed history, including a description of all habitual ictal events, remains the most important initial step in recognizing potential surgical candidates. Neurological examination and psychological, psychiatric, and social evaluations further help to determine whether a patient has epileptic seizures and an epilepsy syndrome that is amenable to surgical treatment. Psychological and social evaluation is essential for determining how the patient will tolerate the presurgical evaluation and whether improvement or cure of the epilepsy condition will have a sufficiently positive impact on quality of life to justify the risks and expense. Psychiatric consultation is also an important part of the presurgical protocol, to identify potential problems and ensure that support is available if needed (Kanner, 2009). Interestingly, depression may predict a poorer surgical outcome with respect to epileptic seizures, but this is certainly not a contraindication to surgery (Kanner, 2009). Psychological and social effects of successful surgery need to be anticipated and discussed with the patient; for instance, elimination of habitual seizures can alter a personality type from passive dependence to assertive independence, which in some cases has serious interpersonal consequences, including divorce. Transient depression is also well documented to occur during the first postoperative year and can be problematic, so it helps to warn patients and their families of this possibility. The only absolute contraindications to surgical treatment are an underlying neurodegenerative disease as the cause of the epilepsy that cannot be altered by surgery or a medical condition that would make surgery an unacceptable risk. In the latter patients, GKS could be an alternative. A typical presurgical evaluation protocol is diagrammed in the flow chart shown in Figure 16–3.

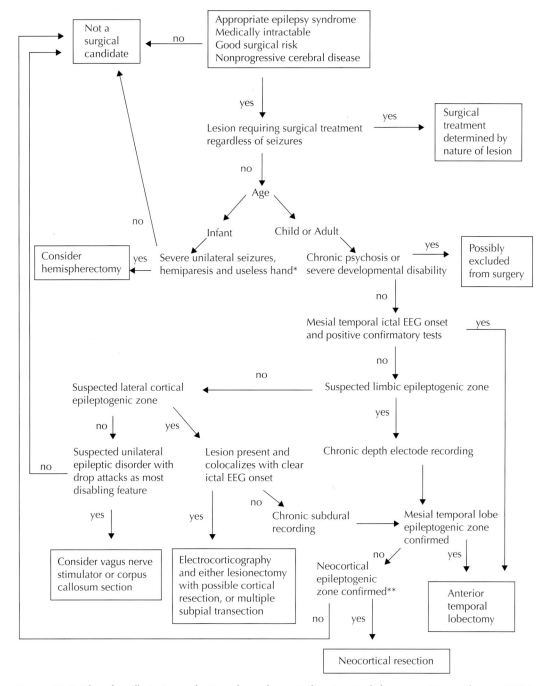

Figure 16–3. Flow chart illustrating evaluation scheme for surgical treatment of pharmacoresistant epilepsy at UCLA. °Young children also may be considered for hemispherectomy, and some patients who do not already have a severe hemiparesis may choose to undergo hemispherectomy and accept the inevitable neurological deficit. °°Identification of extratemporal epileptogenic zones may require two intracranial procedures, with depth electrode recording preceding the subdural electrode recording. (Modified from Engel, 1989, by Stern and Engel, 2012, with permission.)

PHASE I

The term *Phase I* is usually applied to noninvasive presurgical diagnostic testing. Interictal EEG and MRI are invariably performed in all patients with epilepsy who ultimately might be considered surgical candidates. Localization of epileptiform transients and nonepileptiform abnormalities on the interictal EEG are useful, the former particularly when they confirm the epileptogenic nature of a structural lesion seen on MRI, but rarely do the results of these studies rule patients in or out as candidates for a surgical procedure. More often, misconceptions in the community about the results of these tests prevent appropriate referral, as already discussed. MRI identification of hippocampal atrophy or hyperintensity on T2 imaging strongly suggests the presence of hippocampal sclerosis in patients with a history and EEG findings consistent with MTLE, while other structural lesions help determine the presence of a resectable epileptogenic region; however, these studies are most informative when performed according to the epilepsy protocol described in Chapter 12. When routine MRI studies are read as negative, this specialized approach, including additional strategies such as *diffusion tensor imaging (DTI)* to evaluate white matter tracts, surface reconstruction, and other manipulations (Chapter 12), often reveals subtle structural disturbances consistent with hippocampal sclerosis, focal cortical dysplasia, and other malformations of cortical development that are highly epileptogenic but often impossible to see with routine MRI techniques. *Statistical parametric mapping (SPM)* of hippocampus and neocortex with high-resolution MRI permits determination of patterns of atrophy and cortical thickness not apparent on visual analysis of MRI or volumetry (Lin et al., 2005, 2007; Ogren et al., 2009a, 2009b). Even when these specialized high-resolution MRI scans are negative, localized hypometabolism on FDG-PET can still indicate the presence of an epileptogenic lesion (Carne et al., 2004; Chassoux et al., 2010; Fong et al., 2011), and PET ligands other than FDG are occasionally used (Chapter 12).

The next important step is inpatient VEM to capture spontaneous seizures, permit observation of clinical behavior, and, when possible, determine the site of ictal EEG onset (Chapter 12). Electroclinical correlations are important because initial ictal behaviors observed on video can provide lateralizing and localizing clues (Table 6–3). Especially when MTLE is suspected, basilar electrodes are necessary to best identify a mesial temporal ictal EEG onset. Whereas in the past these routinely included sphenoidal electrodes, T_1-T_2 scalp placements are equally useful in most cases, and sphenoidal electrodes are now reserved for resolving equivocal results. The typical scalp-recorded ictal onset pattern of MTLE is a 5- to 7-Hz buildup of activity in one basal electrode as the initial EEG change or within 30 seconds of a more diffuse but not contralateral ictal EEG discharge (Risinger et al., 1989) (see Fig. 6–6). In rare instances, this pattern is initially seen contralateral to the site of ictal onset, usually when the sclerotic hippocampus is so atrophic it is incapable of generating activity with a high enough amplitude to be seen at the scalp, a situation referred to as the *burned-out hippocampus* (Mintzer et al., 2004). Ictal EEG onset is often much more difficult to localize when epileptic seizures originate in the neocortex, and although interictal EEG spikes are notoriously misleading, they can provide more reliable localizing information than ictal EEG in some patients. Quantitative interictal EEG spike data can be obtained using automatic spike detection, when necessary, during inpatient VEM and can be useful for patients with MTLE and bilateral interictal spikes; however, spike frequency is not always greater on the epileptogenic side. In patients with structural lesions on MRI or localized hypometabolism on FDG-PET, inpatient VEM provides largely confirmatory information to establish that the structural lesion is indeed epileptogenic. In patients without abnormalities on neuroimaging, the interictal and ictal data are essential for developing a hypothesis necessary for planning invasive testing, or *Phase II*.

The third critical diagnostic component of the presurgical evaluation is neurocognitive testing, which provides important information concerning the location and extent of the functional deficit zone (Jones-Gotman and Djordjevic, 2009; Wilson and Engel, 2010) (Chapter 12). Tests of material-specific disturbances in memory and learning help to localize as well as lateralize a mesial temporal abnormality, while other test batteries identify disturbances indicating dysfunction in the language-dominant or nondominant hemisphere and in the frontal lobe. In many patients with suspected neocortical epileptogenic zones, fMRI is useful for determining hemisphere dominance for language and for mapping cortical functions to determine the spatial relationship between the suspected epileptogenic zone and essential cortical areas that must not be damaged during surgery.

Functional MRI, however, is not yet capable of replacing the *intracarotid amobarbital procedure (IAP)* for confirming that the temporal lobe contralateral to a proposed mesial temporal resection can support memory by anesthetizing the ipsilateral hemisphere (Jones-Gotman et al., 2008) (Chapter 12). If necessary, contralateral injection can also be performed to determine that the suspected mesial temporal area is dysfunctional, confirming a functional deficit zone consistent with the presence of an abnormality that may not be visible on MRI or FDG-PET and increasing confidence that removal of this area of the brain will not result in an additional, unacceptable memory deficit. Whereas in the past it was considered always necessary to perform IAP prior to an anteromesial temporal resection (you don't remove a kidney without making sure the other kidney works), there is disagreement today over the criteria for requiring this test. Some centers perform IAP only when surgery is planned in the language-dominant hemisphere or when neurocognitive testing or other studies indicate that there may be problems in the contralateral hemisphere. Still other centers do not perform IAP at all, a situation exacerbated by the chronic shortage or unavailability of amobarbital in many countries. *Topiramate* and *zonisamide* interfere with test results and should be discontinued several weeks before an IAP (Bookheimer et al., 2005) (Chapter 12). An alternative approach using *etomidate (the etomidate speech and memory—eSAM—test)* has been proposed as an alternative (Jones-Gotman et al., 2008). This agent has the additional advantage that it can be administered continuously for as long as necessary to carry out the studies.

When necessary, additional information concerning the location of the irritative zone can be obtained with interictal MEG, simultaneous EEG-fMRI, and source localization of EEG spikes (Chapter 12). Interictal functional and structural abnormalities can also be identified with *magnetic resonance spectroscopy (MRS)* and fMRI cortical mapping (Chapter 12). Additional information regarding the location of the ictal onset zone can be obtained with ictal SPECT, it is occasionally possible to obtain ictal MEG, and source localization can be carried out on ictal EEG data (Chapter 12).

Noninvasive diagnostic tests under investigation include α-*methyl-tryptophan (AMT) PET* and *pathological high-frequency oscillations (pHFOs)* (Chapter 4). AMT is preferentially taken up by the epileptogenic tuber in patients with tuberous sclerosis and multiple lesions and might identify other epileptogenic regions such as hippocampal sclerosis and focal cortical dysplasia (Kumar et al., 2011). Pathological HFOs have a high correlation with epileptogenicity when recorded directly from the brain and may, under certain circumstances, be detected with scalp electrodes, MEG, or fMRI, in which case they could provide important localizing information (Worrell and Gotman, 2011) (Chapter 12). Indeed, pHFOs could possibly distinguish red from green spikes.

When noninvasive test results are concordant, they are usually sufficient to permit determination of the location and, where necessary, the extent of the epileptogenic zone, and the patient can proceed to surgery. For MTLE, this usually means that there is evidence implicating one hippocampus based on unilateral hippocampal sclerosis or another lesion on MRI or mesial temporal hypometabolism on FDG-PET, confirmed by material-specific memory dysfunction based on neurocognitive testing, epileptogenicity demonstrated by interictal and ictal EEG, and seizure semiology consistent with seizure generation in this location. At many centers, when structural and functional neuroimaging data are unequivocal, agree with seizure semiology, and the contralateral hemisphere can support memory, a lateralized ictal EEG onset rather than a localized one is sufficient to justify surgery. For tailored neocortical resections, concordance of structural and functional data and ictal and interictal EEG findings can reliably localize the epileptogenic zone but not necessarily determine its boundaries. Chronic invasive studies may not be necessary in most cases, however, when it is safe to remove a structural lesion with margins determined by ECoG (Holmes and Chatrian, 2008). The location and extent of adjacent essential cortex can be identified with fMRI or MEG, and if there is overlap, this can be clarified by intraoperative functional mapping in most cases. This approach is not possible, however, for mapping functions, such as language, that require awakening during the operation, if the patient cannot cooperate, as is the case for young children. Results of noninvasive testing are almost invariably sufficient to permit surgical resection when hemispherectomies, hemispherotomies, or corpus callosotomies are planned. Ablative surgery and response stimulation require localization of the epileptogenic zone, but this is not necessary for deep-brain stimulation.

PHASE II

When the results of Phase I testing are inadequate to allow a patient to go directly to surgery but sufficient to permit a reasonable hypothesis to be made concerning the likely locations of a few possible resectable epileptogenic zones, Phase II, consisting of chronic intracranial recordings, is usually recommended to evaluate the pattern of EEG onset of spontaneous seizures (Spencer et al., 2008, 2009). When an epileptogenic zone is suspected within the mesial temporal regions, stererotactically implanted depth electrodes are preferred, involving bilateral placements in amygdalae, hippocampi and sometimes other limbic structures such as anterior cingulate and orbitofrontal cortex (Fig. 16–4). Electrodes can be placed in other areas when the hypothesis includes a possible epileptogenic zone in other neocortical areas. Stereotactically implanted depth electrodes may also be preferred if an epileptogenic zone is suspected in other deep-brain areas, such as mesial frontal or occipital lobe. Some centers, however, prefer subdural strips. If the potential epileptogenic zone is neocortical, on the lateral surface of the brain, and well lateralized, subdural grid arrays are used, individually designed to cover the suspected cortical areas (Fig. 16–5). These can also be combined with subdural strips inserted under the temporal lobe and between hemispheres. Subdural grids require a craniotomy for insertion and therefore are not used when distinguishing between epileptogenic zones in both hemispheres. In this situation, subdural strips are inserted bilaterally through burr holes. Interpretation of EEG ictal onsets from subdural grid recordings can be difficult; however, a new, dense-array, flexible grid system could greatly enhance the amount of useful information gleaned from this procedure (Viventi et al., 2011). Functional mapping can be carried out easily with chronic subdural grid recordings when this cannot be performed intraoperatively, but is difficult to do with subdural strip or depth electrodes.

So-called *semi-invasive* recording is also performed at some centers, although this practice is falling out of favor. Electrodes are inserted bilaterally through the *foramen ovale* with a technique similar to that used for ablative treatment of *trigeminal neuralgia*. These multicontact electrodes, inserted freehand into the *ambient cistern,* record from the mesial surface of the temporal lobe and can be useful for distinguishing between bilateral potential epileptogenic zones; however, they are inadequate for determining whether activity might be propagated from elsewhere in the brain (Wieser, 2008). *Epidural peg electrodes*, plastic, mushroom-shaped pegs containing a disc electrode that can be inserted through a small burr hole to record from the surface of the brain, are now used only rarely as sentinel electrodes contralateral to a subdural grid (Wieser, 2008).

Several invasive approaches under investigation that might become extremely valuable in the near future for localizing the epileptogenic zone include direct brain recording of *pHFOs* (Worrell and Gotman, 2011), which may be even more reliable than the ictal onset zone in defining the boundaries of epileptogenic tissue (Jacobs et al., 2010); *optical imaging* that uses light reflectance to measure the state of neuronal activation (Haglund et al., 2008); and *microdialysis probes*, which permit extracellular fluid to be sampled during and after seizures (Cavus and Wilson, 2008) (Chapter 12). Although *hypersynchronous* and *low-voltage fast* EEG patterns are typically used to identify the ictal onset zone (Chapter 4), focal *initial ultraslow waves* may also provide important localizing information in the future (Bragin and Engel, 2008).

Chronic invasive VEM for MTLE identifies an epileptogenic region in approximately two-thirds of patients who undergo such evaluations. Most often, these result in standardized anteromesial temporal resections or, at times, tailored resections that include more lateral neocortex. Almost all patients who undergo subdural grid recording for neocortical epilepsy receive a surgical resection; the surgical

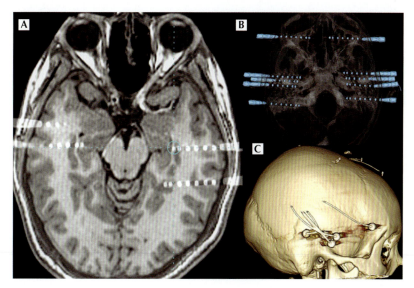

Figure 16–4. Depth electrode implantation **A.** MRI-CT fusion: coregistration of preoperative MRI and post–depth electrode placement computed tomography (CT) of the brain. Position of the electrode is precisely evaluated. **B.** Depth electrodes (*blue*) are demonstrated with transparent skull view. **C.** Surface rendering of the skull with five depth electrode placement locations on the right hemisphere. (Courtesy of Dr. Noriko Salamon.)

team usually decides that it would be reasonable to carry out some resective procedure during the craniotomy required to remove the subdural grid.

PHASE III

Phase III, therapeutic surgery, is determined by the results of Phases I and II and occasionally requires intraoperative ECoG or

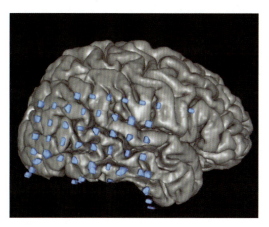

Figure 16–5. Subdural grid array. Surface rendering image of the patient's brain with superposition of the grid placement. This helps to identify anatomical correlation with the location of each grid. (Courtesy of Dr. Noriko Salamon.)

functional mapping. Advances in neuroimaging and microsurgical techniques have greatly improved the safety and efficacy of mesial temporal lobe resections (Vives et al., 2008; Leiphart and Fried, 2009), localized neocortical resections (Comair et al., 2008; Leiphart and Fried, 2009), lesionectomies and surgical resection for specific structural abnormalities (Radhakrishnan et al., 2008; Chern and Comair, 2009; Uff and Kitchen, 2009; Wetjen et al., 2009), multilobar resections and hemispherotomy (Binder and Schramm, 2008; Dorfmüller et al., 2009), corpus callosotomy (Roberts, 2008, 2009), MST (Polkey and Smith, 2008; Smith et al., 2009), approaches to hypothalamic hamartoma (Smith et al., 2009), ablative radiosurgery (Yang et al., 2009), frameless stereotaxic surgery (McEvoy and Arnold, 2009), and awake surgery (Kaufman and Pilcher, 2009). Specialized approaches to anesthesia have also been developed for the various epilepsy surgery procedures (Van de Wiele, 2009). Detailed discussion of surgical procedures is beyond the scope of this text.

Outcome

In recent years, quantitative outcome assessment has become an important aspect of epilepsy surgery research, necessary to evaluate the sensitivity and specificity of presurgical diagnostic tests and the efficacy of surgical interventions. Outcome is measured with respect to epileptic seizures, *health-related quality of life (HRQOL)*, cognitive and social function, and surgical complications. Typically, outcome measures are made only on the population of patients undergoing surgical treatment; however, a much more realistic representation of a surgical center's efficacy would be to measure outcome for the total population referred for surgery. This figure is essential in assessing the cost-effectiveness of surgical therapy (Langfitt, 1997), because cost of presurgical evaluation must be considered whether or not the patient proceeds to surgery.

SEIZURES

The classification of postoperative outcome from the 1993 Palm Desert conference (Table 16–6) is the one most commonly used in reporting results of surgical series and controlled trials (Engel et al., 1993). However, the ILAE classification (Table 16–7) is also used, when accurate documentation of preoperative seizure frequency is available (Wieser et al., 2001). Table 16–8 shows outcome data with respect to seizures for mesial temporal resections, neocortical resections, hemispherectomies, and corpus callosotomies obtained from two worldwide surveys carried out in 1986 and 1991, at the time of the first and second Palm Desert conferences (Engel et al., 1993). These data demonstrate an increase between 1985 and 1990 in the percentage of patients who were seizure-free following limbic resections and, perhaps more importantly, an even greater decrease in the number of patients who were not improved, reflecting advances in presurgical evaluation for MTLE during this interval. Although there was no change in outcome with respect to seizure freedom for patients undergoing neocortical resections, there was a considerable decrease in those not improved, indicating an overall better outcome. The advent of subdural grid recording during this interval perhaps resulted in an increase in patients who underwent resections based on electrophysiological findings alone, less than 50% of whom became seizure-free. On the other hand, when a lesion was present, surgical outcome with

respect to seizures was essentially the same as for those who underwent anteromesial temporal resection. There was an increasing interest in hemispherectomies during this interval. The drop in efficacy of this procedure is most likely explained by the fact that surgical teams were willing to operate on patients with more difficult epileptic encephalopathies.

There have been only two RCTs of epilepsy surgery, both for temporal lobe epilepsy. The first, carried out at the University of Western Ontario, used an intention-to-treat paradigm that randomized patients with long-standing temporal lobe epilepsy before presurgical evaluation; it found that 58% of those randomized to surgery and 8% of those randomized to the medical arm were seizure-free a year later. However, not all patients randomized to surgery actually received a therapeutic surgical procedure (Wiebe et al., 2001). Evaluating only those patients who actually received surgery, the percentage who became seizure-free was 64%, essentially the same value seen in the 1991 Palm Desert survey. The AAN, in association with the AES and the AANS, subsequently carried out a meta-analysis of 24 nonoverlapping surgical series published between 1990 and 2000, which also found two-thirds of patients to be seizure-free after temporal resections for temporal lobe epilepsy (Engel et al., 2003). Based on this finding, a *practice parameter* was issued recommending surgery as the treatment of choice for medically refractory temporal lobe epilepsy (Engel et al., 2003). Although the meta-analysis also found that 50% of patients undergoing neocortical resections became seizure-free, again similar to results obtained in the 1991 Palm Desert survey, the AAN did not permit recommendations, because no RCTs had been performed. These data are confirmed by a more recent review that found 53–84% of patients to be seizure-free after at least one year following temporal lobe surgery and 36–76% after neocortical surgery (Spencer and Huh, 2008). Outcomes for epilepsy surgery in the pediatric population are also improving (Hemb et al., 2010).

The second RCT was the multicenter *Early Randomized Surgical Epilepsy Trial (ERSET)* (Engel et al., 2012). The AAN practice parameter recommended early surgical intervention to reduce the development of irreversible psychological and social disability. ERSET, therefore,

Table 16–6 Classification of Postoperative Outcome

Class I: Free of disabling seizures[°]
  A. Completely seizure-free since surgery
  B. Nondisabling simple partial seizures only since surgery
  C. Some disabling seizures after surgery, but free of disabling seizures for at least 2 years
  D. Generalized convulsions with antiseizure drug discontinuation only

Class II: Rare disabling seizures ("almost seizure-free")
  A. Initially free of disabling seizures but has rare seizures now
  B. Rare disabling seizures since surgery
  C. More than rare disabling seizures since surgery, but rare seizures for the last 2 years
  D. Nocturnal seizures only

Class III: Worthwhile improvement[†]
  A. Worthwhile seizure reduction
  B. Prolonged seizure-free intervals amounting to greater than half the follow-up period, but not <2 years

Class IV: No worthwhile improvement
  A. Significant seizure reduction
  B. No appreciable change
  C. Seizures worse

[°]Excludes early postoperative seizures (first few weeks).
[†]Determination of "worthwhile improvement" will require quantitative analysis of additional data, such as percentage seizure reduction, cognitive function, and quality of life.
From Engel et al., 1993, with permission.

Table 16–7 ILAE Proposal for a New Classification of Outcome with Respect to Epileptic Seizures

Outcome Classification	Definition
1	Completely seizure-free; no auras
2	Only auras; no other seizures
3	One to three seizure days per year; ± auras
4	Four seizure days per year to 50% reduction of baseline seizure days; ± auras
5	Less than 50% reduction of baseline seizure
6	More than 100% increase of baseline seizure days; ± auras

From Wieser et al., 2003, with permission.

was designed to enroll patients within two years after failure of two trials of antiseizure drugs, to compare the effectiveness of surgical intervention with continued pharmacotherapy early in the course of the disease process. In contrast to the Western Ontario RCT, patients were randomized *after* they had undergone detailed presurgical evaluation and were deemed candidates for anteromesial resection. Because the outcome of continued medical treatment at this early time was uncertain, a two-year follow-up was considered ethical. In this study, none of the patients randomized to the medical arm were seizure-free during the second year, while 85% in the surgical arm were seizure-free. The excellent surgical outcome most likely reflects the careful selection process rather than the early intervention, but results for the medical arm demonstrate the futility of continued medical treatment for most patients with MTLE.

Long-term outcome with respect to seizures is difficult to assess. Most patients who become seizure-free after surgery remain seizure-free, and others who are not seizure-free after surgery continue to have seizures, although they are usually improved. However, some patients have seizures that initially "run down" and eventually go away, while others who are initially seizure-free may begin having seizures again many years later (Engel, 1987c; Spencer and Huh, 2008; de Tisi et al., 2011). In the latter situation, it is uncertain whether this always represents a relapse of the initial seizure disorder or whether some patients with a genetic predisposition to epilepsy are likely to develop seizures at a later date for some other reason. To date, there are insufficient data regarding results of surgical treatment other than that performed for MTLE to establish reliable patterns of outcome with respect to seizures, let alone identify risk factors for poor outcome.

QUALITY OF LIFE

With the exception of the classic study of Taylor (1972), who visited the homes of 100 patients operated on by Falconer to determine the effects of surgical treatment and any changes in seizure frequency on their daily lives, a feat that is likely never to be repeated, studies on

Table 16–8 **Outcomes Before 1985 and from 1986 to 1990**

		Number of Patients (%)			
		Seizure-free	Improved	Not Improved	Total
Limbic resections					
Before 1985		1,296 (55.5)	648 (27.7)	392 (16.8)	2,336 (100)
1986–1990	ATL	2,429 (67.9)	860 (24.0)	290 (8.1)	3,579 (100)
	AH	284 (68.8)	92 (22.3)	37 (9.0)	413 (100)
Neocortical resections					
Before 1985		356 (43.2)	229 (27.8)	240 (29.1)	825 (100)
1986–1990	ETR	363 (45.1)	283 (35.2)	159 (19.8)	805 (100)
	L	195 (66.6)	63 (21.5)	35 (11.9)	293 (100)
Hemispherectomies					
Before 1985		68 (77.3)	16 (18.2)	4 (4.5)	88 (100)
1986–1990	H	128 (67.4)	40 (21.1)	22 (11.6)	190 (100)
	MR	75 (45.2)	59 (35.5)	32 (19.3)	166 (100)
Corpus callosotomies					
Before 1985		10 (5.0)	140 (71.0)	47 (23.9)	197 (100)
1986–1990		43 (7.6)	343 (60.9)	177 (31.4)	563 (100)

AH = amygdalohippocampectomy; ATL = anterior temporal lobectomy; ETR = extratemporal resection; H = hemispherectomy; L = lesionectomy; MR = large multilobar resection.
From Engel et al., 1993, with permission.

outcome of surgical treatment for epilepsy focused almost entirely on epileptic seizures until the development in the 1990s of instruments for quantitatively assessing quality of life in patients with epilepsy (Chapter 11). With this important advance, workers now believe that it is not sufficient to demonstrate that a surgical procedure can be successful in eliminating epileptic seizures unless it can also be shown that seizure freedom is accompanied by a significant improvement in quality of life. The original *Epilepsy Surgery Inventory-55 (ESI-55)* (Vickrey et al., 1992) has evolved into the *Quality of Life in Epilepsy (QOLIE)* scales, which were specifically designed to measure HRQOL in surgical series (Devinsky et al., 1995) (Chapter 11). Several versions exist for adults, and there is also a QOLIE for adolescents (Cramer et al., 1999). HRQOL was significantly improved after one year in the surgical group compared with the medical group in the Western Ontario RCT (Wiebe et al., 2001) and at the end of the second year for the ERSET study (Engel et al., 2012). Many noncontrolled studies have also demonstrated improvement in HRQOL when patients become seizure-free following surgery (Engel et al., 2003; Spencer and Huh, 2008), but HRQOL may not be as good if patients continue to have auras (Vickrey et al., 1995a).

COGNITIVE, PSYCHIATRIC, AND SOCIAL OUTCOMES

There was a trend toward improvement in employment and school attendance after one year in patients randomized to surgery in the Western Ontario RCT, and there was improvement in independence and socialization after two years for patients randomized to surgery in the ERSET study. Cognitive testing was not performed in the Western Ontario study, and although there were no statistically significant differences in cognitive function between the two groups in the ERSET study, numbers were too small to permit definitive conclusions. It has been consistently demonstrated, however, that anteromesial temporal resection is not likely to introduce additional disturbing memory deficits in patients who already have memory impairment prior to surgery but that a verbal memory deficit is inevitable following anteromesial temporal resection of the language-dominant hemisphere in patients who have normal memory function preoperatively (Jones-Gotman et al., 2008). Consequently, outcome with respect to memory was an important question for the ERSET study because surgery was performed early, when patients are less likely to have a memory deficit preoperatively and are at greater risk for new cognitive impairment. Although the data in this study were inadequate to definitively demonstrate that surgery did not lead to memory impairment, the robust improvement in HRQOL suggests that even if a new memory disturbance appeared, it was offset by the benefits of seizure freedom.

In a prior study, of patients followed for two to five years after temporal lobe resection, HRQOL improved in the 82% in remission whether or not memory declined and in the 10% who were not in remission but had no memory impairment, but HRQOL decreased in the 8% who were not in remission with memory decline (Langfitt et al., 2007). Although patients who continue to have seizures following a dominant hemisphere anteromesial temporal resection are most likely to be impaired by worsening of verbal memory function, those with preoperative memory deficits can experience improvement in memory and in overall IQ if they become seizure-free postoperatively. The effect occurs even before antiseizure medication is reduced and presumably reflects the fact that the contralateral hippocampus is no longer involved in propagated epileptiform activity. A recent systematic literature review of cognitive outcomes after surgery for MTLE found that although memory and learning abilities were reduced in many patients, particularly after surgery of the language-dominant hemisphere, IQ, executive functioning, and attention declined in only a few patients, and there was substantial improvement in verbal fluency with left-sided temporal lobe surgery (Sherman et al., 2011). Self-reported cognitive gains were more common than declines.

It has been difficult to document postoperative improvements in employment in epilepsy surgery series, most likely because the patients had epilepsy for many years before becoming seizure-free and had already missed the opportunity to gain the interpersonal and vocational skills necessary to obtain employment and live independently. Earlier surgery and formal rehabilitation programs should improve social outcome (Fraser and Thorbecke, 2008; Zarroli et al., 2011). The AAN practice parameter meta-analysis found that 79% of patients were driving postoperatively compared with 20% preoperatively and that 88% were living independently compared with 68% preoperatively (Engel et al., 2003). A recent meta-analysis confirmed improved social outcome after localized surgical resections for epilepsy (Hamiwka et al., 2011). Studies have indicated that mortality rate is reduced in patients who are seizure-free following surgery (Sperling, 2004; Choi et al., 2008), and the one patient that died in the Western Ontario RCT was in the medical arm (Wiebe et al., 2001).

It is well known that depression occurs postoperatively, and this was found to occur in one-quarter to one-half of patients during the first postoperative year in the AAN practice parameter meta-analysis (Engel et al., 2003). Such problems should be anticipated and will resolve in time, while de novo more severe psychiatric symptoms are rare and most common in patients who continue to have seizures (Wrench et al., 2011). A recent meta-analysis found that after surgery psychiatric outcomes generally improve or remain the same (Macrodimitris et al., 2011).

SURGICAL COMPLICATIONS

Complications of surgery have been best documented for anteromesial temporal resection (Engel et al., 2003; Polkey, 2009). Many patients will have a contralateral superior quadrantanopsia following this procedure, but it is rarely noted by the patient and is usually identified only by formal visual field testing. According to the AAN practice parameter meta-analysis, 6% of patients experience other new neurological deficits, consisting of mild aphasias, cranial nerve III and IV palsies, visual field deficits greater than a quadrant, and hemiparesis, but half of these resolve within three months (Engel et al., 2003). Most of the aphasias were receptive and followed temporal resections, while the hemipareses resulted from neocortical resections adjacent to motor cortex. Postoperative infections occurred in 5% of patients, mostly involving the wound, but there was one brain abscess and one case of deep vein thrombosis. Mortality attributed to surgery was less than 0.4% but may be slightly higher in children (Spencer and Huh, 2008). Complications of neocortical resections vary depending on the location and proximity to essential cortex.

Hydrocephalus and *hemosiderosis* are late complications of hemispherectomy but are rarely encountered now with modified hemispherectomies and hemispherotomies. The troublesome disconnection syndromes occasionally encountered with corpus callosotomy are usually avoided when only the anterior two-thirds of the corpus callosum is sectioned, but patients may develop transient language problems postoperatively, most likely due to traction of the mesial frontal lobe.

Development of New Centers

Presurgical evaluation and surgical treatment of epilepsy require a dedicated hospital facility with highly specialized equipment and a team of experienced personnel, including a neurologist; a neurosurgeon; a clinical neurophysiologist; a neuropsychologist; a neuroradiologist; a psychiatrist; paraprofessionals trained in patient education, nursing, and rehabilitation; and appropriate technologists. Guidelines developed by the NAEC for essential services, personnel, and facilities in specialized epilepsy centers can be found at its web site (www.naec-epilepsy.org). These include requirements for *Level 3 epilepsy centers*, which provide basic neurodiagnostic evaluation as well as basic medical, neuropsychological, and psychosocial services and for *Level 4 epilepsy centers*, which provide more complex forms of intensive neurodiagnostic monitoring, more extensive medical, neuropsychological, and psychosocial treatment, and complete evaluation for epilepsy surgery. Surgical treatment of epilepsy should not be attempted on an ad hoc basis in centers without a commitment to this approach. However, more patients with epilepsy require surgery than there are available beds in epilepsy surgery centers. Consequently, hospitals with appropriate resources should be encouraged to develop facilities for epilepsy surgery.

VAGUS NERVE STIMULATION

In 1997, VNS (device by *Cyberonics*) became the first and only FDA-approved device for treatment of epilepsy. It was approved as adjunctive therapy for adults and adolescents over 12 years of age with pharmacoresistant focal seizures. VNS is now approved in many countries and has been proven to be effective, safe, and well-tolerated (Schachter and Boon, 2008; Schachter, 2009). The efficacy profile is similar to that seen with trials of new antiseizure drugs in patients with drug-resistant focal seizures; approximately 50% of patients have a 50% or greater reduction in seizure frequency, and very few become seizure-free. There is a suggestion, however, that efficacy improves over time. Consequently, it may take up to a year to determine whether VNS is having a beneficial effect. To date, no studies have identified clinical features that will predict whether or not VNS will reduce seizures. In addition to its antiseizure effect, there are studies suggesting that VNS can improve mood, anxiety, dysphoria, daytime alertness, and sleep quality. The primary advantage of VNS is that it does not cause the typical central nervous system (CNS) side effects associated with antiseizure drugs. Although VNS does not replace these drugs, it can permit a reduction in dosage. The principal disadvantage is that it requires a surgical procedure for its implantation. Furthermore, the battery life is limited, and surgery is required to replace it every 6 to 11 years.

In VNS, a stimulating electrode in the form of a cuff is placed around the left vagus nerve in the neck, because it has less influence on cardiac activity than the right vagus nerve, and a lead is connected subcutaneously to a pulse generator inserted in a subdermal pouch on the chest. The device is powered by a lithium carbon monofluoride battery and is MRI compatible. If VNS is unsuccessful, the pulse generator and wire can be easily removed, but it can be difficult to remove the cuff electrode without damaging the vagus nerve. Computer software is used to program the pulse generator using radiofrequency signals from a programming wand. Stimulation is ramped up every two weeks to effect and then adjusted periodically as necessary. Typical therapeutic parameters include 1- to 2-mA output current, 30-Hz signal frequency, 500-μsec pulse width, with a signal on time of 30 seconds and off time of 5 minutes. In addition, the patient can use a magnet for on-demand stimulation at the time of seizure onset, which may abort or reduce the severity of seizures. Intermittent stimulation can also be temporarily stopped with a magnet taped over the pulse generator.

Patients can usually feel the stimulation, and approximately a third will experience hoarseness with each stimulus. Other, less common side effects include throat pain, coughing, and shortness of breath, which, if troublesome, might be resolved by reducing the output current, frequency, or the pulse width. Caution should be exercised when using VNS in patients with cardiac conduction disorders as well as asthma and sleep apnea. A safety alert was issued against the use of *diathermy* in patients with VNS devices, as this could heat up the pulse generator or lead and cause tissue damage.

The mechanisms of action of VNS are unknown. The initial work on VNS was based on early studies demonstrating that VNS causes EEG synchronization and desynchronization (Chase et al., 1968) and later work showing that this resulted in inhibition of experimental seizures in dogs (Zabara, 1992). Other than the demonstration that lesions of the *locus coeruleus* in rats prevent the seizure-attenuating effects of VNS (Krahl et al., 1998), no experimental information has identified the fundamental neuronal mechanisms underlying this effect.

A variation on VNS that is currently under investigation is *trigeminal nerve stimulation (TNS)* (DeGiorgio et al., 2009). TNS does not require surgical insertion; electrodes are placed on the face and can be covered by hair or a hat.

HORMONE THERAPY

Natural and synthetic reproductive hormones can increase or decrease neuronal excitability and can influence epileptic activity (Herzog, 2008). *Estradiol* exerts excitatory effects via the N-*methyl-D-aspartate (NMDA) glutamate* receptor, and *progesterone* exerts inhibitory effects via γ-*aminobutyric acid A (GABA$_A$)* receptor mechanisms. Fluctuations in the ratios of these two reproductive steroids are responsible for alterations in seizure threshold during the menstrual cycle, resulting in perimenstrual and periovulatory increases in seizure frequency in women with *catamenial epilepsy* (Chapter 9). There is considerable evidence from noncontrolled trials that hormonal therapies that increase progesterone effects

or decrease estradiol effects can reduce seizure exacerbation in women with *catamenial seizures*. A recent randomized placebo-controlled trial of progesterone therapy found that the responder rate improved in women who experienced perimenstrual seizure exacerbation at least twice that of baseline (Herzog et al., 2012). *Cyclic progesterone* therapy is usually administered during the second half of the menstrual cycle and tapered gradually over three to four days at the end of the cycle. Failure to taper progesterone can cause withdrawal seizures. Adverse effects include sedation, emotional depression, and asthenia, as well as breast tenderness, weight gain, vaginal bleeding, and constipation. An alternative treatment is parenteral *depomedroxyprogesterone* every 6 to 12 weeks in doses large enough to induce *amenorrhea*. Adverse effects of this synthetic progesterone include hot flashes and breakthrough vaginal bleeding. It may take 6 to 12 months for regular ovulatory cycles to return after discontinuation of this parenteral therapy. Other investigational approaches include the estrogen antagonist *clomiphene*, which increases gonadotropin secretion, and *triptorelin*, a synthetic gonadotropin-releasing hormone analog. Sex hormone treatment can be administered in men with epilepsy to treat seizure-related sexual dysfunction.

Melatonin is a hormone commonly used for sleep disorders, particularly jet lag, and is taken by patients with epilepsy who have difficulty sleeping. There is no evidence concerning the effect of melatonin on epileptic seizures per se (Schachter et al., 2008).

IMMUNE THERAPY

Inflammatory processes are involved in epileptogenesis and in many epileptic encephalopathies (Chapter 5); consequently, immunomodulatory therapy can be helpful in pharmacoresistant patients with these conditions. *Intravenous immunoglobulin (IVIg), corticotropin, corticosteroids, plasmapheresis, immunoadsorption with protein A, and interferon (IFN-alpha)* all have been used in the treatment of epilepsy (Villani et al., 2008). IVIg has been used particularly in *Rasmussen syndrome, West syndrome, Lennox-Gastaut syndrome*, and *Landau-Kleffner syndrome*. IVIg is an effective treatment for the newly described *faciobrachial dystonic seizures* associated with *limbic encephalitis* and the *LGI1* antibody (Irani et al., 2011), and undoubtedly immunotherapy will become more important as we better understand the role of autoantibodies in other epilepsy syndromes (Chapter 5).

COMPLEMENTARY AND ALTERNATIVE MEDICINE

Diet

KETOGENIC DIET

Based on knowledge that *ketosis* and *acidosis* have anticonvulsant effects, the ketogenic diet was introduced by Wilder (1921) as a treatment for epilepsy. This diet requires 1 g of protein per kilogram of body weight a day, plus fat to make up the additional needed calories, and only a minimal amount of carbohydrate. The high fat intake and severe carbohydrate restriction make this diet extremely unpalatable. The antiseizure effect depends on the degree of ketosis, which in turn is determined by the fat-to-carbohydrate ratio. The ketogenic diet also results in an increase in plasma cholesterol and a reduction in plasma glucose.

Subsequently, a *medium-chain triglyceride (MCT) diet* was introduced (Huttenlocher et al., 1971) that uses *octanoic* and *decanoic acids* predominantly. With the MCT diet, effective ketosis can be produced with considerably less carbohydrate restriction; hypoglycemia and elevated plasma cholesterol do not occur. The recommended MCT diet derives 60% of calories from octanoic acid and decanoic acid in a ratio of 3 or 4 to 1, 11% from other dietary fat, 19% from carbohydrate, and 10% from protein. MCT oil is given in three divided doses at mealtimes. It can be mixed with twice the volume of skim milk in a blender and served chilled in lieu of milk. It is recommended that the diet be adjusted to maintain urine ketones at 3+ to 4+ as measured by a dipstick.

The mechanisms of action of the ketogenic diet are unknown (Stafstrom et al., 2008; Kossoff and Dorward, 2009). Although the diet produces acidosis, dehydration, and hyperlipidemia, which could conceivably have an antiseizure effect, these are less likely to be responsible for therapeutic efficacy than the ketone bodies themselves. *Acetoacetate, acetone,* and *β-hydroxybutyrate* are formed in the liver when the body is forced to store fats for energy. They are transported via a *monocarboxylic acid transporter* into the brain, where they are metabolized to supply energy. More recent studies suggest that the ketone bodies themselves may not be essential and that other modified diets, such as the *Atkins diet,* may yield similar results. Consequently, mechanisms could include increased fats, decreased glucose, caloric restriction, or any of a number of other consequences of carbohydrate restriction.

Guidelines for the management of children receiving the ketogenic diet have been published (Kossoff et al., 2009). The ketogenic diet should be initiated in the hospital after two nights and one day of fasting (DeVivo, 1983). After 10–14 days of adequate ketosis, the child can be discharged and may remain on the diet for months or years. Beneficial effects may persist after the diet is discontinued. Up to 50% of children experience seizure control. Although the ketogenic diet can be effective in the treatment of all types of seizures, including some in adults, it is the treatment of choice for *GLUT1 deficiency* and is also used particularly in *infantile spasms* and medically refractory *atonic, myoclonic,* and *atypical absence seizures* in patients with the Lennox-Gastaut syndrome. The MCT diet is somewhat more palatable than the original ketogenic diet, but compliance remains the major difficulty with its use. Nausea, vomiting, and lethargy can occur early but are usually transient. Some may find the characteristic breath odor unpleasant (Stafstrom et al., 2008; Kossoff and Dorward, 2009). In addition to hyperlipidemia, the most common side effects include growth retardation, *gastroesophageal reflux disease (GERD),* constipation, osteoporosis and nephrolithiasis. Monitoring is important for treatment, if not always prevention, of unacceptable outcomes (Bergqvist, 2011).

Care must be taken to avoid carbohydrate-based medications, for instance, syrups that contain sugar, because they can precipitate seizure recurrence or status. With long-term use of the ketogenic diet, vitamin supplements are necessary. *Valproic acid* interferes with the determination of urine ketones. If valproic acid is given concurrently, it is not possible to use the dipstick test to monitor the ketotic effect of the diet. Because both valproic acid and the ketogenic diet elevate medium-chain fatty acids, there is a theoretical risk of enhancing *valproic acid–induced hepatotoxicity* (DeVivo, 1983). *Acetazolamide* should be discontinued one to two weeks before initiation of the ketogenic diet, because the combination can lead to severe metabolic acidosis (DeVivo, 1983). This is not necessarily true for *topiramate* and *zonisamide*. Acetazolamide can be safely restarted after the diet is in effect and the patient's metabolic condition has stabilized. The ketogenic diet is contraindicated in patients with *pyruvate carboxylase deficiency*, *porphyria*, *primary carnitine deficiency*, and *fatty acid oxidant defects*.

DIETARY SUPPLEMENTS

Dietary supplements have also been recommended for the treatment of epilepsy. Although some promising animal studies have been performed, clinical trials are lacking and supplements have not gained much support (Whitmarsh, 2009).

Amino Acids

Taurine has inhibitory effects in the CNS, and evidence of decreased taurine levels in patients with epilepsy was responsible for its use as adjunctive treatment for seizures (Barbeau and Donaldson, 1973). Variable results have been reported with taurine administration, and a role for taurine in the treatment of epilepsy has not been accepted (Oja and Kontro, 1983). Because of the demonstration that *L-5-hydroxytryptophan (L-5-HTP)* can reduce posthypoxic action myoclonus (Van Woert et al., 1977), *tryptophan* was recommended as a dietary supplement in patients with these myoclonic jerks (Chapter 7). Effects of this approach have not been well studied, and it is not commonly used. L-5-HTP has also been used as an investigational drug.

Vitamins

Although *pyridoxine* is necessary for the synthesis of the inhibitory neurotransmitter GABA (Chapter 3) and is effective when epileptic seizures are due to *pyridoxine dependency* (Chapter 7), there is no evidence that pyridoxine is useful in the treatment of other forms of epilepsy. *Folic acid*, *vitamin B$_{12}$*, and *vitamin D* deficiencies commonly occur in patients with epilepsy taking a variety of antiseizure drugs (Chapter 14). These deficiencies have been proposed as a mechanism for the development of certain interictal behavioral disturbances (Chapter 11) and some toxic effects of antiseizure drugs. The need for replacement therapy for folic acid, however, remains controversial (Reynolds, 1967; Whitmarsh, 2009). Folic acid is recommended in women of childbearing age taking antiseizure drugs because it reduces the risk of certain birth defects (Chapter 14). Vitamin D has been reported to have some therapeutic effect in epilepsy, which appears to be unrelated to changes in serum calcium or *magnesium* (Christiansen et al., 1974), and *vitamin E* is used by many physicians, but without justification (Whitmarsh, 2009). Studies are under way to examine the beneficial effects of *omega-3 fatty acids* (DeGiorgio et al., 2008). Fish oil supplements not only may raise seizure threshold but could improve cardiac function, perhaps even reducing the risk of *sudden unexpected death in epilepsy (SUDEP)* (Chapter 9).

Minerals

Decreased levels of *calcium* and *magnesium* can predispose to epileptic seizures (Chapters 3 and 9), but there is no evidence that additional calcium or magnesium in the diet has any beneficial effect in the management of epilepsy in general. Elevated *zinc* levels, on the other hand, have been postulated to play a role in the exacerbation of epileptic seizures. One proposed mechanism for the effect of taurine has been the chelation of zinc (Barbeau and Donaldson, 1974). No explanation has been offered for the observation of low *manganese* blood levels among patients with epilepsy (Carl et al., 1986). Zinc and *selenium* have also been suggested to help seizure control (Whitmarsh, 2009), and these minerals can reduce certain toxic effects of antiseizure drugs, such as *alopecia*.

Food Sensitivity

Patients occasionally report that certain foods can precipitate seizures. Most commonly these include coffee, colas, and other caffeinated beverages, but virtually any food can appear to have this effect. Although there have been no controlled trials of food sensitivity (Whitmarsh, 2009), it is possible that allergic reactions to foods lower the seizure threshold in some patients. It is important to take these observations seriously and assist these patients with adjusting their diet to determine whether exclusion of certain foods might improve their seizure control.

Traditional and Folk Medicine

The role of traditional and folk medicine in the management of disease processes should not be overlooked when patients come from cultures that contain strong beliefs in such practices. Not only can these be effective adjunctive measures in the treatment of epilepsy because of the importance of psychological and social factors in the precipitation of ictal events, but certain remedies may possess actual antiseizure properties. Many drugs in our modern pharmacopoeia derive from folk remedies, and there is a need to evaluate and analyze newly recognized herbal treatments and other folk medicines for active ingredients.

There are reports of antiseizure effects of some *Chinese herbal compounds* based on both experimental animal studies and clinical trials (Narita et al., 1982; Takato et al., 1982; Schachter et al., 2008). Unfortunately, these herbal remedies usually consist of a great number of ingredients, and isolation of the active agent would be extremely difficult. One preliminary animal study of *chinaberry juice*, a folk remedy for epilepsy in the southeastern United States, suggested that this substance may contain an ingredient with long-acting antiseizure potency (Wannamaker et al., 1982). A list of Chinese herbs used to treat epilepsy is shown in Table 16–9, and herbs that might make epilepsy worse are shown in Table 16–10.

Marijuana (Cannabis sativa) is an herbal remedy that is widely used for a variety of medical conditions in addition to its recreational use. Many states in the United States now have legalized medical marijuana, and epilepsy is one of the indications for its use. Although there are numerous animal studies indicating that the primary psychoactive component, *tetrahydrocannabinol*, acts on GABAergic interneurons in hippocampus, amygdala, and neocortex, in some cases suppressing experimental seizures, there are no Class I studies

Table 16–9 **Most Frequently Used Herbs in the Far East for Clinical Studies of Epilepsy**

Number of Studies	Botanical Name	Chinese Name
21	*Pinella ternata*	Ban Xia
20	*Arisaema japonicum*	Tian Nan Xing
17	*Acorus calamus*	Shi Chang Pu
14	*Gastrodia elata*	Tian Ma
13	*Buthus martensii*	Quan Xie
12	*Poria cocos*	Fu Ling
12	*Bombyx batryticatus*	Jiang Chan
11	*Citrus reticulata*	Chen Pi
11	*Uncaria rhynchophylla*	Gou Teng
10	*Glycyrrhiza glabra*	Gan Cao
10	*Salvia miltiorrhiza*	Dan Shen
7	*Scolopendra subspinipes*	Wu Gong
7	*Bupleurum falcatum*	Chai hu
7	*Succinum*	Hu Po
7	*Paeonia albiflora*	Bai Shao
6	*Panax ginseng*	Ren Shen
6	*Perichaeta communissma*	Di Long
6	*Curcuma longa*	Yu Jin

From Schachter et al., 2008, with permission.

Table 16–10 **Herbal Products Reported to Have Proconvulsant Properties**

- Wormwood (*artemisia absinthium*)
- Ephedra (*ma huang*)
- Starflower (borage) (*Borago officinalis*)
- Evening primrose oil (*Oenothera biennis*)
- Japanese star anise (*Illicium anisatum*)
- Chinese star anise (*Illicium verum*)
- Pennyroyal (*Mentha pulegium*)
- *Ginkgo biloba*
- Eucalyptus (*Eucalyptus globulus*)
- Shankhapusphi (*Evolvulus alsinoides*)
- Star fruit (*Averrhoa carambola*)
- St. John's wort (*Hypericum perforatum*)
- Grapefruit (*Citrus x paradisi*)
- Sho-seiryu-to/Sho-saiko-to
- Bai Shao (white peony root)
- Hyssop (*Hyssopus officinalis*)
- Fennel (*Foeniculum vulgare*)
- Sage (*Salvia officinalis*)
- Rosemary (*Rosmarinus officinalis*)
- Thyme (*Thymus vulgaris*)
- Savin (*Juniperus sabina*)
- Tansy (*Tanacetum vulgare*)
- Thuja (*Thuja occidentalis*)
- Caffeine

to confirm antiseizure properties in patients (Schachter et al., 2008).

Included in traditional and folk medicine are practices as well as medications. *Acupuncture, acupressure, moxibustion*, and other manipulations have been used for thousands of years in treating epilepsy, but the results have not been adequately examined. Western physicians in China refer medically intractable patients with epilepsy to traditional physicians and feel that acupuncture may at times be effective, particularly for nonconvulsive generalized seizures.

Disdain for traditional and folk experience in the treatment of disease is a particularly unuseful manifestation of the arrogance of Western medicine. Given that most current medical practice is based on serendipitous observations, controlled studies of these potentially useful approaches to the treatment of epilepsy must be undertaken before they can be dismissed as nonscientific; indeed, it would be unscientific to reject them without the benefit of such studies.

In addition to the possibility that traditional and folk medicine might provide unique insights into novel approaches to the treatment of epilepsy in Western cultures, Western physicians must acknowledge that most people in developing countries will seek healers when they are sick, either in addition or in preference to Western doctors. This is also the case for patients from cultures that traditionally use healers who emigrate to industrialized countries. Consequently, it is essential for Western physicians to acknowledge the role of traditional approaches and, where possible, collaborate with traditional healers. A text published by the World Federation of Neurology for neurologists practicing in developing countries states: "Perhaps a bigger problem than the failure of people in developing countries to understand modern medical concepts of epilepsy is the failure of the medical establishment to understand and respect traditional beliefs of their patient population. The perceived arrogance of medical practitioners and cross-cultural mismatches undoubtedly account for a considerable percentage of treatment failures in developing countries. Interpreters are necessary who will not only translate words, but philosophies, and who will ensure that both parties to the discussion are treated with equal respect and understanding" (Engel et al., 2005).

Behavioral Therapies

The seizure threshold can be exquisitely sensitive to psychological conditions (Chapter 11), so it is not surprising that behavioral modification can have a beneficial effect on seizure occurrence (Chapter 11). This provides adjunctive therapy in addition to antiseizure medication but is rarely effective by itself (Wolf, 2008; Whitmarsh, 2009). Situations where behavioral therapy can be effective alone include the treatment of reflex epilepsies and the rare situations where seizures can be aborted by sensory stimulation. EEG biofeedback and a variety of psychological approaches, largely aimed at reducing stress, are practiced with variable results.

TREATMENT OF THE REFLEX EPILEPSIES

Behavioral treatment has been particularly successful for reflex seizures induced by specific sensory stimulation (Chapter 9). Forster (1977) used five approaches for treatment of reflex epilepsies: *avoidance, stimulus alteration, threshold alteration, vigilance inhibition,* and *avoidance conditioning.*

Avoidance is commonly used for photosensitive epilepsy. It may require removing the patient from an environment in which a precipitating stimulus is likely to occur, for instance, a discotheque with stroboscopic lights, but this is not always possible. Protective devices can be effective in some cases, such as patching one eye or wearing colored glasses. Avoidance techniques are also used when seizures are provoked by nonsensory influences such as alcohol withdrawal, sleep deprivation, or hypoglycemia. This is accomplished by establishing more regular living habits that ensure adequate sleep, regularly scheduled meals, and moderation or abstinence in the use of substances that appear to induce seizures directly or by their withdrawal.

Stimulus alteration involves desensitization or induction of tolerance by repeated presentation. This can be used, for instance, to treat *musicogenic epilepsy*. When seizures are produced only by a specific piece of music, patients are repeatedly exposed to a similar piece of music or to the same music altered in such a way that it does not provoke a seizure. Gradual approximation to the effective stimulus may eventually allow it to be presented without inducing a seizure. This type of desensitization is time-consuming, and the process may need to be renewed at regular intervals to prevent relapse; however, it can be a useful therapeutic approach in some patients with reflex epilepsy who are unable or unwilling to avoid the offending stimulus.

Threshold alteration takes advantage of the fact that patients with complex reflex epilepsy (Chapter 9) experience a prolonged refractory period following each sensory-induced seizure. Repeated presentation of the effective stimulus during the refractory period can also result in desensitization, perhaps by elevation of threshold. This approach has the same advantages and disadvantages as stimulus alteration.

Vigilance inhibition is simply voluntary diversion of attention. This form of avoidance is possible when seizures develop after a period of exposure to the offending stimulus and there is sufficient time to interrupt the process.

Classical *avoidance conditioning* can be helpful in some patients with self-induced seizures. Punishment is used as a conditioning stimulus to prevent behavior patterns that lead to epileptic seizures.

ABORTIVE SENSORY STIMULATION

Some patients may be able to abort their own epileptic seizures by various techniques (Chapter 9). Concentration or applying a specific stimulus, such as rubbing the body part involved in ictal onset, can occasionally be effectively employed to improve epileptic seizure control. In other instances, the abortive stimulus may be too complicated to apply quickly enough to prevent the ictal event. Theoretically, it is possible to use classical conditioning to substitute a more readily available stimulus to the same effect. This approach is illustrated by the classic case of Efron (1957). His patient had temporal lobe seizures with a long olfactory aura. A strong olfactory stimulus, such as perfume, could abort her seizures. Using conditioning techniques, the sight of the patient's bracelet was substituted for the strong smell, and eventually merely the thought of the bracelet was effective in aborting seizures. Unfortunately, very few patients are candidates for this type of conditioning.

EEG BIOFEEDBACK

A form of EEG operant conditioning that has been referred to as *biofeedback* has been used effectively in some patients. Practitioners of this technique train patients to maintain a state of cerebral activity presumably associated with an elevated threshold for epileptic seizure generation (Sterman and Friar, 1972; Sterman et al., 1974). Initial investigations were based on observations that a central 12- to 15-Hz EEG rhythm, the *sensory motor rhythm (SMR)*, was present during motor inactivity, disappeared during motor activity, and was deficient in patients with epilepsy. Conditioning a population of patients with epilepsy to increase their SMR resulted in a statistically significant decrease in the occurrence of epileptic seizures.

Despite the clear demonstration of a beneficial effect in some patients, reproduced in several laboratories, this approach has not gained acceptance, for both scientific and practical reasons. Scientifically, it has not been possible to explain this phenomenon satisfactorily on the basis of induction of SMR per se, as EEG frequency analysis has failed to demonstrate persistent enhancement of a 12- to 15-Hz central rhythm in patients in whom conditioning has resulted in seizure reduction. Other mechanisms, involving thalamocortical influences and normalization of sleep, have been proposed (Sterman and Bowersox, 1981). Practically, biofeedback is an extremely labor-intensive form of treatment. The effort required from professional personnel does not appear to be justified by the rather modest and unpredictable benefits.

PSYCHOLOGICAL TREATMENTS

Many psychological approaches to the treatment of epilepsy have been tried, and some positive results have been published. However, these reports are for the most part anecdotal and have not always clearly distinguished epileptic from psychogenic seizure disorders. Psychological approaches mentioned in the literature include *punishment and reward*, *relaxation techniques* (including *meditation*), *hypnosis, psychodynamic psychotherapy*, and *cognitive therapy* (Brown, 1987; Wolf, 2008; Whitmarsh, 2009). Interestingly, meditation appears to increase the size of certain limbic structures (Luders et al., 2009) and may have an effect that antagonizes the atrophic processes induced by epilepsy (Chapter 5), depression, and anxiety (Chapter 11). *Mindfulness-based therapy* and other meditation practices have become increasingly popular as a form of alternative therapy for many conditions. The largely anecdotal literature cites both pro- and antiseizure effects of meditation (Lansky and St. Louis, 2006), but these studies have not controlled for how well patients performed the practice. Perhaps drowsiness rather than meditation accounts for some of the pro-seizure effects. Given the role of psychological influences as precipitating factors in epilepsy, it is not surprising that these approaches might occasionally be successful in individual patients. However, although psychological treatments may be reasonable alternatives for a few patients and useful adjunctive therapy in others, general statements about their indications and utility must await the results of appropriately controlled clinical trials.

Physical Interventions

It has been known since ancient times that epileptic disorders can remit or improve for months or years after particularly stressful physical interventions such as cautery or trephining (Temkin, 1945) (Chapter 2). As a result of observations in the early part of the last century that epileptic seizures often stopped after general surgery or pneumoencephalography, procedures such as *thymectomy* or *air insufflation* were seriously considered as treatments for epilepsy (Penfield, 1936). A major practical lesson from this experience has been the realization that improvement immediately after surgical therapy for epilepsy can be a nonspecific, transient effect (Engel, 1987).

Electroconvulsive shock therapy (ECT) has also been suggested as a treatment for epilepsy. Experimentally, the postictal seizure suppression induced by electroconvulsive shock is known to retard kindling (Post et al., 1984). A single patient report revealed, however, that the total number of seizures occurring during a course of ECT treatments, including those induced by ECT, was no different from baseline (Sackeim et al., 1983). Although there may be some theoretical advantages to the fact that some seizures occurred under controlled conditions rather than spontaneously, at this time ECT must be considered an unaccepted and potentially dangerous intervention.

Transcranial magnetic stimulation (TMS) is a considerably more benign alternative to ECT. TMS has been used experimentally for diagnostic purposes to measure cortical excitability (Chapter 12), but there are studies suggesting that low-frequency *repetitive TMS (rTMS)* applied over the vertex or over the presumed epileptogenic zone might reduce seizure frequency (Theodore and Fisher, 2004; Whitmarsh, 2009). However, at least one study has indicated that this approach may decrease seizure severity but increase frequency (Schrader et al., 2004). A novel technique currently under investigation is *low-intensity focused ultrasound pulsation (LIFUP)* (Bystritsky et al., 2011).

Nonallopathic Medical Systems

Conventional Western medicine is referred to as *allopathic medicine*. Allopathy grew out of other medical traditions in the late 19th and 20th centuries as a result of application of modern concepts of the scientific method to establish the efficacy of medical and surgical interventions. Although the science of allopathic medicine is often imperfect, its foundation in the scientific method distinguishes it from other medical systems. *Ayurveda* is the ancient Indian system of medicine that uses herbal remedies, diet, and lifestyle changes to balance disturbances in three physiological properties: *vata* (air), *pitta* (bile), and *kapha* (phlegm). *Homeopathy*, which is widespread in the Western world, challenges the body with highly diluted solutions of substances believed to exacerbate the illness. *Naturopathy* uses approaches said to stimulate the body to heal itself. *Chiropractic* diagnoses and treats disease by manipulation of the vertebrae column and joints. *Kinesiology* asserts that manual muscle testing can be used to determine how the body will react to drugs and other therapies and to diagnose disease. Although a substantial percentage of people with epilepsy worldwide will adhere to one or more of these and certainly to other, organized systems of medicine, practitioners of these disciplines do not perform the quantitative studies necessary to accumulate evidence-based support for their beliefs. Consequently, there are no studies to either confirm or deny their usefulness in people with epilepsy. Even if positive results are only a placebo effect, there can be benefit and certainly little chance of harm when patients who adhere to one of these medical systems use it for their epilepsy as long as it is adjunctive and does not replace standard Western allopathic medicine.

SUMMARY AND CONCLUSIONS

Surgical treatment for epilepsy is greatly underused, and when patients are referred for surgery it is too often too late to avoid the development of irreversible adverse psychological and social consequences of recurrent seizures and a lifetime of disability.

All patients with seizures that have not been controlled by two appropriate trials of antiseizure medication should be referred to an epilepsy center, because epilepsy specialists at these centers are in the best position to determine whether a patient is a surgical

candidate. Even if the patient is not a surgical candidate, specialists at epilepsy centers can often offer additional alternative treatments that are beneficial. Referral should be made as soon as possible, certainly when seizures begin to interfere with work, school, or interpersonal relationships.

Surgically remediable syndromes are conditions with a known pathophysiological substrate, a poor outcome after failure of two appropriate antiseizure drug trials, and an excellent response to surgical therapy. MTLE is the prototype of a surgically remediable syndrome, but patients with resectable neocortical lesions and infants and young children with epileptic encephalopathies due to diffuse lesions limited to one hemisphere also have a 50–80% chance of becoming seizure-free with surgery.

Corpus callosotomy is a useful palliative surgical treatment for drop attacks, but these disabling pharmacoresistant seizures can also respond to vagus nerve stimulation. VNS is an adjunctive treatment with an efficacy profile similar to that seen with trials for new antiseizure drugs but does not cause CNS side effects. Because very few patients become seizure-free with VNS, it should not be the first choice in patients with pharmacoresistant seizures who might be candidates for more definitive surgical therapy.

Hormonal therapy can be a useful adjunctive treatment for women with catamenial epilepsy, and immunotherapy is an important intervention for seizures with an inflammatory etiology.

The ketogenic diet as well as variations such as the MCT diet can be effective in children with severe pharmacoresistant seizures and is the treatment of choice for GLUT1 deficiency. This approach may also be beneficial in adults. There is evidence that benefit persists even following termination of the diet.

Traditional and folk medicine should not be overlooked as a source of potential adjunctive or alternative therapy in patients receptive to these measures.

Behavioral treatments are successful in some selected patients, particularly those with reflex epilepsies, but are labor intensive and yield inconsistent results. EEG biofeedback has not proved to be an efficient alternative therapy.

Epileptologists have relied heavily on pharmacological therapy, which is usually nonspecific and associated with disturbing side effects.

Both basic and clinical research should investigate whether available complementary and alternative medical therapies may antagonize precipitating and predisposing factors for epileptic seizures without producing adverse side effects.

REFERENCES

Apuzzo, MLJ (1991). Neurosurgical Aspects of Epilepsy. Park Ridge, IL:American Association of Neurological Surgeons.

Bailey, P, and Gibbs, FA (1951). Surgical treatment of psychomotor epilepsy. JAMA 145:365–370.

Baltuch, G, and Villemure, J-G (eds) (2009). Operative Techniques in Epilepsy Surgery. New York: Thieme.

Barbeau, A, and Donaldson, J (1973). Taurine in epilepsy [letter]. Lancet 2: 387.

Barbeau, A, and Donaldson, J (1974). Zinc, taurine, and epilepsy. Arch Neurol 30:52–58.

Bauer, J, Buchmüller, L, Reuber, M, and Burr, W (2008). Which patients become seizure free with antiepileptic drugs? An observational studyin 821 patients with epilepsy. Acta Neurol Scand 117:55–59.

Berg, AT, Langfitt, J, Shinnar, S, Vickrey, BG, Sperling, MR, Walczak, T, Bazil, C, Pacia, SV, and Spencer, SS (2003). How long does it take for partial epilepsy to become intractable? Neurology 60:186–190.

Bergey, GK (2009). Brain stimulation. In The Treatment of Epilepsy, 3rd ed. Edited by S Shorvon, E Perucca, and J Engel, Jr. West Sussex, UK: Wiley-Blackwell, pp. 1025–1033.

Bergqvist, AG (2012). Long-term monitoring of the ketogenic diet: Do's and don'ts. Epilepsy Res 100:261–266.

Binder, DK, and Schramm, J (2008). Multilobar resections and hemispherectomy. In Epilepsy: A Comprehensive Textbook, 2nd ed. Edited by J Engel, Jr, and TA Pedley. Philadelphia: Lippincott Williams & Wilkins, pp. 1879–1889.

Bingaman, WE (guest ed) (2002). Cortical dysplasias. Neurosurg Clin N Am.

Bogen, JE, and Vogel, PJ (1962). Cerebral commissurotomy in man: Preliminary case report. Bull Los Angeles Neurol Soc 27:169–172.

Bookheimer, S, Schrader, LM, Rausch, R, Sankar, R, and Engel, J, Jr (2005). Reduced anesthetization during the intracarotid amobarbital (Wada) test in patients taking carbonic anhydrase-inhibiting medications. Epilepsia 46:236–243.

Boshuisen, K, van Schooneveld, MMJ, Leijten, FSS, et al. (2010). Contralateral MRI abnormalities affect seizure and cognitive outcome after hemispherectomy. Neurology 75:1623–1630.

Bragin, A,and Engel, J, Jr. (2008). Slow waves associated with seizure activity. In Computational Neuroscience in Epilepsy. Edited by ISoltesz and K Staley. San Diego: Elsevier, pp. 440–453.

Brown, SW (1987). Psychological treatments. In Epilepsy. Edited by A Hopkins. New York: Demos, pp. 328–336.

Bystritsky, A, Korb, AS, Douglas, PK, et al. (2011). A review of low-intensity focused ultrasound pulsation. Brain Stimul 4:125–136.

Callaghan, BC, Anaud, K, Hesdorffer, D, Hauser, WA, and French, JA (2007). Likelihood of seizure remission in an adult population with refractory epilepsy. Ann Neurol 62:382–389.

Carne, RP, O'Brien, TJ, Kilpatrick, CJ, et al. (2004). MRI-negative PET-positive temporal lobe epilepsy: Adistinct surgically remediable syndrome. Brain 127:2276–2285.

Carl, GF, Keen, CL, Gallagher, BB, Clegg, MS, Littleton, WH, Flannery, DB, and Hurley, LS (1986). Association of low blood manganese concentrations with epilepsy. Neurology 36:1584–1587.

Cataltepe, O, and Jallo, G (eds) (2010). Pediatric Epilepsy Surgery: Preoperative Assessment and Surgical Treatment. New York: Thieme.

Cavus, I, and Wilson, CL (2008). Microdialysis. In Epilepsy: A Comprehensive Textbook, 2nd ed. Edited by J Engel, Jr, and TA Pedley. Philadelphia: Lippincott Williams & Wilkins, pp. 1031–1039.

Cendes, F (2005). Progressive hippocampal and extra-hippocampal atrophy in drug resistant epilepsy. Curr Opin Neurol 18:173–177.

Chang, EF, Quigg, M, Oh, MC, et al. (2010). Predictors of efficacy after stereotactic radiosurgery for medial temporal lobe epilepsy. Neurology 74:165–172.

Chase, MH, Nakamura, Y, Clemente, CD, et al. (1968). Cortical and subcortical EEG patterns of response to afferent abdominal vagal stimulation: Neurographic correlates. Physiol Behav 3:605–610.

Chassoux, F, Rodrigo, S, Semah, F, et al. (2010). FDG-PET improves surgical outcome in negative MRI Taylor-type focal cortical dysplasias. Neurology 75:2168–2175.

Chern, J, and Comair, YG (2009). Surgery of developmental anomalies causing epilepsy. In The Treatment of Epilepsy, 3rd ed. Edited by S Shorvon, E Perucca, and J Engel, Jr. West Sussex, UK: Wiley-Blackwell, pp. 925–933.

Choi, H, Sell, RI, Lenert, L, et al. (2008). Epilepsy surgery for pharmacoresistant temporal lobe epilepsy: Adecision analysis. JAMA 300:2497–2505.

Choi, H, Carlino, R, Heiman, G, Hauser, WA, and Gilliam, FG (2009). Evaluation of duration of epilepsy prior to temporal lobe epilepsy surgery during the past two decades. Epilepsy Res 86:224–227.

Christiansen, C, Rodbro, P, and Sjo, O (1974). "Anticonvulsant action" of vitamin D in epileptic patients: A controlled pilot study. Br Med J 2:258–259.

Chugani, HT, Shewmon, DA, Peacock, WJ, Shields, WD, Mazziotta, JC, and Phelps, ME (1988). Surgical treatment of intractable neonatal seizures: The role of positron emission tomography. Neurology 38:1178–1188.

Chugani, HT, Shields, WD, Shewmon, DA, Olson, DM, Phelps, ME, and Peacock, WJ (1990). Infantile spasms: I. PET identifies focal cortical dysgenesis in cryptogenic cases for surgical treatment. Ann Neurol 27:406–413.

Comair, YG, Van Ness, PC, Chamoun, RB, and Bouclaous, CH (2008). Neocortical resections. In Epilepsy: A Comprehensive Textbook, 2nd ed. Edited by J Engel, Jr, and TA Pedley. Philadelphia: Lippincott Williams & Wilkins, pp. 1869–1878.

Cooper, IS, Crighel, E, and Amin, I (1973). Clinical and physiological effects of stimulation of the paleocerebellum in humans. J Am Geriatr Soc 21:40–43.

Cramer, J,Westbrook, L, Devinsky, O, Perrine, K, Glassman, MB, and Camfield, C (1999). Development of the

Quality of Life in Epilepsy Inventory for Adolescents: TheQOLIE-AD-48. Epilepsia40:1114–1121.

Crandall, PH (1987). Cortical resection. In Surgical Treatment of the Epilepsies. Edited by J Engel, Jr. New York: Raven Press, pp. 377–404.

Crandall, PH, Walter, RD, and Rand, RW (1963). Clinical applications of studies on stereotactically implanted electrodes in temporal lobe epilepsy. J Neurosurg 20:827–840.

Dam, M, Gram, L, and Schmidt, K (eds) (1988). Surgical treatment of epilepsy. Acta Neurol Scand.117(suppl).

Dam, M, Andersen, AR, Rogvi-Hansen, B, and Jennum, P (eds) (1994). Epilepsy surgery: Non-invasive versus invasive focus localization. Acta Neurol Scand 152(suppl).

Dandy WE (1919). Roentgenography of the brain after injection of air into the spinal canal. Ann Surg 70:397–403.

DeGiorgio, CM, Miller, P, Meymandi, S, and Gornbein, JA (2008). n-3 fatty acids (fish oil) for epilepsy, cardiac risk factors, and risk of SUDEP: Clues from a pilot, double-blind, exploratory study. Epilepsy Behav 13:681–684.

DeGiorgio, CM, Murray, D, Markovic, D, and Whitehurst, T (2009). Trigeminal nerve stimulation for epilepsy: Long-term feasibility and efficacy. Neurology 72:936–938.

deTisi, J, Bell, GS, Peacock, JL, McEvoy, AW, Harkness, WFJ, Sander, JW, and Duncan, JS (2011). The long-term outcome of adult epilepsy surgery, patterns of seizure remission, and relapse: A cohort study. Lancet 378:1388–1362.

Devinsky, O, Vickrey, BG, Cramer, J, Perrine, K, Hermann, B, Meador, K, et al. (1995). Development of the Quality of Life in Epilepsy Inventory. Epilepsia 36(11):1089–1104.

DeVivo, DC (1983). How to use other drugs (steroids) and the ketogenic diet. In Antiepileptic Drug Therapy in Pediatrics. Edited by PL Morselli, CE Pippenger, and JK Penry. New York: Raven Press, pp. 283–292.

Dorfmüller, G, Bulteau, C, and Delalande, O (2009). Hemispherectomy for epilepsy. In The Treatment of Epilepsy, 3rd ed. Edited by S Shorvon, E Perucca, and J Engel, Jr. West Sussex, UK: Wiley-Blackwell, pp. 935–942.

Dow, RS, Fernandez-Guardiola, A, and Manni, E (1962). The influence of the cerebellum on experimental epilepsy. Electroencephalogr Clin Neurophysiol 14:383–398.

Duchowny, M, Resnick, T, and Alvarez, L (eds) (1990). Pediatric epilepsy surgery. J Epilepsy 3(suppl 1).

Duchowny, MS, Cross, JH, and Mathern, GW (2008). Special considerations for pediatric epilepsy surgery. In Epilepsy: A Comprehensive Textbook, 2nd ed. Edited by J Engel, Jr, and TA Pedley. Philadelphia: Lippincott Williams & Wilkins, pp. 1949–1956.

Dymond, AM, Sweizig, JR, Crandall, PH, and Hanley, J (1971). Clinical application of an EEG radio telemetry system. In Proceedings of the8th Annual Rocky Mountain Bioengineering Symposium, Colorado State University, Fort Collins, May 3–5, pp. 16–20.

Efron, R (1957). The conditioned inhibition of uncinate fits. Brain 80:251–262.

Engel, J, Jr (ed) (1987a). Surgical Treatment of the Epilepsies. New York: Raven Press.

Engel, J, Jr (1987b). Approaches to localization of the epileptogenic lesion. In Surgical Treatment of the Epilepsies. Edited by J Engel, Jr. New York: Raven Press, pp. 75–96.

Engel, J, Jr (1987c). Outcome with respect to epileptic seizures. In Surgical Treatment of the Epilepsies. Edited by J Engel, Jr. New York: Raven Press, pp. 553–572.

Engel, J, Jr (1989). Seizures and Epilepsy. Philadelphia: FA Davis.

Engel, J, Jr (ed) (1993). Surgical Treatment of the Epilepsies, 2nd ed. New York: Raven Press.

Engel, J, Jr (1996). Surgery for seizures. N Engl J Med 334:647–652.

Engel, J, Jr (2001a). Finally, a randomized controlled trial of epilepsy surgery. N Engl J Med 345:365–367.

Engel, J, Jr (2001b). A proposed diagnostic scheme for people with epileptic seizures and with epilepsy: Report of the ILAE Task Force on Classification and Terminology. Epilepsia 42:796–803.

Engel, J, Jr (2005a). Natural history of mesial temporal lobe epilepsy with hippocampal sclerosis: How does kindling compare with other commonly used animal models? In Kindling 6. Edited by ME Corcoran andSL Moshé. New York: Springer Science + Business Media, pp. 371–384.

Engel, J, Jr (2005b). The emergence of neurosurgical approaches to the treatment of epilepsy. In From Neuroscience to Neurology: Neuroscience, Molecular Medicine, and the Therapeutic Transformation of Neurology. Edited by S Waxman. Amsterdam: Elsevier, pp. 81–105.

Engel, J, Jr (2008). Surgical treatment for epilepsy: Too little too late? JAMA 300:2548–2550.

Engel, J, Jr (2009). Overview of surgical treatment for epilepsy. In The Treatment of Epilepsy, 3rd ed. Edited by S Shorvon, E Perucca, and J Engel, Jr. West Sussex, UK: Wiley-Blackwell, pp. 743–756.

Engel, J, Jr, and Shewmon, DA (1991). Impact of the kindling phenomenon on clinical epileptology. In Kindling and Synaptic Plasticity: The Legacy of Graham Goddard. Edited by F Morrell. Cambridge, MA: Birkhäuser Boston, pp. 195–210.

Engel, J, Jr, and Shewmon, DA (1993). Overview: Who should be considered a surgical candidate? In Surgical Treatment of the Epilepsies, 2nd ed. Edited by J Engel, Jr. New York: Raven Press pp. 23–34.

Engel, J, Jr, and Wiebe, S (in press). Who is a surgical candidate? In Handbook of Clinical Neurology. Edited by H Stefan and W Theodore. Amsterdam: Elsevier.

Engel, J, Jr, Driver, MV, and Falconer, MA (1975). Electrophysiological correlates of pathology and surgical results in temporal lobe epilepsy. Brain 98:129–156.

Engel, J, Jr, Rausch, R, Lieb, JP, Kuhl, DE, and Crandall, PH (1981). Correlation of criteria used for localizing epileptic foci in patients considered for surgical therapy of epilepsy. Ann Neurol 9:215–224.

Engel, J, Jr, Brown, WJ, Kuhl, DE, Phelps, ME, Mazziotta, JC, and Crandall, PH (1982a). Pathological findings underlying focal temporal lobe hypometabolism in partial epilepsy. Ann Neurol 12:518–528.

Engel, J, Jr, Kuhl, DE, Phelps, ME, and Crandall, PH (1982b). Comparative localization of epileptic foci in partial epilepsy by PCT and EEG. Ann Neurol 12:529–537.

Engel, J, Jr, Kuhl, DE, Phelps, ME, and Mazziotta, JC (1982c). Interictal cerebral glucose metabolism in partial epilepsy and its relation to EEG changes. Ann Neurol 12:510–517.

Engel, J, Jr, Van Ness, P, Rasmussen, TB, and Ojemann, LM (1993). Outcome with respect to epileptic seizures. In Surgical Treatment of the Epilepsies, 2nd ed. Edited by J Engel, Jr. New York: Raven Press, pp. 609–621.

Engel, J, Jr, Wiebe, S, French, J, Gumnit, R, Spencer, D, Sperling, M, Williamson, P, Zahn, C, Westbrook, E, and Enos, B (2003). Practice parameter: Temporal lobe and localized neocortical resections for epilepsy. Neurology 60:538–547.

Engel, J, Jr, Birbeck, G, Diop, AG, Jain, S, and Palmini, A (2005). Epilepsy: Global Issues for the Practicing Neurologist. World Federation of Neurology Seminars in Clinical Neurology. New York: Demos Press.

Engel, J, Jr, Taylor, DC, and Trimble, MR (2008). Neurobiology of behavioral disorders. In Epilepsy: A Comprehensive Textbook, 2nd ed. Edited by J Engel, Jr, and TA Pedley. Philadelphia: Lippincott Williams & Wilkins, pp. 2077–2083.

Engel, J, Jr, McDermott, MP, Wiebe, S, Langfitt, JT, Stern, JM, Dewar, S, Sperling, MR, Gardiner, I, Erba, G, Fried, I, Jacobs, M, Vinters, HV, Mintzer, S, and Kieburtz, K (2012). Early surgical therapy for drug-resistant temporal lobe epilepsy: a radomized trial. JAMA 307:922–930.

Falconer, MA (1953). Discussion on the surgery of temporal lobe epilepsy: Surgical and pathological aspects. Proc R Soc Med 46:971–974.

Falconer, MA (1974). Mesial temporal (Ammon's horn) sclerosis as a common cause of epilepsy: Aetiology, treatment and prevention. Lancet 2:767–770.

Ferrier, D (1874). On the localisation of the functions of the brain. Br Med J 2:766–767.

Fisher, R, Salanova,V, Witt, T, et al. (2010). Electrical stimulation of the anterior nucleus of thalamus for treatment of refractory epilepsy. Epilepsia 51:899–908.

Fisher, RS, McKhann, GM, Stern, JM, et al. (2008). New therapeutic directions. In Epilepsy: A Comprehensive Textbook, 2nd ed. Edited by J Engel, Jr, and TA Pedley. Philadelphia: Lippincott Williams & Wilkins, pp. 1415–1430.

Foerster, O, and Penfield, W (1930). The structural basis of traumatic epilepsy and results of radical operation. Brain 53:99–119.

Fong, JS, Jehi, L, Najm, I, Prayson, RA, Busch, R, and Bingaman, W (2011). Seizure outcome and its predictors after temporal lobe epilepsy surgery in patients with normal MRI. Epilepsia 52:1393–1401.

Forster, FM (1977). Reflex Epilepsy, Behavioral Therapy and Conditional Reflexes. Springfield, IL: Charles C Thomas.

Fraser, RT, and Thorbecke, R (2008). Pre-/postoperative rehabilitation. In Epilepsy: A Comprehensive Textbook, 2nd ed. Edited by J Engel, Jr, and TA Pedley. Philadelphia: Lippincott Williams & Wilkins, pp. 1939–1947.

Gates, JR, Rosenfeld, WE, Maxwell, RE, and Lyons, RE (1987). Response of multiple seizure types to corpus callosum section. Epilepsia 28:28–34.

Goddard, GV, McIntyre, DC, and Leech, CK (1969). A permanent change in brain function resulting from daily electrical stimulation. Exp Neurol 25:295–330.

Goldring, S, and Gregorie, EM (1984). Surgical management of epilepsy using epidural recordings to localize the seizure focus. Review of 100 cases. J Neurosurg 60:457–466.

Haglund, MM, Hochman, D, and Toga, AW (2008). Optical imaging of seizure activity. In Epilepsy: A Comprehensive Textbook, 2nd ed. Edited by J Engel, Jr, and TA Pedley TA. Philadelphia: Lippincott Williams & Wilkins, pp. 1025–1030.

Hamiwka, L, Macrodimitris, S, Tellez-Zenteno, JF, et al. (2011). Social outcomes after temporal or extratemporal epilepsy surgery: Asystematic review. Epilepsia 52:870–879.

Haneef, Z, Stern, J, Dewar, S, and Engel, J, Jr (2010). Referral pattern for epilepsy surgery after evidence-based recommendations: Aretrospective study. Neurology 75:699–704.

Hauptman, JS, and Mathern, GW (2009). Epilepsy surgery in children. In The Treatment of Epilepsy, 3rd ed. Edited by S Shorvon, E Perucca, and J Engel, Jr. West Sussex, UK: Wiley-Blackwell, pp. 967–974.

Hemb, M, Velasco, TR, Parnes, MS, et al. (2010). Improved outcomes in pediatric epilepsy surgery. The UCLA experience, 1986–2008. Neurology 74:1768–1775.

Hermann, BP, Seidenberg, M, Dow, C, Jones, J, Rutecki, P, Bhattacharya, A, et al. (2006). Cognitive prognosis in chronic temporal lobe epilepsy. Ann Neurol 60:80–87.

Herzog, AG (2008). Sex-hormone treatment. In Epilepsy: A Comprehensive Textbook, 2nd ed. Edited by J Engel, Jr, and TA Pedley. Philadelphia: Lippincott Williams & Wilkins, pp. 1387–1394.

Herzog, AG, Fowler, KM, Smithson, SD, Kalayjian, LA, Heck, CN, Sperling, MR, Liporace, JD, Harden, CL, Dworetzky, BA, Pennel, PB, Massaro, JM, and the Progesterone Trial Study Group (2012). Progesterone versus placebo for women with epilepsy: Arandomized clinical trial. Neurology 78:1959–1966.

Holmes, MD, and Chatrian, G-E (2008). Intraoperative electrocorticography. In Epilepsy: A Comprehensive Textbook, 2nd ed. Edited by J Engel, Jr, and TA Pedley,1886: Philadelphia: Lippincott Williams & Wilkins, pp. 1817–1831.

Horsley, V: Brain-surgery. Br Med J 2:670–675.

Huttenlocher, PR, Wilbourn, AJ, and Signore, JM (1971). Medium-chain triglycerides as a therapy for intractable childhood epilepsy. Neurology 21:1097–1103.

Irani, SR, Michell, AW, Lang, B, et al. (2011). Faciobrachial dystonic seizures precede Lgi1 antibody limbic encephalitis. Ann Neurol 69:892–900.

Jackson, GD, Berkovic, SF, Tress, BM, Kalnins, RM, Fabinyi, G, and Bladin, PF (1990). Hippocampal sclerosis can be reliably detected by magnetic resonance imaging. Neurology 40:1869–1875.

Jacobs, J, Zijlmans, M, Zelmann, R, Chatillon, CE, Hall, J, Olivier, A, Dubeau, F, and Gotman, J (2010). High-frequency electroencephalographic oscillations correlate with outcome of epilepsy surgery. Ann Neurol 67:209–220.

Janszky, J, Janszky, I, Schulz, R, et al. (2005). Temporal lobe epilepsy with hippocampal sclerosis: Predictors for long-term surgical outcome. Brain 128:395–404.

Jasper, H, and Kershman, J (1941). Electroencephalographic classification of the epilepsies. Arch Neurol Psychiatr 45:903–943.

Jasper, H, Pertuisset, B, and Flanigin, H (1951). EEG and cortical electrograms in patients with temporal lobe seizures. Arch Neurol Psychiatr65:272–290.

Jayakar, P, and Lesser, RP (2008). Extraoperative functional mapping. In Epilepsy: A Comprehensive Textbook, 2nd ed. Edited by J Engel, Jr, and TA Pedley. Philadelphia: Lippincott Williams & Wilkins, pp. 1851–1858.

Jensen, I (1975). Temporal lobe surgery around the world. Acta Neurol Scand 52:354–373.

Jinnai, D, and Mukawa, J (1970). Forel-H-tomy for the treatment of epilepsy. Confin Neurol 32:307–315.

Jones-Gotman, M, and Djordjevic, J (2009). Neuropsychological testing in presurgical evaluation. In The Treatment of Epilepsy, 3rd ed. Edited by S Shorvon, E Perucca, and J Engel, Jr. West Sussex, UK: Wiley-Blackwell, pp. 851–863.

Jones-Gotman, M, Smith, ML, and Wieser, HG (2008). Intraarterial amobarbital procedures. In Epilepsy: A Comprehensive Textbook, 2nd ed. Edited by J Engel, Jr, and TA Pedley. Philadelphia: Lippincott Williams & Wilkins, pp. 1833–1841.

Kanner, AM (2009). Presurgical psychiatric evaluation. In The Treatment of Epilepsy, 3rd ed. Edited by S Shorvon, E Perucca, and J Engel, Jr. West Sussex, UK: Wiley-Blackwell, pp. 865–874.

Kaufman, CB, and Pilcher, WH (2009). Awake surgery for epilepsy. In The Treatment of Epilepsy, 3rd ed. Edited by S Shorvon, E Perucca, and J Engel, Jr. West Sussex, UK: Wiley-Blackwell, pp. 959–966.

Kossoff, EH, and Dorward, JL. (2009). Ketogenic diets. In The Treatment of Epilepsy, 3rd ed. Edited by S Shorvon, E Perucca, and J Engel, Jr. West Sussex, UK: Wiley-Blackwell, pp. 301–310.

Kossoff, EH, Zupec-Kania, BA, Amark, PE, Ballaban-Gil, KR, Bergqvist, AG, Blackford, R, Buchhalter, JR, Caraballo, RH, Cross, JH, Dahlin, MG, Donner, EJ, Klepper, J, Jehle, RS, Kim, HD, Liu, YM, Nation, J, Nordli, DR, Jr, Pfeifer, HH, Rho, JM, Stafstrom, CE, Thiele, EA, Turner, Z, Wirrell, EC, Wheless, JW, Veggiotti, P, Vining, EP; International Ketogenic Diet Study Group (2009). Optimal clinical management of children receiving the ketogenic diet: Recommendations of the International Ketogenic Diet Study Group. Epilepsia 50:304–317.

Krahl, SE, Clark, KB, Smith,DC, et al. (1998). Locus coeruleus lesions suppress the seizure-attenuating effects of vagus nerve stimulation. Epilepsia 39:709–714.

Krynauw, RA (1950). Infantile hemiplegia treated by removing one cerebral hemisphere. J Neurol Neurosurg Psychiatry 13:243–267.

Kumar, A, Asano, E, and Chugani, HT (2011). α-[^{11}C]-methyl-l-tryptophan PET for tracer localization of epileptogenic brain regions: Clinical studies. Biomark Med 5:577–584.

Kwan, P, Arzimanoglou, A, Berg, AT, Brodie,MJ, Hauser, WA, Mathern, G, Moshé, SL, Perucca, E, Wiebe, S, and French, J (2010). Definition of drug resistant epilepsy: Consensus proposal by the ad hoc Task Force of the ILAE Commission on Therapeutic Strategies. Epilepsia 51:1069–1077,.

Langfitt, JT (1997). Cost-effectiveness of anterotemporal lobectomy in medically intractable complex partial epilepsy. Epilepsia 38:154–163.

Langfitt, JT, Westerveld, M, Hamberger, MJ, Walczak, TS, Cicchetti, DV, Berg, AT, Vickrey, BG, Barr, WB, Sperling, MR, Masur, D, and Spencer, SS (2007). Worsening of quality of life after epilepsy surgery: Effect of seizures and memory decline. Neurology 68:1988–1994.

Lansky EB, and St Louis, E (2006). Transcendental meditation: Adouble edged sword in epilepsy? Epilepsy Behav 9:394–400.

Lee, BI, Markand, ON, Wellman, HN, Siddiqui, AR, Park, HM, Mock, B, Worth, RM, Edwards, MK, and Krepshaw, J (1988). HIPDM-SPECT in patients with medically intractable complex partial seizures. Arch Neurol 45:397–402.

Leiphart, J, and Fried, I (2009). Mesial temporal lobe surgery and other lobar resections. In The Treatment of Epilepsy, 3rd ed. Edited by S Shorvon, E Perucca, and J Engel, Jr. West Sussex, UK: Wiley-Blackwell, pp. 875–885.

Lerner, JT, Salamon, N, Hauptman, JS, Velasco, TR, Hemb, M, Wu, JY, Sankar, R, Shields, WD, Engel, J,Jr, Fried, I, Cepeda, C, Andre, VM, Levine, MS, Miyata, H, Yong, WH, Vinters, HV, and Mathern, GW (2009). Assessment and surgical outcomes for mild type I and severe type II cortical dysplasia: Acritical review and the UCLA experience. Epilepsia 50:1310–1335.

Lesser, RP, Lüders, H, Klem, G, Dinner, DS, Morris, HH, Hahn, JF, and Wyllie, E (1987). Extraoperative cortical functional localization in patients with epilepsy. J Clin Neurophysiol 4:27–53.

Lin, JJ, Salamon, N, Dutton, RA, Lee, AD, Geaga, JA, Hayashi, KM, Toga, AW, Engel, J, Jr, and Thompson, PM (2005). Three-dimensional preoperative maps of hippocampal atrophy predict surgical outcomes in temporal lobe epilepsy. Neurology 65:1094–1097.

Lin,JJ, Salamon, N, Lee, AD, Dutton, RA, Geaga, JA, Hayashi, KM, Luders, E, Toga, AW, Engel, J, Jr, and Thompson, PM (2007). Reduced neocortical thickness and complexity mapped in mesial temporal lobe epilepsy with hippocampal sclerosis. Cereb Cortex1 7:2007–2018.

Luciano, AL, and Shorvon, SD (2007). Results of treatment changes in patients with apparently drug-resistant chronic epilepsy. Ann Neurol 62:375–381.

Luders, E, Toga, AW, Lepore, N, and Gaser, C (2009). The underlying anatomical correlates of long-term meditation: Larger hippocampal and frontal volumes of gray matter. Neuroimage 45:672–678.

Lüders, HO (ed) (1992). Epilepsy Surgery. New York: Raven Press.

Lüders, HO, and Comair, YG (eds) (2001). Epilepsy Surgery, 2nd ed. Philadelphia: Lippincott Williams & Wilkins.

Lüders, HO, Engel, J, Jr, and Munari, C (1993). General principles. In Surgical Treatment of the Epilepsies, 2nd ed. Edited by J Engel, Jr. New York: Raven Press, pp. 137–153.

Lüders, HO, Bingaman, W, and Najm, IM (eds) (2008). Textbook of Epilepsy Surgery. London: Taylor and Francis Medical Books.

Macewen, W (1881). Intra-cranial lesions—illustrating some points in connexion with the localisation of cerebral affections and the advantages of aseptic trephining. Lancet ii:544 and 581.

Macrodimitris, S, Sherman, EMS, Forde, S, et al. (2011). Psychiatric outcomes of epilepsy surgery: Asystematic review. Epilepsia 52:880–890.

Mathern, GW (ed) (1999). Pediatric epilepsy and epilepsy surgery. Dev Neurosci 21:159–408.

McEvoy, AW, and Arnold, FJL (2009). Stereotactic surgery for epilepsy. In The Treatment of Epilepsy, 3rd ed. Edited by S Shorvon, E Perucca, and J Engel, Jr. West Sussex, UK: Wiley-Blackwell, pp. 975–992.

Miller, JW, and Silbergeld, DL (eds) (2006). Epilepsy Surgery: Principles and Controversies. New York: Taylor & Francis.

Milner, B, Branch, C, and Rasmussen, T (1962). Study of short-term memory after intracarotid injection of sodium amytal. Trans Am Neurol Assoc 87:224–226.

Mintzer, S, Cendes, F, Soss, J, Andermann, F, Engel, J,Jr, Dubeau, F, Olivier, A, and Fried, I (2004). Unilateral hippocampal sclerosis with contralateral temporal scalp ictal onset. Epilepsia45:792–802.

Moniz, E (1934). L'Angiographie Cérébrale. Paris: Masson et Cie.

Morrell, F (1959/60). Secondary epileptogenic lesions. Epilepsia 1:538–560.

Morrell, F (1985). Secondary epileptogenesis in man. Arch Neurol 42:318–335.

Morrell, F, Whisler, WW, and Bleck, TP (1989). Multiple subpial transection: A new approach to the surgical treatment of focal epilepsy. J Neurosurg 70:231–239.

Morrell, M, for the RNS System in Epilepsy Study Group (2011). Responsive-cortical stimulation for the treatment of medically intractable partial epilepsy. Neurology 77:1295–1304.

Munari, C, Kahane, P, Francione, S, Hoffman, D, Tassi, L, Cusmai, R, Vigevano, F, Pasquier, B, and Betti, OO (1995). Role of the hypothalamic hamartoma in the genesis of gelastic fits (a video-stereo-EEG study). Electroencephalogr Clinical Neurophysiol 95:154–160.

Narabayashi, H, and Mizutani, T (1970). Epileptic seizures and the stereotaxic amygdalotomy. Confin Neurol 32:289–297.

Narita, Y, Satowa, H, Kokubu, T, and Sugaya, E (1982). Treatment of epileptic patients with the Chinese herbal medicine "aiko-keishi-to." IRCS Med Sci 10:88–89.

Ogren, JA, Wilson, CL, Bragin, A, Lin, JJ, Salamon, N, Dutton, RA, Luders, E, Fields, TA, Fried, I, Toga, AW, Thompson, PM, Engel, J, Jr, and Staba, RJ (2009a). Three-dimensional surface maps link local atrophy and fast ripples in human epileptic hippocampus. Ann Neurol 66:783–791.

Ogren, JA, Bragin, A, Wilson, CL, Hoftman, GD, Lin, JJ, Dutton, RA, Fields, TA, Toga, AW, Thompson, PM, Engel, J, Jr, and Staba, RJ (2009b). Three-dimensional hippocampal atrophy maps distinguish two common temporal lobe seizure-onset patterns. Epilepsia 50:1361–1370.

Oja, SS, and Kontro, P (1983). Free amino acids in epilepsy: Possible role of taurine. Acta Neurol Scand 93(suppl):5–20.

Palmini, A (2009). Epilepsy surgery in countries with limited resources. In The Treatment of Epilepsy, 3rd ed. Edited by S Shorvon, E Perucca, and J Engel, Jr. West Sussex, UK: Wiley-Blackwell, pp. 1051–1056.

Penfield, W (1936). Epilepsy and surgical therapy. Arch Neurol Psychiatry 36:449–484.

Penfield, W, and Erickson,TC (1941). Epilepsy and Cerebral Localization. Springfield, IL: Charles C Thomas.

Penfield, W, and Flanigin, H (1950). Surgical therapy of temporal lobe seizures. Arch Neurol Psychiatr 64:491–500.

Penfield, W, and Jasper, H (1954). Epilepsy and the Functional Anatomy of the Human Brain. Boston: Little, Brown & Co.

Pickard, JD, Trojanowski, T, Maira, G, and Polkey, CE (eds) (1990). Neurosurgical Aspects of Epilepsy. New York: Springer-Verlag.

Polkey, CE (2009). Complications of epilepsy surgery. In The Treatment of Epilepsy, 3rd ed. Edited by S Shorvon, E Perucca, and J Engel, Jr. West Sussex, UK: Wiley-Blackwell, pp. 993–1005.

Polkey, CE, and Smith, MC (2008). Multiple subpial transections and other interventions. In Epilepsy: A Comprehensive Textbook, 2nd ed. Edited by J Engel, Jr, and TA Pedley. Philadelphia: Lippincott Williams & Wilkins, pp. 1921–1928.

Post, RM, Putnam, F, Contel, NR, and Goldman, B (1984). Electroconvulsive seizures inhibit amygdala kindling: Implications for mechanisms of action in affective illness. Epilepsia 25:234–239.

Purpura, DP, Penry, JK, and Walter, RD (eds) (1975). Neurosurgical Management of the Epilepsies. Adv Neurol 8.

Radhakrishnan, K, Fried, I, and Cascino, GD (2008). Lesionectomy: Management of substrate-directed epilepsies. In Epilepsy: A Comprehensive Textbook, 2nd ed. Edited by J Engel, Jr, and TA Pedley. Philadelphia: Lippincott Williams & Wilkins, pp. 1891–1906.

Rasmussen, T (1987). Commentary: Extratemporal cortical excisions and hemispherectomy. In Surgical Treatment of the Epilepsies. Edited by J Engel, Jr. New York: Raven Press, pp. 417–424.

Reynolds, EH (1967). Effects of folic acid on the mental state and fit-frequency of drug-treated epileptic patients. Lancet 1:1086–1088.

Risinger, MW, Engel, J, Jr, Van Ness, PC, Henry, TR, and Crandall, PH (1989). Ictal localization of temporal lobe seizures. Neurology 39:1288–1293.

Roberts, DW (2008). Corpus callosotomy. In Epilepsy: A Comprehensive Textbook, 2nd ed. Edited by J Engel, Jr, and TA Pedley. Philadelphia: Lippincott Williams & Wilkins, pp. 1907–1913.

Roberts, DW (2009). Corpus callosotomy. In The Treatment of Epilepsy, 3rd ed. Edited by S Shorvon, E Perucca, and J Engel, Jr. West Sussex, UK: Wiley-Blackwell, pp. 943–950.

Rogawski, M, and Schwartzkroin, PL (eds) (2009). Nontraditional epilepsy treatment approaches. Neurotherapeutics 6(special issue).

Sackeim, HA, Decina, P, Prohovnik, I, Malitz, S, and Resor, SR (1983). Anticonvulsant and antidepressant properties of electroconvulsive therapy: A proposed mechanism of action. Biol Psychiatry 18:1301–1310.

Sanabria, E, Chauvel, P, Askienazy, S, Vignal, JP, Trottier, S, Chodkiewicz, JP, and Bancaud, J (1983). Single photon emission computed tomography (SPECT) using ^{123}I-isopropyl-iodo-amphetamine (IAMP) in partial epilepsy. In Current Problems in Epilepsy 1:Cerebral Blood Flow, Metabolism and Epilepsy. Edited by M Baldy-Moulinier, D-H Ingvar, and BS Meldrum. London: John Libbey, pp. 82–87.

Sankar, R, Curran, JG, Kevill, JW, Rintahaka, PJ, Shewmon, DA, and Vinters, HV (1995). Microscopic cortical dysplasia in infantile spasms: Evolution of white matter abnormalities. AJNR Am J Neuroradiol 16:1265–1272.

Schachter, SC (2009). Vagal nerve stimulation. In The Treatment of Epilepsy, 3rd ed. Edited by S Shorvon, E Perucca, and J Engel, Jr. West Sussex, UK: Wiley-Blackwell, pp. 1017–1023.

Schachter, SC, and Boon, P (2008). Vagus nerve stimulation. In Epilepsy: A Comprehensive Textbook, 2nd ed. Edited by J Engel, Jr, and TA Pedley. Philadelphia: Lippincott Williams & Wilkins, pp. 1395–1399.

Schachter, SC, Acevedo, C, Acevedo, KA, Lai, C-W, and Diop, AG (2008). Complementary and alternative medical therapies. In Epilepsy: A Comprehensive Textbook, 2nd ed. Edited by J Engel, Jr, and TA Pedley. Philadelphia: Lippincott Williams & Wilkins, pp. 1407–1414.

Schrader, LM, Stern, JM, Koski, L, Nuwer, MR, and Engel J, Jr (2004). Seizure incidence during single- and paired-pulse transcranial magnetic stimulation (TMS) in individuals with epilepsy. Clin Neurophysiol 115:2728–2737.

Schramm, J (2002). Hemispherectomy techniques. Neurosurg Clin N Am 13:113–134.

Semah, F, Picot, M-C, Adam, C, Broglin, D, Arzimanoglou, A, Bazin, B, Cavalcanti, D, and Baulac, M (1998). Is the underlying cause of epilepsy a major prognostic factor for recurrence? Neurology 51:1256–1262.

Sherman, EM, Wiebe, S, Fay-McClymont, TB, et al. (2011). Neuropsychological outcomes after epilepsy surgery: Systematic review and pooled estimates. Epilepsia 52:857–869.

Shields, WD, Shewmon, DA, Chugani, HT, and Peacock, WJ (1990). The role of surgery in the treatment of infantile spasms. J Epilepsy 3(suppl):321–324.

Silbergeld, DL, and Ojemann, GA (eds) (1993). Neurosurgery Clinics of North America. Epilepsy Surg4.

Smith, MC, Byrne, R, and Kanner, AM (2009). Hypothalamic hamartoma and multiple subpial transection. In The Treatment of Epilepsy, 3rd ed. Edited by S Shorvon, E Perucca, and J Engel, Jr. West Sussex, UK: Wiley-Blackwell, pp. 951–957.

Spencer, DD, and Spencer, SS (eds) (1991). Surgery for Epilepsy. Cambridge, MA:Blackwell.

Spencer, DD, Spencer, SS, Mattson, RH, Williamson, PD, and Novelly, RA (1984a). Access to the posterior medial temporal lobe structure in surgical treatment of temporal lobe epilepsy. Neurosurgery 15:667–671.

Spencer, S, and Huh, L (2008). Outcomes of epilepsy surgery in adults and children. Lancet Neurol 7:525–537.

Spencer, SS, Spencer, DD, Glaser, GH, Williamson, PD, and Mattson, RH (1984b). More intense focal seizure types after callosal section: The role of inhibition. Ann Neurol 16:686–693.

Spencer, SS, Gates, JR, Reeves, AR, Spencer, DD, Maxwell, RE, and Roberts, D (1987). Corpus callosum section. In Surgical Treatment of the Epilepsies. Edited by J Engel, Jr. New York: Raven Press, pp. 425–444.

Spencer, SS, Sperling, MR, Shewmon, DA, and Kahane, P (2008). Intracranial electrodes. In Epilepsy: A Comprehensive Textbook, 2nd ed. Edited by J Engel, Jr, and TA Pedley. Philadelphia: Lippincott Williams & Wilkins, pp. 1791–1815.

Spencer, SS, Nguyen, DK, and Duckrow, RB (2009). Invasive EEG in presurgical evaluation of epilepsy. In The Treatment of Epilepsy, 3rd ed. Edited by S Shorvon, E Perucca, and J Engel, Jr. West Sussex, UK: Wiley-Blackwell, pp. 767–798.

Sperling, MR (2004). The consequences of uncontrolled epilepsy. CNS Spectr9:98–109.

Stafstrom, CE, Vining, EPG, and Rho, JM (2008). Ketogenic diet. In Epilepsy: A Comprehensive Textbook, 2nd ed. Edited by J Engel, Jr, and TA Pedley. Philadelphia: Lippincott Williams & Wilkins, pp. 1377–1385.

Stephen, LJ, Kwan, P, and Brodie,MJ (2001). Does the cause of localisation-related epilepsy influence the response to antiepileptic drug treatment? Epilepsia 42:357–362.

Sterman, MB, and Bowersox, SS (1981). Sensorimotor EEG rhythmic activity: A functional gate mechanism. Sleep 4:408–422.

Sterman, MB, and Friar, L (1972). Suppression of seizures in an epileptic following sensorimotor EEG feedback training. Electroencephalogr Clin Neurophysiol 33:89–95.

Sterman, MB, Macdonald, LW, and Stone, RK (1974). Biofeedback training of the sensorimotor EEG rhythm in man: Effects on epilepsy. Epilepsia 15:395–416.

Stern, J, and Engel, J, Jr (2012). Epilepsy surgery. In Encyclopedia of Neurological Sciences. Edited by J Aminoff and R Daroff. Amsterdam: Elsevier, pp. 143–163.

Sutter, B, and Schrottner, O (eds) (2002). Advances in epilepsy surgery and radiosurgery. Acta Neurochir, Suppl 84.

Swarztrauber, K, Dewar, S,and Engel, J, Jr (2003). Patient attitudes about treatments for intractable epilepsy. Epilepsy Behav 4:19–25.

Takato, M, Takamure, K, Sugaya, A, Tsuda, T, and Sugaya, E (1982). Effect of the Chinese medicine "saiko-keishi-to" on audiogenic seizure mice, kindling animals and conventional pharmacological screening procedures. IRCS Med Sci 10:86–87.

Talairach, J, David, M, and Tournoux, P (1958). L'Exploration Chirurgicale Stéréotaxiquedu Lobe Temporaledansl' Épilepsie Temporale. Paris: Masson etCie.

Talairach, J, Bancaud, J, Szikla, G, Bonis, A, Geier, S, and Vedrenne, C (1974). Approche nouvelle de la neurochirurgie de l'épilepsie. Méthodologiestéréotaxiqueetr ésultatsthérapeutiques. Neurochirurgie 20(suppl 1).

Taylor, DC (1972). Mental state and temporal lobe epilepsy: A correlative account of 100 patients treated surgically. Epilepsia 13:727–765.

Taylor, J (ed) (1958). Selected Writings of John Hughlings Jackson, Vol 1. New York: Basic Books.

Temkin, O (1945). The Falling Sickness: A History of Epilepsy from the Greeks to the Beginnings of Modern Neurology. Baltimore: Johns Hopkins University Press.

Theodore, WH (ed) (1992). Surgical Treatment of Epilepsy. Amsterdam: Elsevier.

Theodore, WH, and Fisher, RS (2004). Brain stimulation for epilepsy. Lancet Neurol 3:111–118.

Tuxhorn, I, Holthausen, H, and Boenigk, H. (eds) (1997). Paediatric Epilepsy Syndromes and Their Surgical Treatment. London: John Libbey.

Uff, CE, and Kitchen, ND (2009). Resective surgery of vascular and infective lesions for epilepsy. In The Treatment of Epilepsy, 3rd ed. Edited by S Shorvon, E Perucca, and J Engel, Jr. West Sussex, UK: Wiley-Blackwell, pp. 903–924.

Van de Wiele, B (2009). Anaesthesia for epilepsy surgery. In The Treatment of Epilepsy, 3rd ed. Edited by S Shorvon, E Perucca, and J Engel, Jr. West Sussex, UK: Wiley-Blackwell, pp. 1007–1016.

Van Wagenen, WP, and Herren, RY (1940). Surgical division of commissural pathways in the corpus callosum: Relation to spread of an epileptic attack. Arch Neurol Psychiatry 44:740–759.

Van Woert, MH, Rosenbaum, D, Howieson, J, and Bowers, MB (1977). Long term therapy of myoclonus and other neurological disorders with l-5-hydroxytryptophan and carbidopa. N Engl J Med 296:70–75.

Vickrey, BG, Hays, RD, Graber, J, Rausch, R, Engel, J, Jr, and Brook, RH (1992). A health-related quality of life instrument for patients evaluated for epilepsy surgery. Med Care30:299–319.

Vickrey, BG, Hays, R, Engel, J, Jr, Spritzer, K, Rogers, W, Rausch, R, Graber, J, and Brook, R (1995a). Outcome assessment for epilepsy surgery: The impact of measuring health-related quality of life. Ann Neurol 37:158–166.

Vickrey, BG, Hays, RD, Rausch, R, Engel, J, Jr, Visscher, BR, Ary, CM, Rogers, WH, and Brook, RH (1995b). Outcomes in 248 patients who had diagnostic evaluations for epilepsy surgery. Lancet346:1445–1449.

Villani, F, Bien, CG, and Avanzini, GG (2008). Immunoglobulin and immunomodulatory therapy. In Epilepsy: A Comprehensive Textbook, 2nd ed. Edited by J Engel, Jr, and TA Pedley. Philadelphia: Lippincott Williams & Wilkins, pp. 1741–1746.

Viventi, J, Kim, D-H, Vigeland, L, Frechette, ES, Blanco, JA, Kim, Y-S, Arvin, AE, Tiruvadi, VR, Hwang, S-W, Vanleer, AC, Wulsin, DF, Davis, K, Gelber, CE, Palmer, L, Van der Spiegel, J, Wu, J, Xiao, J, Huang, Y, Contreras, D, Rogers, JA, and Litt, B (2011). Flexible, foldable, actively multiplexed, high-density electrode array for mapping brain activity in vivo. Nat Neurosci 14:1599–1607.

Vives, K, Lee, G, Doyle, W, and Spencer, DD (2008). Anterior temporal resection. In Epilepsy: A Comprehensive Textbook, 2nd ed. Edited by J Engel, Jr, and TA Pedley. Philadelphia: Lippincott Williams & Wilkins, pp. 1859–1867.

Wannamaker, BB, Diamond, BI, Hammond, D, Koonce, JR, and Walter, W (1982). Chinaberry juice: A natural product extract with antiepileptic properties [abstract]. Abstr Soc Neurosci 8:506.

Wetjen, N, Junna, MR, Radhakrishnan, K, et al. (2009). Resective surgery of neoplasms. In The Treatment of Epilepsy, 3rd ed. Edited by S Shorvon, E Perucca, and J Engel, Jr. West Sussex, UK: Wiley-Blackwell, pp. 887–901.

Whitmarsh, T (2009). Non-pharmacological, complementary and alternative treatments for epilepsy. In The Treatment of Epilepsy, 3rd ed. Edited by S Shorvon, E Perucca, and J Engel, Jr. West Sussex, UK: Wiley-Blackwell, pp. 311–322.

Wiebe, S, Blume, WT, Girvin, JP, and Eliasziw, M (2001). A randomized, controlled trial of surgery for temporal lobe epilepsy. N Engl J Med 345:311–318.

Wieser, HG (1986). Selective amygdalohippocampectomy: Indications, investigative technique and results. Adv Tech Stand Neurosurg13:39–133.

Wieser, HG (2008). Foramen ovale and peg electrodes. In Epilepsy: A Comprehensive Textbook, 2nd ed. Edited by J Engel, Jr, and TA Pedley. Philadelphia: Lippincott Williams & Wilkins, pp. 1779–1789.

Wieser, HG, and Elger, CE (eds) (1987). Presurgical Evaluation of Epileptics: Basics, Techniques, Implications. Berlin: Springer-Verlag.

Wieser, HG, Blume, WT, Fish, D, Goldensohn, E, Hufnagel, A, King, D, Sperling, MR, and Lüders, H (2001). Proposal for a new classification of outcome with respect to epileptic seizures following epilepsy surgery. Commission on Neurosurgery of the International League Against Epilepsy (ILAE) 1997–2001. Epilepsia 42:282–286.

Wilder, RM (1921). The effect of ketonemia on the course of epilepsy. Mayo Clin Bull 2:307–308.

Wilson, DH, Reeves, A, and Gazzaniga, M (1978). Division of the corpus callosum for uncontrollable epilepsy. Neurology 28:649–653.

Wilson, DH, Reeves, A, and Gazzaniga, M (1982). "Central" commissurotomy for intractable generalized epilepsy: Series two. Neurology 32:687–697.

Wilson, SJ,and Engel, J, Jr (2010). Diverse perspectives on developments in epilepsy surgery. Seizure 19:659–668.

Wolf, P (2008). Behavioral therapies. In Epilepsy: A Comprehensive Textbook, 2nd ed. Edited by J Engel, Jr, and TA Pedley. Philadelphia: Lippincott Williams & Wilkins, pp. 1401–1405.

Worrell, G, and Gotman, J: High-frequency oscillations and other electrophysiological biomarkers of epilepsy: Clinical studies. BiomarkMed 5:557–566.

Wrench, JM, Rayner, G, and Wilson, SJ (2011). Profiling the evolution of depression after epilepsy surgery. Epilepsia 52:900–908.

Wright, GDS, McLellan, DL, and Brice, JG (1985). A double-blind trial of chronic cerebellar stimulation in twelve patients with severe epilepsy. J Neurol Neurosurg Psychiatry 47:769–774,.

Wyler, AR, and Hermann, BP (eds) (1994). The Surgical Management of Epilepsy. Boston: Butterworth-Heinemann.

Yang, I, Chang, EF, and Barbaro, NM (2009). Stereotactic radiosurgery for medically intractable epilepsy. In The Treatment of Epilepsy, 3rd ed. Edited by S Shorvon, E Perucca, and J Engel, Jr. West Sussex, UK: Wiley-Blackwell, pp. 1035–1041.

Yasargil, MG, Teddy, PJ, and Roth, R (1985). Selective amygdalohippocampectomy. Operative anatomy and surgical technique. Adv Tech Stand Neurosurg 12:93–123.

Zabara, J (1992). Inhibition of experimental seizures in canines by repetitive vagal stimulation. Epilepsia 33:1005–1012.

Zarroli, K, Tracy, JI, Nei, M, Sharan, A, and Sperling, MR (2011). Employment after anterior temporal lobectomy. Epilepsia 52:925–931.

Zentner, J, and Seeger, W (eds) (2003). Surgical Treatment of Epilepsy. New York:Springer-Verlag.

Chapter 17

Social Management

STIGMA

QUALITY OF LIFE

ACTIVITIES OF DAILY LIVING
Driving
Participation in Sports
Alcohol and Drugs
Specific Hazards

FAMILY
The Child with Epilepsy
The Parent with Epilepsy

SCHOOL

EMPLOYMENT

LEGAL RIGHTS

INSURANCE

FINANCIAL AID

RESOURCES

HEALTH CARE DISPARITIES

SUMMARY AND CONCLUSIONS

Persons with epilepsy generally seek the help of a physician because their seizures interfere with daily living or cause concerns about their well-being. These psychosocial consequences of illness have been referred to as the patient's *predicament* (Taylor, 1982). For all medical conditions, the sensitive and effective physician not only attempts to diagnose and treat the disease process but also directs efforts toward resolving the predicament. For patients with epilepsy, this requires understanding the unique predicament created by the threat of recurrent epileptic seizures and the stigma associated with this condition. Maintaining a compassionate support system is most difficult for patients with severe epilepsy disorders who require lifetime care and their families (Douglass, 2011).

Ignorance is the primary obstacle to a positive self-image and a satisfactory life adjustment for the person with epilepsy (Masland, 1985; Jacoby et al., 2008). For this reason, the physician should take care to explain the disorder and its implications in detail to the patient and family, encourage questions, and dispel misconceptions (Table 17–1). Patients

Table 17–1 What Persons with Epilepsy and Their Families Want Most to Know

Diagnosis
    Type of epilepsy
    Cause(s) if known
    Diagnostic test result (why EEG may be normal)
Treatment
    Pharmacokinetics (why specific drug regimen is
        necessary)
    When blood levels are indicated
    Avoidance of precipitating factors (how to raise
        and lower seizure threshold)
First aid
    What to do for different seizure types
    How to recognize status epilepticus
Prognosis
    Chance for seizure control
    Chance for remission
    Risk of death or brain damage

From material gathered by R. Mittan and the Sepulveda Epilepsy Education (SEE) Program, with permission.

or parents often request reading material; excellent brochures are available from the national chapters of the *International Bureau for Epilepsy (IBE)* (www.ibe-epilepsy.org). The *Epilepsy Foundation* is the United States chapter of IBE, which has many local affiliates; a list of excellent books and DVDs for people with epilepsy, parents, children, teachers, health care providers, and first responders is available on the foundation's web site (www.epilepsy-foundation.org). Community education is also important in reducing the prejudice faced by persons with epilepsy; they suffer less disability when family members, teachers, employers, and others who interact with them understand their condition. Dissemination of information has done much to create more favorable public attitudes toward persons with epilepsy, which improved greatly several decades ago (Caveness and Gallup, 1980) (Table 17–2).

Common sense is necessary when deciding whether to limit the activities of daily living of persons with epilepsy. The general philosophy today is to encourage them to lead as normal lives as possible, restricting activities only when there may be serious risk of injuring themselves or others. To provide comprehensive care for their patients, physicians must be familiar with state and federal legal restrictions on persons with epilepsy, legal rights of the disabled, insurance problems that such persons might encounter, community resources, self-help groups, and available educational literature.

STIGMA

Stigma remains a major cause of distress and disability for people with epilepsy whose seizures can be easily and effectively controlled (Jacoby et al., 2008). The concept of stigma has been reformulated for research purposes as a process in which adverse social judgments are made that are medically unwarranted (Weiss and Ramakrishna, 2001). Because stigma varies greatly from culture to culture, even within a single country, it has been difficult to carry out quantitative studies characterizing its features and effects. The culture-bound stigmatizing attitudes of individuals and society toward

Table 17–2 Changing Public Attitudes Toward Epilepsy In The United States

Question	Percent Answering Yes						
	1949	1954	1959	1964	1969	1974	1979
Have you ever heard or read about the disease called "epilepsy" or convulsive seizures (fits)?	92	90	93	95	94	94	95
Would you object to having any of your children in school or at play associate with persons who have seizures?	24	17	18	13	9	5	6
Do you think epilepsy is a form of insanity or not?	13	7	4	4	4	2	3
Do you think epileptics should be employed in jobs like other people?	45	60	75	82	76	81	79

From Caveness and Gallup, 1980, with permission.

people with epilepsy (*enacted stigma*) clearly have negative impact when the epilepsy condition is apparent; however, even when it is not, there is a *felt stigma* associated with impaired self-esteem, self-efficacy, and sense of mastery; perceived helplessness; increased rates of anxiety and depression; increased somatic symptomatology; and reduced life satisfaction (Jacoby et al., 2008). Efforts to change negative public attitudes include education and advocacy, which are worldwide objectives of the *Global Campaign Against Epilepsy (GCAE)*, a joint effort of the *World Health Organization (WHO)*, the *International League against Epilepsy (ILAE)*, and IBE (www.globalcam paignagainstepilepsy.org). The GCAE has carried out a number of demonstration projects in resource-poor countries aimed at increasing health care delivery for people with epilepsy, using educational and other interventions to overcome the misconceptions and stigma that prevent appropriate patient identification and referral. Promoting empathy by increasing contact between people with epilepsy and the general population is another strategy that could reduce stigma. If prominent public figures with epilepsy would make their conditions known, even if they did not take up active advocacy roles on behalf of epilepsy, this could have a major positive impact on reducing the negative impressions our society has about epilepsy.

The negative public image of the person with epilepsy has been largely shaped by the portrayal of seriously flawed fictional characters with this condition. *Dostoyevsky*, who had epilepsy himself as well as a son who died of epilepsy, attempted a positive depiction of someone with epilepsy in *Prince Myshkin*, the hero of his novel *The Idiot*. Although the prince was highly intelligent, to make him realistic, Dostoyevsky developed the character as uneducated and therefore taken to be an idiot. His novels had other, less attractive characters with epilepsy, such as *Smerdyakov* in *The Brothers Karamazov*, *Kirilov* in *The Possessed*, and *Elena* in *The Insulted and Injured*, who were often unaccomplished, depressed, and suicidal. *George Eliot*'s *Silas Marner*, the miserly recluse, is another well-known negative literary portrayal of a protagonist with epilepsy. Suicide and shame were the overriding themes of the 1949 film *Night unto Night*, about a man who overcomes his desire to kill himself when he

learns that the woman he loves knows of his condition and doesn't care. More recently, *Marsha Norman*'s Pulitzer Prize–winning play *'night, Mother* sympathetically portrayed the predicament of a young woman with epilepsy and depression who ultimately commits suicide. The homicidal maniac protagonist of *Michael Crichton*'s novel *The Terminal Man* projected a dangerously misleading image. Crichton's inaccurate depiction of violent epileptic seizures was retracted, with a formal apology, in the paperback edition. Objectionable scenes and references were also deleted from the film version. An Emmy-winning BBC film, *The Lost Prince* (2003), compassionately documents the life of Prince John, the youngest son of King George V of England, who had epilepsy and was hidden from the public. The heroine of the 2004 film *Garden State* was notable because her epilepsy did not particularly compromise her quirky but positive character. Perhaps this film represents a shifting attitude in response to concerted efforts of advocacy groups to combat negative stereotypes.

A review of the portrayal of epilepsy in films and television concluded that the people who craft these depictions are more concerned about what the images can do for plot development and less interested in accurate portrayals that would be helpful, rather than detrimental, to public concepts of epilepsy (Kerson and Kerson, 2006). Given that most people have never seen an epileptic seizure, the public is much more likely to be influenced by negative images in the visual media than by attempts at education by the scientific and medical community. With the advent of the Internet, however, patients with epilepsy are now beginning to share their personal experiences on YouTube and other outlets, which could have an encouraging counterbalancing effect (Kerson et al., 2012).

Epilepsy advocacy groups have walked a fine line between the need to destigmatize epilepsy in order to reduce the disabling impact negative misconceptions have on people with this condition and the need to publicize that epilepsy is a serious, at times life-threatening condition in order to gain public support for research and resources. Fortunately these positions are not mutually exclusive, but constant attention is necessary to make sure that well-meaning statements in favor of one do not detract from the other. A case in point is the tendency of the epilepsy community to tiptoe around the use of the word *epilepsy*, preferring to tell patients that they have a *seizure disorder* and insisting that epilepsy is a *disorder* and not a *disease*. Sadly, persistence in this practice perpetuates the stigma of these words while at the same time belittling the condition and diminishing competitiveness for limited resources (Engel, 2010). Cancer is many diseases, but referring to it in general as a *disease* has neither caused confusion nor stigmatized people with cancer. Although the global burden of disease represented by epilepsy is at least equivalent to that of breast cancer in women, lung cancer in men, and, among primary disorders of the brain, depression, dementia, and substance abuse (Murray and Lopez, 1994) (Chapter 2), epilepsy receives only a small fraction of the media attention and resources devoted to those diseases. This discrepancy likely reflects both the stigma that still surrounds epilepsy and failure to adequately promote epilepsy as a serious, life-threatening disease.

QUALITY OF LIFE

Quantitative instruments to measure *health-related quality of life (HRQOL)* were first introduced to study outcomes following surgery for epilepsy, as discussed in the previous chapter (Vickrey et al., 1992), but the subsequently developed series of scales referred to as the *Quality of Life in Epilepsy (QOLIE)* inventory (Devinsky et al., 1995) (Chapters 11 and 16) are now also widely used to assess quality of life of people with epilepsy under a variety of conditions (Rubin and Wiebe, 2008). The widespread use of these instruments reflects the current understanding that epilepsy is more than epileptic seizures and that its treatment involves more than elimination of epileptic seizures. Health outcomes research, therefore, has shifted its focus from the ictal to the interictal period (Rubin and Wiebe, 2008). Medication toxicity and psychiatric comorbidity, particularly depression, account for the greatest variance in overall HRQOL apart from seizure occurrence (Chapter 11), but other factors discussed in this chapter present potentially remediable problems that contribute greatly to the burden of epilepsy. For research purposes, assessment of HRQOL may be insufficient

when it is important to understand why changes in HRQOL have occurred. Numerous instruments that measure social adjustment are available for this purpose (Austin et al., 2008; Rubin and Wiebe, 2008).

The QOLIE instruments consist of 10, 39, and 81 separate questions sampling, respectively, 7, 7, and 17 domains of quality of life that are differentially affected by epilepsy (Chapter 11). The degree to which patients perceive individual domains as important for quality of life is to a certain extent culturally and politically determined, as was demonstrated by application of the *Washington Psychosocial Seizure Inventory* (Chapter 11) to epileptic patients in four countries: Canada, Finland, East Germany, and the United States. The results of this study indicated that patients in the United States showed more concern than patients in other countries about the areas of vocational adjustment and financial status and also reported the poorest overall psychosocial functioning among the four countries (Dodrill et al., 1984). This finding undoubtedly reflects differences in national attitudes about governmental responsibility for social welfare. Because seizure control is negatively affected by environmental stress, and disability is often imposed by society, the plight of persons with epilepsy might be eased as much by improved social services as by new therapeutic approaches.

ACTIVITIES OF DAILY LIVING

Certain changes in activities of daily life may reduce the probability of seizure occurrence by limiting exposure to predisposing and precipitating factors (Chapters 5 and 9). A general rule for most persons with epileptic seizures is to develop regular eating, sleeping, and working habits, in order to avoid sleep deprivation, unnecessary anxiety, and illness. On the other hand, lifestyle can be severely compromised by knowledge that loss of control could occur at any time, perhaps without warning. In some cases, limitations on activities are advisable to reduce the risk of injury or embarrassment caused by an epileptic seizure. These risks, however, must be balanced against the damaging consequences of dependence, overprotection, and social isolation (Chapter 11).

Side effects of drugs, particularly sedation, also can compromise activities of daily living. Medications, however, may occasionally be manipulated to meet social needs. For instance, a student whose seizures are controlled only by levels of antiseizure medication that produce some sedation may prefer to decrease medication and risk a seizure to be more alert during an important examination. A teacher may allow the examination to be repeated if a seizure occurs, but sedation from medication is rarely accepted as an excuse for poor performance. Reduction or discontinuation of medication after a period of seizure freedom should be considered, but there are reasons why patients are not always accepting of this possibility (Chapter 14).

Driving

In the United States and other industrialized countries, restrictions on driving are among the most serious social constraints imposed on persons with epilepsy as a result of their medical condition. A corollary is that driving is the most commonly cited concern (70%) among persons with epilepsy (Gilliam et al., 2004). Given the importance of driving in modern society, it is not surprising that answers to the question of whether or when a patient with epileptic seizures should drive a car are confusing, contradictory, and controversial from both legal and practical points of view. Nevertheless, patients with new-onset epilepsy are almost always willing to stop driving, no matter how inconvenient it might be, when the subject is reasonably approached. This includes explaining that the restriction on driving is likely to be temporary until diagnosis and treatment results in seizure control and that in the meantime driving endangers not only the patient's life but also the lives of loved ones and strangers who might be affected in any serious accident.

Driving is a privilege, not a right. There is little disagreement that individuals who are at high risk for losing control of an automobile and causing injury to others as well as themselves should not drive. The controversies concern who should determine when a person presents a sufficient risk to warrant withholding a driving license and whether physicians should be responsible for reporting such persons to appropriate authorities. Driving

regulations in individual states and countries change periodically; regulations in the United States are summarized at www.nrsponline.com/resources.html and are also reviewed at www.epilepsyfoundation.org/resources/driving-laws-by-state.cfm. Laws regarding driving for people with epilepsy in individual countries are summarized at www.wikipedia.org/wiki/epilepsy_and_driving#laws_by_country.

PRACTICAL CRITERIA FOR RESTRICTIONS ON DRIVING

Epileptic seizures that recur without warning and result in alteration of consciousness, loss of motor control, or other transient dysfunction that would impair the ability to operate a motor vehicle constitute a sufficient justification for advising someone not to drive. On the other hand, patients who experience only focal seizures without alteration of consciousness or marked motor disturbances are usually not functionally disabled during these events and may not present a hazard when driving (Gastaut and Zifkin, 1987). Furthermore, when persons with epilepsy have prolonged auras that provide time to prepare for a seizure or have seizures that occur only at particular times of the day or in particular situations, it may be possible to determine conditions under which it would be safe to drive. Finally, driving need not be suspended for persons whose seizures occur only during sleep or who had reactive seizures in the past that were clearly due to a transient disturbance that is now resolved (Chapter 5).

Once it has been decided to recommend against driving, it becomes necessary to determine those conditions under which adequate seizure control would allow driving to again be advisable. The most common guidelines adopted by the states have been to consider epileptic seizures under control after three months to one year without a recurrence, either on or off medication. In practice, however, this decision must be made on an individual basis, taking into account several factors. Obviously, it is impossible to be certain that a person whose epilepsy is controlled by medication will never have another seizure (likewise, it is impossible to conclude that someone who has never had a seizure will not someday have one). Statistics on epilepsy syndromes or types of seizures in adults are inadequate to

permit accurate determination of the probability of seizure recurrence following different
seizure-free durations; however, persons with
only generalized tonic-clonic seizures are more
likely to remain seizure-free than persons with
focal seizures (Chapter 6), and those with certain genetic epilepsy syndromes are more likely
to have their disorder resolve completely than
those with epilepsy syndromes due to structural or metabolic causes (Chapter 7). When
seizures are frequent, it is possible to recognize the effectiveness of an antiseizure drug
much more quickly than when seizures are
infrequent. If seizure frequency is once a year
or less, a seizure-free interval of one year provides no information on the degree of control
achieved. In some persons, medication does
not control all epileptic seizures, but those that
remain may be only nocturnal or focal without
impaired consciousness and so present no hazard for driving. It is necessary, therefore, that
the physician take all of these factors into consideration when recommending that a patient
with epilepsy be allowed to resume driving.

Once a person has been seizure-free for a
sufficient time to permit antiseizure medication
withdrawal, that process presents an increased
risk for seizure recurrence. The occurrence of a
seizure during drug withdrawal does not neces-
sitate that driving be restricted until another
prolonged seizure-free interval has passed,
unless state law requires such a restriction. If
seizures come under control with reinstitution
of medication, there is usually no reason to recommend against driving. The more important
question, however, is whether a person should
be driving during the time that medication is
being withdrawn. This issue is not addressed
by law or to much extent in the medical literature. Studies of seizure recurrence following
discontinuation of medication have been concerned predominantly with childhood epilepsies (Chapters 8 and 14) and have indicated
that seizures are most likely to recur during the
withdrawal period or within the first six months
after withdrawal. Consequently, for patients
whose previous seizures could impair the ability to operate an automobile, it is reasonable to
recommend against driving during drug withdrawal and until at least three months after
withdrawal has been completed.

Common sense dictates that persons who are
at increased risk for loss of control as a result of
epileptic seizures should not place themselves
in situations that pose an unusually great danger to others. For instance, the approach to
determining restrictions on driving an automobile discussed in the previous paragraphs is
much more lenient than the approach required
for determining whether it is appropriate for
a person with epilepsy to operate a truck, a
school bus, or an airplane. It can be argued
that persons with an epilepsy disorder should
avoid such situations even if their seizures are
controlled by medication. Indeed, the United
States Department of Transportation will not
allow an individual with a history of seizures of
any kind to hold a commercial pilot's license.
Restrictions are under review that require
interstate commercial drivers to be more than
10 years seizure-free off antiseizure medications or more than 5 years seizure-free after a
single reactive seizure (Krumholz et al., 2008).

DRIVER'S LICENSE REGULATIONS

Governments, in establishing regulations such
as those that determine driving privileges, must
balance competing interests of public safety
and individual opportunity. Governments are
obligated to make laws limiting the privileges
of drivers who present an unacceptable risk
to themselves and others. "Across-the-board"
regulations, however, fail to reflect individual
differences and threaten to restrict the opportunities of some people unnecessarily. In fact,
the accident rate of persons with epileptic seizures who drive automobiles may be less than
the rate of accidents caused by drivers who
come to the attention of licensing authorities
for other reasons, and certainly the incidence
of fatal accidents caused by drivers with epileptic seizures is a small fraction of those caused
by people with other medical disorders who
are not generally restricted as well as by drivers
under the age of 25 (Table 17–3). One study
in the state of Washington revealed a lower
overall accident rate for women with epilepsy
than for men without epilepsy (Crancer and
McMurray, 1968), and alcohol consumption
may be at least a thousand times more likely
to cause an automobile accident than is an epileptic seizure (Masland, 1985). Statistics do not
appear to justify the degree of emphasis many
governments have placed on seizure disorders
when granting driver's licenses. Although some
restrictions are certainly appropriate, withdrawal of driving privileges greatly impairs

Table 17–3 Medical Causes Leading to Death in Motor Vehicle Accidents in the United States (1995–1997)

Causes of Fatal Crashes	No. of Deaths in Fatal Crashes		
	1995	1996	1997
Seizures	82	80	97
Other medical causes	1,873	1,971	1,987
Diabetes mellitus	127	148	156
Cardiovascular and hypertensive disorders	1,746	1,822	1,831
Alcohol related (alcohol abuse and alcoholism)	13,881	13,557	12,870
Young drivers (<25 years)	10,694	10,665	10,379
Total population	43,884	44,186	44,012

From Sheth et al., 2004, with permission.

individual opportunity in most societies and should not be imposed without good cause. Consequently, it is necessary to strive for flexible and reasonable regulations concerning the granting of driver's licenses for persons with active epilepsy.

In most states of the United States it is up to the individual to report an epilepsy condition when applying for a driver's license. However, in a handful of states, physicians are required to report anyone who experiences losses of consciousness or seizures despite medical treatment (Delaware, New Jersey, and Oregon) or who has a diagnosis of epilepsy or has experienced a seizure or loss of consciousness (California, Nevada, and Pennsylvania). Although no court has yet found a physician liable for loss or injury when an unreported patient with epilepsy had an automobile accident as a result of an epileptic seizure, several physicians have experienced considerable legal costs in defending themselves against such claims. These laws unacceptably compromise the doctor-patient relationship and are not necessarily effective in reducing the risk of automobile accidents caused by epileptic seizures. No statistical evidence exists to show that states with such laws have a lower incidence of automobile accidents caused by individuals with epilepsy. A logical result of such laws is that some persons with epileptic seizures will be less likely to seek medical attention or will be less honest with their physicians concerning the recurrence of seizures for fear of losing their driving privileges. Consequently, although in states without physician reporting regulations there may be persons with recurrent seizures driving automobiles because they fail to report themselves to authorities, in states with such laws there are persons with uncontrolled

epileptic seizures who are driving because they fail to seek adequate medical attention. This latter situation is the less acceptable of the two: an individual with recurrent epileptic seizures who fails to consult a physician or to admit to a physician that he or she has had recurrent seizures not only represents a hazard on the road but is denied appropriate medical intervention that might bring the seizures under control. A law that provides a negative incentive for persons to seek treatment for epilepsy is not in the best interests of the person with epilepsy or of society. Patients and physicians should advocate for voluntary reporting with appropriate liability protections and reversal of egregious mandatory reporting laws that breach the physician-patient relationship and constitute a disincentive for appropriate therapy.

It should be noted that a number of states do not provide immunity from liability to physicians who certify to their departments of motor vehicles that, in their good faith judgment, a patient's seizures are adequately controlled under state driving laws. This has led, for example, in Ohio and Michigan, to liability to third parties even when the physician complied with all state laws. The Epilepsy Foundation, the *American Epilepsy Society (AES)*, and the *American Academy of Neurology* have developed consensus statements on driving in the United States that recommend the adoption of physician immunity laws as reasonable advice to state medical advisory boards or departments of motor vehicles (Consensus statements, 1994). Most states have in place an exception to patient confidentiality laws that permits any physician who believes that a patient's driving poses a danger to others (e.g., if the physician knows the patient may drive against medical advice) to report the individual to the authorities without fear of violating patient confidentiality.

Ideally, physicians should advise their patients, based on the features of their seizure disorders, on whether it is safe for them to drive an automobile. Patients should bear the responsibility of reporting their condition to the appropriate authorities. Driving privileges should then be determined on a case-by-case basis according to the advice of the patient's physician and an appropriately experienced physicians' review board. Restricted or probationary driver's licenses should be made available to individuals whose seizure patterns would allow them to drive under certain conditions but not others. Periodic medical reports from the patient's physician should be required only until it is established that in all probability seizures will remain controlled. Departments of motor vehicles should have a medical advisory board that includes at least one neurologist familiar with epilepsy disorders in order to ensure that all factors are adequately and knowledgeably considered. Individuals should also be entitled to hearings, if requested, before licenses are revoked, except under certain emergent circumstances, and to judicial review if there are disagreements.

Participation in Sports

After driving, the next most frequently discussed restriction placed on persons with epilepsy concerns swimming (Austin et al., 2008). Drowning is an unusually common cause of death among those with epilepsy (Chapter 9), and persons with epileptic seizures of any type should be advised never to swim alone. This is the only absolute limitation placed on persons with epilepsy with regard to participation in sports. Although some physicians advise that contact sports should be avoided for fear that head injury might exacerbate an epileptic condition, there is inadequate evidence that this is ever the case (Livingston and Berman, 1973; Austin et al., 2008). The general philosophy today is to encourage the person with epilepsy to lead as active and vigorous a life as possible.

It is appropriate to foster an interest in sports, including those that present some risk of injury or even of provoking seizures (Masland, 1985; Austin et al., 2008). Although a few patients with epilepsy could occasionally experience seizures during participation in sports, less likely due to hyperventilation than to emotional excitement, the heightened attention required for involvement in competitive activities tends to have an antiseizure effect. More often, seizures occur during relaxation after the competition is over. People with epilepsy can become excellent athletes and even champions. Success in sports requires that other participants understand the epilepsy condition and that the person with epilepsy have sufficient self-confidence to overcome embarrassment or defeat due to an inopportune ictal event.

Cycling is a popular activity for children, but in many countries it is also an important means of transportation for the general public. There is no need to restrict cycling for people with epilepsy whose seizures are controlled as long as proper safety precautions are observed, which include use of a helmet and avoidance of busy highways when possible. When seizures are not controlled, supervised cycling away from heavy traffic and the use of three-wheeled bicycles can be considered in individual situations (Austin et al., 2008).

With the increasing interest in high-risk sports among young people, additional precautionary advice may be necessary. A person with epilepsy must recognize the inherent dangers of participating in such sports as skydiving and hang gliding. Scuba diving could present a particularly unacceptable risk for people with epilepsy. In some high-risk sports, such as rock or mountain climbing, where climbers are roped together, an epileptic seizure could also place the lives of others in jeopardy. However, there are people with epilepsy, even those with uncontrolled seizures, who can safely engage in rock and mountain climbing, so even in this arena, blanket rules are not appropriate. When persons with epilepsy attempt such sports, all participants must be made aware of their epilepsy condition.

Alcohol and Drugs

Patients commonly ask whether they can use alcohol and occasionally ask about other legal and illegal drugs. Some drugs, like *cocaine*, may be epileptogenic, while others, including *alcohol* and *tranquilizers*, are anticonvulsant but can induce seizures during withdrawal (Chapter 5). If a person with epilepsy has seizures that are under medical control, there is usually no contraindication to moderate use of alcohol or other pharmacological agents. Unusual susceptibility—for instance, to alcohol withdrawal—is relatively rare (Chapter 9), but when such a susceptibility is identified, it constitutes a reason for complete restriction. In all persons with epilepsy, binge drinking or frequent use of sedative drugs such as tranquilizers greatly increases the risk of seizures on withdrawal. Similarly, heavy use of stimulants such as coffee or potentially epileptogenic street drugs can make seizures more difficult to control, and use of cocaine, even once, can precipitate seizures. *Marijuana*, on the other hand, is reported to have antiseizure potential, and indeed epilepsy is an indication for the use of marijuana in states and countries where medical marijuana is legal (Chapter 16). Although, theoretically, withdrawal seizures might occur if marijuana is discontinued abruptly after heavy usage, there are no data to support this possibility.

In some persons with epilepsy a vicious cycle occurs when sedation due to antiseizure medication leads to an increase in coffee or other stimulant intake. When this produces breakthrough seizures, antiseizure medication is increased, sedation becomes worse, and the person consumes more coffee and highly caffeinated beverages. Occasionally, by greatly reducing coffee or other stimulant intake, seizures can be better controlled with tolerable levels of medication. On the other hand, use of alcohol and sedative drugs can exacerbate the sedation caused by antiseizure medication. Although it is not invariably dangerous to take alcohol or hypnotic drugs in moderation in addition to antiseizure medications that have sedative side effects, such combinations in excess are not recommended. Practitioners should be aware that chronic alcohol abuse and use of certain street drugs, such as narcotics, induce liver enzymes and can greatly enhance the metabolism of antiseizure drugs.

Specific Hazards

Life is filled with hidden dangers for the unwary, and risks posed by common situations such as crossing a street in heavy traffic, emptying a pot of boiling water, or even walking down a flight of stairs become much greater when an epileptic seizure could occur at any time without warning. Depending on the type of seizures, their frequency, and their pattern of occurrence, persons with epilepsy need to be alert to the possibility of certain hazards in their lives. In most cases this requires the simple use of common sense and good judgment. It is, for instance, safer for persons with recurrent epileptic seizures to shower rather than bathe. Occupations that require climbing into high places or continued concentration to operate heavy machinery, explosives, or other dangerous equipment should be undertaken only if adequate safety measures or accommodations are in place to prevent injury in the event of impaired consciousness or loss of motor control. If seizures have known precipitating factors or temporal patterns, these must be taken into account in planning activities of everyday life (Chapter 9).

Other potential hazards can be avoided if anticipated (Austin et al., 2008). For some persons with epilepsy, climbing a tree or leaning out an upstairs window could be taking an unnecessary chance. Learning the proper use of knives, other sharp objects, and firearms along with ordinary safety procedures at home and at work can avert serious consequences should a seizure occur at an inopportune moment. Common sense precautions in the home include shielding open fires and stoves, removing furniture with sharp edges, using unbreakable dishes and glasses, temperature control on hot water taps, doors that will not lock from the inside, and mattresses on the floor for individuals who fall out of bed (Austin et al., 2008). Smoking in bed as well as around other flammable material is hazardous for anyone, but particularly so for persons with epilepsy. Finally, some types of seizures by themselves present such risk for injury that continuous precautions are necessary. For instance, many patients with drop attacks must wear protective helmets, and patients who frequently lacerate their tongues and mouths during generalized tonic-clonic seizures may be fitted with special mouthpieces.

FAMILY

The Child with Epilepsy

The most important social consideration for the child with epilepsy is overprotection

(Austin et al., 2008; Rodenberg et al., 2011). Parents must realistically balance the need to protect their child from injury during a seizure against the need to allow the child to lead as normal a life as possible. It is often very difficult for a child to accept severe limitations on activities in the present because of something that *might* happen in the future. The dependence and self-doubt caused by growing up in an overly restricted environment can become more of a disability than the epileptic seizures themselves. Maintaining a healthy attitude on the part of the child is also important. On the one hand, children may learn to use their illness to manipulate their parents; on the other hand, adolescents not uncommonly become overly reckless or stop taking their medication in an effort to assert their independence or deny their illness. Nonconstructive personality traits can be largely avoided by proper parental attention to psychological and social development. The appropriate approach promotes every opportunity for the child to realize his or her full potential despite the occurrence of epileptic seizures.

When there are other children in the family, special attention to the child with epilepsy can cause sibling resentment and disrupt family structure. Disagreement between parents regarding how the child should be treated is a common cause of avoidable stress. One parent may be overprotective, and the other may choose to deny the problem. It is the physician's responsibility to uncover differences in parental attitudes and help the parents to develop a unified and effective approach, but more professional help is often necessary. Identification and involvement of a multidisciplinary support system including psychologists, social workers, and psychiatrists is valuable. Family counseling should be recommended. Parents should be encouraged to spend time with each other, away from the patient, to strengthen their relationship and thereby create a supportive family environment for the child with epilepsy. A supportive family is one of the most important factors determining good psychological and social rehabilitation when seizures are controlled (Crandall et al., 1987).

Although any seriously ill child creates difficult problems for parents, a child with epilepsy is unique for two reasons. First, the unexpected and paroxysmal nature of epileptic seizures tends to make parents more fearful that children will become injured, even if they have no interictal disability. Consequently, children with epilepsy may be prevented from enjoying life and developing their full potential when they are not sick for fear they might become sick. The opportunity to take advantage of substantial interictal capabilities should not be missed unnecessarily. Second, seizure occurrence is influenced by environmental factors. Inappropriate restrictions that create tension as well as family discord can exacerbate epileptic seizures and make them more difficult to control.

The Parent with Epilepsy

When a person with epilepsy reaches adulthood or when epileptic seizures begin in adulthood, the first question concerning family may be whether it is appropriate to become a parent (Austin et al., 2008; Rodenberg et al., 2011). For most patients, there are no genetic contraindications to having a family. In situations where an epilepsy condition results from a familial disorder (Chapter 5), genetic counseling can be recommended. Although the incidence of birth defects is slightly higher among children of a parent with epilepsy, and antiseizure drugs have some teratogenic effects, these relatively small risks are rarely a reason to decide against having children. Issues of pregnancy and breastfeeding are discussed in detail in Chapter 14. Prospective mothers with epileptic seizures occasionally are concerned that they might drop the baby or otherwise bring harm to the child during an epileptic seizure. They should be properly advised on all medical aspects of pregnancy, birth, and childrearing; on the real risks of having children with epilepsy; on the effects of antiseizure drugs; and on the problems with day-to-day care of a baby. Simple advice can take away the anxiety and reduce many of the risks of caring for infants. For instance, diapers can be changed on the floor, preventing the baby from getting hurt if the mother has a seizure. The baby can be sponged off while lying in its crib (De Boer, 2012). It is actually rather uncommon for a mother to injure a child during a seizure, but it does happen. Advice in this regard requires good judgment based on knowledge of habitual seizure type and frequency of seizure occurrence.

Small children, having none of the basic prejudices about epilepsy in the general population, are usually extremely sympathetic and supportive when a parent has epilepsy. As soon as they are old enough to understand, children should be told the full details of the parent's seizure disorder and be advised about what to do and what not to do when a seizure occurs. One great handicap that uncontrolled epileptic seizures create for a parent in modern society, particularly a mother, results from a loss of driving privileges that makes participation in carpools and other chauffeuring responsibilities impossible. Of course, indirect effects on the family from seizure-related loss of income from unemployment, failure to obtain insurance, and other problems with daily living can be much more serious.

SCHOOL

School is a safer, pleasanter, and more rewarding experience for the child with epilepsy when the teacher and other appropriate school officials fully understand the nature of the child's condition and how to deal with it (Seidenberg and Clemmons, 2008; Rodenberg et al., 2011). If the school itself has not provided adequate educational materials about epilepsy for its teachers and staff, brochures and DVDs are available at www.epilepsyfoundation.org and www.ibe-epilepsy.org. At minimum, the teacher should be familiar with the specific features of the child's seizure disorder; how to recognize a seizure if it occurs and what to do about it; what the child's medication regimen is; how the medication might affect school performance and classroom behavior; and what restrictions on activity are and are not necessary. It may be appropriate for the teacher, together with the child with epilepsy if possible, to discuss these issues with the class. In that event, care must be taken to ensure that the discussion is held in a manner that does not cause embarrassment to the child. Such a situation creates an excellent opportunity to educate children about epilepsy and to correct the negative misconceptions about epilepsy that are commonly held by the general public. A comic book is available from the Epilepsy Foundation for this purpose: *Spider-Man Battles the Myth Monster* (Marvel Comics).

Many children with epilepsy have problems that affect learning (Chapter 11). A physician should be aware of this possibility and refer children with epilepsy for neuropsychological testing when appropriate; special programs or counseling may help when specific learning disabilities or behavior disorders can be documented. Early identification of special needs and multidisciplinary intervention yield the best results (Seidenberg and Clemmons, 2008). Having epilepsy, however, does not automatically mean that a child will need or be entitled to special education services. United States federal law (Pub. L. No. 94-142) provides that only those children whose epilepsy adversely affects their educational performance are entitled to special education and related supportive services. To the maximum extent possible, schools must provide these services in a setting with nondisabled children. Parents who believe their children with epilepsy are not receiving appropriate special education services have the right to a due process hearing to challenge the school's educational decisions. Testimony by neurologists and other professional experts in epilepsy is often important at these hearings. In the United States, the *Rehabilitation Act of 1973*, as amended, and the *Americans with Disabilities Act (ADA) of 1990*, as amended, also give children a right to accommodations to enjoy equal opportunity to participate in school-related activities. It is not unusual for a child who does not require special education services to later require some accommodations to continue to participate in school. In addition to federal laws, some state laws provide children with epilepsy separate rights to receive special education. More information about the educational rights of children with epilepsy can be found at www.epilepsylegal.org.

EMPLOYMENT

Difficulty in finding and maintaining employment is a major cause of disability for persons with uncontrolled epileptic seizures and in some cases even for persons with epilepsy whose seizures are adequately controlled (Thorbecke and Fraser, 2008). The Rehabilitation Act of 1973 prevents federal agencies or employers that receive federal funds from refusing employment to otherwise qualified people solely on the basis of a medical condition unless that condition poses a clear threat to health or safety. Most states have similar laws to prohibit such job discrimination. Nevertheless, employers are often reluctant to hire individuals known to have epileptic seizures, for a variety of reasons: they may fear a lawsuit or insurance problems if the employee is injured during a seizure, they may be concerned about absenteeism or poor job performance if seizures occur frequently, or they may be sensitive to prejudices against epilepsy and fear that an employee with epilepsy could adversely affect their public image. Many people with epilepsy prefer not to tell prospective employers about their epilepsy conditions. On the other hand, there are definite advantages when an employer knows about an employee's epilepsy and can ensure a supportive attitude should an epileptic seizure occur on the job. Persons choosing to admit to epilepsy when seeking a job should answer any questions about disability that might appear on the employment form with "I will discuss this at the interview" rather than writing "epilepsy" directly on the form.

Educating employers about epilepsy in order to eliminate unreasonable concerns about hiring and retaining individuals with epileptic seizures is the ultimate answer to underemployment and unemployment among persons who have epilepsy. Physicians can aid their patients by taking advantage of opportunities to communicate with employers or prospective employers to provide information that could help the patient maintain a steady job. On the other hand, people with epilepsy should also be educated on how to disclose that they have epilepsy in an appropriate manner. Four issues should be kept in mind when disclosing:

- Limit the information to your own epilepsy and seizures.
- Provide the information in a positive way; do not scare the prospective employer.
- Describe the course of your seizures.
- Explain what assistance you may need (De Boer et al., 2007).

Employment for people with disabilities in the United States was greatly enhanced by the passage in 1990 of the ADA, which prohibits employers with 15 or more employees from discriminating on the basis of disability against individuals who can do the essential functions of a job or could do so with reasonable accommodations (Beran et al., 2008). The law requires that accommodations must be made if they would not be an undue hardship on the employer. Unfortunately, the US Supreme Court ruled several years later that the ADA does not apply to persons whose disabilities can be controlled by medication, even if the medication is ineffective, thus nullifying application of the ADA to people with epilepsy. Following the unfortunate experience of many people with epilepsy who were denied jobs due to epilepsy and who then went to court only to be told they were not disabled under the ADA, the law was amended in 2008 to make it clear that people with conditions like epilepsy are indeed covered by the ADA. The *ADA Amendments Act of 2008* placed the emphasis on discrimination rather than disability and ensured that the ADA covers people with disabilities like epilepsy and chronic seizures even if their condition is episodic, treated with medication, or not so severe as to make them unable to function.

Underemployment is particularly demoralizing for persons with epilepsy. Epileptic seizures have prevented many individuals from becoming adequately trained for work they could competently perform. Initial assessment and short-term rehabilitation; vocational training and retraining when needed; placement services; and services aimed at keeping people with epilepsy employed are crucial to addressing unemployment and underemployment of people with epilepsy (Thorbecke and Fraser, 2008). Vocational rehabilitation is often available through state or federal agencies. For help with specific employment problems, a person with epilepsy can be referred to vocational or occupational therapists, local volunteer agencies such as local Epilepsy Foundation affiliates, state vocational rehabilitation programs, or state and federal employment services. Detailed information is available at the Epilepsy Foundation's web site (www.epilepsyfoundation.org) or at www.epilepsylegal.org.

LEGAL RIGHTS

Legislation can be an important means of addressing the problems and challenges raised by having epilepsy. Well-crafted legislation based on internationally accepted human rights standards can prevent discrimination against people with epilepsy and violations of laws addressing their needs, promote and protect their human rights, enhance their autonomy and liberty, and improve equity in access to health care services and community integration (www.globalcampaignagainstepilepsy.org).

However, the reality is that epilepsy raises numerous legal concerns (Beran et al., 2008). For residents of the United States, the Epilepsy Foundation's *Jeanne A. Carpenter Epilepsy Legal Defense Fund* (www.epilepsyfoundation. org/resources/epilepsy/index.cfm) was created to end epilepsy-related discrimination and injustice through education and increased access to legal services for individuals with epilepsy and to advance the rights of people with epilepsy by changing discriminatory practices, policies, and laws. A brochure on legal rights and legal issues affecting people with epilepsy, as well as other useful legal information, is available on its web site. Legal issues relevant to other countries are addressed by the International Bureau for Epilepsy (www. ibe-epilepsy.org) and its national chapters. Until the 1980s some US states still had laws that placed unreasonable restrictions on the lives of persons with epilepsy by allowing their involuntary sterilization, prohibiting them from marrying, and allowing a child's epilepsy to be the basis for adoption annulment. Child custody and licenses to practice professions in some states can still be denied or revoked because of a disability, including epilepsy. Regulations on driver's licenses for persons with epilepsy have already been discussed.

In contrast to the few remaining United States federal and state laws that have a potentially negative impact on persons with epilepsy, most relevant federal and state laws today are aimed at reducing discrimination and increasing benefits and services. Consequently, laws that protect people with disabilities pertain to people with epilepsy, as do laws that provide for developmental disability benefits, vocational rehabilitation, federal financial benefits, and assigned-risk insurance programs. In all states, identification cards can be obtained by individuals who do not have driver's licenses. Of particular concern to persons with epilepsy are the laws that regulate arrest and search, because ictal and postictal behavior can be mistaken for disorderly conduct and are often mistaken for substance abuse. A number of states have adopted the *Uniform Duties to Disabled Persons Act* or similar legislation that requires an arresting officer to search for medical identification on persons found to be semiconscious or unconscious to determine whether they are suffering from the effects of an illness. Persons with epilepsy should carry their antiseizure medication in the original, labeled container or in a container with a copy of the prescription to avoid a mistaken charge of illegal possession of a drug. The Epilepsy Foundation also offers free training in seizure recognition and response for first responders such as emergency medicine technicians, paramedics, firefighters, and law enforcement personnel. More information is available at www. epilepsyfoundation.org/livingwithepilepsy/ firstresponders/index.cfm.

The use of epilepsy as a legal defense for criminal behavior is a controversial issue that has caused negative publicity for persons with epilepsy. Epileptic seizures do not take the form of premeditated, directed violent acts (Chapter 11), and the inappropriate but successful use of epilepsy in some courts as a defense for violent crimes creates a false image of persons with epilepsy as dangerous individuals. On the other hand, damage to property and even personal injury may inadvertently occur on rare occasions as a result of an epileptic seizure or, more likely, postictal confusion, and individuals should not be held accountable for their actions under these conditions (Chapters 9 and 11). The Epilepsy Foundation provides guidance on arrest for seizure-related behavior at www.epilepsyfoundation.org/resources/ epilepsy/legal/legal-fact-sheets.cfm.

INSURANCE

Inability to obtain adequate health, life, and automobile insurance causes major difficulties for persons with epilepsy. Antidiscrimination laws have done little to alleviate this problem, and insurance companies continue to treat those with epilepsy as a class rather than recognize differences among them in their potential for claims. Health insurance is a particular problem in the United States, which does not have a comprehensive national health system. Recent progress in health care legislation that will eliminate denial of insurance due to pre-existing conditions could eventually eliminate these challenges for people with epilepsy.

In the United States, federal health insurance (*Medicare*) and state health insurance (*Medicaid*) are available for some disabled persons with epilepsy, including all children, if they meet certain criteria, but these programs do not always provide adequate reimbursement for certain expensive, highly sophisticated diagnostic and therapeutic procedures. The patients most likely to require these medical services are usually without private insurance and therefore most likely to be on Medicaid or Medicare. Too often either they are denied essential diagnosis and treatment or hospitals lose money and refuse to develop new programs.

Persons with epilepsy in the United States who are unable to retain employment because of poorly controlled epilepsy but who are not found to be eligible for social security disability insurance or supplemental security income are at greatest disadvantage. They are ineligible for state or federal health insurance, do not obtain health insurance through employers, and are often rejected by private insurance agencies. Although health care reform should eventually guarantee eligible individuals the right to purchase health insurance, today many persons with disabilities, especially the marginally employed, simply cannot afford it. Thus many individuals who suffer from epilepsy cannot obtain the specialized medical services needed for their management. For some of them, as well as for society, this is a particular tragedy because appropriate medical or surgical intervention might result in complete seizure control and allow them to return to full employment. For this reason, people who continue to have seizures regularly despite medical treatment should apply for social security disability insurance, and if they are initially turned down, should appeal with the support of an expert in social security disability. Half of all disability determination denials are overturned on appeal.

Patients with epilepsy face similar problems obtaining life insurance, although simple plans are available. According to the Epilepsy Foundation, automobile insurance eligibility in the United States is based on accident record and not medical conditions, so this is not a common concern for people with epilepsy.

FINANCIAL AID

If epileptic seizures prevent an individual from performing "basic work activities," federal financial aid may be available in the United States through three programs: *Supplemental Security Income (SSI)*; *Retirement, Survivors, Disability, and Health Insurance (RSDHI)*; and *Veterans Benefits*. In some cases, persons with epilepsy who are unable to work are denied benefits because they fail to meet other requirements regarding type, frequency, duration, and sequelae of seizures. A more difficult problem arises when persons with epilepsy are not disabled by their seizures and can work but cannot obtain employment because of employer prejudices. At present, such individuals have little recourse. Veterans Benefits are available only if the seizure disorder originated during or was aggravated by active duty in the uniformed services. If an individual's disability is thus service-connected and he or she was other than dishonorably discharged, monthly compensation is granted according to the degree of disability.

Persons in the United States whose mental or physical impairments have substantially limited their ability to learn, communicate, live independently, and be self-supporting since before the age of 22 are entitled to state services funded in part by the federal government through the *Developmental Disability Assistance and Bill of Rights Act*. Although the original act specifically entitled individuals with epilepsy to benefits, the current wording no longer lists individual disorders, and some persons with epilepsy have had difficulty convincing authorities they meet the requirements for benefits.

RESOURCES

To ensure appropriate diagnosis and management of social problems experienced by persons with epilepsy, the responsible physician must be aware of available resources and make appropriate referrals. Hospitals and clinics can provide access to psychiatrists or psychologists, if necessary, as well as to a variety of counseling services, including specialized educational nurses and nurse clinicians, genetic counseling, family counseling, occupational therapy, and social workers. It is important, however, to find counselors who are familiar with epilepsy and the unique predicament this disorder creates. Local self-help groups provide excellent support for people with epilepsy and their families. Table 17–4 lists several organizations committed to service for persons with epilepsy.

The national chapters of the IBE provide crucial assistance to people with epilepsy in many countries. Its United States chapter, the Epilepsy Foundation, and the foundation's local affiliates aid patients and physicians in the identification of available resources, organize support groups, and distribute educational materials. In addition to its own pamphlets covering a wide variety of topics, the Epilepsy Foundation can provide lists of books and educational films on epilepsy, publishes a semimonthly magazine, *epilepsyUSA*, for lay readers, and puts out an *eNewsletter*. The foundation has been instrumental in developing not only the needed patient services mentioned previously but also self-help groups; counseling, recreational and educational programs; legal advocacy services; community education programs; and access to discount antiseizure drugs for members. It also supports research on epilepsy and provides funds for fellowships for medical students, physicians, and workers in the social sciences. Information about lay organizations in other countries dedicated to helping people with epilepsy and their locations can be obtained from the IBE, which coordinates international activities and publishes *International Epilepsy News*. Numerous other *nongovernmental organizations (NGOs)* in the United States are devoted to the support of research and care for people with epilepsy (Table 17–4), and an excellent web site for general information about epilepsy can be found at www.epilepsy.com.

The ILAE (see Table 17–4) is a professional organization committed to the exchange and dissemination of clinical and research information on epilepsy; the AES is its United States chapter. The AES holds annual meetings and promotes research and other professional activities. It also supports postdoctoral fellowship awards, but otherwise there is no overlap between the activities of this society and those of the Epilepsy Foundation. Letters requesting information about epilepsy directed to the AES are automatically forwarded to the Epilepsy Foundation. Chapters of the ILAE

Table 17–4 Important Organizations for Epilepsy

International

International Brain Research Organization (IBRO)
IBRO
255 rue Saint-Honoré
75001 Paris, France
+33 1 46 47 92 92 Telephone
+33 1 46 47 42 50 Fax
www.ibro.org

International Bureau for Epilepsy (IBE)
11 Priory Hall, Stillorgan, Blackrock
Co. Dublin, Ireland
+353 1 210 8850 Telephone
+353 1 210 8450 Fax
ibedublin@eircom.net
www.epilepsy.org

International League Against Epilepsy (ILAE)
324 North Main St.
West Hartford, CT 06117-2507
USA
860-586-7547 Telephone
860-586-7550 Fax
www.epilepsy.org

ILAE/IBE/WHO Global Campaign Against Epilepsy (GCAE)
P.O. Box 540
2130 AM Hoofdorp
The Netherlands
+31 23 55 88 411/412 Telephone
+31 23 55 88 409 Fax
www.globalcampaignagainstepilepsy.org

World Federation of Neurology (WFN)
Hill House
Heron Square
Richmond, Surrey TW9 IEP
UK
+44 208 439 9556/9557 Telephone
+44 208 439 9499 Fax
info@wfneurology.org
www.wfneurology.org

World Health Organization (WHO)
Neurological Disorders and Neuroscience
Avenue Appia 20
CH-1211 Geneva 27, Switzerland
+41 22 791 36 21 Telephone
+41 22 791 41 60 Fax
www.who.int/mental_health/management/globalepilpsycampaign/en/

United States

American Epilepsy Society (AES)
342 North Main St.
West Hartford, CT 06117-2507

(continued)

Table 17–4 Continued

860-586-7505 Telephone
860-586-7550 Fax
www.aesnet.org

Anita Kaufman Foundation
P.O. Box 11
New Milford, NJ 07646
201-655-0420
www.akfus.org

Centers for Disease Control and Prevention (CDC)
Atlanta, GA 30333
800-232-4636 Telephone
888-232-6348 TTY
www.cdc.gov

Citizens United for Research in Epilepsy (CURE)
223 W. Erie, Suite 2SW
Chicago, IL, 60654 |
(800) 765-7118 |
(312) 255-1801
www.cureepilepsy.org/home.asp

Danny Did Foundation
P.O. Box 46576
Chicago, IL 60646
800-278-6101
www.dannydid.org

Dravet Syndrome Epilepsy Action
IDEA League
P.O. Box 797
Deale, MD 20751
443-607-8267
dravet.org

Dup 15q Alliance
P.O. Box 674
Fayetteville, NY 13066
855-387-1572
www.idic15.org

Epilepsy Foundation (EF)
8301 Professional Pl.
Landover, MD 20785
800-332-1000 Telephone
301-577-2684 Fax
www.epilepsyfoundation.org

Epilepsy Therapy Project
www.epilepsy.com/epilepsy_therapy_project

Finding a Cure Against Epilepsy (FACES)
faces.med.nyu.edu
646-558-0900 Telephone
646-385-7163 Fax
FACESinfo@nyumc.org
223 E. 34th Street
New York, NY 10016

Health Resources and Services Administration
5600 Fishers Lane

(*continued*)

Table 17–4 Continued

Rockville, MD 20857
888-275-4772 Telephone
877-489-4772 TTY
www.hrsa.gov

Hemispherectomy Foundation
P.O. Box 1239
Aledo, TX 76008
hemifoundation.org

Hope for Hypothalamic Hamartomas
P.O. Box 721
Waddell, AZ 85355
www.hopeforhh.org

Intractable Childhood Epilepsy (ICE) Alliance
www.ice-epilepsy.org

Lennox-Gastaut Syndrome Foundation
192 Lexington Avenue
Suite 216
New York, NY 10016
718-374-3800 Telephone
www.lgsfoundation.org

My Epilepsy Story
myepilepsystory.org

National Association of Epilepsy Centers
5775 Wayzata Boulevard, Suite 200
Minneapolis, MN 55416
888-525-6232 Telephone
952-525-4526 Telephone
952-525-1560 Fax
www.naec-epilepsy.org

National Institute of Neurological Disorders and Stroke (NINDS)
P.O. Box 5801
Bethesda, MD 20824–800
301-496-5751 Telephone
301-468-5981 TTY
www.ninds.nih.gov

Patients Like Me
PatientsLikeMe Inc.
155 Second Street
Cambridge, MA 02141
www.patientslikeme.com

RE Children's Project
79 Christie Hill Road
Darien, CT 06820
rechildrens.com

Seizure Tracker
www.seizuretracker.com

Tuberous Sclerosis Alliance
801 Roeder Road, Suite 750
Silver Spring, MD 20910
301-562-9890 Telephone
800-225-6872 Telephone
301-562-9870 Fax
www.tsalliance.org/

exist in over 100 countries and can be found on the ILAE web site (www.ilae.epilepsy.org). The official journal of the ILAE is *Epilepsia*, published bimonthly, and the journal of the AES is *Epilepsy Currents*. Other professional journals dedicated to epilepsy include *Epilepsy Research*, the *Journal of Epilepsy*, *Epilepsy and Behavior*, *Epileptic Disorders*, and *Seizure*.

The Epilepsy Foundation and the AES have their own annual meetings, directed predominantly at the lay and professional communities, respectively. Similar annual meetings are held by lay and professional societies in many other countries. An international joint meeting of the ILAE and the IBE is held biennially, and regional meetings in the Latin American, European, Asian-Oceanic, Western Pacific, and African regions are held on alternate years. On alternate years, the AES meeting also serves as the North American ILAE regional meeting. Some of these meetings are held jointly between ILAE and IBE, and some are held separately.

The United States government sponsors research on epilepsy through grants and contracts awarded by the *National Institutes of Health (NIH)*. The institute responsible for identifying areas of research need and overseeing research support in epilepsy is the *National Institute of Neurological Diseases and Stroke (NINDS)*; however, other NIH institutes also fund epilepsy research, as do other federal

agencies such as the *Department of Defense (DOD)*, the *Centers for Disease Control (CDC)*, the *Agency for Healthcare Research and Quality (AHRQ)*, and the *Health Resources and Services Administration (HRSA)*. NINDS also carries out a drug-screening program for potential antiseizure compounds (Chapter 15) and serves as a general information source for professional activities relevant to epilepsy. *Epilepsy Abstracts*, a comprehensive bibliography of the world's literature on epilepsy initiated by NINDS and published through 1993, is an excellent source for papers published before Internet literature searches became generally available. The United States Institute of Medicine recently published a comprehensive assessment of the status of public health for people with epilepsy and recommended future efforts (IOM, 2012).

HEALTH CARE DISPARITIES

This textbook is aimed primarily at neurologists practicing in the industrialized world, where comprehensive epilepsy centers and adequate resources for diagnosis and treatment exist. Over 80% of people with epilepsy in the world, however, live in developing countries, where modern diagnostic and treatment approaches are unavailable (Fig. 17–1). Perhaps 90% of

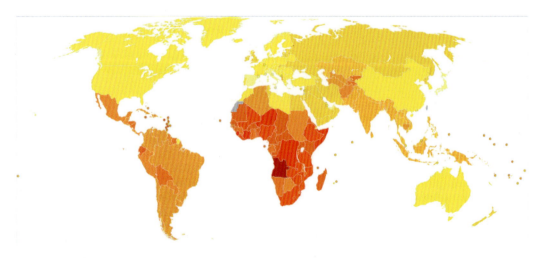

Figure 17–1. World map depicting disability-adjusted life years (DALYs), the number of life years lost due to disability or premature death, by country, as determined by the World Health Organization (2008). Scale ranges from less than 50 (yellow) to over 250 (magenta) per 100,000 inhabitants. (From Wikipedia, derived from data published by the World Health Organization, 2008, with permission.)

people with epilepsy in these areas receive no treatment at all. The global burden of disease is greatest in the developing world (Chapter 2). Not only does this treatment gap exist in developing countries (Meyer et al., 20010; Birbeck and Hesdorffer, 2011; Yemadje et al., 2011), but health care disparities also exist in industrialized countries (Griggs and Engel, 2005; Begley et al., 2011); in the United States epilepsy is a particular problem on Native American reservations (Parko and Thurman, 2009). The WHO, ILAE, and IBE have a major commitment through the GCAE to address problems of epilepsy in the developing world (Engel, 2003; De Boer et al., 2005). This is also part of the mission of the *World Federation of Neurology (WFN)*.

Work to reduce the treatment gap in countries with limited resources must be sustainable to be ethical; that is, it would not be appropriate to bring in drugs and specialists that would be present for a limited period of time and then leave. For this reason, the GCAE has undertaken a series of *demonstration projects* that determine the prevalence of epilepsy and the treatment gap in specific developing countries or regions of developing countries, then undertake steps to reduce this gap. These projects, in general terms, have four aspects:

1) *Educational and social intervention:* assessing whether *knowledge, attitudes,* and *practice (KAP)* of the population are adequate, correcting misinformation, and increasing awareness of epilepsy and how it can be treated
2) *Epidemiological assessment and case finding:* assessing the number of people with epilepsy and estimating how many of them are appropriately treated
3) *Service delivery and intervention:* ensuring that people with epilepsy are properly served by health personnel equipped for their task
4) *Outcome measurement:* analyzing the outcome and preparing recommendations for those who wish to apply the findings to the improvement of epilepsy care in their own country and other countries.

It is anticipated that education will greatly reduce the burden of epilepsy by dispelling negative beliefs about the condition that exist in many cultures of the developing world, but

it is also likely that efforts to provide affordable health care to people with epilepsy in countries with limited resources will lead to more cost-effective approaches to health care delivery for people with epilepsy in the industrialized world. The WHO has published the *Atlas of Epilepsy Care in the World* (WHO, 2005), showing resources available in almost all of the countries of the world, which clearly documents the health care disparities that need to be addressed. Regional reports and demonstration project descriptions are available from the GCAE (Table 17–5).

The WFN has published a textbook for neurologists practicing in countries with limited resources (Engel et al., 2005) that addresses issues related not only to delivery of care in settings with limited resources but also to tropical diseases, malnutrition, and cultural and social conditions that characterize practice in the developing world. This text is available in English and Spanish free of charge on the WFN web site (www.wfneurology.org). Western physicians practicing in developing countries must understand and respect the social and medical cultures of their patients to provide the most effective care, and the same applies to those practicing in the industrialized world who often

Table 17–5 Reports of the Global Campaign Against Epilepsy

Regional Reports on Epilepsy
   Epilepsy in the WHO African Region: Bridging the Gap
   Informe sobre la Epilepsia en Latino América
   Epilepsy in North America: A Report Prepared Under the Auspices of the Global Campaign Against Epilepsy, the International Bureau for Epilepsy, the International League Against Epilepsy, and the World Health Organization
   Epilepsy in the WHO Eastern Mediterranean Region: Bridging the Gap
   Epilepsy in the WHO European Region: Fostering Epilepsy Care
   Epilepsy in the WHO South-East Asian Region: Bridging the Gap
   Epilepsy in the Western Pacific Region: A Call to Attention and Action
Reports on Demonstration Projects
   Brazil
   China
   Georgia

Reports available from www.globalcampaignagainst epilepsy.org.

see patients from developing countries with unfamiliar cultures. Failure to consider the importance of these cultural influences can lead to tragic consequences, as described in excruciating detail by Anne Fadiman (1997) in her book *The Spirit Catches You and You Fall Down*. This book should be required reading for all physicians, particularly those who see patients with epilepsy in communities where the potential for cultural misunderstandings is high.

SUMMARY AND CONCLUSIONS

The psychosocial problems that arise because of an epilepsy condition constitute the patient's predicament. To deal with this aspect of management, a physician must take into account the family groups, social groups, school groups, and work groups to which the patient belongs. Education of family, friends, teachers, and coworkers is the most effective means of ensuring that the person with epilepsy has a safe and supportive environment. Education is the best way to overcome stigma and misconceptions that contribute heavily to reduced quality of life and disability for people with epilepsy. Destigmatizing epilepsy, however, does not require averting public attention from the seriousness of epilepsy. Referring to epilepsy as a disease rather than a disorder, for instance, should not be seen as stigmatizing and could help in the competition for limited health resources.

Some limitations on activities of daily living such as driving and bathing may be appropriate for avoiding injury or death during epileptic seizures, but these limitations should interfere as little as possible with the ability to enjoy a full and satisfying life. Driving restrictions represent a particular handicap for persons with epilepsy and should be a matter of best judgment between patient and physician. Although some epileptic seizures constitute a valid reason to withhold driving privileges, many people with epilepsy are not a hazard on the road. Laws that require physicians to report their patients with epilepsy result in unfair driving restrictions for some individuals, interfere with the doctor-patient relationship, and do not necessarily prevent accidents.

Epilepsy poses serious obstacles to finding or maintaining employment, obtaining adequate insurance coverage, and participating in a variety of necessary or desirable activities. Problems are more likely to be resolved when physicians know how to refer patients to proper counseling facilities, professional and community resources, and the relevant literature and web sites. This also requires an awareness of the legal rights of people with epilepsy, available financial aid, and services. The IBE and its members, including its United States member, the Epilepsy Foundation; the ILAE and its chapters, including its United States chapter, the AES; the WHO; the joint GCAE; and the WFN are dedicated to research on epilepsy and to providing necessary resources for people with epilepsy worldwide.

Ninety percent of the global burden of disease represented by epilepsy exists in the developing world, where most patients with epilepsy receive no treatment at all. Efforts by the ILAE, IBE, and WHO through the GCAE, as well as by the WFN, are addressing interventions aimed at sustainable reduction in treatment gaps in the developing world, including educational programs to eliminate damaging misconceptions about epilepsy. Significant health care delivery disparities as well as stigmatizing beliefs exist in the industrialized world as well. Consequently, work to improve cost-effective health care delivery and the quality of life for people with epilepsy in countries with limited resources undoubtedly will lead to more cost-effective approaches to health care delivery and improved quality of life for people with epilepsy in the industrialized world.

REFERENCES

Austin, JK, de Boer, HM, and Shafer, PO (2008). Disruptions in social functioning and services facilitating adjustment for the child and the adult. In Epilepsy: A Comprehensive Textbook, 2nd ed. Edited by J Engel, Jr, and TA Pedley. Philadelphia: Lippincott Williams & Wilkins, pp. 2237–2245.

Begley, C, Basu, R, Lairson, D, et al. (2011). Socioeconomic status, health care use, and outcomes: Persistence of disparities over time. Epilepsia 52:957–964.

Beran, RG, Devereux, J, McLin, W, et al. (2008). Legal concerns and effective advocacy strategies. In Epilepsy: A Comprehensive Textbook, 2nd ed. Edited by J Engel, Jr, and TA Pedley. Philadelphia: Lippincott Williams & Wilkins, pp. 2277–2282.

Birbeck, G, and Hesdorffer, D (2011). The geography of epilepsy: A fatal disease in resource-poor settings. Neurology 77:96–97.

Caveness, WF, and Gallup, GH, Jr (1980). A survey of public attitudes towards epilepsy in 1979 with an indication of trends over the past thirty years. Epilepsia 21:509–518.

Consensus statements, sample statutory provisions, and model regulations regarding drivers licensing and epilepsy. Epilepsia 35:696–705, 1994.

Crancer, A, Jr, and McMurray, L (1968). Accident and violation ratio of Washington's medically restricted drivers. JAMA 205:272–276.

Crandall, PH, Rausch, R, and Engel, J, Jr (1987). Preoperative indicators for optimal surgical outcome for temporal lobe epilepsy. In Methods of Pre-Surgical Evaluation of Epileptic Patients: Basics, Techniques, Implications. Edited by HG Wieser and CE Elger. Berlin: Springer-Verlag, pp. 325–334.

De Boer, H (in press). Epilepsy, social consequences. In Encyclopedia of Neurological Sciences. Edited by M Aminoff and R Daroff. Amsterdam: Elsevier.

De Boer, H, Engel, J, Jr, and Prilipko, L (2005). Global Campaign against Epilepsy. In Atlas of Epilepsy Care in the World. World Health Organization and World Federation of Neurology. Geneva: World Health Organization, pp. 82–83.

De Boer, HM, de Haa, GJ, and Mulder, OG (2007). Handboek Arbeid en Belastbaarheid. Houten: Bohn Stafleu van Loghum.

Devinsky, O, Vickrey, BG, Cramer, J, et al. (1995). Development of the Quality of Life in Epilepsy Inventory. Epilepsia 36:1089–1104.

Dodrill, CB, Beier, R, Kasparick, M, Tacke, I, Tacke, U, and Tan, S-Y (1984). Psychosocial problems in adults with epilepsy: Comparison of findings from four countries. Epilepsia 25:176–183.

Douglass, L (ed) (2011). Long-term outlook of Lennox-Gastaut syndrome and related epilepsies: Care for a lifetime. Epilepsia 52(suppl 5).

Engel, J, Jr (2003). Bringing epilepsy out of the shadows. Neurology 60:1412.

Engel, J, Jr (2010). Do we belittle epilepsy by calling it a disorder rather than a disease? Epilepsia 51:2363–2364.

Engel, J, Jr, Birbeck, G, Diop, AG, Jain, S, and Palmini, A: Epilepsy (2005). Global Issues for the Practicing Neurologist. World Federation of Neurology Seminars in Clinical Neurology. New York: Demos Press.

Fadiman, A (1997). The Spirit Catches You and You Fall Down. New York: Farrar, Straus and Giroux.

Gastaut, H, and Zifkin, G (1987). The risk of automobile accidents with seizures occurring while driving: Relation to seizure type. Neurology 37:1613–1616.

Gilliam, F, Carter, J, and Vahle, V (2004). Tolerability of antiseizure medications: Implications for health outcomes. Neurology 63:S9–S12.

Griggs, J, and Engel, J, Jr (2005). Epilepsy surgery and the racial divide. Neurology 64:8–9.

IOM (2012). Epilepsy across the Spectrum, Promoting Health and Understanding. Washington: The National Academic Press, pp. 237.

Jacoby, A, Snape, D, and Baker, G: Social aspects: Epilepsy stigma and quality of life. In Epilepsy (2008). A Comprehensive Textbook, 2nd ed. Edited by J Engel, Jr, and TA Pedley. Philadelphia: Lippincott Williams & Wilkins, pp. 2229–2236.

Kerson, TS, and Kerson, LA (2006). Implacable images: Why epileptiform events continue to be featured in film and television. Epileptic Disord 8:103–113.

Kerson, TS, Sewell-Roberts, C, and Kerson, LA (in press). Depictions of epilepsy on YouTube. Social Work in Health Care (in press).

Krumholz, A, Quigg, M, Krauss, G, Fisher, R, and Engel, J, Jr (2008). Assessing US commercial driving restrictions for people with seizures. American Epilepsy Society Abstract 1.107. Available at http://www.aesnet.org/

Livingston, S, and Berman, W (1973). Participation of epileptic persons in sports. JAMA 224:236–238.

Masland, RL (1985). Psychosocial aspects of epilepsy. In The Epilepsies. Edited by RJ Porter and PL Morselli. London: Butterworths, pp. 356–380.

Meyer, AC, Dua, T, Ma, J, Saxena, S, and Birbeck, G (2010). Global disparities in the epilepsy treatment gap: A systematic review. Bull World Health Organ 88:260–266.

Murray, CJL, and Lopez, AD (eds) (1994). Global Comparative Assessment in the Health Sector: Disease Burden, Expenditures, and Intervention Packages. Geneva: World Health Organization.

Parko, K, and Thurman, DJ (2009). Prevalence of epilepsy and seizures in the Navajo Nation 1998–2002. Epilepsia 50:2180–2185.

Rodenberg, R, Wagner, JL, Austin, JK, Kerr, M, and Dunn, DW (2011). Psychosocial issues for children with epilepsy. Epilepsy Behav 22:47–54.

Rubin, ZA, and Wiebe, S (2008). Issues in health outcomes assessment. In Epilepsy: A Comprehensive Textbook, 2nd ed. Edited by J Engel, Jr, and TA Pedley. Philadelphia: Lippincott Williams & Wilkins, pp. 2267–2273.

Seidenberg, M, and Clemmons, DC (2008). Maximizing school functioning and the school-to-work transition. In Epilepsy: A Comprehensive Textbook, 2nd ed. Edited by J Engel, Jr, and TA Pedley. Philadelphia: Lippincott Williams & Wilkins, pp. 2247–2252.

Sheth, SG, Krauss, G, Krumholz, A, and Li, G (2004). Mortality in epilepsy: Driving fatalities vs other causes of death in patients with epilepsy. Neurology 63:1002–1007.

Taylor, DC (1982). The components of sickness: Disease, illness and predicaments. In One Child. Edited by J Apley and C Ounsted. London: William Heinemann Medical Books, pp. 1–13.

Thorbecke, R, and Fraser, RT (2008). The range of needs and services in vocational rehabilitation. In Epilepsy: A Comprehensive Textbook, 2nd ed. Edited by J Engel, Jr, and TA Pedley. Philadelphia: Lippincott Williams & Wilkins, pp. 2253–2265.

Vickrey, BG, Hays, RD, Graber, J, et al. (1992). A health-related quality of life instrument for patients evaluated for epilepsy surgery. Med Care 30:299–319.

Weiss, MG, and Ramakrishna, J (2001). Interventions: Research on reducing stigma. Paper presented at US NIH Conference on Stigma and Global Health: Developing a Research Agenda, Bethesda, MD. Available at http://www.stigmaconference.nih.gov

World Health Organization: Atlas (2005). Epilepsy Care in the World. Geneva: World Health Organization.

World Health Organization (2008). The Global Burden Of Disease, 2004 Update. World Health Organization.

Yemadje, L-P, Houinato, D, Quet, F, Druet-Cabanac, M, and Preux, P-M (2011). Understanding the differences in prevalence of epilepsy in tropical regions. Epilepsia 52:1376–1381.

Index

Note: Page numbers followed by "*f*" and "*t*" refer to figures and tables, respectively.

AAN. *See* American Academy of Neurology
AANS. *See* American Association of Neurological
    Surgeons
Abdominal epilepsy, 210, 455
Ablative surgery, 615
Abnormal brain areas, 616, 616*t*
Abortive sensory stimulation, 634
Abortive stimuli, ictal initiation, 326
Abscess, 305, 347
Absence epilepsy
    CAE
        clinical description, 260–261, 261*t*
        differential diagnosis, 262
        epidemiology, 261
        etiology, 262
        prognosis, 262–263
        treatment, 262
    EEG, 480
    JAE, 263
        medication discontinuation, 522
Absences, 4–5
    atypical, 15
    generalized seizures, 15
    genetic absence epilepsies, 15
    myoclonic, 224–225
Absence seizures, 36
    atypical
        clinical considerations of, 224
        EEG of, 224, 224*f*
        mechanisms of, 222
        phenomenology of, 224
    typical
        clinical considerations, 222
        EEG, 222, 223*f*
        mechanisms, 220–221, 221*f*
        phenomenology, 221
Absence status, 333
Absence status epilepticus, 369
    clinical description of, 358–359
    confusion in, 359
    differential diagnosis of, 359
    etiology of, 359
    incidence of, 359
    prognosis of, 360
    treatment of, 359–360
Absolute refractory period, 60
Absorption, pharmacological, 495–496
Accidents, epileptic driver, 649, 650*t*
Acetaldehyde, 585
(R)-2-acetamido-M-benzyl-3-methocypropramide, 566
Acetaminophen, drug interactions, 568
Acetate, elimination, 499
Acetazolamide, 85, 520, 578–579
    drug interactions, 553

ketogenic diet and, 631
    levels, 330
    tolerance, 501
Acetic acid, 585
Acetylcholine, 65
Acetylcholinesterase, 65
    inhibitors, 72
Acid-base imbalance, 85, 170*t*, 454
Acidemia in early myoclonic encephalopathy, 245
Acidosis, 350
    conditions causing, 454
    lactic, 169, 335
    treatment, 352
Acquired causes of epilepsy disorders, 7, 169–182
    anoxia and trauma, 169, 171–172
    brain tumors as, 174, 174*t*
    cerebrovascular disorders, 172–173
    HS as, 177–182
    immune-mediated diseases as, 176–177
    infectious diseases as, 174–176
    inflammation-mediated diseases as, 176–177
    MCDs as, 177
    metabolic disturbances as, 177
    toxic disturbances as, 177
Acquired epilepsies, 138–139
    susceptibility, 144
Acquired genetic disturbances, 135–138, 138*f*
Acquired immunodeficiency syndrome (AIDS), 176
ACTH. *See* Adrenocorticotropic hormone
Action myoclonus, 225
    of acquired neurological disturbances, 236
    posthypoxic, 284
    with progressive myoclonus epilepsies, 326
    renal failure syndrome, 267
Action potentials, 58–59, 59*f*
Activities of daily living
    alcohol and drugs, 651–653
    driving, 648–651, 650*t*
    limitations, 662
    participation in sports, 651
    social management, 647–652
    specific hazards, 652
Acupressure, 633
Acupuncture, 633
Acute hemispheric disconnection syndrome, 392
Acute models. *See* Models
Acute seizures, in vitro studies of, 107–109
ADA. *See* Americans with Disabilities Act of 1990
ADD. *See* Antiepileptic Drug Development Program
ADEAF. *See* Autosomal dominant epilepsy with auditory
    features
Adenoma, sebaceous, 412, 412*f*
Adenosine, 66
    as neuromodulator, 90

Adenosine (*cont.*)
  in postictal refractory period, 120
Adenosine triphosphate (ATP), 57
ADHD. *See* Attention-deficit hyperactivity disorder
Adhesiveness of language, 381
ADNFLE. *See* Autosomal dominant nocturnal frontal
        lobe epilepsy
Adolescence, epilepsy syndromes of
  ADEAF as, 267
  epilepsy with generalized tonic-clonic seizures only, 265
  familial temporal lobe epilepsies as, 267–268
  JAE as, 263
  JME as, 263–265
  PME and, 265–267
Adrenocorticosteroids, 579–580
Adrenocorticotropic hormone (ACTH), 515, 516f, 577,
        579–580
  WS, 247
Adrenoleukodystrophy, 166
Adulthood, epilepsy syndromes of
  ADEAF as, 267
  epilepsy with GTS only, 265
  familial temporal lobe epilepsies as, 267–268
  JAE as, 263
  JME as, 263–265
  PME and, 265–267
Adversive focal seizures, 249
Adversive movement, 205
Adversive status epilepticus, 360
AES. *See* American Epilepsy Society
Affect, 382–383
Affective symptoms in partial seizure, 210
Afterdischarge
  definition of, 6
  in electrical stimulation, 100
  in kindling, 116
  thresholds, 307
Afterhyperpolarization (AHP), 63–64, 101, 103f
Age, pharmacological treatment and, 523–524
Age-adjusted prevalence, 49–50
Age at onset
  electroclinical syndromes by, 29t
  epilepsies by, 29t
  seizure history and, 408–409, 409t
Agency for Healthcare Research and Quality
        (AHRQ), 660
Age-related incidence, 162
Age-specific incidence
  benign epilepsy of childhood, 47
  rates, 45, 47–50, 47f, 48f
Aggressive behavior
  ictal, 465
  limbic dyscognitive seizures, 270
  postictal, 332
Aggressive personality trait, 381
Agranulocytosis, 514
AHP. *See* Afterhyperpolarization
AHRQ. *See* Agency for Healthcare Research and Quality
Aicardi's syndrome, 166
AIDS. *See* Acquired immunodeficiency syndrome
Ainu imu, 460
Airway obstruction, 217
Akinetic mutism, TIAs and, 456
Alcohol use, 651–653
  blackouts in, 454
Alcohol withdrawal, 6, 528–529

delirium tremens in, 454
  as epilepsy cause, 161
  seizures, 100
  seizures, differential diagnosis, 467–468
Alexander the Great, as epileptic, 43
Alfred the Great, as epileptic, 43
Alkalosis, neuron excitability and, 85
Allergic reactions to food, seizure threshold and, 632
Allopathic medicine, 635–636
Allylglycine, 66
Alopecia, 515
Alpha harmonics, 469, 470f
Alpha rhythm, 86
Alprenolol, drug interactions, 548
Alternating hemiplegia in childhood, 460–461
Alternative therapy, 530
Ambulatory automatisms, 211
Ambulatory recording
  EEG, 530–531
  PNES, 463
  VEM, 423
Amenhotep, as epileptic, 43
American Academy of Neurology (AAN), 606, 650
American Association of Neurological Surgeons
        (AANS), 606
American Epilepsy Society (AES), 606, 650, 658, 658t
Americans with Disabilities Act (ADA) of 1990
  Amendments Act of 2008, 655
  employment and, 655
  school and, 654
Amino acids, 631
  disorders, 166
  receptors, excitatory, 68
(S)-3-(Aminomethyl)-5-methylhexanoic acid, 571
1-Aminomethyl-cyclohexyl-acetic acid, 565
Aminophylline, 66
Amitriptyline, drug interactions, 575
Ammon's horn, 74–78, 75f
Amnesia
  alcoholic blackout, 454
  anterograde, 212, 270
  for ictal event, 203
  in migraines, 456
  postictal, 209, 376, 408
  posttraumatic, 304
  retrograde, 270
  transient global, 456
Amobarbital
  drug interactions, TPM, 575
  EEG, 422
  IAP, 271, 439–440, 604, 621
AMT. *See* α-methyl-tryptophan
Amygdala
  complex, 79–80
  dopamine, 119
  rhythmic stimulation of, 80–81
Amygdala-kindled model, 592
Amygdalotomy, 615
Amyloidosis, 451–452
Analgesics, drug interactions, 556
Anatomical substrates, 194–197, 195t, 197f
Anemia, 514
Anger, 381–382
Angiographic stains, 432
Angiomas
  cavernous, 173, 173f, 608

venous, 608
Animal models, 99–100
  of chronic epilepsy, 298
  of epilepsies, 298
  MES, 591–592
  PTE, 298
  PTZ, 591–592
  research, 143
  rodent, 592, 593*t*
    MES, 591–592
    PTZ, 591–592
  TBI, 298
Animals, epilepsy in, 120–121
Anosmia, 210
Anosognosia, TIAs and, 456
Anoxia, epilepsy and, 169, 171–172
Antacids, 565
Antasabbu, 34
Anterior commissure, 614
Anterior hypothalamus, 326–327
Anteromesial temporal resection, 612, 612*f*
Antiabsence drugs, 5, 10
Anticonvulsant drugs, 5, 10. *See also* Antiepileptic drugs
Anticonvulsant Screening Project (ASP), 591
Antidepressants, 183, 465. *See also* Tricyclic
      antidepressants
Antidromic excitation of neuron, 73
Antiepilepsy treatments, 10. *See also specific treatments*
Antiepileptic Drug Development (ADD) Program,
      590, 596
Antiepileptic drugs, 5, 10, 31, 541–597, 544*t*. *See also
      specific drugs*
  administration, 503, 504*t*
  adverse effects of, 508, 511–512*t*
    behavioral, 389–390, 389*t*
  available, 596
  chronic epilepsy, 305
  clearance, 499
  dyskinesias related to, 515
  elimination, 499
  first-line drugs, 596
  folic acid and, 526
  generalized convulsive status epilepticus, 353–354
  generic preparations, 530
  hematological disorders related to, 514
  history, 409
  under investigation, 594–596
  metabolism, 499
  nervous system effects of, 515
  new-drug development, 590–594
    clinical evaluation of, 592–594
    identification of new compounds and, 591
    preclinical evaluation and, 591–592
  newer drugs
    ESL, 561–562
    EZG, 562–563
    FBM, 563–565
    GBP, 565–566
    LCM, 566–567
    LEV, 569–570
    LTG, 567–569
    OXC, 570–571
    PGN, 571–572
    RUF, 572–573
    TGB, 573–574
    TPM, 574–576
    VGB, 576–577
    ZON, 577–578
  nonepilepsy uses for, 520, 521*t*
  nursing and, 527
  pharmacological interactions, 508, 509*t*
  positive psychotropic effects, 390, 390*t*
  psychotropic effects of, 390, 391*t*
  recognizing potential, 591
  SANAD, 519
  SAR, 542, 591
  second and third-generation, 542, 543*f*
  special and rarely used
    acetazolamide, 578–579
    ACTH, 579–580
    adrenocorticosteroids, 579–580
    barbiturates, 580
    benzodiazepines, 580–582
    bromides, 582
    hydantoins, 582–584
    oxazolidinediones, 584–585
    paraldehyde, 585–586
    phenacemide, 586
    piracetam, 586–587
    progabide, 587
    propofol, 587–588
    stiripentol, 588
    succinimides, 588–589
    sulthiame, 589–590
  spectra of action, 198–199
  standard older
    benzodiazepines, 554–557
    CBZ, 557–559
    ESM, 553–554
    PB, 543–549
    PHT, 550–552
    PRM, 552–553
    VPA, 559–561
  tolerance, 501
  trade names, common abbreviations, and conversion
      factors, 657*t*
Antiepileptogenesis
  complete, 297
  definition, 13
  partial, 297
  terminology, 13–14, 297*t*
Antihistaminics, drug interactions, 556
Antipsychotics, 183
Antipyrine drug interactions, 548
Antiretroviral agents, comorbidity and, 527
Antiseizure drugs. *See also* Antiepileptic drugs
Anxiety, 383–384
  postictal, 377
  prodromal behavioral changes and, 376
Anxiety disorder, 375
Apasmara, 34
Aphasia
  expressive, 212
  in LKS, 260
  in postictal period, 377
Aphasic features, 210, 216*t*
Aphasic seizures, 205
Aphasic status epilepticus, 360
Aplastic anemia, 514
Apnea
  in epileptic seizures, 217
  sleep, 328, 457

Apnea (*cont.*)
   in stiff baby syndrome, 460
   in tonic seizures, 227
Apraxia, acute hemispheric disconnection
      syndrome and, 392
Area tempestas, 105
Arene oxide intermediates, 550, 583
Aretaeus, on epilepsy, 33
Arrest reaction, 209, 307
Arrhythmia, cardiac, 355
   SUD, 336
   syncope caused by, 450
Ashepak, 34
Ash leaf spots, 412
ASP. *See* Anticonvulsant Screening Project
Asterixis, 454
   TIAs and, 456
Asymmetrical dystonic posturing in tonic motor
      seizures, 205
Asystole, 450
Ataxias, episodic, 461
Atazanavir, comorbidity and, 527
Athetosis, 459
Atonic seizures, 4
   generalized
      clinical considerations of, 228
      EEG of, 228, 231*f*
      mechanisms of, 228
      phenomenology of, 228
   myoclonic, 226
ATP. *See* Adenosine triphosphate
Atrial tachycardia, 450
Attention-deficit hyperactivity disorder (ADHD),
      384, 395–396
Attitudes towards epilepsy, 34, 645, 645*t*
Auditory features
   ADEAF, 267
   lateral temporal lobe epilepsy with, 57
Auditory symptoms, 206. *See also* Sensory symptoms
Aura continua, 360
Auras, 9, 203
   fear, 382
   MTLE with HS, 270
   seizure history and, 407
Autism spectrum disorders, 386–387
Automatisms
   limbic seizures and, 209–211
   reactive, 408
Automobile insurance. *See* Driving
Autonomic seizures, diencephalic, 461
Autonomic status epilepticus, 360
Autonomic symptoms
   of limbic seizures, 210
   psychiatric disturbances distinguished
      from, 466
   simple partial seizure, 15
Autosomal dominant epilepsy with auditory features
      (ADEAF), 267
Autosomal dominant nocturnal frontal lobe epilepsy
      (ADNFLE), 253–254, 327, 459
Avoidance, 634
Axillary freckling, 412, 412*f*
Axon, 63*f*
   hillock, 62–64, 100
   terminal, 64–65

Babylonian Law of Hamurabbi, 34
Balthazar, as patron of epilepsy, 42
Baltic myoclonus, 266
Barbiturates, 543
   adverse behavioral effects of, 389–390
   adverse side effects, dose-dependent, 513
   drug interactions, CLN, 556
   EEG, 421–422
   EEG discharges and, 485
   metharbital, 580
   methylphenobarbital, 580
   nursing and, 527
   physical dependence, 501
   pregnancy and, 527
   secondary epileptogenesis, 311
   teratogenic effects of, 526
   withdrawal, 507
Basal electrodes, 418, 419*t*
   and normal phenomena, 471, 472*f*, 477*f*
Basal forebrain nuclei, 81
Basic mechanisms of epilepsy, 99–144
   experimental models and, 100–122
   molecular genetic investigations and, 135–138
   possible mechanisms of human epileptic phenomena,
      138–143
   studies of human epilepsy, 122–135
Basic rest activity cycle (BRAC), 327–328, 329*f*
Basilar artery migraine, 456
Basilar dendrites of neuron, 62
Basket cells of hippocampus, 75
β-Carboline, 555
Bear-Fedio Personality Inventory, 381–382
BECTS. *See* Benign epilepsy with centrotemporal spikes
Beethoven, Ludwig van, as epileptic, 44
Behavioral disturbances
   antiseizure drug, 389–390, 389*t*
   chronic, 374–396
   diagnostic issues, 395
   ictal, 376–378
   interictal, mechanisms of, 387–395
      effects of treatment on, 389–392, 389*t*
      epilepsy-induced neurobiological factors and,
         392–396, 394*f*
      neuropathological factors in, 388–389
      psychosocial factors in, 387–388
   periictal, 376–378
   phenomenology of, 376–387, 377*t*
      ADHD and, 384
      affect and, 382–383
      anxiety and, 383–384
      autism spectrum disorders and, 386–387
      cognitive function and, 380
      intellectual function and, 380
      mood and, 382–383
      neurological function and, 380
      neuropsychiatric disorders in epilepsy, classification
         of, 385–386, 386*t*
      personality and, 380–382
      psychosis and, 384–385
      psychosocial adaptation and, 378–380
   prodromal, 376
   surgery-associated, 391–392
   treatment issues, 395
Behavioral features of epileptic seizures, 4
Behavioral modification, 530

Behavioral therapies, 636
  abortive sensory stimulation, 634
  EEG biofeedback, 634–635
  psychological treatments, 635
  treatment of reflex epilepsies, 633–634
Bel uri, 34
Bemegride, EEG, 421
Benign epilepsy of childhood, 13
  age-specific incidence and, 47
Benign epilepsy of childhood with centrotemporal spikes,
      165
  EEG, 480
  resolution of, 522
  sulthiame for, 590
Benign epilepsy with centrotemporal spikes (BECTS)
  clinical description, 251–252, 253f
  differential diagnosis, 252
  epidemiology, 252
  etiology, 252
  prognosis, 252
  treatment, 252
Benign epileptiform transients of sleep (BETS), 471
Benign essential myoclonus, 236, 284
Benign familial infantile epilepsy (BFIE), 249
Benign familial neonatal epilepsy (BFNE), 244–245
Benign focal epilepsy of childhood, 417
Benign idiopathic neonatal seizures, 278
Benign infantile epilepsy (BIE), 249
Benign infantile spasms, 247
Benign myoclonus of early infancy, 247. *See also*
      Myoclonus
Benign neonatal familial convulsions, 24t
Benign neonatal seizures (BNS), 278
Benign paroxysmal vertigo, 461
Bennu, 34
1,2-Benzisoxazole-3-methanesulfonamide, 577
Benzodiazepines, 460
  adverse side effects
    behavioral, 389, 389t
    dose-dependent, 513
  alcohol and sedative drug withdrawal, 528–529
  BECTS, 253
  CLB, 557
  CLN, 555–556
  clorazepate, 580–581
  comorbidity and, 527
  discontinuation, 523
  DS, 249
  DZP, 555
  EEG discharges and, 485
  EMA, 255
  epileptic seizure types and, 199
  FS, 280
  intermittent explosive disorders, 465
  LGS, 259
  LZP, 556–557
  MEI, 249
  midazolam, 581
  monitoring, 518
  nitrazepam, 581–582
  nursing and, 527
  physical dependence, 501
  positive psychotropic effects, 390, 390t
  pregnancy and, 527
  receptors, 555

subtle status epilepticus, 366
tolerance, 501
trials, 519
withdrawal, 507
Benzoylamino-benzopyran, 595
Berger, Hans, 40, 41f
Beta harmonics, 469
BETS. *See* Benign epileptiform transients of sleep
BFIE. *See* Benign familial infantile epilepsy
BFNE. *See* Benign familial neonatal epilepsy
Bible, epilepsy references in, 41–42
Bicêtre Hospital, Paris, 36
Bicuculline, 90
  effects of GABA and, 71
BIE. *See* Benign infantile epilepsy
Bioavailability, 494–495, 496f
Biofeedback, EEG, 634–635
Biomarkers
  chronic epilepsy, 306, 306t
  diagnostic evaluation, 440–441
  of epileptogenesis, 314–315
  new drug, 594
  risk factors compared with, 440
Biotransformation, 499
Bipolar neuron, 62
Birth defects, 533
Bishydroxycoumarin, drug interactions, 548
Blackouts, alcoholic, 454
Blindness, 206
  in epilepsia partialis continua, 363
  in photosensitive seizures, 323
Blinking
  with absences, 255
  unilateral, 211
Blood, human, as ancient treatment, 35
Blood-brain barrier
  GBP and, 565
  immune responses and, 176
  permeability, 435
Blood glucose, 347–350
Blood oxygen level-dependent (BOLD), 133, 435
Blood pressure
  during seizure, 217, 334–335
  in status epilepticus, 347
Blood volume
  intravascular, 347
  SPECT and, 453
Blue Guide (Le Guide Bleu), 18
BNS. *See* Benign neonatal seizures
BOLD. *See* Blood oxygen level-dependent
Bone disorders, vitamin D deficiency and, 515
Bone marrow suppression, 514
Bouchet, on epilepsy, 36
BRAC. *See* Basic rest activity cycle
Brain
  areas, abnormal, 616, 616t
  hemispheres, epileptic seizures and, 5
  immature
    epileptic susceptibility of, 312, 314
    treatment and, 313–314
  neonatal, 312
  surgery, PTE after, 306
  TBI, 112, 171–172
    animal models, 298
  tumors, 174, 174t

Brain damage
  caused by epilepsy, 143
  diffuse, 203
  epileptic, 368–369
  in LGS, 256
  secondary, 177
  structural, 9
Brain development, 90–91
  epileptic seizures and, 312–314
    migration of interictal EEG spike in, 313
    practical considerations for, 313–314
  models of, 113–115
Brain-mapping, 424
Brain scanning, rectilinear radionuclide, 438–439
Brain stem, excitability and, 81
Bravais, L.-F., on epilepsy, 36
Breast milk, antiseizure drugs in, 527
Breath holding
  cyanotic form, 452–453
  differential diagnosis, 452–453, 453t
Brief epileptic seizure, 6
Bright, R., on epilepsy, 36
Brittanicus, as epileptic, 44
Brivaracetam, 594–595
Brodmann, map of, 78
Bromides, 582
  adverse behavioral effects of, 389t
  comorbidity and, 528
Bromism, 582
The Brothers Karamzov (Dostoyevsky), 646
Bruxism, 458
Buddha, as epileptic, 42
Burden of normality, 379–380
Burmese jauns, 460
Byron, Lord, as epileptic, 44

Cl⁻ channels, 59–60, 70, 70f
  causes of human epilepsy, 157–159
  complex, 90
  GABA and, 71
Ca²⁺ currents, 63–64
Cable telemetry, 423
Ca⁺ channels, 58, 59f
CAE. See Childhood absence epilepsy
Café au lait spots, 412, 412f
Calcium-binding proteins, 137
Calcium channel blockers, 461
Calcium gluconate, 283
Caligula, as epileptic, 43
Calmeil, L. F., on epilepsy, 36
Calmodulin, 64
CAM. See Complementary and alternative medicine
cAMP, 65, 68
Camphor, 454–455
Cannabis, 330, 632
Capote, Truman, as epileptic, 44
Carbachol, 105, 118
Carbamazepine (CBZ), 246, 542, 557–559
  administration, 559
  ADNFLE, 254
  adverse behavioral effects of, 389–390, 389t
  adverse side effects, 516, 558
    dose-dependent, 513
  BECTS, 252
  choosing appropriate drug and, 518–520
  chronic epilepsy, 305

  comorbidity and, 527
  drug combinations, 519
  drug efficacy, 508
  drug interactions, 548, 559
    ESL, 562
    EZG, 563
    FBM, 564
    LEV, 569
    LTG, 568
    OXC, 571
    PHT, 551
    PRM, 553
    RUF, 573
    TGB, 574
    VPA, 561
    ZON, 578
  DS, 249
  dyskinesias related to, 515
  elimination, 499
  EMA aggravated by, 255
  EMAS exacerbated by, 251
  epileptic seizure types and, 199
  hematological disorders related to, 514
  indications, 559
  intermittent explosive disorders, 465
  JME exacerbated by, 265
  LGS, 259
  mechanisms of action, 558
  MEI, 249
  monitoring, 517
  MTLE, 275
  pharmacokinetics, 558
  pharmacoresistance and, 609
  physical dependence, 501
  positive psychotropic effects, 390, 390t
  PS, 251
  psychotropic effects of, 390, 391t
  sensory disorders, 461
  simple reflex seizures, 326
  toxicity, 558
  trials, 519
5-Carbamoyl-5H-dibenz[b,f]azepine, 557
Carbohydrate metabolism disorders, 167
Carbonic anhydrase, 85
  enzyme, 575
  inhibitors, 62, 515
Cardiac arrest, 284
Cardiac causes of syncope, 450–451
Cardiac glycosides, 61
Cardiorespiratory arrest, 251
Cardiovascular disease, 412
Carotid sinus, 450
Castration, as early treatment, 35
Catamenial epilepsy, 86, 557
  seizure susceptibility and, 327
  seizure threshold and, 162
Catamenial exacerbation of epileptic seizures, 519
Cataplexy, 457
Catastrophic epilepsies, 28
Catecholamines, 72, 394
Caudate kindling, 118
Caudate nucleus, 80
Causes of human epilepsy, 157–186
  genetic investigations, 185
  multifactorial approach to understanding, 157
  nonspecific predisposing factors, 157–162

dynamic aspects of threshold and, 162
environmental factors as, 161–162
genetic factors as, 159–161, 159f
precipitating factors, 157, 182–185
Rochester study, 169, 171t
specific epileptogenic disturbances, 157–159
acquired causes of epilepsy disorders as, 169–182
genetic causes of epilepsy as, 163–169
Cauterization, as early treatment, 35
Cavernous angiomas, 173, 173f, 608
Cazauvieilh, on epilepsy, 36
CBZ. *See* Carbamazepine
[11]C-carfentanil, 434
Cecil Textbook of Medicine, 33
Centers for Disease Control (CDC), 660
Centrencephalic source of epileptic seizure, 5
Centrotemporal spikes
BECTS
clinical description, 251–252, 253f
differential diagnosis, 252
epidemiology, 252
etiology, 252
prognosis, 252
treatment, 252
benign epilepsy of childhood with, 165, 480, 522, 590
EEG, 480
resolution of, 522
sulthiame for, 590
childhood epilepsy with, 327
Cerebellar degeneration, 515
Cerebellar fits, 461
Cerebellar stimulation, 82
Cerebellum
degeneration, 515
excitability and, 82
Cerebral cortex
abnormalities, 5
congenital malformations, 169
developmental stages of, 84f
EEG activity, 86
epileptic seizure type diagnosis and, 194
lesions in, 166
Cerebral edema, 347
Cerebral malaria, 279
Cerebral palsy, 45
BECTS differential diagnosis and, 252
as epilepsy risk factor, 161, 388
lesions and, 417
Cerebral structures
abnormalities, 185
genetic factors and, 161
Cerebrospinal fluid (CSF), 361
Cerebrovascular autoregulation, 344–347
Cerebrovascular disorders
differential diagnosis, 455–457
epilepsy caused by, 172–173
Ceroid lipofuscinoses
late infantile, 482
neuronal, 266
C-fos gene, 61–62
cGMP. *See* Cyclic guanosine 3,5-monophosphate
Channels
cl[-], 59–60, 70, 70f
complex, 90
GABA and, 71
ca[+], 58, 59f
HCN, 57
ligand-gated, 56
VGKC, 57
voltage-gated, 56–57, 57t
Chaos theory, 321
Charcot, Jean-Martin, 39, 40f
Charge gradient of ion channel, 57
Charles of Austria, Archduke, as epileptic, 43
Charles V of Spain, as epileptic, 43
Chemical names of drugs and metabolites. *See specific drugs and metabolites*
Chemical synapses, 64–72, 65f
Cherry-red spot, 412f
myoclonus, 266
Chewing, 210. *See also* Automatisms
Child care, by epileptic parents, 653–654
Childhood
alternating hemiplegia in, 460–461
benign epilepsy of, 13
age-specific incidence and, 47
benign epilepsy of childhood with centrotemporal spikes, 13, 165
EEG, 480
resolution of, 522
sulthiame for, 590
benign focal epilepsy of, 417
epilepsy syndromes of
ADNFLE as, 253–254
BECTS as, 251–252
CAE as, 260–263
CSWS as, 259–260
EMA as, 254–255
EMAS as, 251
FS+, 250
late childhood occipital epilepsy (Gastaut type) as, 254
LGS as, 255–259
LKS as, 260
PS as, 250–251
Childhood absence epilepsy (CAE)
clinical description, 260–261, 261t
differential diagnosis, 262
epidemiology, 261
etiology, 262
prognosis, 262–263
treatment, 262
Childhood epilepsy with centrotemporal spikes, 327
Children
adverse side effects in, 514
with epilepsy
overprotection of, 652–653
in school, 654
social management of, 652–653
epileptic seizures in, 300, 300t
pharmacological treatment and, 523–524
seizures in, 7–8
surgical treatment for, 618
Chinaberry juice, as treatment, 632
Chinese herbal compounds, 632
Chiropractic, 636
Chloral hydrate in EEG study, 421
Chloramphenicol, drug interactions, 551
Chlordiazepoxide, alcohol and sedative drug withdrawal, 529
Chloride, 89
channels, 88

Chloride (*cont.*)
    ferric, 109
7-Chloro-1-methyl-5-phenyl-1,5-benzodiazepine-2,
        4-dione, 557
7-Chloro-2,3-dihydro-2-oxo-5-phenyl-1H-1,4-
        benzodiazepine-3-carboxylic acid, 581
7-Chloro-5-(o-chlorophenyl)-1,3-dihydro-3-hydroxy-
        2H-1,4-benzodiazepine-2-one, 556
5-(2-Chlorophenyl)-1,3-dihydro-7-nitro-2H1,
        4-benzodiazepine-2-one, 556
4-([[(4-Chlorophenyl)][(1E)-3-fluoro-6-oxocyclohexa-2,
        4-dien-1-ylidene]methyl]amino)butanamide, 587
Chlorpromazine, ictogenic potential, 161
Chorea, 459
Chromosome disorders, 168
Chronic epilepsy
    animal models, 298
    antiseizure drugs, 305
    biomarkers, 306, 306*t*
    development, 297
    differential diagnosis, 468
    neonatal seizures and incidence, 283, 283*t*
    prophylaxis for, 305–307
    in vitro studies of, 121–122
Chronic hyperventilation syndrome, 453
Chronic models. *See* Models
Chronic recurrent seizures, 358
Chronobiology, 326–329
Cimetidine, drug interactions, 551
Circadian rhythms, 326
    fluctuations, 328
Classification of the Epilepsies and Epileptic
        Syndromes, 244
Classifications, 14–32. *See also specific classifications*
    biologically based, 30
    diagnosis and, 30–31
    of epilepsy, 3, 14, 31
        etiological, 28, 30*t*
        ICD, 18, 19*t*, 20*t*
        1985 International, 18–25, 24*t*
        1989 International, 18–25, 24*t*
        older, 17–25
        proposed diagnostic scheme and, 26, 27*t*
        WHO, 18
    of epilepsy syndromes, 28, 29*t*, 31, 285
        1985 International, 18–25, 24*t*
        1989 International, 18–25, 24*t*
    of epileptic seizures, 3, 14–16
        proposed diagnostic scheme and, 26, 27*t*
    etiological, of epilepsies, 28, 30*t*
    international, 3
        epileptic seizures, 15–16, 16*t*
        revising, 25–28
    older, 3
        of epilepsies, 17–25
        of epileptic seizures, 14–17
    practical considerations, 3, 30–31
    precise, 32
    seizure, 16–17, 28, 28*t*
CLB. *See* Clobazam
Clear consciousness, 16
Clinical laboratory tests, 415, 416*t*
Clinical research on epilepsy, 36
Clinical seizures, 407–408
Clinical studies
    current drugs under investigation, 594–596

new-drug development, 592–594
    Phase I, 592
    Phase II, 592
    Phase III, 592
        brivaracetam trails in, 594–595
        ganaxolone trials in, 595
        perampanel trials in, 595
CLN. *See* Clonazepam
Clobazam (CLB), 555
    elimination, 499
    EMAS, 251
    monitoring, 517
    simple reflex seizures, 326
    trials, 519
Clomiphene, 629
Clomipramine, ictogenic potential, 161
Clonazepam (CLN), 555
    ADNFLE, 459
    drug interactions, 548, 556
        VPA, 561
    LGS, 259
    monitoring, 517
    myoclonus, 237
    reflex epilepsies due to structural lesions, 324
Clonic motor seizures, 205
Clonic seizures
    faciobrachial, 57
    generalized
        clinical considerations for, 227
        EEG of, 227
        mechanisms of, 226–227
        phenomenology of, 227
Clorazepate, 555, 580–581
    alcohol and sedative drug withdrawal, 529
Clozapine, ictogenic potential, 161
Cocaine, 651–652
Coelho, Tony, 44–45
Cognitive deficits, epilepsy disorders associated
        with, 14
Cognitive disturbances
    in partial seizures, 210
Cognitive function, behavioral disturbances and, 380
Cognitive outcomes of surgery, 626–627
Coma
    drug-induced, 171, 357
    due to toxic and metabolic encephalopathies, 455
    epileptic seizures and, 4
    postanoxic, 171, 361
    subtle status epilepticus and, 344
Commission for the Control of Epilepsy and Its
        Consequences, 45
Comorbidity
    pharmacological treatment and, 527–528
    psychiatric, in epilepsy, 375–376, 376*f*
Complementary and alternative medicine (CAM), 603
    behavioral therapies
        abortive sensory stimulation, 634
        EEG biofeedback, 634–635
        psychological treatments, 635
        treatment of reflex epilepsies, 633–634
    diet
        ketogenic diet, 630–631
        supplements, 631–632
    nonallopathic medical systems, 635–636
    physical interventions, 635
    traditional and folk medicine, 632–633, 632*t*, 633*t*

Complex partial status epilepticus. *See* Focal dyscognitive status epilepticus; Focal dyscognitive (complex partial) status epilepticus
Computed tomography (CT)
  SPECT, 134, 434–435, 436*f*
    postictal cerebral dysfunction, specific, 332, 333*f*
    presurgical imaging, 605
  x-ray, 432, 432*f*
Conditioned inefficacy, 307
Conductance, membrane, 56
Conduction, 62
Confusion
  in absence status epilepticus, 359
  corpus callosotomy and, 614
  in focal dyscognitive status epilepticus, 363
  JAE, 263
  phenobarbital and, 548
  phenytoin and, 551
  postictal, 270, 331, 377
Confusional migraine, 456
Congenital malformations
  cerebral, 169
  in children of mothers with epilepsy, 526
  epilepsy-causing, 172–173
  neonatal seizures due to, 281
  vascular, 172–173
Connective tissue disturbances, 515
Connectomics, 87–88
Consciousness, 4
  in absence, 15
  in absence seizures, 221
  in atypical absences, 224
  in childhood disorders, 264
  clear, 16
  definition of, 203
  in focal neocortical seizures, 207
  in hemiclonic seizures, 227
  ictal discharges and, 209
  in ictal events, 332
  impaired, 16, 28, 203
  in partial seizures, 15, 203
  in PS, 250
Consequences of epileptic seizures, 143
  Commission for the Control of Epilepsy and Its Consequences, 45
Continuous spike-and-wave during sleep (CSWS), 310
  epileptic encephalopathy of, 259–260
Contraversive movements, 211
Control, 3
  complete, 11
    duration of, 12
  definition, 11–12
  good, 11, 12
  terminology, 11–13
Convulsant drugs, 185*t*
  proposed mechanisms of action, 100, 102*t*
Convulsions, 203
  benign neonatal familial, 24*t*
  definition, 203
  febrile, 165*t*, 271
  generalized, 453*t*
  generalized, differential diagnosis, 453*t*
  term, 5
  tonic-clonic, 216
Convulsive status epilepticus, generalized
  clinical description of, 344–351

etiology of, 351–352
  incidence of, 351
  other forms of, 350–351
  prognosis, 358
  tonic-clonic, 344–350
  treatment of, 352–358, 353*t*
    alternative, 357
    drug, 354*t*
    DZP, 355–356
    EEG monitoring, 357–358
    follow-up for, 357–358
    fosphenytoin, 355–356
    general anesthesia, 357
    LZP, 355
    other drugs for, 356–357
    paraldehyde, 355–356
    PB, 354–356, 354*t*
    pharmacokinetic properties of drug, 354*t*
    ventilation and, 357–358
Convulsive syncope, 330, 452
Coprolalia, 460
Corpus callosotomy, 604, 614, 636
Corpus callosum
  bilateral synchrony and, 116
  mirror foci, 115
  section, 82, 392
    acute hemispheric disconnection syndrome and, 392
    atonic seizures and, 228
Cortical areas, interictal EEG spikes in various, 300, 300*t*
Cortical development, 82–83, 84*f*
  comparative periods of, 85*t*
  fetal period, 83
  MCD, 83
    as acquired cause of epilepsy disorders, 177
    classification scheme, 177, 178*t*
  ontogeny, 82–83
  perinatal period, 83
  phylogeny, 82–83
Cortical dysplasia, 114
  FCD, 177, 179*t*, 180*f*, 181*f*
Cortical myoclonus, 236
Cortical reflex
  myoclonus, 460
Cortical reflex myoclonus, 460
Cortical thickness of MTLE with HS, 273, 274*f*
Creutzfeldt-Jacob disease, 351
Crossover, pharmacological, 507
Cross-tolerance, 501
Cryptogenic epilepsy, 18
Cryptogenic focal epilepsy, 605
CSF. *See* Cerebrospinal fluid
CSWS. *See* Continuous spike-and-wave during sleep
CT. *See* Computed tomography
Cultural considerations, 661–662
Cure, 3
  definition, 11–12
  diagnosis of, 13
  remission compared with, 13
  terminology, 11–13, 297*t*
Cursive epilepsy, 211
Cyclic guanosine 3,5-monophosphate (cGMP), 65
Cyclic progesterone, 629
Cysts
  polycystic ovary syndrome, 560
  porencephalic, 172, 173*f*
  subarachnoid, 608

Cytochrome P450, drug interactions, VPA, 561
Cytokines, 137

DALYs. *See* Disability-adjusted life years
Dancing amnia, 42
Dante, as epileptic, 44
Daydreaming, differential diagnosis, 466
Deactivating enzymes, 65–66
Deep-brain stimulation, 530
Deepened emotionality, 381
Deep prepiriform cortex, 105
Default mode network (DMN), 89, 436–437
Déjà entendu/vécu/vu, 210. *See also* Memory
Delirium tremens, 454
de Maupassant, Guy, as epileptic, 44
Dementia, 161
    as drug side effect, 515
    hippocampal atrophy in, 178
    PME and, 265
Democritus, as epileptic, 44
Dentate gate, 302
Dentate gyrus (DG), 133, 133*f*
2-Deoxyglucose, 595
Deoxyribonucleic acid (DNA), 61
Department of Defense (DOD), 660
Depersonalization
    disorders, 465
    hyperventilation and, 454
    in ictal cognitive disturbances, 210
Depersonalized dystonia, 383
Depolarization
    excitable membrane and microenvironment, 58–59
    PDS, 64, 101, 103*f*
Depomedroxyprogesterone, 330, 629
Depression, 383*t*, 395
    bipolar, 571
    ictal depressed mood, 382–383
    postictal depressed mood, 383
Dermatitis, exfoliative, 513
Dermatologic abnormalities, 412–413
N-Desmethylclobazam, 557
N-Desmethyldiazepam, 557
Developmental Disability Assistance and Bill of Rights
        Act, 657
DEXA. *See* Dual-energy X-ray absorptiometry
Dexamethasone, 579–580
Dexamethasone suppression test, 515
DG. *See* Dentate gyrus
Diabetes, 451
Diabetic neuropathy, 566
Diagnosis
    classifications and, 30–31
    of cure, 13
    epilepsy, 6, 441–442
        EEG and avoiding inappropriate, 468–483
        EEG and positive, 483–485
    epilepsy disorders, 8
    epilepsy syndromes, 238
    PNES, 464
    syndromic, 31
    of underlying cause, 31
Diagnostic and Statistical Manual of Mental Disorders
        (DSM-IV), 386
Diagnostic evaluation, 405–442, 406*t*
    biomarkers, 440–441
    history and, 405–411

    antiseizure drug, 409
    family, 411
    past medical, 411
    psychosocial, 411
    seizure, 406–409
    laboratory examination and
        clinical laboratory tests, 415, 416*t*
        EEG, 417–425
        functional neuroimaging, 432–439
        MEG, 426–427, 428*f*
        structural neuroimaging, 429–432
        TMS, 427–429
    physical examination and, 411–415
        epileptic seizure observation, 414–415, 414*t*
        general, 412–413, 412*f*, 413*f*
        neurological, 413–414
    psychological evaluation, 439–440, 439*t*
Diagnostic testing, presurgical, 617
3,5-Diamino-6-[2,3-dichlorophenyl]-1,2,4-triazine, 567
Diathermy in VNS, 629
Diazepam (DZP), 555
    alcohol and sedative drug withdrawal, 528–529
    chronic epilepsy, 305
    comorbidity and, 528
    EEG, 421
    elimination, 499
    epilepsia partialis continua, 363
    generalized convulsive status epilepticus, 354, 354*t*,
        355–356
    LZP compared with, 556
    neonatal seizures, 283
    neonatal status epilepticus, 367–368
    psychiatric conditions and, 528
5H-Dibenz[b,f]azepine-5-carboxamide, 557
Dickens, Charles, as epileptic, 44
Dickinson, Emily, as epileptic, 44
Dicumarol, drug interactions, 551
Diencephalic autonomic seizures, 461
Diencephalic influences on excitability, 81
Diet
    ketogenic, 530, 630–631, 636
        drug interactions, VPA, 561, 630–631
    supplements, 631–632
Differential diagnosis, 449–487. *See also specific disorder*
    abdominal epilepsy, 455
    absence status epilepticus, 359
    alcohol withdrawal seizures, 467–468
    BECTS, 252
    breath holding, 452–453, 453*t*
    CAE, 262
    cerebrovascular disorders, 455–457
    chronic epilepsy, 468
    daydreaming, 466
    dissociative states, 465–466
    epilepsia partialis continua, 362–363
    epilepsy
        functional imaging in, 486–487
        use of EEG in, 468–486
    epilepsy syndromes, 487
    epileptic seizures, 237–238
        types of, 487
    focal dyscognitive status epilepticus, 364, 366*t*
    focal seizures, 238
    FS, 279
    generalized convulsions, 453*t*
    generalized seizures, 238

hyperventilation, 453–454, 453t
intermittent explosive disorders, 464–465
JME, 263–265
LGS, 257–259, 258t
metabolic disturbances, 454–455
motor disorders, 459–461
MTLE with HS, 273–275
neonatal seizures due to structural and metabolic
    disorders, 282
nonepileptic paroxysmal events
    abdominal epilepsy and, 455
    breath holding and, 452–453
    cerebrovascular disorders and, 455–457
    daydreaming, 466
    dissociative states, 465–466
    hyperventilation and, 453–454
    intermittent explosive disorders, 464–465
    metabolic disturbances and, 454–455
    motor disorders, 459–461
    neurological disturbances, 455–461
    nonpsychotic psychiatric conditions, 466
    PNES, 461–464
    psychogenic disturbances in, 461–466
    psychoses, 466
    sensory disorders and, 461
    sleep disorders and, 457–459
    syncope and, 450–452
    systemic disturbances in, 450–455
    toxic disturbances and, 454–455
nonpsychotic psychiatric conditions, 466
paroxysmal event, 450, 451t
PNES, 375, 461–464, 487
psychosis, 466
Rasmussen's syndrome, 362
of reactive epileptic seizures
    alcohol withdrawal seizures and, 467–468
    recurrent reactive seizures and, 468
recurrent reactive seizures, 468
sensory disorders, 461
sleep disorders, 457–459
status epilepticus
    absence, 359
    focal dyscognitive, 364, 366t
syncope, 453t
    tonic-clonic epilepsy and, 452
toxic disturbances, 454–455
VEM and, 487
WS, 247
Diffusion tensor imaging (DTI), 89, 133, 620
Digitoxin, drug interactions, 548
Digoxin, drug interactions, 575
Dimethadione, 584
Diphenhydramine, adverse side effects, 513
Dipyrone, drug interactions, 548
Disability
    Developmental Disability Assistance and Bill of Rights
        Act, 657
    epilepsy-associated, 337
        assessing, 380
    RSDHI, 657
Disability-adjusted life years (DALYs), 48–49, 660f
Disease modification, 3, 297
    definition, 13
    terminology, 13–14, 297t
Diseases, 647. See also specific diseases
    epilepsy as, 647

epileptic seizures and, 4
global burden of disease, 660f, 661, 662
    DALYs and, 48
    epilepsy, 45, 48–49, 50
immune-mediated, 176–177
infectious, 174–176
systemic, 169, 170t
Dissociative states, differential diagnosis, 465–466
Distribution, pharmacological, 496–498
Disulfiram, 585
    drug interactions, PHT, 551
Dive reflex, 337
DMN. See Default mode network
DNA. See Deoxyribonucleic acid
DNETs. See Dysembryoplastic neuroepithelial tumors
DOD. See Department of Defense
Dopamine, 355
    amygdala, 119
    as neurotransmitter, 66
Dopaminergic influences on forebrain, 81
Dose
    loading, 501–503
    monotherapy and, 503–507
    trough level, 517
Dose-dependent adverse side effects, 510–513, 533
Dose planning, pharmacological, 501–503, 504t
Dostoyevsky, Feodor Mikhailovich
    as epileptic, 44
    fictional characters with epilepsy, 646
Double cortex syndrome, 166
Dravet syndrome (DS), 247, 249, 311, 322
    treatment, LTG and, 568
Driving, 648–651
    license regulations, 649–650, 650t
    practical criteria for restrictions on, 648–649
Drop attacks, 203. See also Atonic seizures
    during dyscognitive seizures, 212
    in LGS, 255
    treatment for, 228
Drowning, 337
Drug efficacy, 533
    clinical factors influencing, 508
Drug interactions, 501. See also specific drugs
    CBZ, 559
    CLN, 556
    drug efficacy and, 508
    ESL, 562
    ESM, 554
    EZG, 563
    FBM, 564
    GBP, 565
    LCM, 566
    LEV, 569
    LTG, 568
    OXC, 571
    PB, 548
    PGN, 572
    PHT, 551–552
    polytherapy and, 507, 507f, 510f
    PRM, 553
    RUF, 573
    TGB, 574
    TPM, 575
    VGB, 576
    VPA, 561
    ZON, 578

Drug levels, 330
   toxic, 510
Drug resistance, 3. *See also* Pharmacoresistance
   definition, 11–12
   MDR, 61
   terminology, 11–13
Drug-resistant epilepsy, 13, 494
Drugs. *See also* Antiseizure drugs
   antiabsence, 5, 10
   anticonvulsant, 5, 10
   antiepileptic, 10, 31
      positive psychotropic effects, 390, 390*t*
   convulsant, proposed mechanisms of action, 100, 102*t*
   generic, 520
   precipitating generalized tonic-clonic seizures, 183, 185*t*
   psychomimetic, 454–455
   psychotropic, risk of seizures from, 161
   tolerability, 508
   use, 651–652
Drugs under investigation
   Phase III trials
      brivaracetam, 594–595
      ganaxolone, 595
      perampanel, 595
   preclinical development
      huperzine A, 595
      ICA105665, 595
      T2000, 595
      tonabersat, 595
      2-deoxyglucose, 595
      valproic acid derivatives, 595
      VX-765, 596
      YKP3089, 595
Drug withdrawal
   drug tapering and, 507
   sedative, 528–529
Drusus, as epileptic, 43
DS. *See* Dravet syndrome
DSM-IV. *See* Diagnostic and Statistical Manual of Mental Disorders
DTI. *See* Diffusion tensor imaging
Dual-energy X-ray absorptiometry (DEXA), 515
Dupuytren's contractures, 515
Dysautonomia, familial, 451
Dyscognitive focal seizures, pharmacological treatment of, 494
Dyscognitive seizures
   focal, 27, 31, 203
   limbic, 270
Dyscognitive state, 4
Dyscontrol syndrome, episodic, 377
Dysembryoplastic neuroepithelial tumors (DNETs), 174, 175*f*, 389
Dyskinesias, 460
   antiseizure drug-related, 515
   paroxysmal, 459
   TIAs and, 456
Dysmnesic symptoms, 210
Dysphasic status epilepticus, 360
Dysphoria, 383
Dysplasia
   cortical, 114
   FCD, 177, 179*t*, 180*f*, 181*f*
Dystonia, 459, 460
   benign essential myoclonus and, 236

depersonalized, 383
myoclonus, 284
nocturnal paroxysmal, 253
paroxysmal, 326
DZP. *See* Diazepam

Ear lobe electrodes, 417
Early infantile epileptic encephalopathy (EIEE), 245
Early myoclonic encephalopathy (EME), 245
Early Randomized Surgical Epilepsy Trial (ERSET), 625–626
Early seizures, prophylaxis for, 304–305
Eating-induced seizures, 325
Eclampsia, 524–525
ECoG. *See* Electrocorticography
ECS, seizure induction, 106
ECT. *See* Electroconvulsive shock treatment
Ectodermal dysplasias, 389
Edema, cerebral, 347
Education
   health care disparities and, 661
   reading epilepsy, 324
      primary, 269
   school, 654
EEG. *See* Electroencephalogram
Effectiveness, pharmacological, 508
Efflux transporter, 528
EIEE. *See* Early infantile epileptic encephalopathy
Elderly, pharmacological treatment and, 523–524
Electrical stimulation, 100
Electroclinical syndromes, 244
   by age at onset, 29*t*
Electroconvulsive shock treatment (ECT), 307, 635
   generalized convulsive status epilepticus, 357
Electrocorticography (ECoG), 424
Electrodecremental events, 350
Electrodecremental response
   in atonic seizures, 228
   in epileptic spasms, 229, 230*f*
   in myoclonic tonic seizures, 226
Electrodes for EEG, 417*f*, 418*f*, 420*f*
   basal, 418, 419*t*
      and normal phenomena, 471, 472*f*, 477*f*
   ear lobe, 417
   epidural peg, 622
   foramen ovale, 417
   mastoid, 417
   sphenoidal, 418, 418*f*
   T, 417–418
   zygoma, 417–418
Electroencephalogram (EEG), 441
   absence epilepsies, 480
   absence seizures
      atypical, 224, 224*f*
      typical, 222, 223*f*
   activity, neuronal basis of, 86–87, 87*f*
   afterdischarge and, 6
   ambulatory recording, 530–531
      PNES, 463
   anatomical substrates, 194–197, 197*f*
   atonic seizures, generalized, 228, 231*f*
   bilateral discharges, 485
   biofeedback, 634–635
   chaos theory applied to, 321
   clonic seizures, generalized, 227
   CSWS, 310

epileptic encephalopathy of, 259–260
dipoles, 424
electrodes for, 417*f*, 418*f*, 420*f*
    basal, 418, 419*t*
    basal and normal phenomena, 471, 472*f*, 477*f*
    ear lobe, 417
    epidural peg, 622
    foramen ovale, 417
    mastoid, 417
    sphenoidal, 418, 418*f*
    T, 417–418
    zygoma, 417–418
epilepsia partialis continua, 360, 361*f*
epilepsy diagnosis with
    avoiding inappropriate, 468–483
    positive, 483–485
    types and, 485–486
epilepsy differential diagnosis and, 468–486
epileptic seizures on, 4–6
epileptic spike focus determined on, 10
epileptiform events, 31
    focal, 122, 123*f*, 124*f*
epileptiform patterns on, 5–6
EPSP-IPSP complex on, 86
focal spikes, 475–480, 479*f*, 480*f*
frontal mittens, 468, 469*f*
generalized convulsive status epilepticus treatment
    monitoring with, 357–358
GTS, 217–220, 219*f*
3-Hz spike-and-wave discharges, 222, 223*f*
6-Hz positive spikes, 471, 472*f*
6-Hz spike-and-wave pattern, 471, 475*f*
14-Hz positive spikes, 471, 472*f*
harmonics, 469, 470*f*
interictal spikes, 122
    migration of, 313
    in various cortical areas, 300, 300*t*
interictal state on, 9
invention of, 40
JME, 263, 264*f*
limbic seizures, 212–213, 213*f*, 214*f*
midline theta rhythm, 471, 476*f*
MTLE with HS, 271, 271*f*
myoclonic seizures, 226
neocortical seizures, 206–207, 207*f*
neonatal seizures, 232–233, 232*t*, 234*f*
normal phenomena, 468–471, 469*f*, 470*f*, 471*f*
    basal electrodes and, 471, 472*f*, 477*f*
occipital spike driving, 481–482, 483*f*
photomyogenic response, 323, 480–481, 482*f*
photoparoxysmal response, 323, 323*f*, 480, 481*f*
PNES, 462–463
Rasmussen's syndrome, 276, 276*f*
RMTD, 471, 474*f*
SEM, 436
sharp transients of dubious significance, 469–471
simultaneous, 11
sleep spindles, 313
source modeling, 424
special approaches to
    additional electrodes and, 417–419, 417*f*, 418*f*, 420*f*
    computer-enhanced, 424–425, 425*f*, 426*f*, 427*f*
    evoked potentials and, 425
    physiological activation procedures and, 419–421
    VEM, 422–424, 422*f*, 423*t*
spike-and-wave discharges, 5, 86–87, 88*f*, 106, 108*f*

epilepsy types and, 485
spikes, 126, 128*f*
SREDA, 482–483, 484*f*
SSS, 471, 472*f*
studies of human epilepsy with, 122–126, 126*f*
syncope, prodromal period, 452
tonic-clonic status epilepticus, 347*f*, 348*f*, 349*f*
tonic seizures, generalized, 227–228
treatment assessment with, 530–531
VEM, 422–424, 422*f*, 423*t*, 441
    ambulatory recorder, 423
    differential diagnosis and, 487
    PNES, 463
vertex sharp waves, 313
when to use, 415–417
wicket spikes, 471, 473*f*
Electrographic seizures, 6
Electrolyte imbalance, 170*t*, 177
    reactive seizures and, 467
Electrolyte metabolism disorders, 166
Electronic conduction, 62
Electronic synapses, 72
Electroretinogram (ERG), 425
Electroshock-induced seizures, 107
Elementary visual status epilepticus, 360
Elimination, pharmacological, 499, 499*f*, 500*f*
EMA. *See* Epilepsy with myoclonic absences
EMAS. *See* Epilepsy with myoclonic-atonic seizures
EME. *See* Early myoclonic encephalopathy
Empedocles, as epileptic, 44
Employment, 654–655
    ADA and, 655
Encephalitic form of epilepsia partialis continua, 360
Encephalitis, 279
    Rasmussen's, 618
    Russian spring-summer, 361
Encephalitis lethargica, 457
Encephalopathy. *See also specific encephalopathies*
    acidemia in early myoclonic, 245
    epileptic, 10, 14, 26, 308, 375
        of CSWS, 259–260, 310
    metabolic, 455
    toxic, 455
    valproic, 569
    Wernicke's, 352
Endocrine metabolism, 515–516
    disorders, 166
Endogenous opioids, 66, 119, 331
Environmental factors, 161–162
    photosensitive seizures and, 323
Environmental toxins, precipitatory, 184, 185*t*
Enzymes
    deactivating, 65–66
    inhibition
        elimination and, 499, 499*f*, 500*f*
        polytherapy and, 506, 506*f*
Enzymes induction, elimination and, 499, 499*f*, 500*f*
Epidemiology, 33
    CAE, 261
    of epilepsy, 45–49
    FS, 279
    health care disparities epidemiological assessment and
        case finding, 661
    JME, 263
    LGS, 256
    MTLE with HS, 273

Epidemiology (*cont.*)
  neonatal seizures due to structural and metabolic
    disorders, 282
  psychiatric comorbidity in epilepsy, 375–376, 376*f*
  WS, 246
Epidermal necrolysis, 558
Epidural peg electrodes, 622
Epigastric rising in partial seizure, 210
Epilepsia partialis continua, 6, 618
  clinical description of, 360–361
  differential diagnosis, 362–363
  EEG, 360, 361*f*
  encephalitic form, 360
  etiology, 361–362
  FDG-PET, 360, 362*f*
  focal form, 360
  incidence, 361
  prognosis, 363
  treatment, 363
Epilepsy, 3, 6
  acquired, 138–139, 144
  active, 12
  by age at onset, 29*t*
  animal models, 298
  in animals, 120–121
  attitudes towards, 34, 645, 645*t*
  basic mechanisms of, 99–144
    experimental models and, 100–122
    molecular genetic investigations and, 135–138
    possible mechanisms of human epileptic phenomena,
      138–143
    studies of human epilepsy, 122–135
  behavioral disturbances in, phenomenology of,
    376–387, 377*t*
  causes of, 36, 157–186
    genetic investigations, 185
    multifactorial approach to understanding, 157
    nonspecific predisposing factors, 157–162
    precipitating factors, 157, 182–185
    Rochester study, 169, 171*t*
    specific epileptogenic disturbances, 157–159,
      162–182
  chronic
    animal models, 298
    antiseizure drugs, 305
    biomarkers, 306, 306*t*
    development, 297
    differential diagnosis, 468
    neonatal seizures and incidence, 283, 283*t*
    prophylaxis for, 305–307
    in vitro studies of, 121–122
  classification, 14, 31
    etiological, 28, 30*t*
    ICD, 18, 19*t*, 20*t*
    international, revision of, 25–28
    1985 International, 18–25, 24*t*
    1989 International, 18–25, 24*t*
    older, 3, 17–25
    proposed diagnostic scheme and, 26, 27*t*
    WHO, 18
  Classification of the Epilepsies and Epileptic
    Syndromes, 244
  Commission for the Control of Epilepsy and Its
    Consequences, 45
  conditions, 13
  definitions of, 6–7, 8, 31

  depression and, 382–383, 383*t*
  diagnosis, 6, 441–442
    EEG and avoiding inappropriate, 468–483
    EEG and positive, 483–485
  differential diagnosis, 450
    EEG in, 468–486
    functional imaging in, 486–487
  disability associated with, 337
    assessing, 380
  as disease, 647
  drug-resistant, 13
  epidemiological perspective, incidence and prevalence
    definitions, 45–46
  experimental models
    acute, 100–109, 101*t*
    chronic, 109–122
  explaining, 644–645, 645*t*
  with focal seizures, in vivo models of, 109–120
  generalized, 17–18, 25*f*
    in animals, genetic generalized, 120–121
    idiopathic, 31
    IGE, 248
    localization-related epilepsies and, 25
    partial, 26*f*
    primary, 17
    secondary, 17
  with generalized seizures, in vivo models of, 120–121
  genetic, 159, 164–166
    manifestations, 165
    rare single-gene, 165
  genetic disorders with, 166–169, 167*t*, 168*f*
  genius and, 43–45
  global burden of disease, 45, 48–49, 50
  with GTS only, 265
  historical perspectives of, 34–45, 49
  hysteria confused with, 34
  idiopathic, 7, 31, 36
  importance today of, 49
  incidence, 45–48
    WHO, 33
  kindling compared with, 307, 308*t*
  kindling model of, 298
  as legal defense, 377, 656
  literature, 3, 34
    Western, 49
  localization-related, 18
  medical history of
    ancient and medieval periods, 34–36
    modern era, 36–41, 49
  medically intractable, 13
  misdiagnosis, 450
  neuropsychiatric disorders in, classification of,
    385–386, 386*t*
  organizations for, 658*t*
  partial, 17
  perspectives on, 33–49
  predisposing factors, 36
  prevalence, 45–48
    age-adjusted, 49–50
    definitions of, 45–46
    estimates of, 46–48
    methodological considerations, 46
    rates, 49–50
  prognosis, 309
  progressive nature of, 307–312, 609
    clinical evidence for, 308–311

practical considerations for, 311–312
psychiatric comorbidity in, epidemiology of,
   375–376, 376*f*
reflex, 6
religion and, 34–35, 41–42, 43*f*, 44*f*
status epilepticus models of, kindling and, 119
stigma associated with, 45
studies of human
   biochemical investigations, 134–135, 135*f*
   brain imaging technique investigations, 130–134
   electrophysiological investigations, 122–130
   microanatomical investigations, 134
   molecular investigations, 134–135, 135*f*
symptomatic, 31
symptom progression, 309
term, 4
terminology, 8
types, EEG and diagnosing, 485–486
in Western literature, 49
Epilepsy centers
   NAEC, 606
   reference to, 494
Epilepsy development
   character of lesion and, 299–300
   genetic factors in, 302–304
   location of lesion and, 300–302
   phenomenology of, 297–299
   practical considerations in
      prophylaxis for chronic epilepsy and, 305–307
      prophylaxis for early seizures and, 304–305
Epilepsy disorders, 3, 31–32, 647
   acquired causes of, 7, 169–182
      anoxia and trauma, 169, 171–172
      brain tumors as, 174, 174*t*
      cerebrovascular disorders, 172–173
      HS as, 177–182
      immune-mediated diseases as, 176–177
      infectious diseases as, 174–176
      inflammation-mediated diseases as, 176–177
      MCDs as, 177
      metabolic disturbances as, 177
      toxic disturbances as, 177
   cognitive deficits associated with, 14
   cryptogenic, 7
   definition, 6
   diagnosis, 8
   essential, 7
   genetic, 7, 13
   genetic causes of, 163–169
      genetic disorders with epilepsy and, 166–169
      genetic epilepsies and, 164–166
   idiopathic, 7
   neurological deficits associated with, 14
   pathophysiological mechanisms, 8
   presumed idiopathic, 7
   presumed symptomatic, 7
   primary, 7, 17
   recurrent epileptic seizures associated with, 14
   secondary, 17
   secondary symptomatic, 7
   structural/metabolic, 77
   terminology, 6–8
   types, 7
   unknown, 7
Epilepsy of infancy with migrating focal seizures
   (MPSI), 245–246

Epilepsy Surgery Inventory-55 (ESI-55), 379, 626
Epilepsy syndromes, 7, 28, 243–285
   of adolescence-adult
      ADEAF as, 267
      epilepsy with generalized tonic-clonic seizures only,
         265
      familial temporal lobe epilepsies as, 267–268
      JAE as, 263
      JME as, 263–265
      PME and, 265–267
   characterization, 31, 285
   of childhood
      ADNFLE as, 253–254
      BECTS as, 251–252
      CAE as, 260–263
      CSWS as, 259–260
      EMA as, 254–255
      EMAS as, 251
      FS+, 250
      late childhood occipital epilepsy (Gastaut type) as, 254
      LGS as, 255–259
      LKS as, 260
      PS as, 250–251
   classification, 28, 29*t*, 31, 285
      1985 International, 18–25, 24*t*
      1989 International, 18–25, 24*t*
   Classification of the Epilepsies and Epileptic
      Syndromes, 244
   conditions with epileptic seizures not traditionally
      diagnosed as
      BNS as, 278
      FS as, 278–280
      neonatal seizures due to structural and metabolic
         disorders as, 281–283
      reactive seizures as, 280–281
   defining, 31
   diagnosis, 238
   differential diagnosis, 487
   distinctive constellations
      gelastic seizures with hypothalamic hamartoma as,
         277, 277*f*
      head nodding syndrome as, 278
      HHE as, 277–278
      MTLE with HS, 269–275
      Rasmussen's syndrome, 275–277
   evolution, 312–313
   genetic, 311
   of infancy
      BFIE, 249
      BIE, 249
      DS, 249
      MEI, 248–249
      MPSI, 245–246
      myoclonic encephalopathy in nonprogressive
         disorders, 249–250
      WS, 246–248
   with less specific age relationships
      familial focal epilepsy with variable foci as, 268
      reflex epilepsies as, 268–269
   myoclonus syndromes, 283–284
   neonatal period, 244–245
   severe, 28
   surgically remediable, 605, 609–611, 610*t*
      MTLE as prototype of, 610, 611*t*
      pharmacoresistance and, 610
   symptom complex, 285

Epilepsy with myoclonic absences (EMA), 254–255. *See also* Absences
Epilepsy with myoclonic-atonic seizures (EMAS), 251
Epileptic (term), 8. *See also* Person with epilepsy
Epileptic brain damage, 368–369
Epileptic encephalopathies, 10, 14, 26, 308, 375
    of CSWS, 259–260, 310
Epileptic focus (foci), 11
    cortical, 82
    definition, 11
    discrete, 144
    experimental, 11, 103–104, 104*f*
    familial focal epilepsy with variable foci, 268
    penicillin-induced neocortical, 101
    secondary, 115
Epileptic personality, 381, 395
Epileptic phenomena, 5, 144
    genetic characteristics of, 165, 165*t*
    possible mechanisms of human
        epileptogenesis as, 138–139, 139*f*
        ictal termination as, 142
        ictogenesis as, 140–141
        ictus as, 141–142
        interictal state as, 139–140
        postictal period as, 142–143
Epileptic seizures, 3, 193–238
    acute symptomatic, 7
    behavioral features of, 4
    brain development and, 312–314
        migration of interictal EEG spike in, 313
        practical considerations for, 313–314
    brain hemispheres and, 5
    brief, 6
    catamenial exacerbation of, 519
    centrencephalic source of, 5
    in children, 300, 300*t*
    classification
        international, 15–16, 16*t*
        international, revision of, 25–28
        older, 3, 14–17
        proposed diagnostic scheme and, 26, 27*t*
    conditions with, not traditionally diagnosed as epilepsy
        BNS as, 278
        FS as, 278–280
        neonatal seizures due to structural and metabolic disorders as, 281–283
        reactive seizures as, 280–281
    definition, 4
    differential diagnosis, 237–238
        PNES and, 461–462
    diseases/disorders and, 4
    on EEG, 4, 5–6
    focal, 5, 15
        mechanisms of, 27
        onset of, 27
        origin of, 27
    generalized, 5, 15
    ILAE classification of, 193
    intermittent, 6
    local, 15
    neurological disturbances and, 7
    neuronal mechanism, 4
    neuronal synchronization and, 55
    observation, 414–415, 414*t*
    paroxysmal, 6
    partial, 5

pathologic mechanisms, 5
possible consequences of, 143
provoked, 7
    unprovoked seizure distinguished from, 8
provoked acute symptomatic, 6
reactive, 6, 7, 8, 31
recurrent, epilepsy disorders associated with, 14
sleep-wake cycle and, 328
spontaneous, 6
in startle epilepsy, 324
systemic diseases associated with, 169, 170*t*
terminology, 4–6
treatment, 238
types, 4–5, 31, 199–204, 200*t* (*See also specific types*)
    anatomical substrates for diagnosis of, 194–197, 195*t*
    characterization of, 31
    diagnosing, 237
    differential diagnosis, 487
    neurobiological considerations for diagnosis of, 194–199
    pathophysiological mechanisms for diagnosis of, 197–198
    pharmacological considerations for diagnosis of, 198–199
unclassified, 200*t*
    epileptic spasms as, 228–229, 230*f*, 231*f*
    neonatal seizures, 229–233
    reflex seizures as, 229
unprovoked, provoked seizure distinguished from, 8
Epileptic spasms, 230*f*, 231*f*
    types, 228–229
Epileptic spike focus, 3, 31
    definition, 10
    diffuse, 10
    EEG and determining, 10
    multifocal, 10
    terminology, 10–11
Epileptiform discharges, 5–6
    bilateral, 10
    focal, 10
    independent, 10
    PLEDs, 366, 471–475, 478*f*
Epileptiform EEG events, 31
    focal, 122, 123*f*, 124*f*
Epileptiform effect, subcortical structures, 81–82
Epileptiform phenomena, genetic characteristics of, 165, 165*t*
Epileptogenesis, 3, 138–139, 139*f*, 296–315, 440
    antiepileptogenesis
        complete, 297
        definition, 13
        partial, 297
        terminology, 13–14, 297*t*
    biomarkers of, 314–315
    definition, 9–10, 296
    development of epilepsy
        character of lesion and, 299–300
        genetic factors in, 302–304
        location of lesion and, 300–302
        phenomenology and, 297–299
        practical considerations in, 304–307
    epilepsy syndrome and brain development in, 312–314
    hippocampus and, 302, 303*f*
    kindled, 117–118
    progressive nature of epilepsy and, 307–312
        clinical evidence for, 308–311

practical considerations for, 311–312
prophylaxis, 314
research on, 314–315
secondary, 10, 115–120, 117*f*, 307–308
  frontal lobe tumors and, 310
  kindling and, 116–118, 307
  mirror focus and, 307
  terminology, 9–10, 297*t*
types, 314
Epileptogenic activity, 4
Epileptogenic agents, 10
Epileptogenic disturbances, specific, 157–159
  acquired causes of epilepsy disorders as, 169–182
  genetic causes of epilepsy as, 163–169
Epileptogenicity, 3, 440
  definition, 9–10
  neuronal basis of, 144
  terminology, 9–10
Epileptogenic lesion, 3, 31, 617
  definition, 10
  terminology, 10–11
Epileptogenic zone or region, 3, 31, 196–197, 616
  definition, 10
  primary, 11
  secondary, 11
  terminology, 10–11
Episodic ataxias, 461
Episodic dyscontrol syndrome, 377
Epoxide hydrolase systems, drug interactions, 561
EPSP. *See* Excitatory postsynaptic potential
EPSP-IPSP complex, 75
  EEG rhythms, 86
ERG. *See* Electroretinogram
ERSET. *See* Early Randomized Surgical Epilepsy Trial
Erythema multiforme, 513
Erythromycin
  drug efficacy, 508
  drug interactions, CBZ, 559
eSAM. *See* Etomidate speech and memory test
ESI-55. *See* Epilepsy Surgery Inventory-55
ESL. *See* Eslicarbazepine acetate
Eslicarbazepine, elimination, 499
Eslicarbazepine acetate (ESL), 561–562
  administration, 562
  drug interactions, 562
  indications, 562
  mechanisms of action, 562
  pharmacokinetics, 562
  toxicity, 562
ESM. *See* Ethosuximide
Estradiol, 629
Estrogen, 329
Ethanol, drug interactions
  CLN, 556
  PHT, 551
Ethosuximide (ESM)
  absence status epilepticus, 359
  administration, 554
  adverse behavioral effects of, 389*t*, 390
  adverse side effects, 516
  animal models, 298
  CAE, 262
  drug interactions, 554
    LTG, 568
    PHT, 551
    VPA, 561

EMA, 255
EMAS, 251
  epileptic seizure types and, 199
  indications, 554
  JAE, 263
  LGS, 259
  mechanisms of action, 554
  MEI, 249
  monitoring, 517
  nursing and, 527
  pharmacokinetics, 554
  toxicity, 554
  trials, 519
Ethotoin, 550, 583–584
5-Ethyldihydro-5-phenyl-4,6(1H,5H)-pyrimidinedione, 552
Etomidate, IAP, 621
Etomidate speech and memory test (eSAM), 440, 621
Evoked potentials
  EEG, 425
  SEPs, 425
  VEPs, 425
Excessive fragmentary myoclonus in non-REM sleep, 284
Excitability, 55. *See also* Neuronal excitation
  brain stem and, 81
  cerebellum and, 82
  diencephalic influences on, 81
  factors influencing, 321
  hippocampal patterns of, 76–77, 81
  increasing, 72
  interhemispheric influences on, 82
  neocortex, 81
  neurotransmitters, 62
  synapses, 62
Excitable membrane and microenvironment
  action potentials, 58–59
  conductance, 56
  depolarization, 58–59
  equilibrium potentials, 57–58
  membrane physiology, 57–61
  polarization, 57–58, 58*f*
  potential difference, 56–61
  voltage-gated channels, 56–57, 57*t*
Excitatory postsynaptic potential (EPSP), 60*f*, 62
Exercise
  intolerance, 169
  seizures provoked by, 330
Exfoliative dermatitis, 513
Experimental epileptic focus, 11
Experimental models of seizures and epilepsy, 100–122
  acute, 100–109, 101*t*
  ESM and, 554
Explosiveness, 382
Extracellular ionic concentrations, 60–61
Eyelid myoclonia, 225, 324
Ezekiel, as epileptic, 42
Ezogabine (EZG), 562–563
  administration, 563
  drug interactions, 563
  identification of, 591
  indications, 563
  mechanisms of action, 563
  pharmacokinetics, 563
  toxicity, 563

Faciobrachial clonic seizures, 57
Factitious disorders, 14

Falling disease, 34
Falling sickness, 35, 49
Familial dysautonomia, 451
Familial focal epilepsy with variable foci, 268
Familial hemiplegic migraine, 456
Familial paroxysmal dystonic choreoathetosis, 459–460
Familial temporal lobe epilepsies, 267–268
Family
   aggregation, 163
   child with epilepsy and, 652–653
   explaining epilepsy to, 644–645, 645*t*
   history, 302–304, 411
   parent with epilepsy and, 653–654
Fast prepotentials (FPPs), 63, 103
FBM. *See* Felbamate
FCD. *See* Focal cortical dysplasia
fcMRI. *See* Functional connectivity magnetic resonance
   imaging
FDG. *See* 18F-fluorodeoxyglucose
FDG-PET, 307, 433–434, 433*t*, 434*fI*, 435f. *See also*
   Positron emission tomography
   epilepsia partialis continua, 360, 362*f*
   GTS, 220, 220*f*
   limbic seizure, 213, 215*f*
   MTLE with HS, 271, 272*f*
   postictal cerebral dysfunction, specific, 332, 334*f*
Fear
   aura of, 382
   as ictal affective symptom, 210
   in ictal period, 206, 210
   in limbic epilepsy, 377
   in panic attacks, 466
Febrile infection-related epilepsy syndrome (FIRES), 367
Febrile seizures (FS), 165
   benign, 7, 468
   clinical description, 278–279
   differential diagnosis, 279
   epidemiology, 279
   etiology, 279
   later nonfebrile seizure incidence and, 280, 281*f*
   prognosis, 280, 280*f*
   susceptibility to, 184
   treatment, 280, 314
Febrile seizures plus (FS+), 250
   GEFS+, 250
Febrile status epilepticus, 367, 369
Feedback inhibition, 75, 76*f*
Feedforward inhibition, 75, 76*f*, 103, 104*f*
Felbamate (FBM)
   administration, 564–565
   comorbidity and, 527–528
   drug interactions, 564
      PHT, 551
      VPA, 561
   epileptic seizure types and, 199
   hematological disorders related to, 514
   hepatotoxicity induced by, 515
   indications, 564
   LGS, 259
   mechanisms of action, 564
   monitoring, 517
   pharmacokinetics, 564
   toxicity, 564
   trials, 519
Feline generalized penicillin model, 106, 107*f*, 554
Felodipine, 570

Felt stigma, 646
Ferdinand V of Spain, as epileptic, 43
Ferric chloride, 109
Ferrier, David, 37, 38*f*
Fetal hydantoin syndrome, 551
Fetishism, 381
Fever. *See also* Febrile seizures
   convulsions, 165*t*, 271
   as epileptogenic stimuli, 83
   seizure threshold and, 161
18F-fluorodeoxyglucose (FDG), 130–132, 132*f*
Financial aid, 657
FIRES. *See* Febrile infection-related epilepsy syndrome
Fits
   cerebellar, 461
   rum, 467
   uncinate, 326
      with olfactory symptoms, 15
Flaubert, Gustave, as epileptic, 44
Fluconazole, drug interactions, 551
Flumazenil, 132
Fluoroacetate, neuronal excitability and, 61
Fluorocitrate, neuronal excitability and, 61
Fluorothyl, seizure induction, 106
Fluoxetine, ictogenic potential, 161
Fluphenazine, ictogenic potential, 161
fMRI. *See* Functional magnetic resonance imaging
Focal cortical dysplasia (FCD), 177, 179*t*, 180*f*, 181*f*
Focal dyscognitive seizures, 27, 31, 203
Focal dyscognitive (complex partial) status epilepticus
   clinical description of, 363–364, 365*f*
   confusion in, 363
   differential diagnosis of, 364, 366*t*
   etiology of, 364
   incidence of, 364
   prognosis of, 366
   treatment of, 364–366
Focal epilepsies
   cryptogenic, 605
   development, 297–298
   familial, with variable foci, 268
   penicillin model, 125
   symptomatic, 31
Focal form of epilepsia partialis continua, 360
Focal negative myoclonus, 205
Focal seizures, 5, 26, 31, 199
   descriptive factors, 28, 28*t*
   differential diagnosis, 238
   dyscognitive, pharmacological treatment of, 494
   epilepsy with, in vivo models of, 109–113
   Jacksonian march of motor symptoms, 15
   limbic, 209–215
   MPSI, 245–246
   neocortical, 204–209
   psychomotor seizures, 15
   secondarily generalized seizure evolution from
      clinical considerations for, 216
      mechanisms of, 215
      phenomenology of, 216, 216*f*
   uncinate fits with olfactory symptoms, 15
   in vivo models of, 101–105
Focal structural lesions, 310
Focal syndromes, 26
Folic acid, 514, 533
   antiseizure medications and, 527
Folk medicine, 632–633, 632*t*, 633*t*

Food sensitivity, 631–632
Foramen ovale electrodes, 417
Fosphenytoin, 550, 582–583
    elimination, 499
    epilepsia partialis continua, 363
    generalized convulsive status epilepticus, 354*t*, 355–356
    neonatal status epilepticus, 367
FPPs. *See* Fast prepotentials
Frontal lobe tumors, secondary epileptogenesis, 310
Frozen shoulder syndrome, 515
FS. *See* Febrile seizures
FS+. *See* Febrile seizures plus
Fugue states, 333
Functional connectivity magnetic resonance imaging
    (fcMRI), 89, 133–134
Functional deficit zone, 617
Functional imaging, epilepsy differential diagnosis,
    486–487
Functional magnetic resonance imaging (fMRI), 11, 133,
    435–438, 438*f*, 439*f*
    presurgical imaging, 605
Functional neuroimaging
    fMRI, 435–438, 438*f*, 439*f*
    MRS, 438
    PET, 432–434
    rectilinear radionuclide brain scanning, 438–439
    SPECT, 434–435, 436*f*
Funduscopic abnormalities, 412, 412*f*

GABA. *See* γ-Aminobutyric acid
GABA$_A$. *See* γ-Aminobutyric acid A
Gabapentin (GBP)
    administration, 566
    adverse side effects, 516
    BECTS, 253
    choosing appropriate drug and, 518–519
    comorbidity and, 528
    distribution, 498
    drug interactions, 565
        FBM, 564
    EMA aggravated by, 255
    indications, 565–566
    JME exacerbated by, 265
    mechanisms of action, 565
    MEI, 249
    monitoring, 517
    pharmacokinetics, 565
    psychotropic effects of, 390, 391*t*
    toxicity, 565
Galen, 34–35
γ-Aminobutyric acid (GABA), 66
    Cl⁻ channels and, 71
    receptors, 343
    VPA and, 560
γ-Aminobutyric acid A (GABA$_A$), 343
γ-Hydroxybutyrate model, 554, 560
Gamma knife surgery (GKS), 615
Ganaxolone, 595
Ganglioglioma, 389
Gangliosidoses, 166
Gaspar, as patron of epilepsy, 42
Gastrointestinal side effects, 513
Gastrointestinal symptoms
    in partial seizures, 210
GBP. *See* Gabapentin
GCAE. *See* Global Campaign Against Epilepsy

GEFS+. *See* Generalized epilepsy with febrile seizures +
Gelastic seizures, 5, 205–206
    with hypothalamic hamartoma, 277, 277*f*
Gene
    c-fos, 61–62
    discovery, 135–136
    identification, 160, 164, 164*t*
    IEGs, 137
    mutation, SCN5A, 336
    rare single-gene epilepsies, 165
Gene ontology (GO), 136–137
General anesthesia, generalized convulsive status
    epilepticus, 357
Generalization
    genetic factors and, 25
    secondary, 18
Generalized convulsions, differential diagnosis, 453*t*
Generalized convulsive status epilepticus
    clinical description of, 344–351
    etiology of, 351–352
    incidence of, 351
    other forms of, 350–351
    prognosis, 358
    tonic-clonic, 344–350
    treatment of, 352–358, 353*t*
        alternative, 357
        drug, 354*t*
        DZP, 355–356
        EEG monitoring, 357–358
        follow-up for, 357–358
        fosphenytoin, 355–356
        general anesthesia, 357
        LZP, 355
        other drugs for, 356–357
        paraldehyde, 355–356
        PB, 354–356, 354*t*
        pharmacokinetic properties of drug, 354*t*
        ventilation and, 357–358
Generalized epilepsies, 17–18, 25*f*
    in animals, genetic generalized, 120–121
    idiopathic, 31
    IGE, 248
    localization-related epilepsies and, 25
    partial, 26*f*
    primary, 17
    secondary, 17
Generalized epilepsy with febrile seizures +
    (GEFS+), 250
Generalized seizures, 5, 199, 200*t*
    absences, 15
    absence seizures
        atypical, 222–224
        typical, 220–222
    asymmetric, 27
    atonic seizures, 228
    clonic seizures, 226–227
    convulsive, 15
    differential diagnosis, 238
    epilepsy with, in vivo models of, 120–121
    eyelid myoclonia, 225
    hyperthermia-induced, 114
    major motor, 15
    minor motor, 15
    myoclonic absences, 224–225
    myoclonic atonic seizures, 226
    myoclonic seizures, 225–226

Generalized seizures (*cont.*)
   myoclonic tonic seizures, 226
   nonconvulsive, 15
   origin, 27
   secondary, 15
      focal seizure evolution into, 215–216
   subdivision of, 15
   tonic-clonic seizures, 216–220
   tonic seizures, 227–228
   in vivo models, 105–107
Generalized tonic-clonic seizures (GTS), 4–5, 36
   clinical considerations, 220
   drugs precipitating, 183, 185*t*
   EEG, 217–220, 219*f*
   emergency treatment of, 532
   epilepsy with, 265
   FDG-PET, 220, 220*f*
   mechanisms, 216–217
   pharmacological treatment of, 494
   phenomenology, 217, 218*f*
Generic drugs, 520. *See also specific drugs*
Genetic absence epilepsies, 15
Genetic causes of epilepsy disorder, 163–169
   genetic disorders with epilepsy and, 166–169
   genetic epilepsies and, 164–166
Genetic characteristics of epileptic/epileptiform
      phenomena, 165, 165*t*
Genetic disorders
   with epilepsy, 166–169, 167*t*
   inherited, 166, 168*f*
Genetic disturbances, acquired, 135–138, 138*f*
Genetic epilepsies, 159, 164–166
   generalized, 120–121
   manifestations, 165
   rare single-gene, 165
   reflex, ictal initiation and, 322–324
Genetic factors, 159–161, 159*f*
   cerebral structures and, 160–161
   in epilepsy development, 302–304
   generalization and, 25
   inherited differentiated from, 160
Genetics
   causes of epilepsy and, 185
   molecular
      discovery-driven approaches, 136
      hypothesis-driven approaches, 136
      of seizures and epilepsy, 135–138
   seizure types and, 304
Genetic syndromes, 311
Genius, epilepsy and, 43–45
Gestural automatisms, 211
Gilles de la Tourette syndrome, 460
Gingival hyperplasia, 515
GKS. *See* Gamma knife surgery
Glial influences, neuronal excitability, 73
Glibenclamide, drug interactions, 575
Global burden of disease, 660*f*, 661, 662
   DALYs and, 48
   epilepsy, 45, 48–49, 50
Global Campaign Against Epilepsy (GCAE), 645, 661*t*
   demonstration projects, 661
Glucose transporter-1 (GLUT1), 61
Glucuronyl transferase, drug interactions, 561
GLUT1. *See* Glucose transporter-1
Glycine, 66
Glycine receptor, 460

GO. *See* Gene ontology
Grand mal seizures, 14–15. *See also* Generalized
      tonic-clonic seizures
Griseofulvin, drug interactions, 548
GTS. *See* Generalized tonic-clonic seizures
Gustatory symptoms. *See also* Sensory symptoms
   of limbic seizures, 210

Half-life, pharmacological, 499–500, 501, 502*f*, 503, 504*t*
Hallucinations
   complex, 254
   hypnopompic, 457
   ictal formed, 206
   Lilliput, 461
   peduncular, 461
   positive/negative elementary, 254
   schizophrenic, 208
   toxic and metabolic, 454
Haloperidol
   drug interactions, 575
   ictogenic potential, 161
Hamartomas, 388–389
   hypothalamic, 614
      gelastic seizures with, 277, 277*f*
Handel, George Frederick, as epileptic, 44
Hashimoto's disease, 351
HCN channels. *See* Hyperpolarization-activated
      cyclic-nucleotide-gated-cation channels
Head
   drops, 255
   injury
      closed, 172
      early seizures and, 304
      open, 172
   missile wounds, 306
   trauma, 161, 301*f*
      closed, 299
      nonmissile, 298, 299*t*
      withdrawal seizures and, 281
   turning, 205, 211
Headache
   migraine, 456, 461
   postictal, 268
   after seizures, 333–334
Head nodding syndrome, 278
Health care disparities, 660–662, 660*f*
   education and social intervention, 661
   epidemiological assessment and case finding, 661
   outcome measurement, 661
   service delivery and intervention, 661
Health insurance, 656–657
Health-related quality of life (HRQOL), 12, 379, 605,
      626, 647
Health Resources and Services Administration
      (HRSA), 660
Hematological disorders, antiseizure drug-related, 513
Hemiballismus, 459
Hemiconvulsion-hemiplegia-epilepsy (HHE),
      277–278, 351
Hemifacial spasms, 461
Hemimegalencephaly, 174, 175*f*
Hemiplegia
   acute, 358
   alternating, in childhood, 460–461
   familial hemiplegic migraine, 456
   HHE, 277–278, 351

Hemispherectomy, 604, 613–614, 613f
  complications, 628
  modified, 613
Hemispherotomy, 613–614
Hemorrhage
  cerebral, 172
  intracerebral, 350
  intracranial, 420
  intraventricular, 282
  neonatal seizures and, 281
  subarachnoid, 173
Hemosiderosis, surgical complications, 628
Hepatic dysfunction, 514
Hepatosplenomegaly, 412
Hepatotoxicity, 514
Hercules, as epileptic, 42
Heterotopia, 166
HHE. See Hemiconvulsion-hemiplegia-epilepsy
Hippocampal atrophy, 178
Hippocampal commissure, 614
Hippocampal sclerosis (HS), 110, 182f, 367
  as acquired cause of epilepsy disorders, 177–182
  mossy fiber sprouting and, 129–130, 131f
  MTLE with, 178–182, 250
    clinical description of, 269–272
    cortical thickness of, 273, 274f
    differential diagnosis of, 273–275
    EEG of, 271, 271f
    epidemiology of, 273
    etiology of, 273
    FDG-PET of, 271, 272f
    prognosis of, 275
    treatment of, 275
  resulting from cytotoxic agents, 368
Hippocampal seizures, 125
Hippocampus
  Ammon's horn and, 74, 75f
  epileptic, 129–130, 129f
  epileptogenesis and, 302, 303f
  excitability patterns, 76–77, 81
  MRI and changes in, 306
  neuronal circuits, 90
  neurons, oscillatory patterns of, 77–78
  normal, 182, 183f
Hippocrates, 34–35
Historical perspectives, 33–34
  on epilepsy, 34–45, 49
  on surgery, 604–606
History
  medical
    of epilepsy, 34–41, 49
    past, 411
  pharmacotherapy, 39–40
  psychosocial, 411
  seizure, 406–409
    age at onset and, 408–409, 409t
    aura or prodrome and, 407
    clinical, 407–408
    frequency, 408
    postictal period and, 408
    precipitating factors and pattern in, 408
    progression of symptoms and, 409, 410t
History, diagnostic evaluation and, 405–411
  antiseizure drug, 409
  family, 411
  past medical, 411

  psychosocial, 411
  seizure, 406–409
    age at onset and, 408–409, 409t
    aura or prodrome, 407
    clinical, 407–408
    frequency and, 408
    postictal period and, 408
    precipitating factors and pattern in, 408
    progression of symptoms and, 409, 410t
Holoprosencephaly, 166
Homeopathy, 636
Homosexuality, 381
Hormone replacement, 330
Hormone therapy, 629
Horsley, Victor, 38, 39f
Hosea, as epileptic, 42
Hot water epilepsy, 269, 325
HRQOL. See Health-related quality of life
HRSA. See Health Resources and Services Administration
HS. See Hippocampal sclerosis
Huperzine A, 595
Hydantoins
  ethotoin, 583–584
  fosphenytoin, 582–583
  mephenytoin, 583
Hydantoin syndrome, fetal, 551
Hydrocephalus, surgical complications, 628
Hydrochlorothiazide, drug interactions, 575
HYP. See Hypersynchronous ictal onset pattern
Hypercarbia
  in experimental models, 100
Hyperexcitability, 55. See also Neuronal excitation
Hyperglycemia, 516
  nonketogenic, 325
  nonketotic, 362
Hypergraphia, 381
Hyperkinetic automatisms, 211
Hyperparathyroidism, 166
Hyperplasia, gingival, 515
Hyperpolarization, 103, 104f
Hyperpolarization-activated cyclic-nucleotide-gated-
    cation (HCN) channels, 57
Hyperpyrexia, 344
Hyperreligiosity, 381
Hypersensitive adverse side effects, 513–517
Hypersynchronous (HYP) ictal onset pattern,
    125, 125f, 622
Hyperthermia-induced generalized seizures, 114
Hyperventilation
  chronic, 453
  differential diagnosis, 453–454, 453t
  episodes, 454
  systemic symptoms of, 454
Hypnic jerk, 284
Hypocretin, 457
Hypoglycemia, 330, 347, 454
  alcohol withdrawal seizures and, 467
Hypomagnesemia, 166
Hypomania, 383
Hypometabolism, interictal zone of, 130
Hypometamorphosis, 381
Hypoparathyroidism, 166
Hyposexuality, 381
Hypotension, 350
Hypothalamic hamartoma, 614
  gelastic seizures with, 277, 277f

Hypothalamic-pituitary adrenal axis, 375
Hypothalamus, anterior, 326–327
Hypothesis, 528
Hypothesis-driven approaches, molecular genetics, 136
Hypotonia, 460
Hypoxia, 350
    as epileptogenic stimuli, 83
    in experimental models, 100
    perinatal, 113–114
Hypsarrhythmia, 229, 230f, 231f, 313
Hysteria, epilepsy confused with, 34
Hysteroepilepsy, 14, 39, 461
3-Hz spike-and-wave discharges, 222, 223f
6-Hz limbic seizure test, 592
6-Hz positive spikes, 471, 472f
6-Hz spike-and-wave pattern, 471, 475f
14-Hz positive spikes, 471, 472f

IAP. *See* Intracarotid amobarbital procedure
IBE. *See* International Bureau for Epilepsy
ICA. *See* Independent component analysis
ICA105665, 595
ICD. *See* International Classification of Diseases
Ictal (term), 3, 8–9
Ictal initiation, 320–326
    abortive stimuli, 326
    clinical considerations for
        genetic reflex epilepsies and, 322–324
        reflex seizures and, 322, 322t
    mechanisms of, 321
    reflex epilepsies due to structural lesions, 324–325
    reflex myoclonus, 326
    simple *versus* complex reflex epilepsies, 325–326, 325t
Ictal onset
    patterns, 197–198
    sites, 194, 195t
    zone, 616–617
Ictal period
    aggressive behavior in, 465
    behavior in, 376–378
    depressed mood in, 382–383
    events in, 8, 36
        psychiatric symptoms resembled or
            mimicked by, 376
Ictal state, interictal state transition to, 140–141
Ictal termination as possible mechanism of human
        epileptic phenomena, 142
Ictogenesis, 8, 10
    as possible mechanism of human epileptic phenomena,
        140–141
Ictogenic potential, 161
Ictus, 8
    as possible mechanism of human epileptic
        phenomena, 141–142
Idiopathic epilepsy, 7, 31, 36
Idiopathic generalized epilepsy (IGE), 248. *See also*
        Generalized epilepsies
Idiopathic photosensitive occipital lobe epilepsy, 268, 322
Idiopathic seizures, 18
The Idiot (Dostoyevsky), 646
IEGs. *See* Immediate early genes
IGE. *See* Idiopathic generalized epilepsy
iGluRs. *See* Ionotropic glutamate receptors
Ignatius, Saint, as epileptic, 42
ILAE. *See* International League Against Epilepsy
Illusions, 206

Imipramine, sleep disorder, 457
Immature brain
    epileptic susceptibility of, 312, 314
    treatment and, 313–314
Immediate early genes (IEGs), 137
Immune-mediated diseases, 176–177
Immune therapy, 629–630
Immunological side effects, 516
Impaired consciousness, 16, 28, 203
Incidence
    absence status epilepticus, 359
    age-related, 162
    age-specific
        benign epilepsy of childhood, 47
        rates, 45, 47–50, 47f, 48f
    chronic epilepsy, after neonatal seizures, 283, 283t
    cumulative, 46
    definitions of, 45–46
    epilepsia partialis continua, 361
    epilepsy, 45–46
        WHO, 33
    estimates of, 46–48, 47f, 48f
    focal dyscognitive status epilepticus, 364
    generalized convulsive status epilepticus, 351
    methodological considerations, 46
    PTE, late, 301, 301t
    rates, 45, 49–50
    sex-specific, 45–46
Incontinence
    during dyscognitive seizures, 212
    in postictal period, 217
IND. *See* Investigational new drug; Notice of Claimed
        Investigational Exemption for a New Drug
Independent component analysis (ICA), 89, 436–437
Infancy
    benign myoclonus of early, 247
    epilepsy syndromes of
        BFIE, 249
        BIE, 249
        DS, 249
        MEI, 248–249
        MPSI, 245–246
        myoclonic encephalopathy in nonprogressive
            disorders, 249–250
        WS, 246–248
    late infantile ceroid lipofuscinosis, 482
    pharmacological treatment in, 524
    SIDS, 336
    surgical treatment in, 618
Infantile spasms, 228–229, 246, 312
    benign, 247
    treatment, 520
Infantile syncope, 452–453
    pallid form of, 453
Infection
    as acquired cause of epilepsy disorders, 169
    as epileptogenic stimuli, 83
    FIRES, 367
    as risk factor, 161
    viral, 166, 276
Infectious diseases as acquired cause of epilepsy
        disorders, 174–176
Inflammation-mediated disorders as acquired cause of
        epilepsy disorders, 176–177
Inheritance
    factors, genetic differentiated from, 160

genetic disorders, 166, 168*f*
multifactorial, 160–161, 160*f*
Inhibition
  enzymes
    elimination and, 499, 499*f*, 500*f*
    polytherapy and, 506, 506*f*
  feedback, 75, 76*f*
  feedforward, 75, 76*f*, 103, 104*f*
  neuronal, 75–77, 76*f*, 77*f*
  presynaptic, 66
Inhibitory neurotransmitters, 66
Inhibitory postsynaptic potential (IPSP), 60*f*, 62. *See also*
    EPSP-IPSP complex
Initial slow waves (ISWs), 125
Insulin, epilepsia partialis continua, 363
The Insulted and the Injured (Dostoyevsky), 646
Insult models, 109–113, 111*f*, 112*f*, 113*f*, 114*f*, 115*f*
Intellectual function
  behavioral disturbances and, 380
  epilepsy and, 43–45
Intercurrent illness, 508
Interference effect, 116
Interhemispheric influences on excitability, 82
Interictal behavioral disturbances, mechanisms of,
    387–395
  effects of treatment on, 389–392, 389*t*
  epilepsy-induced neurobiological factors and,
    392–396, 394*f*
  neuropathological factors in, 388–389
  psychosocial factors in, 387–388
Interictal period, 8–9
  on EEG, 9
  ictal state and transition from, 140–141
  inhibitors, 140
  as possible mechanism of human epileptic phenomena,
    139–140
  psychosis in, 384–385
  spikes in, 122
    migration of, 313
    in various cortical areas, 300, 300*t*
Interictal zone of hypometabolism, 130
Intermittent explosive disorders, differential diagnosis,
    464–465
International Bureau for Epilepsy (IBE), 645, 658*t*
International Classification of Diseases (ICD), 18
  epilepsy section of ninth, 19*t*
  epilepsy section of tenth, 20*t*
International Classification of Epilepsies, 1970 (ILAE),
    17–18, 17*t*
  revision of, 25
International Classification of Epileptic Seizures (ILAE),
    15, 16*t*, 193
  revision of, 25
International League Against Epilepsy (ILAE), 4, 45, 646,
    658–660, 658*t*
  diagnostic manual, 31
  epilepsy defined by, 6–7
  International Classification of Epilepsies, 1970,
    17–18, 17*t*
  International Classification of Epileptic Seizures,
    15, 16*t*
  terminology revision and, 27
Interneuronal connections
  chemical synapses and, 64–72, 65*f*
  electronic synapses and, 72
  nonsynaptic communication and, 72–73

Interventions
  health care education and social, 661
  health care service delivery and, 661
  physical, 635
  social, health care disparities and, 661
Intracarotid amobarbital procedure (IAP), 271, 439–440,
    604, 621
Intracerebroventricular enkephalin model, 554
Investigational new drug (IND), 591
In vitro studies
  of acute seizures, 107–109
  of chronic epilepsy, 121–122
In vivo models
  of epilepsy with focal seizures
    models of developing brain, 113–115
    secondary epileptogenesis, 115–120, 117*f*
  of epilepsy with generalized seizures, 120–121
  of focal seizures, 101–105
  of generalized seizures, 105–107
Ion channels
  charge gradient of, 57
  coding genes, 57*t*
  concentration gradient of, 57
Ionophores, 56
Ionotropic glutamate receptors (iGluRs), 68, 69*f*
Ions, 57
Ipsiversive movements, 211
IPSP. *See* Inhibitory postsynaptic potential
Irritative zone, 196
Isaiah, as epileptic, 42
Isoniazid, drug interactions, 548
  PHT, 551
ISWs. *See* Initial slow waves

Jackknife seizure, 229
Jackson, John Hughlings, 4, 36–38, 37*f*
Jacksonian march of motor symptoms, 15
JAE. *See* Juvenile absence epilepsy
Jamais entendu/vécu/vu, 210. *See also* Memory
Jeanne A. Carpenter Epilepsy Legal Defense Fund, 656
Jeavons syndrome, 225
Jeremiah, as epileptic, 42
Jesus, epileptic child and, 41–42, 43*f*, 44*f*
Jitteriness, 455
JME. *See* Juvenile myoclonic epilepsy
John, Saint, as patron saint of epilepsy, 42
Johnson, Samuel, as epileptic, 44
Judaism, epilepsy and, 41
Julius Caesar, as epileptic, 43
Jumping Frenchmen of Maine, 460
Juvenile absence epilepsy (JAE), 263
  confusion in, 263
  medication discontinuation, 522
Juvenile myoclonic epilepsy (JME), 351
  clinical description, 263
  differential diagnosis, 263–265
  EEG, 263, 264*f*
  epidemiology, 263
  etiology, 263
  prognosis, 265
  treatment, 265
    LTG and, 568
    VPA and, 265, 561

Kainic acid, 104
  HS and, 368

K⁺ concentration, extracellular, 60–61
K⁺ current, 58, 59f
Ketamine, generalized convulsive status epilepticus, 357
Ketogenic diet, 530, 636
    drug interactions, VPA, 561, 630–631
Kidneys, medical treatment of epilepsy and, 527
Kindled epileptogenesis, 117–118
Kindling, 10, 39, 609
    amygdala-kindled model, 592
    in animals, 118
    caudate, 118
    chemical, 118–119
    clinical relevance of, 310
    epilepsy compared with, 307, 308t
    model of epilepsy, 298
    molecular basis of, 118–119
    rapid, 117
    secondary epileptogenesis and, 116–118, 307
    status epilepticus models of epilepsy and, 119
Kinesiology, 636
Kleine-Levin syndrome, 457–458
Klüver-Bucy syndrome, 380
Kojewnikow syndrome, 360
Krabbe's disease, 166

Laboratory examination, diagnostic evaluation and
    clinical laboratory tests, 415, 416t
    EEG
        special approaches to, 417–425
        when to use EEG, 415–417
    functional neuroimaging
        fMRI, 435–438, 438f, 439f
        MRS, 438
        PET, 432–434
        rectilinear radionuclide brain scanning, 438–439
        SPECT, 434–435, 436f
    MEG, 426–427, 428f
    structural neuroimaging
        MRI, 429–432, 430f, 431f
        radiographs, 432
        x-ray CT, 432, 432f
    TMS, 427–429
Lacosamide (LCM)
    administration, 567
    drug interactions, 566
    generalized convulsive status epilepticus, 357
    indications, 566–567
    mechanisms of action, 566
    pharmacokinetics, 566
    toxicity, 566
Lactic acidosis, 335
Lafora bodies, 265–266
Lafora disease, 166
Lamotrigine (LTG)
    administration, 568–569
    adverse behavioral effects of, 389t, 390
    BECTS, 253
    CAE, 262
    choosing appropriate drug and, 518–519
    comorbidity and, 527
    drug efficacy, 508
    drug interactions, 568
        ESL, 562
        OXC, 570, 571
        RUF, 573
        VPA, 561, 567

DS, 249
EMAS, 251
indications, 568
JAE, 263
JME, 265
LGS, 259
mechanisms of action, 567
monitoring, 517
nursing and, 527
pharmacokinetics, 567
psychotropic effects of, 390, 391t
tapering, 508
toxicity, 567–568
trials, 519
WS, 247
Landau-Kleffner syndrome (LKS), 260, 327
    CSWS, 310
Language, 381
    cortical, 78
    disorders, 195t
    lesion location and, 388
    LKS and, 260
    Rasmussen's syndrome and, 276–277
Language-dominant hemisphere
    aphasic features and, 210, 216t
    MTLE and, 380, 627
    surgical treatment and, 391, 618
Lapp panic, 460
Late childhood occipital epilepsy (Gastaut type), 254
Late infantile ceroid lipofuscinosis, 482
Lateral temporal lobe epilepsy, with auditory features,
        57. See also Temporal lobe epilepsies
LCM. See Lacosamide
Lear, Edward, as epileptic, 44
Learned helplessness, 387
Lee, Anne, as epileptic, 42
Legal defense, epilepsy as, 377, 656
Legal rights, 655–656
Le Guide Bleu. See Blue Guide
Lennox-Gastaut syndrome (LGS), 222, 245, 312, 350, 519
    CLB for, 557
    clinical description, 255–256, 256f, 257f
    differential diagnosis, 257–259, 258t
    epidemiology, 256
    etiology, 256–257
    medication discontinuation, 522
    prognosis, 259
    treatment, 259
Lesionectomies, selective, 608
Lesion models, 109–113, 111f, 112f, 113f, 114f, 115f
Lesions, 198. See also specific lesions
    character, epilepsy development and, 299–300
    epileptogenic, 3, 31, 617
        definition, 10
        terminology, 10–11
    location
        epilepsy development and, 300–302
        hamartomas, 388
    structural
        focal, 310
        reflex epilepsies due to, 324–325
    vascular, 172, 173f
Leukopenia, 514, 558
Levetiracetam (LEV)
    administration, 570
    adverse behavioral effects of, 389t

adverse side effects, dose-dependent, 513
 comorbidity and, 528
 dose planning, 503
 drug interactions, 569
 EMAS, 251
 focal dyscognitive status epilepticus, 364
 generalized convulsive status epilepticus, 357
 indications, 569–570
 JAE, 263
 JME, 265
 LGS, 259
 loading dose, 503
 mechanisms of action, 569
 MEI, 249
 MTLE, 275
 myoclonus, 237
 pharmacokinetics, 569
 psychotropic effects of, 390, 391t
 toxicity, 569
 trials, 519
Levodopa, syncope due to, 452
LGS. *See* Lennox-Gastaut syndrome
Ligand-gated channels, 56
Lilliput hallucinations, 461
Limbic dyscognitive seizures, 270
Limbic epilepsy, 270
Limbic seizures, 16, 79–80, 122
 clinical considerations, 213–215, 216t
 EEG, 212–213, 213f, 214f
 FDG-PET, 213, 215f
 mechanisms, 209
 phenomenology
  automatisms and, 209–211
  autonomic symptoms and signs, 210
  motor symptoms and, 211–212
  psychic symptoms and, 210
  sensory symptoms, 209–210
Limbic system, 375
Limbic temporal lobe seizures, 210
Lipid storage disorders, 166
Lissencephaly, 166
Lithium
 drug interactions
  OXC, 570
  TPM, 575
 HS and, 368
 intermittent explosive disorders, 465
Liver
 antiseizure drugs in
  biotransformation of, 498f, 499
  clinical efficacy of, 508
 disease, 514
 medical treatment of epilepsy and, 527
LKS. *See* Landau-Kleffner syndrome
Loading dose, pharmacological, 501–503
Lobectomy
 anterior temporal, 304, 392
 anteromesial temporal, 530
Localization of lesion
 epilepsy development and, 300–302
 hamartomas, 388
Localization-related epilepsy, 18
 generalized epilepsy and, 25
Local seizures, 15
Locus heterogeneity, 164
Long-term potentiation (LTP), 119

Lopinavir, comorbidity and, 527
Lorazepam (LZP), 555
 alcohol and sedative drug withdrawal, 528
 DZP compared with, 556
 epilepsia partialis continua, 363
 generalized convulsive status epilepticus, 352, 354,
  354t, 355, 356
 neonatal seizures, 283
 neonatal status epilepticus, 367–368
Louis XIII of France, as epileptic, 43
Low-voltage fast (LVF) ictal onset pattern, 125, 125f,
  126–129, 127f
LTG. *See* Lamotrigine
LTP. *See* Long-term potentiation
Lupoid drug reactions, 516
Lupus erythematosus, 516
LVF. *See* Low-voltage fast ictal onset pattern
Lysosomal storage diseases, 166
LZP. *See* Lorazepam

Macewen, William, 38–39
Magnesium, chronic epilepsy, 305
Magnesium sulfate, 525
Magnetic resonance imaging (MRI), 122, 441
 hippocampal changes with, 306
 presurgical imaging, 605
 structural neuroimaging, 429–432, 430f, 431f
Magnetic resonance spectroscopy (MRS), 134, 438, 621
Magnetoencephalography (MEG), 11, 424, 426–427, 428f
 presurgical imaging, 605
Malay latah, 460
Malformations of cortical development (MCD), 83
 as acquired cause of epilepsy disorders, 177
 classification scheme, 177, 178t
Malingering, 14
MAM. *See* Methylazoxymethanol acetate
Mammalian target of rapamycin (mTOR), 167, 298.
  See also Rapamycin
Maprotiline, ictogenic potential, 161
Marijuana, 632–633, 652
Mastoid electrodes, 417
Maturational effects on excitability and synchronization,
  83–84, 85f
Maturational factors, 162
 immature brain
  epileptic susceptibility of, 312, 314
  treatment and, 313–314
Maximal electroshock (MES), 542
 mouse model, 591–592
MCD. *See* Malformations of cortical development
MCT. *See* Medium-chain triglyceride
MDR. *See* Multidrug resistance
3-Mecaptopropionic acid, 66
Medical history
 of epilepsy
  ancient and medieval periods, 34–36
  modern era, 36–41, 49
 past, 411
Medically refractory seizures, 529–530
Medium-chain triglyceride (MCT), 630
MEG. *See* Magnetoencephalography
Megaloblastic anemia, 514
MEI. *See* Myoclonic epilepsy in infancy
Melatonin, 629
Melchior, as patron of epilepsy, 42
Memory. *See also* Amnesia

Memory (cont.)
  deficits, 380
  dysmnesic symptoms, 210
  episodic, 78
Meningitis, 279
  alcohol withdrawal seizures and, 467
  as epilepsy cause, 175
Menopause, 330
Menses, 329
Mental deficiency, 358
Meperidine, surgery and, 528
Mephenytoin, 550, 583
  adverse side effects, 516
Meprobamate, 563
MERRF. See Myoclonus epilepsy with ragged red fibers
MES. See Maximal electroshock
Mesial temporal lobe epilepsy (MTLE), 110–111, 184f,
        302, 367
  familial, 273
  with HS, 178–182, 250
    clinical description of, 269–272
    cortical thickness of, 273, 274f
    differential diagnosis of, 273–275
    EEG of, 271, 271f
    epidemiology of, 273
    etiology of, 273
    FDG-PET of, 271, 272f
    prognosis of, 275
    treatment of, 275
  as surgically remediable syndrome, 610, 611t
  treatment, LEV, 569
Mesial temporal sclerosis, 368
Metabolic disorders
  carbohydrate, 167
  mineral, 515
  neonatal seizures due to
    clinical description of, 281
    differential diagnosis of, 282
    epidemiology of, 282
    etiology of, 282
    prognosis of, 283
    treatment of, 282–283
  neurological dysfunction and, 454–455
Metabolic disturbances
  as acquired cause of epilepsy disorders, 177
  differential diagnosis, 454–455
Metabolic encephalopathy, 455
Metabolic influences, 329–330
Metformin, drug interactions, 575
Metharbital, 543, 580
Methionine sulfoximine, neuronal excitability and, 61
Methohexital, 543
  IAP, 440
Methsuximide, 588–589
  drug interactions
    FBM, 564
    PHT, 551
Methylazoxymethanol acetate (MAM), 114
Methylphenobarbital, 543, 580
Methylprednisolone, 579
α-methyl-tryptophan (AMT), 132, 621
  PET, 306
Metoprolol, drug interactions, 548
Metronidazole, drug interactions, 551
Metyrapone test, 515
MHD. See 10-monohydroxy derivative

Microanatomical investigations, 134
Microarray research, 136
Microdysgenesis, 166
Midazolam, 555, 581
  generalized convulsive status epilepticus, 352, 357
Migraine, 456, 461
Mimetic automatisms, 210–211
Minerals, 631
  metabolism disorders, 515
Minisphenoidals, 419
Minnesota Multiphasic Personality Index (MMPI), 380–381
  PNES on, 462
Mirror focus, 10, 307, 609
Misdiagnosis
  epilepsy, 450
  PS, 250
Mitochondrial disorders, 169
Mixed seizure disorders, 519
MMPI. See Minnesota Multiphasic Personality Index
Models. See also Animal models; In vivo models
  acute, 100–109, 101t
    convulsant drugs, proposed mechanisms of action of,
        100, 102t
    penicillin, 103, 104f, 105f
    in vitro studies of acute seizures, 107–109
    in vivo models of focal seizures, 101–105
    in vivo models of generalized seizures, 105–107
  amygdala-kindled, 592
  chronic, 109–122
    in vitro studies of chronic epilepsy, 121–122
    in vivo models of epilepsy with focal seizures, lesion
        and insult models, 109–113, 111f, 112f, 113f,
        114f, 115f
  experimental, of seizures and epilepsy, 100–122
    acute, 100–109, 101t
    ESM and, 554
  feline generalized penicillin, 106, 107f, 554
  γ-hydroxybutyrate, 554, 560
  insult, 109–113, 111f, 112f, 113f, 114f, 115f
  intracerebroventricular enkephalin, 554
  lesion, 109–113, 111f, 112f, 113f, 114f, 115f
Modification
  behavioral, 530
  disease, 3, 297
    definition, 13
    terminology, 13–14, 297t
  seizure, 13, 297
    terminology, 297t
  syndrome, 297
    terminology, 297t
Mohammed, as epileptic, 42
Molecular genetics
  discovery-driven approaches, 136
  hypothesis-driven approaches, 136
  of seizures and epilepsy, 135–138
Molecular neurobiology, 90
Molière, as epileptic, 44
Molindone hydrochloride, drug interactions, 551
Monitoring
  EEG, generalized convulsive status epilepticus
        treatment, 357–358
  pharmacological treatment, 517–518
  VEM, 422–424, 422f, 423t, 441
    ambulatory recorder, 423
    differential diagnosis and, 487
    PNES, 463

10-monohydroxy derivative (MHD), 570
Monotherapy, pharmacological, 503–508, 533
   advantages of, 507–508
   crossover in, 507
   dose and, 503–507
Mood, 382–383
Moodiness, 381–382
Morbidity, tonic-clonic status epilepticus-associated, 350
Morphine, 331
Morphometry, voxel-based, 132
Morris, William, as epileptic, 44
Mortality
   comorbidity and, 335
   drowning, 337
   SUDEP and, 335–337; 451
   after surgery, 336, 606
Mossy fiber sprouting, 129–130, 131f
Motionless stare, 209
Motor disorders
   differential diagnosis, 459–461
   paroxysmal, of sleep, 458, 458t
Motor events, 15
Motor seizures, 205
   generalized, 15
   supplementary motor area seizures, 324
Motor signs, neocortex seizures, 205–206
Motor symptoms
   Jacksonian march of, 15
   of limbic seizures, 211–212
   simple partial seizure, 15
Motor vehicle accidents, 649, 650t
Movement disorders
   intermittent muscle spasms, 461
   sleep, 458
      PLMS, 284
Moxibustion, 633
Moyamoya disease, 456
MPSI. *See* Epilepsy of infancy with migrating focal
     seizures
MRI. *See* Magnetic resonance imaging
MRS. *See* Magnetic resonance spectroscopy
MSLT. *See* Multiple Sleep Latency Test
MST. *See* Multiple subpial transection
MTLE. *See* Mesial temporal lobe epilepsy
mTOR. *See* Mammalian target of rapamycin
Multidrug resistance (MDR), 61
Multifactorial inheritance, 160–161, 160f
Multiple Sleep Latency Test (MSLT), 328
Multiple subpial transection (MST), 608, 615
Muscle spasms, intermittent, 461
Musicogenic epilepsy, 324–325
Myasthenia gravis-like syndrome, 515
Myelin disorders, 166
Myoclonia, eyelid, 225, 324
Myoclonic absences, 224–225. *See also* Absences
Myoclonic atonic seizures, 226
Myoclonic encephalopathy in nonprogressive disorders,
    249–250, 351
Myoclonic epilepsy in infancy (MEI), 248–249
Myoclonic seizures, 283
   EEG, 226
   mechanisms, 225
   phenomenology, 225–226
Myoclonic syndromes
   benign essential myoclonus, 284
   epilepsy syndromes, 283–284

   nocturnal myoclonus, 284
   posthypoxic myoclonus, 284
Myoclonic tonic seizures, 226
Myoclonus, 5, 203–204, 233–237, 283
   action, 225
      of acquired neurological disturbances, 236
      posthypoxic, 284
      with progressive myoclonus epilepsies, 326
      renal failure syndrome, 267
   Baltic, 266
   benign, of early infancy, 247
   benign essential, 236, 284
   benign myoclonus of early infancy, 247
   cherry-red spot, 266
   classification, 233, 236t, 237
   cortical, 236
   dystonia, 284
   excessive fragmentary, in non-REM sleep, 284
   focal negative, 205
   generalized, 236
   localized, 233
   nocturnal, 284
   nonepileptic, 283
   phenomena, 283
   posthypoxic, 284
   reflex, 236
      ictal initiation, 326
      reticular, 237
   segmental, 236
   sporadic, 233
   among storage disorders, 266, 267t
   syndromes, 283–284
   treatment, 237
Myoclonus epilepsy with ragged red fibers (MERRF),
    166, 266

N-2-glucuronides, 567
N-5-glucuronides, 567
Na$^+$ channels, 57–58, 58f
   absolute refractory period, 60
   action potential, 58, 59f
NAEC. *See* National Association of Epilepsy Centers, US
Naloxone, 331
Napoleon I, as epileptic, 43
Naproxen, drug interactions, 574
Narcolepsy, 457
National Association of Epilepsy Centers,
    US (NAEC), 606
National Institute of Neurological Disorders and Stroke
    (NINDS), 99, 660
   new-drug development, 590
National Institutes of Health (NIH), 660
Naturopathy, 636
Nausea
   as drug side effect, 551
   in syncope, 452
NDA. *See* New Drug Application
N-desmethyl metabolite, 589
Necrolysis, epidermal, 558
Neocortex
   excitability, 81
   intrinsic organization, 78, 79f, 80f
   neuronal circuits, 90
Neocortical seizures
   clinical considerations, 207–209
   EEG, 206–207, 207f

Neocortical seizures (cont.)
  mechanisms, 204
  PET, 207, 208f
  phenomenology, 204–206
    motor signs and, 205–206
    sensory symptoms of, 206
Neonatal brain, 312
Neonatal period epilepsy syndromes
  BFNE, 244–245
  EME, 245
  OS, 245
Neonatal seizures, 229–233, 312–313
  benign, 7–8
  causes, 169, 171t
  chronic epilepsy incidence after, 283, 283t
  classification, 229–232, 232t
  due to structural and metabolic disorders
    clinical description of, 281
    differential diagnosis of, 282
    epidemiology of, 282
    etiology of, 282
    prognosis of, 283
    treatment of, 282–283
  EEG, 232–233, 232t, 234f
  emergency treatment of, 532
  ictal patterns, 229–232
Neonatal status epilepticus, 367–368
Neonates, pharmacological treatment and, 523–524
Nerve stimulation
  TNS, 629
  VNS, 530, 534, 603, 615, 628–629
    diathermy in, 629
Nervous system, antiseizure drug effects on, 515
Neuralgia, 566
Neuraminidase deficiencies, 166
Neurobiological factors, epilepsy-induced, 392–396, 394f
Neurobiology
  epileptic seizure types and, 194–199
    anatomical substrates of, 194–197, 195t
    pathophysiological mechanisms of, 197–198
    pharmacological considerations for, 198–199
  molecular, 90
Neurocysticercosis, 608
Neurofibromatoses, 412, 412f
  as epilepsy cause, 166
Neuroimaging. See also specific imaging techniques
  epilepsy, studies of human, 130–134
  functional
    fMRI, 435–438, 438f, 439f
    MRS, 438
    PET, 432–434
    rectilinear radionuclide brain scanning, 438–439
    SPECT, 434–435, 436f
  structural
    MRI, 429–432, 430f, 431f
    radiographs, 432
    x-ray CT, 432, 432f
Neurological deficits
  epilepsy disorders associated with, 14
  focal, 332
  postictal, 9
Neurological disorders, positive/negative symptoms, 4
Neurological disturbances
  epileptic seizures and, 7
  nonepileptic paroxysmal event differential
    diagnosis and

cerebrovascular disorders, 455–457
  motor disorders, 459–461
  sensory disorders, 461
  sleep disorders, 457–459
Neurological dysfunction, 454–455
Neurological examination, diagnostic evaluation and,
  413–414
Neurological function, behavioral disturbances and, 380
Neurological side effects, 513
Neuromodulators, 66, 67, 91
Neuronal basis of epileptogenicity, 144
Neuronal ceroid lipofuscinoses, 166, 266
Neuronal circuits, 90
Neuronal destruction, 4
Neuronal excitation, 55–91, 321
  EEG activity and, 86–87, 87f
  endogenous factors modulating, 321
  exogenous factors modulating, 321
  glial influences, 73
  interneuronal connections
    chemical synapses and, 64–72, 65f
    electronic synapses and, 72
    nonsynaptic communication and, 72–73
    receptor concentrations, 71–72
  intracellular processes, 61–62
  long-term changes, 61
  maturational effects on, 83–84, 85f
  methodological developments, 87–89
  neuron, 56–73
    excitable membrane and microenvironment, 56–61
    intracellular processes, 61–62
    structure-function relationships of neuronal
      elements, 62–64, 63f
  neuronal networks, 73–82, 74f
    intrinsic organization of Ammon's horn, 74–78, 75f
    intrinsic organization of neocortex and, 78, 79f, 80f
    subcortical and interhemispheric connections, 78–82
  pharmacological agents altering, 61
  phylogeny and ontogeny, species differences in, 82
  plastic changes, 61
  presynaptic, stimulation of, 67
  structure-function relationships of neuronal elements,
    62–64, 63f
  synapses, chemical, 64–72, 65f
  systemic influences on, 85–86
Neuronal inhibition, 75–77, 76f, 77f
Neuronal networks, 73–82, 74f
  computer modeling of, 89
  intrinsic organization of Ammon's horn, 74–78, 75f
  intrinsic organization of neocortex and, 78, 79f, 80f
  subcortical and interhemispheric connections, 78–82
Neuronal storage disorders, 266
Neuronal synchronization, 55–91, 321
  EEG activity and, 86–87, 87f
  glial influences, 73
  interneuronal connections
    chemical synapses and, 64–72, 65f
    electronic synapses and, 72
    nonsynaptic communication and, 72–73
    receptor concentrations, 71–72
  intracellular processes, 61–62
  long-term changes, 61
  maturational effects on, 83–84, 85f
  methodological developments, 87–89
  neuron, 56–73
    intracellular processes, 61–62

structure-function relationships of neuronal elements, 62–64, 63f
neuronal networks, 73–82, 74f
  intrinsic organization of Ammon's horn, 74–78, 75f
  intrinsic organization of neocortex and, 78, 79f, 80f
  subcortical and interhemispheric connections, 78–82
ontogeny, species differences in, 82
pharmacological agents altering, 61
phylogeny, species differences in, 82
plastic changes, 61
presynaptic, stimulation of, 67
structure-function relationships of neuronal elements, 62–64, 63f
synapses
  chemical, 64–72, 65f
  electronic, 72
systemic influences on, 85–86
Neurons, 56–73
  excitable membrane and microenvironment, 56–61
    membrane physiology and, 57–61
    voltage-gated channels, 56–57, 57t
  hippocampal, oscillatory patterns of, 77–78
  mechanism, epileptic seizures, 4
  neuronal excitation and, 56–73
    excitable membrane and microenvironment, 56–61
    intracellular processes, 61–62
    structure-function relationships of neuronal elements, 62–64, 63f
  neuronal synchronization and
    intracellular processes, 61–62
    structure-function relationships of neuronal elements, 62–64, 63f
Neuron-specific enolase (NSE), 358
Neuropathic pain, 566, 571
Neuropathological factors in interictal behavioral disturbances, 388–389
Neuropathy
  diabetic, 566
  peripheral, 515
Neuropeptides, 66, 67t
Neuropsychiatric disorders in epilepsy, classification of, 385–386, 386t
Neurotransmitters, 67. *See also specific neurotransmitters*
  deactivation of, 65
  excitatory, 59, 62
  inhibitory, 62, 66
  receptors, 56
  release of, 64
  synthesis, 61
Neutral-state syndrome, 457
Nevus anemicus, 412
New Drug Application (NDA), 594
New-drug development, 590–594
  biomarkers, 594
  clinical evaluation of, 592–594
  identification of new compounds and, 591
  preclinical evaluation, 591–592
  rodent models, 592, 593t
Newton, Isaac, as epileptic, 44
Night terrors, 458
NIH. *See* National Institutes of Health
Nimodipine, drug interactions, 561
NINDS. *See* National Institute of Neurological Disorders and Stroke
1985 International Classification of epilepsies and epileptic syndromes, 18–25, 24t

1989 International Classification of epilepsies and epileptic syndromes, 18–25, 24t
Nitrazepam, 555, 581–582
  WS, 247
N-methyl-D-aspartic acid (NMDA), 68–69, 564
  receptor channel complex, 90
  receptor encephalitis, 351
  status epilepticus and, 343
Nobel, Alfred, as epileptic, 44
Nocebo effect, 520
Nocturnal myoclonus, 284
Nocturnal paroxysmal dyskinesias, 460
Nocturnal start, 284
Nodding disease, 278
Nonallopathic medical systems, 635–636
Nonepilepsy, recognizing, 450
Nonepileptic events, recognizing, 487
Nonepileptic paroxysmal events, differential diagnosis
  abdominal epilepsy and, 455
  breath holding and, 452–453
  cerebrovascular disorders and, 455–457
  daydreaming, 466
  dissociative states, 465–466
  hyperventilation and, 453–454
  intermittent explosive disorders, 464–465
  metabolic disturbances and, 454–455
  motor disorders, 459–461
  neurological disturbances, 455–461
  nonpsychotic psychiatric conditions, 466
  PNES, 461–464
  psychogenic disturbances in, 461–466
  psychoses, 466
  sensory disorders and, 461
  sleep disorders and, 457–459
  syncope and, 450–452
  systemic disturbances in, 450–455
  toxic disturbances and, 454–455
Nonepileptic paroxysmal phenomena, 449, 451t
Nonepileptic seizures, 3, 4
  PNES, 14, 330
    diagnosis, 464
    differential diagnosis, 375, 461–464, 487
    EEG, 462–463
    features, 462
    on MMPI, 462
    treatment, 464
  psychogenic, 31
  terminology, 14
Nonepileptic signs and symptoms, 5
Nonketogenic hyperglycemia, 325
Nonketotic hyperglycemia, 362
Nonpharmacological therapy, 603–637. *See also specific therapies*
  CAM
    behavioral therapies, 633–635
    diet, 630–632
    traditional and folk medicine, 632–633, 632t, 633t
  hormone therapy, 629
  immune therapy, 629–630
  surgical
    candidates for, 607–609, 607t, 618, 619f
    for children and infants, 618
    cost, 606–607
    development of new centers, 628
    diagnostic testing before, 617–618
    early, arguments for, 609

Nonpharmacological therapy (*cont.*)
    historical perspectives on, 604–606
    mortality rate after, 606
    outcome, 623–628, 626*t*
    pharmacoresistance and, 606–607
    presurgical imaging, 605
    protocols, 616–623
    schizencephaly, 608
    therapeutic procedures, 611–616
    tuberous sclerosis, 608
    underutilization of, 606
    VNS, 628–629
Nonprogressive disorders, myoclonic encephalopathy in, 249–250, 351
Nonpsychotic psychiatric conditions, differential diagnosis, 466
non-REM (NREM), 327. *See also* Rapid eye movement
    Excessive fragmentary myoclonus in, 284
    sleep disorders, 458
Nonspecific predisposing factors, epilepsy, 157–162
    dynamic aspects of threshold and, 162
    environmental factors, 161–162
    genetic factors, 159–161, 159*f*
    threshold and, 186
Nonsynaptic communications, 72–73
Nordazepam, 555
Notice of Claimed Investigational Exemption for a New Drug (IND), 592
NREM. *See* non-REM
NSE. *See* Neuron-specific enolase
Numbness, 4, 206
Nursing, 653
    antiseizure drugs and, 527
Nystagmus, 270, 344
    as drug side effect, 390

Obsessive-compulsive disorder (OCD), 466
Obstructive sleep apnea, 459
Occipital spike driving, 481–482, 483*f*
OCD. *See* Obsessive-compulsive disorder
Oculocephalic reflex, 452
Ohtahara syndrome (OS), 245
Olanzapine, drug interactions, 568
Olfactory symptoms of limbic seizures, 209–210. *See also* Sensory symptoms
Ontogeny
    cortical development, 82–83
    maturational effects on excitability, 83–84, 85*f*
    species differences in, 82
Opioids, endogenous
    in kindling, 119
    in postictal period, 393
    properties, 66
    seizures induction with, 106
Optical imaging, 622
Optogenetics, 88
Oral contraceptives, 520
    drug efficacy, 508
    drug interactions
        PHT, 552
        TPM, 575
Organizations for epilepsy, 658*t*
Oroalimentary automatisms, 210
OS. *See* Ohtahara syndrome
Oscillatory patterns, hippocampal neurons, 77–78
Osteoporosis, 515

Ouabain, neuronal excitability and, 61
Owsei, Temkin, 34
Oxazolidinediones
    paramethadione, 585
    trimethadione, 584–585
Oxcarbazepine (OXC)
    administration, 571
    adverse side effects, 516
        dose-dependent, 513
    BECTS, 253
    choosing appropriate drug and, 518–520
    drug interactions, 571
        LTG, 568
        PHT, 551
    elimination, 499
    EMA aggravated by, 255
    indications, 571
    JME exacerbated by, 265
    mechanisms of action, 570
    MEI, 249
    pharmacokinetics, 570
    positive psychotropic effects, 390
    psychotropic effects of, 390, 391*t*
    toxicity, 570–571
    trials, 519
Oxygen
    BOLD, 133, 435
    hyperbaric, 100
    hypoxia, 350
        as epileptogenic stimuli, 83
        in experimental models, 100
        perinatal, 113–114
    metabolism, 433, 433*t*

Paganini, Nicolo, as epileptic, 44
Pain
    neuropathic, 566, 571
    paroxysmal extreme, 455
Palm Desert Conference on Surgical Treatment of Epilepsies, 604
Panayiotopoulos syndrome (PS), 250–251
    misdiagnosis, 250
Pancuronium bromide, 455
Panic attacks, 466
Panic disorder, 375
Paracelsus, 35
Parageusia, 210
Paraldehyde, 585–586
    alcohol and sedative drug withdrawal, 528–529
    comorbidity and, 528
    elimination, 499
    generalized convulsive status epilepticus, 355–356
Paralysis
    postictal, 9
    Todd's, 143, 332
Paramethadione, 585
Parasomnia, secondary, 459
Parents
    with epilepsy, 653–654
    of epileptic child, 652–653
Paresthesias, 4, 206
    in psychiatric disorders, 466
Parkinson's disease, 451
    synucleinopathy in, 459
Paroxetine, ictogenic potential, 161
Paroxysmal depolarization shift (PDS), 64, 101, 103*f*

Paroxysmal dyskinesias, 459, 461
    acquired, 460
    nocturnal, 460
Paroxysmal dystonia, 326
Paroxysmal events
    differential diagnosis, 450, 451*t*
    nonepileptic, differential diagnosis
        abdominal epilepsy and, 455
        breath holding and, 452–453
        cerebrovascular disorders and, 455–457
        daydreaming, 466
        dissociative states, 465–466
        hyperventilation and, 453–454
        intermittent explosive disorders, 464–465
        metabolic disturbances and, 454–455
        motor disorders, 459–461
        neurological disturbances, 455–461
        nonpsychotic psychiatric conditions, 466
        PNES, 461–464
        psychogenic disturbances in, 461–466
        psychoses, 466
        sensory disorders and, 461
        sleep disorders and, 457–459
        syncope and, 450–452
        systemic disturbances in, 450–455
        toxic disturbances and, 454–455
Paroxysmal exertional dyskinesia, 460
Paroxysmal extreme pain, 455
Paroxysmal high-frequency oscillations, 436
Paroxysmal motor disorders of sleep, 458, 458*t*
Paroxysmal phenomena, nonepileptic, 449, 451*t*
Paroxysmal vertigo, benign, 461
Partial epilepsies, 17, 26*f*
Partial seizures. *See also* Focal seizures
    affective symptoms in, 210
    classification, 200*t*
    cognitive disturbances in, 210
    complex, 15, 16, 16*t*, 20*t*, 26, 31
        EEG in, 195*t*
        FDG-PET, 334*f*
        in infancy, 213
    consciousness in, 15, 203
    epigastric rising in, 210
    epileptic, 5
    gastrointestinal symptoms in, 210
    simple, 15, 16, 16*t*, 20*t*, 26, 31
        autonomic symptoms of, 15
        EEG in, 195*t*
        motor symptoms of, 15
        psychic symptoms of, 15
        sensory symptoms of, 15
Partial status epilepticus. *See* Focal dyscognitive
            (complex partial) status epilepticus
Pascal, Blaise, as epileptic, 44
Past medical history, 411
Pathological high-frequency oscillations (pHFOs),
            111–112, 111*f*, 112*f*, 113*f*, 126–128, 306, 621
Pathologic mechanisms, epileptic seizures, 5
Paul, Saint, as epileptic, 42
PB. *See* Phenobarbital
PDS. *See* Paroxysmal depolarization shift
PE. *See* Phenytoin-equivalent
Peduncular hallucinations, 461
PEMA. *See* Phenylethylmalonamide
Penicillin, 77
    acute models, 103, 104*f*, 105*f*

feline generalized penicillin model, 106, 107*f*, 554
    human focal epilepsy, 125
Penicillin-induced neocortical epileptic focus, 101
Pentobarbital, 543
    generalized convulsive status epilepticus, 357
    neonatal status epilepticus, 367
Pentylenetetrazol (PTZ)
    EEG, 421
    mouse model, 591–592
    neuronal excitation and, 61–62
    seizure induction, 106
        ESM and, 554
    subcutaneous, 542
Perampanel, 595
Perchlorate, neuronal excitability and, 61
Periictal behavioral, 376–378
Periictal phenomena, 320–337
    ictal initiation and, 320–326
    metabolic influences, 329–330
    mortality, comorbidity and, 335
    postictal symptoms, mechanisms, 331
    psychological stress and, 330
    research issues, 337
    sleep-wake cycles, 326–328
    toxic influences, 329–330
Periodic leg movements of sleep (PLMS), 284
Peripheral neuropathy, 515
Personality
    aggressive personality trait, 381
    Bear-Fedio Personality Inventory, 381–382
    behavioral disturbances and, 380–382
    epileptic, 381, 395
    MMPI, 380–381
        PNES on, 462
Personality disorders, 375
Person with epilepsy (PWE), 8
    families of, explaining epilepsy to, 644–645, 645*t*
    negative public image of, 646
    philosophers, artists and scientists as, 44
    in religion, 42
    rulers and warriors as, 43–44
PET. *See* Positron emission tomography
Peter the Great, as epileptic, 43
Petit mal seizures, 14–15. *See also* Absence seizures
Petrarch, Francesco, as epileptic, 44
P-glycoprotein (PGP), 61
PGN. *See* Pregabalin
PGP. *See* P-glycoprotein
Phakomatoses, 412, 412*f*
Pharmacodynamic actions, 500–501, 502*t*
Pharmacogenomics, 596–597
Pharmacokinetics, 495, 497*t*
    tolerance, 500–501
Pharmacological agents, neuronal excitability-altering, 61
Pharmacological studies, 434
Pharmacological treatment
    adverse side effects, 508–517
        chronic, 513–517
        dose-dependent, 510–513
        hypersensitive, 513–517
    bioavailability, 494–495, 496*f*
    choosing appropriate drug, 518–520, 518*t*
    discontinuation of medication, 520–523, 532–533
    drug efficacy, 533
    drug monitoring, 517–518, 517*t*
    epileptic seizure types and, 198–199

Pharmacological treatment (*cont.*)
  of GTS, 494
  history of, 542
  pharmacokinetics, 495, 497*t*
  principles, 494–508
    absorption and, 495–496
    clinical factors influencing drug efficacy, 508
    distribution and, 496–498
    dose planning, 501–503, 504*t*
    elimination and, 499
    half-life, 499–500
    monotherapy, 503–507
    pharmacodynamic actions, 500–501, 502*t*
    polytherapy, 503–507, 505*t*
    protein binding and, 496, 497*f*
    Vd and, 498
    zero-order kinetics, 500, 501*f*
  special considerations
    age and, 523–524
    alcohol withdrawal and, 528–529
    comorbidity and, 527–528
    pregnancy and, 524–527, 525*t*
    psychiatric conditions and, 528
    sedative drug withdrawal and, 528–529
    surgery and, 528
Pharmacoresistance, 12, 45
  proving, 609
  surgery and, 606–607
  surgically remediable syndrome and, 610
Pharmacosensitive, 12
Pharmacotherapy, history of, 39–40
Phenacemide, 586
  adverse behavioral effects of, 390
Phenelzine, ictogenic potential, 161
Phenobarbital (PB), 542, 543
  ACTH and, 579
  administration, 548–549
  adverse behavioral effects of, 389*t*, 390
  adverse side effects, 516
  chronic epilepsy, 305
  connective tissue disturbances with, 515
  discontinuation, 523
  drug combinations, 519
  drug efficacy, 508
  drug interactions, 548
    FBM, 564
    LTG, 568
    OXC, 571
    PHT, 551
    RUF, 573
    TGB, 574
    ZON, 578
  focal dyscognitive status epilepticus, 364
  generalized convulsive status epilepticus, 354–356, 354*t*
  indications, 548
  mechanisms of action, 543, 656
  megaloblastic anemia and, 514
  monitoring, 517
  neonatal seizures, 283
  neonatal status epilepticus, 367
  PET pharmacological studies of, 434
  pharmacokinetics, 548
  sedative effects, 558
  toxicity, 548
  withdrawal, 507
Phenothiazines, 66

  drug interactions, 556
  psychiatric conditions and, 528
  syncope due to, 452
Phensuximide, 516, 553, 589
Phenurone, 586
Phenylacetylurea, 586
Phenylbutazone, drug interactions, 548
  PHT, 551
  VPA, 561
Phenylethylmalonamide (PEMA), 553
Phenylketonuria, 166
Phenytoin (PHT), 39, 542
  ACTH and, 579
  administration, 552
  adverse behavioral effects of, 389*t*, 390
  adverse side effects, 516
    dose-dependent, 513
  allergic reactions with, 514
  choosing appropriate drug and, 519
  chronic epilepsy, 305
  comorbidity and, 527
  connective tissue disturbances with, 515
  development, 590
  drug combinations, 519
  drug interactions, 548, 551–552
    ESL, 562
    EZG, 563
    FBM, 564
    fosphenytoin and, 583
    LTG, 568
    OXC, 571
    PRM, 553
    RUF, 573
    TGB, 574
    VPA, 561
    ZON, 578
  dyskinesias related to, 515
  early seizure, 305
  effects of, 413
  EMA aggravated by, 255
  EMAS exacerbated by, 251
  epileptic seizure types and, 199
  generalized convulsive status epilepticus, 354, 354*t*
  hematological disorders related to, 514
  indications, 552
  JME exacerbated by, 265
  LGS, 259
  mechanisms of action, 550
  megaloblastic anemia and, 514
  monitoring, 517
  myasthenia gravis-like syndrome associated with, 515
  neonatal seizures, 283
  PET pharmacological studies of, 434
  pharmacokinetics, 550–551
  pharmacoresistance and, 609
  physical dependence, 501
  positive psychotropic effects, 390, 390*t*
  psychiatric conditions and, 528
  sedative effects, 558
  seizures induced by, 106
  sensory disorders, 461
  simple reflex seizures, 326
  teratogenic effects of, 526
  toxicity, 551
Phenytoin-equivalent (PE), 355
Pheochromocytoma, 454

pHFOs. *See* Pathological high-frequency oscillations
Philippine mali-mali, 460
Photic stimulation, 322
Photomyogenic (photomyoclonic) response, 323
    EEG changes, 421
    mechanisms of, 480–481, 482f
Photoparoxysmal (photoconvulsive) response, 323, 323f
    EEG epileptiform, 421
    epileptic, 480, 481f
Photosensitive epilepsy
    idiopathic photosensitive occipital lobe epilepsy,
        268, 322
    simple reflex epilepsies and, 326
Photosensitive seizures, 322
    environmentally-induced, 323
    preventing, 324
    variations, 323–324
Photosensitivity, 166, 184, 321
    intermittent-light, 322–323
PHT. *See* Phenytoin
Phylogeny
    cortical development, 82–83
    maturational effects on excitability, 83–84, 85f
    species differences in, 82
Physical dependence, pharmacological, 501
Physical examination, diagnostic evaluation and, 411–415
    epileptic seizure observation and, 414–415, 414t
    general, 412–413, 412f, 413f
    neurological, 413–414
Physical examination, syncope, 452
Physical interventions, 635
Pickwickian syndrome, 458
Picrotoxin, 90
Pilocarpine, 104
    HS and, 368
Pimozide, ictogenic potential, 161
Pioglitazone, drug interactions, 575
Piracetam, 586–587
Pitt, William, as epileptic, 43
PLEDs. *See* Pseudoperiodic lateralized epileptiform
        discharges
PLMS. *See* Periodic leg movements of sleep
Plotinus, as epileptic, 44
Plutarch, as epileptic, 44
PME. *See* Progressive myoclonus epilepsies
PNES. *See* Psychogenic nonepileptic seizure
Polycystic ovary syndrome, 560
Polymorphisms, 163
Polysomnography, 458
Polytherapy, pharmacological, 503–507, 505t
    choosing drugs and, 519
    crossover in, 507
    drug interactions, 507, 507f, 510f
    enzyme inhibition and, 506, 506f
Porencephalic cysts, 172, 173f
Poriomania, 465
Porphyria, 166, 451
    acute intermittent, 454
    antiseizure drugs and, 390
Port wine stain, 412
Positron emission tomography (PET), 122, 432–434
    AMT-, 306
    epilepsy evaluated with, 130–132, 132f
    neocortical seizures, 207, 208f
    pharmacological studies, 434
    presurgical imaging, 605

radiopharmaceuticals, 433, 433t
    tracers, 434
The Possessed (Dostoyevsky), 646
Postherpetic neuralgia, 566
Posthypoxic myoclonus, 284
Postictal (term), 3, 8–9
Postictal cerebral dysfunction
    nonspecific, 332–333
    specific, 331–332
        FDG-PET, 332, 334f
        SPECT, 332, 333f
Postictal paralysis
    neurological deficits in, 9
Postictal period, 8
    aggressive behavior in, 332
    amnesia in, 376, 408, 209
    anxiety in, 377
    aphasia in, 377
    confusion in, 270, 331, 377
    depression in, 383
    dysfunction, 377
        systemic, 333–335
    headache in, 268
    paralysis in, 9
    as possible mechanism of human epileptic phenomena,
        142–143
    seizure history and, 408
Postictal psychosis, 9, 376, 378, 384
Postictal refractory period, 120
Postictal symptoms, 9
    clinical considerations
        nonspecific postictal cerebral dysfunction, 332–333
        specific postictal cerebral dysfunction, 331–332
        systemic postictal dysfunction, 333–334
    mechanisms, 331
Posttraumatic epilepsy (PTE), 112, 172
    animal models, 298
    after brain surgery, 306
    late
        incidence of, 301, 301t
        time of first late seizure in, 299, 299t
Potassium bromide, 542
Potential difference, 56
Precipitants of epileptic activity, 85–86
Precipitating factors, epilepsy, 157, 182–185
    drugs, 183–184, 185t
    identifying, 186
    nonspecific, 183–184, 185t
    seizure history and, 408
    specific, 184–185
the Predicament, 387
Predisposing factors, 161
    epilepsy, 36
    nonspecific, 157–162
        dynamic aspects of threshold and, 162
        environmental factors, 161–162
        genetic factors, 159–161, 159f
        threshold and, 186
Prednisolone, 579
Prednisone, 579
    WS, 247
Pregabalin (PGN)
    administration, 572
    adverse side effects, 516
    distribution, 498
    drug interactions, 572

Pregabalin (PGN) (*cont.*)
    indications, 572
    mechanisms of action, 571
    monitoring, 518
    pharmacokinetics, 571–572
    psychotropic effects of, 390, 391*t*
    toxicity, 572
Pregnancy, 653
    drug efficacy and, 508
    pharmacological treatment in, 524–527, 525*t*
Presynaptic inhibitions, 66
Presynaptic neurons, stimulation of, 67
Prevalence, epilepsy
    age-adjusted, 49–50
    definitions of, 45–46
    estimates of, 46–48
    methodological considerations, 46
    rates, 49–50
Prevention, 3
    definition, 13
    terminology, 13–14, 297*t*
Primary reading epilepsy, 269
Primidone (PRM)
    administration, 553
    adverse behavioral effects of, 389*t*, 390
    adverse side effects, 516
    connective tissue disturbances with, 515
    discontinuation, 523
    drug combinations, 519
    drug interactions, 553
        FBM, 564
        LTG, 568
        TGB, 574
        ZON, 578
    elimination, 499
    indications, 553
    JME, 265
    mechanisms of action, 552
    megaloblastic anemia and, 514
    monitoring, 517
    nursing and, 527
    pharmacokinetics, 552–553
    sedative effects, 558
    toxicity, 553
    withdrawal, 507
Prince, as epileptic, 44
Prine Myshkin (Dostoyevsky), 646
PRM. *See* Primidone
Probenecid-sensitive transport of VPA, 560
Prodromal behavioral changes, 376
Prodromal period in syncope, 452
Prodromes, 9
    seizure history and, 407
Progabide, 71, 587
Progesterone, 329
    cyclic, 629
Progression of symptoms, 409, 410*t*
    epilepsy, 309
Progressive myoclonus epilepsies (PME), 265–267,
        322, 519. *See also* Myoclonus
    conditions causing, 266–267
    treatment, LTG and, 568
Progressive nature of epilepsy, 307–312, 609
    clinical evidence for, 308–311
    practical considerations for, 311–312
Prolactin, 335

PNES and, 463
Prophylaxis
    for chronic epilepsy, 305–307
    for early seizures, 304–305
    epileptogenesis, 314
Propofol, 587–588
    generalized convulsive status epilepticus, 357
    IAP, 440
    infusion syndrome, 587–588
Propoxyphene
    drug efficacy, 508
    drug interactions, CBZ, 559
    surgery and, 528
Propranolol
    drug interactions, 548
        TPM, 575
    intermittent explosive disorders, 465
Propylene glycol, generalized convulsive status
        epilepticus, 355
Prostate-specific antigen (PSA), 440
Protein binding, 496, 497*f*
Protein metabolism disorders, 166
PS. *See* Panayiotopoulos syndrome
PSA. *See* Prostate-specific antigen
Pseudolymphoma, 516
Pseudoperiodic lateralized epileptiform discharges
        (PLEDs), 366, 471–475, 478*f*
Pseudoseizure, 14, 31, 461
Psychiatric comorbidity in epilepsy, epidemiology of,
        375–376, 376*f*
Psychiatric conditions
    nonpsychotic, differential diagnosis, 466
    pharmacological treatment and, 528
Psychiatric outcomes of surgery, 626–627
Psychiatric symptoms, ictal events resembling or
        mimicking, 376
Psychic symptoms
    of limbic seizures, 210
    simple partial seizure, 15
Psychogenic disturbances, nonepileptic paroxysmal event
        differential diagnosis and
    daydreaming, 466
    dissociative states, 465–466
    intermittent explosive disorders, 464–465
    nonpsychotic psychiatric conditions, 466
    PNES, 461–464
    psychoses, 466
Psychogenic epileptic seizures, 325, 330
Psychogenic nonepileptic seizure (PNES), 14, 330.
        See also Nonepileptic seizures
    diagnosis, 464
    differential diagnosis, 375, 461–464, 487
        epileptic seizures and, 461–462
    EEG, 462–463
    features, 462
    on MMPI, 462
    treatment, 464
Psychological evaluation, diagnostic evaluation,
        439–440, 439*t*
Psychological stress, 330
Psychometric testing, 441
Psychomimetic drugs, 454–455
Psychomotor epilepsy, 270
Psychomotor seizures, 15, 210
    surgery, 604
    temporal lobe, 16

Psychosis, 385*t*
  differential diagnosis, 466
  interictal, 384–385
  postictal, 9, 376, 378, 384
Psychosocial adaptation
  evaluating, 378–379
  factors influencing, 379–380
Psychosocial factors
  in interictal behavioral disturbances, 387–388
  treatment, 530
Psychosocial history, 411
Psychosocial management. *See* Social management
Psychotropic drugs, risk of seizures from, 161
PTE. *See* Posttraumatic epilepsy
PTZ. *See* Pentylenetetrazol
PWE. *See* Person with epilepsy
Pyramidal cell, 62, 63*f*
Pyridoxine
  dependency, 166
  neonatal seizures, 283
  WS, 247
Pythagoras, as epileptic, 44

QOLIE. *See* Quality of Life in Epilepsy
Quality of life
  HRQOL, 12, 379, 605, 626, 647
  social management and, 647
  surgery and, 625–626
Quality of Life in Epilepsy (QOLIE), 379, 379*t*, 647
  surgery and, 626
Quetiapine, postictal psychosis, 378
Quisqualate, 132

Radiographs, structural neuroimaging, 432
Radiopharmaceuticals, PET, 433, 433*t*
Radiotelemetry, 423
Rapamycin, 115–116
  TSC treatment with, 167
Rapid eye movement (REM), 327
  sleep disorders, 457–458
Rapid kindling, 117
Rasmussen's encephalitis, 618
Rasmussen's syndrome, 275–277, 360
  differential diagnosis, 362
  EEG, 276, 276*f*
  treatment, 276–277
Raynaud's phenomenon, 454
RBD. *See* REM sleep behavior disorder
Reactive automatisms, 211, 408
  postictal, 212, 270, 332
  violent, 337
Reactive epileptic seizures, differential diagnosis
  alcohol withdrawal seizures and, 467–468
  recurrent reactive seizures and, 468
Reactive seizures, 280–281, 467
Reading epilepsy, 324
  primary, 269
Rectilinear radionuclide brain scanning, 438–439
Recurrent reactive seizures, differential diagnosis, 468
Recurrent seizures, 14
  chronic, 358
Reference range, 501
Reflex epilepsies, 6, 184, 268–269
  behavioral therapies, 633–634
  complex, 325–326, 325*t*
  due to structural lesions, ictal initiation of, 324–325

genetic, ictal initiation and, 322–324
  simple, photosensitive epilepsy and, 326
  simple *versus* complex, 325–326, 325*t*
Reflex myoclonus, 236
  ictal initiation, 326
  reticular, 237
Reflex seizures, 229
  ictal initiation and, 322, 322*t*
Refractory period, postictal, 120
Rehabilitation Act of 1973, 654
Religion
  epilepsy and, 34–35, 41–42, 43*f*, 44*f*
  hyperreligiosity, 381
  treatment and, 35
REM. *See* Rapid eye movement
Remission
  medication discontinuation and, 522
  spontaneous, 522
REM sleep behavior disorder (RBD), 458
Research
  AHRQ, 660
  animal models, 143
  biological, 143
  clinical, 36
  epileptogenesis, 314–315
  microarray, 136
  on patients, 143
  periictal phenomena, 337
Resections
  anteromesial temporal, 612, 612*f*
  standard, 611–614, 612*f*, 612*t*, 613*f*
  surgical, 248
  tailored, 614
Resources, 657–660, 658*t*
Responsive stimulation, 615
Restless leg syndrome (RLS), 284
Reticular reflex myoclonus, 460
Retirement, Survivors, Disability, and Health Insurance (RSDHI), 657
Rett syndrome, 167
Reye's syndrome, 514
Rhythmic midtemporal discharge (RMTD), 471, 474*f*
Ribonucleic acid (RNA), 61
Rickets, 515
Rifampicin, drug interactions, 568
Risk factors, 161
  biomarkers compared with, 440
Risperidone
  drug interactions
    TPM, 575
    ZON, 578
  ictogenic potential, 161
  postictal psychosis, 378
Ritonavir
  comorbidity and, 527
  drug interactions, 568
RLS. *See* Restless leg syndrome
RMTD. *See* Rhythmic midtemporal discharge
RNA. *See* Ribonucleic acid
Rochester, Minnesota, epilepsy study, 169, 171*t*
Rodent models. *See also* Animal models
  MES, 591–592
  new-drug development, 592, 593*t*
  PTZ, 591–592
Rolandic epilepsy, 309

RSDHI. *See* Retirement, Survivors, Disability, and Health Insurance
Rufinamide (RUF), 571–573
    administration, 573
    drug interactions, 573
        VPA, 561
    epileptic seizure types and, 199
    indications, 573
        LGS, 259
    mechanisms of action, 572
    pharmacokinetics, 572–573
    toxicity, 573
    trials, 519
Rum fits, 467
Russian spring-summer encephalitis, 361

Salaam seizures, 229
Salicylates, drug interactions
    PHT, 551
    VPA, 561
Salicylic acid, drug interactions, 574
Salpetrière Hospital, Paris, 36
Saltatory conduction, 62
SANAD. *See* Standard and New Antiepileptic Drug
SAR. *See* Structure-activity relationship
Schizencephaly, surgery, 608
Schizophrenia, 466
    epilepsy compared with, 272
    hallucinations, 208
    in PWE, 375
Schizophreniform paranoid psychosis, 385
School, 654
Schumann, Robert, as epileptic, 44
Sclerosis
    HS, 110, 182*f*, 367
        as acquired cause of epilepsy disorders, 177–182
        mossy fiber sprouting and, 129–130, 131*f*
        MTLE and, 178–182, 250
        resulting from cytotoxic agents, 368
    mesial temporal, 368
    TSC, 166–167, 168*f*
    tuberous, 412, 413*f*
        surgery, 608
SCN5A gene mutation, 336
Scott, Sir Walter, as epileptic, 44
Screening procedures, 542
Secondary generalization, 18
Secondary parasomnia, 459
Sedative drug withdrawal, 528–529
SEEG. *See* Stereotactic depth electrode electroencephalography
Seizure days, 13
Seizure focus, 11
Seizure-free interval
    definition of, 11–12
    drug discontinuation and, 527
    after surgery, 608
Seizure history, 406–409
    age at onset and, 408–409, 409*t*
    aura or prodrome and, 407
    clinical, 407–408
    frequency, 408
    postictal period and, 408
    precipitating factors and pattern in, 408
    progression of symptoms and, 409, 410*t*
Seizure modification, 13, 297

terminology, 297*t*
Seizures. *See also* Epileptic seizures; *specific seizures*
    acute, in vitro studies of, 107–109
    aphasic, 205
    basic mechanisms of, 99–144
        experimental models and, 100–122
        molecular genetic investigations and, 135–138
    chronic recurrent, 358
    classifications, 16–17, 28, 28*t*
    clinical, 407–408
    early, prophylaxis for, 304–305
    eating-induced, 325
    electrographic, 6
    electroshock-induced, 107
    experimental models of, acute, 100–109, 101*t*
    frequency, 408
    grand mal, 14–15
    hippocampal, 125
    induction, 103–106
        electroshock, 107
    jackknife, 229
    local, 15
    medically refractory, 528–529
    nonepileptic, 3, 4
        psychogenic, 31
        terminology, 14
    onset, 312
    patterns, 408
    petit mal, 14–15
    prediction, 424–425
    reactive, 280–281
    salaam, 229
    surgery and outcome, 624–625, 625*t*
    term, 4
    types, 28, 28*t*
        genetics and, 304
Selective amygdalohippocampectomies, 612
Self-induced seizures, 324
Self-sustained status epilepticus (SSSE), 110
SEM. *See* Simultaneous EEG
Sensory disorders, differential diagnosis, 461
Sensory motor rhythm (SMR), 634
Sensory symptoms
    auditory, 206
    gustatory, 210
    of limbic seizures, 209–210
    of neocortex seizures, 206
    olfactory, 209–210
    simple partial seizure, 15
    visual, 206
SEPs. *See* Somatosensory evoked potentials
Sertraline
    drug interactions, LTG, 568
    ictogenic potential, 161
Sex-specific incidence rates, 45–46
Sexual automatisms, 211
Sexual symptoms, 381
Shagreen patch, 412, 413*f*
Sharp transients of dubious significance in EEG, 469–471
Shelley, Percy Bysshe, as epileptic, 44
Shy-Drager syndrome, 451
Sialidosis with macular changes, 266
Siberian ikota, 460
Siberian Shamanism, epilepsy and, 42
Side effects, adverse, 493. *See also specific drugs*
    acute, 508

of antiseizure drugs, 508, 511–512t
  behavioral effects, 389–390, 389t
behavioral, 389–390, 389t
CBZ, 558
in children, 514
chronic, 508, 513–517
dose-dependent, 510–513, 533
gastrointestinal, 513
hypersensitive, 513–517
neurological, 513
of pharmacological treatment, 508–517
Type A, 508
Type B, 508
Type C, 508
Type D, 508
SIDS. *See* Sudden infant death syndrome
Simultaneous EEG (SEM), 436
Single-nucleotide polymorphisms (SNPs), 163–164
Single photon emission computed tomography (SPECT), 134, 434–435, 436f
  postictal cerebral dysfunction, specific, 332, 333f
  presurgical imaging, 605
Skin abnormalities
  in physical examination, 412, 412f
  rash, 513
Sleep apnea, 328, 457
  obstructive, 459
Sleep disorders
  differential diagnosis, 457–459
  major paroxysmal motor, 458, 458t
  movement, 458
    PLMS, 284
  narcolepsy, 457
  REM, 457–458
Sleep spindles, 313
  harmonics, 469
Sleep-wake cycles, 326–328
Small sharp spikes (SSS), 471, 472f
Smell disorders. *See* Olfactory symptoms of limbic seizures
Smith, Joseph, as epileptic, 42
SMR. *See* Sensory motor rhythm
SNPs. *See* Single-nucleotide polymorphisms
Social intervention, health care disparities and, 661
Social management, 644–662
  activities of daily living, 647–652
    alcohol and drugs, 651–653
    driving, 648–651, 650t
    limitations, 662
    participation in sports, 651
    social management, 647–652
    specific hazards, 652
  employment, 654–655
  family
    child with epilepsy in, 652–653
    parent with epilepsy in, 653–654
  financial aid, 657
  health care disparities, 660–662, 660f
  insurance, 656–657
  legal rights, 655–656
  quality of life, 647
  resources, 657–660, 658t
  school, 654
  stigma, 645–647
Social outcomes of surgery, 626–627
Socrates, as epileptic, 44

Sodium oxybate, sleep disorder, 457
Somatosensory evoked potentials (SEPs), 425
Somatosensory seizures, 206
Spasms
  epileptic, 228–229, 230f, 231f
    types, 228–229
  hemifacial, 461
  infantile, 228–229, 246, 312
    benign, 247
    treatment, 520
  muscle, intermittent, 461
Spasticity, 460
SPECT. *See* Single photon emission computed tomography
Speech arrest, 205
Speech disorders. *See also* Language
  antiseizure medications and, 389
  hypometamorphosis, 381
Sphenoidal electrodes, 418, 418f
Spike-and-wave discharges/patterns, 5, 86–87, 88f, 106, 108f. *See also* Electroencephalogram
  epilepsy types and, 485
Spike focus, epileptic, 3, 31
  definition, 10
  diffuse, 10
  EEG and determining, 10
  multifocal, 10
  terminology, 10–11
Spikes. *See also* Centrotemporal spikes
  autonomy, 327–328
  6-hz positive, 471, 472f
  14-hz positive, 471, 472f
  interictal, 122
    migration of, 313
    in various cortical areas, 300, 300t
  occipital, driving, 481–482, 483f
  SSS, 471, 472f
  wicket, 471, 473f
Spike-wave stupor, 6
SPM. *See* Statistical parametric mapping
Spontaneous automatisms, 210
Sport participation, 651
Spreading depression, 100
SQUID. *See* Superconducting quantum interference device
SREDA. *See* Subclinical rhythmic EEG discharges of adults
SSI. *See* Supplemental Security Income
SSS. *See* Small sharp spikes
SSSE. *See* Self-sustained status epilepticus
Standard and New Antiepileptic Drug (SANAD), 519
Startle disease, 324, 460
Startle epilepsy, 269
  CLB for, 557
  epileptic seizures in, 324
  synchronization and, 321
Statistical parametric mapping (SPM), 132–133, 620
Status epilepticus, 342–370
  absence, 369
    clinical description of, 358–359
    differential diagnosis of, 359
    etiology of, 359
    incidence of, 359
    prognosis of, 360
    treatment of, 359–360
  classification, 343, 344t

Status epilepticus (*cont.*)
    clonic, 350
    convulsive, 343
    definition, 342
    electroclinical distinctions, 369
    electrographic, 343
    epilepsia partialis continua, 360–363
    febrile, 367, 369
    focal dyscognitive
        clinical description of, 363–364, 365*f*
        differential diagnosis of, 364, 366*t*
        etiology of, 364
        incidence of, 364
        prognosis of, 366
        treatment of, 364–366
    generalized convulsive
        clinical description of, 344–351
        etiology of, 351–352
        incidence of, 351
        other forms of, 350–351
        prognosis, 358
        tonic-clonic, 344–350
        treatment of, 352–358, 353*t*
    impending, 343
    models of epilepsy, kindling and, 119
    myoclonic, 351
    neonatal, 367–368
    nonconvulsive, 343
    refractory, 357
    SSSE, 110
    subtle, 343, 344, 366
    terminans, 344, 366
    tonic, 350
Status epilepticus terminans, 344, 366
Steady-state condition, 501
Stereotactic depth electrode electroencephalography
        (SEEG), 122, 604
Stevens-Johnson syndrome, 513, 514
    CBZ and, 558
    LTG and, 567
Stiff baby syndrome, 460
Stigma, 645–647
    of epilepsy, 45
    felt, 646
Stimulation, 615–616
Stimulus alteration, 634
Stiripentol, 588
    drug interactions, 551
Stokes-Adams syndrome, 450
Storage disorders
    myoclonus among, 266, 267*t*
    neuronal, 266
Stress
    management, 464
    as precipitating factor, 85, 330
    reducing, 265
    theory, 120
Strokes, 172
    NINDS, 99, 590, 660
Structural disorders, neonatal seizures due to
    clinical description of, 281
    differential diagnosis of, 282
    epidemiology of, 282
    etiology of, 282
    prognosis of, 283
    treatment of, 282–283

Structural lesions
    focal, 310
    reflex epilepsies due to, ictal initiation of, 324–325
Structural neuroimaging
    MRI, 429–432, 430*f*, 431*f*
    radiographs, 432
    x-ray CT, 432, 432*f*
Structure-activity relationship (SAR), 542, 591
Studies
    clinical
        current drugs under investigation, 594–596
        new-drug development, 592–594
        Phase I, 592
        Phase II, 592
        Phase III, 592, 594–595
    of human epilepsy, 122–135
        biochemical investigations, 134–135, 135*f*
        brain imaging technique investigations, 130–134
        electrophysiological investigations, 122–130
        microanatomical investigations, 134
        molecular investigations, 134–135, 135*f*
    pharmacological, PET, 434
    in vitro
        of acute seizures, 107–109
        of chronic epilepsy, 121–122
Sturge-Weber syndrome, 173
    epilepsy differential diagnosis and, 456
    physical examination of, 412, 412*f*
Subarachnoid cysts, 608
Subclinical rhythmic EEG discharges of adults (SREDA),
        482–483, 484*f*
Subclinical seizures, 6
Subcortical structures, epileptiform effect, 81–82
Subtle status epilepticus, 343, 366
    coma and, 344
Succinimides, 542
    methsuximide, 588–589
    phensuximide, 589
SUD. *See* Sudden unexpected death
Sudden infant death syndrome (SIDS), 336
Sudden unexpected death (SUD), 335–337
Sudden unexpected death of epilepsy (SUDEP), 335–337,
        451, 568
Sulfisoxazole, drug interactions, 551
Sulfonamides, drug interactions, 551
Sulthiame, 589–590
    BECTS, 252, 253
    WS, 247
Sumatriptan, drug interactions, 575
Superconducting quantum interference device
        (SQUID), 426
Supplemental Security Income (SSI), 657
Supplementary motor area seizures, 324
Supplementary motor seizures, 205
Surgery, 494, 603
    behavioral disturbances associated with, 391–392
    brain, 306
    candidates for
        misconceptions about, 607–609, 607*t*
        selecting, 618, 619*f*
    for children and infants, 618
    cost, 606–607
    development of new centers, 628
    diagnostic testing before, 617–618
    early, arguments for, 609
    historical perspectives on, 604–606

mortality rate after, 336, 606
outcome, 623–628, 626*t*
    cognitive, 626–627
    complications and, 627–628
    psychiatric, 626–627
    quality of life and, 625–626
    seizures and, 624–625, 625*t*
    social, 626–627
pharmacological treatment and, 528
pharmacoresistance and, 606–607
presurgical imaging, 605
protocols
    candidate selection and, 618, 619*f*
    Phase I, 620–622
    Phase II, 620, 622–623, 623*f*
    Phase III, 623
    strategy for, 616–618, 616*t*
schizencephaly, 608
therapeutic procedures
    ablative surgery, 615
    disconnection surgery, 614–615
    standard resections, 611–614, 612*f*, 612*t*, 613*f*
    stimulation, 615–616
    tailored resections, 614
tuberous sclerosis, 608
underutilization of, 606
Surgically remediable epilepsy syndromes, 605, 609–611, 610*t*, 611*t*
    MTLE as prototype of, 610, 611*t*
    pharmacoresistance and, 610
Surgical resection, WS, 248
Surrogate markers, 440
Susceptibility
    acquired epilepsies, 144
    epileptic, of immature brain, 312, 314
    to FS, 184
    genes, 159
    molecular, 144
Sv2a. *See* Synaptic vesicle protein 2a
Swedenborg, Emanuel, as epileptic, 44
Swift, Jonathan, as epileptic, 44
Swimming, hazards of, 337, 651
Swinburne, Algernon Charles, as epileptic, 44
Symptomatic epilepsy, 31
Symptomatic seizures, 18
Symptomatogenic zone, 204, 617
Symptom complex, 244
    epilepsy syndrome as, 285
Symptoms
    autonomic
        of limbic seizures, 210
        simple partial seizure, 15
    motor
        Jacksonian march of, 15
        of limbic seizures, 211–212
        simple partial seizure, 15
    nonepileptic, 5
    postictal, 9, 331–335
    progression
        epilepsy, 309
        seizure history and, 409, 410*t*
    psychiatric, 376
    psychic
        of limbic seizures, 210
        simple partial seizure, 15
    sensory

auditory, 206
gustatory, 210
of limbic seizures, 209–210
of neocortex seizures, 206
olfactory, 209–210
simple partial seizure, 15
visual, 206
systemic, of hyperventilation, 454
vertiginous, 206
Synapses
    chemical, 64–72, 65*f*
    electronic, 72
    excitability, 62
Synaptic plasticity, 69–70
Synaptic vesicle protein 2a (Sv2a), 569
Synchronization, 4, 55, 321. *See also* Neuronal synchronization
Syncope
    cardiac causes of, 450–451
    convulsive, 330, 452
    differential diagnosis, 450–452, 453*t*
        tonic-clonic epilepsy and, 452
    disorders, characteristics of, 452
    infantile, 452
    noncardiac causes of, 451–452
    phenothiazines and, 452
    physical examination, 452
    prodromal period, EEG during, 452
    tricyclic antidepressants and, 452
    vasodepressor, 450
    vasovagal, 450
Syndrome modification, 297
    terminology, 297*t*
Synucleinopathy, 459
Systemic diseases, epileptic seizure-associated, 169, 170*t*
Systemic disturbances, nonepileptic paroxysmal event differential diagnosis and
    abdominal epilepsy, 455
    breath holding, 452–453
    hyperventilation, 453–454
    metabolic disturbances, 454–455
    neurological disturbances, 455–461
    syncope, 450–452
    toxic disturbances, 454–455
Systemic symptoms, of hyperventilation, 454

T2000, 595
Target hypothesis, 528
Tasso, Torquato, as epileptic, 44
TBI. *See* Traumatic brain injury
Tchaikovsky, Peter Ilyich, as epileptic, 44
T electrodes for EEG, 417–418
Temkin, Owsei, 35, 42
Temporal lobe epilepsies, 304, 309
    characteristics due to interictal behavior in, 381, 381*t*
    familial, 267–268
    lateral, with auditory features, 57
Temporal lobe seizures
    limbic, 210
    psychomotor, 16
Temporal-parietal occipital (TPO) junction, 270
Teratogenicity, 525–526, 533
Teresa of Avila, Saint, as epileptic, 42
Terminology, 3–14
    antiepileptogenesis, 13–14, 297*t*
    changes in, 26

Terminology (*cont.*)
  control, 11–13
Terminology
  cure, 11–13, 297*t*
  disease modification, 13–14, 297*t*
  drug resistance, 11–13
  epilepsy, 8
  epilepsy disorders, 6–8
  epileptic seizures, 4–6
  epileptic spike focus, 10–11
  epileptogenesis, 9–10, 297*t*
  epileptogenicity, 9–10
  epileptogenic lesion, 10–11
  epileptogenic zone or region, 10–11
  ILAE and revision of, 27
  inconsistent, 31
  nonepileptic seizures, 14
  precise, 32
  prevention, 13–14, 297*t*
  revision, 27
  seizure modification, 297*t*
  spike focus, epileptic, 10–11
  syndrome modification, 297*t*
TGB. *See* Tiagabine
Thai bah-tsche, 460
Thalamus, 5
The Falling Sickness (Owsci), 34
Theophylline, drug interactions, 552
Theory of mind, 382
Therapeutic range, 501
Thiamine, generalized convulsive status epilepticus, 352
Thiocyanate, neuronal excitability and, 61
Thiopental, 543
  EEG, 421–422
Thiosemicarbazide, 66
Threshold, 157–158, 158*f*
  alteration, 634
  dynamic aspects of, 162
  factors raising, 186
  nonspecific predisposing factors and, 186
Thrombocytopenia, 514
Tiagabine (TGB), 351
  administration, 574
  drug interactions, 574
  EMA aggravated by, 255
  indications, 574
  mechanisms of action, 573
  MEI, 249
  monitoring, 517
  pharmacokinetics, 573–574
  psychotropic effects of, 390, 391*t*
  toxicity, 574
TIAs. *See* Transient ischemic attacks
Tissot, Simon André, 36
TMS. *See* Transcranial magnetic stimulation
TNS. *See* Trigeminal nerve stimulation
Todd's paralysis, 332
  classical, 143
  definition of, 9
Tolerance, pharmacological, 500
  cross-, 501
Tolstoy, Leo, as epileptic, 44
Tonabersat, 595
Tonic-clonic epilepsy, differential diagnosis, 452
Tonic-clonic seizures. *See* Generalized tonic-clonic
  seizures

Tonic-clonic status epilepticus, 344–350
  EEG patterns of, 347*f*, 348*f*, 349*f*
  morbidity associated with, 350
  recurrent ictal events of, 344
Tonic motor seizures, 205
Tonic seizures, generalized
  clinical considerations for, 228
  EEG of, 227–228
  mechanisms of, 227
  phenomenology of, 227
Topiramate (TPM)
  administration, 576
  ADNFLE, 254
  adverse behavioral effects of, 389*t*, 390
  adverse side effects, 516
    dose-dependent, 513
  choosing appropriate drug and, 518–519
  drug interactions, 575
    ESL, 562
    EZG, 563
    LEV, 569
    LTG, 568
    OXC, 571
  DS, 249
  EMAS, 251
  generalized convulsive status epilepticus, 357
  IAP, 439–440, 621
  indications, 575
  JME, 265
  ketogenic diet and, 631
  LGS, 259
  mechanisms of action, 574–575
  MEI, 249
  monitoring, 517
  myoclonus, 237
  pharmacokinetics, 575
  psychotropic effects of, 390, 391*t*
  toxicity, 575
  WS, 247
Toxic disturbances
  as acquired cause of epilepsy disorders, 177
  differential diagnosis, 454–455
  neurological dysfunction and, 454–455
Toxic encephalopathy, 455
Toxic influences, 329–330
Toxic levels, pharmacological, 510
Toxic states, 330
TPM. *See* Topiramate
TPO. *See* Temporal-parietal occipital junction
Traditional and folk medicine, 632–633, 632*t*, 633*t*
Tramadol, surgery and, 528
Tranquilizers, 651
Transcranial magnetic stimulation (TMS), 635
Transcription, 136
Transient global amnesia, 456
Transient ischemic attacks (TIAs), 455–456
Translation, 136
Transvestism, 381
Tranylcypromine, ictogenic potential, 161
Trauma, epilepsy and, 169, 171–172
  PTE, 112, 172
    animal models, 298
    after brain surgery, 306
    late, 299, 299*t*, 301, 301*t*
Traumatic brain injury (TBI), 112, 171–172
  animal models, 298

Trazodone, ictogenic potential, 161
Treatment, 495t. *See also specific treatments*
    alternative therapy, 530
    ancient and medieval, 35
    antiepilepsy, 10
    EEG and assessing, 530–531
    emergency, 532
    general principles of, 493–534
    medically refractory seizures and, 528–529
    objective, 532
    occult and magical, 35
    pharmacological
        adverse side effects of, 508–517
        principles of, 494–508
        special considerations for, 523–528
    psychosocial considerations, 530
    religious, 35
    side effects, 493
    after single seizure, 531–532
Tricyclic antidepressants
    drug interactions
        CLN, 556
        VPA, 561
    syncope due to, 452
Tricyclic compounds, sleep disorder, 457
Trigeminal nerve stimulation (TNS), 629
Trigeminal neuralgia, 461, 566
Trimethadione, 40, 542, 584–585
    adverse side effects, 516
    teratogenic effects of, 526
Triptorelin, 629
Trough level, 517
TSC. *See* Tuberous sclerosis complex
Tuberous sclerosis, 412, 413f
    surgery, 608
Tuberous sclerosis complex (TSC), 166–167, 168f
Tumors
    brain, 174, 174t
    DNETs, 174, 175f, 389
    frontal lobe, 310
Twilight states, 333

UDP-glucuronosyltransferase, 567
Ultradian cycles, 327
Ultraslow waves, 125
    initial, 144
Uncinate fits, 326
    with olfactory symptoms, 15
Unclassified epileptic seizures, 200t
    epileptic spasms as, 228–229, 230f, 231f
    neonatal seizures, 229–233
    reflex seizures as, 229
Uniform Duties to Disabled Persons Act, 656
Unverricht-Lundborg syndrome, 166
Up-down state, 86
Uremia, 177
    chronic, 508

Vagus nerve stimulation (VNS), 392, 530, 534, 603, 615, 628–629
    diathermy in, 629
Valentine, Saint, as patron saint of epilepsy, 42
Valnoctamide, 595
Valproate, adverse side effects, 516
Valproic acid (VPA), 542, 559–560
    absence status epilepticus, 359

    administration, 561
    adverse behavioral effects of, 389–390, 389t
    adverse side effects, 516
        dose-dependent, 513
    CAE, 262
    children taking, 514
    choosing appropriate drug and, 519
    chronic epilepsy, 305
    comorbidity and, 527–528
    derivatives, 595
    discovery of, 591
    distribution, 498
    dose planning, 503
    drug interactions, 561
        CLN, 556
        EZG, 563
        FBM, 564
        LTG, 567, 568
        OXC, 571
        PHT, 551
        TGB, 574
    DS, 249
    EMA, 255
    EMAS, 251
    epileptic seizure types and, 199
    focal dyscognitive status epilepticus, 364
    generalized convulsive status epilepticus, 356–357
    indications, 561
    JAE, 263
    JME, 265, 561
    ketogenic diet and, 561, 630–631
    LGS, 259
    mechanisms of action, 560
    MEI, 249
    monitoring, 517
    myoclonus, 237
    pharmacokinetics, 560–561
    pharmacoresistance and, 609
    physical dependence, 501
    positive psychotropic effects, 390
    probenecid-sensitive transport of, 560
    PS, 251
    psychotropic effects of, 390, 391t
    reflex epilepsies due to structural lesions, 324
    simple reflex seizures, 326
    teratogenic effects of, 526
    toxicity, 560–561
    trials, 519
    WS, 247–248
Valproic encephalopathy, 569
Valrocemide, 595
Valsalva maneuvers, 450
van Gogh, Vincent, as epileptic, 44
Vascular lesions, 172, 173f
Vascular malformations, 172–173
Vasodepressor syncope, 450
Vasovagal syncope, 450
Vd. *See* Volume of distribution
VEM. *See* Video-EEG monitoring
Venlafaxine, ictogenic potential, 161
Venous angiomas, 608
VEPs. *See* Visual evoked potentials
Verbal automatisms, 211
Versive movements, 205
    limbic seizure, 211
Vertebral basilar insufficiency, 455

Vertex sharp waves, 313
Vertiginous symptoms, 206
Vertigo
    due to epileptic discharges, 461
    paroxysmal, 206, 461
VGB. *See* Vigabatrin
VGKC. *See* Voltage-gated K+ channel
Video-EEG monitoring (VEM), 422–424, 422*f*, 423*t*, 441
    ambulatory recorder, 423
    differential diagnosis and, 487
    PNES, 463
Vigabatrin (VGB), 246, 351
    administration, 577
    adverse behavioral effects of, 389*t*, 390
    adverse side effects, 516
    drug interactions, 576
        PHT, 551
    EMA aggravated by, 255
    EMAS exacerbated by, 251
    indications, 576–577
    infantile spasms, 520
    JME exacerbated by, 265
    mechanisms of action, 576
    MEI, 249
    monitoring, 518
    pharmacokinetics, 576
    reversible asymptomatic changes, 515
    WS, 247
Violence
    epilepsy and, 656
    ictal, 377
Viral infections, 166
    autoimmune mechanisms, 276
Viscosity of language, 381
Visual evoked potentials (VEPs), 425
Visual pattern sensitivity, 324
Visual symptoms. *See also* Hallucinations; Sensory
            symptoms
    focal dyscognitive status epilepticus, 363
    ictal, 206
    photosensitivity, 166, 184, 321
        intermittent-light, 322–323
    in tonic-clonic seizures, 251
    unformed, 206
Vitamin D deficiency, 515
Vitamins, 631
    metabolism disorders, 166
Vitus, Saint, as patron saint of epilepsy, 42
VNS. *See* Vagus nerve stimulation
Voltage-gated channels, 56–57, 57*t*
Voltage-gated K+ channel (VGKC), 57
Volume of distribution (Vd), 498
Voxel-based morphometry, 132
VPA. *See* Valproic acid
VX-765, 596

Warfarin, drug interactions, 548
    ESL, 562
Washington Psychosocial Seizure Inventory (WPSI),
            378–379, 647
Wernicke's encephalopathy, 352

West syndrome (WS), 228, 245, 310
    CBZ, 559
    clinical description, 246
    differential diagnosis, 247
    epidemiology, 246
    etiology, 246–247
    medication discontinuation, 522
    prognosis, 248
    symptomatic subgroups, 246
    treatment, 247–248
WFN. *See* World Federation of Neurology
WHO. *See* World Health Organization
Wicket spikes, 471, 473*f*
Wilding, Michael, as epileptic, 44
William III, as epileptic, 43
Willibrord, Saint, as patron saint of epilepsy, 42
Willis, Thomas, 35
Withdrawal, 501
    alcohol, 528–529
        seizures, differential diagnosis, 467–468
    drug
        drug tapering and, 507
        sedative, 528–529
Wood's lamp, 412
World Federation of Neurology (WFN), 661
World Health Organization (WHO), 646, 658*t*
    epilepsy classifications, 18
    global burden of epilepsy, 45, 48–49
    incidence of epilepsy, 33
WPSI. *See* Washington Psychosocial Seizure Inventory
WS. *See* West syndrome

X-ray
    CT, structural neuroimaging, 432, 432*f*
    DEXA, 515

YKP3089, 595
Young, Neil, as epileptic, 44

Zero-order kinetics, pharmacological,
            500, 501*f*
Zidovudine
    comorbidity and, 527
    drug interactions, 561
Zonisamide (ZON)
    administration, 578
    adverse side effects, 516
    chronic epilepsy, 305
    drug interactions, 578
    IAP, 439–440, 621
    indications, 578
    ketogenic diet and, 631
    mechanisms of action, 577
    monitoring, 517, 518
    myoclonus, 237
    pharmacokinetics, 577
    psychotropic effects of, 390, 391*t*
    toxicity, 577–578
    trials, 519
    WS, 247
Zygoma electrodes for EEG, 417–418